Disease-related Malnutrition

613.2/STR

An Evidence-based Approach to Treatment

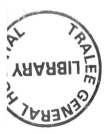

Disease-related Malnutrition

An Evidence-based Approach to Treatment

_____

Rebecca J. Stratton

Institute of Human Nutrition
University of Southampton
UK

Ceri J. Green

Nutricia Healthcare
Zoetermeer
The Netherlands

and

Marinos Elia

Institute of Human Nutrition
University of Southampton
UK

CABI *Publishing*

CABI *Publishing* is a division of CAB *International*

CABI Publishing
CAB International
Wallingford
Oxon OX10 8DE
UK

Tel: +44 (0)1491 832111
Fax: +44 (0)1491 833508
E-mail: cabi@cabi.org
Web site: www.cabi-publishing.org

CABI Publishing
44 Brattle Street
4th Floor
Cambridge, MA 02138
USA

Tel: +1 617 395 4056
Fax: +1 617 354 6875
E-mail: cabi-nao@cabi.org

A catalogue record for this book is available from the British Library,
London, UK.
A catalogue record for this book is available from the Library of Congress,
Washington, DC, USA.

ISBN 0 85199 648 5

Typeset in Melior by Columns Design Ltd, Reading.
Printed and bound in the UK by Biddles Ltd, Guildford and King's Lynn.

Contents

Preface

Malnutrition continues to be a major problem worldwide, particularly in hospitals, care homes and communities, where diseases and disabilities are common. Although the increasing growth of the elderly population represents a major triumph in medicine and social care, aging brings its own problems and challenges that are linked to disease, disability and malnutrition. It is disturbing that, even in developed countries, disease-related malnutrition (DRM) is under-recognized, underestimated and under-treated, adversely affecting both individuals and society. There is also concern about the confusion that exists in relation to what constitutes malnutrition, uncertainties about the types of disabilities produced by malnutrition in the presence of disease, and about the extent to which these disabilities respond to nutritional intervention. Our desire has been to collect, rationalize and highlight a wide range of information to help health care professionals make decisions, from those providing nutritional support to individual patients to those planning policy and research. This has been enabled by the support of the Institute of Human Nutrition, University of Southampton, and Nutricia Healthcare, the latter also being involved in the promotion of the book. However, in undertaking this project we considered it essential that the evidence and conclusions were assembled methodologically with intellectual freedom and no prior agenda. Standard procedures for undertaking systematic reviews and meta-analyses have been used and the data presented in detail so that the evidence and the conclusions are traceable and verifiable. Any serious evidence that might alter the conclusions presented here would be welcomed.

Chapter 1 of this book introduces a new conceptual framework for considering the definition, consequences and treatment of malnutrition. Chapter 2 contributes to this framework by establishing an extensive clinical database, which shows an alarming prevalence of protein-energy malnutrition in a variety of patient groups in different health-care settings. Both the causes and consequences of this widespread problem are discussed in detail in Chapters 3 and 4, in the light of recent findings. Reduced nutritional intake is identified as potentially the most important component of a causal pathway leading to the development of DRM. However, the value of using particular types of nutritional support to increase nutritional intake in specific patient groups remains controversial. Therefore, Chapters 5–9 build on the conceptual framework by establishing a multi-layered evidence base for the treatment of DRM using a series of systematic reviews, including meta-analysis. Chapter 5 discusses the methodology used to establish the evidence base, whilst the next three chapters present new findings relating to the effectiveness of oral nutritional supplements (ONS) and dietary modification (Chapter 6), enteral tube feeding (ETF) (Chapter 7), ONS and ETF in combination (Chapter 8), and parenteral nutrition compared with ETF (Chapter 9). Some remarkable physiological and clinical benefits of nutritional support are highlighted, both generally and specifically, according to patient groups, disease categories and health-care settings. As the literature is extensive, it is likely that some relevant reports were missed in the review process, for which we apologise. From the analysis of the trials included, it is clear that there are limitations in study design and execution, and that evidence is lacking in a number of specific areas, which we have identified throughout the book. Chapter 10 provides a practical guide to planning, undertaking and reporting clinical nutrition trials.

The final chapter (Chapter 11) emphasizes that for some patients the decision as to whether or not to provide nutritional support is clear-cut. A well-nourished individual with no history of weight loss does not need nutritional support, whereas an individual with severe and prolonged catabolic disease, prolonged intestinal failure or a swallowing disorder will almost certainly require nutritional support. However, for other patient groups there is more uncertainty as to the value of nutritional support. Therefore, this book attempts to clarify the role and the effectiveness of nutritional support in clinical practice both in general and in specific groups of patients by establishing a multi-levelled evidence base. At the most specific level, evidence is based on reports of the effects of specific forms of nutritional therapy in specific patient groups with a particular type or phase of illness, which may be of most value to the clinician dealing with such patients. At a more general level, evidence is based on reports that focus on the combined effects of different treatments in a variety of patients with different conditions. Such evidence may influence the care of specific patients but can also be of value to health-care planners implementing evidence-based policies for the nutritional treatment of the patient population. Each of these levels contributes to the knowledge matrix upon which decisions about clinical management and future research can be based. Even when all of the information is taken into account, interpretation of both the strength and the value of the evidence base for the detection and treatment of DRM will vary, and we invite the reader to decide.

R.J. Stratton
Institute of Human Nutrition
University of Southampton, UK

C.J. Green
Nutricia Healthcare
Zoetermeer, The Netherlands

M. Elia
Institute of Human Nutrition
University of Southampton, UK

About the Authors

Dr Rebecca Stratton, Institute of Human Nutrition, University of Southampton, UK
Dr Rebecca Stratton obtained a BSc (Hons) in Nutrition and State Registration in Dietetics from the University of Surrey and a PhD from the University of Cambridge, UK. After working at Hammersmith Hospital, London, she moved to the MRC Dunn Clinical Nutrition Centre in Cambridge where she undertook research in clinical nutrition. She is now employed as a Research Fellow at the University of Southampton and practises clinically within Southampton University Hospitals Trust. Dr Stratton is already firmly established as one of the leading young researchers in the field of clinical nutrition, with many publications in key journals (original research and reviews). She is a member of a number of national committees, including the British Artificial Nutrition Survey (BANS) and the Malnutrition Advisory Group (MAG) of the British Association for Parenteral and Enteral Nutrition (BAPEN), and the Clinical Nutrition and Metabolic Group of The Nutrition Society, UK.

Dr Ceri Green, International Nutritional Sciences Manager, Nutricia Healthcare, Zoetermeer, The Netherlands
Dr Ceri Green obtained a BSc (Hons) in Nutrition and State Registration in Dietetics from the University of Surrey, UK, and a PhD from the University of Liverpool, UK. Following this, Dr Green worked as a dietitian in three UK hospitals. Since then she has worked for Nutricia in The Netherlands for over 10 years, for the first 7 years in the corporate research department, and latterly as International Nutritional Sciences Manager for Nutricia Healthcare. Dr Green has presented on clinical nutrition topics around the world, and published reviews on a number of these issues.

Professor Marinos Elia, Institute of Human Nutrition, University of Southampton, UK
Professor Marinos Elia (MB ChB, BSc (Hons), FRCP) is recognized as one of the key global opinion leaders in Clinical Nutrition. He obtained a BSc (Hons) in Medical Biochemistry and MB ChB degrees in Medicine from the University of Manchester, before undertaking research for an MD at the MRC Metabolic Research Laboratories, Oxford, headed by Sir Hans Krebs. Professor Elia was head of The Clinical Nutrition Group at the MRC Dunn Clinical Nutrition Centre in Cambridge, head of The Nutrition Team at Addenbrooke's Hospital, and Senior Research Fellow at Churchill College, University of Cambridge. He is now Professor of Clinical Nutrition and Metabolism at the Institute of Human Nutrition, University of Southampton, and honorary consultant physician at

Southampton General Hospital, UK. He is an editor of five nutrition journals, and has been editor-in-chief of *Clinical Nutrition*. He has served on many national and international committees, and has chaired a number of them, including the Clinical Nutrition and Metabolism Group of the Nutrition Society in the UK, the British Artificial Nutrition Survey (BANS) and the Malnutrition Advisory Group (MAG) of the British Association for Parenteral and Enteral Nutrition (BAPEN). He has received a number of prestigious awards, including the John Lennard-Jones medal (BAPEN).

Foreword

Clinical nutrition, despite its respectable pedigree going back to such authorities as Hippocrates, John Hunter and Florence Nightingale, has been a Cinderella of modern medicine, not only because it is old technology, but also because of a failure of its practitioners to define it in a way that engages doctors and causes them to take it seriously. We have been somewhat vague over the definition of malnutrition, or at least that degree of it which requires intervention. We have been imprecise and have been perceived to disagree on how to diagnose it and describe its prevalence. We have also been slow to define and teach the adverse clinical consequences of even modest levels of undernutrition. Lastly, until recent times, good quality intervention studies demonstrating clinical benefit and cost effectiveness of nutritional support have been few and far between.

Although evidence-based medicine is not a new concept, recent emphasis upon it has rightly put the onus on nutritionists to prove their case. Unfortunately some systematic reviews on this and related subjects have been written by authors familiar with the technology of trials and statistics, but inexperienced in the clinical problems concerned. This has led to a lumping together of disparate and inappropriate studies and hence to erroneous conclusions, raising the old question: 'Quis custodiet ipsos custodes?' ('Who referees the referee?'). In contrast, the authors of this book bring to it a wealth of clinical and scientific experience and expertise in the field. With immense labour and meticulous attention to detail, they have combined scientific rectitude with clinical judgement and common sense, to produce a reference work of great importance not only to clinicians but also to other health-care disciplines and to managers. They have distilled from an enormous volume of literature a reasoned and practical definition of malnutrition in its various facets; they provide evidence-based guidelines on how to diagnose it and on when its severity merits intervention; from this they proceed to a reasoned account of its prevalence; they also catalogue its functional and clinical consequences, and review the evidence of benefit from various modes of nutritional intervention. In this they distinguish clearly between the various clinical circumstances in which the different modalities of nutritional support – oral, enteral and parenteral – may be useful. At the one extreme is the patient with prolonged gastrointestinal failure who, without parenteral nutrition would die within 2 or 3 months. This is analogous to the management of respiratory failure by ventilation and of kidney failure by dialysis. The end point is the same, only the time scale is different. To suggest that under these circumstances patients should be subjected to a controlled trial is manifestly absurd and flies in the face of all clinical experience. The goal in this situation is survival. On the other hand, in circumstances of moderate undernutrition or even fasting for a few days during illness, the issue is not just survival but maintenance of function, reduction in complications and rate of recovery. Treatment costs are also important end points which can only be tested by appropriate and well-designed studies.

Lastly, the authors provide much needed guidelines on how to design nutritional trials, making them not only statistically valid but clinically relevant. The authors have achieved a global and scholarly survey of the evidence upon which the modern practice of clinical nutrition can and should be based, and are to be congratulated on this important achievement. They also emphasize that this is not the last word, and urge us all to strive for better understanding and more evidence upon which to base further improvements in our nutritional care of patients.

Simon Allison
Professor in Clinical Nutrition, University of Nottingham
and Queen's Medical Centre
Chairman of the European Society of Parenteral and Enteral Nutrition

August 2002

Acknowledgements

We would like to express our gratitude to all of our colleagues at the Institute of Human Nutrition, University of Southampton, and Nutricia Healthcare. In particular, we would like to thank Michael Kliem for his vision for this project, and Mike Stroud, Alan Jackson, Sarka Svobodova and Karin de Hiep for their continued support and for helping to make this book a reality. We are also grateful to Corry de Vries and the libraries at Numico Research, Wageningen, and the University of Southampton for helping with our many reference requests. It has been a pleasure to work with Rebecca Stubbs and Rachel Robinson from CABI *Publishing* who remained helpful throughout. Finally, we would like to thank our families, and in particular our partners James Anderson, Marcel Kras and Irene Elia, for their patience, encouragement and support during the writing of the book.

R.J. Stratton
C.J. Green
M. Elia

Abbreviations

–	no data reported	HGS	hand-grip strength
A	abstract	HIV	human immunodeficiency virus
AAA	aromatic amino acid	% IBW	per cent ideal body weight
ADL	activities of daily living	ICD	International Classification of
AIDS	acquired immune deficiency		Disease
	syndrome	ICU	intensive care unit
ASPEN	American Society for Parenteral	inc.	increase/increased
	and Enteral Nutrition	IU	international units
BANS	British Artificial Nutrition Survey	i.v.	intravenous
BAPEN	British Association for	kcal	kilocalories
	Parenteral and Enteral Nutrition	kg	kilograms
BCAA	branched-chain amino acid	LBM	lean body mass
BEE	basal energy expenditure	LFT	liver function tests
BMI	body mass index ($kg\,m^{-2}$)	LOS	length of stay
BMR	basal metabolic rate	m	male
CHI	creatinine–height index	MAC	mid-arm circumference
CHO	carbohydrate	MAMC	mid-arm muscle circumference
CI	confidence interval	MCT	medium-chain triglyceride
CON	control group	MN	malnourished
COPD	chronic obstructive pulmonary	MS	multiple sclerosis
	disease	n	number/sample size
CVA	cerebrovascular accident	N	nitrogen
DCH	delayed cutaneous	NBM	nil by mouth
	hypersensitivity	NG	nasogastric
DM	dietary manipulation	noMN	not malnourished
DRM	disease-related malnutrition	NRT	non-randomized trial
est.	estimated	NS	not statistically significant
ETF	enteral tube feeding	ONS	oral nutritional supplements/
f	female		supplementation
F	fat	P	protein
GI	gastrointestinal	PEG	percutaneous endoscopic
GIT	gastrointestinal tract		gastrostomy
H	hospital	PEM	protein-energy malnutrition

PN	parenteral nutrition	sig.	statistically significant
Postop.	postoperative	TEI	total energy intake
Prealb.	prealbumin	TPI	total protein intake
Preop.	preoperative	TPP	thiamine pyrophosphate
Pt (pts)	patient(s)	TSF	triceps skin-fold thickness
PVS	persistent vegetative state	US	unsupplemented patients/
RCT	randomized controlled trial		group
RDI	recommended daily intake	VFI	voluntary food intake
REE	resting energy expenditure	vit.	vitamin(s)
S	supplemented patients/group	vs.	versus
SD	standard deviation	?	not clear if statistically evaluated

1
Scientific Criteria for Defining Malnutrition

Introduction

Malnutrition literally means bad or faulty nutrition. Since this implies deviations from normal nutrition, it is necessary to define cut-off points between normal and abnormal nutrition and to establish ways of identifying these deviations. Unfortunately, there are inconsistencies and a certain amount of confusion about both the definition and the recognition of malnutrition. For example, Table 1.1 shows the extraordinarily large range of cut-off values of body mass index (BMI) (weight (kg) height^{-2} (m^2): 17–23.5 kg m^{-2}) that have been recommended or used to identify individuals with chronic protein-energy undernutrition. However,

Table 1.1. Anthropometric cut-off values that include body mass index (BMI) (kg m^{-2}) for detecting underweight or undernutrition in adults.

Anthropometric criteria	Recommended/type of study using criteria	Reference
BMI < 17.0	Elderly	Wilson and Morley, 1988
BMI < 17.5	International classification for anorexia nervosa	World Health Organization, 1992
BMI < 18	Nursing homes	Lowik et al., 1992
BMI < 18.5	Community and hospital	Elia, 2000b; Kelly et al., 2000
BMI < 19.0	Community and hospital	Dietary Guidelines for Americans, 1995; Nightingale et al., 1996
BMI < 20 (< ~90% ideal body weight[a])	Community and hospital	Jallut et al., 1990; Vlaming et al., 1999
BMI < 20 (and < 15th centile for MAMC and/or 15th centile for TSF)	Hospital and community studies	McWhirter and Pennington, 1994; Edington et al., 1996, 1999
BMI < 21	Elderly in hospital	Incalzi et al., 1996
BMI < 22	Free-living elders (> 70 years)	Posner et al., 1994
BMI < ~23.5 (25th centile for BMI)	Community and hospital	Potter et al., 1998; Potter, 2001
BMI < 24 (and other criteria)	Community	Gray-Donald et al., 1995
BMI < 24 (and other criteria)	Recipients of 'meals on wheels'	Coulston et al., 1996

[a]Based on the mid-point of the Metropolitan Life Insurance tables for mid-point of 'ideal' or 'acceptable' weight range. MAMC, mid-arm muscle circumference; TSF, triceps skin-fold thickness.

the most commonly used cut-off values are between 18.5 and 20.0 kg m^{-2} (Table 1.2), both for clinical practice (Consumers' Association, 1996, 1999; Elia, 2000b; Royal College of Physicians, 2002) and for public health (Willett *et al.*, 1999). These cut-off points are of key importance to nutritional science because they determine the incidence and rationale for treatment of malnutrition. Therefore, the principles of establishing these criteria are discussed in more detail below. Another problem concerns the term 'malnutrition', which is used to denote not only deficiency but also excess and imbalance of a wide range of nutrients in both the presence and the absence of disease. This loose terminology provides an explanation for the wide incidence of malnutrition, which has been reported to range from 10–70% in hospitals, 10–90% in nursing homes and 10–100% for specific conditions. It also provides an explanation for the different reported responses to treatment, which are

discussed in subsequent chapters of this book. Here, we begin by briefly considering the malnutrition spectrum in the light of the terminology used by various workers, and the scientific basis for establishing appropriate cut-off values that distinguish between normal and abnormal nutrition. In doing so, we explore a new conceptual framework for considering malnutrition, which places more emphasis on the function of tissues rather than on their mass. It also considers potential windows of opportunity during growth, development and disease that permit nutritional modulation of function over periods that may range from days to decades (see subsequent sections in this chapter).

The Malnutrition Spectrum

Although there is no universally accepted definition of malnutrition, the following has been suggested (Elia, 2000b):

Table 1.2. Categories of BMI for identifying risk of chronic protein-energy malnutrition in adults.

BMI category (kg m^{-2})	Weight category	Interpretation
< 18.5	Underweight	Chronic malnutrition probable
18.5–20	Underweight	Chronic malnutrition possible
20–25	Desirable weight	Chronic malnutrition unlikely (low risk)
25–30	Overweight	Increased risk of complications associated with chronic overnutrition
> 30	Obese	Moderate (30–35 kg m^{-2}), high (35–40 kg m^{-2}) and very high risk (> 40 kg m^{-2}) of obesity-related complications

1. The adult BMI categories apply to both men and women of different ages. The categorization can be overridden by clinical judgement, e.g. the presence of oedema can be misleading by producing a higher BMI, and there are some perfectly healthy adults, especially young adults, with a BMI of 18.5–20 kg m^{-2}.
2. The categories provide a simple but approximate indication of malnutrition risk, which is also influenced by other factors, such as the presence of diseases/disabilities, family history of diseases, diet, physical activity and body composition.
3. BMI also gives an indication of body composition (% fat and fat-free mass), but at a given BMI body composition varies with gender (more % fat in women than in men), age (more % fat in older than in younger adults, especially in men), muscularity (less % fat in muscular individuals) and fluid status (oedema, dehydration).
4. The cut-off values for overweight and obesity are largely based on risk of premature death in initially healthy individuals, but they are also related to morbidity. The cut-off values for undernutrition are largely based on loss of pathophysiological function in individuals with and without disease, but they are also related to mortality in previously healthy individuals. They may be affected by race. There is general international consensus for choosing cut-off values of 18.5–20 kg m^{-2}. Amongst the considerations are the following: reduced work capacity and muscle strength; the effect of low maternal BMI in producing low-birth-weight babies, who are more prone to neonatal problems and mortality and to increased risk of cardiovascular disease in adult life; and response to nutritional therapy.

Malnutrition is a state of nutrition in which a deficiency or excess (or imbalance) of energy, protein, and other nutrients causes measurable adverse effects on tissue/body form (body shape, size and composition) and function, and clinical outcome.

This broad definition implies that malnutrition may arise from a wide range of conditions that differ in severity and cause, as well as the type of nutrient(s). Therefore, it is not surprising that malnutrition has been subdivided in different ways and these are discussed below.

Malnutrition of macronutrients and micronutrients

When the incidence of malnutrition or risk of malnutrition is being established, it is necessary to specify both the type of nutrient(s) under consideration and the cut-off values that are used to distinguish between the normal and abnormal range or between low and high risk of malnutrition.

Nutrients can be divided into micronutrients and macronutrients. There is universal agreement that fat, protein and carbohydrate are macronutrients and malnutrition due to these nutrients is generally referred to as protein-energy malnutrition.

However, more than one classification system exists for both macronutrients and micronutrients. This means that certain other nutrients, such as iron and zinc and even sodium and potassium, are sometimes classified as micronutrients (Baumgartner, 1991) and sometimes as macronutrients (Jeejeebhoy *et al.*, 1988). One classification system defines a micronutrient as a nutrient present in the body in less than 1 part per million (1 mg kg^{-1} body weight) (Thomas, 1994). According to this criterion, sodium, potassium, iron and zinc are not micronutrients. On the other hand, some workers apply this criterion to ultra-trace elements and suggest that trace elements are measured in mg per kg body weight (Nielsen, 1998) (1 mg kg^{-1} = 1 part per million). Another classification system defines a micronutrient as a nutrient that has a daily average requirement for a healthy adult of less than 1 mg day^{-1} (Thomas, 1994). Iron and zinc would again not qualify as micronutrients according to this criterion because their requirements are well above 1 mg day^{-1}.

In yet another classification system, only fat, protein and carbohydrate (and fibre and alcohol) are macronutrients (Jeejeebhoy *et al.*, 1988), which means that minerals, including sodium, potassium and iron, are micronutrients (Jeejeebhoy *et al.*, 1988; Baumgartner, 1991). Trace elements and vitamins are normally regarded as micronutrients but, since there are various definitions for a micronutrient, it is not surprising that some authorities regard some nutrients, such as iron and zinc, as trace elements (National Research Council, 1989) and others do not, referring to them simply as minerals.

Since the amount of carbohydrate in the human body is only 0.2–0.5 kg, the term protein-energy status generally refers to protein and fat. In general, large energy reserves are associated with an increased amount of protein and low energy reserves with a reduced amount of protein. This is because accumulation of adipose tissue is associated with increased mass of muscle (containing myofibrillar proteins) and bone (containing collagen), both of which support the extra weight of adipose tissue, as well as extra protein in tissues such as the heart, which pumps more blood, and skin, which covers a larger surface area. The BMI has been widely used as a simple reproducible index of chronic protein-energy status, in both obesity (BMI > 30 kg m^{-2}), which is associated with increased fat and lean tissues containing protein, and underweight (BMI < 20 kg m^{-2}), which is associated with reduced fat and lean tissues. This classification implies that a BMI of less than 20 kg m^{-2} is associated with some detrimental effect, such as increased risk of mortality (Metropolitan Life Insurance Company, 1959), morbidity (Elia, 2000b) or loss of physiological function (Shetty and James, 1994; Elia, 2000b). However, the incidence of specific nutrient deficiencies (e.g. micronutrients or macronutrients) varies widely in different circumstances, and their presence does not necessarily reflect chronic protein-energy status. For example, it is possible for an individual to have an acceptable whole-body protein-energy status, or even be obese, while manifesting overt clinical deficiencies of specific vitamins, such as vitamin D or thiamine (vitamin undernutrition). The National Diet and Nutrition Survey (Finch et al., 1998) for people aged 65 years and over in the UK revealed that the incidence of individual vitamin deficiencies varied from less than 2% to more than 25% (Table 1.3), while underweight (BMI < 20 kg m^{-2}) was present in about 5% of the free-living subjects and 16% of those living in institutions (the corresponding figures for those with a BMI of less than 18.5 kg m^{-2} were 2–3% and 10%, respectively). A secondary analysis of the National Diet and Nutrition Survey showed that there are no significant relationships between the status of many trace elements or vitamins, on the one hand, and BMI or BMI categories (< 20 and > 20 kg m^{-2}; or $<$ 18.5, 18–20 and > 20 kg m^{-2}), on the other.

Malnutrition of single and multiple nutrients

Malnutrition may refer to the abnormal status of a specific nutrient or to any one of a number of nutrients or combination of nutrients. It may also refer to an abnormal pattern of nutrient status, even when the status of individual nutrients falls in the acceptable reference range. The incidence of identifiable nutritional abnormalities, indicating 'malnutrition', may increase considerably when the status of multiple nutrients is assessed. In a study of lung cancer patients (Kramer, 1999), blood was taken to assess the status of a large range of vitamins, using cut-off points employed by the National Diet and Nutrition Survey. Table 1.4 shows that the incidence of selected individual vitamin deficiencies in cancer patients ranged from $< 2\%$ to 45%, but the presence of one or more deficiencies was as high as 76%. These values represent the 'average' frequency of deficiencies between diagnosis and death, but, as the disease progressed, the proportion of deficiencies increased even further. Such observations can help explain why the incidence of malnutrition has been reported to approach 100% in some patient groups. However, none of these subjects with lung cancer were considered to have vitamin A and E deficiencies, since their plasma retinol and tocopherol (and tocopherol/cholesterol ratio) concentrations were within the acceptable reference range (not shown in Table 1.4). Furthermore, none of the patients had specific clinical manifestations of vitamin deficiencies, despite the fact that

Table 1.3. Proportion of subjects 65 years and over with selected vitamin deficiencies and body mass index of less than 20 kg m^{-2} (based on Finch et al., 1998).

	Free-living (%)	Institutions[a] (%)	Criteria	
Vitamin deficiencies				
Folate: deficiency	29	35	Red-blood-cell concentration	< 345 μmol l^{-1}
severe deficiency	8	16		< 230 μmol l^{-1}
Thiamine deficiency	9	14	Erythrocyte transketolase activation coefficient	< 1.25
Vitamin B$_{12}$ deficiency	6	9	Plasma concentration	< 118 pmol l^{-1}
Vitamin D deficiency	1–2	1–5	Plasma OH-vitamin D	< 12 μmol l^{-1}
Vitamin C: deficiency	14	40	Plasma concentration	< 11 μmol l^{-1}
severe deficiency	5	16		< 5 μmol l^{-1}
Body mass index < 20 kg m^{-2}	3	16		

[a]Registered residential homes (57%), nursing homes (30%), dual-registration homes (9%) and other facilities (4%).

Table 1.4. Proportion and cumulative proportion of patients with circulating vitamin concentrations below cut-off values (Kramer, 1999).

Number of vitamins with concentrations below cut-off points	% of patients with deficiency ($n = 59$)	Cumulative % with deficiency ($n = 59$)
1	24	24
2	27	51
3	17	68
≥ 4	8	76

15% were underweight (BMI < 20 kg m^{-2}), some with cachexia or clinically obvious protein-energy undernutrition.

The situation is complex, since nutrient deficiencies may occur together and interact with each other. Such interactions may occur between macronutrients (fat, carbohydrate and protein) (e.g. nitrogen (N) balance depends not only on protein intake but also on the energy intake from fat and carbohydrate) and between micronutrients (e.g. iron may compete with other trace elements for absorption). Interactions may also occur between micro- and macronutrients. For example, thiamine deficiency affects the metabolism of glucose by acting as a cofactor in the first irreversible step in the oxidation of glucose carbon (pyruvate dehydrogenase), and vitamin E affects fat metabolism. Furthermore, deficiencies of specific trace elements (e.g. zinc) and vitamins (e.g. several B-complex vitamins) may reduce appetite (Shils, 1979) and predispose to other nutrient deficiencies. Such deficiencies can lead to other nutritional problems independently of anorexia, as shown by a study of patients with liver disease receiving intravenous nutrition (parenteral nutrition (PN)) (Rudman *et al.*, 1975). During the 6-day baseline period the subjects were in substantial positive N balance, partly because they were depleted and likely to have anabolic potential, and partly because their PN provided copious amounts of amino acids and energy, which were well above those required to maintain energy balance. During the next 6-day period, when phosphate was removed from the PN regimen while the other components were unaltered, the N balance rapidly became negative. It became positive again when phosphate was reintroduced into the regimen (Fig. 1.1). A similar phenomenon was observed with potassium (Fig. 1.1). In contrast, temporary withholding of sodium, a predominantly extracellular constituent, had relatively little effect on the N balance. Since both potassium and phosphate are predominantly intracellular constituents, it has been argued that the accretion of cell mass depends on the availability of not only protein and energy but also other constituents predominantly present in lean tissues, including certain trace elements, such as zinc. Therefore, a limiting nutrient may affect the metabolism of other nutrients and both the mass and the function of tissues. This can explain why specific nutrient deficiencies can produce a wide range of non-specific symptoms.

Primary and secondary malnutrition

There are different classification systems for primary and secondary malnutrition. Since response to nutritional support is usually affected by the presence of disease, clinicians often use the term 'secondary' malnutrition to refer to malnutrition due to disease (disease-related malnutrition) and primary malnutrition to refer to malnutrition arising in the absence of disease (e.g. lack of food due to poverty and/or social isolation). Both of these forms of malnutrition develop when intake does not meet demands. However, when nutrient deficiencies occur as a result of the increased demands of pregnancy, lactation or physical activity, in otherwise healthy individuals, the malnutrition is primary malnutrition because it is not caused by disease. This is not the case according to another classification system that is advocated in *The Encyclopaedia of Human Nutrition* (Solomons, 1998). This alternative classification attempts to distinguish between malnutrition arising from reduced nutrient intake, which is referred to as primary malnutrition, and from other causes,

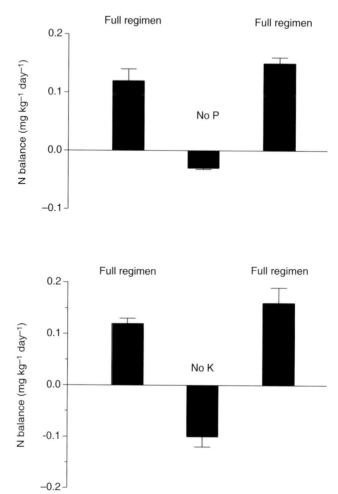

Fig. 1.1. Effect of omitting potassium (K) and phosphate (P) from a parenteral nutrition regimen on the nitrogen (N) balance in depleted patients receiving hypercaloric feeding (based on Rudman *et al.*, 1975).

which is referred to as secondary malnutrition. Here, malnutrition arising from increased requirements, such as those due to lactation, pregnancy or hot environments that produce increased evaporative water and salt losses, is regarded as secondary malnutrition. Disease-related factors, such as malabsorption, decreased utilization of nutrients, antagonism by drugs (e.g. anticoagulants antagonize the effect of vitamin K) or increased demand for nutrients (e.g. due to vomiting or diarrhoea), lead to secondary malnutrition. But, since a wide range of diseases cause such effects while producing anorexia and reduced dietary intake, they

are responsible for both primary and secondary malnutrition, according to this classification system. There is scope for considerable confusion and therefore clarification is required whenever the terms primary malnutrition and secondary malnutrition are used.

Undernutrition and overnutrition

The incidence of malnutrition due to specific nutrients varies considerably depending on whether deficiency, excess or both are used as the defining criteria for malnutrition. The same applies to protein-energy malnutrition. For example, if underweight (BMI < 20 kg m^{-2}), overweight (BMI 25–30 kg m^{-2}) and obesity (BMI > 30 kg m^{-2}) are taken to represent a suboptimal protein-energy status, then the distribution of the BMI curve in English adults in 1998 (Erens and Primatesta, 1999) suggests that most of the population has some form of malnutrition (5.3% underweight, 38.3% overweight and 19.4% obese). Such a situation is also illustrated diagrammatically in Fig. 1.2, which also shows a decrease in underweight and an increase in overweight/obesity over time. Although both under- and overnutrition are forms of malnutrition, the term 'malnutrition' is often used to refer only to undernutrition. This convention will be used in this book, so that the term 'disease-related malnutrition' refers only to disease-related undernutrition.

Clinical and subclinical malnutrition

The earliest attempts to recognize malnutrition were based on clinical observations. A patient was classified as thin or malnour-ished on clinical grounds. Substantial loss of muscle and subcutaneous fat suggests undernutrition, whereas excess adiposity suggests overweight and obesity. Hippocrates stated that 'in the face of disease thin people do badly', but he did not define thinness, which was assessed subjectively. Whereas severe under- or overnutrition is easily recognized, less severe forms of malnutrition may be difficult to identify with confidence. Formal attempts to define or recognize protein-energy malnutrition or risk of malnutrition have not been entirely successful. However, bedside or field methods that take into account both chronic protein-energy status (e.g. current weight-for-height or BMI) and recent unintentional weight loss, which if unchecked will produce chronic protein-energy malnutrition, are useful indicators (Elia, 2000b).

Specific nutrient deficiencies can also be detected clinically, for example, by ecchymosis and gingivitis, due to scurvy, night-blindness, due to vitamin A deficiency, and goitre, due to iodine deficiency. However, clinical detection usually occurs only in the advanced stages of such deficiencies. Biochemical or other tests can

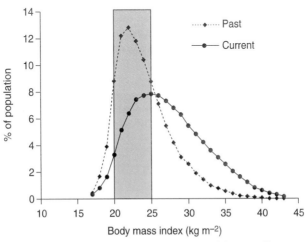

Fig. 1.2. A comparison of current and past distribution of BMI in adults typically seen in developed countries. The percentage values refer to the proportion of subjects who fall within 1 BMI unit. The values indicated on the graph represent the lower end of each BMI unit, e.g. the value for 20 kg m^{-2} represents the proportion of individuals with a BMI between 19.1 and 20.0. The majority of individuals in the 'current' distribution fall outside the range of 20–25 kg m^{-2}, predominantly in the overweight and obese range.

identify the deficiency before the specific clinical manifestations become apparent – pre- or subclinical malnutrition. For example, a low circulating concentration of vitamin C occurs before scurvy becomes apparent. Similarly, visual function tests and retinograms may detect abnormalities due to vitamin A deficiency before night-blindness develops. Detection of preclinical or subclinical malnutrition has the obvious advantage that the condition(s) can be identified and treated at an early stage to improve function or prevent progression of the condition. In most circumstances the incidence of subclinical undernutrition is considerably higher than that of clinical undernutrition.

Adult and childhood malnutrition

Although many of the basic principles associated with defining, detecting and managing malnutrition in adults and children are similar, growth in children makes some of the issues more complex. Wasting (low weight-for-height) is a relatively recent manifestation of malnutrition (although even this can take a considerable time to develop) and generally reflects a severe form of malnutrition. Stunting often occurs before wasting becomes obvious. Various classification systems have been used to 'define' malnutrition in children (Gomez et al., 1956; McLaren and Read, 1972, 1975; Waterlow, 1972; Cole and Stanfield, 1981), which include kwashiorkor and marasmus. These terms were originally established to describe syndromes of protein-energy malnutrition in children in developing countries. For example, kwashiorkor is a severe form of undernutrition, which produces oedema, depigmentation of skin and hair (World Health Organization, 1992) and other features, such as an enlarged liver. In contrast, marasmus is characterized by severe wasting with little or no oedema. However, the terms are sometimes used to describe the nutritional state of children and adults in developed countries. This may be confusing and inappropriate. Consider the low

circulating concentration of essential amino acids, which is one of the characteristic biochemical manifestations of kwashiorkor and which is probably involved in the aetiology of some of the classic manifestations of the condition. The low availability of these blood amino acids for hepatic protein synthesis, including hepatic export proteins, probably contributes to the characteristic hypoalbuminaemia and oedema of children with kwashiorkor (Waterlow et al., 1992). The reduced availability of essential amino acids may also contribute to the low circulating concentration of lipoproteins by limiting the synthesis of the apoprotein component. This reduced capacity of the liver to synthesize and export lipoproteins may contribute to both the low circulating concentrations of triglycerides/lipoproteins and the accumulation of lipid in the liver (steatosis), another characteristic feature of kwashiorkor (Waterlow et al., 1992). In contrast, undernourished adults with oedema due to heart failure do not typically have reduced circulating concentrations of essential amino acids, albumin or lipoproteins, which may actually be elevated and predispose to the development of ischaemic heart disease; nor do they typically have other classic features of kwashiorkor, such as massive amounts of fat in the liver, easily pluckable hair and poorly pigmented skin. In our view it is better to avoid the indiscriminate and routine use of such terms in clinical practice in developed countries. Descriptive terms, such as wasting with oedema due to heart failure, or nephrotic syndrome, will reduce the overabundant confusion that already exists in the field of malnutrition.

Residential/non-residential malnutrition and institutionalized/non-institutionalized malnutrition

These descriptive terms refer to the location of individuals with malnutrition. Non-institutionalized malnutrition normally refers to malnutrition in free-living individuals. Hospital malnutrition is an example of institutionalized malnutrition, which also includes malnutrition in nursing and/or residential homes. Table 1.3 shows the prevalence of vitamin deficiencies and underweight in elderly free-living and residential subjects in the UK. The incidence and pattern of vitamin deficiencies in hospitalized patients can be different from those shown in Table 1.3. Similarly, the incidence of protein-energy malnutrition and underweight is much greater in hospitalized patients (10–40% in the UK; see Chapter 2) than in the community as a whole (about 5% in the UK).

From the above discussion it is clear that the incidence of malnutrition depends on the method used to identify it. It is also determined by the cut-off values or thresholds used by each method to distinguish between normality and abnormality. The factors involved in establishing the cut-off values differ with the nutrient, but the principles are similar. These are discussed in some detail below, using protein-energy malnutrition as an example. In subsequent chapters, the cut-off points are used to establish national and international variations in the incidence of malnutrition and

to show how intervention with food, oral nutritional supplements and artificial nutrition (enteral tube feeding (ETF) and PN) can be used to improve body structure and/or function and clinical outcome.

Establishing Cut-off Values for Protein-energy Malnutrition

General considerations

Risk of deficiency and toxicity

Figure 1.3 shows that, above and below certain cut-off points of nutrient status, the risk of metabolic derangements and of 'deficiency' or 'toxicity' increases rapidly. The same framework can be used to consider the effects of inadequate and excess intake of nutrients (FAO/WHO/UNU, 1985). The safe range varies widely with the nutrient, e.g. there is a wide range between recommended dietary allowances and toxicity levels for vitamin C and B_{12}, but this range is much narrower for vitamin D, which at high concentrations may produce symptoms due to hypercalcaemia

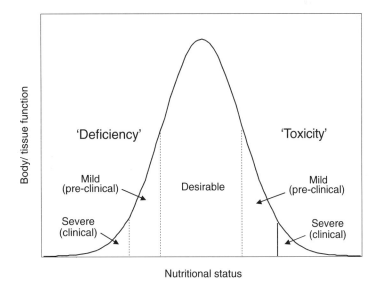

Fig. 1.3. Desirable range of nutritional status in relation to risk of undernutrition (deficiency) and overnutrition (toxicity). The graph applies to protein-energy status as well as individual nutrients. Deviations from the desirable range of nutritional status are often detected earlier using laboratory tests or tests of body function (pre-clinical) than clinical procedures.

(Department of Health, 1991b). Subclinical manifestations may occur considerably earlier (sometimes years) than the clinical manifestations, especially for nutrients that have large stores. For example, a low circulating concentration of vitamin B_{12} often occurs many months before pernicious anaemia becomes clinically apparent. Similarly, visual function tests and retinograms may detect abnormalities due to vitamin A deficiency many months before night-blindness becomes clinically detectable. Biochemical tests of nutrient status have the advantage that no adjustment is usually necessary for individuals of different weight or height. This contrasts with some anthropometric indices, such as weight, which may be adjusted for height (typically BMI in adults (weight height^{-2}) or ponderal index in newborns (weight height^{-3})).

Normal, acceptable and ideal reference ranges

Both the distribution and the mean values for anthropometric characteristics, such as weight, height or BMI, can vary considerably from one population to another and in the same population at different times (Fig. 1.2). Therefore, what is average or 'normal' in one population is not 'normal' for another. The reference range for BMI established from the obese population of Pima Indians in Arizona, USA, is obviously higher than for other populations. In contrast, the 'normal' range or the distribution of the circulating vitamin A concentration for a population living in a geographical region where vitamin A deficiency is endemic is lower than in non-endemic regions. Although it is obvious that the average observed reference range for biochemical or anthropometric indices of a patient population is not necessarily ideal for that population, this distinction is not always made. Furthermore, it is possible for a patient population to have similar nutritional status to that of a reference population and for substantial malnutrition to be present in both populations. Table 1.5 shows that, in the same group of patients with lung cancer mentioned above, the incidence of vitamin deficiencies was generally no different from the free-living control population, although both groups showed evidence of significant vitamin deficiencies. On the other hand, the incidence of underweight inpatients with lung cancer was three times more than in the reference population.

The *International Statistical Classification of Diseases and Related Health Problems* (World Health Organization, 1992) used weight, expressed as standard deviation scores (z scores), to define probability of malnutrition (Fig. 1.4 and Table 1.6). This statistical approach does not use a weight-for-height index and does not define the reference population, either for adults or for children.

Table 1.5. Proportion of patients with circulating vitamin concentrations below cut-off values (Kramer, 1999).

	Cut-off for 'inadequate' status	Free-living 'control' (%)	Cancer patients (%)	
Retinol (μmol l^{-1})	< 0.7	0	0	NS
Vitamin D (nmol l^{-1})	< 25	8	10	NS
Vitamin C (μmol l^{-1})	< 11	14	22	NS
Iron (% saturation)	< 15	11	32	$P < 0.001$
Riboflavin (activation ratio)	< 1.3	41	45	NS
One or more 'deficiency'[a]		–	76	–

[a]Other vitamins measured included thiamine, pyridoxine, vitamin B_{12} and folic acid.
NS, not significant.

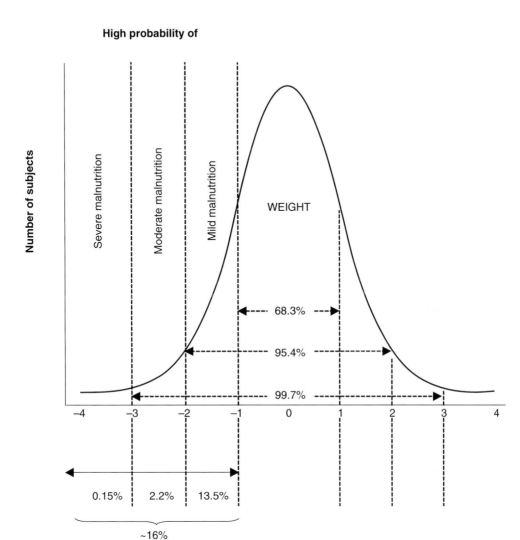

Fig. 1.4. The risk of malnutrition according to the International Statistical Classification of Disease (ICD10) (World Health Organization, 1992).

Table 1.6. Classification of malnutrition (undernutrition) in adults and children by standard deviation scores (z scores) below the mean of the weight of the reference population (International Classification of Disease (ICD) (World Health Organization, 1992)).

Type and degree of malnutrition (ICD code)	Definition (high probability of malnutrition)
No malnutrition	z score −1 to +1
Mild malnutrition (E 44.0)	z score −1 to −2
Moderate malnutrition (E 44.1)	z score −2 to −3
Severe malnutrition (E 43)	z score < -3
Kwashiorkor (E 40)	Severe malnutrition with nutritional oedema and depigmentation of skin and hair
Nutritional marasmus (E 41)	Severe malnutrition with marasmus wasting
Marasmic kwashiorkor (E 42)	Severe malnutrition with signs of both kwashiorkor and marasmus

To understand some of the controversies and confusion that continue to exist about different classification systems for protein-energy malnutrition, it is helpful to consider the establishment of normal, acceptable and ideal reference ranges from a historical perspective. Anthropometric cut-off values from malnutrition have been derived and discussed separately below from mortality statistics and physiological considerations based on loss of body function. Mortality statistics are considered first, using BMI as a marker of chronic protein-energy status.

BMI cut-off points in relation to mortality in adults

Despite the existence of malnutrition since prehistoric times, it is only relatively recently that health professionals have attempted to establish 'ideal' or acceptable weight ranges. The ultimate aim of establishing these reference ranges is to identify individuals with a high risk of developing a disease or condition, so that preventive measures can be instituted at an early stage to reduce the risk and/or improve clinical outcome. The first attempt to establish acceptable weight-for-height tables was made in 1846 by an English surgeon, John Hutchinson, who produced a weight-for-height table for Englishmen aged 30 years. He recommended that censuses should include such information to predict disease and mortality and that the information should be used to establish public health policy (Weigley, 1984). When insurance companies became interested in the weights and heights of individuals, they used average weight-for-height as the reference standards. It was soon recognized that these standard average weights were not the best predictors of premature death. In 1942 and 1943 Metropolitan Life Insurance Company in the USA introduced the concept of 'ideal weight'. The potential health benefits of maintaining a lower than average weight were described in the 1959 Metropolitan Life Insurance tables (Metropolitan Life Insurance Company, 1959). The Metropolitan tables published in 1983, which were based on the

actuary *Build Study* (Society of Actuaries and Association of Life Insurance Medical Doctors of America, 1980), increased the reference weight-for-height values after considering recent mortality data, and referred to them as 'acceptable' rather than 'ideal' reference ranges. Other data were also in general agreement with the above ranges. The U-shaped BMI–mortality curves typically suggested that a BMI of 20–25 kg m^{-2} was acceptable, since this was associated with the lowest mortality. Mortality was increased both below a BMI of 20 kg m^{-2} (underweight or 'undernourished') and above a BMI of 25 kg m^{-2} (overweight or 'overnourished'). The mid-point of the reference range has been referred to as the ideal body weight for height, and generally corresponds to a BMI of about 22.5 kg m^{-2}, although this varies somewhat depending on gender and height (according to the Metropolitan Life Insurance tables, it is slightly lower for women than for men and in taller than in shorter individuals). The Office of Population Censuses and Surveys (1993, 1994) in England also classified adults with a BMI less than 20 kg m^{-2} as 'underweight', and those with a BMI more than 25 kg m^{-2} as overweight. However, the validity of the Metropolitan Life Insurance tables for general application to the population of the USA and other developed countries has been questioned, for three main reasons:

- The mortality data of individuals taking life insurance may not reflect the mortality characteristics of the rest of the population.
- The tables included only a small proportion of individuals over 60 years (even the standard 1983 tables were intended for individuals aged 25 to 59 years) and therefore there is uncertainty about the extent to which they apply to older subjects.
- The effect of race on the BMI–mortality curves was inadequately considered

Since then a variety of studies have examined the role of weight and height (or BMI) and age in relation to mortality. A recent review (Elia, 2001b) identified four key features of the BMI–mortality curves.

1. The curves move upwards (greater mortality) with age, with no abrupt rise between 20 and 85 years.

2. The curves tend to become attenuated with increasing age and may become totally flat in advanced old age. If these mortality curves are to be used to define malnutrition, then one interpretation of the flat curves is that there is no malnutrition (undernutrition or overnutrition) in advanced age. It is possible that individuals sensitive to the effects of underweight and overweight have already died, leaving a group of individuals that are resistant to the adverse effects of underweight and overweight. Another possible explanation is that there are cohort effects, since the curves were often established cross-sectionally in individuals with different lifestyles brought up in different environments and at different times, some of which were in the pre-antibiotic era. However, some longitudinal studies have shown attenuated BMI–mortality curves, suggesting that this may not be a specific feature of cross-sectional studies. Yet another explanation for the attenuated BMI–mortality curves concerns a ceiling effect for survival. Since very elderly individuals have a limited time to survive, long-term studies (often 10 or more years) will result in a very high mortality irrespective of initial BMI. Therefore, an analysis over shorter periods of time is required.

3. Some, but by no means all, BMI–mortality curves obtained in Caucasians have been reported to shift to the right with increasing age, implying that it is more acceptable to be heavier at an older than at a younger age. In 1989 the National Research Council (USA) recommended age-specific BMI ranges. The acceptable reference BMI range was considered to be 19–24 kg m^{-2} for those aged 19–25 years and 20–25 kg m^{-2} for those aged 25–35 years, with further increments by 1 BMI unit for every decade until the age of 65 years. This meant that, for those aged over 65 years, the desirable reference range was as high as 24–29 kg m^{-2}. By analogy with previous U-shaped curves, individuals aged 75 to 85 with a BMI below 24 kg m^{-2}

could be regarded as underweight or undernourished. In 1990 the edition of the US Department of Agriculture (USDA) report, *Dietary Guidelines for Americans* recommended age-specific BMI reference ranges, e.g. by providing separate cut-off values for those aged below and above 35 years. A strong reaction against the use of age-specific ranges arose from the scientific community, on the basis that much of the data had not taken into consideration confounding variables, such as pre-existing disease and smoking, which are known to reduce weight and increase the risk of premature death. The 1995 edition of *Dietary Guidelines for Americans* withdrew the age-specific BMI recommendations and reverted to older reference ranges, which always included a lower boundary of 19 kg m^{-2} and an upper boundary of about 25 kg m^{-2}. Presumably, at this time the USDA reconsidered the evidence and could not make a strong enough case for the age-specific BMI recommendations. Since then, individual workers have summarized the reasons for retaining the earlier reference ranges (Willett *et al.*, 1999). By this time, the idea that older individuals were undernourished even when they had a BMI between 20 and 24 kg m^{-2} had become widespread, and was largely responsible for the high BMI cut-off points that have found their way into some nutrition screening tools and papers on nutritional assessment for the purpose of nutritional intervention (Posner *et al.*, 1993; Gray-Donald *et al.*, 1995; Coulston *et al.*, 1996). In the meantime, several recent studies have shown that, within the BMI range of about 19–25 kg m^{-2}, there is a direct positive relationship between BMI and morbidity (Ford *et al.*, 1997; National Institutes of Health, 1998; Ashton *et al.*, 2001), mortality (Stevens *et al.*, 1998; Willett *et al.*, 1999) and biochemical risk factors (Ashton *et al.*, 2001), implying that a better or healthier BMI might be less than 25 kg m^{-2}.

4. Most of the mortality statistics and BMI–mortality curves have been established in Caucasians in the USA and Europe. The results do not necessarily apply to other racial groups. Indeed, the BMI–mortality curves are shifted substantially upwards (greater mortality) in black Americans compared with Caucasians, even after controlling for confounding variables, such as smoking and social class. In Asia, results of BMI–morbidity/mortality curves have led to a demand to lower the acceptable range of BMI to 18.5–23 kg m^{-2} (shift to the left) (James *et al.*, 2001). A reduction in the upper BMI cut-off to a value between 23 and 24 kg m^{-2} has also been suggested for the Chinese (Ko *et al.*, 1999).

The BMI–mortality curves and the cut-off points used often emerged from studies that excluded individuals with overtly serious disease at the outset (Elia, 2001b). Many also began analysing mortality data after a 'wash-out' period of up to several years (Elia, 2001b). Since many individuals with serious illness were expected to have died during this period, they were excluded from the analysis. Both of these approaches have their limitations, especially in studies of the elderly, who frequently suffer from a range of disabilities and diseases (Elia *et al.*, 2000c). Nevertheless, the BMI–mortality curves were intended to apply to initially healthy subjects without serious overt diseases. Many studies also controlled for smoking or included only those subjects that did not smoke (Elia, 2001b).

In summary, the traditional lower and upper cut-off points of BMI for predicting the lowest mortality are 20 and 25 kg m^{-2}, respectively, but there is still some uncertainty about the universal application of these cut-off values to different racial groups, ages and genders. Lower boundary BMI values of 23 or 24 kg m^{-2}, which have been incorporated into nutrition screening tools that aid detection and clinical management of malnutrition in the elderly, are considered by many to be inappropriate. This is not only because of the theoretical reasons outlined above, but also for practical clinical reasons, since the use of such cut-off points will result in large segments of the elderly population in developed countries being included in the undernourished category. For example, a study of

older men living in an urban area in America reported that 63% had a BMI < 24 kg m^{-2} (Ritchie *et al.*, 1997). Furthermore, although the BMI cut-off points discussed above were intended to provide a 'long-term' guide to mortality over several years for initially healthy individuals, many clinicians and other health professionals are more interested in the 'shorter-term' detriments of malnutrition. Such health professionals deal with established malnutrition, which is often present in association with diseases that were specifically excluded, when recognized, in many of the epidemiological studies. Therefore, there is a need to consider the BMI cut-off points from a different perspective that takes into account the adverse physiological and clinical effects of malnutrition. Furthermore, some workers feel that epidemiological approaches have not clearly defined a lower BMI boundary cut-off (Willett *et al.*, 1999).

BMI cut-off points in relation to loss of body function in adults

In contrast to mortality, which represents a single clear-cut event, loss of body function involves loss of multiple functions, such as physiological, behavioural and psychological functions (Table 1.7). Even within each one of these categories, there are multiple functions that may deteriorate at different rates. For example, as BMI declines, sensory functions, such as sight, hearing and smell, generally tend to be preserved more than motor functions, such as strength. Despite these theoretical difficulties, reports from a wide range of national or international organizations and agencies that have taken into account physiological function have generally been consistent in recommending a lower BMI cut-off point between 18.5 and 20 kg m^{-2} (FAO/WHO/UNU, 1985; Shetty and James, 1994; Shenkin *et al.*, 1996; Elia, 2000b). Cut-off values between 18.5 and 20 kg m^{-2} are also recommended by a variety of other bodies, including the Royal College of Physicians (London) (2002) and other independent review bodies (Consumers' Association,

Table 1.7. Some adverse consequences of undernutrition (based on Elia, 2000b).

	Potential consequence
Physical function	
Impaired immune function (Chandra, 1988)	Predisposes to infection
Reduced respiratory muscle strength	Poor cough pressure, predisposing and delaying recovery from chest infection
Reduced sensitivity of the respiratory centre to oxygen	Predisposes to or delays weaning from artificial ventilation in patients with respiratory disease
Reduced muscle strength and fatigue	Contributes to inactivity, reduced work output and poor self-care (Leyton, 1946; Keys *et al.*, 1950; Elia, 1993, 1997a). Falls may result from abnormal muscle function
Inactivity (Leyton, 1946), especially in bedridden patients	Predisposes to pressure sores and thromboembolism
Impaired thermoregulation (Allison, 1997)	Leads to hypothermia, especially in the elderly
Impaired wound healing (Haydock and Hill, 1986)	Prolonged recovery from illness, increased length of hospital stay and delayed return to work
Reduced cushioning effects of subcutaneous fat	Predisposes to fractures in those who have accidental falls
Fetal and infant programming (Henry and Ulijaszek, 1996; O'Brien *et al.*, 1999; United States Department of Agriculture, 2002)	Predisposes to common chronic diseases, such as cardiovascular disease, cerebrovascular accident, hypertension and diabetes in adult life
Psychosocial function	
Apathy, depression and hypochondria (Keys *et al.*, 1950; Elia, 1993)	Reduces well-being
Impaired social interactions and impaired mother–child bonding (Brozek, 1990)	Poor family relations and poor child rearing
Loss of libido (Keys *et al.*, 1950; Elia, 1993)	Reduces reproductive competence
Self-neglect (Keys *et al.*, 1950; Elia, 1993)	Predisposes to other detrimental physical and psychological effects

1996, 1999; National Prescribing Centre, 1998; Elia, 2000b) and individual workers from various parts of the world (Garrow, 1988; James *et al.*, 1988; Thomas and Gill, 1998). The following functional outcome measures have been taken into account to establish the cut-off values for BMI (Shetty and James, 1994; Elia, 2000b).

1. Maternal BMI, birth weight and early growth. Maternal BMI is related to birth weight, which is associated with increased risk of infection, respiratory problems and neonatal mortality. Thus, studies in various countries show that low-birth-weight babies are more likely to be born to mothers with a BMI < 18.5 than to those with BMI > 18.5 kg m^{-2} (Allen *et al.*, 1994). In Kenya and Mexico, all low-birth-weight infants were born to mothers with a BMI < 21 kg m^{-2}. Furthermore, in the USA, the National Natality Survey showed that low

maternal BMI in early pregnancy (BMI < 19.8 kg m^{-2}) led to the lowest-birth-weight infants (Institute of Medicine, 1990). In India, where chronic protein-energy malnutrition is more common, the relative risk of low-birth-weight babies gradually increases from 1.0 in mothers with a BMI of 20–25 kg m^{-2}, to 1.05, 1.37, 1.58 and 2.02 in mothers with a BMI of 18.5–20.0, 17.0–18.5, 16.0–17.0 and < 16.0 kg m^{-2}, respectively (Naidu and Rao, 1994). Similar trends have been observed in other countries (Kusin *et al.*, 1994). Furthermore, babies tend to have lower weights at 3 and 6 months when born to women with a BMI < 18.5 kg m^{-2} compared with those with a BMI > 18.5 kg m^{-2}. In The Gambia, where there are seasonal variations in BMI (~10% variation around a BMI of 20 kg m^{-2}) (Ferro-Luzzi *et al.*, 1994), there is seasonal variation in birth weight. Nutritional supplementation (protein and energy) of underweight pregnant women leads to increased birth weight and, in some cases, reduction in infant mortality in those born to underweight mothers (Ceesay *et al.*, 1997; De Onis *et al.*, 1998) but not normally nourished mothers (Rush, 1989).

2. Disease. The frequency of illnesses has been found to increase considerably in individuals with a low BMI in a variety of countries. In Rwanda, a major increase in sickness has been reported in adults with a BMI of less than 17.6 kg m^{-2} (Shetty and James, 1994; Elia, 2000b) and, in Bangladesh, time off work due to illness increases considerably in fathers with a BMI of less than 18 kg m^{-2}. Similar observations have been made in more developed countries. In the USA, there is a relationship between BMI and the functional capabilities of community-dwelling elderly (Galanos *et al.*, 1994). In the UK, free-living individuals in the community with a BMI < 20 kg m^{-2} are more likely to consult their general practitioners, to need medication, to function badly and to be admitted to hospital (Martyn *et al.*, 1998; Stratton *et al.*, 2002), where they have more complications and take longer to recover (Consumers' Association, 1996, 1999). Causal relationships between nutritional status and function have not always been established, although it is known that a low BMI predisposes to and delays recovery from illness by a variety of mechanisms, including effects on the immune system and the muscular system (Table 1.7). Furthermore, particularly in the community (but not in hospital), several studies have reported that functional benefits from nutritional support are more likely to occur in those with a BMI < 20 kg m^{-2} than those with BMI > 20 kg m^{-2} (Stratton and Elia, 1999a; see Chapter 6).

3. Physical activity, exercise and work output. Physical work capacity, which is often measured as maximum oxygen consumption (VO_2 max.), has been repeatedly reported to be reduced in underweight individuals, who have reduced muscle mass. There does not appear to be a single cut-off value since there is a gradual deterioration in VO_2 max. as BMI decreases.

Nevertheless, studies in young Colombian adults found that only the severely undernourished with a BMI < 18.5 kg m^{-2} had a marked reduction in VO_2 max. (Spurr *et al.*, 1977; Spurr, 1987), even when adjusted for body weight (other studies do not necessarily show a reduction in VO_2 max. per kg body weight). Experimental studies also show a reduction in VO_2 max. during weight loss and improvement after weight regain (Keys *et al.*, 1950; Gibney, 2002). Studies in various parts of the world also show that BMI or other weight-to-height indices are linked to labour productivity, farm output, industrial tasks and ability to maintain work output (Shetty and James, 1994). Furthermore, studies in India and Ethiopia have reported that individuals with a BMI < 18.5 kg m^{-2} work fewer hours per day than those with a BMI > 18.5 kg m^{-2}, after adjusting for sociological and cultural factors. In addition, a low BMI increases the time taken to perform hard physical tasks. For example, individuals in Guatemala with a mean BMI of 20.1 kg m^{-2} took about 70% longer to complete the same agricultural task than those with a BMI of 23.2 kg m^{-2} (Torun *et al.*, 1989). Supplementation studies in Guatemala resulted in improved productivity (Spurr, 1987). In the Minnesota study (USA), in which healthy individuals with a mean initial BMI of > 20 kg m^{-2} lost about 25% of their body weight over 6 months to achieve a final BMI of 16.5 kg m^{-2}, there was a marked reduction in activity and motivation to undertake physical activity (Keys *et al.*, 1950). Other experimental studies in the USA have shown that, in healthy individuals with reduced intake, there is a change in the pattern of activities, with a preference for discretionary activities that require less effort (Gorsky and Calloway, 1983). In developing countries, substantial work output can be maintained at the expense of body weight and discretionary social activities (Torun *et al.*, 1989). It can also be increased by supplementation. However, work performance, physical activity and body weight can be affected by motivation to earn money and by health status.

On the basis of physiological and clinical considerations, a BMI cut-off value between 18.5 and 20 kg m^{-2} has been commonly incorporated into nutrition screening tools (Pinchcofsky-Devin and Kaminski, 1985a; Keller, 1993; McWhirter and Pennington, 1994; Lennard-Jones *et al.*, 1995; Reilly, H.M. *et al.*, 1995; Edington *et al.*, 1996, 2000; National Prescribing Centre, 1998; Elia, 2000b; Kelly *et al.*, 2000) that are used clinically to screen for risk of nutritionally related morbidity and to identify subjects for more detailed assessment of nutritional status (for example, see Fig. 1.5). It also corresponds closely to the lower BMI cut-off point established from mortality statistics in apparently healthy subjects (see above). Much less attention has been given to establishing an upper BMI cut-off point for adverse physiological effects and clinical outcome (other than mortality).

Merits and limitations of using the BMI to establish cut-off points for risk of malnutrition

BMI is a simple and reproducible measurement (Fuller *et al.*, 1991) that reflects body composition (Elia, 1992b) and function (Shetty and James, 1994). It has been recorded in a wide range of studies in relation to mortality and body function in a variety of circumstances. This makes possible a comparison of an extensive amount of data obtained from different parts of the world and different health-care settings. It is, of course, necessary to investigate possible causal links when there are relationships between BMI, on the one hand, and mortality, morbidity and physiological function, on the other. However, in some circumstances, randomized clinical controlled trials may be difficult to undertake for ethical reasons (see Chapter 10). Randomized controlled studies involving nutritional interventions are discussed in detail in Chapters 6 and 7.

Since taller individuals are generally heavier than shorter individuals, it is obviously necessary to establish a weight-for-height index to control for this source of

variation. Naturally, the ratio of weight/height was proposed for this purpose. Unfortunately, the ratio is related to height, so that taller individuals have a higher index than shorter individuals. This means that the index does not totally control or adjust for height. To improve the situation the height term can be raised to the power of 2 (weight for height^2) to establish the BMI. However, the BMI is not necessarily ideal for use in different countries, where exponents greater or less than 2 are theoretically more appropriate, due to differences in the proportions (weight and height) of body segments. However, for simplicity and for comparative purposes, international agencies have favoured the use of BMI.

BMI is an attractive index to use because it is linearly related to fat and inversely related to the proportion of body weight due to lean tissues, which carry out a variety of physiological functions, and the proportion of body weight due to body fat, which is a risk factor for premature death. However, the relationship between BMI and body composition is only approximate and is affected by gender, age and race. For example, there are constitutional differences between individuals, who have different frames and muscularity and different segmental proportions of length and mass. The Chinese tend to have lower leg-to-height ratios than Africans. In addition, after 30–40 years of age, subjects tend to lose lean tissue and replace it with fat. This implies that, for the same BMI, older individuals tend to have more fat and less muscle than younger individuals (Elia, 2001b). This 'wasting' of muscle with increasing age is more marked in men than in women, probably because muscle accounts for a greater proportion of body weight and lean body mass in men than in women. However, since the overall effects are not striking, especially in women, in whom it can be difficult to demonstrate an age effect, the same BMI cut-off values are often used throughout the adult lifespan. However, it should be appreciated that one of the confounding variables is kyphosis, which tends to occur with increasing age as a result of osteoporosis. A 5 cm decrease

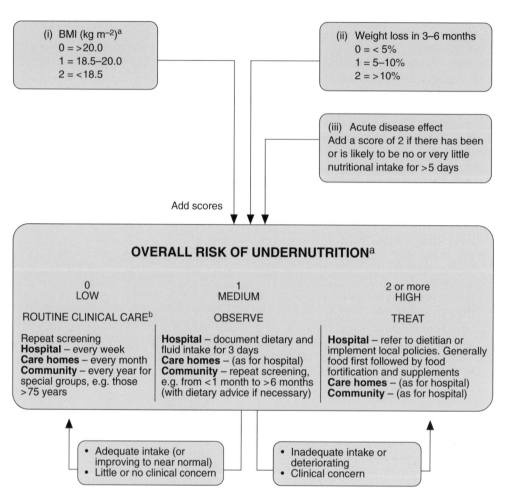

Fig. 1.5. The malnutrition universal screening tool (MUST). The tool has validity (content and face validity as well as concurrent and predictive validity) and very good to excellent reliability when examined in a variety of health-care settings by different types of health workers (nurses, health-care assistants, students, doctors) (Elia, 2000b; Stratton and Elia, 2002; Stratton *et al.*, 2002; Weekes and Elia, 2002). It has also been found to be practical in hospitals and nursing homes and in the community (general practice surgeries) (Elia, 2000b). The tool is accompanied by charts to allow rapid categorization of patients into BMI and weight-loss categories and for converting knee height to stature. The care plan shown is a general one, but care plans for different health-care settings/patient groups are suggested and amenable to adaptation and modification according to local needs. The documentation sheets allow identification and recording of obesity (BMI > 30 kg m^{-2}), which follows a different management pathway, and special diets received by patients, which are considered in both pathways.

[a] **If height, weight or weight loss cannot be established**, use documented or recalled values (if considered reliable). When measured or recalled height cannot be obtained, use knee height as a surrogate measure. **If neither can be calculated**, obtain an overall impression of malnutrition risk (low, medium, high) using the following:
 (i) Clinical impression (very thin, thin, average, overweight).
(ii) • Clothes and/or jewellery have become loose-fitting.
     • History of decreased food intake, loss of appetite or dysphagia up to 3–6 months.
     • Disease (underlying cause) and psychosocial/physical disabilities likely to cause weight loss.
[b] Involves treatment of underlying condition and help with food choice and eating when necessary (also applies to other categories).
© British Association for Parenteral and Enteral Nutrition (BAPEN).

in height (about 2 inches) in individuals with an initial BMI of 20–25 kg m^{-2} will generally decrease the BMI by 1.1–1.5 kg m^{-2}. Another difficulty concerns the interpretation of BMI measurements in the presence of fluid disturbances, such as oedema, dehydration and ascites. About 2–3 kg of fluid accumulates before oedema can be detected clinically, and several times more fluid can accumulate in some clinical conditions. In such situations, clinical judgement about protein-energy malnutrition, based on the presence of wasted muscles or excess fat, can be very valuable.

Body composition analysis has clearly demonstrated that at a given BMI, women have more body fat than men. However, the same cut-off point for men and women can be justified on the basis of the following: (i) additional energy required by women to sustain late pregnancy and lactation and child rearing; (ii) women are shorter and lighter than men and therefore disadvantaged in weight-bearing activities (more relevant in developing countries, where women undertake heavy manual work); and (iii) simplicity in having a single cut-off value for both sexes. Nevertheless, in view of this difference and the relative resistance of women compared with men to cardiovascular disease for the same per cent body fat, outcome measures such as mortality are analysed separately for men and women.

It is difficult to establish a single BMI cut-off point for identifying undernutrition for at least two reasons. First, the constitutional, racial and gender- and age-related factors mentioned above make interpretation of relationships between BMI and body composition or body function more difficult. For example, older individuals with the same BMI will generally have less muscle, less strength and less capacity to work than younger individuals. In addition, Behnke, a physician in the US navy demonstrated in a classic paper (Behnke *et al.*, 1942) the limitations of weight-to-height indices for predicting fatness. He demonstrated that a number of American football players who were found to be functionally unfit for military service during the Second World War because of their

excess body weight actually had less fat than control subjects who were suitable for military service. Conversely, some individuals below a BMI of 18.5 kg m^{-2} may be perfectly healthy. For example, 2–3% of apparently fit and healthy soldiers in the British army were found to have a BMI less than 18.5 kg m^{-2} (James *et al.*, 1988). It should also be appreciated that some individuals with a BMI between 18.5 and 20 kg m^{-2} may be chronically malnourished. Methods for distinguishing undernourished from healthy individuals within the BMI range of 18.5–20.0 kg m^{-2} would be valuable.

Secondly, as indicated above, different physiological functions are affected to a different extent as BMI decreases. Sensory functions (Keys *et al.*, 1950) and lactational performance (Prentice *et al.*, 1994) are generally well preserved during undernutrition. In contrast, birth weight and maximum capacity for work are lower in individuals with a BMI < 18.5 kg m^{-2} than in those with BMI > 18.5 kg m^{-2}. Physiological function can be affected by disease, drugs and the rate of weight loss, independently of BMI, a topic that will be considered in more detail below.

In summary, it appears that a single BMI cut-off value for detecting chronic protein undernutrition has the advantage of simplicity and reproducibility. The use of the same reference standards also allows comparisons between and within different countries and health-care settings. However, the index should generally be used to provide only an approximate guide to the probability or risk of protein-energy malnutrition rather than to identify malnutrition *per se*. Furthermore, the use of a single BMI measurement gives no indication of recent weight changes or likelihood of future weight changes. Several clinical studies have demonstrated that recent weight change is one of the most important components, of malnutrition screening tools when used on particular groups of patients (Hirsch *et al.*, 1991). It also contributes to the overall malnutrition risk score and to clinical outcome independently of BMI (Murphy *et al.*, 2000). Therefore, it is not surprising that a number of nutrition screening tools use both BMI and weight loss to predict risk of malnutrition (see Fig. 1.5 for an example).

Weight loss cut-off points in relation to loss of body function in adults

Whereas BMI indicates chronic protein-energy status, recent unintentional weight loss (to distinguish it from intentional weight loss due to dieting for overweight and obesity) indicates more acute changes in protein-energy status. Such measurements are valuable because significant unintentional weight loss suggests the presence of an underlying disease, which if unchecked is likely to produce further weight loss, undernutrition and deterioration in body function. Therefore, it is important to define significant weight loss so that cut-off values can be used to separate those at risk of malnutrition from those in whom the weight loss is part of the normal physiological fluctuations in weight. Unfortunately, there are no internationally agreed cut-off values, either for adults or for children, and clinicians have often used their judgement and experience. A more scientific approach to establishing cut-off values for weight loss, which can complement clinical judgement and vice versa, involves consideration of the following.

1. *Normal intra-individual variation in weight change.* Information on the normal variability in weight over time is needed to establish an appropriate reference range, e.g. 95% reference range, corresponding to 2 standard deviations (SD) on either side of the mean or median. In individuals who unintentionally lose more weight than the lower cut-off point, there is a substantial probability that an underlying pathological cause will produce malnutrition, if it has not already done so. Normal individual weight changes increase with time, and therefore the period over which the weight loss occurs needs to be specified. Various national reports and organizations and individual workers have provided a range of cut-off values, which generally fall within the 5–10% range of weight loss over the previous 3–6 months (or 10% of pre-illness weight) (Blackburn *et al.*, 1977; Blackburn and Harvey, 1982; Detsky *et al.*, 1987; Morley *et al.*, 1988; American Society for Parenteral and Enteral Nutrition, 1989; Morley, 1991; ASPEN, 1993a; British Dietetic Association, 1994; Allison, 1995; Caroline Walker Trust, 1995; Nikolaus *et al.*, 1995; Elia, 1996a; Klein *et al.*, 1997; Moore, A.A. *et al.*, 1997; White, 1997; National Prescribing Centre, 1998; Elia, 2000b). There is a remarkable paucity of information as to why these cut-off values were chosen, but it seems that clinical judgement was important. The Malnutrition Advisory Group (MAG) of the British Association for Parenteral and Enteral Nutrition (BAPEN) summarized information on intra-individual variability in weight (Elia, 2000b) and went on to assess the detrimental effects associated with weight loss. There is little information on normal unintentional weight variability in weight loss over 3–6 months, but the available information tentatively suggested that it is approximately 5% for middle-aged to elderly subjects (–2 SD). Studies over longer periods (6 months to 10 years) are more numerous and, as expected, show greater intra-individual variability.

2. *Detriments associated with weight loss.* It is necessary to establish at what point(s) within or outside the normal intra-individual range of weight loss functionally important detriments develop. The extent of weight loss associated with detrimental physiological or clinical effects varies between studies with the outcome variable under consideration. However, when healthy subjects lose 5% of their body weight rapidly through dietary restriction, they feel less energetic, reduce their voluntary physical activity and develop fatigue more easily. These as well as other changes in muscle function (Keys *et al.*, 1950; Jeejeebhoy, 1988b), disturbances in thermoregulation (Fellows *et al.*, 1990) and poor response to or outcome of surgery (Studley, 1936; Seltzer *et al.*, 1982; Windsor and Hill, 1988) and chemotherapy (DeWys *et al.*, 1980) are present at 10% weight loss and become more severe at 20% weight loss. It is obviously important to distin-

guish between nutritional and non-nutritional contributions to outcome. Nutritional intervention studies, which are a major focus of this book, provide a means of making this distinction. Another way is to study weight loss in the absence of disease. For example, in studies preliminary to the Minnesota experiment (Keys *et al.*, 1950), a 10% weight loss over 3 months in healthy lean men reduced grip strength by 8–9% and maximum capacity for work (*VO*$_2$ max.) and reduced will-power for undertaking strenuous physical exercise. They also became more sensitive to cold, felt weaker and more fatigued and lost libido.

3. *Common reference criteria for men and women.* If possible, it would be an advantage to provide cut-off points that are common to men and women, irrespective of body weight or age. Since body weight varies considerably between individuals and between sexes, it is appropriate to use per cent unintentional weight loss as a practical common denominator to compare the magnitude of the 'nutritional stress'. However, some nutrition screening tools use absolute weight. For example, the Nutrition Screening Initiative in the USA and a number of individual workers (Moore, A.A. *et al.*, 1997; Matarese and Gottschlich, 1998) have suggested that an unintentional weight loss of 10 lbs (4.5 kg, corresponding to 5.3–9.0% weight loss in individuals weighing 50–85 kg) over 6 months should be used as a warning signal for malnutrition. Even so, there is limited information as to whether the same per cent weight loss affects older and younger individuals in the same way. A further theoretical difficulty is that the composition of weight loss may vary between individuals. For example, starvation (Elia, 1992a; Elia *et al.*, 1999) and semi-starvation in the absence of disease (Elia, 1992a; Ferro-Luzzi *et al.*, 1994; Dulloo *et al.*, 1996) produce loss of a considerably greater proportion of lean tissue in thin than in obese individuals. In chronic conditions, such as human immunodeficiency virus (HIV), the proportion of weight loss due to lean tissue is also greater in thinner than in fatter individuals (Mulligan *et al.*, 1997). This means that slow weight loss in lean

individuals is more likely to detrimentally affect many of the functions of the body, such as muscle strength, that strongly depend on the mass of lean tissue.

4. *Unintentional weight loss as an indicator of underlying pathology.* In a study of unintentional weight loss of 5% or more over a period of 6 months in adults of various ages, individuals were followed up as either hospital out-patients or in-patients. In the majority of cases, their weight loss was found to have an identifiable treatable physical cause (Marton *et al.*, 1981). Another study of elderly subjects found in the majority of individuals with a 5% weight loss over 12 months an underlying physical problem when investigated in hospital (Rabinovitz *et al.*, 1986).

Although there are obvious limitations to using a single cut-off value for detecting clinically relevant weight loss (as for BMI), there is general agreement that unintentional weight loss of more than 10% over 3–6 months is significant. Furthermore, weight loss in excess of the normal intra-individual variation (tentatively suggested to be 5% over 3–6 months) can be used as a warning signal for the development of malnutrition. The pattern of change is also important. For example, an individual who has unintentionally lost 10% body weight over 3 months and is continuing to lose weight is more at risk of developing functional deficits due to undernutrition than an individual who has just lost the same amount of weight but is now regaining it.

Combination of BMI and weight loss

There are well over 50 published nutritional screening tools and many more unpublished tools. Some use only BMI as a criterion for undernutrition (Kelly *et al.*, 2000), others use only changes in anthropometry (e.g. weight and upper-arm anthropometry (Guo, 1994)) and several others combine BMI (or another weight-for-height index) and weight loss (Pinchcofsky-Devin and Kaminski, 1985a; Keller, 1993; Lennard-Jones *et al.*, 1995; Reilly, H.M. *et* al., 1995; National Prescribing Centre, 1998; Edington et al., 2000; Elia, 2000b). Some also include likely future changes in weight. These are also often related to loss of appetite and the underlying disease likely to have caused the changes. An example of a screening tool that uses such a combination is shown in Fig. 1.5. When measurements of weight or height cannot be made, less objective measures can be used. Such tools can identify patients who are at risk of malnutrition and who can be referred for more detailed assessment of nutritional status. The screening tools should be linked to care plans.

Malnutrition in Children

Anthropometric cut-off points for malnutrition in children (single measurements)

The international statistical classification of disease and related health problems used weight, expressed as SD scores (z scores) to define probability of malnutrition (Fig. 1.4 and Table 1.6). For example, a z score between −1 and −2 (representing 13.5% of the reference population) indicates a probability of mild malnutrition, and a z score of less than −2 indicates a probability of severe malnutrition (2.3%). This statistical approach does not use a weight-for-height index and does not define the reference population. The World Health Organization (WHO) (1995) has also recommended an additional classification for malnutrition in children, which has become widely used. It differs from the International Classification of Disease (ICD) classification in four ways:

1. The likelihood of malnutrition is defined according to a cut-off of a z score of −2. No longer is a child with a z score between −1 and −2 defined as malnourished.
2. The z scores refer to deviations from the median rather than the mean. This has a statistical advantage for populations with skewed distributions.
3. The reference population is defined as

the National Centre for Health Statistics (USA) (NCHS)/WHO reference standard.
4. It describes three manifestations of malnutrition, two of which involve height. Low height-for-age reflects long-term growth faltering (stunting). Low weight-for-height (wasting) reflects more short-term growth failure because weight is sensitive to recent growth disturbances. Low weight-for-age, which is a manifestation of both of the above, can be used to diagnose children who are underweight, which is usually more common than wasting or stunting. Obviously, difficulties arise when oedema is present. Alternative classifications are available, including the Waterlow classification, which considers oedema (Waterlow, 1972). Long debates have occurred as to the relative practical advantages and theoretical validity of these classifications.

The NCHS/WHO standard seems to have been widely adopted for international use (World Health Organization, 1995). However, there are also French, American, Swedish and UK reference charts, which are often preferred for use in their country of origin. The latest UK reference charts (Cole et al., 1995, 1998) were based on measurements made on 9282 children in 1990, and they have increasingly replaced the Tanner–Whitehouse charts (Tanner et al., 1966), which were published over 30 years ago.

The same standard reference charts may not be appropriate for all circumstances, since growth is affected by feeding practices, parental stature, altitude, gender (sex-specific references are available) and racial/ethnic differences. There has been a long-standing debate about whether a single standard is appropriate for both developed and developing countries, as in developing countries the mean heights and weights of children are lower than in developed countries. One of the arguments in favour of using a single reference standard is that, when children of different ethnic origins are allowed to express their genetic potential, the variation is much less than that related to geographical and socio-economic differences in different parts of the world (World Health Organization, 1995). Another advantage of using a single reference is its simplicity, which can be of great value for comparisons between countries and in the same country over time (e.g. to reflect the effects of famine or affluence). However, it is recognized that there are anomalies with the NCHS/WHO reference standard, which are partly technical and partly biological in nature (World Health Organization, 1995). Therefore, new international reference standards are being developed. In the UK, it is appropriate to use the recent reference standards (Cole *et al.*, 1995, 1998), which were primarily developed for children in the UK.

It has been suggested that the lowest centile line (0.4th centile, corresponding to −2.67 SD) on the UK reference charts should be used as a practical 'cut-off' for surveillance, instead of the 3rd centile (the lowest centile curve) on the previously used Tanner–Whitehouse charts (Tanner *et al.*, 1966) or the 2nd centile curve, corresponding to a z score of about −2, on the NCHS/WHO chart. Although this recommendation may increase specificity and reduce referral rates (Cole, 1994; Hall, 1996; Mulligan *et al.*, 1998), a significant proportion of children with treatable abnormalities will not be identified using this cut-off. For example, 41% of children with growth hormone deficiency were reported to be above the 0.4th centile for height (Cotterill *et al.*, 1996). Therefore, it has been suggested that the 2nd centile be used as a cut-off, which is the same centile cut-off recommended by the WHO (−2 SD) for management of severe malnutrition (World Health Organization, 1995). Patterns of growth are also important but there are no internationally agreed recommendations.

As in adults, there are difficulties in establishing anthropometric cut-off points to identify children who are at risk of malnutrition. However, the principles are similar and involve establishing relationships, especially causal relationships, between the anthropometry and the outcome measures (mortality or other functional outcome measures). The following are taken into account.

1. Anthropometric cut-off values and mortality in children. A meta-analysis of six large longitudinal studies (Pelletier *et al.*, 1993) suggests an exponential association between the extent of weight-for-age (below 80% of ideal weight-for-age, corresponding to a z score less than −2) and mortality. Causality has not been established, but there is a clear clinical need for early detection and management of such patients.

2. Anthropometric cut-off values in relation to body function in children (malnutrition):

- Child development and school performance. Several studies suggest that children with a z score of less than −2 for weight-for-age have impaired development (Pollitt *et al.*, 1993) and school performance (McGuire and Austin, 1987). Food supplementation studies suggest some improvement, but the issue of mental development is very complex and influenced by social and environmental factors, including intellectual stimulation (Pollitt, 1995). However, studies suggest that, in children receiving suboptimal nutrient intake, exploratory behaviour is reduced before growth faltering occurs (Elia, 1997a). Although this may be regarded as an adaptation, it may contribute to long-term detrimental effects on development.
- Mechanical consequences in adult life. Childhood stunting predisposes to small adult size, which in turn results in reduced work capacity (Spurr *et al.*, 1977). Short women have a greater risk of obstetric problems due to a small pelvis (an effect independent of maternal weight) (Kramer, 1987). They also produce low birth weight babies, who are more likely to become small adults (Klebanoff and Yip, 1987; Binkin *et al.*, 1988).
- Childhood morbidity. Undernourished children have more diarrhoeal episodes and a greater risk of dehydration, hospital admissions and growth faltering

(World Health Organization, 1995). They also have an increased risk of pneumonia. However, causality is not clearly established.

• Early origins of adult disease. Increasing evidence suggests that many common adult diseases have their origins in fetal and early life. It is suggested that poor nutrition during fetal life and early infancy can increase the risk of developing type II diabetes, hypertension and cardiovascular disease in adult life (Barker and Fall, 1993; Henry and Ulijaszek, 1996; O'Brien *et al.*, 1999). If this hypothesis is correct, attention to early nutritional and other environmental factors could have major consequences several decades later. Specific cut-off points have not been defined and recent studies suggest that rapid growth in childhood may be associated with long-term detrimental effects (see below).

In treating malnutrition in both adults and children, it is obvious that the underlying causes should also be identified and dealt with.

New Perspectives on Malnutrition: Critical Periods and the Time Dimension

In the screening tool for the identification of malnutrition that is shown in Fig. 1.5, 3–6 months was chosen as a convenient period to assess weight loss, but others have suggested both shorter and longer periods. For example, cut-off values for weight loss over a year (10%) and a month (5%) (Blackburn *et al.*, 1977; Blackburn and Harvey, 1982) have been proposed. There is no reason why even shorter (Blackburn *et al.*, 1977; Blackburn and Harvey, 1982; Nagel, 1993) or longer periods (National Prescribing Centre, 1998) cannot be used, especially if nutritional treatment can be shown to influence important physiological functions or clinical outcome. Malnutrition can develop very rapidly in hospitalized patients, partly because of the catabolic effects of the

injury and partly because of the effects of partial or total starvation, which are frequently associated with severe disease. Starvation (water only) for 5 days, even when uncomplicated by disease, produces a weight loss between 5% of body weight, which typically occurs in obese individuals with a BMI of 35 kg m^{-2}, and 10% of body weight, which occurs in thin individuals with a BMI of about 18 kg m^{-2}. In the presence of severe disease, weight loss can occur even faster and lead to malnutrition within days rather than months. However, it appears that nutrition can influence physiological and clinical outcome independently of gross changes in body weight and gross body composition, as indicated below. In addition, some effects appear to develop in the medium term, long term and ultra-long term, which span as much as a lifetime. The implications of these issues to nutritional science are enormous. Therefore, each of the above periods is considered in turn, and then an attempt is made to synthesize the information into a new conceptual framework for considering malnutrition.

Short-term effects

Many of the short-term effects described here suggest that nutrients can affect body function while there is little or no change in gross body composition. Furthermore, in some cases, attenuation of weight loss or negative N balance appears to be associated with a worse prognosis.

Septic models of injury

Since lean tissues are responsible for many of the functions of the body, changes in N balance (rather than changes in body weight) have been used to assess both alterations in nutritional status and adequacy of nutritional support. However, animal studies involving septic models of injury suggest that reduced nutrient intake early after induction of sepsis can dramatically improve survival (two- to fourfold) (Wing and Young, 1980; Yamazaki *et al.*,

1986; Alexander *et al.*, 1989). The improvement produced by lower intake was observed both above (Alexander *et al.*, 1989) and below the maintenance level of energy intake (Wing and Young, 1980; Alexander *et al.*, 1989), i.e. intake below maintenance is better than intake at maintenance, which is better than intake above maintenance. Furthermore, in a *Listeria monocytogenes* model of peritonitis, not only did the animals that received the low nutrient intake have a twofold greater final survival, but the survival time of those that ultimately died was twofold longer than that of the control animals that had a normal intake. Administration of more nutrients may improve N balance or maintain a better weight, but survival is reduced (Alexander *et al.*, 1989). The dissociation between accretion of lean tissue mass (N retention) and function (reduced survival) is of considerable importance to nutritional science, but the mechanisms responsible for these dissociations are unclear. One possibility concerns the detrimental effects of administering in the feed more iron, which is a pro-oxidant and favours generation of free radicals, which in turn damage the structure and function of body tissues. Another possibility concerns the hyperglycaemia that results from the administration of carbohydrate to glucose-intolerant septic animals (diabetes of 'injury'). Since hyperglycaemia favours the growth of bacteria, it is possible that sepsis becomes more rampant when carbohydrate intake is increased. Glucose may also affect the function of immune cells (Rayfield *et al.*, 1982; Losser *et al.*, 1997; Geerlings and Hoepelman, 1999; Rassias *et al.*, 1999). Although the above animal experiments should not be directly extrapolated to humans, it is known that in clinical practice excess administration of nutrients in the early phases of critical illness, when patients are metabolically unstable, can produce hyperglycaemia, hyperosmolarity and more metabolic instability. The benefits of good glycaemic control in critically ill patients are discussed below. Therefore, the traditional methods for detecting and treating malnutrition by focusing specifically on the mass of lean tissues may not always be appropriate in acute situations.

Acute-phase responses in animals and humans

Further insights into the interactions between nutrition and acute disease can be obtained by considering studies on the acute-phase protein response to aseptic abscesses induced by subcutaneous injections of turpentine in rats (Jennings and Elia, 1991, 1994; Jennings *et al.*, 1992a,b). Compared with the well-nourished animals, those that were malnourished were found to have both delayed healing of the abscess and reduced acute-phase protein response, reflected by changes in the circulating α_2-macroglobulin concentration. This response can help limit damage and aid repair at the abscess site (Cruickshank *et al.*, 1991), at least partly by the antiprotease activity of acute-phase proteins, which prevents proteolysis beyond the margins of the injury. It was also demonstrated that malnourished humans undergoing gastrointestinal surgery had an attenuated acute-phase protein response (Cruickshank *et al.*, 1991) and further studies in animals were undertaken to examine whether the attenuation was due to malnutrition *per se* or the associated reduction in recent food intake (Jennings and Elia, 1994). The diets of rats were restricted to varying degrees so that they lost weight at different rates. When they had all lost the same target weight, they were injected with turpentine and their weight was clamped by administering a weight-maintenance diet. If a difference in the acute-phase protein response were to be observed, it would reflect differences in dietary intake prior to the turpentine injection and not to the magnitude of the weight loss or the dietary intake after the injection. This is exactly what was found. The acute-phase protein response was much higher in the animals that had lost weight slowly over a more prolonged period of time than in those that had lost it rapidly over a shorter period of time

(Jennings and Elia, 1994). Intermediate dietary intake and rate of weight loss were associated with intermediate acute-phase protein responses. The acute-phase protein response, assessed using α_2-macroglobulin, was several-fold lower than in rats that had lost weight rapidly, implying that there was a 'carry-over' effect produced by recent dietary intake or rate of weight loss prior to the insult (turpentine injection). These and other observations suggested that animals that lost weight rapidly had a metabolic response to 'injury' that might make them worse off for healing and recovery than those that had lost just the same amount of weight but more slowly.

Muscle function and physical activity in humans

It is well known that muscle function tests, such as grip strength, deteriorate as malnutrition with muscle wasting becomes progressively more severe. However, there is evidence to suggest that nutrition exerts effects on muscle function independently of muscle mass. For example, starvation for a few days may detrimentally affect muscle function tests, such as by fatigue, while producing little change in muscle mass. This may be mediated by changes in volition (central fatigue) but studies involving direct electrical stimulation of the adductor pollicis longus muscle in the hand also demonstrate abnormal muscle function (Lennmarken *et al.*, 1986). Other studies suggest that, during nutritional repletion of patients with anorexia nervosa, improvement in muscle function (muscle stimulation tests (Russell *et al.*, 1983) and bicycle ergometer tests (Rigaud *et al.*, 1997)) occur independently of muscle mass. Furthermore, subjective energy levels and objective measurements of physical activity were reported to be significantly reduced in healthy individuals receiving severe dietary restriction compared with less severe restriction, which produced very similar degrees of weight loss over longer periods of time (Gibney *et al.*, 2002a).

Independent effects of rate of weight loss on body functions in healthy humans

The importance of recent dietary intake for body function has also been explored in humans in both the presence and the absence of disease. For example, the dietary intake of healthy subjects was restricted to varying degrees in a series of human studies (Gibney, 2002). When target body weight was reached (5 or 10% lower than initial body weight), a weight-maintaining diet was administered. Two important observations emerged. First, metabolic function and certain psychological and physical function tests, such as muscle fatigue, depended much more on recent dietary intake than on the extent of tissue loss. Secondly, although there was loss of function during the starvation period, there was a major improvement during the weight maintenance period, when the mass of the fat and the fat-free body remained essentially the same as at the end of the starvation period.

Wound healing after abdominal surgery in humans

Studies in humans suggest that recent dietary intake prior to the stress of elective surgical injury can produce functionally important effects after the injury, just as in the animal studies. A provocative paper entitled 'Wound healing response in surgical patients: recent food intake is more important than nutritional status' (Windsor *et al.*, 1988) examined the effect of preoperative food intake. Patients whose food intake was reduced to less than half in the week prior to surgery had significantly less collagen deposition in wounds, assessed by accumulation of hydroxyproline in Gore-Tex tubes, than those whose intake was greater than half the normal intake. The same group of workers also reported that artificial nutritional support for up to a week before elective abdominal surgery did not produce obvious changes in nutritional status but dramatically increased collagen deposition after surgery, to values that were even greater than normally nourished subjects (Haydock and Hill, 1987). Appendectomy studies are also consistent with this concept. A brief preoperative illness of 12–72 h before appendectomy, which was associated with reduced dietary intake, decreased wound collagen deposition after surgery to an extent that was proportional to the duration of the illness (Goodson *et al.*, 1987). Furthermore, there was less collagen deposition after appendectomy than after traditional (non-laparoscopic) cholecystectomy, which is not preceded by a brief preoperative illness. Other studies in humans have shown that collagen deposition in wounds can be modulated by nutrition. A PN regimen containing a high-energy, high-N content and administered for the first 5 days after abdominal surgery increased the collagen content of wound granulomas 1.8-fold compared with a low-energy, low-N PN regimen administered over the same period of time (Bozzetti *et al.*, 1975).

Glucose administration in surgical patients and glycaemic control during critical illness

There is also evidence that individual nutrients administered preoperatively may influence postoperative course. For example, there is little doubt that glucose administered before abdominal and orthopaedic operations improves glucose tolerance after surgery. There may be complete attenuation of the insulin resistance that occurs shortly after surgery and 50% attenuation the day after surgery, although the mechanisms remain poorly understood. The effect of preoperative glucose infusions in reducing or abolishing the incidence of arrhythmias and hypotension after cardiac surgery (Lolley *et al.*, 1985; Oldfield *et al.*, 1986) may be explained partly by an increase (almost twofold) in cardiac glycogen (Oldfield *et al.*, 1986), which can act as a fuel during hypoxic conditions, and partly by a reduction in the circulating concentration of non-esterified fatty acids, which may induce arrhythmias under hypoxic conditions. Other reports suggesting that oral glucose administration before elective abdominal surgery improves well-being in the pre- and postoperative period, improves postoperative glucose tolerance and

reduces length of hospital stay are of considerable clinical interest (Lindahl, 2001; Ljungqvist *et al.*, 2001; Nygren *et al.*, 2001). During the last decade several countries (Norway, Great Britain, the USA, Sweden and Denmark (Eriksson and Sandin, 1996)) have established new guidelines for administering fluids to surgical patients. In some countries, glucose drinks are recommended up to 2 h before anaesthesia, with the aim of reducing the postoperative incidence of thirst and headaches, and possibly nausea, and increasing the sense of well-being.

Furthermore, a large randomized controlled study involving 1548 critically ill patients treated in intensive care units for more than 5 days demonstrated the advantages of strict control of the blood glucose concentration within the physiological range (4.4–6.1 mmol l^{-1}) (Van den Berghe *et al.*, 2001). The results were compared with those obtained using conventional treatment, which involved administering insulin only when the blood glucose concentration exceeded 11.9 mmol l^{-1}, with the aim of reducing the concentration to between 10.0 and 11.1 mmol l^{-1}. Strict glucose control reduced mortality in the intensive care unit by 44% (from 8.0% to 4.6%), bloodstream infections by 46%, haemodialysis or haemofiltration by 41%, the median number of transfusions by 50% and critical illness polyneuropathy by 44%. The length of stay in the intensive care unit was halved.

Amino acids and hypothermia

Preoperatively, administration of amino acids, which produce more diet-induced thermogenesis than fat or glucose, can prevent postoperative hypothermia (Sellden *et al.*, 1994, 1996), just as thermal insulation does (Kurz *et al.*, 1996). However, as far as we are aware, no clinical trials have reported whether or not such infusions reduce postoperative complications. In contrast, in a study of thermal insulation, a drop of 1°C for only 4–6 h after colorectal surgery produced dramatic effects on complication rates and both biochemical and clinical markers of recovery. The hypothermic group showed a threefold increase in the incidence of postoperative sepsis, a twofold difference in the asepsis score and reduced collagen deposition (Kurz et al., 1996). The hypothermic group also approached the clinical landmarks of recovery more slowly, so that days to first solid food, days to suture removal and days of hospitalization were all significantly prolonged compared with the normothermic group. It seems that the biochemical and clinical outcome measures were dependent on small differences in body temperature that occurred over only a few hours in the immediate postoperative period.

Nutritional support after elective surgery

In contrast to supplementation studies in chronic conditions in the community, where nutritional support is likely to benefit only those with chronic protein-energy malnutrition, nutritional support in acute disease in hospitalized patients may produce benefit independently of chronic protein-energy status. Randomized clinical controlled trials that assess this are discussed in Chapter 6. Here, two well-controlled clinical trials involving gastrointestinal surgery will be considered (Rana et al., 1992; Keele et al., 1997), in order to illustrate an issue about 'malnutrition'. The mean BMI of the patients was close to 25 kg m^{-2} and therefore did not indicate chronic protein-energy malnutrition. However, the supplements significantly reduced the rate of postoperative weight loss, without producing large differences in the extent of weight loss. Remarkably, the supplements in both studies produced a threefold reduction in the incidence of postoperative complications. These differences cannot be easily explained by the effect of the supplement on gross body composition, which can be estimated to affect fat-free mass by only about 1–2%. However, they could result from effects on the function of particular components of the fat-free mass during a critical period after elective gastrointestinal surgery. This issue is discussed further in Chapter 6.

An important biological issue concerns the mechanisms by which nutrients pro-vided during short critical periods of an illness might produce such effects. They cannot be readily explained by gross changes in body composition, which has traditionally been used as a marker of malnutrition and as a guide for the need for nutritional support. However, changes in body temperature or nutrient provision at critical periods might affect the function of cells involved in inflammation, immunity and repair, which are probably responsible for the reduction in complication rates reported in studies of postoperative supplements. If nutritional support during critical periods of illness produces beneficial clinical effects, then withholding nutritional support can be regarded as a form of malnutrition, irrespective of whether or not muscle or lean body mass is depleted.

Medium-term effects

The above discussion has focused on the effects of nutritional intervention during critical periods on short-term clinical and biochemical outcome measures. Few studies have explored the effects of nutritional intervention in an acute illness on medium-term outcome, i.e. several months later. One such study involved 84 intensive care patients, who were randomized to receive either PN supplemented with glutamine or an isonitrogenous mixture of amino acids. Mortality was lower in the glutamine group, but this did not become significant until after discharge from hospital (67% vs. 43% at 6 months; $P < 0.05$) (Griffiths et al., 1997). Other studies with larger numbers of patients are required to examine the medium-term effects of nutritional intervention.

Long-term effects

Programming of cardiovascular diseases, hypertension and diabetes

There are more reports suggesting putative long-term effects of nutritional programming that manifest themselves decades after an identifiable event, than medium-term effects that manifest themselves over months. Indeed, reports of the fetal and infant 'origins' of adult diseases, such as cardiovascular disease, hypertension and diabetes, are well known (United States Department of Agriculture, 2002). An analysis of 80 reports linking low birth weight to hypertension in later life (Huxley *et al.*, 2000) suggests that nutrition during critical periods of development may have major public-health implications several decades later. It is also known that obese children over 10 years of age tend to become obese adults (BMI > 30 kg m^{-2}), whereas most obese children under 10 years do not become obese adults. However, recent work suggests that it is not so much the actual weight of children aged 5–10 years that predicts obesity-related complications in adult life (cardiovascular disease, hypertension), but the growth pathway that led to the weight gain (Eriksson *et al.*, 1999; Huxley *et al.*, 2000). Low-birth-weight children who have an accelerated increase in weight and BMI between age 1 year and school age to within the normal range of BMI are more likely to develop 'obesity'-related complications in adult life than overweight children who have not had accelerated growth. Normally, accelerated growth towards the normal range would be regarded as beneficial, but, if such changes are responsible for the detrimental long-term effects, they can be considered to represent a form of malnutrition. Such a scenario would imply that the same nutritional intervention can be regarded as good nutrition in the shorter term and bad nutrition, or 'malnutrition', in the longer term.

Programming of the immune system

There is also evidence that the immune system of animals and humans can be programmed. Several animal studies have reported that undernutrition in fetal or early postnatal life produces programming effects on humoral and cell-mediated immunity (Jose *et al.*, 1973; Gebhardt and Newberne, 1974; Chandra, 1975; Beach *et al.*, 1982; Calder and Yaqoob, 2000), as

well as acute-phase protein responses that continue into adult life (Langley *et al.*, 1994). In humans the evidence comes from observational (Aref *et al.*, 1970; Chandra, 1975; Hattevig *et al.*, 1989; Ferguson, 1994; Godfrey *et al.*, 1994; Moore, S.E. *et al.*, 1997; Prentice *et al.*, 1999) and intervention studies involving allergic and infective conditions (Chandra *et al.*, 1977; Chandra, 1986, 2000). For example, several observational studies have established a relationship between early life events, such as disproportionate growth, on the one hand, and raised immunoglobulin E (IgE) concentration or incidence of asthma in children up to 16 years of age, on the other (Godfrey *et al.*, 1994). Furthermore, the incidence of allergic disorders in children up to 18 years of age is increased in bottle-fed compared with breast-fed infants (Hattevig *et al.*, 1989; Chandra, 2000) by up to six times according to some studies (Chandra, 2000). In addition, a variety of nutritional interventions during pregnancy, lactation and early infancy have been reported to reduce the incidence of eczema and other allergic disorders by two- to threefold in high-risk children 1.5–5 years later (Chandra *et al.*, 1977; Chandra, 1986, 2000).

There is also evidence that babies that suffered intrauterine growth retardation are more susceptible to infection. For example, such children are reported to have a two- to threefold higher incidence of upper and lower respiratory tract infections, when followed up for 3 years (Chandra, 2000). Furthermore, a variety of immunological defects persist for months or years after intrauterine growth retardation (Chandra, 1975, 2000) or after refeeding children with severe kwashiorkor (Aref *et al.*, 1970). Some interesting recent data about programming of the immune system come from The Gambia (Moore, S.E. *et al.*, 1997). There are marked seasonality effects there due to shortage of food in certain seasons of the year, with the result that the mean body weight of adults is 10% lower in the hungry than in the harvest season. Birth weight is 200–300 g lower during the hungry season, and the incidence of low-birth-weight babies increases up to 25% in the worst months. The first piece of work reporting programming of the immune system of Gambians (Moore, S.E. *et al.*, 1997) was updated subsequently (Prentice *et al.*, 1999). Surprisingly, children born in the hungry season had a similar survival rate up to the age of about 15 years compared with those born in the harvest season. Only after then did differences begin to emerge. The hazard ratio (relative survival or mortality of two groups) for mortality was about 4 after the age of 14.5 years and about 10 after the age of 25 years. Most of the deaths were considered to be due to infections, suggesting that some event related to season of birth had programmed the immune system and that the effects were manifested by premature death decades later.

Ultra-long-term effects

The most intriguing observations are those from animal studies, undertaken mainly in the 1970s and 1980s (Table 1.8). They suggest that nutritional and other variables operating *in utero* or in early life produce programming effects that carry over into more than one generation. Abnormalities in cell-mediated and humoral immunity can be induced by Zn deficiency in pregnant mothers and transmitted to the next two generations, F1 and F2, even if the

original offspring of the F0 generation are nursed by well-nourished mothers. Intergenerational effects have also been described following nutritional deprivation after birth. The intergenerational effects induced by streptozotocin may persist not for only one or two generations but for five generations (seven generations if both the mother and father are affected) (Table 1.8). These intergenerational effects can occur even if the offspring are nursed by normal females and, even more extraordinarily, if only the father is affected. These observations raise fundamental issues about the mechanism of transmission, which are relevant to Darwinism, Neo-Darwinism and even Lamarckism (Steele *et al.*, 1998).

In summary, there may be critical periods during early life (or prenatal life), as well as during adult life, when environmental influences, including nutritional influences, may have major effects on cellular/biochemical function, clinical outcome and public health (Fig. 1.6). In some cases the effects may last for days or weeks, as for example during hospital stay. In others it may last for months, as in a journey of patient care from hospital to home, while in others it may last for a lifetime or more (if the intergenerational effects observed in animals can be confirmed in humans). If this is the case, the key questions that arise are: what is the nature of

Table 1.8. Intergenerational effects produced by nutritional and other insults.

Insult	Outcome	Generation	Reference
Zn-deficient pregnant mice[a]	Cell-mediated immunity; reduced circulatory IgM concentration	F0, F1, F2	Beach *et al.*, 1982
Nutritionally deprived young rats	Impaired antibody-forming cells and responses	F0, F1	Gebhardt and Newberne, 1974
6 weeks' energy restriction in young rats	Impaired humoral immunity	F0, F1, F2	Chandra, 1975
Low-protein diet in pregnant rats[a]	Low body weight	F0, F1, F2	Stewart *et al.*, 1980
Maternal diabetes with streptozotocin in rats[a,b]	Glucose intolerance	F0, F1, F2, F3, F4, F5 (F7)	Goldner and Spergel, 1972
Chemically induced thyroid dysfunction[a,b]	Hormonal disorders	F0, F1, F2	Bakke *et al.*, 1975

[a]Nursed on well-nourished females.
[b]Transmission also via male (i.e. occurs when father is affected).

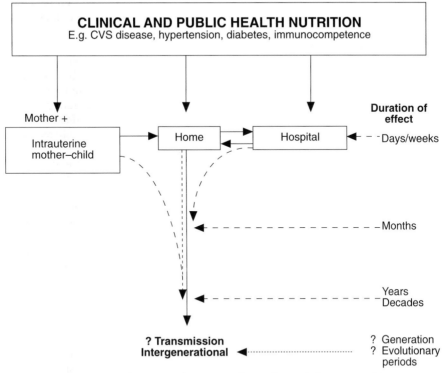

Fig. 1.6. The time dimension in relation to malnutrition and critical periods for nutritional intervention. CVS, cardiovascular.

the signals that mediate these cellular and metabolic 'memory' effects and are they different for short-term, intermediate-term and long-term effects? Currently these questions are largely unanswered. However, if body function in health and disease is the defining criterion for 'malnutrition', then a conceptual framework is needed to consider all of these functions irrespective of the time taken for the manifestations to appear.

A Summary and Synthesis of New and Old Information

A conceptual framework for malnutrition in relation to changes in nutritional status and critical periods of illness

National and international agencies have chosen anthropometric indices (BMI in adults) as the main criteria for identifying protein-energy malnutrition or risk of such malnutrition. These indices frequently reflect gross body composition. However, the information presented above suggests that it is possible to alter the function of tissues independently of mass, using both nutritional and non-nutritional interventions. The agencies have not provided criteria for considering malnutrition using changes in anthropometric measurements over time, e.g. changes in growth, which may reflect this function. However, in the absence of disease, both the rate and the magnitude of weight loss affect body function. In the presence of disease, nutritional support appears to produce clinical benefits (reduced mortality, fewer complications) even in some groups of individuals with normal or acceptable BMI and in those who show little change in BMI relative to the control group during the treatment. Presumably nutritional support affects the function of tissues or cells, such as those of the immune and inflammatory system, which play a key role in the acute phase-response to 'injury'. Chapters 6 and 7 summarize the studies that provide support for this concept. Some of these studies have their limitations, but, if administration of nutrients during short periods before, during and after the onset of an acute condition improves clinical outcome, then withholding such nutrients, even in individuals with a 'normal' or 'acceptable' BMI, would represent a form of 'malnutrition' or 'bad nutrition'.

The 'fetal' or early origins of adult disease hypothesis in relation to malnutrition

Figure 1.6 provides a framework for considering the time dimension, which includes periods ranging from a few days or less to more than a lifetime. There is little doubt that such long-term effects occur in small mammals, since they have been demonstrated by carefully controlled animal experiments. There is also little doubt that in humans the availability of folic acid during the first few weeks of pregnancy reduces the risk of neural tube defects in babies. If many common human conditions can also be programmed by nutritional or other factors during fetal or early postnatal life, then this could form the basis of a strategy for preventing important clinical and public health problems later in life.

The Barker hypothesis about the 'fetal origins' of disease states that common conditions, such as cardiovascular disease, result from adaptations made by the fetus when it is malnourished. According to this hypothesis, these adaptations permanently change the structure and function of the body to allow the fetus to grow and survive, but at the price of morbidity and a shortened lifespan. It is proposed that these problems are more likely to occur when the permanent adaptations made during the early malnourished period are followed by excess nutrition in later life. This provides a tentative explanation for the adverse long-term effects of acceler-

ated growth during early childhood and development of more 'obesity-related complications' in individuals with low weight and low ponderal index at birth. Such considerations suggest that 'malnutrition' is contextual, a topic that is briefly considered below.

Can 'malnutrition' or nutrient deficiencies be beneficial in some circumstances?

Traditionally, it was thought that 'malnutrition' was always detrimental. However, this concept has been intermittently challenged in respect of certain diseases or conditions. Possible benefits of deficiencies are suggested below:

- Vitamin K deficiency and the use of anticoagulants to antagonize the action of vitamin K are beneficial to patients with a tendency to thrombosis.
- It has been suggested by a number of workers, but especially by Murray and colleagues (Murray and Murray, 1977, 1979a,b; Murray et al., 1978, 1995), that poor nutritional state may protect against certain types of infections in both animals and humans (Murray and Murray, 1979b). They noted that in humans the greatest mortality from the influenza pandemic following the First World War apparently occurred in well-fed subjects. They also noted from historical observations in English prisons in the 1830s that significantly greater morbidity and mortality was experienced in well-fed than in less well-fed prisoners and that in the Keys study of semi-starvation (Keys et al., 1950), in which subjects lost 25% of their body weight over a 6-month period, there was no increase in infections, respiratory or otherwise, compared with matched controls (Murray and Murray, 1977). Furthermore, a study in 1995 involving over 4000 famine victims who had lost more than 25% of their body weight concluded that the incidence of overt malaria was 5% before refeeding and 29% 2 weeks after refeeding (Murray et

al., 1995). It has also been suggested on the basis of other observations (Murray *et al.*, 1978) that iron deficiency may suppress infections, such as malaria, while administration of iron may precipitate it. From a historical perspective, it is interesting to note that as long ago as 1872 Trousseau was alerting medical students in Paris to the dangers of giving iron to patients with quiescent tuberculosis (Trousseau, 1872). However, at least some of the human studies are controversial, partly because they are observational and open to various interpretations and partly because subsequent work has not always confirmed the results. This may be because of the confounding effects of the severity of the disease and malnutrition, e.g. severity of iron or protein deficiency, and the dose of nutrients administered. However, there is substantial support for the concept that undernutrition may be a mechanism of host defence against certain types of infections in experimental animals. For example, underweight animals have been reported to be more resistant to foot-and-mouth disease, vaccinia and poliomyelitis. Protein deficiency also protects experimental animals from severe malaria infection. Furthermore, *Plasmodium burghei* malaria in mice is suppressed during vitamin E deficiency and is slowly activated after vitamin E administration. It has been suggested that vitamin E deficiency reduces the antioxidant status of the host, so that the red cells rupture before the dividing parasites become infective and able to invade other cells (Murray and Murray, 1977). Furthermore, a series of studies in mice and rats – already discussed under the section Short-term effects (Septic models of injury) – have also confirmed that reduced dietary intake improves survival in experimental models of peritonitis.

- It has been argued that undernutrition is adaptive in some non-inflammatory diseases, such as severe heart failure, since it reduces cardiac output and oxygen consumption. Rapid refeeding can precipitate heart failure (Heymsfield *et al.*, 1988; Jeejeebhoy and Sole, 2001), in keeping with the well-recognized adage that 'the heart is closer to failure during recovery than in starvation' (Keys *et al.*, 1947). Refeeding places more demands on the heart (increased cardiac output and oxygen consumption), but other suggested mechanisms for the development of heart failure during refeeding include disturbances in electrolytes and micronutrients and in the electrical activity of the heart. Slower rates of refeeding are less likely to precipitate heart failure.

- Reduced dietary intake has been shown to be one of the strongest factors that reduce the incidence of cancer in experimental animals (Rous, 1914; Weindruch and Walford, 1988). In humans, obesity has been reported to be associated with an increase in the risk of non-smoking-related malignancies (Lew and Garfinkel, 1979). Although controlled clinical trials involving reduced energy intake from an early age are not feasible, natural experiments of nature can give some insights. For example, wartime food deprivation in girls during puberty led to a reduced incidence of breast cancer for the remainder of their lives, compared with younger and older individuals not subjected to wartime food deprivation (Tretli and Gaard, 1996). The mechanism is unknown but may involve effects on cumulative cell proliferation and its effects on the mass of specific stem-cell populations (Albanes, 1998).

- Undernutrition in small mammals has been consistently reported to prolong lifespan (Weindruch and Walford, 1988). Ongoing studies are addressing the same issue in primates.

- The fetal origins of adult disease hypothesis also raises the theoretical possibility that maintaining the underweight state in individuals who were adapted to undernutrition *in utero* could reduce morbidity and mortality in later life (Eriksson *et al.*, 1999; Huxley *et al.*, 2000).

In summary, the 'malnutrition' framework presented here raises important possibilities for establishing short-term and long-term policies for public health and clinical practice, although the context should be considered. For example, there is no doubt about the benefits of administering iron to an individual with isolated severe iron-deficiency anaemia due to menorrhagia. However, some centres routinely omit the inclusion of iron during the first few days of PN to patients with severe inflammatory diseases, because of concerns that its pro-oxidant activities might increase free-radical generation, with consequent tissue damage. Such centres include iron in the PN only after the acute phase of disease has resolved. Similarly, vitamin K deficiency may be beneficial in some circumstances and detrimental in others. It is also obvious that the provision of large amounts of salt is necessary in some patients with large intestinal effluent losses, but detrimental to other individuals. Furthermore, a high-energy-density, high-fat diet may be detrimental to healthy subjects but beneficial to malnourished individuals, who are more likely to increase their energy intake using such a diet than when using a low-energy-density, low-fat diet (see Chapter 6). Therefore, what constitutes malnutrition or 'bad nutri-tion' for one individual may be beneficial for another individual, and what is appropriate for one phase of a disease may be inappropriate for another. The observational studies that accelerated growth in initially underweight children is associated with detrimental effects in adult life raise questions about causality. Another problem that relates to the definition of malnutrition is the interplay between physiology, psychology and pathology. When should the measurable psychological and behavioural functional changes arising from dietary deprivation during the transition from the fed to the fasted state be referred to as 'malnutrition'?

Conclusion

It is clear that, whenever the terms 'malnutrition' or 'risk of malnutrition' are used, they should be defined or explained. Such explanations should include the nutrient(s) they refer to, the cut-off values used to identify malnutrition and the type of individual and clinical circumstances to which they relate. Without such clarification, the terms are of limited scientific value and, at worst, can mislead and confuse workers both within and outside the field of nutrition.

2
Prevalence of Disease-related Malnutrition

Introduction

It is believed that malnutrition produces adverse functional effects that have clinical and public-health consequences, with considerable associated economic demands, which should be reversible by appropriate nutritional intervention. In order to obtain an insight into the magnitude of the malnutrition problem and the potential effects of nutritional support, it is necessary first to consider the prevalence of the underlying diseases in the general population and the extent to which they are associated with malnutrition.

Prevalence of malnutrition in the general population of developed countries

A summary of the prevalence of such diseases in Europe and other established market economies (EME) (USA, Australia and New Zealand) is given in Table 2.1. It is clear that both the incidence and outcome of diseases varies in different countries, with implications for the prevalence of disease-related malnutrition.

It has been suggested that malnutrition is a public-health problem in developed countries, at least in some groups of individuals (Elia, 2000b). About 5% of the English population has been classified as underweight, using a body mass index (BMI) of < 20 kg m^{-2} as the criterion (Gregory et al., 1990; Office of Population Censuses and Surveys, 1994), and at risk of malnutrition because of chronic protein-energy deficiency. Other national surveys from Britain (Cox et al., 1993), Ireland (Lee and Cunningham, 1990) and Scotland (Scottish Office, 1995) suggest that the proportion of these populations with a BMI $<$ 20 kg m^{-2} is similar. However, there are other individuals who are not 'underweight' but are at risk of malnutrition (including impairment of body function) associated with substantial unintentional weight loss (e.g. $> 10\%$ in 3–6 months) (Stratton and Elia, 2000). In contrast, some healthy individuals who have a BMI $<$ 20 kg m^{-2} (especially young adults) will function perfectly well (Elia and Lunn, 1996).

In addition to the problems of chronic protein-energy deficiency ('underweight') in the population as a whole, micronutrient deficiencies are also common. National surveys in the UK of the elderly (over 65 years) (Finch et al., 1998) and of children (aged 4–18 years) (Gregory et al., 1994) have highlighted that a significant proportion have deficiencies of one or more micronutrients (including iron, vitamin C, thiamine, folate, vitamin B$_{12}$, vitamin D). The elderly living in institutions (residential homes, nursing homes and other facilities) are particularly

Table 2.1. Disease and disorder incidence for established market economies (EME)[a], listed in alphabetical order (from Harvard School of Public Health, 1996).

Disease/disorder	Incidence[b] (number '000s in 1990)	Incidence rate (per 100,000 in 1990)	Prevalence[c] (number '000s in 1990)	Prevalence rate (per 100,000 in 1990)	Average age at onset[d] (years)	Average duration[e] (years)
AIDS	74	9.3	125	15.6	38.7	2.0
Cancer: bladder	224	28.1	1,050	131.6	67.2	4.7
Cancer: breast	523	66	2,262	283.6	60.3	4.3
Cancer: colon/rectum	499	62.5	1,926	241.5	67.5	3.9
Cancer: leukaemia	85	10.7	385	48.3	56.8	4.6
Cancer: liver	42	5.3	74	9.3	64.3	1.77
Cancer: lymphoma /multiple myeloma	185	23.1	699	87.7	58.5	3.8
Cancer: mouth and oropharynx	121	15.2	517	64.8	59.4	4.3
Cancer: oesophagus	46	5.8	85	10.7	66.2	1.8
Cancer: pancreas	89	11.1	110	13.8	67.7	1.24
Cancer: prostate	452	56.7	2,020	253.2	69.8	4.5
Cancer: stomach	210	26.4	629	78.9	66.6	3.0
Cancer: trachea, bronchus, lung	430	54.0	874	109.6	66.7	2.0
Cerebrovascular disease – first-ever stroke	1,282	160.7	9,467	1,187	70.1	7.8
COPD	670	83.9	4,271	535	67.6	6.6
Dementia	959	120.2	7,082	888	77.4	7.8
Diabetes mellitus (insulin- and non-insulin-dependent)	2,308	289.3	37,850	4,744	60.4	17.8
Edentulism	4,836	606	95,036	11,912	59.4	21.9
End-stage renal disease	105	13.2	415	52	59.4	3.9
Fractured neck of femur – short-term[f]	1,255	157	175	21.9	64.5	0.14
Fractured neck of femur – long-term[f]	90	11.3	1,617	203	64.4	18.7
HIV	138	17.3	1,303	163.3	31.3	9.9
Liver cirrhosis	168	21.0	1,238	155.2	58.7	7.8
Multiple sclerosis	16	2.0	461	58	32.8	35.2
Parkinson's disease	136	17	1,849	232	67.9	14.4

[a]EME include UK, Austria, Belgium, Denmark, Finland, France, Germany, Greece, Iceland, Ireland, Italy, The Netherlands, Norway, Portugal, Spain, Sweden, Switzerland, Australia, New Zealand and the USA (region developed by the World Bank in 1993 to include countries of similar levels of socio-economic development).

[b]Incidence: this indicator measures the occurrence of new cases of disease or injury in 1990. The estimated number of new cases in the EME region (in thousands) is shown, along with the estimated incidence rate in the EME region, expressed as the number of new cases per 100,000 population per year.

[c]Prevalence: the estimated number (in thousands) of cases of disease or injury present in 1990 in the EME region is shown, as is the point prevalence rate, expressed as the number of prevalent cases per 100,000 population.

[d]Average age at onset: the average age (in years) at which new cases of disease or injury occurred in 1990.

[e]Average duration: the average duration of time (in years) that new cases can be expected to spend in a state of ill health as a result of disease or injury.

[f]Falls due to fractured neck of femur. An estimate is made of the duration of the disabling sequelae from injury as either short- or long-term, although the duration is not quantified.

AIDS, acquired immune deficiency syndrome; COPD, chronic obstructive pulmonary disease; HIV, human immunodeficiency virus.

at risk of such deficiencies (Finch *et al.*, 1998; see Chapter 1).

A complete picture of the prevalence of malnutrition in any country is not possible for at least three reasons:

- Lack of information on specific conditions.
- Lack of a comprehensive comparison of malnutrition prevalence in different disease conditions using common criteria.
- Use of different criteria by various workers to define the prevalence of malnutrition.

Use of different criteria to define malnutrition can produce widely different results, as will be illustrated below. Even when a similar prevalence is reported by two independent methods, it is theoretically possible for each method to identify different subjects as at risk of malnutrition. The use of simple and consistent criteria for application in different health-care settings avoids confusion and establishes continuity of nutritional care during a patient's journey from one health-care setting to another. It also allows regional and geographical differences to be established and appropriate resources to be directed to areas with high needs. Furthermore, it allows health planners and policy makers to use internally consistent benchmarks for judging performance. One of the most widely available indicators of chronic protein-energy status is BMI. Therefore in this book an attempt is made to describe the prevalence of BMI < 20 kg m^{-2} where available in studies that have assessed the prevalence of malnutrition with different criteria. Although the use of BMI to assess the prevalence of malnutrition has its limitations (see Chapter 1), it does provide a common benchmark for comparisons.

For example, Fig. 2.1 shows that the prevalence of underweight individuals in Britain (BMI < 20 kg m^{-2}) can be several times greater in hospitals and care homes than in free-living individuals with particular diseases. Figure 2.2 shows a similarly high prevalence of underweight in hospitals and care homes in developed countries generally, with considerable variation across disease categories. BMI

can also be used to obtain insights into the effect of age on both overweight and underweight.

Variation in the prevalence of malnutrition according to age

There appears to be little difference in the proportion of adults who are underweight at different ages. A national UK survey reported that between 3.0 and 7.7% of women and 1.7 and 3.9% of men were underweight (BMI < 20 kg m^{-2}; 25–75-year-olds) (Erens and Primatesta, 1999). A national survey of the elderly across Britain has suggested that 3% of men and 6% of women are underweight (BMI < 20 kg m^{-2}) (Finch *et al.*, 1998), which is similar to other estimates of free-living elderly European populations, including those in Sweden (Thorslund *et al.*, 1990; Cederholm and Hellström, 1992), Belgium (Griep *et al.*, 2000), Italy (Perissinotto *et al.*, 2002) and across Europe (De Groot *et al.*, 1991). However, the reported prevalence of malnutrition in the elderly living in retirement homes and institutions or who are housebound is greater (Finch *et al.*, 1998; Griep *et al.*, 2000). In Britain, 16% of men and 15% of women in institutions have been classified as underweight (Finch *et al.*, 1998) and in Belgium ~40% of elderly living in retirement homes have been classified as at risk of malnutrition (using Mini Nutritional Assessment (MNA) (see Appendix 1; Griep *et al.*, 2000)). Elderly people receiving 'meals on wheels' (who account for ~4% of the population over 65 years in the UK) are another high-risk group (Lipschitz *et al.*, 1985).

Malnutrition can also be a problem in infants and children. A national survey of children in Britain (aged 4–18 years) indicated that 15% of boys and girls were lower than the 5th percentile for BMI (Gregory *et al.*, 1994). Furthermore, data from the National Centre for Health Statistics suggested that ~2.5% of children have z scores below -2.0 and ~14% have z scores between -1.0 and -2.0 for weight-for-age, height-for-age and weight-for-

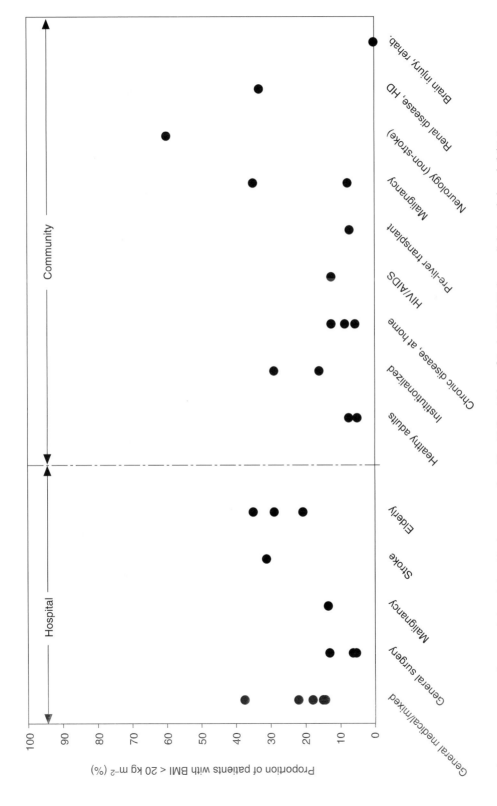

Fig. 2.1. Proportion of patients in hospital and in the community with a BMI < 20 kg m^{-2} in the UK. HD, haemodialysis; rehab., rehabilitation.

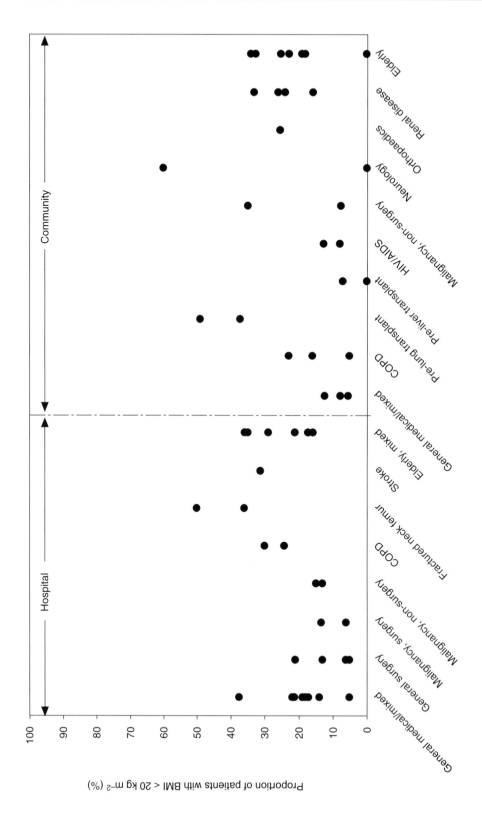

Fig. 2.2. Proportion of patients with a BMI < 20 kg m^{-2} in hospital and in the community across countries.

height (with a normal distribution ~14% of children would be expected to have a z score between −1.0 and −2.0 (see Chapter 1)) (Dibley *et al.*, 1987). However, this may simply suggest that the current percentiles no longer reflect the current population and need to be revised. Some age-specific potential causes and possible consequences of malnutrition have been summarized in Appendix 1.

Malnutrition and health-care expenditure

The availability of BMI in a number of studies has also provided some insights into the economic impact of malnutrition. Data from the USA indicate that individuals with a BMI outside the 'ideal' range have greater health-care expenditure, including those who are 'underweight' and 'overweight' or 'obese'. An analysis performed in 1993 suggested that annual health-care expenditure increased progressively as BMI decreased, from $1850 for a woman with a BMI of 21 kg m^{-2} to $2350 for a woman with a BMI of 15 kg m^{-2}. The increase in annual health-care expenditure was much more marked in men ($1300 for a BMI of 21 kg m^{-2} to ~$3250 for a BMI of 15 kg m^{-2}) and far outweighed the expenditure for overweight or obese men ($1700 for a BMI of 39 kg m^{-2}) (Heithoff *et al.*, 1997). In the UK an informal assessment of expenditure on malnutrition has been estimated to be £15–20 billion per year (Wynn and Wynn, 2001), compared with a formal assessment of expenditure on obesity, which has been estimated to be £2.5 billion per year (National Audit Office, 2000). However, the effects of disease/illness often associated with malnutrition need to be taken into account.

Prevalence of diseases

The primary cause of malnutrition in developed countries is disease (National Audit Office, 2000) – for example, malig-

nancy, diseases of the gastrointestinal (GI) tract, kidney, liver and heart, neurological disease and infective and traumatic disorders (including fractures and surgical procedures). Disease-specific potential causes and possible consequences of malnutrition have been summarized in Appendix 1. A summary of the prevalence of such diseases in Europe and other EME (USA, Australia and New Zealand) can be seen in Table 2.1.[1] The incidence and death rates of diseases vary somewhat between European countries. Taking death rates from stroke and cancer as examples (two of the main diseases associated with increased risk of malnutrition), it has been shown that, in women, the incidence of death from stroke ranges from 5.4 (in France) to 8.3 (in The Netherlands), 9.2 (in England) and 16.1 (in Portugal) per 100,000 population (age standardized, 1995) (Department of Health, 1999). Similarly, for cancer, death rates range from 63 (Finland) to 80 (England), 83 (The Netherlands) and 95 (Denmark) per 100,000 population (age standardized, 1995) (Department of Health, 1999). Patients with fractured neck of femur are also particularly prone to malnutrition and the incidence of this disorder also varies within Europe, from 82 (in the UK) (Lewis, 1981) to 97 (in Belgium) (De Deuxchaisnes and Devogelaer, 1988) and 201 (in Norway) (Falch *et al.*, 1985) per 100,000 population. Substantially higher incidences are noted if only women are considered (e.g. 354/100,000 in the UK) (Boyce and Vessey, 1985).

Despite disease being the primary cause of malnutrition in developed countries, malnutrition is often unrecognized and untreated in hospital in-patients and outpatients (up to 75%), nursing homes (up to 100%) and community (variable but up to 50% in children with failure to thrive) (Elia, 2000b). In order to assess the overall potential effects of intervention, it is first necessary to assess the frequency of malnutrition, its consequences and the extent to which nutritional therapy reverses its adverse effects. The remaining sections of this chapter focus on the prevalence of malnutrition in different clinical conditions in adults and children. Subsequent chapters will deal with the causes (Chapter 3) and consequences of malnutrition (Chapter 4) and the effects of nutritional intervention (Chapters 5–9).

Prevalence of Disease-related Malnutrition According to Disease or Condition, Health-care Setting or Assessment Criteria Used

This section highlights the fact that disease-related malnutrition is a significant problem in patients with a variety of different diseases/conditions. Furthermore, the prevalence of malnutrition varies according to the health-care setting of patients (out-patients, in-patients, nursing home residents) and the criteria used to define it.

Variation in the prevalence of malnutrition according to disease/condition

The studies reviewed suggest that disease-related malnutrition is a significant problem generally across Europe and other developed countries (e.g. the USA). The prevalence of malnutrition varies according to the type and severity of the illness/trauma. Figures 2.1 and 2.2 highlight the fact that up to ~60% of adult patients in hospital and community settings have been identified as underweight (using BMI < 20 kg m^{-2} as the criterion), including patients with cancer and neurological disease and elderly, orthopaedic and surgical patients. Similarly, Fig. 2.3 indicates that > 10% to ~40% of paediatric patients are at risk of malnutrition if weight-for-height < 90% and height-for-age < 95% are used as the criteria. Other groups in whom malnutrition has been identified as a significant problem using other indices include those with respiratory disease, GI and liver disease, human immunodeficiency virus (HIV) infection and acquired immune deficiency syndrome

(AIDS), malignancy, neurological diseases, renal disease, critical illness, orthopaedic and surgical patients (see following sections).

Variation in the prevalence of malnutrition according to health-care setting

The studies reviewed suggest that the prevalence of malnutrition varies across hospital and community settings, typically being greater in hospitalized patients than in those in the community (Elia, 2000b). Although hospitals accommodate only about 0.5% of the population (in the UK), a large proportion of the population are admitted and discharged from hospitals annually. In 1994, the number of admissions to hospital corresponded to ~10% of the adult population (≥ 16 years) in Europe, although the proportion was much greater in the elderly (~15% in 65–74 years; ~20% in 75–84 years; ~24% in > 85 years) (European Commission, 2001). The proportion admitted to hospital also varies across countries within Europe, ranging from 10% in Spain to 25.7% in Finland (UK 23.1%, The Netherlands 11.1%, Germany 20.9%; 1996 data) (European Commission, 2001). Furthermore, this number is growing (National Audit Office, 2000; European Commission, 2001), despite falls in the number of hospital beds. Although the number of hospital beds per 100,000 inhabitants across European countries varies from 401.9 (Norway) to 919.5 (Austria) (UK 445.6, The Netherlands 517.2, Germany 725.7; 1996 data), there is a consistent downward trend, with hospital bed numbers decreasing across all countries for which data exist (European Commission, 2001).

Although the prevalence of malnutrition is greatest in hospitals, most exists in the community, where the majority of the population resides (~99.5% in the UK) (Elia, 2000b). This proportion is likely to increase as hospital bed numbers fall and care in the community is encouraged. At present, within the community, the preva-

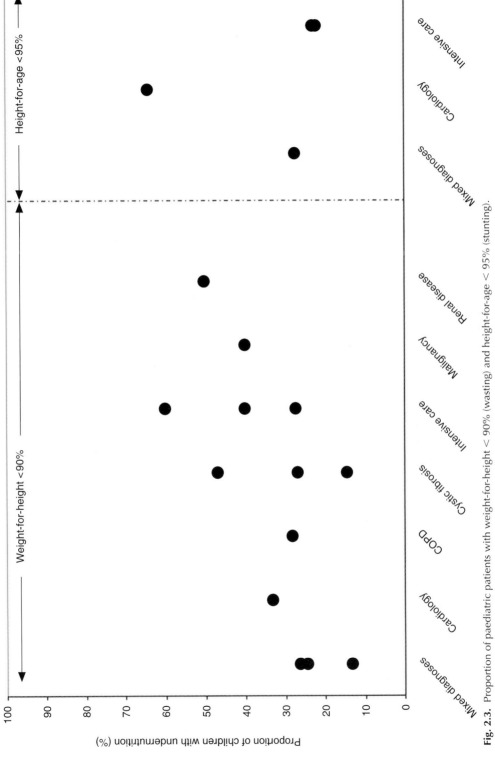

Fig. 2.3. Proportion of paediatric patients with weight-for-height < 90% (wasting) and height-for-age < 95% (stunting).

lence of malnutrition is highest in patients in nursing homes (~233,000 beds in British nursing homes in 1997) (Shaver *et al.*, 1980; Pinchcofsky-Devin and Kaminski, 1986; Tomorrow's Guides Limited, 1997) and in people living in sheltered accommodation (> 500,000 units in the UK) (Caughey *et al.*, 1994a,b; McCafferty, 1994).

The following sections address in greater detail the prevalence of malnutrition in patients with mixed diagnoses (predominantly adults), across different age groups (elderly and paediatric) and different disease groups. The studies reviewed have been summarized in detail in table form for each section and are given in Appendix 1. The likely causes and consequences of malnutrition in each setting are also summarized in table form in Appendix 1. The causes and consequences of disease-related malnutrition in general are addressed in Chapters 3 and 4.

Variation in the prevalence of malnutrition according to the assessment criteria used

A large number of different criteria have been used to identify malnutrition in the studies reviewed in this book. These can be divided into three main categories and are summarized in Tables 2.2–2.4. Further information on criteria used to define malnutrition is given in Appendix 1. In general, the criteria used are not disease-specific, although some trends in preferred methods can be seen in some disease groups; for example, < 90% ideal body weight (IBW) has typically been used in chronic obstructive pulmonary disease (COPD), and weight loss has commonly been used in HIV infection and AIDS. When different criteria are used to identify malnutrition in the same group of patients, widely different estimates of incidence can be obtained (e.g. 20% versus 79% in a group of hospitalized patients) (Cotton *et al.*, 1996).

One approach is to use markers of body mass and composition to determine the extent of malnutrition or risk of malnutri-

tion (Table 2.2). The most common single parameters are an IBW of < 90% or a BMI of < 20 kg m^{-2}. However, many other cut-off points and/or combinations of different anthropometric measures have been used (see Chapter 1). The extent of deviation from normal is sometimes used to define the degree of (or risk of) malnutrition. The reference ranges with which measurements are compared (e.g. if reporting figures in relation to percentiles of population references) may influence the reported extent of malnutrition. Furthermore, there is some debate about the 'ideal' or 'desirable' BMI range for the elderly, with suggestions that mortality in the elderly is lowest in the higher BMI ranges (24–28 kg m^{-2}) (Mattila *et al.*, 1986; Potter *et al.*, 1988; Beck and Ovesen, 1998). However, many of the studies suggesting an increase in the desirable BMI range are confounded by other variables, such as smoking and coexistent disease (see Chapter 1). Also, although the average BMI of the groups studied may be within the 'ideal' range (20–25 kg m^{-2} for adults), the variability within each group can be extensive. For example, in a study of acutely ill hospitalized elderly patients in Germany, mean BMI was ~23 kg m^{-2}, but the range was 11.9–39.1 (Volkert *et al.*, 1992).

All patients are also at risk of malnutrition if involuntary weight loss substantially exceeds the normal intra-individual weight loss that occurs as part of the normal fluctuation in weight over time. Therefore, a second and complementary approach to assessing protein-energy status using BMI is to use recent unintentional weight loss as an index of changes in nutritional status (see Table 2.3). This may simply be a record of whether or not patients report weight loss, or may be a calculation based on current weight compared with recalled usual or pre-illness body weight. The criteria for defining malnutrition based on weight loss range from simply a report of any amount of weight loss, to an established amount of weight lost, often over a given period, e.g. 3–6 months. In some cases, the degree of malnutrition has been

Table 2.2. Criteria for establishing the prevalence of malnutrition in adults[a] (markers of body mass and composition).

Category	Cut-off points used[b]	References
Body weight	< 80% of age and sex mean	Silver *et al.*, 1988; Abbasi and Rudman, 1993; Mühlethaler *et al.*, 1995
% IBW (weight index)[c]	< 100%	Senapati *et al.*, 1990
	< 90%	Brown *et al.*, 1982; Gray-Donald *et al.*, 1989; Wilson *et al.*, 1989; Mowé and Bøhmer, 1991; Süttmann *et al.*, 1991; Laaban *et al.*, 1993; Schols *et al.*, 1993; Dannhauser *et al.*, 1995a; Aparicio *et al.*, 1999; Godoy *et al.*, 2000; Jagoe *et al.*, 2001b; Nezu *et al.*, 2001; Roongpisuthipong *et al.*, 2001
	80–90%	Aoun *et al.*, 1993
	80–90% (mild)	Van Bokhorst-de van der
	70–79% (moderate)	Schueren *et al.*, 1997
	< 69% (severe)	
	85–95%	Deeg *et al.*, 1995
	< 85%	
	< 80%	Aoun *et al.*, 1993
	< 60%	Braun *et al.*, 1984b
	< 80th percentile	Thuluvath and Triger, 1994
% IBW and/or FFM IBW	IBW < 90% and/or FFM IBW < 67(F)/69(M)%	Engelen *et al.*, 1994
% IBW and/or CHI	IBW < 90% and/or CHI < 60%	Schols *et al.*, 1989
Mindex (weight/demispan)	< 50th percentile	Lumbers *et al.*, 2001
	< 10th percentile	Lumbers *et al.*, 2001
BMI	'Low'	Mazolewski *et al.*, 1999
	< 24 kg m^{-2} (and other criteria) – recipients of 'meals on wheels'	Coulston *et al.*, 1996
	< 24 kg m^{-2} (and other criteria) – community	Gray-Donald *et al.*, 1995
	< ~23.5 kg m^{-2} (25th centile for BMI) – community and hospital	Potter *et al.*, 1998; Potter, 2001
	< 22 kg m^{-2} – free-living elders (> 70 years)	Posner *et al.*, 1994
	< 21 kg m^{-2} – elderly in hospital	Incalzi *et al.*, 1996
	18.5–21.7 kg m^{-2}	Landi *et al.*, 2000
	< 18 kg m^{-2}	Maffulli *et al.*, 1999; Weekes, 1999
	< 17.5 kg m^{-2} – international classification for anorexia nervosa	World Health Organization, 1992
	< 17.0 kg m^{-2} – elderly	Wilson and Morley, 1988
	< 5th percentile	Potter *et al.*, 1995
BMI in combination with anthropometry	BMI + TSF + SSF < 25th percentile	Bashir *et al.*, 1990
	BMI < 20 kg m^{-2} + MAMC or TSF < 15th percentile	Edington *et al.*, 1996; Audivert *et al.*, 2000; Corish *et al.*, 2000a
	BMI < 20 kg m^{-2} + MAMC or TSF < 10th percentile	Watson, 1999
	BMI < 20 kg m^{-2} and TSF < 10 mm (M), 15 mm (F)	Comi *et al.*, 1998
	BMI < 20 kg m^{-2} + MAMC or TSF < 15th percentile (mild)	McWhirter and Pennington, 1994; Edington *et al.*, 1997; Harrison, 1997; Thomson *et al.*, 2001
	BMI < 18 kg m^{-2} + MAMC or TSF < 5th percentile (moderate)	
	BMI < 16 kg m^{-2} + MAMC or TSF < 5th percentile (severe)	
	BMI, weight loss % UBW, TSF and/or MAMC < 80% of reference	Davidson *et al.*, 1999

Table 2.2. *continued*

Category	Cut-off points used[b]	References
BMI in combination with weight loss	BMI < 20 kg m^{-2} and $> 5\%$ weight loss in 3 months	Bruun *et al.*, 1999
	BMI < 20 kg m^{-2} and > 3 kg weight loss in 3 months	Tessier *et al.*, 2000
	BMI < 18.5 kg m^{-2} or BMI 18.5–20 kg m^{-2} and weight loss > 3 kg in 3 months	Kelly *et al.*, 2000
BMI in combination with weight loss and/or anthropometry	Weight loss $> 10\%$, BMI < 20 kg m^{-2} or BMI $<$ 20 + kg m^{-2} TSF or MAMC < 15th percentile	Edington *et al.*, 2000
	BMI < 18–20 kg m^{-2} and TSF/ MAMC < 10th percentile and/or weight loss 0–9% (mild)	Strain *et al.*, 1999
	BMI < 18 kg m^{-2} and TSF/MAMC < 5th percentile and/or weight loss 10–15% (moderate)	
	BMI < 16 kg m^{-2} and TSF/MAMC < 5th percentile and/or weight loss $> 15\%$ (severe)	
TSF	< 10 mm (F); < 6 mm (M)	Paillaud *et al.*, 2000
	$< 60\%$ of reference	Braun *et al.*, 1984b
	< 10th percentile	Roongpisuthipong *et al.*, 2001
	< 5th percentile	Mühlethaler *et al.*, 1995; French and Merriman, 1999
MAC	< 23 cm	Paillaud *et al.*, 2000
	< 10th percentile	Dardaine *et al.*, 2001
	< 5th percentile	French and Merriman, 1999
MAMC	$< 60\%$ of reference	Braun *et al.*, 1984b
	< 2 SD below normal range	Brown *et al.*, 1982
	< 15th percentile	Weekes, 1999
	< 5th percentile	French and Merriman, 1999
MAMA	< 5th percentile	Thuluvath and Triger, 1994; Mühlethaler *et al.*, 1995; Plauth *et al.*, 1998
MAMA and/or MAFA	< 5th percentile	Merli *et al.*, 1996
TSF and/or MAC	< 5th percentile	Wicks *et al.*, 1995
TSF and/or MAMC	< 15th percentile	McWhirter *et al.*, 1994b
	< 10th percentile	Alberino *et al.*, 2001
	< 5th percentile	Jackson *et al.*, 1996; Harrison *et al.*, 1997
CAMA	< 16 cm^2 (M); < 16.9 cm^2 (F)	Potter *et al.*, 1995
Lean mass	Depletion	Engelen *et al.*, 1999
	BCM $< 35\%$ of IBW	Plauth *et al.*, 1998
	Observed vs. expected $< 90\%$	Aparicio *et al.*, 1999
	FFM < 10th percentile	Kyle *et al.*, 2001
BCM and ECM	BCM $< 30\%$ body weight and ECM $> 50\%$ body weight	Süttmann *et al.*, 1991
Fat mass	$< 20\%$ body weight	Süttmann *et al.*, 1991
Arm fat area	< 5th percentile	Thuluvath and Triger, 1994

[a]As recommended by various authors.

[b]For further details and results obtained in most of the studies using the cut-off values shown, see Appendix 1.

[c]Typically refers to end-point of the Metropolitan Life Insurance tables for acceptable weight (generally corresponding to BMI 22–23 kg m^{-2}).

BCM, body cell mass; BMI, body mass index; CAMA, corrected arm muscle area; CHI, creatinine–height index; ECM, extracellular mass; FFM, fat-free mass; IBW, ideal body weight; MAC, mid-arm circumference; MAFA, mid-arm fat area; MAMA, mid-arm muscle area; MAMC, mid-arm muscle circumference; SSF, subscapular skin-fold thickness; TSF, triceps skin-fold thickness; UBW, usual body weight.

Table 2.3. Criteria for establishing the prevalence of malnutrition in adults (weight loss).[a]

Category	Cut-off points used[b]	Time period	Studies
Involuntary weight loss	No cut-off	–	Hill *et al.*, 1977; Chlebowski *et al.*, 1989; Dworkin *et al.*, 1990; Senapati *et al.*, 1990; Aoun *et al.*, 1993; Parisien *et al.*, 1993; Engelen *et al.*, 1994; Galanos *et al.*, 1994; Luder *et al.*, 1995; Baarends *et al.*, 1997; Wigmore *et al.*, 1997; Andreyev *et al.*, 1998; Corish *et al.*, 1998; Collins *et al.*, 1999; Lees, 1999; Schols *et al.*, 1999; Daly *et al.*, 2000; Thompson *et al.*, 2001
	No cut-off	Previous 12 months	Persson *et al.*, 1999
	1–2%	1 week	Blackburn *et al.*, 1977
	5%	1 month	Blackburn *et al.*, 1977
	> 5%	3 months	Ovesen *et al.*, 1993
	7.5%	3 months	Blackburn *et al.*, 1977
	> 5%	6 months	DeWys *et al.*, 1980; Engel *et al.*, 1995
	> 5%	12 months	Braun *et al.*, 1984b
	> 10%	3 months	Windsor and Hill, 1988
	> 10%	6 months	Dannhauser *et al.*, 1995a; Van Bokhorst-de van der Schueren *et al.*, 1997; Corish *et al.*, 1998
	0–10%	–	Guenter *et al.*, 1993
	< 10%	–	Chlebowski *et al.*, 1989
	> 5%	–	Bruun *et al.*, 1999
	5–10%	–	Niyongabo *et al.*, 1997; Bosaeus *et al.*, 2001; Jagoe *et al.*, 2001b
	> 10%	–	Anderson *et al.*, 1984; Schols *et al.*, 1989; Parisien *et al.*, 1993; Trujillo, 1993; Luder *et al.*, 1995; Bruun *et al.*, 1999; Bosaeus *et al.*, 2001; Jagoe *et al.*, 2001b; Malvy *et al.*, 2001
	10–20%	–	Chlebowski *et al.*, 1989; Guenter *et al.*, 1993; Niyongabo *et al.*, 1997
	> 20%	–	Chlebowski *et al.*, 1989; Trujillo *et al.*, 1992; Guenter *et al.*, 1993; Niyongabo *et al.*, 1997
	> 2.3 kg	–	Morley and Kraenzle, 1994
	> 4.5 kg	–	Anderson *et al.*, 1985
	Combination of above		Beaver *et al.*, 2001; Kim *et al.*, 2001
Weight loss and organ dysfunction	> 10% plus dysfunction of two or more organ systems		Windsor and Hill, 1988

[a]As recommended by various authors.
[b]For further details and results obtained in most of the studies using the cut-off values shown, see Appendix 1.

graded with, for example, 5–10% representing mild/moderate risk of malnutrition and > 10% as severe risk of malnutrition (see Chapter 1).

Yet another approach is to use a variety of nutritional markers in an effort to determine risk and/or extent of malnutrition (Table 2.4). These include reviews of indices related to anthropometry, biochemistry, immune function and dietary intake, in various combinations and in comparison with various reference values and assigning patients as malnourished or not depending on the number of abnormal values. Combinations of measured values into a previously determined equation or index

Table 2.4. Other combinations of indices used to assess prevalence of malnutrition.[a]

Category	Type	Cut-off points used[b]	Studies
At least one abnormal value of a variety of different indices, e.g. anthropometry, biochemical indices (e.g. albumin, prealbumin, haemoglobin), immune function indices (e.g. total lymphocyte count, delayed hypersensitivity), dietary intake, etc.		Various	Shaver et al., 1980; Symreng et al., 1983; Mendenhall et al., 1984b; Warnold and Lundholm, 1984; Sandström et al., 1985; Haydock and Hill, 1986; Kamath et al., 1986; Meguid et al., 1986; Robinson et al., 1987; Axelsson et al., 1988; Reilly et al., 1988; Sullivan et al., 1989; Larsson et al., 1990; Aoun et al., 1992; Cederholm and Hellström, 1992, 1995; Constans et al., 1992; Pedersen and Pedersen, 1992; Cederholm et al., 1993; Shaw-Stiffel et al., 1993; Sidenvall and Ek, 1993; Larsson et al., 1994a; Mowé et al., 1994; Unosson et al., 1994, 1995; Dannhauser et al., 1995b; Engel et al., 1995; Finestone et al., 1995; Davalos et al., 1996; Giner et al., 1996; Lumbers et al., 1996; Chima et al., 1997; Hammerlid et al., 1998; Christensson et al., 1999; Hanger et al., 1999; Ponzer et al., 1999; Thorsdottir et al., 1999, 2001; Dardaine et al., 2001; Koch et al., 2001; Thorsdottir and Gunnarsdottir, 2002
Composite nutrition scores based on comprehensive nutrition assessment, including anthropometry, biochemical indices (e.g. albumin, prealbumin, haemoglobin), immune function indices (e.g. total lymphocyte count, delayed hypersensitivity), dietary intake, etc.	Maastricht index	> 0 (malnourished)	Naber et al., 1997; Huang et al., 2000
	Mini Nutritional Assessment (MNA)	< 17	Saletti et al., 2000
		17–23.5 (at risk)	Cohendy et al., 1999; Saletti et al., 1999; Wissing and Unosson, 1999
		< 17 (malnourished)	
	Nutrition index	Grade unclear	Compan et al., 1999; Murphy et al., 2000; Van Nes et al., 2001
		< 1.31 (malnourished)	Van Bokhorst et al., 1997
	Nutritional risk index (NRI)	NRI > 97.5 (mild)	Naber et al., 1997; Rey-Ferro et al., 1997; Corish et al., 1998
		NRI 83.5–97.5 (moderate)	
		NRI < 83.5 (severe)	
	Prognostic nutritional index (PNI)	PNI < 40%: low risk	Buzby et al., 1980
		PNI 40–50%: intermediate risk	
		PNI > 50%: high risk	
	Subjective global assessment (SGA)	Grade B (moderate)	Detsky et al., 1987; Hasse et al., 1993; Larsson et al., 1994a; McLeod et al., 1995; Ulander et al., 1998; Covinsky et al., 1999; Persson et al., 1999; Braunschweig et al., 2000; Pirlich et al., 2000; Sacks et al., 2000; Dechelette et al., 2001; Gungor et al., 2001; Karlsson and Nordstrom, 2001; Perman et al., 2001; Roongpisuthipong et al., 2001; Waitzberg et al., 2001
		Grade C (severe)	

Grade 2 (mild) Grade 3 (moderate) Grade 4 (severe) Grades unclear	Heimburger *et al.*, 2000
	Young *et al.*, 1991; Cianciaruso *et al.*, 1995; Hartley *et al.*, 1997; Naber *et al.*, 1997; Audivert *et al.*, 2000; Lawson *et al.*, 2001; Middleton *et al.*, 2001; Planas *et al.*, 2001; Stephenson *et al.*, 2001
Other scores Various	Brookes, 1982; Agradi *et al.*, 1984; Pinchofsky-Devin and Kaminski, 1986; Marckmann, 1988; Thomas *et al.*, 1991; Volkert *et al.*, 1992; Gamble *et al.*, 1993; Laaban *et al.*, 1993; Nielsen *et al.*, 1993; Reilly, J.J. *et al.*, 1995; Azad *et al.*, 1999; Charles *et al.*, 1999; Herselman *et al.*, 2000; Murray *et al.*, 2000; Peake *et al.*, 2000; Nordenram *et al.*, 2001

[a] As recommended by various authors.
[b] For further details and results obtained in most of the studies using the cut-off values shown, see Appendix 1.

to give a 'nutritional score' have also been used. In this case, the most common score to be used is the subjective global assessment (SGA), but several other scores are in existence (see Appendix 1).

Apart from the selection of measures and criteria to be used, there are a number of other points that must be considered as they may also influence the determination of the extent of nutritional impairment. In many studies, certain patients are excluded, such as those who are too sick, cognitively impaired or unconscious, have other diseases or are taking certain medications. Examples have included studies in the elderly (Sidenvall and Ek, 1993; Klipstein-Grobusch *et al.*, 1995), fractured neck of femur patients (Unosson *et al.*, 1995), children (Moy *et al.*, 1990), renal disease (Marckmann, 1988), stroke (Davalos *et al.*, 1996), surgical (Detsky *et al.*, 1987) and general medical patients (Weekes, 1999; Edington *et al.*, 2000). Consequently, the prevalence of malnutrition in such patient groups remains uncertain, although individuals who have been excluded are likely to have the highest risk of malnutrition.

Accurate measurements of nutritional status (e.g. height, weight) are often difficult to obtain in sick patients. In such cases, these patients may have been excluded or estimates or surrogate methods (e.g. knee height, arm span) used, for example, in fractured neck of femur patients (Jallut *et al.*, 1990), the elderly (Shaver *et al.*, 1980; Klipstein-Grobusch *et al.*, 1995), stroke (Unosson *et al.*, 1994; Gariballa *et al.*, 1998b) and general medical patients (Agradi *et al.*, 1984; Coats *et al.*, 1993; McWhirter and Pennington, 1994; Corish *et al.*, 2000a; Edington *et al.*, 2000). This introduces an element of error. In particular, the use of equations to predict height from knee height needs to be validated in European countries (Chumlea *et al.*, 1985; Stratton and Elia, 2000). Different predictor equations exist for other racial groups, such as black Americans (Chumlea *et al.*, 1994), Hispanics (Bermudez *et al.*, 1999) and Japanese (Myers *et al.*, 1994) in the

USA. Furthermore, in the elderly, measurements of height can be misleading due to curvature of the spine. The use of demispan as a surrogate measure for height (demiquet and mindex equivalent to BMI in men and women, respectively) may be more appropriate (Department of Health, 1992), but it has not been formally evaluated in those with curved spines.

The side used for upper-arm anthropometry varies between studies (e.g. right versus left arm; dominant versus non-dominant) or within studies (e.g. right arm followed by left arm in stroke patients (Axelsson *et al.*, 1988)) may affect the interpretation of nutritional status and the comparisons made with reference data. Few studies describe which arm is used for such measurements (Herselman *et al.*, 2000). It seems that there is generally no significant difference between skin-fold thickness obtained on the right and left arm, but mid-arm muscle circumference (calculated from triceps skin-fold thickness and mid-upper-arm circumference) is greater in the dominant, which is normally the right arm.

Some studies use percentiles that require calculation from the original data (e.g. 15th percentile values for upper-arm anthropometry do not appear to be provided by Bishop *et al.*, 1981). It is not clear if all authors used the same methods to calculate the values at the 15th percentile and yet this has been used to assess risk of malnutrition by different authors (e.g. McWhirter and Pennington, 1994; Corish *et al.*, 2000a).

Very few studies take into account the confounding effects of oedema/fluid retention on measurements of body weight. In some studies such patients were excluded – for example, in the elderly (Volkert *et al.*, 1992) and general medical patients (Agradi *et al.*, 1984; Weekes, 1999; Corish *et al.*, 2000a). In other studies, fluid weight was corrected for or the confounding effects of fluid disturbance were ignored – e.g. in general medical patients (Strain *et al.*, 1999).

The above examples illustrate the challenging nature of attempting to compare nutritional risk or malnutrition within and across different patient groups. Nevertheless, the studies reviewed clearly suggest that malnutrition is a significant problem, whatever indices are used to assess or define it. One simple measurement used across many studies of malnutrition in adults is BMI. Table 2.5 and Figs 2.1 and 2.2 give an indication of the proportion of adult patients in hospital with a BMI < 20 kg m^{-2} (designated 'underweight' in the UK by the Office of Population Censuses and Surveys (1994)) from studies across disease groups from a variety of countries. Table 2.6 and Figs 2.1 and 2.2 illustrate the proportions of patients outside the hospital setting with a BMI < 20 kg m^{-2}. These figures highlight the fact that significant proportions of adult and elderly patients across different disease groups are at risk of malnutrition (up to ~60%). As an example of the prevalence of underweight (BMI < 20 kg m^{-2}) adults across different settings in one country (the UK), see Fig. 2.1. Figures 2.4 and 2.5 also provide an indication of the proportion of patients identified as malnourished from trials that have used a variety of criteria, in hospital and community settings.

In paediatrics, a weight-for-height index has been used to assess malnutrition, using $< 90\%$ weight-for-height and $< 95\%$ height-for-age as cut-offs for different degrees of malnutrition. Such criteria suggest that a significant proportion of paediatric patients are at risk of malnutrition (Fig. 2.3).

The following sections address in greater detail the prevalence of malnutrition in patients with mixed diagnoses (predominantly adults), across different age groups (elderly and paediatrics) and different disease groups. The studies reviewed have been summarized in detail in table form for each section, and are given in Appendix 1. The likely causes and consequences of malnutrition in each setting are also summarized in Appendix 1 and discussed in Chapters 3 and 4.

Prevalence of Disease-related Malnutrition in Different Patient Groups

Adults

General medical, surgical and mixed diagnoses

Malnutrition commonly occurs in a wide variety of diseases. Despite earlier reports of the problems of malnutrition in a significant proportion of general hospital patients in the 1970s (Bistrian *et al.*, 1976; Weinsier *et al.*, 1979), the evidence suggests that malnutrition is still a considerable problem across Europe and other parts of the world. The reported prevalence varies widely, depending on the location of patients (hospital, out-patients, general practice), the criteria used to define malnutrition and the diagnoses of patients. As Tables A1.2 (mixed diagnoses, hospital), A1.3 and A1.4 (general medical, hospital) and A1.5 (mixed diagnoses, community) in Appendix 1 illustrate, the diagnostic mix of patients in these studies is broad and the findings are typically presented for the group as a whole. For patients with a variety of diagnoses, reports indicate that up to 62% may be considered at risk of malnutrition or frankly malnourished on admission to hospital (see Figs 2.4 and 2.5), with rates of up to 12.5% in the community (Fig. 2.5 and Table 2.7; see Appendix 1, Table A1.5). Studies specifically in general medical patients indicate a possible prevalence rate of up to 56% on admission to hospital (Fig. 2.4; see Appendix 1, Tables A1.3 and A1.4). Part of the variability is due to the use of different criteria for detecting malnutrition in the studies of patients with general medical, surgical and mixed diagnoses (see Tables 2.2–2.4 and 2.8).

A number of studies have shown that the prevalence of malnutrition will differ if different criteria are used on the same patient group (e.g. 33% versus 42% (Audivert *et al.*, 2000); 24% versus 30% (Strain *et al.*, 1999); 45% versus 62% (Naber *et al.*, 1997); 9% versus 31% (Weekes, 1999) and 20% versus 79% (Cotton *et al.*, 1996)) (Table 2.7; see Appendix 1, Tables A1.3–A1.4).

Table 2.5. Prevalence of underweight (BMI < 20 kg m^{-2}) in adults admitted to hospital, according to patient group and country, from recent studies.

Country	Number of subjects	BMI < 20 kg m^{-2} (%)	Sector of hospital	Reference
General medical/mixed diagnoses				
Iceland	82	5	Mixed	Thorsdottir *et al.*, 1999
Ireland	594	13.5	GM, GS, R, E, O	Corish *et al.*, 2000a
Italy	705	19.1	GM, GS	Comi *et al.*, 1998
Switzerland	995	17.3	GM, GS	Kyle *et al.*, 2001
UK (Luton and Dunstable)	83	14	Mixed	Arnold *et al.*, 2001
UK (Cambridge)	57	21	GM, GS	M. Elia (unpublished data)
UK (Glasgow)	219	18	GM, GS	Kelly *et al.*, 2000
UK (Dundee)	500	37.4	GM, GS, R, O, E	McWhirter and Pennington, 1994
UK (London)	423	15 (M) 18 (F)	GM, GS, O	Vlaming *et al.*, 1999
UK (London)	186	22	GM	Weekes, 1999
Elderly				
Belgium	151	17	E (mixed)	Joosten *et al.*, 1999
Ireland	21	21	E (GM)	Corish *et al.*, 2000b
Ireland	218	16	E (mixed)	Corish *et al.*, 2000b
Sweden	337	36	E (mixed)	Flodin *et al.*, 2000
UK (Leeds)	20	35	E (mixed, acute)	Klipstein-Grobusch *et al.*, 1995
UK (Cambridge)	100	21	E	J. Tharakan, R.J. Stratton and M. Elia (unpublished data)
UK (London)	65	29	E (mixed)	Watson, 1999
COPD				
Iceland	34	24	R	Thorsdottir *et al.*, 2001
Iceland	10	30	R	Thorsdottir and Gunnarsdottir, 2002
Malignancy, prior to surgery				
Ireland	59	6	ON (mixed)	Corish *et al.*, 1998
UK	60	13.3	ON (R)	Jagoe *et al.*, 2001b
Malignancy, non-surgery				
Germany	40	15	ON (Gynae)	Wolf *et al.*, 2001
UK	61	13	ON (ENT)	Collins *et al.*, 1999
Neurology				
UK	201	31	N	Gariballa *et al.*, 1998b
Orthopaedics				
Sweden	42	36	O	Ponzer *et al.*, 1999
Switzerland	20	50	O	Jallut *et al.*, 1990
Surgery				
Norway	244	21	S (GI, O)	Bruun *et al.*, 1999
South Africa	52	13	S (GI, CV)	Dannhauser *et al.*, 1995a
UK	175	5 (M) 13 (F)	GS (mixed)	Fettes *et al.*, 2001b
UK	808	6	GS (mixed)	Harrison, 1997

CV, cardiovascular; E, care of the elderly; ENT, ear, nose and throat; GI, gastrointestinal; GM, general medicine; GS, surgery; Gynae, gynaecology; N, neurology; O, orthopaedics; ON, oncology; R, respiratory medicine; S, surgery.

Table 2.6. Prevalence of underweight (BMI < 20 kg m^{-2}) in adults in the community, according to patient group and country, from recent studies.

Country	Number of subjects	BMI < 20 kg m^{-2} (%)	Sector of community	Reference
General medical/mixed diagnoses				
UK	10,317	7.7 (ON)	Home (GP)	Edington *et al.*, 1999
		5.3 (CV)		
UK	11,357	12.5	Home (GP)	Martyn *et al.*, 1998
Elderly				
Denmark	61	23	Home (GP)	Beck *et al.*, 2001a
Sweden	28	0	–	Faxén Irving *et al.*, 1999
Sweden	872	18	SF	Saletti *et al.*, 2000
		25	OPH	
		19	GLD	
		33	NH	
Sweden	80	34	NCH	Saletti *et al.*, 1999
COPD				
Denmark	2,132	5 (M)	Home	Landbo *et al.*, 1999
		16 (F)		
USA	126	23	Home	Sahebjami *et al.*, 1993
Gastrointestinal and liver disease				
UK	41	7	Home (LTL)	Jackson *et al.*, 1996
USA	20	0	Home (LTL)	Hasse *et al.*, 1993
HIV infection and AIDS				
UK	162	12.6	Home	Hodgson *et al.*, 2001
USA	633	8	Home	Kim *et al.*, 2001
Malignancy, non-surgery				
UK	20	35	Home	Wigmore *et al.*, 1997
UK	5,074	7.7	Home (GP)	Edington *et al.*, 1999
Neurology				
UK	33	0	Rehabilitation	French and Merriman, 1999
UK	417	> 60	C (*n* 99)	Kennedy *et al.*, 1997
			H (*n* 318)	
Orthopaedics				
Sweden	88	25.5	Rehabilitation	Bachrach-Lindström *et al.*, 2001
Renal disease				
France	7,123	24	Home (HD)	Aparicio *et al.*, 1999
Netherlands	250	16	Home (HD and PD)	Jager *et al.*, 2001
UK	57	33	Home (HD)	Engel *et al.*, 1995
USA	58	25.9	Home (HD)	Thunberg *et al.*, 1981
Surgery				
Canada	229	37	Home (LuTL)	Madill *et al.*, 2001
France	74	49	Home (LuTL)	Schwebel *et al.*, 2000

C, community; CAPD, continuous ambulatory peritoneal dialysis; GLD, group living for the demented; GP, general practice; H, hospital; HD, haemodialysis; LTL, liver transplant waiting list; LuTL, lung transplant waiting list; NCH, nursing care at home; NH, nursing home; ON, oncology; OPH, old people's home; PD, peritoneal dialysis; SF, service flats (sheltered accommodation).

Furthermore, these criteria should really be used to indicate risk of malnutrition (Stratton and Elia, 2000) and not the presence of malnutrition *per se*, due to constitutional differences between individuals (see Chapter 1).

In order to overcome some of the problems that are due to the use of different criteria, a common indicator of risk of malnutrition (% of patients with a BMI < 20 kg m^{-2}, also defined as underweight) can be used to compare studies (Stratton

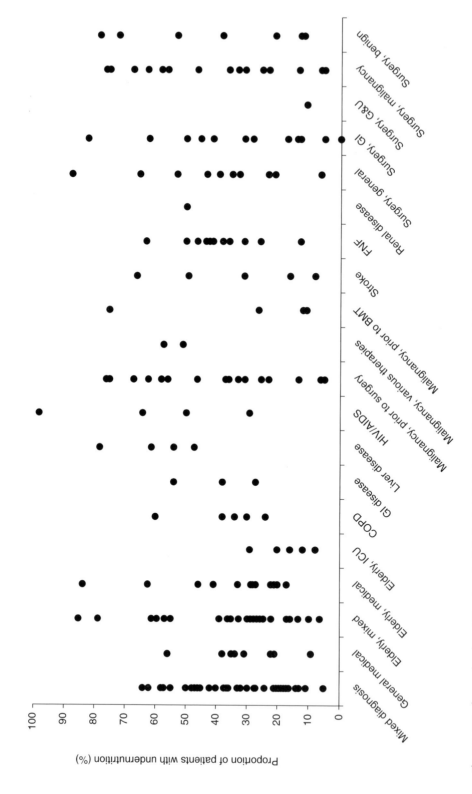

Fig. 2.4. Prevalence of undernutrition in patients in the hospital using a variety of assessment methods. BMT, bone marrow transplant; FNF, fractured neck of femur; GI, gastrointestinal; G&U, gynaecological and urological.

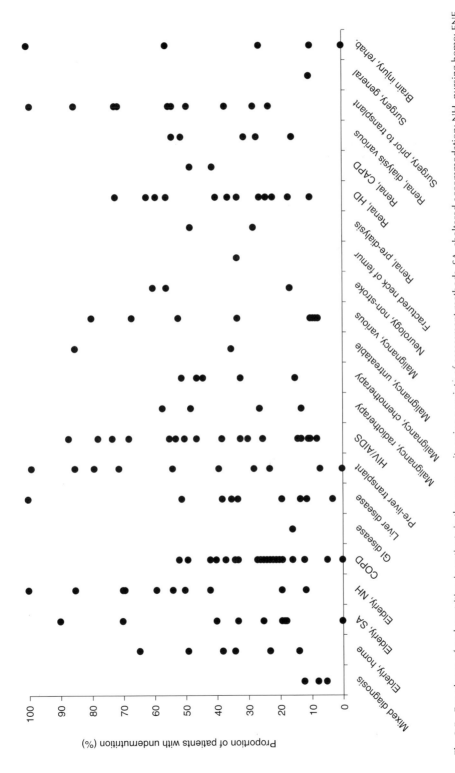

Fig. 2.5. Prevalence of undernutrition in patients in the community using a variety of assessment methods. SA, sheltered accommodation; NH, nursing home; FNF, fractured neck of femur; GI, gastrointestinal; HD, haemodialysis; CAPD, continuous ambulatory peritoneal dialysis; rehab, rehabilitation.

Table 2.7. Prevalence of malnutrition using a variety of criteria and BMI < 20 kg m^{-2} in mixed groups of patients in hospital and the community from different countries.

Country	Number of subjects	Prevalence of malnutrition (risk) (%)[a]	BMI < 20 kg m^{-2} (%)	Sector	Reference
Hospital					
Argentina	1,000	47.4	–	–	Perman et al., 2001
Australia	819	36	–	Mixed	Middleton et al., 2001
Brazil	4,000	48.1	–	GM, GS	Waitzberg et al., 2001
France	1,230	41.9	–	GM, GS	Dechelotte et al., 2001
Iceland	82	21	5	Mixed	Thorsdottir et al., 1999
		5			
Ireland	594	11	13.5	Mixed	Corish et al., 2000a
		13.5			
Italy	705	19.1	19.1	GM, GS	Comi et al., 1998
Italy	9,170 (M)	18.8 (M)	–	Mixed	Landi et al., 2000
	9,145 (F)	27.3 (F)			
Netherlands	155	45	–	Mixed, non-GS	Naber et al., 1997
		57			
		62			
Spain	300	33	–	–	Audivert et al., 2000
		41.6			
Spain	404	46	–	Mixed, non-T	Planas et al., 2001
Sweden	205	20	–	Mixed, acute	Cederholm et al., 1993
Sweden	382	27	–	Mixed	Larsson et al., 1994b
Switzerland	995	17.3	17.3	GM, GS	Kyle et al., 2001
		31			
UK	83	14	14	–	Arnold et al., 2001
UK	850	20	–	Mixed	Edington et al., 2000
UK	219	13	18	GM, GS, acute	Kelly et al., 2000
UK	500	40	37.4	GM, GS, R, O, E	McWhirter and Pennington, 1994
UK	553	64	–	Mixed	Peake et al., 2000
UK	153	50	–	Mixed, incl. P	Reilly, H.M. et al., 1995
UK	326	24	–	Mixed	Strain et al., 1999
		30			
UK	423	15 (M)	15 (M)	GM, GS, O, acute	Vlaming et al., 1999
		18 (F)	18 (F)		
USA	404	54	–	Mixed	Braunschweig et al., 2000
USA	173	32	–	Mixed	Chima et al., 1997
USA	3,047	58	–	Mixed	Kamath et al., 1986
		16.2			
USA	771	55	–	GM, GS	Reilly et al., 1988
Community					
UK	441	8	–	R, GI, N, O	Edington et al., 1996
UK	10,317	7.7 (ON)	7.7 (ON)	ON, CV	Edington et al., 1999
		5.3 (CV)	5.3 (CV)		
UK	11,357	12.5	12.5	Mixed	Martyn et al., 1998

[a]When more than one result is provided for a given study (unless specifically explained) the results have been obtained by applying different criteria to the same group of patients. For more details, refer to Appendix 1.
CV, cardiovascular; E, care of the elderly; GI, gastrointestinal; GM, general medicine; GS, surgery; O, orthopaedics; ON, oncology; N, neurology; P, paediatrics; R, respiratory medicine; T, trauma.

Table 2.8. Prevalence of disease-related malnutrition according to different criteria in general medical and surgical patients.

Criterion	Prevalence of malnutrition (%)	Author
Weight loss > 4.5 kg	34	Anderson *et al.*, 1985
Comparison with IBW	16.2	Kamath *et al.*, 1986
BMI < 21.7 kg m^{-2}	27.3	Landi *et al.*, 2000
BMI < 20 kg m^{-2}	5–22	McWhirter and Pennington, 1994; Comi *et al.*, 1998; Martyn *et al.*, 1998; Edington *et al.*, 1999; Thorsdottir *et al.*, 1999; Vlaming *et al.*, 1999; Weekes, 1999; Arnold *et al.*, 2001; Kyle *et al.*, 2001
BMI < 18 kg m^{-2}	9	Weekes, 1999
Index of fat-free mass (FFM)	31	Kyle *et al.*, 2001
A combination of anthropometric indices	11–45	Agradi *et al.*, 1984; Kamath *et al.*, 1986; McWhirter and Pennington, 1994; Comi *et al.*, 1998; Strain *et al.*, 1999; Weekes, 1999; Audivert *et al.*, 2000; Corish *et al.*, 2000a; Edington *et al.*, 2000; Kelly *et al.*, 2000; Kyle *et al.*, 2001
A combination of anthropometric, biochemical and/or immunological indicators	20–58	Kamath *et al.*, 1986; Robinson *et al.*, 1987; Reilly *et al.*, 1988; Aoun *et al.*, 1992; Cederholm *et al.*, 1993; Coats *et al.*, 1993; Chima *et al.*, 1997; Thorsdottir *et al.*, 1999
Subjective global assessment (SGA)	21–54	Larsson *et al.*, 1994a; Naber *et al.*, 1997; Audivert *et al.*, 2000; Braunschweig *et al.*, 2000; Pirlich *et al.*, 2000; Dechelotte *et al.*, 2001; Middleton *et al.*, 2001; Perman *et al.*, 2001; Planas *et al.*, 2001; Waitzberg *et al.*, 2001
A variety of nutrition risk scores	50–64	Reilly, H.M. *et al.*, 1995; Naber *et al.*, 1997; Peake *et al.*, 2000

and Elia, 2000). Using this simple method, the estimated mean prevalence of underweight in patients admitted to hospital with mixed diagnoses is ~18%, ranging from 5% (Iceland) (Thorsdottir *et al.*, 1999) to 37.4% (UK) (McWhirter and Pennington, 1994). In the community, two large studies from the UK indicate that up to 12.5% of patients with chronic disease are underweight (Martyn *et al.*, 1998; Edington *et al.*, 1999; Fig. 2.2).

Another explanation for differences in the prevalence of malnutrition between studies is the profile of patients studied. Although the majority of studies present data for a group of patients with mixed diagnoses as a whole (see Appendix 1, Table A1.2), some of these investigations have presented information for the prevalence of malnutrition in specific patient subgroups, according to disease/disorder. Reported prevalence using a variety of different criteria for specific patient groups is shown in Table 2.9. For information on the

prevalence of malnutrition in specific age-groups (elderly and paediatric) and in specific patient groups, see the following sections in this chapter.

There are a number of other factors that may explain the differences in reported prevalence of malnutrition. Location of patients with respect to health-care setting may also be a factor. For example, the prevalence appears to be greater in university/teaching hospitals than in general/district hospitals (Edington *et al.*, 2000). Furthermore, as discussed in the introductory part of this chapter, the following affect the interpretation of malnutrition risk:

- The use of surrogate measures for height, including arm span (Coats *et al.*, 1993; Edington *et al.*, 2000) and knee height (McWhirter and Pennington, 1994; Corish *et al.*, 2000a), and for weight (Corish *et al.*, 2000a) may affect the calculations of BMI and per cent weight-for-height.

Table 2.9. Prevalence of malnutrition in different diagnostic groups from studies of mixed groups of patients using a variety of criteria.

Diagnostic group[a]	Prevalence of malnutrition[b] (%)	References
Hospital		
Cardiovascular disease	0–5	Cederholm *et al.*, 1993
Congestive heart failure	20	Cederholm *et al.*, 1993
Gastrointestinal	46–60	Reilly *et al.*, 1988; Chima *et al.*, 1997
General medical	46–59	Reilly *et al.*, 1988; McWhirter and Pennington, 1994
General surgical	27–48	Reilly *et al.*, 1988; McWhirter and Pennington, 1994
Infectious disease	59	Chima *et al.*, 1997
Multiple organ failure	36	Cederholm *et al.*, 1993
Neurology	0	Cederholm *et al.*, 1993
Orthopaedics	39–45	Reilly *et al.*, 1988; McWhirter and Pennington, 1994
Respiratory	33–63	Reilly *et al.*, 1988; Cederholm *et al.*, 1993; McWhirter and Pennington, 1994; Chima *et al.*, 1997
Rheumatology	13	Cederholm *et al.*, 1993
Community		
Malignancy	7.7	Edington *et al.*, 1999
Cardiovascular	5.3	Edington *et al.*, 1999

[a]The results often include patients with a variety of diagnoses within the diagnostic category group, which represent subgroups within the overall population of the main study (see Appendix 1).
[b]As the sample sizes of patient subgroups are small in some studies, the results may not provide a true picture of the prevalence of malnutrition in that particular disease group. Diagnostic groups are broad, they may be differently defined by individual studies and there may be overlap between groups. Criteria used are shown in Appendix 1. For more information on specific disease groups, refer to the individual sections in this chapter.

- The use of arm circumference as a surrogate measure for BMI.
- Calculation of cut-off values from the original reference data (e.g. 15th percentile for upper-arm anthropometry (Bishop *et al.*, 1981)).
- Use of different reference standards.
- Exclusion of patients with gross fluid retention (Comi *et al.*, 1998; Weekes, 1999; Corish *et al.*, 2000a). One study documented the inclusion of such patients and noted that weight measurements were not corrected for fluid retention (Strain *et al.*, 1999). However, this could affect the interpretation of BMI and per cent weight loss data.
- Exclusion of the sickest patients due to failure to give consent and to communicate effectively or due to an inability to weigh (Weekes, 1999; Edington *et al.*, 2000).

Many of the studies reviewed have indicated that various patient groups show a deterioration in nutritional status during hospital stay (Weinsier *et al.*, 1979; Agradi *et al.*, 1984; Coats *et al.*, 1993; McWhirter and Pennington, 1994; Comi *et al.*, 1998; Strain *et al.*, 1999; Braunschweig *et al.*, 2000; Corish *et al.*, 2000a; Arnold *et al.*, 2001). In particular, a substantial proportion (up to 70%) lose weight, including those who are undernourished (McWhirter and Pennington, 1994; Corish *et al.*, 2000a) or well nourished (Corish *et al.*, 2000a) on admission to hospital (Fig. 2.6; see Appendix 1, Tables A1.2, A1.4). Patients with sepsis, malignancy, GI disease and renal disease have been found to be at greatest risk of developing malnutrition during hospitalization (Agradi *et al.*, 1984; Perman *et al.*, 2001; Waitzberg *et al.*, 2001).

Deficiencies of vitamins are also common in patients admitted to hospital. For example, Jamieson *et al.* (1999) showed that 21% of an acutely admitted population (*n* 120) was deficient in thiamine, 32% in

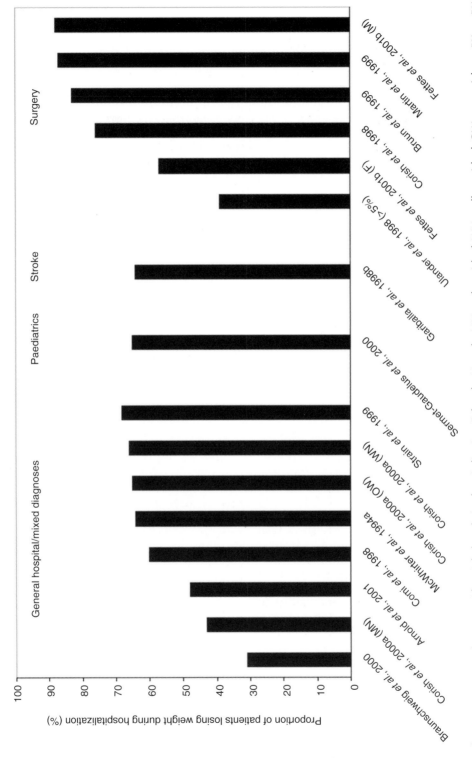

Fig. 2.6. Proportion of patients with weight loss during hospitalization. F, female; M, male; MN, malnourished; WN, well nourished; OW, overweight; > 5%, > 5% weight loss.

pyridoxine and 2.7% in riboflavin. Almost 50% of patients were deficient in at least one of these vitamins. Hypovitaminosis D has also been identified in 57% of general medical patients in the USA (n 290) (Thomas, M.K. *et al.*, 1998). Although it has been demonstrated that the acute-phase response and inflammation can have an impact on circulating micronutrient levels (Louw *et al.*, 1992; Galloway *et al.*, 2000; McMillan *et al.*, 2000), in both of the above studies poor intake was suggested to be of central importance in the development of the deficiencies.

The potential causes and possible consequences of malnutrition in these groups of patients are summarized in Appendix 1 (see Table A1.6).

Elderly

The average age of the population in developed countries is increasing, due to both declining birth rates and increasing longevity. In Europe over recent decades, the population has increased from 340 million (in 1970) to 375.3 million (in 1999) (European Commission, 2001). In that time, the proportion of the old (> 65 years) and very old (> 80 years) has increased steadily, as shown in Table 2.10. Recent estimates indicate that the number of older people worldwide is likely to increase from 600 million to 2 billion by 2050, with 80% of these in developing countries (Bosch, 2002).

Since disease prevalence generally increases with age, it is not surprising that malnutrition or risk of malnutrition is common in the elderly (Appendix 1, Tables A1.7–A1.10). Many elderly people are at

risk of being underweight and undernourished (Clarke *et al.*, 1998) and some of the potential causes and possible consequences of disease-related malnutrition are summarized in Appendix 1 (see Table A1.11). An analysis of a survey of free-living and institutionalized elderly subjects in the UK (n 1355), using a modification of the Malnutrition Advisory Group (MAG) tool, indicated that 7.3% were at medium risk and 6.5% at high risk of malnutrition (Margetts *et al.*, 2002; Stratton *et al.*, 2002). Logistic regression analysis demonstrated that, in men, several factors increased the risk of malnutrition, including having a long-standing illness, living in an institution, being older than 85 years, being in hospital in the last year and living in the north of Great Britain rather than the south. In women, the most notable risk factors were long-standing illness and reported health status. Health-care utilization rose significantly with increasing risk of malnutrition (Stratton *et al.*, 2002). A secondary analysis of the same national data suggests that ~14% of individuals 65 years and over are at medium/high risk of malnutrition, with those living in residential accommodation having a higher incidence of risk (21 vs. 12%). In addition, those living in the north of England have a higher risk than those living in the south of England (19.4 vs. 11.8), mirroring and potentially contributing to other health inequalities (M. Elia, R.J. Stratton, B.M. Margetts and R.M. Thompson, 2002, unpublished). Some studies suggest that poor nutritional status may even precede disease in the elderly and could contribute to its development (Mowé *et al.*, 1994).

Table 2.10. Percentage of the population in various age bands in the European Union-15 countries from 1970 to 1998 (from European Commission, 2001).

Year	0–14 years	15–24 years	25–49 years	50–64 years	65–79 years	80+ years
1970	24.7	14.8	32.6	15.8	10.2	2.0
1980	21.8	15.8	32.9	15.6	11.5	2.4
1990	18.3	15.2	35.1	16.8	11.1	3.4
1995	17.6	13.5	36.7	16.8	11.5	3.9
1998	17.1	12.8	37.1	17.0	12.2	3.7

The elderly account for a high proportion of acute admissions to hospital and of occupied bed days (Tierney, 1996). The evidence reviewed in this section suggests that malnutrition occurs in a significant proportion of elderly people with a variety of diseases across health-care settings. Even though a variety of indices have been used to identify malnutrition in different studies (see Table 2.11), it is evident that malnutrition is a problem in patients living in their own homes (out-patients), in sheltered accommodation and, to a greater extent, in patients with acute or chronic diseases in hospitals and nursing homes. In elderly patients with mixed diagnoses, the studies reviewed indicate that up to 85% may be considered at risk of malnutrition or frankly malnourished on admission to hospital (Fig. 2.4; see Appendix 1, Tables A1.7–

A1.9). Elderly patients living in the community, particularly those in nursing homes, are at risk of malnutrition, with up to 100% of patients being at nutritional risk according to some studies in nursing homes (Fig. 2.5; see Appendix 1, Table A1.10).

As in other patient groups, a variety of different criteria have been used to define malnutrition or risk of malnutrition in elderly patients (see Tables 2.2–2.4). A number of these studies have applied different techniques in the same group of patients and shown considerable differences in results (Cederholm and Hellström, 1992; Mühlethaler *et al.*, 1995; Joosten *et al.*, 1999; Corish *et al.*, 2000b; Dardaine *et al.*, 2001; Faxén Irving *et al.*, 2002). A consensus is required to establish the most appropriate indices to use to identify risk of malnutrition in the elderly across differ-

Table 2.11. Prevalence of disease-related malnutrition according to different criteria in elderly patients.

Criterion	Prevalence of malnutrition (%)	Author
Weight loss	19–40	Morley and Kraenzle, 1994; Faxén Irving *et al.*, 1999
BMI < 21	8–27	Incalzi *et al.*, 1996; Dardaine *et al.*, 2001
BMI < 20 kg m^{-2}	0–36	Klipstein-Grobusch *et al.*, 1995; Faxén Irving *et al.*, 1999; Corish *et al.*, 2000a,b; Flodin *et al.*, 2000; Andersson *et al.*, 2001
BMI < 5th percentile	22	Potter *et al.*, 1995
IBW < 90%	42–61	Shaver *et al.*, 1980; Mowé and Bøhmer, 1991; Sidenvall and Ek, 1993
IBW < 80%	11.8	Abbasi and Rudman, 1993
A combination of anthropometry	6.5–62	Silver *et al.*, 1988; Mowé and Bøhmer, 1991; Morley and Kraenzle, 1994; Mühlethaler *et al.*, 1995; Potter *et al.*, 1995; Incalzi *et al.*, 1996; Joosten *et al.*, 1999; Watson, 1999; Corish *et al.*, 2000a; Dardaine *et al.*, 2001
A combination of anthropometry and biochemical indicators	12–85	Shaver *et al.*, 1980; Sandström *et al.*, 1985; Pinchcofsky-Devin and Kaminski, 1986; Sullivan *et al.*, 1989; Larsson *et al.*, 1990; Cederholm and Hellström, 1992, 1995; Constans *et al.*, 1992; Sidenvall and Ek, 1993; Mowé *et al.*, 1994; Azad *et al.*, 1999; Charles *et al.*, 1999; Christensson *et al.*, 1999; Joosten *et al.*, 1999; Dardaine *et al.*, 2001
Subjective global assessment (SGA)	18–69.8	Covinsky *et al.*, 1999; Faxén Irving *et al.*, 1999; Sacks *et al.*, 2000
Mini Nutritional Assessment (MNA)	26–78.6	Compan *et al.*, 1999; Joosten *et al.*, 1999; Saletti *et al.*, 1999, 2000; Wissing and Unosson, 1999; Van Nes *et al.*, 2001; Beck *et al.*, 2001a
Other nutrition scores	50–54	Thomas *et al.*, 1991; Nordenram *et al.*, 2001
Physician's grading	22	Volkert *et al.*, 1992

ent health-care settings. Until such criteria are established, comparisons between studies and conclusions about the prevalence of malnutrition in different groups of elderly patients are limited. The MAG has provided suggestions for using a universal scoring system across different health-care settings (Elia, 2000b). To enable a cross-comparison of study findings, the per cent of patients with a BMI < 20 kg m^{-2} has been calculated (where possible) as a simple indicator of risk of malnutrition. The results have been presented in Figs 2.1 and 2.2 (see also Tables 2.5 and 2.6). Between 0% (sheltered accommodation (Faxén Irving *et al.*, 2002)) and 36% (mixed diagnoses in hospital (Flodin *et al.*, 2000)) of the elderly have a BMI < 20 kg m^{-2}.

The studies reviewed in this section are undertaken in groups of elderly patients with a wide variety of conditions, including neurological, orthopaedic and surgical patients and those with cancer. Typically the findings of these studies have been presented for the group as a whole and not for specific diagnoses. However, a few trials have identified the prevalence of malnutrition in specific groups of elderly patients. In patients with leg or foot ulcers, living at home, Wissing and Unosson (1999) suggested that 46% were at risk of malnutrition. In a nursing home setting, all of the patients with pressure ulcers were identified as undernourished, although this was only a small group (n 17) (Pinchcofsky-Devin and Kaminski, 1986). In hospitalized patients in Sweden, those with COPD and malignancy were found to have the lowest BMI and the greatest risk of malnutrition (Flodin *et al.*, 2000), while significant proportions of patients in a number of diagnostic groups have been identified as undernourished (cardiovascular disease 32%; respiratory disease 36%; malignancy 56%; multiple organ disease 67%), although sample sizes were small ($n < 34$) (Cederholm and Hellström, 1992).

Studies using different criteria for detecting malnutrition (Fig. 2.5) have identified around 3% (Sweden) (Saletti *et al.*, 1999; Wissing and Unosson, 1999) and 14% (Norway) (Mowé *et al.*, 1994) of

elderly patients living in their own homes as undernourished, with as many as 62% being at risk of malnutrition (Saletti *et al.*, 1999; Wissing and Unosson, 1999). However, estimates of the prevalence of malnutrition in elderly patients in health-care settings (nursing homes, hospitals) are even greater. Reports from nursing homes in Europe and the USA suggest that between 12% (Abbasi and Rudman, 1993) and 85% (Shaver *et al.*, 1980) of patients are undernourished. There appears to have been little change with time as a review of older studies in nursing homes (pre-1980s) suggested that between 30% and 60% of patients were undernourished (Rudman and Feller, 1989). In hospitals across Europe, the reported prevalence of malnutrition or risk of malnutrition in elderly patients ranges from 22% (Germany) (Volkert *et al.*, 1992) to 84% (Ireland) (Charles *et al.*, 1999). A study of elderly patients across different settings indicated that patients in the acute setting, in long-term care and visiting day hospitals were at greater nutritional risk than free-living elderly and those visiting day centres (Morgan *et al.*, 1986).

In addition to the significant proportion of elderly patients who are undernourished, particularly in hospitals, many studies have highlighted that deterioration in nutritional status also occurs while patients are in hospitals and nursing homes across Europe (see Appendix 1, Tables A1.8–A1.10). Loss of weight and/or a reduction in other anthropometric measures have been commonly observed in patients with both acute (Cederholm and Hellström, 1995; Klipstein-Grobusch *et al.*, 1995; Potter *et al.*, 1995; Incalzi *et al.*, 1996; Charles *et al.*, 1999) and chronic (Sandström *et al.*, 1985; Larsson *et al.*, 1990; Constans *et al.*, 1992; Sidenvall and Ek, 1993) health problems. Similar deterioration in nursing homes has been observed in chronically ill patients in the USA (Silver *et al.*, 1988; Thomas *et al.*, 1991; Morley and Kraenzle, 1994). Even in a group of medically stable out-patients, 13% lost $\geq 4\%$ of weight involuntarily over 1 year (Wallace *et al.*, 1995; Fig. 2.6).

Micronutrient status is often poor in the free-living elderly (Keane *et al.*, 1995; Haller, 1999; Ravaglia *et al.*, 2000), which may deteriorate further in geriatric patients (Fenton *et al.*, 1995; Volkert and Stehle, 1999).

COPD

COPD primarily includes chronic bronchitis and emphysema. It is a chronic disease, characterized by progressive, irreversible air-flow obstruction, fibrosis and distortion of the small airways and destruction of the alveolar–pulmonary capillary interface (Congleton, 1999). This leads to dyspnoea, muscle weakness, recurrent bronchial infections and frequently weight loss associated with muscle wasting (Schols and Wouters, 1995). COPD is a leading cause of death, estimated by the World Health Organization (WHO) to be the sixth most common cause of death worldwide in 1990 and predicted to rise to third place by 2020 (cited in Jones, 2001).

As in most other chronic diseases, patients with COPD will spend most of their time outside hospital in the community. However, acute exacerbations of the disease, which may occur between one and eight times per year, frequently necessitate admission to hospital (Rossi and Confalonieri, 2000). COPD is the most common respiratory disease in the developed world, accounting for about 12% of all hospital admissions (Jones, 2001). In Europe, for those countries reporting figures, the average length of stay (LOS) in hospital for patients with respiratory diseases ranged from 5.2 days in Sweden (1995) to 10.9 days in Finland (1995) (European Commission, 2001). More specifically, in a prospective cohort of over 1000 patients with COPD in the USA, the median LOS was 9 days (interquartile range (IQR) 5–15 days) (Connors *et al.*, 1996). Exacerbations can cause life-threatening respiratory failure, often leading to admission to the intensive care unit (ICU) for mechanical ventilation (Rossi and Confalonieri, 2000). These events are associated with poor outcome and high costs (Connors *et al.*, 1996). About 40% of patients with respiratory failure die within 1 year (Rossi and Confalonieri, 2000). In survivors, quality of life is poor (Connors *et al.*, 1996; Monso *et al.*, 1998; Jones, 2001).

COPD represents a significant cost burden on health-care systems, accounting for a large proportion of all general practitioner (GP) consultations (Jones, 2001). In 1996 it was estimated that COPD accounted for $14.5 billion in annual direct costs in the USA (Wilson, L. *et al.*, 2000). In 1998, the indirect cost of morbidity and premature mortality associated with COPD was estimated to be $4.7 billion and $4.5 billion, respectively. In the UK, £1.5 billion was lost as a result of loss of working days and lower productivity in 1996 (Rossi and Confalonieri, 2000). Median costs per patient episode for hospital admission have been estimated to be $7100 (IQR $4100–$16,000) (Connors *et al.*, 1996).

INCIDENCE AND PREVALENCE OF COPD

Worldwide estimates of the prevalence of COPD for all ages indicate figures in the region of 0.7% for men and 0.4% for women (Rossi and Confalonieri, 2000). This is regarded as an underestimate of the true prevalence in those over 50 years, which is when COPD becomes clinically relevant. Indeed, in the UK, it has been estimated that approximately 4% of men and 2% of women over the age of 45 years have been diagnosed with COPD (cited in Jones, 2001). In the EME, prevalence figures for 1990 were 4.2 million, with a rate of 535 per 100,000 of population (Harvard School of Public Health, 1996). The incidence of COPD in the same period was reported to be 670,000, with an incidence rate of 83.9 per 100,000 of population (see Table 2.1).

PREVALENCE OF MALNUTRITION IN PATIENTS WITH COPD

Several studies have examined the prevalence of nutritional depletion in stable outpatients, including those admitted to pulmonary rehabilitation programmes (Fig. 2.5; see Appendix 1, Tables A1.12 and A1.13). Recent involuntary weight loss was noted in 22–52% of patients (Braun *et al.*,

1984b; Schols *et al.*, 1989, 1999; Baarends *et al.*, 1997; Engelen *et al.*, 1999) with more pronounced weight loss seen in those with emphysema compared with chronic bronchitis (Baarends *et al.*, 1997; Engelen *et al.*, 1999; Schols *et al.*, 1999). A cut-off point of < 90% of IBW has been commonly used as a means of defining malnutrition in patients with COPD, with prevalences in the range 19–34% reported (Gray-Donald *et al.*, 1989; Schols *et al.*, 1989, 1993; Wilson *et al.*, 1989; Engelen *et al.*, 1994; Godoy *et al.*, 2000). Using a BMI of < 20 kg m^{-2} as a cut-off, prevalence rates of between 5% (for men) and 23% have been noted (Sahebjami *et al.*, 1993; Landbo *et al.*, 1999; see Fig. 2.2.)

In patients admitted to hospital with acute exacerbations of COPD, prevalence of malnutrition appears to be higher (see Appendix 1, Tables A1.12 and A1.13). Using nutritional indices with multiple components, rates of between 30 and 60% have been reported (Laaban *et al.*, 1993; Thorsdottir *et al.*, 2001; Thorsdottir and Gunnarsdottir, 2002). Using a BMI of < 20 kg m^{-2} as a cut-off, prevalence rates of between 24 and 30% have been noted (Thorsdottir *et al.*, 2001; Thorsdottir and Gunnarsdottir, 2002).

Schols's group has shown that body weight may not be an appropriate index of depletion in COPD, since there is a subgroup of COPD patients that demonstrates depletion of fat-free mass (FFM) despite maintaining normal weight (Schols *et al.*, 1993; Engelen *et al.*, 1994). Furthermore, there are substantial differences in body composition between patients with emphysema and those with chronic bronchitis (Engelen *et al.*, 1999), with more pronounced reductions in both lean mass and fat mass in emphysema. Depletion of FFM may have a more profound impact on function, such as walking distance and respiratory function, than depletion of body weight *per se* (Schols *et al.*, 1989; Engelen *et al.*, 1994; Yoshikawa *et al.*, 1999; Kobayashi *et al.*, 2000; Mostert *et al.*, 2000). This may explain why some studies have failed to show an association between indices of body weight and measurements of function and quality of life (Gray-Donald *et al.*, 1989).

Possible causes and potential consequences of disease-related malnutrition in COPD are summarized in Appendix 1 (see Table A1.14).

GI and liver disease

Any disorders of the GI tract that interfere with the normal processes of eating, chewing, swallowing, digestion and absorption have the potential to cause a deterioration of nutritional status. Likewise, in view of the extensive role of the liver in metabolism and maintenance of homeostasis, liver disorders also predispose to malnutrition. This section will focus on studies that have examined the prevalence of malnutrition in GI diseases, such as inflammatory bowel disease (IBD) and various liver disorders. The prevalence of malnutrition in patients waiting for liver transplantation is also addressed in the section on surgery.

INCIDENCE AND PREVALENCE OF IBD AND LIVER DISEASE
The term IBD covers at least three clinical conditions: ulcerative colitis (UC), Crohn's disease (CD) and indeterminate colitis (Gassull, 2001). Both CD and UC result in chronic inflammation of the bowel wall. CD can affect any part of the GI tract, although is typically found in the lower part of the small intestine, while UC is confined to the large bowel (Thomas, 2001). The aetiology of IBD has not been fully elucidated, although it is thought that environmental factors trigger genes in susceptible individuals (Gassull, 2001). The reported incidence of CD and UC varies from country to country and over time; incidence appears to have been increasing since the 1950s, particularly in Western Europe (Gassull, 2001). Population-based studies indicate an incidence rate of CD of between 3.9 per 100,000 (The Netherlands, 1979–1983) to 9.8 per 100,000 (Scotland, 1985–1987) (Gower-Rousseau *et al.*, 1994). Reported incidence of UC varies from 1.5 per 100,000 (Germany, 1970–1984) to 14.8 per 100,000 (Norway, 1984–1985) (Gower-Rousseau *et al.*, 1994).

Liver disease may be acute or chronic, or an acute episode may be superimposed on chronic disease (Thomas, 2001). Acute liver disease may be caused by viral or non-viral infections, alcohol, drugs, poison or other causes, such as Wilson's disease. Development of rapid severe hepatic dysfunction (within 8 weeks) is known as fulminant hepatic failure. Similar agents may also cause chronic liver disease, as may other conditions such as autoimmune disorders (chronic active hepatitis, primary biliary cirrhosis), biliary obstruction (e.g. due to gallstones or strictures) and vascular disorders (Thomas, 2001). Alcohol accounts for the majority (70–80%) of cases of chronic liver disease (Gopalan *et al.*, 2000). Cirrhosis is a fibrosing chronic liver condition that causes irreversible liver damage. Further insults to the liver at this stage can lead to decompensation, fluid retention and encephalopathy. Ultimately, a liver transplant may be indicated for acute or chronic end-stage liver failure. The incidence of liver cirrhosis in the EME in 1990 was estimated to be 168,000, with an incidence rate of 21 per 100,000. In the same period, the prevalence was 1,238,000, with a prevalence rate of 155.2 per 100,000 (see Table 2.1). In 1998, absolute figures for liver transplants performed in the European Union (EU)-15 countries was 4232 and in the USA 4339 (European Commission, 2001). Within Europe there is wide intercountry variation in the numbers of liver transplants performed, ranging in 1998 from 18 in Greece (1.7 per million population) to 899 in Spain (22.8 per million population) (European Commission, 2001).

PREVALENCE OF MALNUTRITION IN PATIENTS WITH GI AND LIVER DISEASE

Studies of nutritional status using a variety of measures in patients with GI and liver disease (Fig. 2.4; see Appendix 1, Tables A1.15 and A1.16) suggest that malnutrition is a problem in up to 54% of those admitted to hospital with general GI disease (Hirsch *et al.*, 1991; McWhirter and Pennington, 1994; Pirlich *et al.*, 2000). Using SGA criteria, this reflects a higher prevalence than seen in general medical patients in the same centre (27% vs. 21%) (Pirlich *et al.*, 2000), although, using anthropometric criteria alone, others have shown a higher prevalence in medical admissions (38% vs. 46%) (McWhirter *et al.*, 1994b). In the community, 16% of patients with GI disease were regarded as malnourished using anthropometric criteria (McWhirter *et al.*, 1994b). Others have demonstrated, using more comprehensive nutritional assessments, that patients with CD and UC commonly have nutritional deficits soon after diagnosis (Geerling *et al.*, 2000a), as well as after more long-standing illness (Geerling *et al.*, 1998a). In view of the chronic nature of these diseases, many studies have been performed in out-patients rather than in hospitalized patients.

For patients with chronic liver disease, several studies have reported a prevalence of malnutrition of more than 50% using anthropometric criteria (Plauth *et al.*, 1998; Davidson *et al.*, 1999; Alberino *et al.*, 2001; Figs 2.4 and 2.5). Furthermore, the prevalence of malnutrition increases as disease severity increases, both in alcoholic hepatitis (Mendenhall *et al.*, 1984b) and in cirrhosis (Wicks *et al.*, 1995; Alberino *et al.*, 2001; Roongpisuthipong *et al.*, 2001), but particularly in those with alcohol-related disease (Roongpisuthipong *et al.*, 2001).

In patients accepted for liver transplant or being considered for liver transplant, anthropometric indices have revealed a prevalence of malnutrition of up to 54% (Jackson *et al.*, 1996; Harrison *et al.*, 1997; Davidson *et al.*, 1999) or even higher, depending on the percentiles chosen as cut-off values (Harrison *et al.*, 1997). Using SGA criteria, this figure may be as high as 99% (Stephenson *et al.*, 2001; see Fig. 2.5).

One of the problems in assessing nutritional status in patients with liver disease is the variability of body weight associated with ascites and its treatment (Wicks *et al.*, 1995). For example, a German study in liver transplant patients has shown that highly variable changes in weight occur during hospital admission and after transplantation that are not related to outcome. The changes may be largely due to changes in fluid balance associated with alterations in ascitic volume, the severity of oedema and steroid treatment (Möller *et al.*, 1994). Hence, in patients with liver disease, correction of body weight for the presence of ascites is necessary if BMI and indicators of per cent weight loss are to be used as indicators of malnutrition (Mendenhall *et al.*, 1984b). Upper-arm anthropometry may be more appropriate (Wicks *et al.*, 1995), since this part of the body is less likely to be affected by oedema.

Very few studies have assessed changes in nutritional status prospectively over the course of GI and liver disease (see Appendix 1, Table A1.16). In one study that did repeat measures of nutritional status after liver transplant (mean 432 days, range 103–1022), there was an overall improvement in anthropometric measures, although with wide inter-individual variability (Müller *et al.*, 1994). However, for FFM, assessed by bioelectrical impedance, there was an overall, albeit non-significant, decline. Similar findings were reported in a more recent study (Richardson *et al.*, 2001). Measurements at 3-monthly intervals post-liver transplant showed a steady gain in body weight and fat mass until the end of the study period (9 months post-transplant), resulting in 87% of recipients being overweight or obese. This study highlighted the fact that liver transplant patients are not typical of other patients because resting energy expenditure (REE) falls after surgery. It was suggested that this may be due to a loss of hepatic metabolic integration, resulting in energy economy, which is compounded by an overall increase in food intake, and specifically an increase in the percentage of energy derived from fat. In contrast to previous thinking, this study failed to demonstrate a relationship between dose of immunosuppressive drugs and weight gain.

Possible causes and potential consequences of disease-related malnutrition in GI and liver disease are summarized in Appendix 1 (see Table A1.17).

HIV infection and AIDS

HIV is the virus known to cause AIDS (Adler, 2001). Two distinct types of the virus have been identified: type 1 (HIV-1) is responsible for the majority of infections worldwide, while type 2 (HIV-2) is rare outside West Africa (Grant and De Cock, 2001). The most common mode of transmission of the virus in adults is through sexual contact. Other modes of transmission are through receipt of contaminated blood or blood products, donated organs, semen and sharing or reuse of contaminated needles by drug users or for therapeutic procedures and from mother to child (Adler, 2001). The latter is the most common mode of transmission in infants and children (see section on paediatrics, this chapter). The relative importance of different modes of transmission varies according to geographical region (Adler, 2001; Grant and De Cock, 2001).

Primary HIV infection is also known as the seroconversion illness or acute HIV infection. Not all persons have symptoms at the time of seroconversion, and when symptoms do occur they are usually mild (Mindel and Tenant-Flowers, 2001). There is a wide spectrum of clinical manifestations of infection with HIV, and the definition of AIDS has changed over the years as this has become more widely appreciated. AIDS is currently defined as an illness characterized by one or more indicator diseases (Adler, 2001): the AIDS-defining conditions differ somewhat depending on whether or not laboratory evidence of HIV infection is available. It may take 10 years or more for AIDS to develop after seroconversion (Mindel and Tenant-Flowers, 2001).

In recent years, the availability of highly active antiretroviral therapy (HAART) in industrialized countries has meant that the life expectancy of persons with AIDS has increased dramatically. However, in combination with the increase in new HIV infections, this means that the prevalent pool of those who are potentially infectious is increasing (Adler, 2001).

By the end of 2000, it was estimated by the joint United Nations Programme on AIDS (UNAIDS) that there were 36.1 million people living with HIV/AIDS (1.4 million of these being children < 15 years), with 5.3 million new HIV infections occurring in 2000 (Adler, 2001). The vast majority (95%) of all infections occur in developing countries, predominantly sub-Saharan Africa and South-East Asia. For example, at the end of 2000, it was estimated that there were 25.3 million adults and children living with HIV/AIDS in sub-Saharan Africa (population 640 million), with an adult prevalence rate of 8.8% (for adults aged 15–49 years). For the same period in Western Europe, figures were 540,000, with an adult prevalence rate of 0.24%, and in North America, 920,000, with an adult prevalence rate of 0.6% (Adler, 2001).

At any one time, there are five times as many people infected with HIV as having AIDS. By June 1999, the cumulative total of adult AIDS cases reported in the USA was 702,748 and, by June 2000, 236,406 cases had been reported in Europe (Adler, 2001). Within Europe the prevalence rate of AIDS varies between countries. The highest incidence rates per million population are reported in Spain, Portugal, Italy and Switzerland (Adler, 2001; European Commission, 2001) where sharing needles and equipment during injecting drug use is the most common mode of transmission (Adler, 2001). Even within countries there will be regional differences in seroprevalence for HIV and the most common modes of transmission (Adler, 2001).

The annual death rate due to AIDS was estimated to be 2.4 million in sub-Saharan Africa in 2000, compared with 10,100 in the USA in 1999. The latter figure (together with a decrease in morbidity) has declined steeply since 1996 due to the introduction of HAART (Palella *et al.*, 1998; Weiss, 2001).

PREVALENCE OF MALNUTRITION IN PATIENTS WITH HIV
INFECTION AND AIDS

It is well known that patients in developing countries suffer a high degree of malnu-

trition associated with HIV infection and AIDS, often compounded by infections such as tuberculosis, which, independent of HIV, have a significant impact on nutritional status (Castetbon *et al.*, 1997; Niyongabo *et al.*, 1999; Shah *et al.*, 2001). This section, however, will focus on the situation in developed countries.

Most studies examining the prevalence of malnutrition in HIV and AIDS in developed countries were performed in the late 1980s to mid-1990s, in the pre-HAART era, although in some studies the use of some antiretroviral medications was documented. The majority of these studies were cross-sectional, performed in stable outpatients, and defined malnutrition in terms of weight loss, either self-reported or through retrospective analysis of medical notes (see Appendix 1, Tables A1.18 and A1.19). This is probably because HIV wasting syndrome was defined as the unintentional loss of more than 10% body weight (Grunfeld, 1995). In these studies, weight loss of any degree was reported at examination (prior time course of disease often unspecified) in up to 78% of patients with HIV infection and AIDS (Dworkin *et al.*, 1990; Guenter *et al.*, 1993; Parisien *et al.*, 1993; Luder *et al.*, 1995; Niyongabo *et al.*, 1997; Malvy *et al.*, 2001; see Appendix 1, Table A1.18). More specifically, weight loss of greater than 10% usual body weight was reported in up to 31% of patients (Guenter *et al.*, 1993; Parisien *et al.*, 1993; Luder *et al.*, 1995; Niyongabo *et al.*, 1997; Kim *et al.*, 2001; Malvy *et al.*, 2001). Süttmann *et al.* (1991) reported that 53% of a group of patients at different stages of disease but without opportunistic infections weighed less than 90% of IBW. Several studies have reported that weight loss is greater and/or other indices of nutritional status appear more impaired with more advanced disease (Dworkin *et al.*, 1990; Parisien *et al.*, 1993; Ockenga *et al.*, 1997; Woods *et al.*, 2002). Not surprisingly, therefore, the rate of weight loss in patients hospitalized with AIDS is even higher than that reported in the community, with up to 98% reporting some degree of weight loss, up to 68% reporting weight loss of > 10% usual body weight, and up to 29% reporting loss of > 20% usual body weight (Chlebowski *et al.*, 1989; Trujillo *et al.*, 1992; Figs 2.4 and 2.5; see Appendix 1, Tables A1.18 and A1.20).

Few studies have reported longitudinal changes in weight. One reported that 66.5% of a large cohort of patients experienced weight loss over a median 43-month period of follow-up after recruitment (Malvy *et al.*, 2001). A more in-depth study of longitudinal changes in weight in 30 males with stage IV HIV infection revealed two distinct patterns of weight loss: acute episodes, associated predominantly with non-GI opportunistic infections, and chronic episodes, predominantly associated with GI disease (Macallan *et al.*, 1993). However, in this study, periods of both weight stability and weight gain were also reported, showing that weight loss was neither inevitable nor unremitting.

Assessments of weight alone may underestimate the true picture of nutritional status in HIV. It has been shown that patients often lose a relatively greater proportion of lean body mass than would be expected in simple starvation (Kotler *et al.*, 1985). Such changes may occur early in the course of disease, even before symptoms are noted (Ott *et al.*, 1993).

The advent of HAART has had a dramatic impact on morbidity and mortality associated with HIV infection and AIDS, and it has been suggested that concomitant changes in the evolution of nutritional status in association with the disease would be seen. HAART regimens are combination therapies, usually comprised of two nucleoside analogue reverse transcriptor inhibitors (e.g. abacavir, lamivudine, zidovudine) in combination with one or two HIV-1 protease inhibitors (e.g. indinavir, ritonavir, saquinavir) and/or a non-nucleoside analogue reverse transcriptor inhibitor (e.g. efavirenz, nevirapine) (Mooser and Carr, 2001). In non-randomized studies, HAART has been shown to reduce diarrhoeal disease and enteric infections (Foudraine *et al.*, 1998; Maggi *et al.*, 2000), reduce opportunistic infections (Semba *et al.*, 2001), increase appetite in children (cited in Miller *et al.*, 2001a) and

reduce REE (Pernerstorfer-Schoen *et al.*, 1999), all of which may help to improve nutritional status. Indeed, components of HAART therapy have been shown to improve nutritional status, e.g. in an uncontrolled study, indinavir significantly improved nutritional status in patients with HIV-related wasting (Carbonnel *et al.*, 1998), although weight trends were not improved with protease inhibitors (Schwenk *et al.*, 1999a). In uncontrolled studies, HAART improved body weight in patients with chronic diarrhoea (Foudraine *et al.*, 1998) and improved body composition in HIV-infected and AIDS patients without wasting (Pernerstorfer-Schoen *et al.*, 1999) and, in a larger study in children, several growth parameters were improved (Miller *et al.*, 2001a). HAART has also been shown to improve anaemia in HIV-infected injection drug users compared with a control (non-randomized) group not receiving HAART (Semba *et al.*, 2001). However, Wanke *et al.* (2000) reported that wasting may still be significant, despite HAART. In a recent cross-sectional study of outpatients in the UK in whom the majority were receiving HAART, the level of wasting was reported to be relatively low (5.6% with a BMI of < 18.5 kg m^{-2} and 7% with a BMI of 18.5–20 kg m^{-2}) (Hodgson *et al.*, 2001). However, as few other studies in the pre-HAART era reported BMI in this way, it is difficult to make comparisons.

HAART is not without side-effects, including:

- diarrhoea, nausea, mouth ulcers and tiredness (Thomas, 2001);
- lipodystrophy syndrome, including fat redistribution (accumulation and reduction in fat at specific body sites), dyslipidaemia, glucose intolerance/diabetes and lactic acidaemia (Carr and Cooper, 2000; Mooser and Carr, 2001);
- osteopenia (Carr and Cooper, 2000);
- mitochondrial toxicity, drug hypersensitivity (Carr and Cooper, 2000).

These side-effects suggest that additional nutritional challenges will now be faced in patients with HIV infection and AIDS (Ware *et al.*, 2002).

Possible causes and potential consequences of disease-related malnutrition in HIV infection and AIDS are summarized in Appendix 1 (Table A1.21).

Malignancy

Cancer is a major cause of morbidity and mortality worldwide. It is the second most frequent cause of death in Europe and is becoming the leading cause of death in old age. The term 'cancer' is a general one, covering an enormous range of different types of malignant tumours, which can affect virtually every body tissue (Thomas, 2001).

INCIDENCE AND PREVALENCE OF CANCER

Most cancers occur in older adults (European Commission, 2001). Table A1.22 shows the age-standardized incidence rate of cancer in males and females in 15 European member states (EU-15: Austria, Belgium, Denmark, Finland, France, Germany, Greece, Ireland, Italy, Luxembourg, The Netherlands, Portugal, Spain, Sweden, the UK) (European Commission, 2001). In men in 1995, 19.5% of all cancers occurred in the lung, followed by prostate (14.2%), colon/rectum (12.7%) and bladder (8.3%). In women in the same year, breast cancer was the most common cancer (28.5%), followed by colon/rectum (12.7%), bladder (8.3%) and lung (5.9%). In 1995 in the EU-15, the absolute (total) number of incident cancer cases was 785,793, with a 1-year prevalence of 515,761 and a 5-year prevalence of 1,956,589. In women in the same period, the total number of cases was 694,317, with a 1-year prevalence of 509,275 and a 5-year prevalence of 2,092,488 (European Commission, 2001). The incidence and prevalence of various types of cancer in the EME are shown in Table 2.1.

Worldwide, the most common cancers in men (lung) and women (breast) reflect the European situation (Boyle, 1997). However, there are marked geographical variations in cancer risk. For example, there is a high incidence of oesophageal cancers in parts of Iran, China and southern republics of the former USSR and a high incidence of gastric cancer in the former USSR, parts of Japan, China, Latin America and Central/Eastern Europe. Primary liver cancer is most common in South-East Asia and Africa, and melanoma has its highest rates in northern Australia (Boyle, 1997).

Most patients with cancer will spend the majority of their time outside hospital in the community. In Europe, for those countries reporting figures, the average LOS in hospital for patients with neoplasms ranged from 7.1 days in Denmark (1993) to 12.7 days in Italy (1994).

PREVALENCE OF MALNUTRITION IN PATIENTS WITH CANCER

Cancer is often associated with protein-energy malnutrition (Lipman, 1991). A series of studies between 1932 and 1974, summarized by Strain (1979), highlighted the phenomenon of cachexia in patients with cancer. The prevalence of cachexia (criteria not defined) ranged from 8% to 84%, depending on the cancer site, with the highest proportion in patients with gastric (*n* 1112) or pancreatic (*n* 449) cancers (84% and 73%, respectively). Although many of these studies were undertaken in the early part of the 20th century, investigations in cancer patients in the 1980s and 1990s show that malnutrition is still a considerable problem. From the more recent studies reviewed, using a variety of different methodologies including weight loss as the sole parameter (see Appendix 1, Tables A1.23–A1.25, for details), estimates of the prevalence of malnutrition in specific groups of cancer patients include:

- 9% in urological cancer patients (Persson *et al.*, 1999);
- up to 15% in gynaecological cancers (DeWys *et al.*, 1980; Wolf *et al.*, 2001);
- up to 46% in lung cancer patients (DeWys *et al.*, 1980; Bashir *et al.*, 1990; Jagoe *et al.*, 2001b);
- up to 80% in patients with GI cancer (DeWys *et al.*, 1980; Persson *et al.*, 1999);
- up to 67% in head and neck cancer (Brookes, 1982; Van Bokhorst-de van der Schueren *et al.*, 1997; Hammerlid *et al.*, 1998; Collins *et al.*, 1999; Lees, 1999; Beaver *et al.*, 2001);

- 57% in oesophageal cancer (Daly *et al.*, 2000);
- 58% in oesophageal/gastric cancer (Martin *et al.*, 1999);
- up to 65% in gastric cancer (DeWys *et al.*, 1980; Rey-Ferro *et al.*, 1997);
- up to 85% in pancreatic cancer patients (DeWys *et al.*, 1980; Wigmore *et al.*, 1997);
- up to 33% in patients with colorectal cancer (Meguid *et al.*, 1986; Ulander *et al.*, 1998).

Most of the trials reviewed have been undertaken in patients prior to chemotherapy or surgery (see Appendix 1, Table A1.24). Three studies were undertaken prior to radiotherapy (Collins *et al.*, 1999; Lees, 1999; Beaver *et al.*, 2001). In addition, patients with GI cancer undergoing surgery have also been included in studies of mixed groups of surgical patients (see section on surgery, this chapter), although the findings of these studies are typically presented for the group as a whole. Similarly, elderly patients with cancer have been included as part of the studies of mixed groups of elderly patients discussed in the section on the elderly (this chapter).

If expressed in terms of mode of treatment (Figs 2.4 and 2.5; see Appendix 1, Tables A1.23–A1.25), estimates of the prevalence of malnutrition are as follows:

- up to 75% prior to surgery;
- up to 57% prior to radiotherapy;
- up to 65% prior to chemotherapy;
- up to 75% prior to bone-marrow transplant;
- 85% in untreatable cancer.

Although most patients with cancer will spend the majority of their time with disease at home, most studies that have examined nutritional status have done so in hospital prior to therapy (Fig. 2.4). Only a few studies have examined patients at times more remote from treatment. Of these, the largest (Edington *et al.*, 1999) showed that, of a sample of cancer patients from general practice (*n* 5074), 8% had a BMI < 20 kg m^{-2}. In another study of unselected cancer patients with solid tumours,

43% had a weight loss of greater than 10% of usual body weight and 24% had a more moderate weight loss of between 5 and 10% (Bosaeus *et al.*, 2001). In a smaller study in more specific types of cancer, Persson *et al.* (1999) demonstrated a prevalence of malnutrition of 9% in urological cancers and 52% in GI cancers a median 6 months after diagnosis. Thirty-three per cent of those with urological cancer and 80% of those with GI cancer had lost weight in the previous 12 months.

The criteria used to define malnutrition in malignancy vary widely (see Appendix 1, Tables A1.24 and A1.25) and are part of the reason for the wide variance in reported values. They include the following:

- history of weight loss (DeWys *et al.*, 1980; Ovesen *et al.*, 1993; Van Bokhorst-de van der Schueren *et al.*, 1997; Wigmore *et al.*, 1997; Andreyev *et al.*, 1998; Collins *et al.*, 1999; Lees, 1999; Daly *et al.*, 2000; Beaver *et al.*, 2001; Bosaeus *et al.*, 2001; Jagoe *et al.*, 2001b);
- arm anthropometry and/or low BMI or IBW (Bashir *et al.*, 1990; Deeg *et al.*, 1995; Van Bokhorst-de van der Schueren *et al.*, 1997; Wigmore *et al.*, 1997; Corish *et al.*, 1998; Collins *et al.*, 1999; Edington *et al.*, 1999; Beaver *et al.*, 2001; Bosaeus *et al.*, 2001; Gungor *et al.*, 2001; Jagoe *et al.*, 2001a; Wolf *et al.*, 2001);
- subjective global assessment (Ulander *et al.*, 1998; Persson *et al.*, 1999; Gungor *et al.*, 2001);
- nutrition risk index (Rey-Ferro *et al.*, 1997; Corish *et al.*, 1998; Gungor *et al.*, 2001);
- other nutritional status assessments involving multiple measures (Brookes, 1982; Meguid *et al.*, 1986; Hammerlid *et al.*, 1998).

Weight loss has been commonly identified in patients with cancer. At least some degree of weight loss has been reported in up to 75% of cancer patients prior to surgery, 57% prior to radiotherapy, 51% prior to chemotherapy, 85% in unresectable pancreatic cancer and 80% of general cancer patients living in the community. Changes in fluid balance/oedema have not been recorded in any of the studies, although it is likely to have a confounding effect on body-weight measurements in such patients (Kramer *et al.*, 1998).

A large study of cancer patients (by the Eastern Cooperative Oncology Group (USA), *n* 3047 (DeWys *et al.*, 1980)) indicated a relationship between weight loss and tumour site. The lowest frequency of weight loss (31–40% of patients) was in those with non-Hodgkin's lymphoma, breast cancer, acute non-lymphocytic leukaemia and sarcomas. In patients with colon, prostatic and lung cancer and unfavourable non-Hodgkin's lymphoma, between 48 and 61% of patients lost weight. The highest frequency of weight loss (83–87% of patients) was in those with pancreatic or gastric cancer. These findings suggest that the extent of malnutrition varies according to the cancer site. However, it is likely that other factors, such as the severity of the cancer (stage and type), the treatment (chemotherapy, radiotherapy, surgery) and the age of patients, will also be important. Gender may also play a role (Palomares *et al.*, 1996).

Fewer studies have reported the BMI of patients with cancer. In general, between 6 and 15% of patients have a BMI < 20 kg m^{-2} (Corish *et al.*, 1998; Collins *et al.*, 1999; Edington *et al.*, 1999; Jagoe *et al.*, 2001b; Wolf *et al.*, 2001), except in unresectable pancreatic cancer, where the figure is considerably higher (35%) (Wigmore *et al.*, 1997; see Figs 2.1 and 2.2). However, the proportion of underweight individuals frequently increases with time as the tumour becomes more widespread.

A few studies have examined changes in nutritional status during treatment. In all cases, a large proportion of patients showed deterioration in their nutritional status while receiving radiotherapy (Collins *et al.*, 1999; Beaver *et al.*, 2001) and after surgery (Corish *et al.*, 1998; Ulander *et al.*, 1998; Fig. 2.6). In one study in surgical patients, 70% continued to lose weight for up to 3 months after discharge

(Corish *et al.*, 1998). In non-small-cell lung cancer patients receiving a variety of treatments, mean weight loss over the disease course was 5.5 kg in men and 2.5 kg in women (Palomares *et al.*, 1996). In unresectable pancreatic cancer, 85% had already lost weight at the time of diagnosis, which increased to 100% at the time of death. At this point, 65% had a BMI < 20 kg m^{-2} (Wigmore *et al.*, 1997).

The possible causes and potential consequences of disease-related malnutrition in cancer patients are summarized in Appendix 1 (Table A1.26).

Neurological disease

The studies reviewed suggest that malnutrition can be a problem in patients with a variety of neurological disorders, including those with a cerebrovascular accident (CVA) (commonly referred to as a stroke) and other neurological disorders (see Appendix 1, Tables A1.27–A1.29). Most work has been done in the area of stroke, and this will form the focus of this section.

About 80% of strokes are due to cerebral infarction (ischaemic stroke, usually due to a blood clot causing a blockage in blood flow to the brain) and about 10% are due to primary intracerebral haemorrhage (haemorrhagic stroke, due to a ruptured bloodvessel in the brain) (Gariballa, 2000). Stroke is the most important cause of severe disability in the Western population (Gariballa, 2000). About 35% of survivors still require significant help with daily tasks after 1 year (Department of Health, 2001). The cost of strokes to health and social services in the UK has been estimated to be £1.36 billion per year (Department of Health, 2001).

INCIDENCE AND PREVALENCE OF STROKE
Stroke is one of the commonest causes of death after coronary heart disease and cancer (Gariballa, 2000). In the UK, approximately 140,000 new or recurrent strokes occur each year (Department of Health, 2001). This figure is four to five times higher in the USA (Gariballa, 2000). In the EME, 1,282,000 first strokes occurred in

1990, with a prevalence rate of 9,467,000 (Harvard School of Public Health, 1996). The incidence rate per 100,000 of population was 160.7, with an average age of onset of 70.1 years (see Table 2.1).

PREVALENCE OF MALNUTRITION IN STROKE PATIENTS
Studies from the UK (Gariballa *et al.*, 1998b), Spain (Davalos *et al.*, 1996), Sweden (Axelsson *et al.*, 1988; Unosson *et al.*, 1994) and Canada (Finestone *et al.*, 1995) indicate the prevalence of malnutrition in patients admitted to hospital with acute stroke to be about 24%, ranging from 8% (Unosson *et al.*, 1994) to 49% (Finestone *et al.*, 1995) (Fig. 2.4; see Appendix 1, Tables A1.27 and A1.28). This difference may be due to genuine differences in the body composition of the national populations. However, other factors are more likely, including the following:

- Differences in the criteria used to determine malnutrition. These have ranged from the use of BMI < 20 kg m^{-2} (Gariballa *et al.*, 1998b) to a mix of anthropometric, biochemical and/or immunological parameters (Axelsson *et al.*, 1988; Unosson *et al.*, 1994; Finestone *et al.*, 1995; Davalos *et al.*, 1996; Murray *et al.*, 2000).
- Differences in the types of patients (age range, male-to-female ratio).
- Misleading results from small sample sizes, e.g. $n < 50$ (Unosson *et al.*, 1994; Finestone *et al.*, 1995) versus n 201 (Gariballa *et al.*, 1998b).

Surrogate measures for height are frequently used in this patient population, e.g. arm span (Gariballa *et al.*, 1998b), supine height (Unosson *et al.*, 1994) and knee height (Finestone *et al.*, 1995). Although patients with other diseases or those taking ongoing medication are often excluded in such studies, Davalos *et al.* (1996) were able to show that the prevalence of malnutrition in such a group (16.7%) was the same as in the population studied (16.3%).

Stroke patients remaining in hospital show marked and significant deterioration in nutritional status over 2 (Davalos *et al.*, 1996; Gariballa *et al.*, 1998b), 4 (Gariballa

et al., 1998b) and 9 weeks (Unosson *et al.*, 1994) (Fig. 2.6; see Appendix 1, Table A1.28).

The possible causes and potential consequences of disease-related malnutrition in stroke patients are summarized in Appendix 1 (Table A1.30).

PREVALENCE OF MALNUTRITION IN OTHER NEUROLOGICAL DISORDERS
Patients with other chronic neurological disorders are also at high risk of malnutrition (Kennedy *et al.*, 1997; Poehlman and Dvorak, 2000; Thomson *et al.*, 2001; Figs 2.4 and 2.5; see Appendix 1, Table A1.29). A survey of patients with intellectual and neurological diseases across community (n 99) and hospital (n 318) settings has found $> 60\%$ of these patients to have a BMI < 20 kg m^{-2} (Kennedy *et al.*, 1997). (This study also included children, although no data were presented for this group specifically.) Furthermore, the degree of malnutrition appears to be related in part to the severity of feeding problems (Kennedy *et al.*, 1997). In a much smaller sample (n 43) of patients undergoing rehabilitation following brain injury, 56% were identified as undernourished (using a combination of BMI and arm anthropometry) (Thomson *et al.*, 2001). This study also identified that those patients not given nutritional support post-brain injury experienced substantially greater weight loss (mean 12.6%) than those patients given nutrition (5%) (Thomson *et al.*, 2001). Neither of these studies reported the use of surrogate measures or the presence of fluid retention.

Ultimately, there is a need for further investigation of the nutritional status of patients with neurological disease. Although patients with such conditions may have been considered in studies of mixed groups of patients (e.g. in the elderly), specific information about the extent of malnutrition in patients with different types of neurological disease needs to be gathered. Similarly, more research is needed to address the efficacy of nutritional support in those patients who are at risk of malnutrition (see Chapters 6–8).

Orthopaedics

Fractured neck of femur constitutes the greatest problem associated with poor nutritional status in the area of orthopaedics. This section will therefore focus mainly on fractured neck of femur.

Osteoporosis, defined as a reduction in bone mass that increases susceptibility to fracture, is common in Western countries, particularly in elderly females (Cummings *et al.*, 1985). Osteoporosis predisposes to a wide variety of fractures (hip, vertebrae, distal forearm, humerus, pelvis and others). Fractures of the hip, however, are associated with more deaths, disabilities and medical costs than all other osteoporotic fractures combined (Cummings *et al.*, 1985). The burden of hip fractures on health-care systems is enormous. Fracturing a hip is one of the most common reasons for an elderly person to be admitted to hospital (Lumbers *et al.*, 2001). Recent estimates for total annual fracture costs were $10 billion in the USA, $960 million in England and Wales and $740 million in France (excluding vertebral fracture) (Barrett-Connor, 1995).

INCIDENCE AND PREVALENCE OF FRACTURED NECK OF FEMUR

Data from the European Commission (2001) indicate that the incidence of hip fractures is increasing in Europe, and this trend is likely to increase in future years. Others have confirmed that the number of osteoporotic fractures will increase dramatically worldwide in the next 50 years, reflecting population growth, increasing life expectancy and a rising elderly population (Barrett-Connor, 1995).

Total rates of fractured neck of femur are considerably higher for women than for men. For example, in Germany, total incidence rate per 10,000 of population in 1995 was projected to be 89 for women and 19 for men and, in the UK, 55 for women and 13 for men. The incidence rate increases exponentially with age, e.g. in Germany, women aged 50–54 years have an incidence rate of 3 per 10,000, rising to 351 per 10,000 for women aged over 85 years (European Commission, 2001). In the EME,

the incidence rate of fractured neck of femur with short-term sequelae in 1990 was estimated to be 1,255,000, and 90,000 with long-term sequelae (Harvard School of Public Health, 1996). From the same survey, the incidence rate per 100,000 in 1990 was 157 (short-term) and 11.3 (long-term). Average age of onset was about 64.5 years in both types (see Table 2.1).

PREVALENCE OF MALNUTRITION IN FRACTURED NECK OF FEMUR

In an epidemiological follow-up study of a cohort of 2879 white men in the USA, weight loss and bone density were significantly related to hip fracture risk (Mussolino *et al.*, 1998). Malnutrition is also a common problem in hospitalized patients across Europe with fractured neck of femur. Indeed, a simple, large anthropometric survey in the UK has indicated that hospitalized fractured neck of femur patients are significantly thinner than elderly hospital patients and healthy elderly (Mansell *et al.*, 1990b).

The estimated average prevalence of risk of malnutrition from the studies reviewed typically ranges from 13% (Lumbers *et al.*, 2001) to 63% (Murphy *et al.*, 2000) (Fig. 2.4; see Appendix 1, Tables A1.31 and A1.32). It is important to note that the sample sizes of patients tend to be relatively small (*n* 20–119).

The criteria used in studies to determine prevalence of malnutrition in fractured neck of femur included:

- anthropometry (Jallut *et al.*, 1990; Brown and Seabrook, 1992; Maffulli *et al.*, 1999; Paillaud *et al.*, 2000; Bachrach-Lindström *et al.*, 2001; Lumbers *et al.*, 2001);
- a mix of anthropometric and biochemical indices (Unosson *et al.*, 1995; Lumbers *et al.*, 1996; Ponzer *et al.*, 1999; Bachrach-Lindström *et al.*, 2001);
- the MNA (Murphy *et al.*, 2000).

Comparing the studies that have quantified those patients with a BMI < 20 kg m^{-2}, the prevalence of malnutrition ranges from 26% (Bachrach-Lindström *et al.*, 2001) to 50% (Jallut *et al.*, 1990) (see Fig. 2.2).

There may be subgroups of patients in whom malnutrition occurs with greater frequency. Patients with intracapsular fractures of the femur are more malnourished than those with a trochanteric location of the fracture (Maffulli *et al.*, 1999). The prevalence of malnutrition appears to be lower in patients admitted for an elective total hip replacement than in patients admitted with fractured neck of femur (4% total hip replacement, 41% fractured neck of femur using the same criteria) (Lumbers *et al.*, 1996). In addition, women may be more likely to be undernourished than men. In Paillaud *et al.*'s study (2000), 33% of patients were identified as undernourished, and all were women.

In addition to a significant proportion of patients being undernourished on admission to hospital with fractured neck of femur, studies suggest that an increasing proportion of patients become undernourished during their hospital stay. In particular, those who are identified as undernourished on admission often experience further deterioration in their nutritional status (Jallut *et al.*, 1990; Brown and Seabrook, 1992; Unosson *et al.*, 1995; Paillaud *et al.*, 2000; Bachrach-Lindström *et al.*, 2001; see Appendix 1, Table A1.32).

In addition to trials undertaken specifically in orthopaedic patients reviewed in this section, a number of studies in mixed groups of patients have included orthopaedic patients (see sections on the elderly and surgery for details). The possible causes and potential consequences of disease-related malnutrition in patients with fractured neck of femur are summarized in Appendix 1 (see Table A1.33).

OTHER GROUPS OF ORTHOPAEDIC PATIENTS
Compared with fractured neck of femur, there is relatively little information about the nutritional status of other groups of orthopaedic patients. One trial in a mixed group of adult orthopaedic patients identified 48% of patients with one or more indices suggestive of malnutrition (< 90% IBW, low albumin, total iron-binding capacity, triceps skin-fold thickness or mid-arm muscle circumference). This study also indicated that LOS might be greater in patients with poor nutritional status (three abnormal indices) (Dreblow *et al.*, 1981). Similarly, Jensen *et al.* (1982) reported a mean prevalence of subclinical and clinical malnutrition of 42% in 129 patients undergoing orthopaedic surgical procedures, using a variety of criteria (triceps skin-fold thickness, mid-arm muscle circumference, creatinine–height index, transferrin, albumin, total lymphocyte count and skin antigen testing). Furthermore, they identified a significant correlation between subnormal nutritional indices and the development of complications.

Renal disease

Renal diseases include chronic renal failure (predialysis period), end-stage renal disease (ESRD) (dialysis or transplant required), acute renal failure, nephrotic syndrome and renal malignancy. This section will focus on chronic renal failure and ESRD requiring dialysis.

Chronic renal failure is a state of progressive and irreversible renal impairment. There are a large variety of causes of chronic renal failure, including glomerulonephritis, diabetic nephropathy, renal vascular disease/hypertension, chronic pyelonephritis and obstruction (Thomas, 2001). Impaired renal function gives rise to uraemia, a term that encompasses a wide range of symptoms. When renal function has declined to negligible levels (ESRD), renal replacement therapy (dialysis) becomes necessary. Ultimately, a renal transplant may be indicated.

INCIDENCE AND PREVALENCE OF CHRONIC RENAL FAILURE, DIALYSIS AND TRANSPLANTATION
Little information is available on the incidence and prevalence of chronic renal failure in the period prior to need for dialysis, but it is known that the prevalence of chronic renal disease is increasing worldwide. In the USA over the last decade, it has been estimated that the number of patients treated for uraemia is increasing by 6% per year, with a total of 650,000 patients forecast in 2010 (Ruggenenti *et al.*,

2001). The prevalence of ESRD requiring renal replacement therapy can also be used as an indicator of the burden of renal disease in a country (Ruggenenti *et al.*, 2001). In the USA, there were more than 372,000 patients receiving renal replacement therapy at the end of 2000, which was double the number recorded in 1991 (Ruggenenti *et al.*, 2001).

Since 1970, there has been a huge increase in the number of patients receiving dialysis across Europe, although there does seem to be some discrepancy between reported figures. The most recent data from the European Commission (1994) suggested that between 60.9 (Norway) and 481.6 (Greece) per million of population received dialysis (UK 147.3, The Netherlands 263.8, Germany 230.9) (European Commission, 2001). Prevalence data compiled from a variety of different national renal registries giving figures for treated ESRD in 1996 range from 511 per million of population in The Netherlands to 695 per million in Italy. Lowest rates were reported from Romania (57 per million) and highest from Japan (1328) and the USA (1072) (Anon., 1998). Data from the EME indicated an incidence of ESRD of 105,000 in 1990, with a rate per 100,000 of population of 13.2 (Harvard School of Public Health, 1996). Prevalence in 1990 was 415,000 (52 per 100,000) (see Table 2.1). Demographic data from the International Federation of Renal Registries (incorporating registry data from Asia–Pacific, Australia, New Zealand, Canada, Europe, Japan, Latin America and the USA) in 1996 showed that approximately 1 million patients with ESRD received renal replacement therapy and 200,000 new patients started to receive it (Schena, 2000). Treatment of ESRD represents a considerable burden on health-care budgets; in the USA, expenditure is expected to double in this decade to reach a total of more than $28 billion by 2010 (Ruggenenti *et al.*, 2001).

Maintenance dialysis therapy has been in routine practice for almost 40 years, but the mortality rate remains high (Bergstrom and Lindholm, 1998). The main cause of death

is cardiovascular disease, followed by infection. Malnutrition may exacerbate pre-existing heart failure and increase the risk of infection, but might also be a consequence of cardiac failure, infection and inflammation (Bergstrom and Lindholm, 1998).

Relative to the number of patients receiving dialysis, the number of patients receiving kidney transplants is rather low. In the EU-15 countries in 1998, the rate was 31.2 per million of population (European Commission, 2001). Rates per country varied from 16.1 (Greece) to 50.7 (Spain) (UK/Ireland 28.1, The Netherlands 30.9, Germany 28.5).

PREVALENCE OF MALNUTRITION IN PATIENTS WITH CHRONIC RENAL FAILURE AND ESRD

Most studies that have examined malnutrition in renal disease have done so in patients receiving dialysis (see Appendix 1, Tables A1.34 and A1.35). A limited number of studies have examined nutritional status in the predialysis period, suggesting that between 28–48% of patients may be at least mildly malnourished as measured by SGA (Heimburger *et al.*, 2000; Lawson *et al.*, 2001; Fig. 2.5). These studies indicate that patients may often be undernourished at the time of starting renal replacement therapy.

A number of studies have indicated that a significant proportion of outpatients with ESRD receiving chronic ambulatory peritoneal dialysis (CAPD) or haemodialysis are undernourished (Marckmann, 1988; Young *et al.*, 1991; Harty *et al.*, 1993; Cianciaruso *et al.*, 1995; Engel *et al.*, 1995; Aparicio *et al.*, 1999; Herselman *et al.*, 2000; Laws *et al.*, 2000; Chazot *et al.*, 2001; Jager *et al.*, 2001). Prevalences range from 9 to 72%, depending on the criteria used to define malnutrition (Fig. 2.5; see Appendix 1, Tables A1.34 and A1.35). The prevalence of malnutrition seems to increase with age (27% in patients aged 18–40 years and up to 51% in those over 65 years) (Cianciaruso *et al.*, 1995). Some suggest that the extent of malnutrition is greater in patients during the early months of dialysis (Marckmann, 1988), while others indicate the opposite (Chazot *et al.*, 2001). However, the studies reviewed suggest that the frequency of malnutrition differs little according to the dialysis method (CAPD or haemodialysis) (Marckmann, 1988; Cianciaruso *et al.*, 1995; Jager *et al.*, 2001). In most studies, oedema-free weight has been measured (Marckmann, 1988; Cianciaruso *et al.*, 1995), recorded immediately after haemodialysis or without the dialysate in CAPD patients (Marckmann, 1988; Young *et al.*, 1991).

Micronutrient deficiencies (e.g. vitamin C, riboflavin, zinc, selenium, lycopene, β-carotene) and oxidative stress have also been found in patients with ESRD (Kelleher *et al.*, 1983; Ha *et al.*, 1996; Bonnefont-Rousselot *et al.*, 1997; Roob *et al.*, 1998; Salgueiro and Boccio, 2001), which may be due to the losses of these nutrients with dialysis or to limited food intake.

Some studies document loss of weight/deterioration of nutritional status in patients with renal disease undergoing dialysis (Marckmann, 1988; Herselman *et al.*, 2000), although this is not a consistent observation (Thunberg, 1981; Engel *et al.*, 1995; Herselman *et al.*, 2000; Jager *et al.*, 2001; see Appendix 1, Table A1.35). One study examined body composition, and indicated that improvements in BMI were due to a rise in fat mass with no change in lean tissue, particularly in patients receiving peritoneal dialysis (PD) (Jager *et al.*, 2001). Similar findings have been documented after kidney transplant (Ulivieri *et al.*, 2002), although others have shown an improvement in lean body mass over time in similar patients (Steiger *et al.*, 1995).

The possible causes and potential consequences of disease-related malnutrition in renal patients are summarized in Appendix 1 (Table A1.36).

Overall it seems pragmatic to recommend the use of nutritional support in this nutritionally vulnerable group to prevent or treat malnutrition in patients with chronic renal disease (Druml, 1993; Toigo *et al.*, 2000). However, there is limited information about the benefits of using nutritional support in patients with renal disease. Information about the impact of oral nutritional supplementation (ONS) and enteral tube feeding (ETF) in this patient group can be found in Chapters 6–8.

Surgery

Surgery is the branch of medicine that treats diseases, injuries and deformities by manual or operative methods. It can therefore be regarded as a form of treatment that cuts across many areas of medicine. Surgery may be minor or major, may last less than an hour up to many hours and may require from a few hours to a few days in hospital. In some cases, in particular if complications develop, days, weeks or even months in hospital may be required, sometimes in the ICU. The majority of surgical patients will not be at nutritional risk, particularly if surgery is minor. However, there are groups of surgical patients who, as a result of their disease process, the stress of the surgical insult and possible prolonged rehabilitation, may indeed be at great risk of malnutrition.

INCIDENCE AND PREVALENCE OF SURGERY

Table A1.37 in Appendix 1 shows the number of patients who underwent specific types of surgery in The Netherlands in 1992 (Statistics Netherlands, 1995). Assuming a population of approximately 15 million, this indicates that, in 1992, 4.5% of the Dutch population underwent some form of surgery. As indicated above, not all of these patients will be at nutritional risk, but subgroups of them will be, in particular those undergoing moderate to major GI surgery or lung volume reduction surgery, transplant patients and those undergoing surgery for malignancy or emergency repair of fractured neck of femur.

PREVALENCE OF MALNUTRITION IN SURGICAL PATIENTS

Malnutrition can be a significant problem in patients undergoing surgery (see Appendix 1, Table A1.38). Studies of mixed groups of hospital patients have suggested that up to 48% of patients admitted for a variety of surgical procedures are undernourished (Reilly *et al.*, 1988; McWhirter and Pennington, 1994; see section on mixed diagnoses, this chapter). Studies that have investigated the prevalence of malnutrition in specific groups of surgical patients (reviewed in this section) also suggest that a significant proportion of them are at risk of malnutrition (see Appendix 1, Tables A1.38 and A1.39).

Using a variety of different methods, including any degree of weight loss alone (Figs 2.4 and 2.5; see Appendix 1, Tables A1.38 and A1.39), estimates of the prevalence of malnutrition in groups of surgical patients include:

- up to 87% of general surgical patients;
- up to 82% of general surgical patients undergoing GI procedures;
- 11% in general gynaecology/urology surgery;
- up to 38% in benign GI or cardiovascular surgery;
- 18% in major vascular surgery;
- up to 78% in lung volume reduction surgery for COPD;
- up to 85% in patients on transplant waiting lists;
- up to 75% in surgery for malignancy (see also section on malignancy);
- up to 46% in lung cancer surgery;
- up to 67% in head and neck cancer surgery;
- 58% in oesophagogastrectomy;
- 62% in gastric cancer surgery;
- up to 33% in colorectal cancer;
- 72% in patients undergoing lower-leg amputation for ischaemia;
- up to 50% in patients undergoing emergency surgery for fractured neck of femur (see section on orthopaedics for more information on this type of surgery);
- up to 48% in patients undergoing a variety of orthopaedic surgical procedures (see section on orthopaedics).

The large variation in reported prevalence may partly be due to the different diagnoses of patients, whether they are admitted for elective or emergency surgery and the criteria that are used to define mal-

nutrition. Comparisons across studies and surgical groups are hindered by the use of different criteria to define malnutrition. They include:

- weight loss (self-report/comparison with usual body weight) (Hill *et al.*, 1977; Anderson *et al.*, 1984; Windsor and Hill, 1988; Senapati *et al.*, 1990; Aoun *et al.*, 1993; Dannhauser *et al.*, 1995a; Van Bokhorst-de van der Schueren *et al.*, 1997; Corish *et al.*, 1998; Bruun *et al.*, 1999; Martin *et al.*, 1999; Jagoe *et al.*, 2001b);
- comparison with IBW (Brown *et al.*, 1982; Bashir *et al.*, 1990; Senapati *et al.*, 1990; Aoun *et al.*, 1993; Dannhauser *et al.*, 1995a; Van Bokhorst-de van der Schueren *et al.*, 1997; Schwebel *et al.*, 2000; Jagoe *et al.*, 2001b; Nezu *et al.*, 2001);
- BMI < 20 kg m^{-2} (Jackson *et al.*, 1996; Harrison, 1997; Corish *et al.*, 1998; Bruun *et al.*, 1999; Schwebel *et al.*, 2000; Fettes *et al.*, 2001a,b; Jagoe *et al.*, 2001b; Madill *et al.*, 2001);
- BMI < 20 kg m^{-2} in combination with weight loss (Bruun *et al.*, 1999);
- use of anthropometric, biochemical and/or dietary parameters (Hill *et al.*, 1977; Brookes, 1982; Brown *et al.*, 1982; Symreng *et al.*, 1983; Warnold and Lundholm, 1984; Haydock and Hill, 1986; Meguid *et al.*, 1986; Bashir *et al.*, 1990; Pedersen and Pedersen, 1992; Aoun *et al.*, 1993; Shaw-Stiffel *et al.*, 1993; Larsson *et al.*, 1994a; Madden *et al.*, 1994; Dannhauser *et al.*, 1995a; Jackson *et al.*, 1996; Harrison, 1997; Harrison *et al.*, 1997);
- SGA (Detsky *et al.*, 1987; Hasse *et al.*, 1993; McLeod *et al.*, 1995; Ulander *et al.*, 1998; Stephenson *et al.*, 2001);
- nutrition index (Van Bokhorst-de van der Schueren *et al.*, 1997);
- prognostic nutritional index (Buzby *et al.*, 1980);
- nutrition risk index (Rey-Ferro *et al.*, 1997; Corish *et al.*, 1998).

In two of the reviewed studies the same criteria were used in different surgical groups. Using BMI < 20 kg m^{-2} in combination with $> 5\%$ weight loss in 3 months, Bruun et al. (1999) found the prevalence of malnutrition to be greater in GI surgical patients (43%) than in orthopaedic surgical patients (27%). Using several parameters of nutritional status, Warnold and Lundholm (1984) reported a prevalence of malnutrition of 18% in major vascular surgery, 4% in minor vascular surgery and 13% in abdominal surgery.

Weight loss of at least some degree in the months prior to surgery has been commonly identified in a variety of patient groups (see Appendix 1, Table A1.39). More specifically, weight loss of $> 10\%$ usual body weight has been reported in up to 58% of general GI surgical patients (Windsor and Hill, 1988; Bruun et al., 1999), 11% in gynaecological and urological surgery (Anderson et al., 1984), 21% in benign GI and cardiovascular surgery (Dannhauser et al., 1995a), 37% in a variety of malignancies (Corish et al., 1998), 31% in advanced head and neck cancer (Van Bokhorst-de van der Schueren et al., 1997) and 5% in lung cancer (Jagoe et al., 2001b). Using a BMI < 20 kg m^{-2} as a cut-off, percentages of patients range between 0% (prior to liver transplant) to 49% (prior to lung transplant) (Fig. 2.2; see Appendix 1, Tables A1.38 and A1.39).

Notably, during hospitalization, weight loss and deterioration in the nutritional status of surgical patients also occurs (Corish et al., 1998; Ulander et al., 1998; Bruun et al., 1999; Martin et al., 1999; Fettes et al., 2001a,b; Fig. 2.6; see Appendix 1, Table A1.39). A survey of orthopaedic and GI surgical patients indicated that 83% lost weight and 33% lost more than 5% of their admission weight (Bruun et al., 1999). Similarly, 39% of a group of colorectal patients lost $\geq 5\%$ weight during their hospital stay (Ulander et al., 1998). Furthermore, the average weight loss 10 days postoperatively in a group of GI surgical patients was found to be almost 5% (Christensen and Kehlet, 1984). However, few studies note the potential confounding effects of changes in oedema (Bruun et al., 1999).

Few studies have examined the longer-term effects of surgery on nutritional status post-discharge, but, in those that have, long-lasting detriments are indicated. Corish et al. (1998) reported that, in the 3 months following discharge, 70% lost weight. Others have also shown that poor nutritional status may persist for a considerable period after surgery (Beattie et al., 2000). One study examined nutritional status within 6 weeks after major surgery (nutritional status prior to surgery was not reported) (Edington et al., 1997). Using BMI indices in combination with anthropometry, this study demonstrated that 8.1% were mildly malnourished and 2.4% were severely malnourished. In contrast, patients following liver transplant tend to gain weight (Müller et al., 1994; Richardson et al., 2001). Possible reasons for this are discussed in the section on GI and liver disease (this chapter).

The possible causes and potential consequences of disease-related malnutrition in surgical patients are summarized in Appendix 1 (Table A1.40).

Critical illness

Patients admitted to ICU include those who have suffered accidental injury or trauma, medical patients with overdoses or severe exacerbations of a disease (e.g. acute exacerbations of COPD may require mechanical ventilation during a period of respiratory failure) and surgical patients with complications (e.g. severe sepsis). Specialist ICUs are available in some centres that cater for specific groups of patients, such as burns and head injury. A typical overview of patients seen on the general ICU is shown in Table A1.41 in Appendix 1. These data were obtained from a survey on 1 day in 1992 in England and Wales of 256 general ICUs and cardiac units, of which 170 responded, representing 659 patients (Hill et al., 1995). Patients on the ICU as a result of major surgical stress, severe medical problems or trauma, are at high risk of poor oral intake and nutritional depletion, the rate of which will be enhanced by the severity of their metabolic stress. Many of these patients will also be at risk of developing sepsis or systemic inflammation, which can in turn lead to multiple organ dysfunction syndrome (MODS). These patients consume a disproportionate amount of hospital resources and still have a high mortality. Sequential organ system failure was first described in 1973 (Livingston and Deitch, 1995). Despite advances in therapeutic interventions, mortality has remained high. In a prospective study of 60 ICUs at 53 hospitals in the USA (17,440 ICU admissions between 1988 and 1990, and 5677 between 1979 and 1982), the incidence of organ system failure was similar (48% and 44%, respectively) and an identical proportion (14%) developed MODS (Zimmerman *et al.*, 1996). Mortality from MODS has remained very stable over the last 20 years at around 75%, rising to 85–100% once three or more organs have failed (Livingston and Deitch, 1995).

Some patients may remain on the ICU only for a brief period, e.g. routine overnight stay following major surgery, while others may remain on the unit for days, weeks and occasionally even months. A 10-year survey of nutritional support on a surgical ICU from 1986 to 1995 in Switzerland (Berger *et al.*, 1997) indicated that almost 50% of patients stay 24–48 h, 28% stay 48–72 h and 30% require more than 3 days of ICU treatment. A smaller prospective survey, which focused on patients requiring more than 3 days of ICU stay in 1994 on the same unit (*n* 171) described a mean length of stay of 7.8 days (range 4–28 days) (Berger *et al.*, 1997). In a Spanish survey in one hospital over a 15-month period, 152 of 198 patients stayed longer than 3 days (median 16 days; range 4–144) (Grau Carmona *et al.*, 1996). As critical care technology advances, allowing more critically ill patients to be kept alive for longer periods of time, the desire to speed recovery and prevent progression of critical illness to MODS is becoming more urgent. It is not yet clear whether nutritional support can help to prevent this progression, either by minimizing losses to physiological reserves or by providing nutrients that may have a specific pharmacological effect (e.g. modulation of inflammation and immune function), but it is not unlikely that appropriate nutritional support, particularly via the enteral route, can make a contribution.

Patients suffering from critical illness are at high risk of malnutrition as a result of ongoing severe inflammatory and catabolic processes and as a result of inadequate nutritional intake, particularly when patients are cardiovascularly unstable and may have severe fluid overload. Few studies have reported the prevalence of malnutrition in intensive care patients, presumably partly because of the difficulties in making relevant measurements in this difficult population (see Appendix 1, Tables A1.42 and A1.43). Galanos *et al.* (1997) reported that 59% of a large cohort of seriously ill patients (43% who required intensive care) had lost weight prior to admission. Only three studies were found where estimates of the prevalence of malnutrition in patients on ICUs were attempted. A combination of anthropometric and biochemical parameters were used in two studies: the Maastricht index (Huang *et al.*, 2000) or low albumin and per cent IBW < 100% (Giner *et al.*, 1996). Furthermore, both studies included a range of patients with differing diagnoses. The reported rates of malnutrition were 43% (*n* 129) (Giner *et al.*, 1996) and 100% (*n* 49) (Huang *et al.*, 2000). No records were made of the confounding effects of changes in fluid balance on body composition in these studies. One study (Ravasco *et al.*, 2002) used a variety of different anthropometric criteria to assess nutritional status in medical ICU patients requiring mechanical ventilation. They showed that oedema significantly increased per cent IBW and BMI, leading to overestimates of the proportion of well-nourished/overweight patients. Of the methods tried, mid-arm circumference was simple and feasible and appeared to have prognostic value.

It has been suggested that poor nutritional status in ICU patients may compromise gut barrier function, prolong ventilator dependency and increase morbidity and mortality (Huang, 2001). It is clear from the above studies that patients who are undernourished do less well than those who are 'well nourished'. In particular, it was found that patients who were defined as 'undernourished' or at risk of malnutrition stayed in ICU longer (Huang *et al.*, 2000), had longer hospital stays (not significant (NS)) (Giner *et al.*, 1996), had a significantly higher incidence of complications (Giner *et al.*, 1996; Ravasco *et al.*, 2002) and had a higher mortality (Galanos *et al.*, 1997; Ravasco *et al.*, 2002). Furthermore, the number of patients not discharged from hospital was significantly greater among the undernourished than among the well nourished. Although it is difficult to separate out the effect of malnutrition from the role of disease severity, Giner *et al.* (1996) indicated that undernourished patients had a worse clinical outcome than those who were well nourished with greater illness severity.

There is also a paucity of information regarding what happens to nutritional status in survivors of critical illness after discharge from the ICU (see Appendix 1, Tables A1.38, A1.42 and A1.43). Two studies were found which reported measurements of nutritional status during rehabilitation following brain injury (French and Merriman, 1999; Thomson *et al.*, 2001; see Table A1.43). In Thomson *et al.*'s study (2001), patients entered rehabilitation a median of 29 days after initial injury. All had lost a significant amount of weight and, using BMI and anthropometric indices, 56% had evidence of at least mild malnutrition. Nutritional status improved in many of these patients over the course of rehabilitation with appropriate application of nutritional support. In contrast, patients surveyed several years after brain injury were reasonably well nourished, although there was some evidence of muscle depletion in 26% (French and Merriman, 1999). This suggests that, perhaps over a considerable time period, head-injured patients may be able to recover nutritional status to a good degree with appropriate nutritional intervention.

Children

Variation in prevalence of malnutrition in children according to the assessment criteria used

The criteria used to define malnutrition in children are more complex than for adults, as growth needs to be considered. A number of different indices and screening tools are currently used. Although fewer methods are used than in adults, differences in expressing the data and in the percentiles used still make cross-comparisons between studies difficult (Tables 2.12 and 2.13). At present, there is little agreement about the best methods to assess malnutrition in children (Elia, 2000b). Nevertheless, it seems that disease-related malnutrition is a considerable problem in paediatrics (see Appendix 1, Table A1.44). The importance of screening for malnutrition in children is substantial, considering the potential for impaired physical and mental/intellectual development (see Chapter 4).

As the nutritional status of a child clearly affects growth, anthropometric indices are normally used for assessment of paediatric patients. Acute malnutrition (or wasting) is most commonly assessed by measuring weight-for-height. The degree of wasting can thus be graded by comparing actual weight with the 50th percentile of weight-for-current-height (or -length). Weight-for-age and BMI-for-age may also be used for this purpose. Height-for-age indicates chronic malnutrition, or stunting. Similarly, stunting can be graded by comparing the actual height with the 50th percentile of height for current age. The equations for these calculations are given in Appendix 1. Various grading systems have been used, one of the best known of which is the Waterlow classification (Waterlow, 1972). This is also summarized in Appendix 1. Children may thus be classified as normal, stunted (i.e. height deficit for age), wasted (i.e. weight deficit for height) or both. Other classifications to indicate acute malnutrition (wasting) include a weight-for-height (or

Table 2.12. Criteria for establishing the prevalence of malnutrition (wasting) in children.

Category	Cut-off points used	References
Weight-for-height (%)	< 95	Kurugöl *et al.*, 1997
	90–95	
	85–90	
	< 85	
	< 90	Almeida Santos *et al.*, 1998; Westwood and Saitowitz, 1999; Viola *et al.*, 2000; Wiedemann *et al.*, 2001
	< 90	Hendricks *et al.*, 1995
	81–90 mild	
	70–80 moderate	
	< 70 severe	
	< 90	Cameron *et al.*, 1995
	80–89 mild	
	70–79 moderate	
	< 70 severe	
	< 90	Pollack *et al.*, 1981
	80–90	
	70–79	
	< 70	
	70–89 at risk	Briassoulis and Hatzis, 2001
	< 70 severe	
	< 80	Smith *et al.*, 1990, 1991; Pons Leite *et al.*, 1993; Hendrikse *et al.*, 1997; Pietsch and Ford, 2000
	80–90 (Waterlow criteria)	McCarthy and McIvor, 2001
	< 80 (Waterlow criteria)	
	80–90 (after Hendrikse)	McCarthy and McIvor, 2001
	< 80 (after Hendrikse)	
	−1.0 to −2.0 SDS	Moy *et al.*, 1990
	−2.0 SDS	
	< −2.0 SDS	McNaughton *et al.*, 2000
	z score < −1	Pietsch and Ford, 2000
	z score < −2	
	< 50th percentile	Pietsch and Ford, 2000
	< 20th percentile	
Weight-for-age (%)	< 90	Almeida Santos *et al.*, 1998
	< 85	Sermet-Gaudelus *et al.*, 2000
	80–84 mild	
	75–79 moderate	
	< 75% severe	
	−1.0 to −2.0 SDS	Hendrikse *et al.*, 1997
	−1.0 to −2.0 SDS	McCarthy and McIvor, 2001
	−2.0 SDS	
	< −2.0 SDS	Dahl and Gebre-Medhin, 1993; McNaughton *et al.*, 2000; Pereira *et al.*, 2000
	< 5th percentile	Stallings *et al.*, 1993; Hendrikse *et al.*, 1997; Lai *et al.*, 1998
	< 3rd percentile	Venugopalan *et al.*, 2001
Weight-for-age (%) and anthropometry and/or energy intake	W/A < 2.5th percentile	Thommessen *et al.*, 1991
	TSF < 5th percentile	
	EI < 70% RDA	
BMI-for-age (%)	80–90	McCarthy and McIvor, 2001
	< 80	
BMI	< −2.0 SDS	Reilly *et al.*, 1999; Hankard *et al.*, 2001
	z score < −1	Pietsch and Ford, 2000
	z score < −2	
	< 16	Pietsch and Ford, 2000

Table 2.12. *continued*

Category	Cut-off points used	References
Ideal body weight (%)	85–95 < 85	Deeg *et al.*, 1995
Mid-arm circumference	< 5th percentile	Smith *et al.*, 1990, 1991
Triceps skin-fold	< –2.0 SDS	Smith *et al.*, 1990, 1991
thickness	< 5th percentile	Stallings *et al.*, 1993
Mid-arm muscle circumference-for-age	< –1.65 SDS	Pereira *et al.*, 2000
Parent's view	–	Sullivan *et al.*, 2000

EI, energy intake; SDS, standard deviation score; TSF, triceps skin-fold thickness; W/A, weight-for-age; RDA, recommended daily allowance.

Table 2.13. Criteria for establishing the prevalence of malnutrition (stunting) in children.

Category	Cut-off points used	References
Height (or length)-for-age (%)	< 95 90–95 mild 85–89 moderate < 85 severe	Pollack *et al.*, 1981; Hendricks *et al.*, 1995
	< 95 91–94 mild 86–90 moderate < 86 severe	Cameron *et al.*, 1995
	85–95 at risk < 85 severe	Briassoulis and Hatzis, 2001
	< 90	Pons Leite *et al.*, 1993; Almeida Santos *et al.*, 1998
	< 5th percentile	Hendrikse *et al.*, 1997; Lai *et al.*, 1998; Westwood and Saitowitz, 1999
	< 3rd percentile	Venugopalan *et al.*, 2001
	< 2.5th percentile	Thommessen *et al.*, 1991; Dahl *et al.*, 1997
	–1.0 to –2.0 SDS	Hendrikse *et al.*, 1997
	–1.0 to –2.0 SDS –2.0 SDS	Moy *et al.*, 1990
	< –2.0 SDS	Smith *et al.*, 1990, 1991; Dahl and Gebre-Medhin, 1993; McNaughton *et al.*, 2000; Pereira *et al.*, 2000
Upper-arm length-for-age	< 5th percentile	Stallings *et al.*, 1993
Lower-leg length	< 2.5th percentile	Dahl *et al.*, 1997
Bone age delay	> 1 year	Kong *et al.*, 1999

SDS, standard deviation score.

weight-for-age) below the 5th percentile or at least 2 standard deviations (SD) below the mean (referred to as the standard deviation score (SDS)). Weight-for-height between the 5th and 10th percentiles or between 1 and 2 SD is often regarded as indicating a risk of malnutrition requiring further assessment. Similarly, height-for-age below the 5th percentile or at least 2 SD below the mean is often used to indicate the presence of severe malnutrition, while values between the 5th and 10th percentile, or between 1 and 2 SD below the mean, may indicate risk of chronic malnutrition. Combinations of indices of wasting and stunting may be used to determine the presence of both types of malnutrition in children.

Prevalence of disease-related malnutrition in children with different conditions

MIXED DIAGNOSES

From the studies reviewed, the reported prevalence of acute malnutrition (wasting) in infants and children with mixed diagnoses admitted to hospital ranges from 8 to 33%, the reported rate of stunting ranges from 15 to 38% and the prevalence of stunting and wasting in one study was shown to be 16% (Figs 2.3 and 2.7 and Table 2.14; see Appendix 1, Table A1.44). The prevalence rates of different types of malnutrition will depend on the criteria that were used to assess malnutrition, the diagnoses and the age of patients (infants or children). For example, in infants under 2 years, the prevalence of malnutrition appears to be greater than in children aged 2–18 years using the same criteria (Hendricks *et al.*, 1995). Others have also reported a greater prevalence of malnutrition in the youngest age groups in a variety of patient groups (Pollack *et al.*, 1981; Cameron *et al.*, 1995; Lai *et al.*, 1998). Furthermore, as children who are too sick or immobile are often excluded from such studies (Hendrikse *et al.*, 1997), the true prevalence of malnutrition in children with disease may well be underestimated.

Using a common indicator of < 90% weight-for-height, the reported prevalence of malnutrition in children with a variety of diseases ranges from 13% to 26% (Hendricks *et al.*, 1995; McCarthy and McIvor, 2001). Using < 95% height-for-age as an indicator of stunting, one study reported a prevalence of 27% (Hendricks *et al.*, 1995; Fig. 2.3). Although there is little information about changes in children's nutritional status over time, a recent French study in 296 children admitted to hospital has found that ~65% lose weight, with 45% losing > 2% of their admission weight (Sermet-Gaudelus *et al.*, 2000). This study has also highlighted that there is a risk of nutritional deterioration for all children during their stay in hospital, not just those who are undernourished.

The studies described above assessed the extent of malnutrition in consecutive admissions to hospital or visits to a clinic and do not provide information about the extent of malnutrition in diagnostic subgroups. High-risk groups include children with diseases of the GI tract (IBD, coeliac disease), cardiac problems, chronic lung disease including cystic fibrosis, critical illness, cancer, cerebral palsy, HIV infection and AIDS and renal disease. Some examples of studies are given in Table 2.14 and in Appendix 1 (Table A1.44) and some additional information is given below.

CARDIAC DISEASE

In children, most heart disease is congenital, and it represents the most common group of structural malformations in infants. It has been estimated that significant malformations occur in 6–8 per 1000 live-born infants, while some abnormalities are present in greater frequency (e.g. a bicuspid aortic valve in 10–20 per 1000 live births (Lissauer and Clayden, 1999)).

In studies of patients with a variety of diagnoses, Moy *et al.* (1990) indicated that 42% of cardiac patients were severely wasted (weight-for-height < 2 SDS). Similarly, in the USA, 46% of children undergoing cardiac surgery were diagnosed as being severely undernourished (weight-for-age or height-for-age < 5th percentile, weight-for-height < 70% of median or height-for-age < 85% of median) (Hendricks *et al.*, 1995). In a group of paediatric patients admitted specifically for cardiac problems in the USA, 33% were acutely undernourished (low weight-for-height, wasted) and 64% were chronically undernourished (low height-for-age, stunted) (Cameron *et al.*, 1995). In particular, infants and children with cardiomyopathy, congenital heart disease, left-to-right intracardiac shunts and complex heart disease have been indicated as being at high risk of acute or chronic malnutrition (Cameron *et al.*, 1995). In Oman, 27% of children with congenital heart defects were wasted (weight-for-age < 3rd percentile) and 24% were stunted (weight-for-age and height-for-age < 3rd percentile), with prevalence increasing with increasing symptoms (Venugopalan *et al.*, 2001; Figs 2.3 and 2.7 and Table 2.14).

Table 2.14. Prevalence of wasting and stunting in paediatric patients using a variety of criteria.

Location	Number of subjects	Prevalence of wasting (%)[a]	W/H < 90% (%)	Prevalence of stunting (%)[a]	H/A < 95% (%)	Prevalence of stunting and wasting (%)[a]	References
General hospital admissions/mixed diagnoses							
France	52	12	–	–	–	–	Hankard et al., 2001
France	296	26	–	–	–	–	Sermet-Gaudelus et al., 2000
UK	226	8 16	–	15	–	16	Hendrikse et al., 1997
UK	31	13 16 23 26	13 26	–	–	–	McCarthy and McIvor, 2001
UK	255	33	–	38	–	–	Moy et al., 1990
USA	268	24.5	24.5	27.3	27.3	–	Hendricks et al., 1995
Cardiology							
Oman	152	27	–	–	–	24	Venugopalan et al., 2001
USA	160	33	33	64	64	6	Cameron et al., 1995
Cerebral palsy							
Hong Kong	62	–	–	68	–	–	Kong et al., 1999
Norway	42	15	–	48	–	–	Thommessen et al., 1991
Sweden	44	38	–	30	–	–	Dahl and Gebre-Medhin, 1993
Sweden	35	49	–	43	–	–	Dahl et al., 1997
UK	271	38	–	–	–	–	Sullivan et al., 2000
USA	154	30	–	23	–	–	Stallings et al., 1993
Chronic lung disease							
France	50	28	28	–	–	–	Viola et al., 2000
Cystic fibrosis							
Australia	226	7.5 (M) / 1.7 (F) 6.8 (M) / 8.3 (F)	–	7.7 (M) / 7.3 (F)	–	–	McNaughton et al., 2000
Germany	2,325	26.8	26.8	–	–	–	Wiedemann et al., 2001
South Africa	38	14.3 (< 10 years) 47 (> 10 years)	14.3 (< 10 years) 47 (> 10 years)	16	–	–	Westwood and Saitowitz, 1999

Country	Number						Reference
USA	13,116	10.9 (0–1 years) / 3.8 (1–10 years) / 9 (11–18 years)	–	8.3 (0–1 years) / 9.6 (1–10 years) / 8 (11–18 years)	–	27.3 (0–1 years) / 8.5 (1–10 years) / 17 (11–18 years)	Lai *et al.*, 1998
Intensive care							
Brazil	46	17	–	22	–	26	Pons Leite *et al.*, 1993
Greece	71	27	27	23	23	–	Briassoulis and Hatzis, 2001
The Netherlands	51	16 / 29	–	0 / 23	–	–	Hulst *et al.*, 2001
Spain	65	60 / 63	60	13	–	–	Almeida Santos *et al.*, 1998
USA	50	40	40	22	22	–	Pollack *et al.*, 1981
Malignancy							
Turkey	45	51.1	40	–	–	–	Kurugöl *et al.*, 1997
Turkey	47	19.2	–	2.1	–	8.5	Yariş *et al.*, 2002
UK	1,019	8 (M) / 7 (F)	–	–	–	–	Reilly *et al.*, 1999
UK	48	2 / 30	–	–	–	–	Smith *et al.*, 1990
UK	100	20 / 23	–	–	–	–	Smith *et al.*, 1991
USA	576	16	–	–	–	–	Deeg *et al.*, 1995
USA	127	1–47	–	–	–	–	Pietsch and Ford, 2000
Renal disease							
Brazil	30	43 / 53	~50	63	–	–	Pereira *et al.*, 2000

aWhen more than one result is provided for a given study (unless specifically explained) the results have been obtained by applying different criteria to the same group of patients. For more details, refer to Appendix 1.
W/H, weight-for-height; H/A, height-for-age.

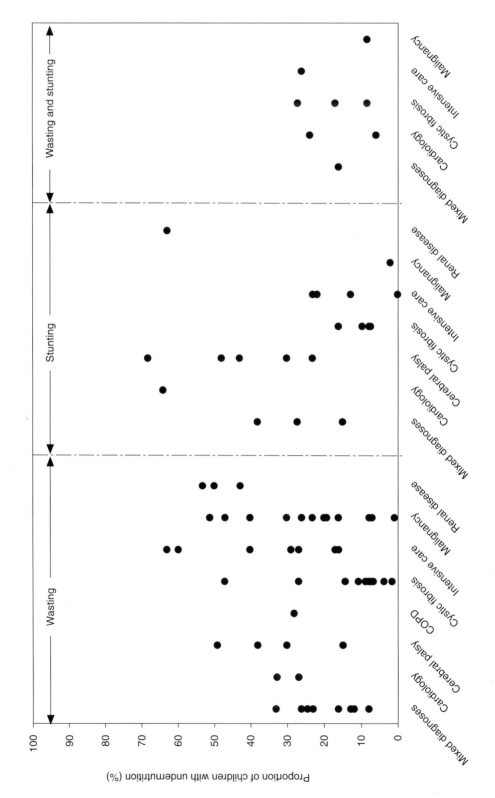

Fig. 2.7. Prevalence of wasting, stunting, and both wasting and stunting in paediatric patients in the hospital and community using a variety of assessment methods.

CEREBRAL PALSY

Cerebral palsy is defined as a disorder of movement and posture due to a non-progressive lesion of the motor pathways in the developing brain (Lissauer and Clayden, 1999). The term includes a variety of non-degenerating neurological disabilities caused by abnormal central nervous system (CNS) development or injuries in the prenatal and perinatal period (Behrman and Kliegman, 1998). Often the aetiology is unknown. The reported incidence is between 2 and 7 per 1000 live-births, with a prevalence of about 500 per 100,000 of population (Behrman and Kliegman, 1998; Lissauer and Clayden, 1999). Cerebral palsy is the most common cause of motor impairment in children. Oromotor dysfunction is typical – it leads to feeding difficulties in up to 90% of patients (Thommessen *et al.*, 1991; Dahl and Gebre-Medhin, 1993; Reilly *et al.*, 1996; Dahl *et al.*, 1997; Sullivan *et al.*, 2000; Fung *et al.*, 2002). Other GI tract dysfunction as a result of damage to the developing CNS, such as gastro-oesophageal reflux, delayed gastric emptying and constipation, may also contribute to feeding difficulties (Sullivan *et al.*, 2000).

Poor nutritional status and growth are often seen in children with cerebral palsy (Fig. 2.7; Thommessen *et al.*, 1991; Dahl and Gebre-Medhin, 1993; Stallings *et al.*, 1993; Dahl *et al.*, 1997; Kong *et al.*, 1999; Sullivan *et al.*, 2000); these are associated with the degree of feeding dysfunction (Krick and Van Duyn, 1984; Fung *et al.*, 2002). Furthermore, children with cerebral palsy frequently have large decrements in FFM accretion (Stallings *et al.*, 1995) and bone mineral density (Shaw *et al.*, 1994; Henderson and Saavedra, 1995). Poor micronutrient status is probably also common (Ramage *et al.*, 1997). As Table 2.14 and Appendix 1 (Table A1.44) show, the prevalence of wasting (15–49%) and stunting (23–68%) in children with cerebral palsy is high.

CHRONIC LUNG DISEASE

Chronic pulmonary insufficiency can lead to growth failure and delayed develop-ment in children. The most common lung diseases in children are cystic fibrosis, bronchopulmonary dysplasia, asthma and congenital lung malformations (Abrams, 2001). More details on cystic fibrosis are given below. One trial in children with chronic lung disease indicated that 28% had a weight-for-height < 90% (Viola *et al.*, 2000; Table 2.14; see Appendix 1, Table A1.44).

CYSTIC FIBROSIS

Cystic fibrosis is the most common lethal genetic disorder in Caucasian populations. It is an inherited, autosomal-recessive disease of exocrine gland secretion, characterized by chronic pulmonary disease and recurrent chest infections, pancreatic enzyme deficiency, resulting in maldigestion and malabsorption, and abnormally high concentrations of electrolytes in sweat (Richardson *et al.*, 2000; Thomas, 2001). Longer-term consequences may include liver disease, diabetes, pancreatitis, impaired fertility and bone and joint disorders (Thomas, 2001). The incidence of cystic fibrosis in Caucasians is approximately 1 in 2000–2500 live-births (Corey *et al.*, 1988; Thomas, 2001). Four per cent of the population are carriers of the cystic fibrosis gene. The incidence of cystic fibrosis in non-Caucasians is much lower; approximately 1 in 20,000 in black populations and 1 in 100,000 in Oriental populations (Corey *et al.*, 1988). Symptoms usually become apparent in infancy, but may not be detected until later in life. Cystic fibrosis tends to be thought of as a childhood disease, particularly as, in the past, survival time was limited to a few years. However, in recent decades, life expectancy has improved tremendously, and currently life expectancy at diagnosis is approximately 40 years and continuing to rise (Richardson *et al.*, 2000; Thomas, 2001). Enhanced survival is a consequence of improved detection and treatment, including improved antibiotics, pancreatic enzymes, physiotherapy and dietary man-agement (Richardson *et al.*, 2000).

In studies of mixed groups of patients, a significant proportion (42%) of hospitalized children with cystic fibrosis have been diagnosed as being severely undernourished (weight-for-age or height-for-age < 5th percentile) (Hendricks et al., 1995) (see Figs 2.3 and 2.7, Table 2.14 and Appendix 1, Table A1.44, for a summary of the results from trials in children with cystic fibrosis). Children with cystic fibrosis spend most of their life outside the hospital setting, and therefore it is relevant to examine studies performed in the community. Children with cystic fibrosis are often reported to be shorter and lighter than non-cystic fibrosis counterparts (Stapleton et al., 2001). In the UK, the mean weight and height of children with cystic fibrosis (survey of 3056 outpatients) have been reported to be 0.5 SD below the norm in the first 10 years of life (Morison et al., 1997). Stature and weight maintenance in children post-puberty are also deficient (Morison et al., 1997). In the USA, it has been highlighted that 73% of cystic fibrosis patients are < 50th percentile for height, 20% are < 5th percentile for height and 24% are < 5th percentile for weight (Anthony et al., 1999). Age differences in stunting and/or wasting have been shown in a very large study in the USA (n 13,116), demonstrating that children less than 1 year and greater than 10 years appear to be at more risk of wasting, with or without stunting, than children aged 1–10 years (Lai et al., 1998). Similar findings for children above and below 10 years of age were demonstrated in a much smaller (n 38) South African study (Westwood and Saitowitz, 1999), although age-related findings were less obvious in a large German study (Wiedemann et al., 2001).

Body composition may also be adversely affected in cystic fibrosis. A recent study of cystic fibrosis out-patients from Australia, using total body potassium as an indicator of body cell mass (BCM), has suggested that 30% of boys and 22% of girls are < 80% of predicted BCM for age (McNaughton et al., 2000; Table 2.14; see Appendix 1, Table A1.44).

Similar findings of a pronounced deficit of muscle using anthropometry have also been demonstrated in children with cystic fibrosis aged 6–11 years (Stapleton et al., 2001). A longitudinal study over 3 years comparing changes in growth, body composition and nutritional status in 25 children aged 5–10 years with cystic fibrosis and 26 healthy controls showed that the growth of boys with cystic fibrosis was impaired on the basis of height, FFM and fat mass, despite comprehensive care (Stettler et al., 2000). The authors cautioned that cross-sectional measurements may not detect suboptimal growth. In this study, the pattern of change in growth was less striking for girls than for boys. However, in a larger 4-year longitudinal survey (968 patients aged 5–8 years, of whom 507 were boys) by the same group, it was the girls who appeared to do less well in terms of z scores for height and weight (Zemel et al., 2000). Others also suggest that girls appear to do less well than boys (Stapleton et al., 2001).

One recent study has examined the nutritional status of adults with cystic fibrosis (n 43, age range 19–43 years for 19 women and 19–45 years for 24 men) (Richardson et al., 2000). Compared with a similar survey in 1983 also cited in this paper, the prevalence of malnutrition (BMI < 20 kg m^{-2}) had decreased from 62% to 9%. Significant improvements were seen in both men and women in terms of weight, height, BMI, mid-arm circumference, triceps skin-fold thickness and percentage body fat. Growth arrest appeared to have been eliminated, as mean height was comparable to the Australian average. Multiple linear regression analysis indicated that nutritional management was the main factor explaining the improvements in nutritional status.

HIV INFECTION AND AIDS

Paediatric HIV infection is the leading cause of death in children worldwide, with Africa and Asia accounting for the majority of cases (Miller, 2000). In late 1994, the WHO estimated that about 1.5 million children had been infected worldwide; this was predicted to increase to between 5 and 10 million by the year 2000 (Scarlatti, 1996). In 2000, 600,000 children were newly infected with HIV, of whom over 90% were in sub-Saharan Africa (Saloojee and Violari, 2001). Actual figures for children less than 15 years of age living with HIV/AIDS at the end of 2000 were estimated to be 1.4 million (Adler, 2001). Vertical transmission of HIV infection from mother to child is the most common route of paediatric HIV infection (Newell and Peckham, 1994; Saloojee and Violari, 2001). Transmission of the infection can occur during pregnancy, in the intrapartum period or postnatally, through breast-feeding (Leroy *et al.*, 1998). Nearly half of all HIV-infected adults are women of childbearing age (Scarlatti, 1996). The rate of transmission from mother to child has been estimated from epidemiological surveys to be between 7 and 42% (Newell and Peckham, 1994; Scarlatti, 1996). In the early 1990s, transmission rates in Europe were estimated to be between 15 and 20% (Newell and Peckham, 1994), with rates of almost double this in Africa (Newell and Peckham, 1994; Scarlatti, 1996). The incidence of perinatally acquired HIV infection in developed countries is now decreasing (estimated now to be in the region of 6–7% (Miller, 2000)), due to improved prenatal screening and treatment during pregnancy. Nevertheless, substantial numbers of cases have been reported in the USA (9000) and Europe (over 7000) (cited in Miller, 2000). Paediatric HIV infection remains the fourth to seventh leading cause of death of children aged 1–4 years in the USA (Miller, 2000).

In developing countries, babies born to HIV-infected mothers often have lower birth weights than those born to non-infected mothers (Henderson and Saavedra, 1995; Dreyfuss *et al.*, 2001). In developed countries, other factors, such as intravenous drug use, appear to be more predictive of birth weight than HIV status of the mother (Henderson and Saavedra, 1995; Miller *et al.*, 2001b). A study in Uganda showed no difference in birth

weight and length between HIV-positive and control babies. However, mean weight-for-age and length-for-age curves were significantly lower from birth to 25 months in infants with HIV infection (*n* 84) compared with HIV-negative children (*n* 251) born to HIV-positive mothers ('seroreverters') and control infants (*n* 124) without HIV infection born to HIV-negative mothers, demonstrating that HIV infection is associated with early and progressive decrements in weight and length. Similarly, in the USA, HIV-infected babies (*n* 18) had comparable weight and length to those of non-infected babies (*n* 29) born to HIV-positive mothers, but, over the first 6 months of life, linear growth was consistently less than that of uninfected infants (Pollack *et al.*, 1997). The adverse effect on growth may be correlated with viral load (Pollack *et al.*, 1997; Miller *et al.*, 2001b). In another study in the USA, HIV-infected infants (*n* 59) were lighter and shorter at birth than non-infected infants (*n* 223) born to HIV-positive mothers, an effect that was sustained until 18 months of age (Moye *et al.*, 1998). A decrement in head circumference was also sustained over this period. After adjustment for covariates, HIV infection was associated with significant decrements in mean *z* scores for weight, length, weight-for-length and head circumference. Weight and height standards are frequently not met in older children as well (Miller *et al.*, 1997, 2001b).

Other authors in the USA have shown that catch-up growth is limited in HIV-infected infants. Although mean birth weights were below the 50th percentile in HIV-infected (*n* 59) and non-infected (*n* 50) infants born to HIV-positive mothers, weight gain was significantly better in the non-infected group by 36 months (Saavedra *et al.*, 1995). Linear growth diverged earlier than weight, with significant differences already evident by 15 months. This may have long-lasting consequences; in a cohort of boys aged 6–19 years with haemophilia, those with HIV infection (*n* 207) had significantly impaired linear growth compared with those without HIV infection (*n* 126) (Gertner *et al.*, 1994).

Body composition changes may also be evident in older children with HIV infection, even in the absence of growth failure. In children aged 4–11 years, those with HIV infection and growth failure (n 18) had reduced FFM and BCM compared with HIV-infected children with normal growth (n 16) and healthy controls (n 52) (Arpadi et al., 1998). In contrast, the fat compartment was normal. Boys infected with HIV with normal growth also had reduced FFM, but girls did not, suggesting that there may be gender differences. Others have also described triceps skinfold and mid-arm muscle circumference measures that are significantly below standards for healthy children (Miller et al., 1997). Cardiac mass may also be impaired (Miller et al., 1997).

Other nutritional deficiencies may be common in HIV disease. For example, 48% of children (n 71) with symptomatic HIV infection have been reported to be deficient in iron, largely due to intestinal iron malabsorption (Castaldo et al., 1996).

The prevalence of malnutrition in paediatric HIV infection may thus be considerable, although this will vary between centres and countries, depending on availability of health-care services. Few studies have attempted to identify absolute figures for prevalence of malnutrition, but it has been estimated that 30–50% of children following HIV programmes in the USA have evidence of protein-energy malnutrition (Miller, 2000). As in adult HIV disease, however, the availability of HAART has had a significant impact on malnutrition in children (Miller, 2002). In an uncontrolled study of children with HIV infection aged between 0.4 and 16.3 years (n 24), HAART had a positive influence on growth, an effect that was sustained for at least 96 weeks (Verweel et al., 2002).

CONDITIONS REQUIRING INTENSIVE CARE

Patients admitted to paediatric ICUs constitute a high-risk group for developing acute malnutrition. Depending on the reasons for admission, acute and/or chronic malnutrition may already be present and, if treatment is prolonged, chronic malnutrition may develop. The studies reviewed demonstrated acute malnutrition in up to 63%, chronic malnutrition in up to 23% and both stunting and wasting in 26% of paediatric patients admitted to intensive care (Table 2.14 and Figs 2.3 and 2.7; see Appendix 1, Table A1.44). None of these studies followed up measures of admission nutritional status over the course of ICU stay or after discharge.

MALIGNANCY

Malignancy in childhood is relatively rare. Approximately 8000 new cases occur in the USA each year, which represents less than 1% of the total incidence of malignancy (Abelson, 1998). About 1400 new cases occur each year in the UK (Lissauer and Clayden, 1999). It has been estimated that one child in 650 develops cancer by the age of 15 years, with about 120–140 new cases per million children aged < 15 years per year (Lissauer and Clayden, 1999). Types of childhood cancers differ from those seen in adults. Table A1.45 in Appendix 1 shows the most common types of cancers seen in children in the UK. Although the incidence of cancer in childhood is increasing, the survival rate for many cancers has improved tremendously over recent years, mainly due to multimodal approaches to care (Lissauer and Clayden, 1999; Ward, 2001).

Up to 50% or more of paediatric patients with malignancy may be acutely undernourished (Table 2.14 and Figs 2.3 and 2.7; see Appendix 1, Table A1.44). Stunting has hardly been investigated in this patient group and, in the one study in which it was measured, the prevalence rate was very low (2.1%) (Yariş et al., 2002). Similarly, stunting and wasting combined has been reported in only one study (8.5%) (Yariş et al., 2002; Fig. 2.7; see Appendix 1, Table A1.44). However, as most studies have been performed at diagnosis, these figures may underestimate the situation at later stages of disease. Treatment of cancer will also influence nutritional status, e.g. chemotherapy has been shown to play a major role in inhibiting catch-up growth in children with acute lymphoblastic leukaemia (Groot-Loonen *et al.*, 1995). Cranial irradiation during childhood will also impair growth (Ogilvy-Stuart and Shalet, 1995). One study (Smith *et al.*, 1990) demonstrated that prevalence of malnutrition increased almost twofold during therapy, despite a third of patients receiving nutritional support. In survivors of treatment for acute lymphoblastic leukaemia, obesity is often a problem in the longer term (Davies *et al.*, 1995; Ventham *et al.*, 1998).

The use of body weight as a means of assessing nutritional status in paediatric cancer patients has been challenged as potentially misleading because of the confounding effects of tumour mass (Smith *et al.*, 1991). Indeed, this may explain why other authors have suggested that children with cancer (Moy *et al.*, 1990) and those undergoing chemotherapy or a bone-marrow transplant are at a lower risk of malnutrition than children with other conditions (Moy *et al.*, 1990; Hendricks *et al.*, 1995). Using upper-arm anthropometric criteria, a study undertaken specifically in children with newly diagnosed cancer in the UK indicated that ~20% are undernourished (Smith *et al.*, 1991). Other authors have indicated that anthropometry may not be sensitive enough to detect reduced muscle protein reserves in children with solid tumours; other techniques, such as regional ultrasonography, may be necessary (Taskinen and Saarinen-Pihkala, 1998).

OTHER DIAGNOSES OR CONDITIONS

In hospitalized children, a high prevalence of severe malnutrition (weight-for-age or height-for-age < 5th percentile) has also been reported for neonatology (71%), subspeciality medical (59%) and general medical (36%) patients (Hendricks *et al.*, 1995), with lower-risk groups including children admitted for elective surgery (Hendricks *et al.*, 1995). A small study of children undergoing CAPD indicated that height retardation and poor nutritional status are common in children with renal insufficiency (Salusky *et al.*, 1983). This has been confirmed in a more recent study (Pereira *et al.*, 2000; Table 2.14 and Figs 2.3 and 2.7; see Appendix 1, Table A1.44). In predialysis patients, nutritional status has been shown to deteriorate with worsening renal function (Norman *et al.*, 2000). CD is associated with impaired growth in children (Sentongo *et al.*, 2000) and wasting and stunting are common in chronic liver disease and those awaiting liver transplants (Sokol and Stall, 1990; Chin *et al.*, 1992) As in those with solid tumours, weight-for-height may underestimate the degree of acute malnutrition in children with chronic liver disease due to increased body weight as a result of organomegaly. The nutritional status of children has also been assessed in other studies of mixed groups of adult and paediatric patients (e.g. Reilly, H.M. *et al.*, 1995; Kennedy *et al.*, 1997), although data are often reported for the group as a whole (see section on mixed diagnoses, this chapter).

The potential causes and possible consequences of disease-related malnutrition in children are summarized in Appendix 1 (Table A1.46).

BEHAVIOURAL PROBLEMS

Malnutrition can also be a common problem in children with behavioural problems (see Chapter 3).

Ultimately, more research is required to determine the most suitable criteria to use to define malnutrition in children in different health-care settings and with different diseases. These criteria can then be used to effectively assess the changes in nutritional status over a period of time (e.g. during hospitalization) or to measure the impact of nutritional intervention. For information about the effects of ONS and ETF in paediatric patients, see Chapters 6–8.

Conclusion

This chapter has demonstrated the difficulties in obtaining accurate values for the prevalence of disease-related malnutrition for comparative purposes. Nevertheless, despite the use of widely different criteria, the general conclusion is that disease-related malnutrition is common in hospital (10–60%), in care homes (up to 50% or more) and in free-living individuals with severe or multiple diseases (> 10%). The use of BMI to compare chronic protein-energy status demonstrates that the prevalence of underweight varies considerably between countries. For example, in India almost half the population has a BMI less than ~18.5 kg m^{-2}, whereas in Britain half the population has a BMI less than ~25 kg m^{-2} (World Health Organization, 1995; Erens and Primatesta, 1999). It also varies considerably between different health-care settings in the same country and is also affected by the type and severity of disease. In the treatment of disease-related malnutrition, it is obviously important to treat the underlying disease and disabilities caused by disease.

Since the consequences of disease-related malnutrition vary with the type of disease, it is necessary to consider these in some detail, since they form the end-points of nutritional intervention trials. Therefore, the causes and consequences of malnutrition are assessed in Chapters 3 and 4, respectively.

Note

[1] For more detailed information about the incidence of diseases and disease-specific mortality rates across Europe, refer to Chapters 4 and 5 of European Commission (2001). Diseases/conditions reported include cancer, human immunodeficiency virus (HIV) infection and acquired immune deficiency syndrome (AIDS), tuberculosis, hip fractures, myocardial infarction, diabetes and neurodegenerative diseases.

3
Causes of Disease-related Malnutrition

Introduction

Hunger and disease, usually in close combination and often precipitated by natural disasters or war, have plagued humankind throughout history (Elia, 2000a). In developed countries, sophisticated methods of food supply and economic access to food ensure a continued year-round availability of virtually all types of produce, enabling a balanced intake of macro- and micronutrients. Environmental hygiene and safe drinking water permit optimal absorption and retention of nutrients. On a worldwide scale, however, hunger and disease continue to be a tremendous problem. In a recent report to the Subcommittee of Nutrition (ACC/SCN) of the United Nations, seven of the eight major global nutritional challenges identified related to correcting undernutrition (Commission on the Nutrition Challenges of the 21st Century, 2000).

The problem of malnutrition, however, is not confined to developing countries. Although malnutrition arising as a result of impaired access to food is relatively uncommon in developed countries, it may be seen in subgroups of the population who live in poverty or who rely on others for nourishment, e.g. infants, children, elderly people, disabled people, the mentally ill and prisoners. In some circumstances, food intake is deliberately reduced, e.g. because of obesity, in anorexia nervosa, or for political reasons (hunger strikes). In most others, it is due to anorexia, but it may also be due to difficulties in eating and swallowing or in the digestion and absorption of food.

There is now increasing evidence to support the contention that insufficient intake of food is of central importance in the development and progression of disease-related malnutrition (DRM). This chapter will focus on the evidence for poor food intake in patients with a variety of disorders and conditions, and indicate the reasons for this situation. It will also briefly consider the importance of this in respect of nutrients whose requirements are altered as a consequence of disease. In view of the key importance of reduced dietary intake, it is surprising that there has been no comprehensive review of it across diseases, health-care settings and different ages (adults/children) until now.

The effect of disease on dietary intake and energy expenditure

The primary cause of malnutrition in developed countries, particularly in adults, is disease: hence the term 'disease-related malnutrition'. In children, behavioural problems might also be an important cause of malnutrition (Batchelor, 1999). Effects of the disease itself are compounded by factors associated with the treatment of disease, inadequate provision of appropriate nutrition for patients with disease, lack of recognition of the existence and consequences of malnutrition in disease and psychosocial factors.

For many years it was assumed that the primary cause of weight loss in patients was increased energy expenditure and catabolism associated with metabolic stress. This was mainly due to the use of inappropriate methods of assessing energy requirements, but changes in clinical practice may also have made a contribution to decreasing energy requirements (Elia, 1995). Although it does appear that resting energy expenditure is increased in a number of patient groups (e.g. human immunodeficiency virus (HIV), pancreatic cancer, small-cell lung cancer, chronic obstructive pulmonary disease (COPD), Crohn's disease), even when expressed according to fat-free mass (Falconer et al., 1994; Gibney et al., 1997; Jebb, 1997; Nguyen et al., 1999; Al-Jaouni et al., 2000) this can in part be explained by the fact that the weights of organs such as brain and liver are preserved even when skeletal muscle mass is lost, and these organs contribute disproportionately (approx. 60%) to resting energy expenditure (Elia and Jebb, 1992; Elia, 1997a; Jebb, 1997). Until recently, measurements of total energy expenditure (TEE) have been confined to critically ill, ventilated patients, in whom inspired and expired air could be accessed continuously. In such patients, TEE has been shown to vary widely from individual to individual, but median values are not raised compared with healthy populations (Green et al., 1995). The advent of stable-isotope technology has enabled measurements of TEE to be made in a variety of other patient groups, including the elderly chronically mentally ill, Parkinson's disease, Huntingdon's chorea, small-cell lung cancer, pancreatic cancer, HIV disease and COPD (Prentice et al., 1989; Macallan et al., 1995; Baarends et al., 1997; Gibney et al., 1997; Elia et al., 2000b; Moses et al.,

2000; Tang et al., 2002). Convincing evidence is now emerging to demonstrate that TEE is not raised in most patient groups; although there may be some exceptions to this rule (e.g. in COPD (Baarends et al., 1997), this has not been shown in all studies (Tang et al., 2002)). On the contrary, in most disease states, TEE is frequently lower than normal, due to a decrease in physical activity level (Prentice et al., 1989; Elia et al., 2000b; Moses et al., 2000), which is a major contributor to TEE (Gibney et al., 1997; Kramer et al., 1998; Elia et al., 2000b; Fig. 3.1).

Although raised TEE is probably not a factor in weight loss in the majority of cases, other consequences of the metabolic response to trauma, infection and inflammation are central in modifying the drive to eat, the assimilation of nutrients and the conservation of body composition. These include the release of cytokines, glucocorticoids, catecholamines, insulin and insulin-like growth factors, the balance of which may be crucial in regulating the ability to generate an anabolic response (Chang et al., 1998). Whether these factors may also influence absorption is not clear. Any factors that serve to reduce digestion or absorption of food in the gastrointestinal (GI) tract, and therefore result in an increased loss of nutrients, can potentially give rise to malnutrition. In most circumstances, however, severe compromise of gut function must occur before losses become clinically significant (Silk, 2001). Causes of malabsorption have been reviewed and classified by the location of the main abnormality in the GI tract (Silk, 2001). Certain drugs may also have an influence on absorption. However, even in diseases typically associated with malabsorption, weight loss may be due to reduced food intake rather than malabsorption per se. For example, in a study of colonic Crohn's disease, where malabsorption is probably of little relevance, food intake was reduced in weight-losing compared with weight-stable patients (Rigaud et al., 1994). This was suggested to be due to anorexia, depression and medical advice to avoid certain foods.

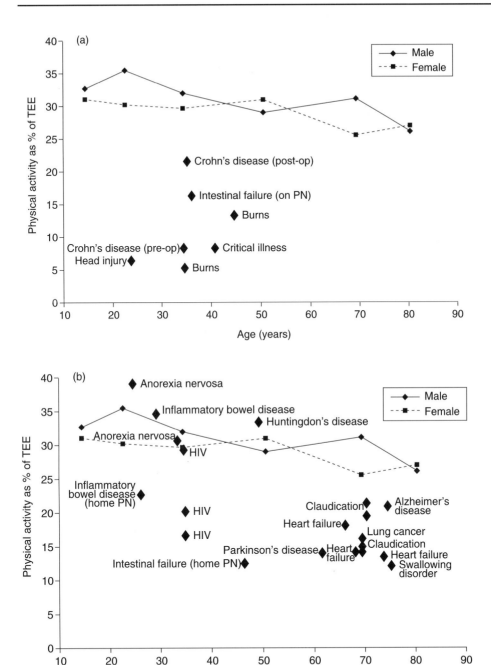

Fig. 3.1. Contribution of physical activity total energy expenditure in healthy male and female subjects and in patients with acute (a) and chronic (b) disease (adjusted for weight). Based on Elia *et al.*, 2000b, and Elia, unpublished. Each point represents a mean result of an individual study. All of these studies involved measurement of total energy expenditure with doubly labelled water, except in three studies of acute conditions (burns, critical illness, head injury) which employed continuous indirect calorimetry in ventilated patients.

Assessment of Food Intake in Patients

Of the studies reviewed, a variety of methods have been used to assess food intake, including assessments of typical intake (e.g. food frequency questionnaires), past food intake (e.g. 24 h dietary recalls), current food intake (e.g. dietary records and weighed food intakes) and combinations of these techniques (see Table 3.1). The most common methods employed have been prospective dietary records and weighed food intakes (3 days being the most typical time period). Comprehensive critiques of the advantages, disadvantages and limitations of all these different methods can be found elsewhere (Bingham, 1987; Stubbs and Elia, 2001; Thomas, 2001). Although it is known that methods of dietary assessment tend to underestimate true intake, particularly energy intake, in healthy free-living populations (Thomas, 2001), it is not clear whether or not this finding also applies to patients, especially in the hospital setting, where health-care staff are likely to be involved in the recording and weighing of food intake. Possible limitations of the various dietary intake methods should therefore be borne in mind when reviewing the data on food intake in patients in different circumstances. In the following section on dietary intake, emphasis is placed on protein and energy, partly because they represent central components of dietary assessment and because there is more information about them than about other dietary constituents. However, in situations where protein and energy intake are reduced, it is likely that overall food intake, including other dietary components will also be reduced.

Food intake in patients in hospitals

A number of studies have examined food intake in hospitalized adult patients, both in general (patients with mixed diagnoses) and in specific age (elderly) or disease groups. These studies are summarized in Appendix 2 (Tables A2.1–A2.13). Figure 3.2 illustrates measured energy intakes from those studies where daily intakes were reported. It can be seen from this figure that mean daily energy intakes in almost all patient groups studied failed to meet estimated average requirements of energy (Department of Health, 1991) or recommended dietary intakes for hospital patients (1800–2200 kcal day^{-1} (Allison, 1999)). This is particularly striking in elderly women with fractured neck of femur.

Many of the studies that reported energy intakes also measured protein intakes in hospitalized patients. Those that reported daily intakes (g day^{-1}) are illustrated in Fig. 3.3, in comparison with recommended reference nutrient intakes (RNI) and typical average intakes of protein in the healthy population (Department of Health, 1991). Although protein intakes on the whole seem to meet recommended requirements better, in many patient groups they still fall considerably short, e.g. in postoperative patients and elderly women with fractured neck of femur. Furthermore, if protein intakes are compared with typical intakes in the healthy population (84 g day^{-1} for men and 64 g day^{-1} for women (Department of Health, 1991) and 77 g day^{-1} for elderly men and 59 g day^{-1} for elderly women (Finch et al., 1998)), the shortfall in protein intake is even more significant. Intakes may be even more compromised if allowance is made for increased requirements due to an already depleted state or as a result of the disease process. Protein requirements for patients with disease are increased compared with the normal healthy situation, typically falling in the range of 1.25–2.5 g kg^{-1} body weight (75–150 g protein day^{-1} for a 60 kg patient) (Elia, 1996a; McAtear, 1999).

Poor intake not only results in an inadequate intake of energy and protein to meet requirements for maintenance or repletion of nutritional status, but also in an inadequate intake of vitamins, minerals and trace elements, and other nutrients, such as fibre. Few studies have examined the full spectrum of nutrient intake in patients. Of those that have examined intakes of other nutrients, most have selected just a few. Nevertheless, findings have frequently demonstrated that intakes are often defi-

Table 3.1. Overview of methods of dietary assessment used in the studies reviewed which measured food intake.

Dietary assessment method	References
Assessments of typical food intake	
Food-frequency questionnaire	Sharkey *et al.*, 1992; Lasheras *et al.*, 1999
3-day food-frequency questionnaire	Chazot *et al.*, 2001
4-day food-frequency questionnaire	Broadhead *et al.*, 2001a
Semi-quantitative food-frequency questionnaire	Charlton, 1997; Klipstein-Grobusch *et al.*, 1999
Semi-structured interview	Mowé *et al.*, 1994
Assessments of past food intake	
Dietary history	Sandström *et al.*, 1985; Rigaud *et al.*, 1994; Staal-van den Brekel *et al.*, 1994; Jackson *et al.*, 1996; Baarends *et al.*, 1997
Modified dietary history method	Van der Wielen *et al.*, 1996; Inelman *et al.*, 2000
Dietary history with cross-check	Geerling *et al.*, 1998a; Schols *et al.*, 1999
24 h dietary recall questionnaire	Hogg *et al.*, 1995; Rea *et al.*, 1998
24 h dietary recall	Nielsen *et al.*, 1993; Caughey *et al.*, 1994a; Smit *et al.*, 1996
24 h dietary recall for 3 days	Trick, 2000
24 h dietary recall for 3 days with menu card prompts	Murphy *et al.*, 2000; Lumbers *et al.*, 2001
24 h dietary recall for 4 days	Lumbers *et al.*, 1998
24 h parental dietary recall	Smith *et al.*, 1991
3-day dietary history	Kurugöl *et al.*, 1997; Lengyel *et al.*, 2001
7-day dietary history	Dowling *et al.*, 1990; Choileáin *et al.*, 1995
Assessments of current food intake	
Patient observations and records	Meguid *et al.*, 1988; Mancey-Jones *et al.*, 1994; Sullivan *et al.*, 1999
7-day observation	Johnson *et al.*, 1995
7-day assessment (no details)	Thuluvath and Triger, 1994
Dietary record (unspecified period)	Trujillo *et al.*, 1992; Gariballa *et al.*, 1998a; Tang *et al.*, 2002
1-day dietary record	Lawson *et al.*, 2000
2-day dietary record	Beaugerie *et al.*, 1998
3-day dietary record	Dworkin *et al.*, 1990; Dahl and Gebre-Medhin, 1993; Lorenzo *et al.*, 1995; Luder *et al.*, 1995; McCargar *et al.*, 1995; de Jong *et al.*, 1998; Gall *et al.*, 1998a; Macqueen and Frost, 1998; Saini *et al.*, 1998; Davidson *et al.*, 1999; Fraser *et al.*, 1999; Pereira *et al.*, 2000; Kim *et al.*, 2001; Richardson *et al.*, 2001
4-day dietary record	Thommessen *et al.*, 1991; Keithley *et al.*, 1992; Cooper and Beaven, 1993; Beck *et al.*, 2001a; Bosaeus *et al.*, 2001
5-day dietary record	Jagoe *et al.*, 2001b
5-day dietary record (by dietitian)	Paillaud *et al.*, 2000
7-day dietary record	Rana *et al.*, 1992; Parisien *et al.*, 1993; Keele *et al.*, 1997; Ockenga *et al.*, 1997; Gretebeck and Boileau, 1998; Persson, M. *et al.*, 2000a; Bachrach-Lindström *et al.*, 2001
9-day dietary record	Elmstahl *et al.*, 1997
14-day dietary record	Sanders *et al.*, 1991
22-day dietary record	Murphy *et al.*, 2001
Weighed food intake (unspecified period)	Sandström *et al.*, 1985; Gegerie *et al.*, 1986
1-day weighed food intake	Brynes *et al.*, 1998; McCollum, 2000
2–3-day weighed food intake	Klipstein-Grobusch *et al.*, 1995
3-day weighed food intake	Older *et al.*, 1980; Holmes and Dickerson, 1991; Ovesen *et al.*, 1991; Chin *et al.*, 1992; Pattison *et al.*, 1997a; Browne and Moloney, 1998; Barton *et al.*, 2000a; Shirley and Moloney, 2000

Continued

Table 3.1. *continued*

Dietary assessment method	References
4-day weighed food intake	Elmstahl, 1987; Finch *et al.*, 1998; Eastwood *et al.*, 2001; Thorsdottir and Gunnarsdottir, 2002
7-day weighed food intake	Foskett *et al.*, 1991; Sharkey *et al.*, 1992; Rigaud *et al.*, 1994; Anthony *et al.*, 1998; Maskell *et al.*, 1999; Hollis and Henry, 2001
Calculation of average portions provided and weighing of plate waste	Barton *et al.*, 2000a; Lawson *et al.*, 2000; Valla, 2000
3-day partially weighed food record	Nicolas *et al.*, 2000; Norman *et al.*, 2000
Part weighed food intake/part questionnaire food record	Hankard *et al.*, 2001
Part weighed food intake/part dietary record	Jallut *et al.*, 1990
3-day weighed food intake and chemical analysis	Levine and Morgan, 1994
Weighed food intake (unspecified period) and vitamin C analysis	Jones *et al.*, 1988
Combination of types of assessments of food intake	
Dietary history and 5-day dietary record	Lewis *et al.*, 1993
Semi-quantitative food-frequency questionnaire and 3-day dietary record	Woods *et al.*, 2002
3-day dietary record plus interview	Jensen and Hessov, 1997

cient (see Appendix 2, Tables A2.1–A2.13). Processing losses that may occur during the preparation and provision of food may further compromise intake (Allison, 1999).

Few studies have examined food intake in hospitalized children (see Appendix 2, Table A2.14). Hankard *et al.* (2001) reported that, in children aged over 6 months with mixed diagnoses, mean energy intake was approximately 50 kcal kg^{-1}, with 66% of those studied having intakes of less than 75% of the recommended daily allowance (RDA). Mean protein intake was approximately 2 g kg^{-1}. It is difficult to interpret this finding without knowing the age of the children studied and the specific diseases involved. Protein requirements of healthy children range from 1.5 g kg^{-1} day^{-1} for infants aged 7–9 months, to 1.1 g kg^{-1} day^{-1} for those aged 4–6 years, but may increase considerably in some diseases (up to 4 g kg^{-1} day^{-1} according to some authors (Shaw and Lawson, 2001)). A more detailed analysis of dietary intake in hospitalized children aged 1–18 years with a variety of malignancies showed that 95% had energy intakes less than the RDA and 36% consumed less protein than the RDA (Kurugöl *et al.*,

1997). Those with active disease appeared to have poorer intakes than those in remission.

Food intake in patients in the community

A number of studies have investigated energy intake in patients at home or in institutions, illustrated in Fig. 3.2 and summarized in Appendix 2 (see Tables A2.4–A2.13). Also included in Fig. 3.2 are energy intakes reported for healthy elderly subjects living at home or in sheltered accommodation. Although overall energy intakes seem to be better than in hospitals, there are still considerable shortfalls seen in several patient groups, notably COPD, liver disease (mainly patients awaiting a liver transplant), renal disease and patients with malignancy. In the latter case, this is most notable in patients during treatments, e.g. chemotherapy or radiotherapy (Ovesen *et al.*, 1991; Macqueen and Frost, 1998; Broadhead *et al.*, 2001a), or in advanced cancer without active treatment (Pattison and Young, 1997). Even in patients who appear overall to be meeting

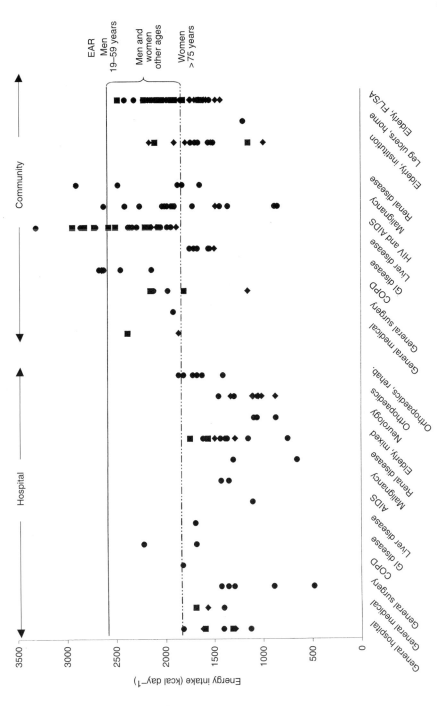

Fig. 3.2. Mean or median energy intake in a variety of patient groups in hospital and community settings in relation to estimated average requirement (EAR) for energy for healthy adults of all ages. Diamond symbols represent women, square symbols represent men and circles represent patient groups of both sexes. The horizontal solid line indicates the EAR for energy for men aged 19–59 years (2550 kcal day⁻¹; value for men 75+ years 2100 kcal day⁻¹). The horizontal dotted line represents the EAR for women aged 75+ years (1810 kcal day⁻¹; value for women 19–50 years 1940 kcal day⁻¹) (Department of Health, 1991). For more details on the studies, refer to the tables in Appendix 2. FL, free-living; SA, sheltered accommodation; AIDS, acquired immune deficiency syndrome; rehab., rehabilitation.

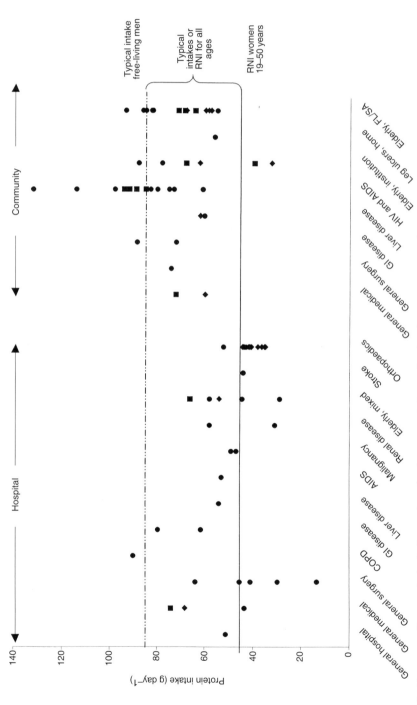

Fig. 3.3. Mean or median protein intake in a variety of patient groups in hospital and in the community in relation to the reference nutrient intake (RNI) and typical intakes for healthy adults of all ages. Diamond symbols represent women, square symbols represent men and circles represent patient groups of both sexes. The horizontal solid line indicates the RNI for protein for women aged 19–50 years (45 g day[-1]; value for men aged 19–50 years 55.5 g day[-1], for men age 50+ years 53.3 g day[-1], for women aged 50+ years 46.5 g day[-1]) (Department of Health, 1991). The horizontal dotted line represents typical daily intakes of protein in free-living men (84 g day[-1] for men; value for women 64 g day[-1]) (Department of Health, 1991); for elderly free-living men 77 g day[-1] and women 59 g day[-1] (Finch *et al.*, 1998). For more details on the studies, refer to the tables in Appendix 2. FL, free-living; SA, sheltered accommodation; AIDS, acquired immune deficiency syndrome.

energy needs, e.g. in GI disease, it can be seen that those who are losing weight have lower intakes than those who are weight-stable (Rigaud *et al.*, 1994). Apparently normally satisfactory intakes may be inadequate to counteract the effects of maldigestion and malabsorption (Geerling *et al.*, 1998a). In addition, dietary intake in patients with impaired GI function may be assessed during remission (Geerling *et al.*, 2000a). Energy intake in clinically stable patients with HIV infection and acquired immune deficiency syndrome (AIDS) has been extensively investigated (Fig. 3.2). Overall energy intakes are reasonable, although several studies appear to show trends for declining energy intake with increasing stage of disease (Dowling *et al.*, 1990; Keithley *et al.*, 1992; Parisien *et al.*, 1993; Ockenga *et al.*, 1997). The patients included in these studies were unlikely to be suffering from ongoing opportunistic infections, when a dramatic decrease in food intake may occur (Grunfeld *et al.*, 1992).

In elderly subjects in nursing homes and other institutions, and in those with leg ulcers being treated at home, energy intakes often fall short of recommendations (Fig. 3.2). However, it should be noted that quite a few of the studies of the elderly living at home or in sheltered accommodation also reveal that intake frequently does not meet recommendations.

Protein intakes on the whole appear to be less compromised than energy intakes in patients in the community (see Fig. 3.3). Most patients appear to meet the RNI for protein (Department of Health, 1991), although whether these levels are appropriate for individuals with disease is, of course, unlikely, as discussed earlier in this chapter. In HIV infection and AIDS, clinically stable patients appear to have comparable intakes with the healthy population. Other patient groups, such as those with liver disease and malignancy, fall short of typical intakes in healthy people. Protein intakes also appear to be less affected than energy intakes by chemotherapy or radiotherapy (Ovesen *et al.*, 1991; Broadhead *et al.*, 2001a).

Relatively few studies have reported protein intakes in institutionalized elderly and, in those that have, there is considerable variation in intake. This is an area worthy of more in-depth evaluation. In the free-living elderly and those in sheltered accommodation, protein intakes are generally adequate in comparison with the RNI, although, in a number of studies, intakes in men fall short of those calculated from reported energy intakes and energy per cent from protein of persons aged 65 years and older in the *National Diet and Nutrition Survey* (77 g day^{-1} for men; 59 g day^{-1} for women (Finch *et al.*, 1998)).

Several studies assessed intakes of some micronutrients (see Appendix 2, Tables A1.1–A1.13 for details). Of particular note is the fact that, even in stable patients with HIV infection, whose energy and protein intakes were generally adequate (often because patients were asymptomatic), poor intakes of micronutrients were frequently noted (Dworkin *et al.*, 1990; Keithley *et al.*, 1992; Luder *et al.*, 1995; Smit *et al.*, 1996; Ockenga *et al.*, 1997; Kim *et al.*, 2001; Woods *et al.*, 2002). Many of the studies in institutionalized elderly also reported low intakes of a variety of micronutrients, although free-living elderly may also often have poor intakes (see Chapter 1, Table 1.6 and Appendix 2, Tables A2.4 and A2.5). This suggests that many patients, particularly the elderly, may already have low physiological reserves of many micronutrients before they are admitted to hospital.

Of the few studies that measured fibre intake in the community, many reported poor intakes (Smit *et al.*, 1996; Geerling *et al.*, 1998a; Broadhead *et al.*, 2001a; Eastwood *et al.*, 2001; Lengyel *et al.*, 2001).

Food intake in paediatric patients living in the community is a rather neglected field (see Appendix 2, Table A2.14). The few studies that have been performed demonstrate that energy intake may be a cause for concern in cerebral palsy, liver disease, malignancy and renal disease. Of the studies reviewed, only two reported on protein intakes. In malignancy, the median per cent of the RDA was 107%, but with a wide range of values, indicat-

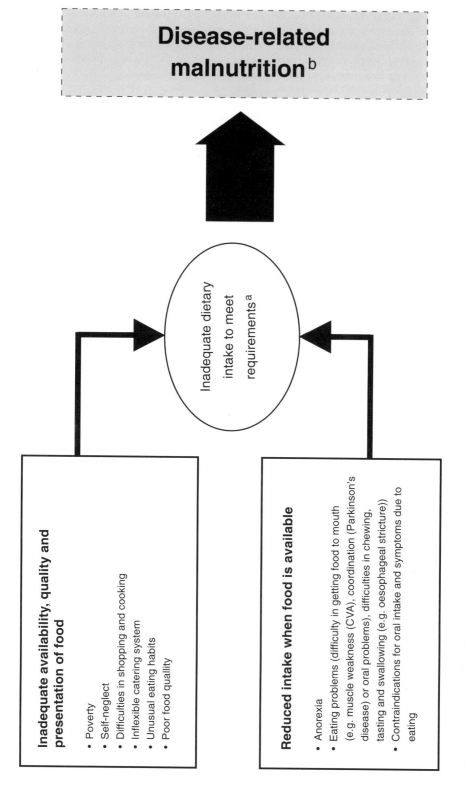

Fig. 3.4. Reasons for insufficient energy and nutrient intake as a cause of disease-related malnutrition. [a] Requirements for some nutrients may be increased due to malabsorption, metabolism and excess losses. [b] Lack of awareness and recognition of malnutrition and its causes by health workers contributes to the problem (for details, see text). CVA, cerebrovascular accident.

ing that many patients will have inadequate intakes (Smith *et al.*, 1991). In chronic renal insufficiency (predialysis), there was a trend to a reduction in protein intake with increasing severity of renal insufficiency, which did not simply reflect dietary advice to reduce protein intake (Norman *et al.*, 2000). However, at 2 g kg^{-1}, this was still approximately twice that recommended for healthy children of the same age. Micronutrient and fibre intakes have been barely investigated in paediatric patients.

Causes of Inadequate Dietary Intake in Disease

There are multiple reasons why individuals suffering from disease, illness or trauma are at high risk of poor nutritional intake and consequently of malnutrition. These can broadly be divided into two main causes: lack of food (or adequate food quality) and a variety of disease-related factors that reduce intake when food is available. Many of these are obvious (e.g. anorexia, difficulties in eating and swallowing), but it is surprising that malnutrition is frequently unrecognized and untreated. Therefore, the causes are summarized in Fig. 3.4 and discussed in more detail below.

Inadequate availability, quality and presentation of food

Inadequate availability of food

Outside the hospital setting, health and social factors identified as affecting food choice and nutritional intake in elderly people with restricted mobility (Wylie *et al.*, 1999) are likely to apply to other types of patients in the community. These include inadequate resources (finances, food storage facilities, cooking facilities), poor access to shops and/or difficulties in undertaking shopping, physical disabilities affecting food preparation, and other psychosocial factors, such as loneliness and bereavement.

Unusual eating habits, poor food choices and lack of assistance with shopping, cooking and eating may compound these problems. In some individuals, poverty, social isolation and self-neglect are mainly responsible for the poor dietary intake.

Within the hospital setting and other institutions, the quality of food supply may also be an issue. Although some of the studies that have examined the quality of food supplied to hospital patients have demonstrated that energy and protein contents are in line with recognized guidelines (Barton *et al.*, 2000a), there are a number of exceptions (Simon, 1991; Fenton *et al.*, 1995; Johnson *et al.*, 1995; Hankey and Wynne, 1996; Browne and Moloney, 1998; Shirley and Moloney, 2000). These data indicate that often patients may simply be offered insufficient food with appropriate nutrient density. Palatability of food served may also be an issue. Furthermore, an inflexible catering service may limit the availability of food. If meals are missed, it is often not possible to obtain a meal or snack until the next mealtime. This is of particular relevance to patients who readily become satiated with small amounts of food and feel hungry between set meal periods, when food is not available.

Inadequate quality of food

Inappropriate food choices may be a further factor limiting food intake. For example, foods that cannot be easily chewed or swallowed, foods that are unfamiliar or low-energy foods may result in impaired nutrient intake. High-fibre, low-energy foods, such as those recommended for healthy eating, may be unsuitable for many patients who are at risk of malnutrition. A greater intake of nutrients is likely to be achieved with high-energy density food items (see Chapter 6).

Inadequate presentation of food

Apart from the nutritional quality of the food, the way in which it is served may also have an impact on food intake. These factors include the following:

SYSTEM OF FOOD DELIVERY TO THE WARD

A plated service in hospital wards has been reported to have disadvantages in terms of food intake compared with a bulk trolley service (Allison, 1999; Shatenstein and Ferland, 2000; Wilson, A. *et al.*, 2000a).

PORTION SIZE OF MEALS

It has been suggested that portion sizes that are too large may result in less food being consumed in hospitalized patients than if smaller serving sizes are used (Barton *et al.*, 2000a); however, this remains controversial (Cluskey and Dunton, 1999).

Reduced intake when food is available

Anorexia

Loss of appetite is probably the most common overall cause of reduced food intake in disease. It results from both physical and psychosocial problems.

INFLAMMATORY DISEASE

Anorexia is a major feature of many acute and chronic inflammatory disorders (e.g. infective, malignant, traumatic conditions) (Plata-Salaman, 1996) and is a significant factor leading to reduced food intake. It is beyond the scope of this book to address the mechanisms of the anorexia of disease; these have been extensively reviewed elsewhere (Plata-Salaman, 1996; Langhans, 2000; MacIntosh *et al.*, 2000; Ballinger and Clark, 2001; Stubbs and Elia, 2001). Modified secretion of cytokines, peptides, neurotransmitters and leptin, changes in GI sensory and motor function and the presence of microbial products associated with disease, inflammation, infection and injury are at least in part responsible. Anorexia has been quantified using subjective appetite parameters in a number of disorders, including advanced malignancy (Hawkins, 2000), sepsis (Cherubini *et al.*, 2000), active Crohn's disease (Bannerman *et al.*, 2001) and orthopaedic patients (Stratton *et al.*, 1997).

NAUSEA AND VOMITING

Certain diseases, drugs and treatments (e.g. opioids, chemotherapy and radiotherapy) may have a profound effect on appetite by causing nausea, vomiting (sometimes in association with mucositis) and taste changes. For example, it has been reported that 50–60% of patients with advanced cancer suffer from nausea, vomiting and/or retching, which may at least in part be due to drugs and treatments (Baines, 1997). This may lead to avoidance of foods for fear of nausea, vomiting and/or diarrhoea, and may even result in the development of food aversions. There are also other ways in which drugs can influence nutrient intake and availability (see Table 3.2). This area has been subject to a recent extensive review (White and Ashworth, 2000). Pain, abdominal or otherwise, may also decrease appetite, especially when it is initiated by eating.

PSYCHOSOCIAL PROBLEMS

Psychological causes. The effects of depression and anxiety in suppressing appetite and the desire to eat are common in disease and should not be overlooked. Anorexia itself may also give rise to anxiety (Hawkins, 2000). In some cases, food aversion can reduce dietary intake; for example, an individual may have had an unpleasant reaction to food at a particular time and may continue avoiding ingestion of that food or avoid eating it at a particular time, even though the cause is no longer present. Some patients with severe dementia may 'forget' how to eat but whether the cause is to be classified as psychological or organic is debatable. Rest *per se* (i.e. bed rest/immobility) reduces spontaneous food intake (Ritz *et al.*, 1999).

Social causes. A non-inviting meal environment can have a negative impact on appetite and food intake, as demonstrated for institutionalized patients (Elmstahl *et al.*, 1987; Hartwell and Edwards, 2001; Mathey *et al.*, 2001a). Timing of meals may also influence appetite and food intake (e.g. ward rounds or cleaning bedpans and bowel evacuations during ingestion of snacks or meals, particularly on hospital wards). For non-institutionalized individuals who may be retired and socially isolated, eating in food clubs or canteens,

Table 3.2. Mechanisms by which drugs may influence nutritional status (adapted from White and Ashworth, 2000).

Category	Effect	Example	Nutrients of most concern
Reduction in oral intake	Need to modify food intake or timing in relation to drug intake	Tetracycline (antibiotic) Protease inhibitors (HIV infection)	Energy, protein, micronutrients
	Nausea and vomiting (central action)	Cytotoxics (cancer) Fluoxetine (antidepressive) Opiates (pain relief) Levodopa (PD)	Energy, protein, micronutrients
	Nausea and vomiting (local irritant action)	Potassium salts Iron salts	Energy, protein, micronutrients
	Influence on gastrointestinal motility (delayed gastric emptying)	Drugs with anticholinergic activity Opiates (pain relief)	Energy, protein, micronutrients
	Anorexia	Spironolactone (diuretic) Digoxin (anti-arrhythmic) Amantadine (PD) Fluoxetine (antidepressive)	Energy, protein, micronutrients
	Taste disturbances	Metronidazole (antibiotic) Griseofulvin (antifungal) Rifampicin (antituberculous) Allopurinol (antigout)	Energy, protein, micronutrients
	Diarrhoea	Metoclopromide (prokinetic) Erythromycin (prokinetic) Acarbose Misoprostol (anti-ulcer, RA) Antibiotics Non-steroidal anti-inflammatories	Energy, protein, micronutrients
Decreased nutrient absorption	Direct binding of certain micronutrients	Antacids containing Al, Mg or Ca salts Tetracycline (antibiotic) Cholestyramine (cholesterol lowering) Phosphate binders (renal disease)	Se, Cr, Fe, Ca, Zn, folate, vitamin B_{12}, magnesium Ca Fe P
	Alteration of gastric/ luminal pH	Antacids Phenytoin (anti-arrhythmic, anticonvulsant)	Se, Cr, Fe, Ca, Zn, folate, vitamin B_{12}, magnesium
	Binding of bile salts Influence on intestinal mucosal proliferation Steatorrhoea	Cholestyramine (cholesterol lowering) Colchicine Methotrexate (antineoplastic) Neomycin (antibiotic) Tetracyclines (antibiotic) Allopurinol (xanthine oxidase inhibitor) Methyldopa (antihypertensive)	Vitamins A, D, K, Fe, folate All nutrients Fat, fat-soluble vitamins, carotenoids
	Intestinal bacterial overgrowth/changes in bacterial flora	Proton pump inhibitors Antibiotics	All nutrients
	Interference with intrinsic factor	Cholestyramine (cholesterol lowering) Neomycin (antibiotic) Methyldopa (antihypertensive) Cimetidine (antisecretory)	Vitamin B_{12}, folate
Altered nutrient metabolism	Altered storage, utilization and/or excretion	Frusemide (diuretic) Chlorpromazine (antipsychotic) Amitryptyline (antidepressant) Isoniazid (antituberculous) Sodium valproate (anticonvulsant) Isoniazid (antituberculous)	Thiamine Riboflavin Riboflavin Nicotinic acid Nicotinic acid Pyridoxine, folate

Continued

Table 3.2. *Continued*

Category	Effect	Example	Nutrients of most concern
		Penicillamine (RA)	Pyridoxine, folate
		Theophylline (bronchodilator)	Folate
		Phenytoin (anti-arrhythmia, anticonvulsant)	Folate
		Methotrexate (antineoplastic)	Vitamin D
		Sulphasalazine (colitis, RA)	Vitamin K
		Anticonvulsants (epilepsy)	Vitamin K
		Warfarin (anticoagulation)	Vitamin K
		Antibiotics	Carnitine
		Laxatives	Copper, iron
		Sodium valproate (anticonvulsant)	
		Penicillamine (RA)	

PD, Parkinson's disease; RA, rheumatoid arthritis.

which are available for past employees of some companies, may improve both social well-being and appetite.

Eating problems

GETTING FOOD TO MOUTH

Patients may have disabilities that prevent them from accessing their meals; for example, arthritis can impair the use of cutlery. Adapted cutlery may help to alleviate this problem, but this is often not available. Food may sometimes simply be placed out of reach of the patient. In some cases, more intensive feeding assistance may be required but is not available. In other cases, the food may be placed in the reach of a patient who cannot see the food (e.g. a stroke patient with hemianopia).

Fatigue and muscle weakness will make it difficult to eat, and the disease or injury itself may further compromise the ability to cut and eat food (e.g. fractured arm, loss of use of arm following stroke) or chew food (e.g. fractured jaw). Certain diseases such as stroke, Parkinson's disease and dementia may also give rise to aberrant eating behaviour that will impede food intake (Athlin *et al.*, 1989; Axelsson *et al.*, 1989; Sidenvall and Ek, 1993).

There may be a number of iatrogenic reasons why food intake is reduced. These include fasting prior to and/or after certain investigations or procedures (e.g. surgery)

(Sullivan *et al.*, 1999), missed meals due to investigations (Eastwood, 1997) or prescription of a restricted diet, e.g. energy-, protein- and/or mineral-restricted – for example, for weight-reducing or renal diets (Cooper and Beaven, 1993; Buckler *et al.*, 1994).

DIFFICULTIES IN CHEWING, TASTING AND SWALLOWING
Lack of teeth. Lack of teeth or poorly fitting dentures are a very widespread problem, particularly in the elderly (Fiske, 1999), and can be a major factor limiting food intake (Lamy *et al.*, 1999; Mojon *et al.*, 1999; Sheiham *et al.*, 2001).

Changes in taste and smell. Taste and smell changes may also occur in disease and compromise nutrient intake through effects on appetite, satiety and, most importantly, enjoyment of food (Hess, 1997). In one study in advanced cancer, patients had a significantly lower bitter detection threshold than age-matched controls without malignancy, as well as subjective alterations in taste perception in a high percentage (68%) and a significantly lower energy intake (Pattison *et al.*, 1997a). This was linked with the production of tumour necrosis factor alpha (TNF-α) and the acute-phase response (Pattison *et al.*, 1997b). In a separate study in similar patients, 70% reported subjective alterations in taste sensation and food choices (Moody *et al.*, 1998). Taste changes are not confined to cancer patients, but may be noted in other diseases as well, such as liver disease (Madden *et al.*, 1997), COPD (Chapman-Novakofski *et al.*, 1999) and patients with chronic renal failure on continuous ambulatory peritoneal dialysis (Middleton and Allman-Farinelli, 1999). A more thorough review of the taste changes in clinical malnutrition states is given elsewhere (Davidson *et al.*, 1998). In addition to taste changes, some patients may experience a loss of sense of smell, which is intimately involved with taste (Hess, 1997). Loss of taste and smell has been shown in patients with HIV infection and AIDS (Heald and Schiffman, 1997). Impaired sense of smell has been demonstrated in renal patients undergoing haemodialysis and peritoneal dialysis. In non-dialysed patients, odour perception correlated with creatinine clearance and appeared to start to decline at an early stage of renal impairment (Griep *et al.*, 1997). Aging *per se* can also have an impact on chemosensory losses (MacIntosh *et al.*, 2000; Schiffman and Graham, 2000). Flavour enhancers have been reported to increase food intake in the elderly. Limited trials with flavour enhancers have been undertaken in specific diseases.

Dry mouth. Dryness of the mouth (xerostomia) as a result of inadequate or sticky saliva production can occur particularly during radiotherapy for cancer (Broadhead *et al.*, 2001b).

Painful mouth conditions. Actual pain on eating may also be a factor, due to the disease or injury itself or due to the side-effects of treatment, such as mucositis during chemo- or radiotherapy, which may also cause bleeding. Mouth ulcers and malignancy can also cause problems.

Respiratory problems. Breathlessness as a result of severe respiratory disease (e.g. severe acute exacerbations of COPD) may impair the ability to eat adequately.

Disorders of swallowing. Swallowing difficulties are a feature of many disorders

(Barer, 1989), e.g. neurological disorders (such as cerebrovascular accident, motor neurone disease, multiple sclerosis) and obstructive lesions of the upper GI tract (such as benign or malignant oesophageal stricture). Xerostomia will also impede swallowing. Semi-solid or viscous foods/feeds are often tolerated better than 'runny' or non-viscous liquid foods/feeds.

Contraindications and symptoms due to eating. Dietary intake is obviously reduced when eating is contraindicated (e.g. GI obstruction or ileus such as postoperative ileus, pancreatitis and peritonitis). Eating under such circumstances may not only exacerbate the disease but also produce distress by causing nausea, vomiting and pain. Eating may induce symptoms in other conditions, such as peptic ulcer, gallstones and short-bowel syndrome, and the patient responds by eating less.

Nutrient Requirements in Disease and the Effects of Reduced Dietary Intake

The requirement for many dietary nutrients may increase in disease, which means that even a normal intake may be inadequate for patients with disease. Some examples of increased oral dietary requirements are given below.

Protein

Requirements increase in many diseases, including short-bowel syndrome or other GI conditions that lead to abnormal GI losses (abnormal digestion and absorption), burns, which lead to loss of protein through the damaged skin, and many catabolic conditions that lead to an increased net tissue breakdown from metabolic disturbances, even when a normal protein intake is provided.

Minerals and trace elements

Increased intakes of sodium, magnesium and potassium are often necessary in patients with GI fluid effluent and diarrhoea. Trace elements, such as zinc, are required in increased amounts in individuals with GI effluents and diarrhoea. Iron requirement increases in patients with GI bleeding.

Vitamins

Increased intakes of antioxidant vitamins (vitamins C and E and vitamin A-related substances, such as carotenoids) are often required in disease to counteract the adverse effects of excess free radical generators. Other vitamins may also be required in increased amounts in disease (e.g. several B vitamins and vitamin D). There is little or no dietary requirement for vitamin D in individuals who are exposed to adequate amounts of sunlight. However, house-bound and elderly patients who have little or no exposure to direct sunlight have increased dietary vitamin D requirements (about 10 mg day^{-1}).

Increased intakes of nutrients are also necessary to replete the 'stores' that have become depleted during the development of DRM. This could apply to energy (fat), protein and individual micronutrients. The extent of depletion, and therefore the need for extra nutrients, varies with the type, duration and severity of disease, as well as the pattern of nutrient depletion produced by disease.

Disease does not always result in an increase in nutrient requirements and in some situations it may actually decrease them. For example, potassium and phosphate requirements may be reduced in renal failure and sodium requirements may be reduced in patients with heart failure and other conditions associated with salt overload. Energy requirements are also frequently reduced in inactive, house-bound patients or other groups of patients whose disease or disabilities severely limit physical activity. Despite the complexity of the situation that exists in different diseases, the following general points can be made.

- Reduced dietary intake is one of the most important, if not the most important, cause of protein-energy malnutrition.

- Total energy requirements are typically not increased in acute and chronic diseases. In inactive patients, they may be decreased. However, a reduction in energy intake is usually associated with a reduction in the intake of protein and other nutrients.
- The dietary requirements of a number of nutrients (e.g. protein, certain vitamins) are increased in many diseases. A reduction in dietary intake in such circumstances leads to rapid development of DRM.

Since reduced intake plays a key role in the development of DRM, increasing dietary intake might be expected to improve nutritional status and to counter the detrimental effects produced by malnutrition. Improvement of dietary intake may be achieved by a variety of methods, including dietary counselling, oral nutritional supplements, artificial nutrition (enteral and parenteral nutrition), drugs and behavioural therapy. However, it is necessary to demonstrate the extent to which these succeed in improving both nutritional status and clinical outcome in different diseases. This is the focus of subsequent chapters of this book. Of course, control of the disease process is of critical importance in dealing with DRM.

Lack of Recognition and Treatment of DRM

Causes for lack of recognition and treatment of DRM

Lack of awareness and recognition of the problem is likely to be part of the reason why DRM develops and why undernourished patients are frequently not identified or treated appropriately in hospital and community settings. This can arise for a number of reasons, as discussed below.

Lack of interest in nutrition and/or poor recording in patient notes

Despite the growing recognition that attention must be given to nutritional status and adequate provision of nutrition, there is still a widespread failure to regard this as important (Payne-James and Silk, 1990; Abbasi and Rudman, 1993; Garrow, 1994; McWhirter and Pennington, 1994; Miller and Miller, 1994; Lennard-Jones *et al.*, 1995; Moran and Jackson, 1995; Davison and Stables, 1996; Bunting and Weaver, 1997; Kelly *et al.*, 2000; Peake *et al.*, 2000; Perman *et al.*, 2001; Waitzberg *et al.*, 2001). This may lead to poor recording in hospital notes and care plans and inadequate referral for specialist input.

Inadequate referral to dietitian/use of nutritional support

Many studies have demonstrated that patients at risk of or with frank malnutrition are not referred to the dietitian and/or, if nutritional support is prescribed, it is inappropriate or insufficient to meet requirements (Roubenoff *et al.*, 1987; George, 1994; Lock and Vald, 1994; McWhirter and Pennington, 1994; Miller and Miller, 1994; Royce and Taylor, 1994; McWhirter *et al.*, 1995; Davison and Stables, 1996; Sullivan *et al.*, 1999; Kelly *et al.*, 2000; Kruizinga *et al.*, 2001; Waitzberg *et al.*, 2001).

Inadequate training and knowledge of medical and nursing staff

A possible reason for the lack of recognition and treatment of DRM is the poor nutritional knowledge of medical and nursing staff (Roubenoff *et al.*, 1987; Payne-James and Silk, 1990; Allison, 1992; Garrow, 1994; Moran and Jackson, 1995; Lean, 1996; Duff and Livingstone, 1997; McDowell, 1997; Nightingale and Reeves, 1999; Rollins *et al.*, 2001; Waitzberg *et al.*, 2001). This is at least in part due to the historical situation, which has given rise to inadequate attention to nutrition at undergraduate level (Jackson, 2001). A European-wide survey by the Federation of European Nutrition Societies (FENS) found that the medical faculties of only seven out of 16 European countries offered nutrition education (Widhalm *et al.*, 1997). Similarly, in the hospital setting, a survey in a UK teaching hospital has indicated that knowledge about the assessment and management of malnutrition among doctors, medical students, nurses and pharmacists is poor (Nightingale and Reeves, 1999). More specifically, a survey of Danish hospitals has highlighted that only 24% of doctors and nurses routinely perform some kind of nutritional assessment on patients at admission and that 40% find it difficult to identify at-risk patients (Rasmussen *et al.*, 1999). Furthermore, this survey has highlighted the lack of treatment of undernourished patients, with more than one-quarter of doctors and nurses not using any active nutritional treatment at all (Rasmussen *et al.*, 1999). Hence, patients at risk of malnutrition may be overlooked and left untreated.

In the community setting, the Malnutrition Advisory Group (MAG) of the British Association for Parenteral and Enteral Nutrition (BAPEN) commissioned a poll of general practitioners (GPs) about malnutrition in the UK in 1998 (M. Elia, personal communication). This survey found that:

- 74% of GPs had received no undergraduate training in nutrition;
- 61% indicated that GPs needed further training in malnutrition;
- 67% of GP practices did not have a dietitian;
- 85% of GPs followed no protocols or guidelines for the treatment of DRM.

Lack of specialist clinical nutrition posts

Although some countries have the benefit of specialist clinical nutrition posts (e.g. The Netherlands), thus lending greater credibility to and raising awareness of the subject, many countries (e.g. the UK) do not (Payne-James and Silk, 1990; Avenell, 1994).

Inadequate management policies with appropriate resources

It has been stated that appropriate management is the first essential for ensuring that nutrition is regarded as an important component of the quality of patient care (Allison, 1996). Unfortunately, there are a number of barriers to achieving this, which will have consequences for nutritional care throughout the facility (Booth et al., 1995; Dhoot et al., 1996).

Poor organization of nutritional services

Although many facilities have an active dietetic department, there is often a lack of organization of nutritional services linking relevant disciplines within hospitals, lack of a nutrition team and/or lack of continuity in responsibility for nutritional support both internally and between hospital and community (Payne-James and Silk, 1990; Garrow, 1994; Rademaker et al., 1996; Daniels and Wright, 1997; Corish et al., 1998).

A recent survey of the current status of artificial nutritional support in Europe was carried out by the European Society of Parenteral and Enteral Nutrition (ESPEN) (Howard et al., 1999). This indicated that 60% of respondents from university teaching hospitals in 11 countries had access to a nutrition team. However, the response rate was rather low, suggesting that this figure is likely to be a gross overestimate of the actual numbers in hospitals (teaching and general) throughout Europe.

Lack of practice guidelines and nationally agreed standards

The lack of guidelines and standards is also a factor in inadequate and inappropriate handling of nutrition issues (Payne-James and Silk, 1990; Farthing, 1994; Silk, 1994).

Strategies for improving recognition and treatment

Improved provision of food in institutions

The discrepancy between an adequate nutrient content of hospital menus and inadequate nutritional intakes indicates that food wastage is high. Indeed, several studies have shown food wastage of served

food to be 40% or even higher (Allison, 1999; Kelly, 1999; Barton et al., 2000a; Valla, 2000), which has serious financial consequences (Barton et al., 2000a). It has been estimated that the monetary value of hospital food wasted annually in England can be calculated as £45 million, rising to £144 million if labour and overheads are included. This does not include the hidden costs associated with increased morbidity as a result of malnutrition (Allison, 1999).

It has been suggested that greater energy provision allows greater percentages of patients to meet their requirements for energy, protein and a number of micronutrients (Heffernan and Maloney, 2000). It has also been shown that, when patients with chronic liver disease and general medical patients were allowed to devise a 3-day menu for themselves from a wide selection of foods, intakes of energy and protein, assessed by weighing, were comparable with recommendations for healthy populations (Levine and Morgan, 1996). Data from patients with cirrhosis suggest that it may be possible to maintain improved intakes over a longer period of time (Nielsen et al., 1995). Other experiences from Denmark also demonstrate that expected weight gain can be achieved in patients without malignant disease when food provision is tailored more individually (Kondrup, 2001). This, of course, carries a higher cost. The cost of ingredients for food provision for hospital patients in the UK was approximately £2 day^{-1} (Allison, 1999) in 1999, although this may have improved with recent government initiatives (see later). Budget constraints have been identified as a factor in limiting the improvement of hospital food quality (Shirley and Moloney, 2000). Lack of availability of familiar foods for ethnic groups in hospitals has also been suggested to be a factor explaining poor food intake (McArdle et al., 1985; McGlone et al., 1996, 1997). This warrants further investigation.

Some local, national and international initiatives are now striving to improve the quality of food provided for patients. For example, the Rigshospitalet in Denmark has instituted a more tailored approach to hospital food (Kondrup, 2001), and a new UK initiative, called 'Better Hospital Food', has recently been implemented. The latter is part of a £40 million government scheme to improve catering in hospitals, and includes a more sophisticated menu designed by celebrity chefs, more choice, more flexibility (24 h snack box for patients who miss meals), more fresh food and more options for vegetarians and others with special diets (Miller and Schencker, 2000; Schenker, 2001). A European initiative has also recently been undertaken in which eight of the Partial Agreement member states of the Council of Europe participated in reviewing the current practice in Europe regarding hospital food provision. Based on a survey, deficiencies have been highlighted and guidelines have been issued to improve the nutritional care and support of patients in hospitals (Beck *et al.*, 2001b; Council of Europe, 2001).

Other factors that should be considered in improvement initiatives include the following:

MORE ASSISTANCE AT WARD LEVEL

Audits and pilot ward hostess schemes suggest that assistance at ward level with respect to ensuring appropriate menu ordering, assistance with eating where necessary, recording of nutritional intake and improved liaison between ward and catering departments can improve patient satisfaction and could lead to improved food intake (Anderson, 2000; Miller and O'Hara, 2000; Waite *et al.*, 2000).

SYSTEM OF FOOD DELIVERY TO THE WARD

A bulk trolley service has been shown to have advantages in terms of food intake compared with a plated service (Allison, 1999; Shatenstein and Ferland, 2000; Wilson, A. *et al.*, 2000).

PORTION SIZE OF MEALS

It has been suggested that portion sizes that are too large may result in less food being consumed than if smaller serving sizes are used (Barton *et al.*, 2000b); however, this remains controversial (Cluskey and Dunton, 1999) and therefore warrants further investigation.

MEAL ENVIRONMENT

Making mealtimes a more pleasurable experience can have a positive impact on food intake, e.g. making the dining area more familiar and encouraging communal eating (Elmstahl *et al.*, 1987; Hartwell and Edwards, 2001; Mathey *et al.*, 2001a). Playing music at mealtimes may also enhance food intake in demented patients, although whether this is through influence on the patients or on the staff is unclear (Ragneskog *et al.*, 1996).

AVAILABILITY OF SNACKS AND FOOD FORTIFICATION

Providing snacks between meals (Lord, 2002) and/or fortifying foods with energy and/or protein, using normal foods, e.g. cream or butter (Gall *et al.*, 1998a; Odlund-Olin *et al.*, 1998; Barton *et al.*, 2000b), or commercially available supplements (Parkinson *et al.*, 1987; Morris *et al.*, 1990), has been demonstrated to improve energy intake and, to a lesser extent, protein intake. Impact on body weight, function and outcome using these strategies has been little investigated. The possible further dilution of micronutrient density of foods when protein and energy contents are enhanced needs to be further investigated.

OTHER STRATEGIES

Other strategies for enhancing nutrient intakes, particularly in elderly persons in long-term care, have been suggested, such as using tactile and verbal prompts, pantomiming desired eating behaviour and providing praise or reinforcement for eating (Cluskey and Kim, 2001). Flavour enhancement may also be of benefit in those with taste and smell loss, e.g. the elderly (Henry *et al.*, 2001; Mathey *et al.*, 2001b).

Overall, there seems to be growing recognition that meals in institutions, especially hospitals, should be seen as an important part of clinical care, rather than just as a 'hotel' function (Allison, 1999; Davis and Bristow, 1999).

Improved education and training

Steps are now being taken in some countries to try to improve the currently poor situation with respect to knowledge and interest of health-care professionals regarding nutrition. For example, in the UK, a core curriculum on nutrition (covering the principles of nutritional science, public-health nutrition, clinical nutrition and nutritional support) has been designed by the National Nutrition Task Force and has been accepted by all undergraduate medical schools in the UK (Jackson, 2001). Postgraduate training is also being addressed. This is the responsibility of the Royal Colleges, who have formed an Intercollegiate Group on Nutrition (Shenkin, 2000). On an international level, FENS has initiated the development of a programme for nutrition education in medical schools (Widhalm *et al.*, 1999).

Nutrition support teams

The benefits of multidisciplinary nutrition teams have been repeatedly demonstrated (Roberts and Levine, 1992; Gales and Gales, 1994; Dhoot *et al.*, 1996; Maurer *et al.*, 1996; Schwartz, 1996; Daniels and Wright, 1997; Pattison and Young, 1997; Fettes, 2000; Ng *et al.*, 2000; Ochoa *et al.*, 2000; Ward *et al.*, 2000a,b; Newton, 2001; Scott *et al.*, 2001), in terms of:

- improved assessment of nutritional risk, nutritional status and assessment of requirements;
- increased number of patients fed successfully;
- increased number of patients fed appropriately (i.e. avoidance of over- or underfeeding, most appropriate route of feeding selected);
- reduced need for unnecessary nutrition support;
- decreased complication rates/improved safety of delivery of nutritional support;
- cost savings;
- education of other nutrition teams;

- development of protocols and standardization;
- overall improvement in quality of care.

Hospital/community liaison nurses may also be an important factor in improving clinical care (Hall and Myers, 2000).

Practice guidelines and nationally agreed standards

Many national and international societies are now taking steps to produce and implement these, e.g. BAPEN (Elia *et al.*, 1994; Silk, 1994; Wood, 1995; Pennington, 1996; Sizer, 1996; Lennard-Jones, 1998; Allison, 1999; McAtear, 1999; Elia, 2000b), the Parenteral and Enteral Group of the British Dietetic Association (Hart and Reeves, 1996; McAtear and Wright, 1996) and the American Society for Parenteral and Enteral Nutrition (ASPEN, 1993a, 2002). Implementation of guidelines can contribute to improving appropriate provision of nutrition support (Chima *et al.*, 1998; Morais *et al.*, 2000), resulting in cost savings (Chima *et al.*, 1998).

Conclusion

Dietary intake is frequently reduced in disease, especially severe disease, and is a major cause of DRM (see Fig. 3.3). In addition to the reduction in dietary intake, the variability in nutrient intake is greater than in health, which further increases the proportion of individuals who do not meet their requirements. The combination of reduced nutrient intake and increased requirements for some nutrients in disease accelerates the development of malnutrition. Extensive information on the physiological and the clinically relevant effects of providing appropriate nutritional support to increase dietary intake is discussed in subsequent chapters of this book.

4
Consequences of Disease-related Malnutrition

Introduction

An inadequate intake of food over time will result in the metabolic, body composition, physical (functional) and psychosocial changes that together constitute a state of malnutrition. In itself, this can give rise to an increased risk of disease. However, malnutrition can also be a consequence of disease, either purely as a result of impaired food intake or compounded by metabolic stress and inflammation.

Malnutrition has a diversity of effects, influencing every system of the body. Disease itself may also have an impact on body structure and function. In order to understand whether or not disease-related malnutrition (DRM) may be responsive to nutritional intervention and to underpin the rationale for providing appropriate nutritional support, it is necessary to try to dissect out and understand the specific effects of malnutrition. In theory, there are a number of models that could be used to help in understanding the process of development of DRM. To examine the effects of disease, it would be necessary to study two groups with the same degree of malnutrition: one otherwise healthy and one with disease. To examine the effects of malnutrition, it would be necessary to compare two groups with the same disease: one with normal nutritional intake/status and the other with malnutrition. In clinical practice, it is difficult to achieve such clear-cut models. However, wherever possible, an attempt has been made in this chapter to examine the effects of malnutrition in otherwise healthy individuals (uncomplicated starvation) and the associations between malnutrition and clinical outcome in the presence of disease. The main focus is on studies in humans wherever available, although in some instances it has been necessary to look at animal models where clinical data are lacking.

Of importance is the fact that malnutrition is more than a reduction in nutritional status. As already outlined in Chapter 1 of this book, there is growing recognition that nutritional intake *per se* may be at least as important as body mass and structure in maintaining normal function. Where feasible, therefore, an attempt has been made to distinguish between those studies that have examined reduced nutritional intake and those that have examined impaired nutritional status. The magnitude of nutritional intake is also important, as this will have a bearing on the extent of impairment in function and rate of weight loss.

Micronutrient intake and status may also play an important role in determining the consequences of malnutrition, although, until now, these aspects have been rather neglected. This is at least in part due to the relative complexity of assessing intakes and interpreting measures of status. This chapter will focus predominantly on protein-energy malnutrition.

Although it may be possible to determine associations between malnutrition and clinical outcome in different disease states, such data alone can never be used to describe cause and effect. Intervention studies are necessary to investigate whether or not the provision of nutritional support can reduce or avoid the potential consequences of malnutrition. Intervention studies are addressed in detail in Chapters 6–8. In these chapters, a variety of functional and clinical end-points are used. Some are rather general, such as quality of life (QOL), and others are more specific, such as respiratory function tests in patients with chronic obstructive pulmonary disease (COPD). This chapter attempts to illustrate the diversity of physical and psychological functions affected by malnutrition (many of which are used as end-points in clinical trials involving nutritional intervention) and complements Chapter 1, which primarily aims to define anthropometric cut-off points between a healthy nutritional state and the undernourished state. Furthermore, since it is sometimes difficult to separate the impact of malnutrition from disease, this chapter also attempts to describe the effects of malnutrition in the absence of disease (or in mild disease) as well as in the presence of disease.

Body Weight, Composition, Growth and Survival

Body weight and composition

The metabolic response to simple starvation (uncomplicated by disease) has been reviewed elsewhere (Elia, 2000a, 2001a). Often, the most obvious sign of poor intake is loss of body weight. Weight loss is due to loss of fat and muscle mass, including organ mass, and is characterized by shifts in body fluids. In patients with anorexia nervosa (voluntary food restriction), a decrease of both fat-free mass and fat mass has always been reported (Scalfi et al., 2002). The pattern of change in body composition during weight loss will depend on initial adiposity (Scobie, 1987; Elia, 2000a; Henry, 2001) and gender (Henry, 2001). This is probably due to differences in metabolic changes, depending on whether individuals are lean or obese at the outset of food shortage (Elia, 2000a), gender differences in the relative use of fat and protein as an energy source, and the ability to mobilize fat stores for energy, probably related to differences in adiposity between the sexes (Scobie, 1987; Umpleby et al., 1995; Dulloo, 1997a; Henry, 2001).

Calculations with the original Keys data (Keys et al., 1950) showed that the inter-individual variability in P ratio (protein energy as a proportion of the total energy gained or lost from the body) during weight loss was large, but was constant within individuals (Dulloo, 1997a). Initial percentage fat mass appeared to be the most important determinant of the P ratio (higher initial fat mass, lower proportion of protein and higher amount of fat mobilized for energy). Rate of weight loss will also be influenced by initial adiposity, with lean subjects having a higher rate of weight loss than obese subjects during fasting (Scobie, 1987; Umpleby et al., 1995) and a greater proportion of the weight lost is lean tissue (Elia, 2000a). The rate of weight loss will also influence function during food shortage, and thus the extent and nature of functional changes will be modulated according to the extent of recent dietary intake (Elia, 2000a).

A recent study found that total starvation for 4–5 days in healthy lean males resulted in a mean weight loss of 5.2% (Gibney et al., 2002a), similar to that documented in a wide range of studies in lean subjects previously summarized (Elia, 1992a). In obese subjects who fasted for 14 days, mean weight loss was 5.6% after 7 days and 9% after 14 days (Sobotka et al., 1999). Fat mass was reduced by 6.9% after 1 week and 12.6% after 2 weeks. In eight hunger strikers in Brazil (seven women, one man, mean body mass index (BMI)

26.1 kg m^{-2}) who fasted for 43 days, weight loss of 18% was observed (Soriano *et al.*, 1999; Faintuch *et al.*, 2001). Partial starvation results in a more gradual weight loss. In lean males, a very low-energy diet (595 kcal day^{-1}) over a period of 19–21 days resulted in a mean weight loss of 9% (Gibney *et al.*, 2002a). In the Keys study in the 1950s, when 32 healthy men underwent partial starvation for 24 weeks, each lost approximately 25% of initial body weight (Keys *et al.*, 1950; Dulloo, 1997a). Overall, fat mass declined to about 30% of baseline value and fat-free mass to about 82% of baseline by the end of the semi-starvation period (Dulloo, 1997b).

When intake is poor or absent for a long time (weeks), weight loss is associated with organ failure and death. A weight loss of about 18% during complete starvation has been suggested to be the point at which major physiological disturbances can be expected (Peel, 1997). Studies reviewed by Elia (2000a, 2001a) suggest that, in lean individuals, the lethal level of weight loss is about 40% during acute starvation and 50% during semi-starvation. For example, nine lean Irish hunger strikers survived for between 57 and 73 days without any food, with a mean weight loss of 38% of initial body weight (Elia, 2001a). Autopsy studies in subjects who died of starvation have shown that there is a virtual total depletion of body fat (Elia, 2001a), particularly in women (Henry, 2001), while there is a loss of only 25–50% of most other tissues and organs. The brain and skeleton are relatively well preserved (Elia, 2001a).

There have been a few case reports of obese persons undergoing a successful 'total' fast (no energy) with much longer survival times (even over a year in one case) and much larger weight loss (65–80% or more of initial body weight in severely obese individuals) (Elia, 1992a, 2000a, 2001a; Henry, 2001). Obesity can thus be of benefit for survival in situations of severe food shortage (Elia, 2000a). Even modest increases in fat stores, such as in women compared with men, can have survival advantages. A BMI below 13 kg m^{-2} in males and below 11 kg m^{-2} in females has

been suggested to be incompatible with life (Henry, 2001), although values as low as 9 have been reported in recent Somali famines (Collins, 1995). Hypothetical values of body composition, fuel availability and survival time in a lean and obese person have been proposed (Elia, 2001a).

Growth and development

In children, malnutrition will have the additional consequence of impeding growth and development, leading to stunting and/or wasting as well as possibly leading to long-term consequences for mental function (see following section). Malnutrition during fetal development and in early childhood may also predispose to chronic disease much later in life, such as cardiovascular disease, stroke and diabetes (Barker and Fall, 1993; O'Brien *et al.*, 1999). Smaller body stores in early childhood mean that the time period of survival during complete starvation is considerably shorter (approximately 32 days for a full-term baby and only 5 days for a preterm infant (Thomas, 1994)) than it is for adults (approximately 70 days (Allison, 1992; Elia, 2001a)).

Chronic malnutrition results in deficits in height-for-age (stunting), whereas acute malnutrition will result in deficits in weight-for-height (wasting) (Moy *et al.*, 1990). Children may be both stunted and wasted (Moy *et al.*, 1990). Weight-for-age is also used as an index of nutritional status in children. Results can be presented either as z scores (number of standard deviations from the mean) or as percentiles compared with published standards. There is currently no consensus with regard to the preferred method (Hendrikse *et al.*, 1997). However, it would seem that a combination of measurements, describing the different aspects of protein-energy malnutrition, would be advantageous. In the presence of oedema, conventional assessment of weight-for-height may in fact underestimate the severity of wasting. The same may apply to children with solid tumours, as the tumour may contribute 3–15% of true body weight (Smith *et al.*, 1990). Arm anthropometry may therefore be of value in nutritional assessment of some children with disease.

A number of studies have demonstrated that children with newly diagnosed cancer and a range of other diseases may be stunted and/or wasted (see Chapter 2). A few studies have described significant associations between poor nutritional status and mortality in a number of diseases in children, e.g cystic fibrosis (Corey *et al.*, 1988), human immunodeficiency virus (HIV) infection and acquired immune deficiency syndrome (AIDS) (McKinney *et al.*, 1994; Berhane *et al.*, 1997; Fontana *et al.*, 1999; Amadi *et al.*, 2001) and cancer (Deeg *et al.*, 1995; Mejia-Arangure *et al.*, 1999). Reduced duration of remission has also been linked with poor nutritional status in neuroblastoma prior to chemotherapy (see section on complications and outcome later in this chapter). Extrapolation from studies in adults and information from Third World countries also indicate that malnourished children with disease are a high-risk group for poor outcome. Timing of refeeding is an important consideration with respect to achieving adequate catch-up growth and the possibility of development of chronic disease in the longer term.

Skeletal Muscle Mass and Function

Poor food intake or total starvation leads to weight loss, of which a proportion is lean tissue. In healthy subjects, muscle function, as assessed by grip strength, is directly proportional to indices of body muscle mass (Martin *et al.*, 1985). It may therefore be expected that losses of body mass will be associated with impaired muscle function. However, although muscle mass is a major factor in determining muscle function, it is not the only factor. Of particular relevance to the rationale for nutritional support is the observation that muscle function in patients is sensitive to reductions in nutritional intake before any change in muscle mass occurs (Brough *et al.*, 1986), and return of function and strength on refeeding is more rapid than can be accounted for by tissue replacement (Jeejeebhoy, 1988a; Bourdel-Marchasson *et al.*, 2001).

In a study in which healthy women underwent 5 days of starvation, significantly lowered skeletal muscle function, assessed by grip strength and adductor pollicis muscle function, was noted, even though anthropometric indices of arm muscle did not change (Lennmarken *et al.*, 1986). In chronically starved, malnourished individuals with anorexia nervosa, electrical stimulation of the ulnar nerve demonstrated markedly abnormal muscle function compared with normal subjects (increased force of contraction at 10 Hz, slowing of maximal relaxation rate and increased muscle fatigue) (Russell *et al.*, 1983). Muscle relaxation rate and fatiguability were restored by refeeding for 4 weeks, with full restoration of function by 8 weeks, even though total body nitrogen was well below predicted normal levels. Also, the workload achieved on an ergometric bicycle by patients with anorexia nervosa was 49% lower than that achieved by age-, sex- and physical activity level (PAL)-matched healthy controls (Rigaud *et al.*, 1997). Performance was correlated with body weight, fat-free mass and leg muscle circumference. However, after 45 days of refeeding, muscle performance appeared to be restored completely, even though normal nutritional status was not achieved. Even after 8 days of refeeding, improvements in exercise capacity were noted, despite no measurable changes in fat-free mass, creatinine index or muscle circumferences.

These findings suggest that impaired muscle function during low energy intake and malnutrition could be related to several factors, apart from reduced muscle mass, and a number of possibilities have been suggested (Russell *et al.*, 1983; Church *et al.*, 1984; Legaspi *et al.*, 1988; Rigaud *et al.*, 1997; Madapallimkattam *et al.*, 2000; Bourdel-Marchasson *et al.*, 2001; Rooyackers *et al.*, 2001):

- Alterations in intracellular concentrations of electrolytes, micronutrients (e.g. carnitine) or energy-rich compounds (e.g. ATP) and/or ratios of muscle metabolites.
- Decreased insulin-stimulated glucose uptake.
- Defects in the sodium–potassium ATPase pump.
- Defects in calcium channels.
- Alterations in skeletal muscle membrane potential.
- Defects in the activity of the electron-transfer chain in muscle mitochondria due to abnormalities in complexes I, II and III.
- Partial atrophy of non-aerobic type II muscle fibres.
- Changes in the number of muscle fibres.
- Changes in activities of muscle enzymes.
- Slowing of muscle relaxation rate.

The rate of weight loss may have an influence on levels of physical activity and fatigue. In healthy lean men subjected to different rates of weight loss (total starvation for 4–5 days or a very low-energy diet for 19–21 days), physical activity energy expenditure was significantly reduced at 5% weight loss in the totally starved group, but was no different from baseline in the semi-starved (Gibney *et al.*, 2002a). In the same experiment, hand-grip fatigue, subjective feelings of fatigue and sleepiness and energy levels were reduced at 5% weight loss in both groups, with subjective feelings of fatigue and sleepiness being more pronounced in the starved group. Central fatigue (measured with critical flicker fusion) did not change in either group (Gibney *et al.*, 2002b). A reduction in PAL is probably the most important mode of energy sparing during starvation. However, this in itself may have adverse consequences for growth, exploratory behaviour and development in children, and immobility resulting in a predisposition to pressure ulcers in all age-groups, but especially the elderly.

These changes, leading to muscle weakness, impaired physical activity, poor self-care and predisposition to falls (Elia, 2001a), will have detrimental consequences in patients with disease, where a number of factors may further compound the adverse effects of poor intake and poor nutritional status. These factors include bed rest and muscle disuse (Gosker *et al.*, 2000), old age (Thorngren and Werner, 1979), inflammation and infection (Martin *et al.*, 1985; Rigaud *et al.*, 1997; Gosker *et al.*, 2000; Wagenmakers, 2001), hypoxia and oxidative stress (Gosker *et al.*, 2000) and use of sedatives and corticosteroids (Martin *et al.*, 1985; Gosker *et al.*, 2000).

Poor muscle function has been identified in a number of patient groups:

- In medical patients without malignancies, those who were malnourished had reduced grip strength, peak expiratory flow and time of ambulation (Cederholm *et al.*, 1993).
- In patients with gastrointestinal (GI) disease, grip strength was a sensitive measurement of the degree of protein loss (assessed by mid-arm muscle circumference and *in vivo* neutron activation analysis) (Windsor and Hill, 1988).
- Poorly nourished COPD patients had lower respiratory muscle and hand-grip strength, abnormal contractility and increased fatiguability of the sternomastoid muscle compared with well-nourished COPD patients (Efthimiou *et al.*, 1988).
- Preoperative patients with carcinoma of the GI tract and weight loss had reduced muscle function (force–frequency relationship in adductor pollicis muscle of the thumb) compared with patients without weight loss (Zeiderman and McMahon, 1989).
- In postoperative patients following elective abdominal surgery, those with the most pronounced weight loss and decrease in triceps skin-fold thickness had the greatest postoperative fatigue (Christensen and Kehlet, 1984).
- Nutritional status was an important predictor of muscle strength in patients undergoing chronic ambulatory peritoneal dialysis and haemodialysis (Fahal *et al.*, 1995).

- Bruce *et al.* (1989) demonstrated that, although malnourished patients (*n* 11) with chronic non-malignant diseases had normal muscle force (adductor pollicis), relaxation rate was significantly slower than in the well-nourished healthy controls tested. Similar results were documented by Lopes *et al.* (1982) in malnourished patients (*n* 10), whereby malnutrition resulted in increased muscle fatiguability and an altered pattern of contraction and relaxation.
- Malnourished elderly patients (*n* 11) had significantly lower muscle mass, inorganic phosphorus (Pi) : ATP ratio and phosphocreatine : ATP ratio than well-nourished control patients, and tended to have lower muscle strength (Bourdel-Marchasson *et al.*, 2001).
- Patients with chronic renal failure had significantly lower grip strength than that predicted by their forearm muscle area (Martin *et al.*, 1985).
- Numerous studies have shown that COPD and chronic heart failure are commonly associated with muscle weakness due to morphological and metabolic abnormalities, and poor skeletal muscle performance in these patients contributes markedly to exercise intolerance (Gosker *et al.*, 2000).

Low grip strength and arm muscle circumference have been shown to be predictive of postoperative complications in patients admitted for GI surgery (*n* 225) (Klidjian *et al.*, 1980), elective surgery (*n* 205) (Hunt *et al.*, 1985) and fractured neck of femur (*n* 76) (Twiston Davies *et al.*, 1984). Fat-free mass has been shown to be an important determinant of peripheral skeletal muscle function (Engelen *et al.*, 1994), maximum exercise performance (Kobayashi *et al.*, 2000) and walking distance (Schols *et al.*, 1993) in patients with COPD. In acute admissions to an elderly geriatric ward, lower grip strength was correlated with mortality (Phillips, 1986).

Cardiac Muscle Mass and Function

Malnutrition results in loss of cardiac muscle. Cardiac weights, measured at autopsy and size estimated radiographically, have been shown to be reduced in starvation (Heymsfield *et al.*, 1978). More recently, reduced BMI and increased age have been shown to be independently related to decreased left ventricular mass (Miján *et al.*, 2000). This in turn results in a decrease in cardiac output, bradycardia (abnormally slow heart rate) and hypotension (low blood pressure). Such physiological findings were documented by physicians in subjects who had lost up to 35% of their body weight in the Warsaw ghettos between 1940 and 1942 (Winick, 1994). Oedema and increased risk of venous thrombosis were also observed. Bradycardia, hypotension, a 45% reduction in cardiac output and other electrocardiogram (ECG) abnormalities, including prolongation of the QT interval[1] (reviewed by Winter, 2001), were also observed in the semi-starvation studies conducted by Keys *et al.* (1950). In eight Brazilian hunger strikers who fasted totally for 43 days (Ladeira *et al.*, 1999), bradycardia and syncope developed in 25% of the subjects.

Heart volume decrease is proportional to body weight loss, and is explained partly by reduced cardiac muscle mass and partly by reduced internal chamber volume (Heymsfield *et al.*, 1978). This will have an impact on exercise tolerance and renal function (by reducing renal plasma flow and glomerular filtration rate). Severe depletion may lead to peripheral circulatory failure. Specific electrolyte and vitamin deficiencies (e.g. thiamine) as a result of poor intake may also play a role in cardiac failure or arrhythmias. Once fat stores are depleted, gross fragmentation of cardiac myofibrils can occur, leading to cardiac failure and arrhythmias (Winter, 2001). Cardiac failure has been suggested to be the possible final cause of death in severe malnutrition (Winter, 2001).

Malnourished general medical patients (BMI < 18.5 kg m^{-2}) had longer corrected QT (QTc) lengths than non-malnourished patients (Cunha *et al.*, 2001). These patients also had lower serum levels of sodium, phosphorus and potassium. Malnourished patients, with a variety of underlying diagnoses leading to weight loss of > 25% of body weight, had a reduction in heart volume (measured by radiography and echo) that was proportional to the loss of body weight. Cardiac output was also reduced (Heymsfield *et al.*, 1978). Changes were reversed by nutritional support, but at different rates. Cardiac problems are also potential hazards of refeeding following severe food deprivation, due to precipitation of hypokalaemia, a sudden increase in fluid volume, overshoot of recovery of bradycardia and hypotension and prolonged QT interval/dispersion (Peel, 1997; Todd, J.A. *et al.*, 2000).

Cardiac failure can also cause weight loss and malnutrition, with the most extreme examples of cardiac cachexia arising in patients with right heart failure and tricuspid incompetence (Jeejeebhoy and Sole, 2001). It has recently been suggested that wasting in these patients is adaptive, with the key to rehabilitation lying in repletion of micronutrients rather than refeeding energy and protein (Jeejeebhoy and Sole, 2001). Further elucidation of this concept is required.

Respiratory Muscle Mass and Function

Protein depletion will adversely affect respiratory muscle structure and function, resulting in reduced mass of the diaphragm, maximal voluntary ventilation and respiratory muscle strength. Autopsy studies showed patients who had lost weight as a result of disease had significantly lower diaphragm muscle mass, thickness, area and length than persons who were clinically well until sudden death (Arora and Rochester, 1982a). Disease alone (without weight loss) did not affect these measures in this study. The diaphragm is the princi-

pal muscle of respiration, and therefore deficits in its mass can be clinically and physiologically important. Arora and Rochester (1982a) confirmed a significant linear correlation between body weight and diaphragm weight. These changes have been correlated with pulmonary function (strength, endurance and vital capacity) in patients without lung disease (Arora and Rochester, 1982b). Loss of inspiratory muscle strength has been shown to correlate with loss of body muscle in patients receiving parenteral nutrition (PN) (Kelly *et al.*, 1984). In severely malnourished subjects with anorexia nervosa, diaphragmatic contractility was severely depressed, but this impairment was completely reversed during refeeding (Murciano *et al.*, 1994). Morphological changes in the lung itself and alterations in its defence mechanisms may also occur in malnutrition (Ghignone and Quintin, 1986).

Neural ventilatory drive is also adversely affected by malnutrition. This factor can lead to an altered breathing pattern and reduced exercise tolerance, as well as altering responses to hypoxia (low oxygen levels in blood) and hypercapnia (excess carbon dioxide in blood). Doekel *et al.* (1976) semi-starved normal subjects by providing 500 kcal of carbohydrate plus electrolytes per day for 10 days. Hypoxic ventilatory response and metabolic rate were significantly reduced by day 10 and, in two subjects, hypoxic ventilation was virtually abolished. It was suggested that this may contribute to the hypoxaemia and respiratory failure seen during energy restriction. These changes reversed towards normal with refeeding.

Measures of lung function have been significantly correlated with BMI or other indices of nutritional status (particularly fat-free mass) in several patient groups, including those with cystic fibrosis (Bell *et al.*, 1998) and COPD (Engelen *et al.*, 1994; Viola *et al.*, 2000; Braulio *et al.*, 2001). Impaired respiratory function and muscle strength will have implications for cough pressure, which may predispose to and delay recovery from chest infections, reduce exercise capacity and tolerance, and delay weaning from mechanical ventilation.

Gastrointestinal Tract Structure and Function

Apart from its role in digestion, absorption and substrate redistribution, the GI tract constitutes a major immune organ, acting as a barrier to prevent entrance of microorganisms into the body. The components of the gut barrier include an intact gut mucosa, mucin, symbiotic microflora, specific secretory antibodies (e.g. secretory immunoglobulin A (IgA)) and macrophages and other immune cells in the lamina propria of the gut and other organs, such as the mesenteric lymph nodes. Adequate nutrition is important for preserving all components of gut structure and function, including digestion, absorption and the gut barrier. Methods of assessing gut absorptive and barrier function are reviewed in detail elsewhere (Debnam and Grimble, 2001; Gabe, 2001).

The intestinal mucosa is nourished from the lumen and from the circulation (Roediger, 1994). Its epithelial cells are completely renewed every 2–3 days and are thus markedly affected by the availability of nutrients, the hormonal environment (e.g. growth hormone, thyroid hormones, glucocorticoids and insulin), GI peptide release, pancreaticobiliary secretions, intestinal blood flow, innervation, changes in motility and intracellular polyamine mobilization (Jackson and Grand, 1991; Raul and Schleiffer, 1996). The most important stimulus for mucosal cell proliferation is the presence of nutrients in the lumen, which has both direct or mechanical effects (e.g. desquamation of cells) and indirect effects (e.g. stimulation of hormones, growth factors and intestinal secretions).

The lining of the gut is sensitive to changes in nutrient supply in the lumen. The healthy GI tract appears capable of responding to large increases in nutrient supply – for example, under conditions of extreme endurance when energy needs may be tremendously increased (Debnam and Grimble, 2001). However, changes may also occur when food intake is limited or completely absent. Partial or complete starvation may have different effects on the gut, as may the duration of the period of food deprivation and the resulting impairment of nutritional status. Furthermore, luminal and systemic starvation can occur separately, e.g. a patient may receive complete nutritional support via the intravenous route to maintain nutritional status, but may receive no nutrients via the enteral route. Alternatively, a subject may be chronically depleted, but may maintain a minimal enteral intake. In addition, the diet may not contain all the necessary nutrients to maintain the health of the length of the GI tract. Finally, the presence or absence of disease may also have an impact on the gut. These are all factors that should be borne in mind when reviewing studies that have examined the effects of inadequate intake on the gut.

Effects of acute and chronic food deprivation in the absence of disease

Changes in GI structure are much less apparent in situations of chronic energy restriction (Ferraris and Carey, 2000). Even though body weight may be decreased dramatically, effects on intestinal structure are relatively modest. This suggests that effects on intestinal structure are closely linked to loss of luminal nutrition rather than to the metabolic consequences of malnutrition *per se*.

Few studies on the effects of acute or chronic food deprivation have been performed in human subjects, presumably because of the relatively inaccessible nature of the GI tract, and perhaps because the possible consequences of lack of use of the gut have not been fully appreciated until relatively recently. In otherwise well-nourished healthy volunteers, short-term lack of luminal nutrition resulted in reduced absorption in the small intestine (measured using D-xylose and 3-0-methyl glucose), which was already detectable after 36 h (Maxton *et al.*, 1989). Absorption was also progressively reduced in two obese patients starved for 11 days (Maxton *et al.*, 1989). Similar findings (measured using mannitol) were seen in lean and obese subjects starved for 4–5 days (Elia *et al.*, 1987). Changes in intestinal permeability were seen in one study (Elia *et al.*, 1987) but not in the other (Maxton *et al.*, 1989). Total starvation for 4–5 days did not have a significant effect on transit time (Elia *et al.*, 1987). Eight Brazilian hunger strikers, who fasted totally for 43 days (Ladeira *et al.*, 1999), all reported nausea and vomiting, one developed haemorrhagic gastritis of moderate severity and three developed diarrhoea.

Adverse effects of malnutrition may not be confined to the stomach, small intestine and colon. In elderly people, atrophic glossitis (absence of papillae in more than 50% of the tongue) has been correlated with a number of measures of nutritional status (Bøhmer and Mowé, 2000). Furthermore, specific micronutrient deficiencies, such as riboflavin, may have an influence on morphology in the small intestine. Rat studies have shown that this may be particularly profound and difficult to reverse if the deficiencies occur during the early stages of development of the GI tract (Williams *et al.*, 1995, 1996; Yates *et al.*, 1997).

Most information on this topic has been derived from animal models and is the subject of a recent extensive review (Ferraris and Carey, 2000). The most apparent effect of acute food deprivation in the small intestine is a reduction in absorptive surface area. This seems to be linked to changes at the villus level, including decreased villus height and decreased number of cells along the crypt–villus axis, probably due to reduced cell proliferation and migration rates and increased rate of cell loss and apoptosis. Paradoxically, under these circumstances, rates of nutrient absorption are enhanced when normalized to absorptive cell mass. Ferraris and Carey (2000) speculated that this may be a benefit to survival by reducing the proportion of energy and nutrients required to maintain a fully functional gut (under normal circumstances, the small intestine is responsible for 17–25% of total body oxygen consumption), thereby

sparing these resources for other more important needs. Meanwhile, adaptive mechanisms come into play that are able to maximize nutrient absorption, possibly including an increase in the proportion of transporting to non-transporting cells along the shortened crypt–villus axis, an increase in expression of nutrient transporters and alterations in electrochemical gradients across the brush-border membrane.

An increase in intestinal secretion of ions and fluid and in intestinal permeability is also characteristic of food deprivation. Ferraris and Carey (2000) proposed that the secretory effect could be a secondary (deleterious) effect resulting from the adaptive response to increase nutrient absorption, ensuring that, even with reduced concentrations of certain luminal nutrients and loss of absorptive surface area, nutrient uptake could still occur against substantial concentration gradients. The increased secretion and permeability (which could allow passage of bacteria and endotoxin from the gut lumen) could help to explain the diarrhoea and higher incidence of diarrhoeal diseases that are seen in areas where malnutrition is common. The large bowel also appears to lose its ability to reabsorb water and electrolytes during starvation (Rolandelli *et al.*, 1990; Roediger, 1994; Lara and Jacobs, 1998), and there is also stimulation of colonic secretion. Diarrhoea is associated with a high mortality rate in severe starvation (Roediger, 1994).

Effects of acute and chronic food deprivation in the presence of disease

In developing countries, inadequate food availability is frequently associated with gut disorders, although how much of this is due to poor nutrition and how much to poor hygiene, infection and inflammation are difficult to determine. Studies of gut function in asymptomatic volunteers from different countries have shown that intestinal permeability is significantly higher and absorptive capacity significantly lower in subjects in the tropics compared with subjects in subtropical and temperate countries (Menzies *et al.*, 1999). In the UK, Indian and Afro-Caribbean immigrant groups have been shown to have higher intestinal permeability and lower villus height/mucosal thickness ratios than the native white population living in the same area (Iqbal *et al.*, 1996). In both studies, environmental rather than genetic factors were suggested to be the cause.

In The Gambia, 43% of observed growth faltering in the first 15 months of life was related to the presence of a mucosal enteropathy in the small intestine (Lunn, 2000). Factors involved in its initiation and persistence are unclear, but pathogens, food allergens or toxins are thought to be a more likely explanation than nutritional deficiencies. There is also a relationship between the presence of the enteropathy and the circulating concentration of endotoxin antibodies and acute-phase proteins. This raises the possibility that a breakdown in the gut barrier function allows endotoxin and other 'toxins' to enter the systemic circulation to produce an inflammatory response and growth failure. The enteropathy is characterized by villus atrophy, reduced absorption and digestion of lactose and possibly of other nutrients and increased translocation of macromolecules into the mucosa and blood, triggering local and systemic inflammation. In children with diarrhoea in Brazil, the *z* score for weight-for-age and weight-for-height indices showed a positive correlation with small intestinal villus height, total mucosal thickness and villus/crypt ratio (Pires *et al.*, 1999). In Jamaica, severely malnourished children have been shown to have impaired hydrolysis of retinyl palmitate and malabsorption of dietary lipid, both of which improve with refeeding (Murphy *et al.*, 2001a,b).

Injury or stress may compound the adverse effects of inadequate food intake on the GI tract. The gut is acutely damaged by a decrease in mesenteric blood flow, a situation that occurs in association with operative procedures and injury. Susceptibility to ischaemia–reperfusion injury and reduced vitality of kidney, heart and liver are dramatically increased by overnight

fasting compared with *ad libitum* feeding in animal models (Boelens *et al.*, 2001; Bouritius *et al.*, 2001), although longer fasts may have a protective effect (Langkamp-Henken *et al.*, 1995a). Other factors occurring as a result of trauma also negatively influence intestinal structure, including altered mucus output, acid secretion, bile secretion and gut motility (Rolandelli *et al.*, 1990). Damaged villi expose underlying intracellular structures to the damaging effects of pancreatic enzymes (Bounous, 1989), leading to further abnormalities. Such changes lead to alterations in the normal endogenous gut flora and allow small intestinal Gram-negative overgrowth (Berg, 1983).

Several studies have been performed in undernourished patients with a variety of underlying pathologies. Probably the most extensive study to date in severely malnourished patients (average BMI 13.4 kg m^{-2}) has recently been reported (Winter *et al.*, 2000). The strength of this study lies in its comparison with healthy controls using the same techniques and in its examination of the effects of refeeding in the undernourished patients. Of the 14 patients, duodenal histology showed various degrees of villus blunting and atrophy in six (43%). Xylose absorption was impaired, and stool frequency and faecal fat were raised compared with controls. Mean maximal gastric acid output and mean amylase, lipase and trypsin outputs were all significantly reduced. Pancreatic endocrine function, however, appeared to be preserved. Although some of the patients did have underlying primary intestinal pathology, this did not appear to explain the results seen when compared with patients without underlying gut pathology. Furthermore, improvements with refeeding were seen in all patients for all measures, except for trypsin output, which remained significantly impaired. More details on pancreatic secretion in severely malnourished patients have been reported separately (Winter, 2001). In another study, patients with moderate nutritional depletion had a dramatic reduction in pancreatic exocrine function after major abdominal surgery, which was thought to be related to the postoperative fasted state rather than the surgical procedure (Sagar *et al.*, 1994). Furthermore, malnourished patients (*n* 31) have been demonstrated to have increased intestinal permeability in association with mucosal immunological activation and raised circulating interleukin 6 (IL-6), compared with well-nourished controls. There was no evidence of increased endotoxin exposure (Welsh *et al.*, 1997). Similar findings with regard to intestinal permeability were demonstrated by Van der Hulst *et al.* (1998), although in this study depletion was not associated with the number of immune cells or proliferating index. Villus height was decreased and correlated with percentage of ideal weight and percentage of fat-free mass.

Effect of route of feeding

The effect of lack of oral intake on gut structure and function during PN is controversial (Spitz *et al.*, 1993; Lipman, 1998; MacFie, 2000b). In healthy volunteers receiving total PN for 14 days, Buchman *et al.* (1995a) demonstrated significant decreases in total mucosal thickness (related to villus height) and villus cell count and increased intracellular oedema and gut permeability, but no effect on intestinal immune function (Buchman *et al.*, 1995b). In two adult patients requiring long-term PN, duodenal villus height and crypt depth were decreased compared with those in control subjects (Pironi *et al.*, 1994). In patients with chronic pancreatitis receiving PN compared with similar patients receiving enteral nutrition (EN), Groos *et al.* (1996) showed a decrease in thickness of the jejunal mucosa as a result of decreased villus height and a remodelling of the epithelium and lamina propria. In contrast, Guedon *et al.* (1986) could not detect gross morphological changes in duodenal mucosa after 21 days of PN, and Sedman *et al.* (1995) showed no difference in mucosal atrophy between patients who received PN or EN preoperatively.

In healthy volunteers, intravenous nutrients do not appear to stimulate the synthesis of pancreatic and mucosal proteins (O'Keefe *et al.*, 1998), but others have shown that PN preserves pancreatic exocrine function in patients (Sagar *et al.*, 1994).

Gall bladder sludge or gallstone formation has been linked to route of feeding, probably related to insufficient stimulation of gall bladder contraction with PN (Onizuka *et al.*, 2001). However, in this respect, the mode of enteral feeding also seems to be important; in infants, continuous enteral feeding led to an enlarged noncontractile gall bladder, which emptied immediately on bolus feeding (Jawaheer *et al.*, 2001). Lack of enteral stimulation may also lead to profound decrements in biliary lipid concentrations, which have been hypothesized to impair hepatic lipid metabolism (de Vree *et al.*, 1999).

Similar controversy surrounds the effects of enteral formulations on gut morphology, with some human studies showing that EN can restore impaired morphology (Buchman *et al.*, 1995a) and maintain normal morphology (Maxton *et al.*, 1989), while others have failed to show an improvement (Cummins *et al.*, 1995) or have even demonstrated an inability to maintain a normal situation (Hoensch *et al.*, 1984). A comprehensive review of this subject concluded that there was no evidence to suggest that PN is detrimental compared with EN in this respect (Lipman, 1998). In this case, composition of formulas (enteral and parenteral) may be of greater importance than the route of feeding, e.g. inclusion of glutamine in parenteral solutions (Van Acker *et al.*, 2000) and fibre in enteral formulas (Green, 2001b).

The concept of 'minimal EN' (i.e. small amounts of EN in conjunction with PN) as a means of maintaining gut structure and function during PN is growing in popularity for adult patients (Spitz *et al.*, 1993; Babineau and Blackburn, 1994; Sax *et al.*, 1996) and for preterm infants and neonates (Spitz *et al.*, 1993; Jawaheer *et al.*, 1996; Okada *et al.*, 1998; McClure and Newell, 2000). However, the amount of

EN that is necessary to maintain adequate gut morphology and function in these circumstances is not yet known. Elia et al. (1987) suggested that as little as 300 kcal day^{-1} of a mixed diet in obese individuals was necessary to prevent the change in intestinal permeability produced by total starvation. In rats, a replacement of 25% of nutrient needs by EN in conjunction with PN failed to demonstrate any appreciable benefit on jejunal atrophy or immunity of the gut assessed by CD2+ cell count and CD4/CD8 ratio (Heel et al., 1998). In piglets, a minimum of 40% of total nutrient intake needed to be given via the gut to increase jejunal mucosal mass, while > 60% EN was needed to sustain normal proliferation and growth (Burrin et al., 2000). Whether this level could be decreased by provision of a more appropriate enteral formula containing polymeric nutrients and fibre is unclear from these animal studies. In neonates requiring PN, 1 ml kg^{-1} milk boluses (frequency not indicated) resulted in a significant reduction in gall bladder size after 2 days (Jawaheer et al., 1996). Small milk boluses also stimulated surges in plasma concentrations of gut hormones in preterm infants receiving PN (Lucas et al., 1986).

Clinical significance of changes in gut structure and function during malnutrition and nutritional support

The clinical significance of changes in intestinal morphology and function seen during starvation and nutritional support remains unclear in view of the large reserve in GI function even in patients with moderately impaired GI function due to bowel disease (Rees et al., 1992). However, audits of the use of nutritional support in hospitals suggest that diarrhoea is the most common complication associated with enteral feeding (Payne-James et al., 1990, 1992). Enteral feeding-related diarrhoea is multifactorial in origin, and it is not known how much it can be attributed to alterations of the GI tract due to prior intralumi-

nal starvation. In light of the above, however, it is not unreasonable to consider this as a possibility in patients who have undergone a period of inadequate intake (Winter et al., 2000).

It has also been suggested that changes in gut structure may result in increased permeability and subsequent translocation of endotoxin and bacteria, defined as the passage of viable indigenous bacteria or bacterial products from the GI tract to the mesenteric lymph nodes and other organs (Berg, 1983). Changes in intestinal permeability have been noted in patients in the following groups:

- burns (Ziegler et al., 1988);
- sepsis (Johnston et al., 1996);
- critical illness (Harris et al., 1992; Hadfield et al., 1995; Gabe et al., 1998a,c; Kohout, 2001);
- multiple trauma (Pape et al., 1994; Langkamp-Henken et al., 1995b);
- acute liver failure (Gabe et al., 1998b, c);
- liver transplant (Wicks et al., 1994);
- upper gastrointestinal surgery (Dave et al., 1996; Davies et al., 1997; Reynolds et al., 1997; Kanwar et al., 1998a; Brooks et al., 1999);
- cardiopulmonary bypass (Ohri et al., 1993);
- major vascular surgery (Roumen et al., 1993);
- inflammatory bowel disease (Hollander et al., 1986; Van der Hulst et al., 1993; Oriishi et al., 1995; Teahon et al., 1996; Arnott et al., 2000);
- malignancy (Van der Hulst et al., 1993; Ryan et al., 1995);
- neonates on extracorporeal membrane oxygenation (ECMO) (Piena et al., 1998);
- children with acute shigellosis (Alam et al., 1994).

Of the studies that examined the effects of nutritional support on intestinal permeability, these changes have been shown to be influenced by route of nutritional support in some studies (Davies et al., 1997) but not in others (Wicks et al., 1994; Reynolds et al., 1997; Piena et al., 1998; Brooks et al., 1999). Furthermore, intestinal permeability may be influenced by fluid balance (Bruins *et al.*, 1998; Hallameesch *et al.*, 1998). Changes in permeability have been associated with the development of sepsis and systemic inflammation in some studies (Ziegler *et al.*, 1988; Pape *et al.*, 1994) and in heightened exposure to endotoxin (Gabe *et al.*, 1998a,c; Reynolds *et al.*, 1997), but not in all (Kanwar *et al.*, 1998b). Bacterial translocation has been shown to occur in clinical situations where the gut is damaged, especially in the presence of GI obstruction, and in this study its presence was associated with increased incidence of septic complications (O'Boyle *et al.*, 1997). However, as yet there is no evidence for direct relationships between altered morphology and increased permeability or between increased permeability and translocation (Saadia, 1995; Dave *et al.*, 1996; Buchman, 1998; O'Boyle *et al.*, 1998). Furthermore, the mechanisms and clinical significance of translocation remain unclear (Lipman, 1995; Buchman, 1998). There is no evidence to suggest that EN is more or less beneficial than PN with respect to preventing or promoting bacterial translocation in patients (Lipman, 1998). However, the presence of nutrients in the gut lumen resulting in a range of physiological responses, including hormone secretion, is thought to be the most important stimulus for intestinal mucosal growth and function (Lara and Jacobs, 1998).

Immune System and Function

The immune system is a highly complex and interactive network of lymphoid organs (lymph nodes, spleen, mucosal-associated lymphoid tissues), cells, humoral factors and cytokines, the primary function of which is to protect the body against foreign invaders. These are known as antigens and include bacteria, viruses, fungi, parasites or portions of products of these antigens (non-self cells) and self cells that have been modified by viruses, cancer or autoimmune disease. The immune system can essentially be divided into two parts, namely the innate and the adaptive responses (see Table 4.1), although in practice there is much interaction between them (Kuby, 1992; Parkin and Cohen, 2001).

Innate immunity includes four types of defensive barriers:

- Anatomical barriers, which include physical barriers (skin and mucous membranes, ciliated epithelial cells) and microbiological factors (i.e. the intestinal flora, which acts as 'colonization resistance' to pathogens).
- Physiological barriers, which include temperature, oxygen tension and secretions (e.g. saliva, tears, gastric and mucous secretions containing lysozyme, gastric acid, peroxidases and/or hydroxylases).
- Endocytosis and phagocytosis, which refer to the ingestion of extracellular macromolecules. In endocytosis, macromolecules contained within the extracellular tissue fluid are internalized by cells, through either pinocytosis or receptor-mediated endocytosis. Endocytosis is carried out by practically all cells. Phagocytosis is the ingestion of particulate material, including whole pathogenic microorganisms. Only specialized cells are capable of phagocytosis. Phagocytic cells include blood monocytes, neutrophils and tissue macrophages.
- The inflammatory response, which is induced if tissue damage occurs. Blood flow to the affected area increases, capillary permeability is increased and influx of phagocytic cells occurs. These events are initiated by a complex series of interactions involving several chemical mediators.

Acute-phase proteins (see subsequent section) and cytokines also play an important role in innate defences.

Acquired immunity is characterized by specificity, diversity, memory and self/non-self recognition. The major groups of cells involved are lymphocytes (mainly B and T cells) and antigen-presenting cells (see Table 4.1).

Table 4.1. An overview of components of the immune system (adapted from Shronts, 1993; Parkin and Cohen, 2001).

Category	Elements	Characteristics
Innate response (non-adaptive or natural immunity) • First line of defence • Not antigen-specific, i.e. does not require sensitization • Can discriminate foreign molecules from self • Requires exposure to the surface of the microbe • Of main value in eradicating extra-cellular organisms, mostly bacteria • Rapid but non-specific, poorly targeted response • Not enhanced by repetition • Can lead to indiscriminate tissue damage	Phagocytes (monocytes, macrophages and granulocytes)	Large cells that engulf and digest antigens. There are several types, including monocytes, macrophages and granulocytes (also known as polymorphonuclear leucocytes). Monocytes migrate to the tissues via the circulation, where they develop into macrophages. Both of these types of cells are activated via lymphokine receptors on their surface. After digestion and processing of antigens, macrophages can present antigens to T cells. Macrophages are present in many organs, including lung, liver, kidney and brain. Neutrophils, eosinophils, mast cells and basophils are all examples of granulocytes (see below)
	Neutrophils	Mobile cells that home to a site of infection aided by proinflammatory mediators, adhesion molecules, chemoattractants and chemokines, resulting in phagocytosis and killing of pathogenic organisms. Opsonization of the particle with specific antibody or complement improves ingestion and killing 100-fold
	Eosinophils	Main role is in protection from parasitic (mainly nematode) infection. Antigen-specific IgE produced in response to infection coats the organism, to which eosinophils bind. Large granules, which are highly cytotoxic, are released on to the organism. Tend not to have a major role in innate immunity in developed countries
	Mast cells and basophils	Relatively few in number but are involved in some of the most severe immunological reactions. Mast cells are found in the mucosa (T mast cells, containing trypsin) and in the connective tissue (containing trypsin and chymotrypsin). Basophils are morphologically similar, are found in blood and bear high-affinity receptors for a subtype of IgE. Cross-linking to these receptors results in degranulation and release of preformed mediators, e.g. vasoactive amines, histamine and serotonin, and membrane-derived mediators, such as leucotrienes and prostaglandins
	Complement	At least 20 serum glycoproteins activated in a cascade sequence, with amplification steps. There are three pathways of complement activation (classical pathway, started by antibody binding to antigen, alternative pathway, started by C3b binding to activating surface, and mannan-binding lectin pathway, started by binding of mannan–binding lectin to mannose residues). All three converge to a final common pathway, resulting in a number of actions, including cell lysis, opsonic action and a targeting role within the specific immune response
	Natural killer cells	Have the morphology of lymphocytes but do not have a specific antigen receptor. Recognize abnormal cells by binding antibody-coated targets (leading to antibody-dependent cellular toxicity) or by binding to cells which do not bind to their surface receptors for MHC class I (host cells are MHC class I-positive). In the event that this receptor is not bound, perforins are secreted, which cause breaks in the cell membrane, through which granzymes are injected, which cause apoptosis in the target
	Cytokines	Low-molecular-weight messengers secreted by virtually all cells and which send intracellular signals to modify cell behaviour by binding to specific cell-surface receptors. Different cytokines have different functions, including effects on white cells (interleukins), chemoattractant activity (chemokines), differentiation and proliferation of stem cells (colony-stimulating factors) and interference with viral cell replication (interferons)
	Acute-phase proteins	Proteins that are synthesized in the liver in response to tissue injury. Play an important role in limiting tissue damage, encouraging and enhancing the scavenging process and promoting repair and healing

| Specific (adaptive) immunity
• Antigen-specific
• More precise
• Slower response (days or weeks)
• Retains 'memory' of previous exposure, allowing a more vigorous and effective response on second exposure to an antigen | T cells (cell-mediated immunity) | T cells begin their development in the bone marrow and undergo further development and selection in the thymus. Cells with a T-cell receptor that recognizes self MHC are positively selected, while T cells that react with self antigens are deleted by apoptosis (negative selection). Presentation and recognition of antigen lead to cell priming, activation and differentiation, which normally occur in the lymphoid tissue. The effector response takes place by the T cells leaving the lymphoid tissue and homing to the disease site. The armed effector cells are CD4 Th1 inflammatory cells, which activate macrophages, CD4 Th2 cells, which help antibody responses, and CD8 cytotoxic cells |
| | B cells (humoral immunity, or antibody-related immunity) | B cells develop in the bone marrow, and then most remain in the lymphoid tissue, where they are presented with antigens. These lymphocytes have membrane-bound antibody receptors and they can bind specific antigens that have entered the body. Binding of a specific antigen to these receptors finally results in differentiation of the cell into memory cells and plasma cells. Subsequently, these plasma cells can produce and secrete specific antibodies. The effector response is either T-cell-dependent or independent, but in both cases involves secretion of antibody (immunoglobulin) into blood and tissue fluids, which ultimately reaches the infective focus. Antibodies neutralize toxins, immobilize bacteria, prevent organisms adhering to or penetrating mucosal surfaces, agglutinate or opsonize bacteria for phagocytosis, sensitize tumour and infected cells for antibody-dependent cytotoxic attack by killer cells, and activate complement. There are different classes of antibody that predominate at different sites of the body (IgM in the intravascular compartment, IgG in the serum and tissues and IgA in secretions such as saliva, tears, GI and respiratory secretions, IgE in small quantities in plasma and tissues and on surface membranes of basophils and mast cells) |

MHC, major histocompatibility complex.

Innate immunity constitutes the immediate and first line of defence against invading organisms and is characteristic of even the simplest animals (Parkin and Cohen, 2001). In contrast, the adaptive response is more precise, slower to develop and retains a memory resulting in a more vigorous and rapid response on second exposure to an antigen. This aspect of immunity is seen only in higher animals (Parkin and Cohen, 2001). The immune system regulates itself by means of T lymphocytes (helper and suppressor cells) and soluble products (cytokines) and through interaction with other bodily systems, such as the neuroendocrine system, and via behavioural factors (Ader *et al.*, 1995).

Effects of acute and chronic food deprivation in the absence of disease

Malnutrition affects nearly all aspects of the immune defence system (Dominioni and Dionigi, 1987; Christou, 1990), but seems to have particular impact on the cellular immune system (Cunningham-Rundles, 1998). Apart from work in animal models, in the human setting much of this information has been derived from studies in malnourished children in developing countries, and some in patients with anorexia nervosa. Although it is not always possible to exclude the impact of a certain amount of disease activity, effects that have been ascribed to malnutrition *per se* include (Dominioni and Dionigi, 1987; Lesourd and Mazari, 1997; Rikimaru *et al.*, 1998; Chandra, 1999; Nagata *et al.*, 1999; Prentice, 1999; Bodger and Heatley, 2001):

- Increased binding of bacteria to nasopharyngeal and buccal epithelial cells *in vitro*.
- Altered quantity and quality of mucus maintained on epithelial surfaces.
- Altered expression of membrane glycoprotein receptors.
- Altered monocyte phagocytic activity.
- Impairments of phagocytosis, chemotaxis and intracellular destruction of bacteria.

- Reduced polymorphonuclear function.
- Reduced complement activity.
- Reduced natural killer cell activity.
- Suppressed acute-phase response.
- Involution of the thymus.
- Reduced weight, size, structure and cellular components of other lymphoid tissues, e.g. tonsils, lymph nodes, spleen.
- Reduced number of T lymphocytes, reduced proliferation and reduced responses to mitogens.
- Reduced production of T-cell and proinflammatory cytokines.
- Altered proportions of critical subsets of lymphocytes, e.g. CD4/CD8 ratio.
- Reduced proportion of B cells.
- Reduced secretory antibody response and antibody affinity.
- Anergy to vaccinations, poor primary recall and delayed cutaneous hypersensitivity responses.

Much of the information examining the link between malnutrition and immune function has focused on energy and protein. However, many specific nutrient deficiencies may also have an impact on immune function, shown mainly in animal models (Kubena and McMurray, 1996; Chandra, 1999; Lesourd and Mazari, 1999; Bodger and Heatley, 2001). This not only may have an impact on the host immune response, but may even predispose to viral mutagens, which could increase viral pathogenicity (Beck, 2001). The effect of short-term food deprivation on parameters of immune function has not been well researched. Production of several cytokines (IL-1, IL-6, tumour necrosis factor alpha (TNF-α), granulocyte colony-stimulating factor (G-CSF) and interferon gamma (IFN-γ)) was impaired in patients with anorexia nervosa, and refeeding was able to restore most of these deficits, although this was not correlated with weight gain. This suggested that actual food intake, or other factors, may be more important than body weight *per se* (Nagata *et al.*, 1999). Others have also shown reversal of impairments in T-lymphocyte subpopulations and cell-mediated immunity with nutritional supplementation in elderly subjects (Chandra *et al.*, 1982).

Effects of acute and chronic food deprivation in the presence of disease

In patients, there are many other factors apart from nutritional status that may influence immune function. These include the specific disease state, which may have a primary effect on aspects of immune function, infection and inflammation, tissue trauma, burns, sepsis, anaesthetic/surgical procedures, stress hormones, malignancy and drug therapy (Januszkiewicz *et al.*, 1998; Bodger and Heatley, 2001). Age itself may also have an impact on immune status, although how much of this is linked to nutritional deficits is unclear (Lesourd, 1999; Lesourd and Mazari, 1999). Animal studies also indicate that hyperglycaemia may have an impact on some phagocytic cells (Kwoun *et al.*, 1997). In some cases, even application of nutritional support in the form of PN may have an adverse effect on aspects of the immune response (Alverdy and Burke, 1992; Okada *et al.*, 1997).

Impairments in immune function associated with nutritional status have been demonstrated in a variety of patient groups:

- Malnourished patients with inoperable carcinoma of the oesophagus had a negative skin-test reaction to dinitrochlorobenzene (DNCB), signficantly depressed absolute lymphocyte counts and T-lymphocyte numbers and depressed mitogenic response to phytohaemagglutinin. IgA levels were raised but serum complement levels were normal (Haffejee and Angorn, 1979).
- Malnourished patients with hepatocellular carcinoma (*n* 16) had lower phagocytic and bacterial activities of neutrophils and a lower percentage of natural killer cells than healthy controls (Iida *et al.*, 1999). Within the patient group the greatest deficits were seen in the most severely malnourished.
- Patients with squamous-cell carcinomas of the head and neck (*n* 53) displayed a highly significant positive correlation between nutritional status and both delayed hypersensitivity response to an antigen and pretreatment total lymphocyte count levels (Brookes and Clifford, 1981).

- In similarly malnourished patients (*n* 32), others have shown significantly lower human leucocyte antigen (HLA)-DR expression on monocytes (class II major histocompatibility antigens, which play a crucial role in mounting antigen-specific immunoresponses to microorganisms) compared with well-nourished patients (*n* 34) and healthy controls (*n* 43) (Van Bokhorst-de van der Schueren *et al.*, 1998).
- In patients undergoing elective major laparotomy (*n* 166), anergy and relative anergy were more often associated with abnormal anthropometric measurements than was normal skin-test reactivity (Ausobosky *et al.*, 1982).
- In patients undergoing elective major surgery (*n* 244), significant associations were found between depressed skin reactions (found in 28% of patients) and increasing age, anaemia, hypoalbuminaemia, low arm-muscle circumference and low weight (Brown *et al.*, 1982).
- Malnourished surgical patients had reduced monocyte major histocompatibility complex class II expression in response to IFN-γ and a significant reduction in the number of bacteria phagocytosed per cell compared with well-nourished age- and disease-matched control patients. Expression of monocyte major histocompatibility complex class II was directly correlated with the severity of malnutrition (Welsh *et al.*, 1996).
- In a small pilot study of malnourished patients with upper GI obstruction, apoptosis of T lymphocytes in peripheral blood was significantly increased compared with that in well-nourished patient controls (Kalfarentzos and Tsamandas, 1999).
- Malnourished men (*n* 26) admitted to general medical/surgical services had a significantly depressed lymphocyte response to phytohaemagglutinin than a well-nourished group. Those who were older than 65 years (*n* 10) also had lower neutrophil chemotaxis (Linn, 1984).

- Malnourished patients (n 16) had lower mitochondrial enzyme activity in lymphocytes than in healthy controls (Twomey *et al.*, 1999). Complex 1 activity was correlated with body weight, BMI and percentage weight loss. Implementation of nutrition support resulted in a rapid rise in complex 1 activity without any measurable change in nutrition assessment parameters, indicating that food intake is more relevant to this parameter than body weight *per se* (Briet *et al.*, 1999; Twomey *et al.*, 2000). The relationship between complex 1 and markers of nutritional status seems to be preserved even in the presence of active disease (Briet *et al.*, 2000).
- In elderly in-patients (n 482), there was a significant correlation between the hypersensitivity skin test and anthropometric measurements (Ek *et al.*, 1990).
- Chronically ill malnourished elderly patients (n 19) had significantly lower polymorphonuclear neutrophil superoxide anion formation than age-matched healthy controls (Cederholm and Gyllenhammar, 1999).
- Monocytes from chronically malnourished patients (n 18) cultured *in vitro* with *Staphylococcus epidermidis* were less able to produce cytokines and induce a febrile response when injected into rabbits when compared with those from healthy controls (Kauffman *et al.*, 1986).

In contrast to the above studies, Dowd *et al.* (1986) failed to show an effect of severity of overall malnutrition on several aspects of the cellular immune response in malnourished patients (n 70) with a variety of malignant and non-malignant diseases, although they suggested that certain individual nutrients, such as vitamin C and zinc, may influence the immunoreactivity of lymphocyte subpopulations. In patients with chronic renal failure receiving haemodialysis, there was no correlation between cutaneous anergy and malnutrition, although this could perhaps in part be explained by inadequate techniques for assessing malnutrition in this population (Bansal *et al.*, 1980). Furthermore, dialysis itself may have an impact on cutaneous anergy (Mattern *et al.*, 1982).

Clinical consequences of impaired immune function

Changes in immune function result in a reduced ability to prevent, fight and recover from infection. Typical infections in undernourished populations include tuberculosis, herpes, *Pneumocystis carinii* pneumonia and measles, which are all caused by intracellular pathogens (Cunningham-Rundles, 1998). In eight previously healthy subjects who fasted totally for 43 days (Ladeira *et al.*, 1999), white blood cell count dropped below 4.0 g l^{-1} and lymphocytes dropped below 1.0 g l^{-1} in 87.5% of the subjects. Overt respiratory infection occurred in one subject, herpes simplex in two and herpes zoster in one.

Despite the large body of evidence suggesting that malnutrition has detrimental effects on immune function and susceptibility to infection, there are some who challenge this concept, arguing that when seen on an evolutionary basis, this would seem counterproductive and that depressed immune function in undernourished states might be caused by concomitant infection (Morgan, 1997). A recent study in a large cohort of moderately malnourished Gambian children failed to show any correlation between weight-for-age z scores and various parameters of immune function (cell-mediated immunity, response to T-cell- or B-cell-mediated vaccination or mucosal immunity as assessed by gut permeability) (Moore *et al.*, 2001). Interestingly, in patients with eating disorders such as anorexia nervosa, existence of multiple impairments of the immune system similar to those seen in simple malnutrition have been described, although, in general, these are less severe and less frequent than would be expected considering the extent of impairment of nutritional status. Furthermore, these patients remain relatively free of severe infection (Marcos, 1997). Possible explanations for these findings include individual variability of actual intake of macro- and micronutrients, and the concept that starvation may suppress certain infections (Murray and Murray, 1977; Marcos, 1997).

Some studies have attempted to link measures of immune function with outcome. In patients with biliary lithiasis (*n* 216), there was a close correlation between relatively anergic or anergic state and development of postoperative septic complications (Cainzos *et al.*, 1989). Nutritional status was not assessed in this study. In elderly in-patients, anergy was associated with a higher mortality rate and more pressure ulcers (Ek *et al.*, 1990). In patients undergoing arthroplasty (hip or knee replacement), those with low total lymphocyte counts (TLC < 1200 cells μl^{-1}) had longer anaesthetic and surgical times, longer hospital stays and higher hospital charges than patients with TLC > 1200 cells μl^{-1} (Lavernia *et al.*, 1999). In patients with hip fractures (*n* 490), a TLC of < 1500 cells μl^{-1} was predictive of 1-year mortality (Koval *et al.*, 1999). However, others were unable to demonstrate a correlation between immune function and outcome in surgical patients (Ausobosky *et al.*, 1982; Brown *et al.*, 1982).

Acute-phase protein response

Tissue injury (e.g. due to major trauma, burns, surgery, damage to cardiac muscle during a myocardial infarction, infection, exacerbations of inflammatory diseases, malignant neoplasia) results in a complex series of systemic metabolic and physiological processes, including fever, leucocytosis, metabolism of muscle proteins and a large increase in the *de novo* synthesis of a number of plasma proteins. The latter is known as the acute-phase response or acute-phase protein response. Most of these proteins are synthesized by the hepatocytes in the liver. The plasma levels of most are increased, but, in some cases, a decrease is observed (see Table 4.2).

Levels of acute-phase proteins start to change around 6–8 h after trauma and peak (or dip) a few days later, e.g. 2–4 days after elective surgery (Stahl, 1987; Elia, 2001a). IL-6 is thought to be important in mediating this process; levels of this cytokine rise and peak before the acute-phase proteins change (Elia, 2001a). The magnitude of the acute-phase protein response is proportional to the extent of tissue injury (Stahl, 1987), although it should be recognized that plasma levels reflect the net result of synthesis, release, degradation, binding and excretion. Hydration status and distribution will also influence plasma levels (Vanek, 1998). In contrast to previous thinking, synthesis rates of albumin in situations such as surgical trauma and in weight-losing cancer patients are the same as in controls or even increased (Barber *et al.*, 1998; Barle *et al.*, 1998; Fearon *et al.*, 1998; Van Acker *et al.*, 1998). In ongoing infection, inflammation and other types of severe illness, the acute-phase response generally persists for much longer, even until death if hepatocellular function is maintained (Pepys and Baltz, 1983).

The full significance and functions of these proteins and the changes in their levels are still not fully understood, but in general it is assumed that they perform a useful role by limiting tissue damage, encouraging and enhancing the scavenging process and promoting repair and healing (Cruickshank, 1989; Elia, 2001a). However, the value of the acute-phase response may be limited if it is prolonged and ongoing. In patients with unresectable pancreatic cancer, the presence of an acute-phase response was the most important predictor of shortened survival time (Falconer *et al.*, 1995).

Animal studies have shown that a limited availability of amino acids because of protein or protein-energy malnutrition attenuates the acute-phase protein response (Elia, 2001a). These findings are partly supported by observations in humans. The clinical syndrome of the stress response during depletion has been described by Soeters *et al.* (2001), namely the absence of fever, leucocytosis, hyperdynamic circulation, pus production and impaired wound healing. Some of the findings reported in humans in relation to the acute-phase response in undernourished states are briefly described below.

Table 4.2. The acute-phase proteins (adapted from Pepys and Baltz, 1983; Chadwick *et al.*, 1986; Stahl, 1987).

General function	Specific function	Positive acute-phase proteins[a]	Negative acute-phase proteins[a]
Coagulation proteins	Essential to the clotting process and therefore to the maintenance of normal haemostasis	Fibrinogen (factor I) Prothrombin (factor II) Antihaemophilic factor (factor VIII) Plasminogen	
Complement proteins	Participation in the complement cascade, resulting in a number of actions, including cell lysis, opsonic action and a targeting role within the specific immune response	C1s, C2, B, C3, C4, C5, C56, C1, 1NH	
Protease inhibitors	Control action of proteolytic enzymes to prevent damage to healthy tissues	α_1-antitrypsin α_1-antichymotrypsin	
Transport proteins	Binding of free haemoglobin, preventing damage to renal tubules	Haptoglobulin	
	Inhibition of prostaglandin synthesis		
	Binding of copper	Ceruloplasmin	
	Antioxidant		
	Antioxidant		Albumin
	Contribution to plasma oncotic pressure		
	Carry thyroxine and form a complex with retinol-binding protein to prevent loss of vitamin A by renal filtration		Prealbumin
	Transport of vitamin A from the liver to peripheral tissues as complex with prealbumin		Retinol-binding protein
	Iron absorption and transport		Transferrin
Miscellaneous	Opsonization of DNA and cell membrane debris for subsequent scavenging	C-reactive protein (CRP)	
	Complement activation		
	Speculative	Serum amyloid A protein	
	Opsonization of noxious agents, thereby enhancing phagocytosis by the reticuloendothelial system		Fibronectin (α_2-glycoprotein)
	Promotion of fibroblast growth	Orosomucoid (α_1-acid glycoprotein)	

[a]Positive acute-phase proteins increase in concentration in response to inflammatory stimuli and negative acute-phase proteins decrease in concentration (Pepys and Baltz, 1983; Elia, 2001a).

In non-infected children, prealbumin levels were lower in the undernourished group than in controls (Malavé *et al.*, 1998). In this study, significant positive correlations were found between prealbumin and z scores for weight-for-age, height-for-age and weight-for-height. These correlations disappeared in children with clinical infections. However, the capacity to produce IL-6 and C-reactive protein (CRP) during infection was preserved in the undernourished children (Malavé *et al.*, 1998).

In healthy volunteers starved for 4.5 days, plasma levels of fibronectin were rapidly reduced, and recovered on refeeding. Albumin levels rose, thought to be related to a loss of extracellular water. Plasma transferrin did not change during starvation, but was significantly reduced by the beginning of the refeeding period and remained low during this time. C3 complement levels did not change (Chadwick *et al.*, 1986). This study did not examine the effects of starvation on ability to mount an acute-phase response to an insult. Fibronectin may also be reduced in healthy volunteers undergoing partial starvation (Van der Linden *et al.*, 1986). Others have confirmed that malnutrition or food deprivation *per se* is unlikely to have an effect on reducing albumin levels (Jeejeebhoy, 1984; Scalfi *et al.*, 1990; Smith, G. *et al.*, 1994), whereas food restriction is likely to reduce prealbumin and retinol-binding protein levels (Scalfi *et al.*, 1990).

In patients undergoing elective gastric or colorectal surgery, undernourished patients (body weight < 80% of ideal and triceps skin-fold thickness < 65% of standard) were matched with well-nourished controls. CRP, α_1-antitrypsin, α_1-acid glycoprotein, albumin, prealbumin and transferrin were measured prior to surgery and each day for 5 days afterwards. Prior to surgery there was a trend towards lower transferrin levels in the undernourished group. After surgery, only CRP was significantly lower in the undernourished patients (Cruickshank, 1989). In obese women, CRP was positively correlated with BMI and was reduced in proportion to weight loss (Heilbronn *et al.*, 2001).

Until recently, albumin has been the most studied component of the acute-phase response. A number of factors have been proposed to explain post-traumatic hypoalbuminaemia, of which perhaps the most important are transcapillary escape rate as a result of increased vascular permeability and increased interstitial distribution space (Fleck *et al.*, 1985; Gosling *et al.*, 1988; Elia, 2001a; Franch-Arcas, 2001). Other factors that influence albumin metabolism include cytokines, hormones, certain drugs, acidosis and possibly hypoxia and exercise (Ballmer, 2001). Nutrition (amino acid availability) may also influence albumin metabolism and, because of this, albumin is still frequently suggested as a suitable marker of nutritional status. It seems overwhelmingly clear by now that this is not the case, in view of the studies of simple starvation and partial food deprivation that have failed to show an effect on plasma albumin concentrations. However, as a prognostic indicator of complications, length of stay (LOS) in hospital or mortality, albumin may indeed have a valuable role in a variety of different patient groups (Whicher and Spence, 1987; Vanek, 1998; Franch-Arcas, 2001), including:

- nursing home patients (Rudman *et al.*, 1987);
- arthroplasty (Lavernia *et al.*, 1999);
- hip fracture (Burness *et al.*, 1996; Koval *et al.*, 1999);
- stroke (Gariballa, 2001);
- end-stage renal disease (Kaysen, 1999);
- AIDS (Chlebowski *et al.*, 1989);
- surgery (Al-Hudiathy and Lewis, 1996);
- patients with a percutaneous endoscopic gastrostomy (PEG) (Friedenberg *et al.*, 1997);
- patients receiving parenteral nutrition (Llop *et al.*, 2001).

Not all studies have demonstrated associations between serum albumin and outcome (Quasim *et al.*, 2000). Possible explanations for a link between serum albumin and mortality have been discussed extensively (Soeters *et al.*, 1990).

In contrast to albumin, other acute-phase response proteins may be more suitable as indices of nutritional status and response to nutritional support, e.g. prealbumin (Tuten *et al.*, 1985; Feitelson Winkler *et al.*, 1989; Bernstein *et al.*, 1995; Mears, 1996; Nataloni *et al.*, 1999; Potter and Luxton, 1999), fibronectin (Kirby *et al.*, 1985; Van der Linden *et al.*, 1986) and retinol-binding protein (Feitelson Winkler *et al.*, 1989). However, this may not be the case in all types of patients, e.g. severe sepsis and multiple injury (Clark *et al.*, 1996), and it must be borne in mind that these proteins are also influenced by the acute-phase response.

Wound Healing

The skin is a main barrier against infection. Therefore, a defence system has evolved to repair any damage or breach in the continuity of the skin as effectively and rapidly as possible.

There are two main areas with respect to development of wounds and wound healing where nutrition may play an important role. The first is in the development of wounds, most notably pressure ulcers, and the second is in healing of wounds, such as pressure ulcers and surgical wounds. Following surgery or trauma, non-skin-related wound healing is also important, e.g. healing of intestinal anastomoses, but this will not be dealt with here.

Wound healing is a complex physiological process. A detailed description of this process is beyond the scope of this text. However, a summary of the four main dynamic phases, which often have considerable overlap, is shown in Fig. 4.1 (Flanagan, 2000). Any alteration in the balance of the complex wound healing process may result in delay or even failure of wound healing or maturation or, in some instances, excess wound healing

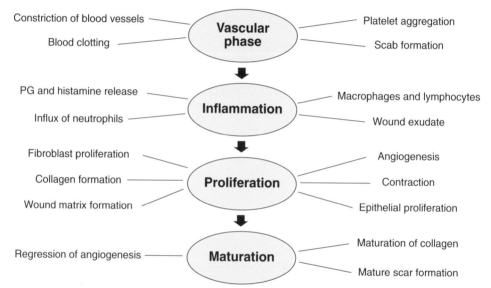

Fig. 4.1. Phases of wound healing. In the first (vascular) phase, constriction of blood vessels and blood clotting stop the bleeding. A fibrin mesh is formed which acts as a temporary closure of the wound, and blood and serous fluid produced by the wound help to keep it clear of surface contaminants. Mediators such as prostaglandins (PGs) and histamine are released as a result of tissue damage and activation of clotting factors. This leads to an inflammatory response (inflammatory phase) due to increased permeability of adjacent blood vessels and influx of first neutrophils and later macrophages. This phase is characterized by redness, heat, swelling and wound exudate. The exudate helps to bathe and cleanse the wound and serves as a growth medium for phagocytic cells. Macrophages produce growth factors and other mediators, which help to regulate the healing process. Slough (dead cellular material consisting of large amounts of leucocytes) formation is common during this phase. Once the wound bed has been cleansed by the inflammatory process, proliferation of new tissue is stimulated by growth factors released from macrophages (proliferative phase). Wound size is reduced by a combination of:

- granulation (formation of a matrix of collagen and ground substance);
- angiogenesis (formation of new blood vessels in the wound matrix, stimulated by growth factors and cytokines produced by macrophages and hypoxia due to reduced blood flow at the time of injury, which leads to the formation of connective tissue that fills the wound);
- contraction (stimulated by fibroblasts around the wound margin, which help to bring the edges together);
- epithelialization (growth of epithelial cells across the wound surface, which is aided by a moist wound environment and inhibited by the presence of necrotic tissue or a scab).

The maturation phase usually begins about 20 days after injury and can last for months or even years, during which time remodelling of scar tissue occurs to maximize tensile strength.

(Clark *et al.*, 2000). A number of factors that can influence the process of wound healing and maturation have been proposed and in many cases confirmed (Meyer *et al.*, 1994; Kiecolt-Glaser *et al.*, 1995; Stotts and Wipke-Tevis, 1996; Richards *et al.*, 1997; Sessler, 1997; Buggy, 2000; Clark *et al.*, 2000; Flanagan, 2000; Table 4.3).

Although there are many factors that can affect wound healing, nutritional status and particularly recent nutritional intake seem to be important (Clark *et al.*, 2000). In comparison with well-nourished patients, impaired or prolonged wound healing has been documented not only in malnourished patients with deep pressure ulcers, but also in those undergoing amputations (Pedersen and Pedersen, 1992) and in surgical patients (Haydock and Hill, 1986). In the latter study, this was assessed by incorporation of hydroxyproline into Gore-Tex tubes (inserted in the arm at the time of surgery) 7 days postoperatively. The investigators ruled out the possible influences of age, severity of surgical procedure and presence of malignancy. Of particular interest was that these changes were evident even in mild depletion, when patients had poor intake but were

Table 4.3. Factors influencing wound healing (from Meyer *et al.*, 1994; Kiecolt-Glaser *et al.*, 1995; Scott *et al.*, 1996; Richards *et al.*, 1997; Sessler, 1997; Buggy, 2000; Clark *et al.*, 2000; Flanagan, 2000).

Categories	Examples
Local factors	Wound infection
	Mechanical stress
	Use of toxic cleaning agents
	Presence of foreign bodies
	Low oxygen tension in the wound due to poor tissue perfusion at certain stages of healing can impair the healing process by impairing bactericidal ability of neutrophils and the amount of scar formation (although in the early stage hypoxia and anaerobic metabolism are beneficial for stimulating angiogenesis, fibroblast proliferation and collagen formation)
	Neural innervation
General health	Age (although it remains controversial whether age *per se* has an impact on wound healing)
	Nutritional status
	Psychological (stress-related) factors
	Smoking
	Alcoholism
Presence of chronic disease or severe illness	Severe trauma (adverse effects possibly linked to lymphocyte function)
	Major surgery (in turn influenced by site, duration and complexity, presence of suture/foreign body, suturing quality, pre-existing local or systemic infection, prophylactic antibiotics, haematoma and mechanical stress on wound)
	Type of anaesthetic management (tissue perfusion, maintenance of normovolaemia, perioperative body temperature, concentration of inspired oxygen, quality of pain relief, and possibly blood transfusion and type of anaesthesia)
	Presence of infection elsewhere in the body, septic complications or systemic sepsis (large wounds themselves may have systemic as well as local effects by generating and maintaining a systemic inflammatory response and possibly even contributing to multiple organ failure)
	Diabetes
	Chronic renal failure
	Jaundice
Drug therapy	Glucocorticoids (e.g. dexamethasone, hydrocortisone) are known to reduce wound healing, probably through interference in the inflammatory phase
	Chemotherapy following surgery

anthropometrically indistinguishable from the normally nourished group. This led the investigators to suggest that impaired wound healing occurs early in the course of malnutrition and is perhaps less dependent on the degree of tissue lost than on the metabolic state (related to recent nutritional intake) of the patient at the time of wounding. Further studies by the same group using the same method to assess wound healing confirmed that preoperative food intake has a greater influence on wound healing than absolute losses of body protein and fat (Windsor *et al.*, 1988) and that intravenous nutrition (Haydock and Hill, 1987) or early postoperative feeding improves wound healing (Schroeder *et al.*, 1991).

Clinical consequences of delayed wound healing

Wound infections are both a consequence and a cause of delayed wound healing (Kurz *et al.*, 1996). They can prolong hospitalization by 5–20 days and substantially increase hospital costs (Kurz *et al.*, 1996; Melling *et al.*, 2001). Infections have been estimated to occur in up to 10% of patients undergoing 'clean surgery' (Melling *et al.*, 2001) and up to 22% in patients undergoing colonic surgery (Kurz *et al.*, 1996). This results in discomfort and pain and will necessitate extra expenditure in terms of staff time, dressings and drug therapies.

Pressure ulcers

Pressure ulcers (decubitus ulcers or pressure sores) constitute a degenerative change that occurs between skin and bones. They occur most commonly on the lower half of the body, and especially on areas of the body where bones protrude, such as the sacrum, hip and buttocks, heel, ankle and elbow. These are the bony prominences supporting the weight of the body during lying, sitting and standing (Versluyen, 1985; Vohra and McCollum, 1994). There are four stages of pressure ulcer development, according to a widely accepted classification system devised by the American National Pressure Ulcer Advisory Panel (NPUAP, 1989), summarized in Table 4.4.

The pathogenesis of pressure ulcers is multifactorial, influenced by both local factors and systemic factors (Vohra and McCollum, 1994; Allman, 1997). The main local risk factors contributing to the development of pressure ulcers are sustained pressure on the skin (causing ischaemia), friction, shear forces (causing mechanical stress to tissues) and moisture (Vohra and McCollum, 1994; Peerless *et al.*, 1999; Whitfield *et al.*, 2000). These are summarized in Table 4.5.

There are many systemic risk factors for the development of pressure ulcers, including nutritional intake and status, age, physical condition, presence of arterial disease or hypotension, activity/mobility (e.g. bedbound, chair-bound) and incontinence

Table 4.4. Pressure ulcer staging (adapted from National Pressure Ulcer Advisory Panel, 1989).

Stage	Characteristics
Stage I	Non-blanchable erythema (redness) of the intact skin. This appears as a defined area of persistent redness on light skin or red, blue or purple hues on dark skin. Changes in skin temperature and tissue consistency and sensations of pain or itchiness can occur
Stage II	Partial-thickness skin loss involving the epidermis and/or the dermis. The ulcer is superficial and presents as an abrasion, blister or shallow ulcer
Stage III	Full-thickness skin loss with damage or necrosis of the subcutaneous tissue, which may extend to the underlying fascia (connective-tissue layer sheathing muscle and protecting organs near the skin). The ulcer presents as a deep crater, which may or may not affect the adjacent tissue
Stage IV	Full-thickness skin loss with extensive destruction, tissue necrosis or damage to muscle, bone or supporting structures (e.g. tendon, joint capsule)

Table 4.5. Main local risk factors for pressure ulcer development (adapted from Vohra and McCollum, 1994; Peerless *et al.*, 1999; Whitfield *et al.*, 2000).

Factor	Characteristics
Pressure	The compression of or repeated trauma to tissue covering bony prominences causes pressure ulcers. Unlike healthy individuals, people with disease who are bed- or chair-bound may be unable to adjust their posture to avoid sustained pressure. Tissue damage is thought to occur when pressures exceeding 9.3 kPa are sustained for more than 2–3 h. Repeated pressure leads to capillary occlusion, which disrupts the microcirculation and impairs the lymphatic drainage of the subcutaneous tissues. The result is that waste products accumulate and oxygen and nutrients cannot reach the tissues
Shearing force	Shearing occurs when a patient in a bed or chair slides downwards or moves while the skin and superficial tissue adhere to the bedclothes and are pulled tightly over the deep fascia. This stretches and traumatizes the underlying blood vessels, leading to thrombosis and subsequent tissue necrosis
Friction	Friction occurs when the movement of a patient against the bed sheets or a chair causes the stratum corneum (top protective layer of the epidermis of the skin) to be removed and the epidermis to be separated from the basal cells. Blistering and erosions result
Increased temperature and moisture	Increases in temperature lead to sweating. The resulting moisture alters the integrity of the skin through maceration and compromises the barrier to infection. Maceration of the skin also occurs with urinary and faecal incontinence, wound drainage and fistulas

(Pinchcofsky-Devin and Kaminski, 1986; Berlowitz and Wilking, 1989; Shannon and Skorga, 1989; Ek *et al.*, 1991; van Rijswijk and Polansky, 1994; Vohra and McCollum, 1994; Meaume and Senet, 1999). The elderly are particularly prone to pressure ulcer development because of aged skin (decreased proliferation in the epidermis, sensory loss, reduced elasticity), loss of subcutaneous tissue, reduced pain perception, decreased cell-mediated immunity and slower wound healing, often combined with long periods of immobility, arterial disease and poor nutritional status (Versluyen, 1985; Pinchcofsky-Devin and Kaminski, 1986; Waltman *et al.*, 1991; Vohra and McCollum, 1994).

Malnutrition is recognized as one of the major systemic risk factors for pressure ulcer development (Bobel, 1987; Berlowitz and Wilking, 1989; Breslow, 1991; Vohra and McCollum, 1994; Levine and Totolos, 1995; Gupta, 1999; Peerless *et al.*, 1999). Both poor nutritional intake and poor nutritional status play a role in increasing risk. There are a number of reasons why poor nutritional intake increases the risk of pressure ulcer development. In addition to reduced nutrient availability in the body for energy metabolism, maintenance and

repair, malnutrition is also accompanied by losses of fat, decreases in skin resistance, physical weakness, decreased mobility and oedema. One or a combination of all of these factors increases the risk of pressure ulcer formation, as shown in Fig. 4.2.

Poor nutritional intake has been shown to correlate with the development of pressure ulcers by a number of investigators (Berlowitz and Wilking, 1989; Weiler *et al.*, 1990; Ek *et al.*, 1991; Bergstrom and Braden, 1992; Breslow and Bergstrom, 1994; Green *et al.*, 1999). Poor nutritional status has also been shown to be associated with development of pressure ulcers (Allman *et al.*, 1986; Pinchcofsky-Devin and Kaminski, 1986; Berlowitz and Wilking, 1989; Ek *et al.*, 1991; Altman, 1995). Furthermore, multivariate analysis has revealed factors such as BMI, body weight, feeding activity and food intake to be independent risk factors for the development of pressure ulcers (Thomas, 1997). However, it should be noted that causality has not yet been established (Mathus-Vliegen, 2001). Deficiencies of specific micronutrients may also increase the risk of pressure ulcer development (Bobel, 1987; Breslow *et al.*, 1991; Utley, 1992; Trujillo, 1993).

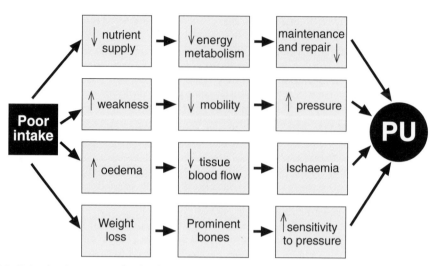

Fig. 4.2. Role of malnutrition in the development of pressure ulcers (PU).

Specifically, deficiencies of vitamin C, vitamin A, carotenes, vitamin E and zinc have been reported in patients with pressure ulcers and leg ulcers (Abbott *et al.*, 1968; McBean *et al.*, 1974; Williams *et al.*, 1988; Goode *et al.*, 1992; Rojas and Phillips, 1999).

Clinical and financial consequences of pressure ulcers

Reports of pressure ulcer prevalence in hospital patients range from 3 to 23% (Allman *et al.*, 1986; Ek *et al.*, 1991; Vohra and McCollum, 1994; O'Dea, 1995; Bours *et al.*, 1999; Whitfield *et al.*, 2000). This has been termed a 'silent epidemic' because pressure sores are not considered by medical staff to be a priority (Kulkarni, 1994). It is widely believed that the prevalence of pressure ulcers in community settings is higher than in hospitals (Vohra and McCollum, 1994; Allman, 1997), with estimates ranging from 3 to 54% (Preston, 1991; Joy and Halling, 1998; Thomas, S. *et al.*, 1998; Bours *et al.*, 1999; Haalboom, 2000a). Although it has been estimated that ~17% of patients cared for in their own home have pressure ulcers (Bours *et al.*, 1999; Haalboom, 2000a), the prevalence is much greater in patients cared for in other community

settngs, such as nursing homes and other long-term care institutions. Estimates for such settings range from 7 to 54% of patients (Smith, 1995; Joy and Halling, 1998; Thomas, S. *et al.*, 1998; Bours *et al.*, 1999; Haalboom, 2000a).

Estimates suggest that the majority (> 70%) of all pressure ulcers occur in patients > 70 years old (Versluyen, 1985; Young and Dobrzanski, 1992; Vohra and McCollum, 1994). Other at-risk groups include orthopaedic patients, particularly those with hip fractures (estimated incidence of 19–30% (Versluyen, 1985; Jensen and Juncker, 1987; Stotts *et al.*, 1998)), the critically ill (incidence of 33–56% of patients in intensive care settings (Peerless *et al.*, 1999)), the physically disabled (up to 85% of paraplegics develop a pressure ulcer (Vohra and McCollum, 1994)), postoperative patients and those receiving palliative care for cancer (Longe, 1986; Vohra and McCollum, 1994). Amongst high-risk patients, the incidence of pressure ulcers is estimated to be 14 per 1000 patient-days (Smith, 1995).

Pressure ulcers are associated with substantial excess morbidity and mortality (Vohra and McCollum, 1994; Levine and Totolos, 1995; Allman *et al.*, 1999). Local and systemic infections (e.g. cellulitis, osteomyelitis, sepsis) commonly occur

(Allman *et al.*, 1986; Allman, 1989). In addition, patients with pressure ulcers frequently suffer from dehydration, anaemia, electrolyte imbalance and malnutrition. Pressure ulcers and the associated morbidity lead to sustained pain and suffering, prolonged hospitalization and a loss of independence (Versluyen, 1985). A four-fold increased risk of death has been reported in geriatric patients and those in nursing homes who develop a pressure ulcer, and the failure of a pressure ulcer to heal in this group has been associated with almost a six times higher death rate (Allman *et al.*, 1986).

Pressure ulcers are a huge financial burden on national health-care systems. The annual cost of treating pressure ulcers has been estimated to be in excess of $3 billion in the USA and £150 million in the UK (with more recent estimates suggesting figures in the region of £750 million (1998 prices) (M. Elia, personal communication)), with the total cost for a patient with a full-thickness sacral sore estimated to be ~£30,000 (Vohra and McCollum, 1994; Hey, 1996). In The Netherlands, pressure ulcers are the fourth most expensive condition to treat after cardiovascular disease, cancer and AIDS (Mathus-Vliegen, 2001), accounting for > 1% of total health-care costs (Haalboom, 2000a). This expenditure is attributable to the costs of medication, surgical procedures, dressing materials, special pressure-relieving devices and the substantial expenditure on complex, intensive nursing care during prolonged hospital stays and community care (Vohra and McCollum, 1994; Hey, 1996; Haalboom, 2000b). The lengthening of hospital waiting lists due to prolonged hospital stays has further financial implications (Haalboom, 2000b). Another financial implication is the potential threat of litigation associated with pressure ulcers. Patients and carers are increasingly attempting to recover costs from health authorities by litigation for the loss of independence, productivity and income caused by pressure ulcers (Vohra and McCollum, 1994).

Energy Homeostasis

During starvation or semi-starvation, energy stores determine survival time (Elia, 1992a). Therefore, a reduction in energy expenditure is expected to reduce the rate of loss of body energy stores and prolong survival time. Reductions in energy expenditure during starvation are well recognized. A detailed analysis undertaken by Elia (1997a) indicated that several independent processes may be involved which can affect all three components of total energy expenditure: physical activity, resting energy expenditure (REE) and dietary-induced thermogenesis. The reduction in dietary-induced thermogenesis is largely due to decreased processing of dietary nutrients (which are reduced or absent during starvation/semi-starvation). The other two components are discussed separately below, partly because they are generally quantitatively more important and partly because of the potential clinical implications.

REE and thermoregulation

Apart from a transient early rise in basal metabolic rate (BMR) during the first few days of total starvation, there is a reduction in BMR during both starvation and semi-starvation. REE during weight loss may be lower than during weight stability after loss of an equivalent amount of body weight. The reduced tissue mass in underweight individuals is responsible for much of the reduction in REE, but there may also be a reduction in the REE of the available tissues (e.g. reduction in REE per kg of body weight, fat-free mass or body cell mass). However, these changes can be confounded by alterations in the proportions of metabolically active to less active tissues with respect to oxidative metabolism, which may sometimes lead to elevations in REE kg^{-1} tissue (Elia, 1997a). Parenthetically, different methods of expressing REE (Elia, 1997a) may also result in different interpretations.

REE can also be affected by changes in thermoregulation. Body temperature (core temperature) tends to be lower in many malnourished individuals, especially children. By itself, this does not indicate that it is the cause or a consequence of the low REE. However, experimental studies in humans (Fellows et al., 1985; Mansell et al., 1990a) and animals (Severinsen and Munch, 1999) suggest that there are important changes in thermoregulation. Some of these changes may prevent shivering from occurring in malnourished individuals at temperatures that produce shivering in normally nourished individuals. The malnourished individual has been likened to the reptilian poikilotherm ('cold-blooded' animal). This can be regarded as an 'adaptation' that results in reduced energy expenditure, preservation of energy stores and prolongation of survival. However, the price is an increased risk of hypothermia (Elia, 1997a).

Core body temperature is usually maintained near 37°C. Under normal circumstances, body temperature is maintained by three components (Sessler, 1997):

- Afferent thermal sensing: heat and cold receptors are widely distributed over the body, signals from which are sent to the central nervous system and spinal cord, where they are integrated.
- Central regulation: the hypothalamus is the primary thermoregulatory control centre in mammals.
- Efferent responses: the major autonomic defences against heat are sweating and active cutaneous vasodilatation and those against cold are vasoconstriction in arteriovenous shunts, located mainly in the fingers and toes. Non-shivering thermogenesis is important in infants but is of little importance in adults. Shivering is an involuntary activity of muscle that can increase metabolic rate to two to three times the normal level. The most effective thermoregulatory response is behavioural change, such as putting on additional clothes or opening a window.

Substantial deviations from the normal constant internal temperature lead to a deterioration of metabolic functions. Factors that can influence normal thermal regulation include ageing, removal of a patient's ability to regulate body temperature through behaviour, general and regional anaesthesia and deliberate cooling, e.g. during cardiac or brain surgery (Sessler, 1997). Other important factors are nutritional intake and nutritional status.

Starvation, weight loss and severe chronic malnutrition predispose to hypothermia. A 1–2°C drop in core temperature can cause confusion, muscle weakness and poor coordination, predisposing to falls and injury, especially in the elderly. Reduced core temperature during surgery has also been shown to have an impact on development of surgical wound infections (Sessler, 1997; Buggy, 2000). Studies have shown that warming during colorectal surgery (Kurz et al., 1996; Sessler and Kurz, 1996) and prior to 'clean' (breast, varicose vein and hernia) surgery (Melling et al., 2001) has significant outcome advantages. These have included a lower rate of surgical wound infections (Kurz et al., 1996; Melling et al., 2001), lower wound scores (Melling et al., 2001), more rapid removal of sutures (Kurz et al., 1996), less need for postoperative antibiotics (Melling et al., 2001) and reduced length of hospital stay (Kurz, 1996).

Physical activity

In experimental conditions, short-term starvation (water only) (Gibney, 2002; Gibney et al., 2002a) and prolonged semi-starvation have been reported to reduce physical activity. In the Keys study of semi-starvation, in which subjects lost 25% of their body weight over 6 months, there was a reduction in both REE and physical activity. However, it was the reductions in physical activity energy expenditure that were responsible for most of the reduction in total energy expenditure (Keys et al., 1950). Feelings of tiredness and lethargy can contribute to this. The marked decreases in physical activity that can occur in severe malnutrition in the presence of disease may predispose to pressure ulcers, thromboembolism and reduced capacity to mobilize and undertake work. However, financial and other rewards can increase physical activity and work performance to normal levels (Gibney, 2002). In children, dietary restriction may also lead to reduced physical activity. This again can be regarded as an adaptation, but long-term reductions in exploratory behaviour may lead or contribute to impaired mental development (Elia, 1997a).

Psychological Function

Mental function may be influenced by nutrition in several ways and at different periods of life. In childhood, protein-energy, iron and iodine deficiencies all have the capacity to produce adverse effects on learning and behaviour. At certain critical time points, the effects of deficiency may be irreversible (Scrimshaw, 1998). Long-term deficits in cognition (awareness, perception, thinking, memory) and school achievement have been associated with these deficiencies, as well as with reduced breast-feeding and small-for-gestational-age birth weight (Grantham-McGregor *et al.*, 2000). The causal nature of these relationships has recently come under some scrutiny, as all these conditions are also linked with poverty and poor health (Grantham-McGregor *et al.*, 2000). Data from multivariate analyses (Mendez and Adair, 1999; Ivanovic *et al.*, 2000) and intervention studies (Grantham-McGregor *et al.*, 2000) do seem to indicate that protein-energy deficits, stunting and specific micronutrient deficiencies, such as iodine, have a long-term effect. The presence or absence of some other nutrients, e.g. omega-3 fatty acids, may influence optimal mental development of the preterm infant and neonate (Scrimshaw, 1998).

Brief fasting may also have an impact on cognition. This has been examined extensively in children in relation to breakfast consumption in both developing (Simeon and Grantham-McGregor, 1989) and developed (Pollitt *et al.*, 1981; Benton and Parker, 1998; Pollitt and Mathews, 1998) countries. Overall, the data suggest that omitting breakfast may interfere with cognition and learning, and this is more obvious in children who are malnourished or at nutritional risk (Pollitt and Mathews, 1998).

Starvation and partial food deprivation in adults lead to anxiety, depression and other mental changes, which may in part be linked to specific micronutrient deficiencies. Cognitive function may also be adversely affected. In Keys's study (Keys *et al.*, 1950), healthy volunteers who underwent partial starvation for 24 weeks, resulting in loss of 25% of body weight, had a concomitant increase in depression score. Although this started to return towards normal on refeeding, pre-experiment levels were not reached even after 20 weeks of refeeding (Allison, 1992). In 30 Irish hunger strikers, severe vitamin deficiencies became apparent over the period of starvation, with severe thiamine deficiency (or Wernicke's encephalopathy[2]) developing in some cases (Allison, 1992).

Specific dietary components may have an influence on risk of depression, cognitive impairment and cognitive decline (Rogers, 2001). Over the past decade, much attention has been given to the possibility that diet may play an important role in influencing cognition and the development of dementia in the elderly. There are two main types of dementia: Alzheimer's disease, which is the most common cause, and 'vascular' dementia, which is the second most frequent cause. Stroke is a major cause of vascular dementia (González-Gross *et al.*, 2001). Various large-scale epidemiological studies have shown associations between quality of diet and prevalence of cognitive impairment (Corrêa Leite *et al.*, 2001; Lee *et al.*, 2001), and that weight loss precedes Alzheimer's-type dementia (Barrett-Connor *et al.*, 1998). Subclinical deficiencies of certain micronutrients (antioxidants, such as vitamins C and E, β-carotene, vitamins B_{12}, B_6 and folate) and nutrition-related disorders

(e.g. hypercholesterolaemia, hypertriglyc-
eridaemia, hypertension, diabetes) have
been identified as possible nutrition-
related risk factors (Calvaresi and Bryan,
2001; González-Gross et al., 2001;
Meydani, 2001; Rosenberg, 2001; Wang et
al., 2001). However, these findings do not
indicate a causal association. Although
preliminary data suggest a benefit of intervention, e.g. with B vitamin supplements
(Calvaresi and Bryan, 2001; Van Asselt et
al., 2001), larger intervention studies are
required (Calvaresi and Bryan, 2001;
Rogers, 2001). Furthermore, sensitive measures of cognitive performance are essential (Salmon, 1994; Calvaresi and Bryan,
2001).

In elderly women with hip fractures,
cognitive function assessed using the short
portable mental status questionnaire was
correlated with BMI (Ponzer et al., 1999).
Using the mini mental test, similar correlations of cognitive function with BMI,
weight loss and age were demonstrated in
elderly people living in sheltered accommodation (Faxén Irving et al., 1999). In
elderly patients with various cognitive dys-
functions (n 102) given energy-enriched
hospital food, improvements in body
weight were correlated with improvements
in cognitive function measured by the mini
mental state examination, especially in
patients with Alzheimer's disease (Faxén
Irving et al., 2000). In acute admissions to
an elderly geriatric ward, a lower mental
test score was correlated with mortality
(Phillips, 1986). However, not all studies
have demonstrated correlations between
nutritional status and cognitive impairment (Burns et al., 1989), and providing
tube feeding for patients with advanced
dementia remains an ethical dilemma
(Finucane et al., 1999; Gillick, 2000;
McNamara and Kennedy, 2001).

Quality of Life

Overall, QOL depends on both physical
and psychological well-being, both of
which can be influenced by nutrition. In
the last 15 years, there has been a tremendous growth in interest in health-related
QOL (Fallowfield, 1996; Testa and
Simonson, 1996; Muldoon et al., 1998). It
is now becoming widely acknowledged
that psychosocial factors, such as pain,
apprehension, restricted mobility and other
functional impairments, difficulty fulfilling
personal and family responsibilities, financial burden and diminished cognition,
must also be included in the description of
the personal burden of illness (Muldoon et
al., 1998). Despite this awareness, there has
been considerable scepticism and confusion regarding measuring QOL
(Fallowfield, 1996; Muldoon et al., 1998),
not aided by the lack of consensus on a
definition. In general, health-related QOL
can be considered as the gap between
expectations of health and actual experience of it (Carr et al., 2001).

QOL assessment aims to measure general well-being based on objective and
subjective changes in physical, functional, mental and social health (Testa
and Simonson, 1996; Muldoon et al.,
1998). There are three main problems
with measuring QOL (Carr et al., 2001):
different individuals have different
health expectations, individuals may be
at different time points in the trajectory
of their illness when measurements are
made and expectations may change over
time. Numerous scales exist, such as the
EuroQOL, SF-36, Nottingham health profile, quality of well-being scale and well-
being in surgical patients (WISP), but all
seem to have additional inherent problems. Many are several pages long, they
may not be validated in more than one
target group or may be too generic (i.e.
not condition-specific), they may not be
relevant to all individuals, they may not
be valid in other languages, they may not
be single-index measures and/or they
may be influenced by the mode of administration. The best mode of assessment of
QOL in children and adolescents is even
less clear. In clinical practice, the simpler, shorter and less ambiguous the questionnaire the better, as patients will not
all be willing or able to cooperate with
more complex surveys.

There is growing awareness that poor nutritional status may have an impact on QOL, and a number of ways of explaining how this could arise have been suggested (Vetta *et al.*, 1999). Good nutrition is essential for adequate function and survival, but eating *per se* satisfies other needs, including pleasure, satisfaction, conviviality and provision of a structure to the day (McKenna and Thörig, 1995).

Bearing in mind the difficulties in measuring QOL and the various methods employed to assess nutritional status, close associations between malnutrition and impaired QOL have nevertheless been reported in 605 healthy free-living elderly (Maaravi *et al.*, 2000) and in 155 free-living subjects over 60 years participating in a meal programme (Vailas *et al.*, 1998). Similar associations have been identified in a number of patient groups, including the following:

- General admissions to an acute hospital (Ferguson and Capra, 1998).
- Weight-losing patients with cancer of the lung, breast and ovary (Ovesen *et al.*, 1993).
- Patients with cancer and weight loss prior to chemotherapy (Andreyev *et al.*, 1998).
- Surgical patients (Larsson *et al.*, 1994a, b).
- Elderly women with hip fractures (Ponzer *et al.*, 1999).
- Patients with COPD (Congleton, 1999; Mostert *et al.*, 2000).
- Patients with end-stage renal disease receiving haemodialysis.

Restitution of body weight and lean body mass during nutritional support has been shown to be associated with significant improvement in QOL indices in chronic illness (Jamieson *et al.*, 1997). In severely malnourished head and neck cancer patients, preoperative nutritional support improved QOL (Van Bokhorst-de van der Schueren *et al.*, 2000b), even though nutritional status was not improved (Van Bokhorst-de van der Schueren *et al.*, 2001), suggesting that improving nutrient intake

per se may have a valuable role. It has been suggested that detailed psychological testing could be a useful parameter for monitoring outcome of treatment (Young *et al.*, 1992; Field *et al.*, 2001), although this may not be realistic, especially in the elderly (Schlettwein-Gsell, 1992).

Complications and Clinical Outcome

Although many of the adverse effects of malnutrition on physical and psychological function have been described in individual sections of this chapter, here an overview is provided of the potential impact of malnutrition on clinical outcome, particularly in relation to utilization of health-care resources.

In disease, the consequences of malnutrition for GI, immune and muscle function are important, because inadequacies in these organ systems may have an even clearer impact on the incidence of complications and clinical outcome (morbidity and mortality). Impaired wound healing will also contribute to poorer clinical outcome (Campos and Meguid, 1992; Pedersen and Pedersen, 1992). These factors may have major implications for LOS in hospital, convalescence and health-care costs. An association between preoperative weight loss and incidence of postoperative complications (in particular, chest infections and impaired wound healing) and mortality was documented more than 60 years ago (Studley, 1936). Since then, numerous publications have provided strong evidence to support these associations in patients undergoing a variety of surgical procedures (see Table 4.6). In addition, poor nutritional status has also been correlated with increased LOS and increased mortality in surgical patients (see Table 4.6).

Associations between malnutrition and poor outcome are not confined to surgical patients (see Table 4.6). Similar findings of increased complications, increased LOS and/or increased mortality have also been demonstrated in a variety of other patient groups including:

Table 4.6. Studies demonstrating significant associations between malnutrition and complication rates, length of stay (LOS), mortality and/or increased health-care costs. Malnutrition assessed by a variety of means, but all methods included anthropometric indices.

Disease	Nutritional status assessment	Increased complications	Increased LOS	Increased mortality/decreased survival	Increased hospital costs	Investigators
General hospital admissions/mixed diagnoses/medical						
General hospital admissions	SGA	✓			✓	Braunschweig et al., 2000: USA
	SGA	✓		✓	✓	Correia and Waitzberg, 1999: Brazil (abstract)
	BMI		✓	✓		Landi et al., 2000: Italy
	SGA	✓	✓			Larsson et al., 1994a: Sweden
	SGA		✓	✓		Middleton et al., 2001: Australia
	SGA	✓	✓			Perman et al., 2001: Argentina (abstract)
	SGA		✓			Planas et al., 2001: Spain (abstract)
	BMI		✓	✓		Potter et al., 1988: USA
Surgical/medical	Composite malnutrition score (albumin, TLC, ideal W/H)	✓		✓	✓	Reilly et al., 1988: USA
Medical	Recent weight loss or inability to eat for 1 week		✓			Anderson et al., 1985: USA
	Ideal W/H, weight loss or albumin		✓		✓	Chima et al., 1997: USA
	SGA, NRI or MI	✓				Naber et al., 1997: The Netherlands
	Weight loss > 10% or composite malnutrition score		✓		✓	Robinson et al., 1987: USA
	Composite malnutrition score (eight parameters)		✓	✓		Weinsier et al., 1979: USA
General diagnoses, community						
Chronic respiratory, GI and neurological disease	BMI < 20 kg m^{-2}	✓ (increased GP consultations, prescriptions and hospital admissions)		✓	✓ (increased use of health-care resources)	Martyn et al., 1998: UK

Group	Index	Consequence	Reference
Cardiovascular disease and cancer	BMI < 20 kg m^{-2}	√ (increased GP consultations, prescriptions; increased hospital admissions in CVD); √ (increased use of health-care resources)	Edington et al., 1999: UK
Elderly			
Hospitalized elderly	BMI < 20 kg m^{-2}	√	Flodin et al., 2000: Sweden
	Not stated	√	Mowé and Bøhmer, 2000: Norway (abstract)
	MNA	√	Van Nes et al., 2001: Switzerland
	Clinical judgement	√	Volkert et al., 1992: Germany
Elderly, medical	Composite malnutrition score	√ (in CHF)	Cederholm and Hellström, 1995: Sweden
	MAC, TSF	√	Constans et al., 1992: France
	SGA	√	Covinsky et al., 1999: USA
	Grip strength, MAMC	√	Phillips, 1986: Australia
	MAC $<$ 10th percentile	√	Dardaine et al., 2001: France
Elderly, ICU	Mid-arm muscle area, body weight	√ (mortality and survival at home)	Mühlethaler et al., 1995: Switzerland
Elderly, assessment unit	Weight loss in year prior to admission	√	Sullivan et al., 1990: USA
Elderly, rehabilitation	Weight loss	√	Sullivan et al., 1991: USA
	SGA	√	Sacks et al., 2000: USA
Elderly, long-term care	Composite malnutrition score	√ (↓ chance of discharge)	Thomas et al., 1991: USA
Paediatrics			
Cystic fibrosis	Growth (weight and height)	√	Corey et al., 1988: USA
HIV infection	Marasmus (Wellcome classification)	√	Amadi et al., 2001: Zambia
	W/A, L/A	√	Berhane et al., 1997: Uganda
	Wt z score < -2	√	Fontana et al., 1999: Italy
	W/A z score < -2, wt gain $<$ 25th percentile rate over first 6 months of zidovudine	√	McKinney et al., 1994: USA

Continued

Table 4.6. *Continued*

Disease	Nutritional status assessment	Increased complications	Increased LOS	Increased mortality/ decreased survival	Increased hospital costs	Investigators
Acute lymphoblastic leukaemia	W/H < 80%			✓		Mejia-Arangure et al., 1999: Mexico
Cancer prior to BMT	< 95% IBW			✓		Deeg et al., 1995: USA
Neuroblastoma prior to chemotherapy	Nutritional status	✓ (duration of remission)		✓ (trend)		Rickard et al., 1983: USA
Chronic obstructive pulmonary disease						
COPD, stable	TSF	✓ (need for hospitalization)				Braun et al., 1984a: USA
	BMI			✓		Gray-Donald et al., 1996: Canada
	BMI			✓		Landbo et al., 1999: Denmark
	BMI, weight gain			✓		Schols et al., 1998: The Netherlands
	% IBW			✓		Wilson et al., 1989: USA
COPD, acute exacerbation	BMI			✓		Connors et al., 1996: USA
				✓		Incalzi et al., 2001: Italy
COPD, lung reduction surgery	BMI	✓ (need for ventilation)	✓			Mazolewski et al., 1999: USA
	% IBW, BMI, FFM, FFMI	✓				Nezu et al., 2001: Japan
Gastrointestinal and liver disease (see also malignancy and surgery sections)						
Liver cirrhosis	MAMC and/or TSF < 10th percentile			✓		Alberino et al., 2001: Italy
	MAMA and/or MAFA < 5th percentile			✓ (univariate analysis only)		Merli et al., 1996: Italy
HIV infection and AIDS						
HIV infection	< 90% UBW			✓		Guenter et al., 1993: USA
	Involuntary weight loss, > 10% weight loss, BMI	✓ (progression to AIDS)				Malvy et al., 2001: France

Continued

HIV infection (early)	Weight loss, LBM ht^{-2}; Involuntary weight loss; Phase angle α (BIA)		✓	Melchior *et al.*, 1999: France; Palenick *et al.*, 1996: USA; Ott *et al.*, 1993: Germany
HIV infection (in-patients)	Nutritional assessment	✓		Mijàn *et al.*, 1998: Spain (abstract)
Advanced HIV infection	Nutritional assessment		✓	Mijàn *et al.*, 1997: Spain (abstract)
HIV infection and AIDS	BMI < 25 kg m^{-2}		✓	Kim *et al.*, 2001: USA
AIDS	Weight loss; BCM, body weight		✓	Chlebowski *et al.*, 1989: USA; Kotler *et al.*, 1989: USA
Malignancy (see also surgery section)				
Prior to chemotherapy	Weight loss		✓	DeWys *et al.*, 1980: USA
Prior to chemotherapy (solid tumours)	Weight loss	✓ (dose-limiting toxicity)		Andreyev *et al.*, 1998: UK
Prior to BMT (haematological cancer)	< 95% IBW		✓	Deeg *et al.*, 1995: USA
Autologous BMT	BMI		✓	Dickson *et al.*, 1999: USA
Solid tumours	Nutritional status		✓	Gogos *et al.*, 1998: Greece
GI and UR cancers	SGA		✓	Persson *et al.*, 1999: Sweden
Head and neck cancer	Nutritional status		✓	Hammerlid *et al.*, 1998: Sweden
Non-small-cell lung cancer	Initial rate of weight loss		✓	Palomares *et al.*, 1996: USA
Neurology				
Amyotrophic lateral sclerosis	BMI < 18.5 kg m^{-2}		✓	Desport *et al.*, 1999: France
Stroke (cerebrovascular accident)	Nutritional assessment; Nutritional assessment after 1 week	✓ (infection); ✓ (infection, trend for more pressure ulcers)		Axelsson *et al.*, 1988: Sweden; Davalos *et al.*, 1996: Spain

Table 4.6. *Continued*

Disease	Nutritional status assessment	Increased complications	Increased LOS	Increased mortality/ decreased survival	Increased hospital costs	Investigators
	Nutritional assessment		√	√		Gariballa *et al.*, 1998b: UK
	Nutrition risk screening tool		√	√		Murray *et al.*, 2000: UK (abstract)
Orthopaedics						
Orthopaedic surgery, mixed	Nutritional assessment		√			Dreblow *et al.*, 1981: USA
	Nutritional assessment	√				Jensen *et al.*, 1982: USA
Orthopaedic surgery, FNF and THR	Nutritional assessment		√ (in rehab)			Lumbers *et al.*, 1996: UK
Orthopaedic surgery, FNF	MAC and TSF		√ (rehab)	√		Bastow *et al.*, 1983: UK
	Low W/H, TSF and MAC		√			Brown and Seabrook, 1992: UK (abstract)
Renal disease						
Chronic renal failure, predialysis	SGA	√ (need for acute hospitalization)		√		Lawson *et al.*, 2001: Australia
End-stage renal disease, dialysis	Nutritional assessment	√ (number of hospital admissions)		√		Engel *et al.*, 1995: UK
	Composite malnutrition score					Herselman *et al.*, 2000: South Africa
	Reactance (BIA)	√ (number of hospital admissions)				Ikizler *et al.*, 1999: USA
	W/H			√		Kopple *et al.*, 1999: USA
	Composite malnutrition score			√		Marckmann, 1989: Denmark
Surgery and intensive care						
Surgery, mixed						
Major surgery, mixed	MAMC, body weight			√		Brown *et al.*, 1982: UK
	PNI	√		√		Buzby *et al.*, 1980: USA

Condition	Nutritional criteria	Outcome	Outcome	Reference
Major GI surgery mixed	Nutritional assessment	✓		Symreng *et al.*, 1983: Sweden
	Weight loss of > 10% and dysfunction of two or more organ systems	✓		Windsor and Hill, 1988: NZ
	Weight loss > 10%, history of poor intake, low albumin or low prealbumin	✓	✓	Shaw-Stiffel *et al.*, 1993: USA
Surgery, benign				
General surgery	Nutritional assessment	✓	✓	Warnold and Lundholm, 1984: Sweden
Abdominal surgery	Nutritional assessment	✓		Dannhauser *et al.*, 1995a, b: South Africa
	Nutritional assessment	✓		Mughal and Meguid, 1987: USA
Cardiac surgery	BMI < 22 kg m^{-2} and albumin < 35 g l^{-1}	✓ (incl. need for MV, time on ICU)	✓	Desseigne *et al.*, 2001: France (abstract)
Liver transplant	Low BMI and albumin	✓ (bacterial infection)	✓	Sagar and Macfie, 1994: UK (abstract)
	MAC and TSF < 25th percentile	✓ (trend)	✓ (trend)	Harrison *et al.*, 1997: UK
	Nutritional assessment			Madden *et al.*, 1994: UK (abstract)
	SGA	✓ (↑ blood products during surgery)	✓	Stephenson *et al.*, 2001: USA
Lung surgery	BMI	✓ (need for ventilation)	✓	Mazolewski *et al.*, 1999: USA
Lung transplant	% IBW, BMI, FFM, FFMI	✓	✓	Nezu *et al.*, 2001: Japan
	BMI < 17 kg m^{-2} or > 25 kg m^{-2} IBW and CHI	✓ (duration ventilation, time on ICU)	✓	Madill *et al.*, 2001: Canada; Schwebel *et al.*, 2000: France
Surgery, malignancy				
Major surgery, oncology	Weight loss > 10% in 6 months	✓		Corish *et al.*, 1998: Ireland (abstract)
Gastrointestinal cancer surgery	Weight loss > 10%	✓		Gianotti *et al.*, 1995: Italy
Head and neck cancer surgery	Weight loss > 10% in 6 months	✓		Van Bokhorst-de van der Schueren *et al.*, 1997: The Netherlands

Continued

Table 4.6. *Continued*

Disease	Nutritional status assessment	Increased complications	Increased LOS	Increased mortality/ decreased survival	Increased hospital costs	Investigators
	Preoperative weight loss > 5%			√ (men only)		Van Bokhorst-de van der Schueren *et al.*, 1999: The Netherlands
	Weight loss of > 12%			√		Van Bokhorst-de van der Schueren *et al.*, 2000a: The Netherlands
Oesophago-gastrectomy	Postoperative weight loss	√				Martin *et al.*, 1999: USA (abstract)
Gastric cancer surgery	Weight loss			√ (trend)		Rey-Ferro *et al.*, 1997: Colombia
Colorectal cancer surgery	Composite malnutrition score	√		√		Meguid *et al.*, 1986: USA
Lung-cancer surgery	Postoperative weight loss		√			Ulander *et al.*, 1998: Sweden
	FFMI, % IBW, BMI	√ (need for ventilation)		√		Jagoe *et al.*, 2001b: UK
Intensive care ICU	W/H and albumin	√	√ (not discharged)[a]			Giner *et al.*, 1996: USA
	BMI < 15th percentile			√		Galanos *et al.*, 1997: USA
	Composite malnutrition score		√ (on ICU)			Huang *et al.*, 2000: Taiwan
	MAC < 15th percentile	√ (major complications)		√		Ravasco *et al.*, 2002: Portugal
Other diseases Chronic heart failure	Involuntary weight loss of > 7.5%			√		Anker *et al.*, 1997: UK

[a]Included those who died, remained in hospital for > 99 days or required readmission to ICU after discharge to the ward.

BCM, body cell mass; BIA, bioelectrical impedance analysis; BMT, bone marrow transplant; CHF, congestive heart failure; CHI, creatinine height index; CVD, cardiovascular disease; FFM, fat-free mass; FFMI, fat-free mass index; FNF, fractured neck of femur; GP, general practitioner; IBW, ideal body weight; ICU, intensive care unit; L/A, length-for-age; LBM, lean body mass; MAC, mid-arm circumference; MAFA, mid-arm fat area; MAMA, mid-arm muscle area; MAMC, mid-arm muscle circumference; MI, Maastricht index; MNA, Mini Nutritional Assessment; MV, mechanical ventilation; NRI, nutrition risk index; PNI, prognostic nutritional index; rehab, rehabilitation; SGA, subjective global assessment; THR, total hip replacement; TSF, triceps skin-fold thickness; UBW, usual body weight; UR, urological; W/A, weight-for-age; W/H, weight-for-height.

- general hospital admissions;
- medical patients;
- the elderly in a variety of health-care settings;
- paediatric patients;
- chronic heart failure;
- COPD;
- GI and liver disease;
- HIV infection and AIDS;
- a number of types of cancer;
- neurological patients;
- intensive-care patients;
- chronic renal failure prior to dialysis;
- end-stage renal disease patients receiving dialysis.

Apart from in-hospital complications and mortality, poor nutritional status has also been linked with a number of adverse consequences both pre- and post-discharge from hospital. These include the following:

- A trend for increased need for hospitalization during follow-up in elderly subjects at nutritional risk compared with well-nourished controls, as assessed by the Mini Nutritional Assessment (MNA; Beck *et al.*, 2001a).
- Significantly higher mortality, higher consultation rate with their general practitioner, higher prescription rate and greater rate of hospital admission in patients with chronic disorders of the respiratory, GI and neurological systems living in the community with a BMI < 20 kg m^{-2} compared with those with a BMI in the ideal range (Martyn *et al.*, 1998).
- Longer rehabilitation time in thin elderly females after orthopaedic hip surgery (Bastow *et al.*, 1983).
- Significantly longer convalescence periods, greater dependence on walking frames at 6 months and a lower rate of return to independent living in elderly females classified as high-risk based on nutritional indices on admission to hospital for orthopaedic hip surgery (Lumbers *et al.*, 1996).
- Reduced ability to be dependent in activities of daily living 3 months after discharge and increased need for admission to a nursing home in the year after

discharge in elderly medical patients (Covinsky *et al.*, 1999).
- Increased likelihood of requiring home health care after discharge in medical patients (Chima *et al.*, 1997).
- Increased rate of discharge to a nursing home in elderly patients (Van Nes *et al.*, 2001).
- Shorter survival time following discharge from a geriatric assessment unit (Mühlethaler *et al.*, 1995).
- Reduced Barthel index 30 days after acute stroke (Davalos *et al.*, 1996).
- Higher risk of non-elective readmission in patients hospitalized previously for medical or surgical reasons (Friedman *et al.*, 1997).
- More diagnostic problems (particularly infections) in the year post-discharge after hospitalization for general medical/surgical reasons (Linn, 1984).
- Increased mortality risk in geriatric patients in the year post-discharge (Sullivan *et al.*, 1991).
- Higher risk of non-elective readmission in patients hospitalized previously for exacerbation of COPD (Pouw *et al.*, 2000).

Furthermore, admission of free-living individuals into hospital and nursing homes is related to nutritional status:

- Elderly individuals at high risk of malnutrition have a greater risk of being admitted to hospital than those at low risk of malnutrition (Stratton *et al.*, 2002).
- In free-living frail elderly, weight loss of ≥ 5 kg has also been shown to be an important predictor of early institutionalization after controlling for social network, health and functional status (Payette *et al.*, 2000).

It is difficult to draw clear conclusions from these findings, and there are a number of limitations to the interpretation of these studies. None of them describe causal relationships between poor nutritional status and outcome and it is very difficult from these studies to separate effects of malnutrition *per se* and the underlying disease process (Anderson *et al.*, 1984). They merely describe associations that can be used to generate the hypothesis that, by improving nutritional status, outcome could be improved. Randomized, controlled intervention studies are necessary to test such a hypothesis. These are discussed in Chapters 6–8. Another limitation is that the method of defining nutritional status varies widely between studies, making direct comparisons difficult. However, in all the studies mentioned in Table 4.6, anthropometric indices were included in the definition of nutritional status (rather than relying on blood biochemistry, e.g. serum albumin and total lymphocyte count), as has been done in some studies that have also tried to suggest a link between poor nutritional status and outcome (Koval *et al.*, 1999; Lavernia *et al.*, 1999).

Few of the studies examined nutritional intake, which could also have an impact on many aspects of function (and therefore outcome), as described earlier in this book. However, a few studies have shown an association between inadequate nutritional intake and poor outcome:

- Reduced energy and nutrient intake may increase risk of hospitalization in the elderly (Mowé *et al.*, 1994).
- Low nutrient intake was associated with increased in-hospital mortality and 90-day mortality in elderly hospitalized patients, even though patients were initially assessed as having reasonable nutritional status (Sullivan *et al.*, 1999).
- Poor intake has been associated with the development or presence of pressure ulcers in studies in the community (Green *et al.*, 1999) and long-term care (Berlowitz and Wilking, 1989; Weiler *et al.*, 1990; Ek *et al.*, 1991; Bergstrom and Braden, 1992).
- Prolonged inadequate intake was associated with increased LOS in general medical patients (Anderson *et al.*, 1985).
- Insufficient spontaneous energy intake in normally nourished patients was associated with prolonged LOS in elderly patients with recent hip fracture (Paillaud *et al.*, 2000).

- A prolonged period of inadequate oral intake was associated with increased complications in patients following abdominal surgery (Meguid *et al.*, 1988).
- Duration of postoperative period without oral nutrient intake was correlated with LOS after major GI surgery (Shaw-Stiffel *et al.*, 1993).
- Cumulative energy deficit due to inadequate intake in survivors of multiple organ dysfunction syndrome on the intensive-care unit (ICU) was independently associated with the number of days with systemic inflammatory response syndrome (SIRS) and LOS on the ICU (Reid and Campbell, 2001).
- Starvation of more than 5 days in acute patients requiring nasogastric feeding was associated with increased mortality, most notably in patients over the age of 65 years (Taylor, 1993).

The definition of complications varies between studies and, with respect to mortality, the period of follow-up may vary from a few weeks to several years. Length of hospital stay can be criticized as an outcome parameter because of the many non-nutritional factors that can influence it. However, it is an outcome measure that captures the possible effects of poor wound healing, infections and impaired functional status, and an estimate of cost (including hotel and treatment costs) can be attached to it (Booth *et al.*, 1995).

Financial Aspects

As already described, many studies have identified associations between DRM and poor outcome, in terms of minor and major complications and mortality. Furthermore, several studies have identified associations between DRM and LOS. Of those studies that have examined the impact of poor clinical outcome and increased LOS on hospital costs, significant effects have been calculated (see Table 4.6).

The earliest reports examined medical (Robinson *et al.*, 1987) or mixed surgical and medical groups (Reilly *et al.*, 1988).

Robinson *et al.* (1987) prospectively audited 100 medical admissions to determine the relationship between initial nutritional status, LOS and actual hospital charges. Patients defined as malnourished on admission had an average LOS of almost 6 days longer than patients identified as well-nourished or borderline. Actual hospital charges were also significantly greater in both the malnourished ($16,691 ± 4389) (pre-1987 prices) and borderline ($14,118 ± 4962) patients compared with the well-nourished group ($7692 ± 687). In a retrospective review of 771 patient records (medical and surgical) in two acute-care hospitals, Reilly *et al.* (1988) determined patients with a likelihood of malnutrition on admission, and assessed the effect of this on rate of complications, LOS and costs and charges. Each item on each patient's itemized bill was ascribed to a cause category (usual and ordinary services, treating of complication, nutrition support and/or treatment of complication of nutrition support), with an appropriate adjustment made to categorization for increased LOS due to treatment of complications. Cost-to-charge ratios were then calculated to derive an estimate of the direct variable cost. Strong associations were demonstrated between likelihood of malnutrition and risk of complications, death and prolonged LOS (range 1.1–12.8 excess days). Likelihood of malnutrition significantly increased excess costs and charges per patient by $1738 (pre-1988 prices) and $3557, respectively, with even greater increases if complications occurred ($2996 and $6157 excess, respectively). These differences were observed in all diagnoses-related groups. For surgical patients with a likelihood of malnutrition, the differences in costs and charges compared with the well-nourished group were mainly related to increased LOS, whereas, in medical patients, raised costs were due to both increased LOS and higher costs per day. The average costs and charges for a well-nourished patient with no complications were $2968 and $6858, whereas for a malnourished patient with a major complication costs and charges were $12,683 and $26,359, respectively.

The cost of surgical infectious complications has been calculated in patients with cancer (Shulkin *et al.*, 1993). Using multivariate analysis, this study showed that the cost of a surgical infection added $12,542 to the cost of patient care. Fever alone, without documented infection, added $9145 to the cost of care.

More recently, Chima *et al.* (1997) demonstrated in a prospective study that patients admitted to the medical service who were classified as at risk of malnutrition (56 of the 172 studied) had significantly longer median LOS (6 vs. 4 days), significantly higher mean hospital costs ($6196 vs. $4563 (pre-1997 prices)) and increased likelihood of requiring home health care after discharge (31% vs. 12%) than the patients regarded as not at risk. In 404 adults admitted to the in-patient service of a university hospital for more than 7 days, patients who declined nutritionally during hospital stay, regardless of nutritional status on admission, had significantly higher mean hospital charges ($28,631 vs. $45,762) compared with those who remained normally nourished throughout (Braunschweig *et al.*, 2000). Preliminary results from a large multicentre study in 25 public hospitals in Brazil (*n* 600) suggest that, based on daily charges for length of hospitalization, hospital costs were increased by 50% in malnourished patients (Correia and Waitzberg, 1999).

In the community setting, a large epidemiological survey of patients attending general practitioners (GPs) in the UK found that those who were underweight (BMI < 20 kg m^{-2}) had higher rates of consultation with a GP, higher rates of prescription, higher hospital admission rates and higher death rates compared with those who were not underweight (BMI > 20–< 25 kg m^{-2}) (Martyn *et al.*, 1998; Edington *et al.*, 1999). More recently, an analysis of data from the National Diet and Nutrition Survey of people aged 65 years and over in the UK showed that healthcare utilization (based on GP visits and hospital admissions) rose significantly with increasing risk of malnutrition (Stratton *et al.*, 2002). In the USA, health-care expenditure has also been shown to increase considerably as BMI deviates from the ideal (Heithoff et al., 1997). It has been estimated that the extra cost of treating patients that have a BMI < 20 kg m^{-2} may be around £7.3 million per year per 100,000 patients in the UK (Martyn et al., 1998; Elia, 1999). If it can be demonstrated that DRM does have a direct impact on costs in hospitals, then it could be argued that patients who are malnourished in the community (i.e. on admission to hospital) will contribute to increased costs.

A number of broad estimates have been made of the financial impact of DRM and, by inference, the amount of money that could be saved if appropriate nutritional support were instituted. In the USA, one review suggested that hospital costs for undernourished patients were 35–75% higher than for well-nourished patients (Gallagher-Allred et al., 1996). Meguid (1993) estimated that increased LOS in malnourished patients at a cost of $5000 per patient amounted to annual costs of $18 billion (pre-1993 prices). Using more complicated techniques in 20 specific diagnosis-related groups in the US Medicare system, the Nutrition Screening Initiative calculated a reduction in spending of $156 million in 1994 if appropriate nutritional support, resulting in reduced LOS, were applied. Over the 1996–2002 period, this would amount to cumulative savings of $1.3 billion (Nutrition Screening Initiative, 1996). Tucker (1996) calculated potential annual savings of over $1 million per average institution if patient stay in hospital could be reduced by nutritional support. Similarly, in the UK in 1992, calculations showed that nutritional support could result in annual savings of £266 million in the National Health Service (NHS) if hospital stay was reduced by 5 days in 10% of in-patients (Lennard-Jones, 1992).

These costs (and therefore potential cost savings) are impressive, and most of the studies that have documented associations between malnutrition and increased costs have called for early, aggressive nutritional support as a means of reducing hospital costs. It is oversimplistic, however, to deduce from these studies that provision of nutritional support will improve outcome and reduce hospital costs, as demonstration of a causal association between DRM and complications, LOS and thus costs was not sought in these studies. Indeed, some argue that DRM is simply a secondary phenomenon of disease and not an important cause of morbidity in itself (Ofman and Koretz, 1997). Despite their limitations (Wolfe and Mathiesen, 1997), prospective, randomized, controlled studies in patients with or at risk of DRM are necessary to determine whether nutritional intervention can positively influence clinical outcome and hospital costs, and ideally clusters of similar studies should be subjected to systematic review to distil the most important findings (see Chapters 6–8).

Conclusion

Malnutrition produces a wide range of physiological and clinically relevant effects, ranging from mortality to impaired function of specific tissues, which are affected to varying degrees by different diseases. Malnutrition can also increase requirements for health care, with economic implications. Therefore, clinical nutrition trials often consider more than one outcome measure (functional, clinical, financial) and these may differ from study to study. Examples of the use of different outcome measures as end-points in clinical nutrition intervention trials are illustrated in Chapters 6–9. These chapters aim to highlight the potential benefits of nutritional support in different patient groups across health-care settings. In some patient groups, the benefits of using nutritional support (e.g. enteral tube feeding) are clear-cut and clinical trials are not required. In other patient groups, particularly where there is controversy about the relative contribution of disease and malnutrition to the outcome variables, and about the benefits and complications of the method of feeding used, nutrition intervention trials can be valuable (see Chapters 6–9).

Notes

[1] The QT interval is measured from the beginning of the QRS complex to the end of the T wave and represents the total time taken for depolarization and repolarization of the ventricles. It is normally between 0.35 and 0.45 s. The QT interval lengthens as the heart rate slows, and therefore heart rate must be taken into account.

[2] A neurological disorder characterized by confusion, apathy, drowsiness, ataxia (failure of muscular coordination), nystagmus (involuntary rapid movement of the eyeball) and opthalmoplegia (paralysis of the eye muscles). It is caused by thiamine deficiency, and is usually associated with chronic alcohol abuse.

5
Framework for Establishing an Evidence Base for Nutritional Intervention

In previous chapters of this book, we discussed the prevalence of disease-related malnutrition (DRM) and its adverse effects on body structure and function and clinical outcome. In Chapter 3, we highlighted the fact that these are frequently caused by reduced dietary intake. Therefore, increasing nutritional intake may be one of the most effective methods for treating DRM. By definition, the impairments in structure, function and clinical outcome that form malnutrition are nutritionally responsive (see Chapter 1). Therefore it is not surprising that one of the key aims of clinical nutrition practice is to increase nutritional intake in patients at risk of DRM. However, some patients with poor appetite or persistent difficulties with eating or swallowing may be unable to maintain or increase their food intake. In such cases, there are a number of ways available clinically to facilitate or increase nutritional intake. Methods of nutritional support include the following:

- Dietary manipulation using fortification and counselling.
- Oral nutritional supplements (ONS).
- Enteral tube feeding (ETF).
- Parenteral nutrition (PN).
- Combinations of the above.

However, how effective is nutritional support?

As Fig. 5.1 indicates, there is little doubt that nutritional support in most patients with obvious, clinical undernutrition will improve structure, physiological function,

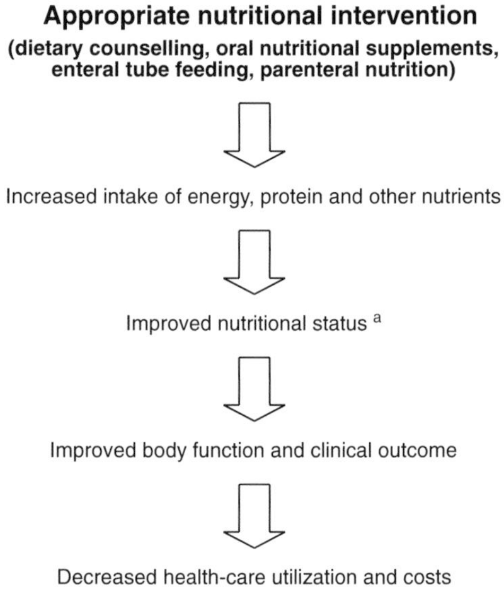

Appropriate nutritional intervention
(dietary counselling, oral nutritional supplements, enteral tube feeding, parenteral nutrition)

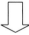

Increased intake of energy, protein and other nutrients

Improved nutritional status [a]

Improved body function and clinical outcome

Decreased health-care utilization and costs

Fig. 5.1. A proposed causal pathway between nutritional intervention in malnourished individuals and functional and clinical outcome.
[a] An improvement in body weight and fat-free mass generally reflects an improvement in protein–energy status. Theoretically, it may also be possible to improve function and clinical outcome, with little or no associated changes in gross body composition (see Chapters 6 and 7).

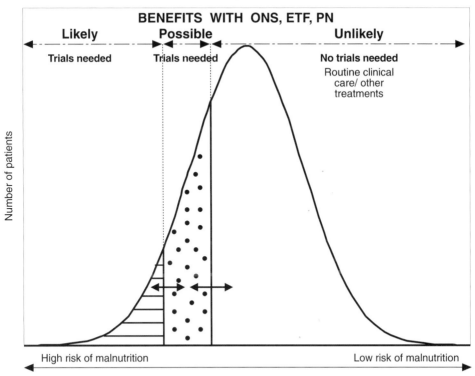

Fig. 5.2. Benefits of nutritional support according to risk of malnutrition and the need for clinical trials.

well-being and clinical outcome. In such cases, increased intake of an appropriate mixture of nutrients by a variety of different methods is likely to be beneficial (left side of distribution curve, Fig. 5.2), unless there are detriments or side-effects of particular feeding methods that outweigh the benefits (e.g. increased septic rate in patients receiving intravenous feeding). It is also obvious that providing nutritional support in well-nourished patients who are eating well is unlikely to be of any value (right side of distribution curve, Fig. 5.2). However, at the interphase between these two groups of patients, there is uncertainty about the benefits of nutritional support. This 'grey area' exists partly because of the difficulties in establishing a single cut-off point to distinguish between malnutrition and health (see Chapter 1) and partly because of the confounding effects of disease, which may alter the interrelationship between nutritional status and efficacy of

nutritional support. The need for nutritional support and the responsiveness to it may differ in the presence of disease/injury (indicated by the arrows (◄─►) on Fig. 5.2) and may vary with the type of disease or injury (e.g. acute or chronic, cancer, chronic obstructive pulmonary disease (COPD)).

The aim of the subsequent four chapters (Chapters 6–9) is to address the effectiveness of nutritional support (oral nutritional support, ETF and PN). However, with the increasing use of ONS and ETF in recent years (Department of Health, 1991–1998; Elia *et al.*, 2001b), particularly in the community setting (see Figs 5.3 and 5.4), there is a greater demand for an evidence base to support their use. Therefore, the rest of this chapter provides a framework for how the evidence base for nutritional intervention (specifically ONS and ETF) has been established. Chapters 6–8 present the findings.

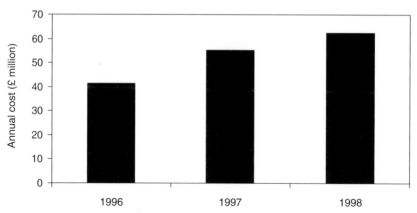

Fig. 5.3. Growth in expenditure on oral nutritional supplements and enteral feeds in the community in England (net ingredient cost, *British National Formulary*, Section 9.4.2) (data from Prescribing Support Unit, Department of Health, Leeds).

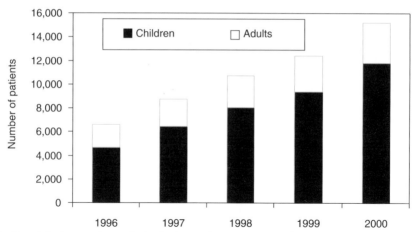

Fig. 5.4. Growth in the use of enteral tube feeding in the community in the UK (point prevalence of patients registered on home enteral tube feeding with British Artificial Nutrition Survey) (Elia *et al.*, 2001b).

Framework for Developing an Evidence Base

An evidence base is established using various levels of evidence (Table 5.1). The systematic review and meta-analysis are often considered the strongest type of evidence upon which to base recommendations for clinical practice. Therefore, there has been an increase in the number of published meta-analyses in recent years, including those on nutrition (see Fig. 5.5). There has also been growth in the number of systematic reviews and meta-analyses of nutritional support.

These have included a number of different approaches:

- Combined analyses of studies of different methods of nutritional support compared with routine clinical care (e.g. oral nutritional support, ETF, PN) across hospital and community settings (e.g. Potter *et al.*, 1998; Ferreira *et al.*, 2000).
- Combined analyses of studies of a mix of diagnostic groups comparing one or more methods of nutritional support with routine clinical care across settings (e.g. Potter *et al.*, 1998; Baldwin *et al.*, 2002).

Table 5.1. Levels of evidence for clinical effectiveness (Cochrane Library Training Guide). RCT, randomized controlled trial(s).

I	Strong evidence from at least one systematic review of well-designed RCT
II	Strong evidence from at least one properly designed RCT of appropriate size
III	Evidence from well-designed trials without randomization: single group pre-post; matched case-controlled
IV	Evidence from well-designed non-experimental studies from more than one centre or research group
V	Opinions of respected authorities, based on clinical evidence, descriptive studies or reports of expert committees
VI	Someone once told me

- Combined analysis of studies at one stage in the course of a disease/injury comparing nutritional support (ETF and oral support) with routine clinical care (e.g. Lewis *et al.*, 2001) or early versus late intervention (e.g. Marik and Zaloga, 2001).
- Comparative analyses of two different forms of nutritional support, e.g. ETF versus PN (Bozzetti *et al.*, 2001; Braunschweig *et al.*, 2001) or ONS versus dietary counselling (Baldwin *et al.*, 2002).
- Comparative analyses of different feed formulations, e.g. standard versus 'immune-enhancing' ETF (Beale *et al.*, 1999; Heys *et al.*, 1999; Heyland *et al.*, 2001b).

A single overall summary result of outcome obtained by combining and analysing the results of a range of studies involving different groups of patients receiving different modalities of nutritional support (ONS, PN, ETF) may be justified on the grounds that they all aim to improve intake when it is inadequate. In this way, nutritional requirements are more likely to be met, with the aim of preventing or reversing the detrimental effects of malnutrition. The combined analysis of a large number of studies is also statistically more powerful than the results of smaller, individual studies (one of the rationales for undertaking a meta-analysis). Therefore, the main advantages of this type of procedure are to increase power and allow generalizability of results across patient groups or test conditions (see Fig. 5.6). An example of this approach is the meta-analysis by Potter *et al.* (1998), who have assessed the effects of oral nutritional support and ETF in patients with variable degrees of malnutrition suffering from acute and chronic conditions in hospital and the community. However, a single result obtained by analysis of a heterogeneous group of studies may be of limited value, because it may not identify the subgroups of studies producing benefit and those that do not. It does not allow the clinician to decide whether to provide treatment for the specific groups or individual patients under his/her care on the basis of the findings (both clinical and economic) obtained from such general analyses.

Critics of the above approach argue that there could be important interactions between disease, degree of malnutrition (nutritional status) and type of nutritional support and that analyses should be carried out in a much more homogeneous group of patients (e.g. a specific form of nutritional support for a particular disease (Fig. 5.6)). Therefore, meta-analyses with more restrictive entry criteria have been undertaken (e.g. in patients undergoing surgical resections receiving ETF (Lewis *et al.*, 2001) or critically ill patients receiving PN (Heyland *et al.*, 2001b)). However, even these studies involve patients suffering from different phases of illness and various degrees of malnutrition.

An extension of this line of argument is to direct the analysis towards individual trials. However, even individual studies may be heterogeneous in certain respects. Purists may argue for preplanned subgroup analysis of studies with sufficient numbers of patients or the design of new studies

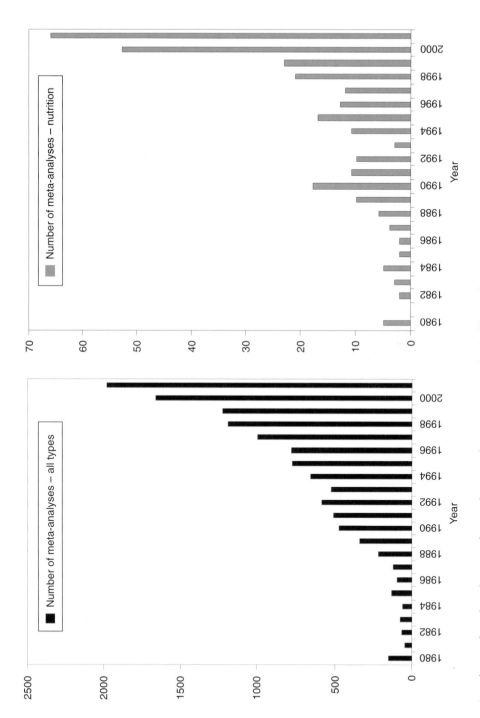

Fig. 5.5. Growth in total number of meta-analyses and meta-analyses on nutrition identified by Medline between 1980 and 2000 (search words: meta-analysis, meta-analyses and nutrition).

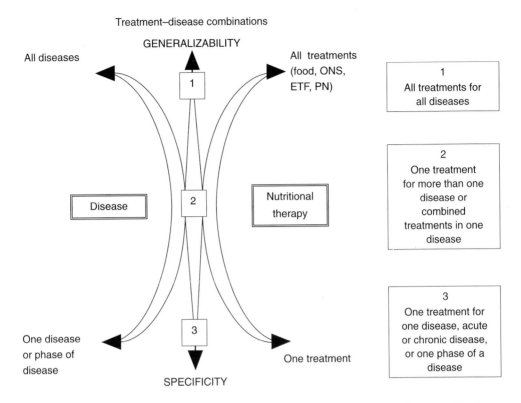

Fig. 5.6. Multi-layer approach to establishing the evidence base using various treatment–disease combinations.

with more restrictive entry criteria. This approach may increase confidence in the results of an intervention in a particular group of patients studied under a restrictive set of conditions (greater specificity). Although such studies have specificity, they lack 'generalizability', which may be necessary when establishing policies about nutritional intervention in general (see Fig. 5.6). Other workers take intermediate views between the two extremes indicated above (e.g. one modality of treatment for a group of related diseases).

In addition to the selection of studies on a clinical basis for meta-analysis, quality criteria can also be used, which can be assessed using a variety of scales. Therefore, it is of no great surprise that meta-analyses addressing the same question may come up with different and sometimes opposite conclusions (e.g. effectiveness of low-molecular-weight heparins in prevent-

ing postoperative thrombosis (Leizorovicz *et al.*, 1992; Nurmohamed *et al.*, 1992) and antirheumatic drugs in the treatment of rheumatoid arthritis (Felson *et al.*, 1990; Götzsche *et al.*, 1992)). There is no perfect single solution and it seems that there are advantages in building an evidence base using multiple approaches. The need to provide meta-analyses that are transparent and enable the reader to form their own clinical conclusions is also important.

In an attempt to provide both generic and specific insights into the effectiveness of enteral nutritional support (ONS and ETF) compared with routine clinical care, a multilayer systematic approach to establishing the evidence has been undertaken and is presented in this book. An overview of the concept of this analysis can be seen in Fig. 5.6. To obtain specificity and 'generalizability', the framework for this multilayer, systematic review is as follows:

- Individual randomized controlled trial(s) (RCT) and non-randomized trial(s) (NRT) arranged according to patient group, type of intervention (ONS or ETF) and setting (see Appendices 3 and 4 (ONS) and Appendices 5 and 6 (ETF)).
- Summary and analysis of RCT, NRT and other evidence (e.g. other reviews, meta-analyses and committee recommendations) for specific patient groups arranged according to the type of intervention (ONS or ETF) and the setting (hospital or community) (see Appendices 3 and 4 (ONS) and Appendices 5 and 6 (ETF)).
- Summary and meta-analysis of all trials according to type of intervention (ONS and ETF) and setting (hospital and community) (see Chapters 6 (ONS) and 7 (ETF)).
- Summary and meta-analysis of all trials (both hospital and community settings) according to the type of intervention (ONS or ETF) (see Chapters 6 (ONS) and 7 (ETF)).
- Summary and meta-analysis of all trials (both ONS and ETF, hospital and community settings, across patient groups) (see Chapter 8).

An overall summary, by combining a diverse group of studies or different patient groups or different modalities of nutritional support (ONS, ETF and PN), may be justified on the basis that they all aim to improve intake when it is low. In this way, nutritional requirements are more likely to be met and therefore prevent the detriments that would otherwise occur in such patients are prevented.

The rest of this chapter provides more details about the systematic review framework undertaken to establish the evidence base for ONS and ETF.

Establishing the Evidence Base: Review Processes

Undertaking systematic reviews

Systematic reviews are critical, objective appraisals of evidence, conducted according to explicit and reproducible methodology. A systematic review has been defined as a review that has been prepared using a systematic approach to minimize biases and random errors, which is documented in a methods section. A systematic review may or may not include a meta-analysis. The quality of reporting of meta-analyses (QUORUM) statement provides guidelines for assessing the methodology of systematic reviews. The steps undertaken in this systematic review process and described below followed this.

Step 1

The first step in the systematic review process is to define the question(s) that need to be addressed. For this review, four main questions were defined:

(I) What effect do ONS and ETF have on the voluntary food intake and total energy intake of patients in hospital and the community?
(II) What effect do ONS and ETF have on the body weight and composition of patients in hospital and the community?
(III) What effect do ONS and ETF have on the body function of patients in hospital and the community?
(IV) What effect do ONS and ETF have on the clinical and financial outcome of patients in hospital and the community?

Questions III and IV assessed the main outcome measures of nutritional intervention and questions I and II were included to provide possible explanations of the mechanisms by which outcome may be improved. In all cases, the efficacy of ONS and ETF was assessed relative to routine clinical care/no nutritional support. Whenever possible, information about dietary or other treatment was extracted for subsequent analysis (see Chapters 6 and 7 and Appendices 3–6).

Step 2

The second step is to define the inclusion and exclusion criteria for the selection of studies before beginning the review process. These criteria specify the types of intervention (e.g. for this review ONS, ETF), types of patients (e.g. adults and children), types of studies (e.g. randomized, controlled) and the outcomes for studies to be included in the review process. In this systematic review, different inclusion criteria were set for analysis of the systematic review of ONS and ETF (Chapters 6 and 7) and are shown in Table 5.2. Once gathered, studies were selected or excluded on the basis of the inclusion and exclusion of criteria specified at the start of the review process. This process should be undertaken by two investigations independently. The exclusion criteria were similar for both reviews: studies investigating the use of specialized enteral formulas (e.g. disease-specific formulations), studies of feeds containing only a single macronutrient or only micronutrients, studies of supplements used for the preoperative preparation of bowels, studies in developing countries and retrospective studies (which were only briefly considered where relevant).

Step 3

The third step is the comprehensive gathering of studies. The search strategies and sources of information used for this systematic review (presented in Chapters 6 and 7) included:

1. Electronic databases. These included MEDLINE, Bath Information and Data Services (BIDS), EMBASE, CINAHL, the Cochrane Library, Cancerlit, British Nursing Index, National Health Service (NHS) Research and Development Evidence-Based Medicine, NHS Centre for Reviews and Dissemination and NHS Economic Evaluation Database.
2. Cross-referencing from reference lists of published papers, reviews and industrial information.
3. Hand searching of abstracts and earlier nutrition journals not included on databases (*Proceedings of the Nutrition Society, Journal of Human Nutrition and Dietetics, Clinical Nutrition*).

Table 5.2. Inclusion criteria for systematic reviews of oral nutritional supplements and enteral tube feeding.

Oral nutritional supplement review: inclusion criteria	Enteral tube feeding review: inclusion criteria
Studies using oral nutritional supplements that: • Contain a mix of macronutrients (carbohydrate, fat, protein), including nutritionally complete and nutritionally incomplete supplements • Are of any form (sip feeds, drinks, bars, puddings, powders) • Are commercially produced, 'hospital-made' or 'home-made' • Are prescribable or non-prescribable	Use of enteral tube feeding: • Using nasoenteric tubes and other enteral access routes (including all types of gastrostomy and jejunostomy) • Using commercially produced, 'hospital-made' or 'home-made' tube feeds that contain a mix of macronutrients (carbohydrate, fat, protein), with or without micronutrients
Studies of oral nutritional supplementation in patients who are hospital-based or community-based (out-patients, nursing and residential homes, own homes)	Studies of enteral tube feeding in patients who are hospital-based or community-based (out-patients, nursing and residential homes, own homes)
Studies of patients of all ages who are not pregnant	Studies of patients of all ages
Studies that are a randomized, controlled design. Non-randomized trials will also be gathered and summarized briefly	Studies that are a randomized, controlled design. Non-randomized trials will also be gathered and summarized briefly
Studies including one or more of the following outcomes: total energy/nutrient intake, voluntary food intake, anthropometry, functional outcomes, clinical outcomes, financial assessments	Studies including one or more of the following outcomes: total energy/nutrient intake, voluntary food intake, anthropometry, functional outcomes, clinical outcomes, financial assessments

4. Discussion with health professionals and academic researchers working in the specialist areas.
5. Professional bodies – dietetic and disease-related groups (USA, Canada and UK).

Step 4

The fourth step is to categorize and code all the studies according to their methodology. For this review, randomized trials were assessed using the Jadad scoring system (Jadad *et al.*, 1996), which includes five criteria (Table 5.3).

NRT were categorized as non-randomized, controlled trials (systematic allocation, non-random concurrent trials) (code B) and prospective, non-randomized, non-controlled trials (code C). Any trials that were clearly reported by the same author twice as an abstract and a full paper were reviewed only once, using data from the full paper.

Step 5

The fifth step is retrieval of the data that will allow answers to the questions posed at the start of the review. This will include

information about: (i) the population studied (e.g. patients' age, diagnosis, body mass index (BMI)); (ii) the intervention used (e.g. type, composition, amount and duration of ONS); and (iii) the outcome measures (e.g. weight, hand-grip strength and mortality rate).

POPULATIONS AND INTERVENTIONS
For this systematic review, information was gathered from each of the trials reviewed in each disease grouping of: the number of patients studied (both intervention and controls), their initial nutritional status, the duration of supplementation or ETF, information on the type, composition and amount of feed prescribed and taken and the type of tube used (if relevant). The timing of ONS or ETF was also recorded. This included any documentation of the time of day ONS or ETF was given and the time of their introduction during treatment. The toleration of ONS or ETF (where reported) was also noted. Any information on the provision of dietary counselling for either intervention or control groups or any other treatments that patients received was briefly summarized.

Table 5.3. Jadad scoring of randomized controlled trials (Jadad *et al.*, 1996).

Jadad criteria	Score	
	Yes	No
Was the study described as randomized? (Includes the use of words such as randomly, random, randomization)	1	0
Was the method to generate the sequence of randomization described and was it appropriate (e.g. table of random numbers, computer-generated)?		
• Described and appropriate or	1 or	0
• Described and inappropriate	−1	
Was the study described as double-blind?	1	0
Was the method of double-blinding described and appropriate (identical placebo, active placebo, dummy)?		
• Described and appropriate or	1 or	0
• Described and inappropriate	−1	
Was there a description of withdrawals and drop-outs?	1	0

The maximum score is 5 and the minimum score 0. The scores for each of these categories for each study are summarized in the relevant tables as a five-digit number (e.g.11001) (see Appendices 3–6). For example, a coding of 11001 (total score 3) means that the study was described as randomized (score 1), the method used to randomize was appropriate (score 1), the study was not double-blind (score 0), did not involve a placebo (score 0) and described the number of drop-outs (score 1).

All the information extracted from the individual studies is summarized in table form in Appendices 3–6. Within these tables, studies are arranged in alphabetical order. Where relevant information was not provided in a paper, a dash '–' is used in the table.

OUTCOME MEASURES

Changes in the following outcome measures after intervention with ONS or ETF, were recorded where information was available, and summarized in table form:

Total energy intake and voluntary food intake. Changes in total energy intake observed during the study were recorded and quantified. The impact of ONS or ETF on voluntary food intake in patients able to eat was assessed whenever possible. Within the ONS review, estimation of the % of supplement energy that was additive to food energy was also made, using one of the following three methods, depending on the data available in each study:

1. In RCT involving matched groups of patients, the % of supplement energy intake that was additive to food intake was calculated as:

$$100 - \left(\frac{\text{S} + \Delta \dfrac{\text{EIF during S} - \text{EIF before}}{\text{EIF in control US group}} \times 100}{\text{ONS energy intake}} \right)$$

where EIF is energy intake from food, S is supplementation and US is unsupplemented. Studies in which patients were not matched (e.g. different disease severity, different treatments) were excluded. Studies involving a crossover design were amenable to this methodological approach.

2. This method was used when baseline information on energy intake in supplemented patients was not available, but results of the food energy intakes in the supplemented and unsupplemented groups during the study were. This assessment was only made in RCT in which patients in supplemented and unsupplemented groups were well matched. Errors arising from inadequate matching of patients are reduced when the energy intake from the supple-

ments is large. The % of supplement energy intake that was additive to food intake was calculated as:

$$\frac{\text{TEI of S group} - \text{TEI of US group}}{\text{ONS energy intake}} \times 100$$

where TEI is total energy intake, S is supplemented and US is unsupplemented.

3. This method was used when data from a control group were unavailable. It involved longitudinal assessment of energy intake from food before and during supplementation. This assessment can be of some value in patients with relatively stable disease but may be subject to errors associated with spontaneous changes in food intake resulting from a change in disease activity, or as a result of the interest and attention provided by the study investigators/health professionals (placebo effect). The extent of error with this method is again likely to be smaller when the energy intake from the supplement is large. The % of supplement energy intake that was additive to food intake was calculated as:

$$\frac{\text{EIF during S} - \text{EIF before S}}{\text{ONS energy intake}} \times 100$$

where EIF is energy intake from food and S is supplementation.

In view of the methodological limitations associated with ingestion of small amounts of ONS, only studies that involved the ingestion of > 350 kcal from the supplement were assessed using the above methods. This effectively excluded four studies (Rana *et al.*, 1992; Volkert *et al.*, 1996; Jensen and Hessov, 1997; Keele *et al.*, 1997). Longitudinal studies involving patients with cancer or Crohn's disease, in which disease activity changed during the course of the study, were also excluded from this analysis (e.g. Harries *et al.*, 1984).

Body weight and composition and growth. The outcome measures recorded included: changes in body weight/BMI (kg m^{-2}); lean body mass (LBM); fat mass; arm anthropometry (mid-arm muscle circumference, skin-folds); and growth in children. The presence of confounding factors, such as oedema or use of steroids, was noted.

Functional outcome. General functional outcome measures were noted but these varied with the studies, e.g. quality of life and hand-grip strength, and disease-specific outcome measures (i.e. respiratory muscle strength in COPD patients) were noted.

Clinical and financial outcome. Information on changes in clinical outcome (e.g. length of hospital stay, mortality, complication rates, prescription use) and any financial data relating to the cost-effectiveness of ONS or ETF use were collected (including prospective and retrospective calculations and estimates).

Step 6

The sixth step is the critical analysis and synthesis of the findings. For this review, in addition to presenting information on individual studies, summaries of the efficacy of the two different forms of enteral nutritional support (ONS and ETF) were made separately for all studies as a whole, for each disease/condition-specific group and for hospital and community locations. In addition, some combined analyses of the effects of both ONS and ETF were undertaken. The findings are presented in Chapters 6–8.

Undertaking meta-analysis

As part of the systematic review, meta-analysis was performed. Meta-analysis has been defined as 'a statistical procedure that integrates the results of several independent studies considered to be "combinable"' (Altman, 1995).

Meta-analysis facilitates a more objective assessment of the evidence than a narrative review. It can provide a single quantitative estimate of a treatment effect and can highlight the heterogeneity between the results of individual studies.

A number of packages are available for analysing results of meta-analyses (Egger *et al.*, 2001), but, for this analysis, MetaWin statistical package (Version 2.0, Sinauer and Associates, Massachusetts)

was used. Meta-analysis was undertaken to gain an indication of the treatment effect (of ONS or ETF) on a number of outcome measures. These were % weight change, mortality rates and complication rates. For continuous data (e.g. mean and standard deviation of % weight change), mean weighted difference between intervention (ONS or ETF) and control groups was calculated for each trial. For binary data (e.g. dead or not dead), odds ratios were used. A 'fixed effects' model for meta-analysis was used to calculate the overall effect size. This assumes that the true effect of treatment is the same value in each study (fixed), with the differences between study results being due to chance. A test of homogeneity was used to test the assumption of a fixed effect. A 'random effects' model was also applied as appropriate. This model assumes different underlying effects for each study, which contribute an additional source of variation. As yet, there is no consensus about which model (fixed or random effects) should be used (Egger *et al.*, 2001) but the random-effects model will normally give a more conservative result. It is also desirable to only include data from intention-to-treat analysis in the meta-analysis, although it was not always possible to do this in the present analysis due to limitations in the data sets provided. Part of the meta-analytic procedure can also include an estimate of the heterogeneity of the studies included and an assessment of publication bias. Publication bias can be defined as the publication or non-publication of research findings, depending on the nature and direction of the results (Egger *et al.*, 2001). Studies with statistically significant results are more likely to get published than those with non-significant results. A variety of graphical and statistical methods have been developed for evaluating publication bias (Sterne *et al.*, 2001). For this review, the possibility of publication bias was assessed in two ways. First, the effect size was plotted against the sample size of the individual studies to assess any 'funnel' effects, whereby the smallest trials show the largest treatment effects and vice versa. As a graphical display can be difficult to interpret with small numbers of trials, Rosenthal's method of fail-safe numbers was also used (Rosenthal, 1979). The fail-safe number is the number of non-significant, missing or unpublished studies that would need to be added to a meta-analysis in order to change the results from significance to non-significance. If this number is large relative to the number of trials included in the meta-analysis, there is greater confidence that the observed result, even with some publication bias, is likely to be a reliable estimate of the true effect. A score of $(5n + 10)$ or more (n = number of trials) is a conservative value against which the fail-safe number was tested (Rosenthal, 1979). For the present analysis, these procedures were undertaken using the MetaWin v2.0 statistical package.

Step 7

The final step in the systematic review process is the formation of conclusions and recommendations for clinical practice and for further research. Conclusions relating to the present analysis can be found in Chapters 6–8.

This book does not provide detailed information on how to undertake a systematic review and meta-analysis, but a complete guide by Egger *et al.* (2001) is recommended.

Decision Making

When considering the treatment of individual patients, it is important to balance clinical judgement and expertise of the treatment of specific patients and of specific conditions with the available evidence base (see Fig. 5.7). Practising evidence-based nutrition means combining the best available clinical evidence from systematic research with clinical expertise and the practicalities of undertaking the treatment (e.g. resources available). The knowledge

matrix is incomplete and the limitations of different approaches to assessing the evidence base, ranging from individual studies to meta-analyses of heterogeneous groups of patients, have been highlighted. Each approach has specific advantages and can contribute to the overall evidence base. Ultimately, judgement will be based not only on this knowledge base but also on previous clinical experience and available resources.

In undertaking this systematic review, it became clear that inadequacies in planning, undertaking and reporting clinical trials were common. Therefore, a separate chapter is included in this book to provide a practical guide to undertaking clinical nutrition trials (Chapter 10). In some situations, the evidence base for using a particular nutrition intervention in the treatment of a specific condition may be lacking. The clinician will then base decisions primarily on clinical expertise, assuming adequate resources. In other situations, there may be good evidence for the use of a particular nutritional intervention in certain groups of patients (e.g. long-term use of PN in chronic intestinal failure) but inadequate resources to fund it.

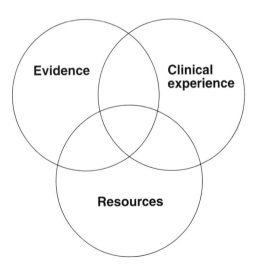

Fig. 5.7. Decision making for nutritional intervention.

6
Evidence Base for Oral Nutritional Support

Systematic Review of Oral Nutritional Supplements

This chapter provides a detailed evidence base for the use of oral nutritional supplements (ONS) in clinical practice. The systematic review and meta-analysis presented indicate that marked and significant improvements in clinical outcome may follow ONS. In particular, significant reductions in mortality and complication rates are achieved by using ONS compared with routine clinical care in patients at risk of disease-related malnutrition (DRM). Reductions in hospital length of stay (LOS) are also consistently observed. The use of ONS can lead to a range of functional benefits, many of which are specific to particular diagnostic groups. The mechanisms by which ONS produce benefits in body function and clinical outcome are uncertain, but they probably involve improvements in both the mass and function of body tissues. The extent to which these are mediated by individual nutrients or combinations of nutrients is unclear. For a summary of the key findings from the evidence base, see Box 6.1 (hospital setting) and Box 6.2 (community setting).

The efficacy of dietary methods to increase nutritional intake (e.g. dietary fortification and counselling) is also considered later in this chapter.

Types of ONS

One of the main strategies for increasing nutritional intake orally is by the use of nutritional supplements. ONS can be used to improve patients' total intakes of energy and a variety of nutrients, including protein, vitamins, trace elements and minerals, in clinical practice. They are typically used as a supplement to the diet to increase total nutritional intake. There are a number of different types of ONS (Table 6.1), including ready-made milk-, juice- and yoghurt-based or savoury drinks (sip feeds), which are available in a wide variety of flavours. Some ONS are 'nutritionally complete', meaning that they contain all essential nutrients in proportions that make them suitable for use as a sole source of nutrition if a certain amount is consumed. They may contain fibre. A variety of puddings are also available to supplement food intake. Powder supplements come in two forms: (i) those that can be made up into a drink and may contain added vitamins and minerals; and (ii) those that can be added to drinks and food, which are usually energy or protein sources only (Table 6.2).

Some ONS have been specifically formulated for children (see Table 6.1). In addition, a number of ONS are available which have been especially formulated for

Box 6.1. Key findings from the evidence base for oral nutritional supplements in the hospital setting (58 trials, 34 RCT, *n* 3883). RCT, randomized controlled trials; COPD, chronic obstructive pulmonary disease; CI, confidence interval; BMI, body mass index.

ONS can improve energy and nutrient intake
ONS increased total energy intake in all RCT (*n* 25 assessed intake, 70% of which were significant increases) in a variety of patient groups (COPD, elderly, post-surgical, orthopaedic, liver disease, cancer). This effect was observed, irrespective of whether the mean BMI of the group was < 20 kg m^{-2} or > 20 kg m^{-2}. ONS had little suppressive effect on food intake and in some groups (e.g. post-surgical patients) appeared to stimulate appetite and food intake. Although the effectiveness of ONS at increasing total energy intake may be limited during the peak of the acute-phase response in some conditions, overall there is uncertainty about the optimal timing or composition for oral nutritional supplementation.

ONS can improve body weight or attenuate weight loss
ONS improved weight in 81% of trials (*n* 35 assessed weight), of which 46% were significant. Average % weight change between supplemented and control patients was +3% (17 RCT) across a variety of patient groups (surgery, elderly, COPD) and was similar in trials in which mean BMI was < 20 kg m^{-2} or > 20 kg m^{-2}. Meta-analysis (ten RCT, *n* 1187) showed a mean effect size with ONS of 0.65 (95% CI 0.52–0.79), with considerable heterogeneity between studies. Changes in body composition and fluid balance (presence or absence of oedema or ascites) were often not assessed.

ONS can improve functional outcomes
Most RCT assessing function (76%, *n* 17) reported benefits, of which 71% were significant. Benefits included increased muscle strength, walking distances, well-being, physical and mental health and activity levels, depending on the patient group. Greater % weight change in supplemented relative to control patients was observed in trials showing functional benefit (+3.9%) than in those that did not (+1.3%). Functional benefits were reported in trials in which the mean BMI of patients was < 20 kg m^{-2} or > 20 kg m^{-2}. The impact of ONS may be limited in patients with severe disease who have become severely undernourished. No significant functional detriments were reported.

ONS can improve clinical outcomes
Most RCT (88%, *n* 15) assessing clinical outcome showed improvements, more than 50% of which were statistically significant.

- Mortality rates were significantly lower in supplemented (19%) than unsupplemented (25%) patients (elderly, liver disease, surgery and orthopaedics, *P* < 0.001; odds ratio 0.61 (95% CI 0.4–0.78), meta-analysis of 11 trials, *n* 1965; no significant heterogeneity between individual studies). The reduction in mortality with ONS tended to be greater in patient groups in which the average BMI was < 20 kg m^{-2} than in those with BMI > 20 kg m^{-2}.
- Complication rates were significantly lower in supplemented (18%) than in unsupplemented (41%) hospital patients (surgical, orthopaedic, elderly, neurology, *P* < 0.001; odds ratio 0.31 (95% CI 0.17–0.56), meta-analysis of seven trials, *n* 384; no significant heterogeneity between individual studies). Complication rates were similarly reduced in patient groups with a BMI < 20 kg m^{-2} and > 20 kg m^{-2}.
- Length of hospital stay in supplemented compared with control patients was reduced in all nine RCT that presented results, either as means or medians (9/9 trials; binomial test, *P* < 0.002). The reduction in length of stay appeared to be greater in patient groups with a BMI < 20 kg m^{-2} than when BMI was > 20 kg m^{-2}.

In trials that reported a positive effect on clinical outcome, the accompanying weight change was relatively small (< 1% to 5%), often as the duration of ONS was short.

Methodology
The methodological limitations of the reviewed trials included lack of randomization (59% RCT), lack of double-blinding and placebo controls and small sample sizes. Larger, well-designed RCT in specific patient groups are needed in the hospital setting to fully characterize the clinical and cost-effectiveness of ONS.

Box 6.2. Key findings from the evidence base for oral nutritional supplements in the community setting (108 trials, 44 RCT, *n* 3747). COPD, chronic obstructive pulmonary disease; RCT, randomized controlled trials; BMI, body mass index; HIV, human immunodeficiency virus; CI, confidence interval.

ONS can improve energy and nutrient intake
ONS increased total energy, protein and micronutrient intakes across a variety of patient groups in the community (including COPD, elderly, cystic fibrosis, Crohn's disease). Ninety-one per cent of RCT (*n* 29) assessing energy intake showed improvements, of which > 70% were significant. Despite some suppression in food intake with ONS, the mean increase in total energy intake was equivalent to 69% of the ONS energy but the increase was greater in studies of patients with a mean BMI < 20 kg m^{-2} (~83%) than > 20 kg m^{-2} (~45%). During long-term use of ONS in those with chronic disease, food and total energy intake may decrease.

ONS can improve body weight and growth
Improvements in body weight were documented in 90% of RCT assessing weight, of which 60% were significant increases. Mean weight change in supplemented relative to unsupplemented patients (+1.87%; 30 RCT) varied considerably between patient groups and individual trials and tended to be greater in trials of patients with a mean BMI < 20 kg m^{-2} than those with > 20 kg m^{-2} (+3.1% and +1.3%; 24 RCT; consistent with findings of non-randomized trials reviewed). Meta-analysis of % weight change data 13 RCT (in COPD, elderly, HIV, liver disease, cancer, post-surgical patients) suggested a mean effect size with ONS of 0.61 (95% CI 0.50–0.71), with considerable heterogeneity between trials.

Improvements in growth in growth-retarded children were evident in all the trials that made such assessments (*n* 14, only two RCT). Improvements in body composition (increases in muscle and/or fat mass, mostly measured using upper-arm anthropometry) were reported in 56% (*n* 25) of trials that made such assessments and appeared to be more likely in trials in which patients had an average BMI < 20 kg m^{-2}.

ONS can improve functional outcomes and may improve clinical outcome
Functional improvements were observed in most RCT (63%, *n* 22), of which 45% were significant. These varied according to the patient group and included improvements in respiratory muscle function and walking distances in COPD patients, skeletal muscle strength in those with liver disease and increases in activities of daily living and fewer falls in the elderly. Although % weight increase was similar in trials with and without significant functional benefits (+3.73%, *n* 11 and +3.25%, *n* 12 respectively), in some patient groups (e.g. underweight COPD patients and the elderly) functional benefits were only observed when weight gain was ≥ 2 kg. Functional benefits were more likely in trials in which patients had a mean BMI < 20 kg m^{-2} than those with > 20 kg m^{-2} (*P* < 0.009). No significant functional detriments were reported.

ONS may improve clinical outcomes, reducing rates of infection and the frequency of hospitalization and reducing hospital stays, but there is a scarcity of information about the clinical and cost-effectiveness of ONS use in the community setting.

Methodology
Inadequate randomization (only 41% of trials) and poor study designs (low Jadad scores, small sample sizes and lack of statistical power) were common limitations of the data set reviewed. Larger, well-designed RCT, where appropriate, are required to assess the impact of ONS on outcome in community-based patients.

use in patients with specific diseases, disorders or conditions, such as inflammatory bowel disease and other gastrointestinal conditions, pressure ulcers, renal disease and respiratory disease.

The availability of ONS in terms of types of products and whether or not they are reimbursed varies from country to country. In some countries, e.g. the UK, some types of ONS are available on prescription and are

Table 6.1. Examples of oral nutritional supplements.

Oral nutritional supplement	Presentation	Energy content (kcal 100 ml^{-1})	Protein content (g 100 ml^{-1})
Oral supplements suitable as a sole source of nutrition ('nutritionally complete')			
Milk-based liquid sip feeds			
Biosorb Drink (Nutricia)	Bottle (500 ml)	100	4
Nutridrink / Fortisip Multi Fibre* (Nutricia)	Tetra (200 ml)	150	6
Nutridrink / Fortisip (Nutricia)	Tetra (200 ml)	150	6
Clinutren Iso (Nestle)	Cup (200 ml)	100	3.8
Clinutren 1.5 (Nestle)	Cup (200 ml)	150	5.6
Fresubin Original (Fresenius)	Tetra (200 ml)	100	3.8
	Bottle (500 ml)		
Fresubin Energy* (Fresenius)	Tetra (200 ml)	150	5.6
Ensure Fibre with FOS* (Abbott)	Can (8 fl.oz)	106	3.8
Ensure (Abbott)	Can (8 fl.oz; 32 fl.oz)	106	3.7
Enrich Plus Drink* (Abbott)	Tetra (200 ml)	150	6.25
Ensure Plus Drink (Abbott)	Tetra (220 ml)	150	6.25
Yoghurt-based liquid sip feeds			
Fortifresh (Nutricia)	Tetra (200 ml)	150	6
Ensure Plus Yoghurt style (Abbott)	Tetra (220 ml)	150	6.25
Milk-based liquid sip feeds suitable for children			
Fortini Multi Fibre* (Nutricia)	Tetra (200 ml)	150	3.4
Fortini (Nutricia)	Tetra (200 ml)	150	3.4
Resource Junior Drink (Novartis)	Tetra (200 ml)	150	3
Frebini MiniMax (Fresenius)	Tetra (200 ml)	150	3.8
Paediasure with Fibre* (Abbott)	Tetra (200 ml)		
	Can (8 fl.oz)	101	2.8
Paediasure (Abbott)	Tetra (200 ml)	101	3
	Can (8 fl.oz)		
Paediasure Plus (Abbott)	Tetra (200 ml)	150	4.2
Oral supplements not suitable as a sole source of nutrition			
Milk-based liquid sip feeds			
Fortimel (Nutricia)	Tetra (200 ml)	100	10
Resource 1.5 (Novartis)	Carton (200 ml)	150	5.6
Resource 1.7 Energy/Shake (Novartis)	Carton (175 ml)	170	5.1
Resource 2.0 (Novartis)	Carton (200 ml)	200	9
Resource Protein (Novartis)	Carton (200 ml)	125	9.4
Resource Meritene (Novartis)	Bottle (250 ml)	95	8
Clinutren HP (Nestle)	Cup (200 ml)	125	7.5
Protenplus Drink (Fresenius)	Tetra (200 ml)	125	9
'Juice'-based liquid sip feeds			
Fortijuce (Nutricia)	Tetra (200 ml)	150	4
Resource Fruit (Novartis)	Carton (200 ml)	90	4
Clinutren Fruit (Nestle)	Cup (200 ml)	125	4
Provide Xtra (Fresenius)	Tetra (200 ml)	125	3.75
Enlive (Abbott)	Tetra (200 ml)	125	4.16
Desserts			
Forticreme (Nutricia)	Cup (125 g)	161 kcal 100 g^{-1}	10 g 100 g^{-1}
Resource Dessert Energy (Novartis)	Cup (125 g)	160 kcal 100 g^{-1}	4.8 g 100 g^{-1}
Clinutren Dessert (Nestle)	Pot (125 g)	125 kcal 100 g^{-1}	9.5 g 100 g^{-1}
Formance (Abbott)	Pot (113 g)	148 kcal 100 g^{-1}	3.5 g 100 g^{-1}

Continued

Table 6.1. *Continued*

Oral nutritional supplement	Presentation	Energy content (kcal 100 ml^{-1})	Protein content (g 100 ml^{-1})
Powders for reconstitution into a drink			
Scandishake Mix (Nutricia)	Powder (85 g) reconstituted with 240 ml whole milk	598 kcal/serving (2 kcal ml^{-1})	11.7 g/serving
Build-Up (Nestle)	Powder (38 g) reconstituted with 284 ml whole milk	330 kcal/serving (1.1 kcal ml^{-1})	18.2 g/serving
Calshake Powder (Fresenius)	Powder (87 g) reconstituted with 240 ml whole milk	598 kcal/serving (2 kcal ml^{-1})	12 g/serving

* Contains fibre.
This table was compiled based on information available to the authors at the time of writing (July 2002). This is not a complete overview of all products available on the market, but is intended to give examples of the main products. Not all products/presentations are available in all countries. Furthermore, product names, presentations and compositions may vary between countries, and may be subject to change. For more accurate information, contact individual manufacturers.

Table 6.2. Examples of energy and protein modules for oral nutritional supplementation.

Energy modules		Protein modules	
Name	Type	Name	Type
Nutrical / Polycal liquid (Nutricia)	Glucose polymer, liquid	Protifar (Nutricia)	Powder
Fantomalt / Polycal (Nutricia)	Maltodextrin, powder	Maxipro (SHS)	Powder
Maxijul (SHS)	Glucose polymer, liquid and powder		
Calogen (SHS)	Fat emulsion		
Duocal (SHS)	Fat and glucose emulsion, liquid, powder and bar		

This table was compiled based on information available to the authors at the time of writing (July 2002). This is not a complete overview of all products available on the market, but is intended to give examples of the main products. Not all products/presentations are available in all countries. Furthermore, product names, presentations and compositions may vary between countries, and may be subject to change. For more accurate information, contact individual manufacturers.

reimbursed in the community for specific indications (e.g. disease-related malnutrition, preoperative preparation of undernourished patients, inflammatory bowel disease, dysphagia, intractable malabsorption). In other countries, some types of ONS are available to the public to buy from pharmacies.

Evidence Base for ONS

As highlighted in Chapter 5, ONS are a commonly used method of nutritional support in the prevention or treatment of DRM. ONS are used in a wide range of patients (from young children to the elderly) suffering from different diseases or conditions (chronic obstructive pulmonary disease (COPD), trauma, cystic fibrosis, cancer, human immunodeficiency virus/acquired immune deficiency syndrome (HIV/AIDS), liver and gastrointestinal (GI) disease) or undergoing procedures (e.g. surgery) that affect body weight and nutritional status (Schurch and Scrimshaw, 1987; James and Ralph, 1992; Ramsey *et al.*, 1992; Elia and Lunn, 1996). They are used in the treatment of acute and chronic disease in patients in both hospital and community settings, but their use has particularly increased in the community setting (Department of Health, 1991–1998) in countries such as England (see Fig. 5.3, Chapter 5). Figure 6.1 suggests that ONS are likely to be of some value in patients who are at high risk of malnutrition (left side of distribution curve) and are not eating well, usually as a result of severe acute or chronic disease. However, evidence of benefit is often lacking. For other patients who have a lower risk of malnutrition and are eating more, there is greater uncertainty about the benefits of using ONS. Clinical trials are usually undertaken in these two groups of patients. Patients who are well nourished and have an adequate intake (right side of distribution curve, Fig. 6.1) do not require ONS and are unlikely to

benefit from them. Such patients are generally not included in clinical trials. Therefore the effectiveness of ONS requires clarification in patient groups at risk of malnutrition.

The lack of a consensus about the value of ONS in certain patient groups in different settings has meant that there are no generally agreed recommendations for their use. It is difficult to make such recommendations without fundamental information about the effects of ONS on habitual food intake, body weight and/or composition and, most importantly, body function and clinical outcome in different clinical situations. One key issue is whether the energy consumed as ONS merely suppresses appetite and food intake, replacing the energy habitually taken from food and so failing to substantially increase total energy or nutrient intake. If this occurs, then improvements in body weight, composition and function may not follow. If the

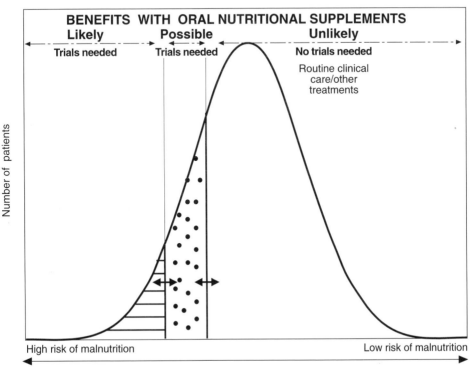

Fig. 6.1. Benefits of ONS according to risk of malnutrition and the need for clinical trials (oral intake feasible in this population).

ONS replaces normal food intake, then the cost of the ONS is effectively equivalent to 'purchasing' food. In contrast, if the energy of the ONS is additional to that from habitual food intake, then improvements in body weight and possibly function and clinical outcome are more likely. Another issue is whether any improvements resulting from supplementation are maintained or rapidly lost when the supplements are no longer consumed.

A number of meta-analyses have attempted to address the efficacy of this mode of nutritional support (Potter *et al.*, 1998; Ferreira *et al.*, 2000; Avenell and Handoll, 2001; Potter, 2001; Poustie *et al.*, 2002; Smyth and Walters, 2002), some in specific patient groups (e.g. COPD (Ferreira *et al.*, 2000), fractured neck of femur (Avenell *et al.*, 2001), elderly (Potter, 2001)) and others across a variety of patient groups (e.g. Potter *et al.*, 1998). However, as Table 6.3 highlights, some of these analyses have included trials of patients with a mix of diagnoses and of a variety of different interventions (e.g. food, ONS or enteral tube feeding (ETF)). Very few analyses have provided detailed information on individual trials. Analyses have also commonly failed to address the impact of ONS in different health-care settings or to consider their potential mechanisms of action (e.g. in relation to changes in weight and to nutritional status). What is lacking is a complete overview and analysis of the impact of ONS *per se* on a spectrum of outcomes (functional, clinical and financial) in specific patient groups (according to age, disease, nutritional status) and across different settings (hospital and community). Consideration of the mechanisms by which ONS may affect outcome (including their effects on nutritional intake and body weight and composition) is also required.

Therefore, a systematic and critical analysis of the available evidence on the efficacy of ONS in patients in the hospital and the community (update of previous analysis (Stratton and Elia, 1999a) of community studies) has been undertaken. For this systematic review, ONS have been compared to routine clinical care and, as

stated in Chapter 5, four main questions are addressed:

(I) What effect do ONS have on the voluntary food intake and total energy intake of patients?
(II) What effect do ONS have on the body weight and composition of patients?
(III) What effect do ONS have on the body function of patients?
(IV) What effect do ONS have on the clinical and financial outcome of patients?

In following our multilayer approach to assessing the evidence (Fig. 5.6, Chapter 5) for specificity, the efficacy of ONS has been addressed in individual randomized controlled trials (RCT) and non-randomized trials (NRT) in specific patient groups (according to age, disease or condition) and in hospital and community settings (see Fig. 6.2). Details of individual studies and summaries of the efficacy of ONS in different patient groups (according to disease or age) can be found in Appendix 3 (hospital studies) and Appendix 4 (community studies). The main findings of the systematic review are presented in this chapter, according to hospital and community setting. For generalizability (Fig. 5.6, Chapter 5), a combined analysis of all ONS studies has been undertaken and is presented later in this chapter. Also, in Chapter 8, a combined analysis of trials looking at the impact of ONS and ETF can be found.

Evidence Base for ONS in the Hospital Setting

Summary characteristics of hospital trials in the ONS review

Study design

Fifty-eight trials (3883 patients) comparing the effects of ONS with no nutritional support in hospital patients were systematically reviewed. Thirty-four trials (59%, *n* 2475 patients) were a randomized, controlled design (RCT) and 24 trials (40%,

Table 6.3. Previous meta-analyses including trials of oral nutritional supplements.

Author	Patient group(s)	Intervention	Setting	Findings	Potential limitations
Potter *et al.*, 1998 27 trials	Mixed	ONS, ETF, diet	Hospital and community	Consistent improvement in body weight and upper-arm anthropometry (standardized mean difference 0.50 (95% CI 0.40–0.60) for weight). Reduction in mortality (odds ratio 0.66 (95% CI 0.48–0.91))	Incomplete data set Unable to separate the effects of the different modes of intervention (ETF, ONS, diet) in specific patient groups Studies in hospital and community settings No details of individual studies
Ferreira *et al.*, 2000 9 trials	COPD	ONS, ETF	Hospital and community	Small (+1.65 kg) non-significant increases in body weight, upper-arm anthropometry, 6 min walking distance, FEV and $P_I$max	Interventions < 2 weeks excluded Unable to separate the effects of the different modes of intervention (ETF, ONS, diet) Studies in hospital and community settings No analysis according to nutritional status No details of individual studies Specific to patients with COPD
Avenell and Handoll, 2001 15 trials	Fractured neck of femur	ONS, ETF, vitamin supplements	Hospital and community	ONS may reduce unfavourable outcome (death or complications; relative risk 0.52 (95% CI 0.32–0.84) but no effect on mortality (RR 0.85 (95% CI 0.42–1.70))	Studies in hospital and community settings No analysis according to nutritional status Specific to fractured neck of femur patients
Potter, 2001 18 trials	Elderly (mixed diagnoses including orthopaedics, excluding malignancy and surgical patients)	ONS	Hospital and community	Significantly lower mortality (odds ratio 0.61 (95% CI 0.45–0.82))	Mix of conditions Studies in hospital and community settings No analysis according to nutritional status No details of individual studies
Smyth and Walters, 2002 2 trials	Cystic fibrosis	ONS	Community only	Insufficient data to undertake meta-analysis	
Poustie *et al.*, 2002 2 trials	Children with a variety of chronic diseases	ONS > 1 month	Community only	Insufficient data to undertake meta-analysis	

CI, confidence interval; FEV, forced expiratory volume; $P_I$max, maximal inspiratory pressure; RR, relative risk.

Evidence base for oral nutritional supplements

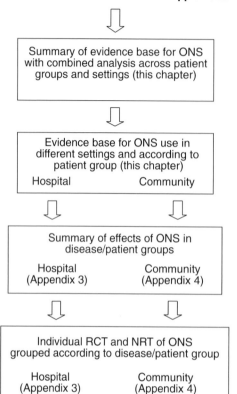

Fig. 6.2. Multilayer approach to establishing the evidence in the ONS systematic review.

n 1408 patients) were non-randomized (NRT). All trials were reviewed in patient-specific groups and are summarized in Tables 6.4 and 6.5. (For some diseases, no

studies in the hospital setting were found (e.g. HIV/AIDS).) Table 6.6 shows the Jadad scores for grading RCT (Jadad *et al.*, 1996).

ONS used in hospital trials

CONSISTENCY AND TYPE OF ONS

Liquid ONS were used in 91% (31/34) of RCT. These included commercial, liquid sip feeds (24 studies) or powders reconstituted to form drinks (seven studies) (both sweet and savoury flavours, nutritionally complete and incomplete). Puddings were used in only one study (COPD patients (Saudny-Unterberger *et al.*, 1997)) and powders were used in combination with liquid supplements in two studies (in COPD (Schols *et al.*, 1995) and elderly patients (Hankey *et al.*, 1993)). In NRT of hospital patients, the majority of ONS used were liquids (20 studies). These included commercial, liquid sip feeds (13 studies) or powders reconstituted to form drinks (e.g. Demling and DeSanti, 1998). In one study in cancer patients, a variety of ONS were used but not described (Cohn *et al.*, 1982) and, in another study (in children with cancer), neither the name nor the type of ONS was documented (Rickard *et al.*, 1983). Further details of the ONS used in studies can be found in Appendix 3.

Only four reports documented the use of juice-based sip feeds (brands: Fortijuice, Enlive, Rynkeby) in orthopaedic (Doshi *et al.*, 1998; Lawson *et al.*, 2000) and surgical

Table 6.4. Summary of randomized controlled trials of oral nutritional supplement use in hospital patients.

Disease/patient group	Number of randomized controlled trials reviewed	Total number of patients in trials reviewed
Chronic obstructive pulmonary disease	2	127
Elderly	12	1146
Liver disease	3	391
General medical	1	61
Neurology	1	42
Orthopaedic	6	296
Oral/maxillofacial surgery	3	65
Surgery	6	347
Total	34 (59% of total)	2475

Table 6.5. Summary of non-randomized trials of oral nutritional supplement use in hospital patients. RCT comparing groups of patients receiving different types of ONS (with no unsupplemented group) were also reviewed as non-randomized longitudinal data.

Disease/patient group	Number of non-randomized trials reviewed	Total number of patients in trials reviewed
Burns	2	90
Elderly	5	759
HIV/AIDS	2	48
Liver disease	4	82
Malignancy	5	82
Orthopaedic	3	230
Surgery	3	117
Total	24 (41% of total)	1408

Table 6.6. Summary of the Jadad scores for hospital randomized controlled trials (Jadad *et al.*,1996). Individual codes relating to the design of each study can be seen in the summaries in Appendix 3. For an explanation of the Jadad scoring system, refer to Chapter 5.

Jadad score	Number of trials (%)	Patient group (number of trials)
1	11 (32%)	Elderly (4), oral surgery (1), surgery (2), orthopaedics (4)
2	14 (41%)	COPD (2), elderly (4), liver disease (1), medical (1), orthopaedic (1), oral surgery (2), surgery (3)
3	7 (21%)	Elderly (4), liver disease (1), neurology (1), surgery (1)
4	2 (6%)	Orthopaedic (1), liver disease (1)
5	–	–

–, no data.

(Wara and Hessov, 1985; MacFie *et al.*, 2000) patients.

COMPOSITION OF ONS

Most ONS contained a mixture of macro-nutrients and micronutrients and some were nutritionally 'complete'. In some studies, peptide or elemental ONS were used, and occasionally ONS were enriched with fish-oil, medium-chain triglycerides or branched-chain amino acids. Disease-specific ONS have not been considered in any depth in this review. The energy density of ONS ranged from 0.45 kcal ml^{-1} to 2.1 kcal ml^{-1} (1.9 kJ ml^{-1} to 8.8 kJ ml^{-1}), although the most common energy densities for ONS were 1 kcal ml^{-1} and 1.5 kcal ml^{-1}. The energy densities of ONS used in studies of different patient groups are shown in Table 6.7.

AMOUNT OF ONS PRESCRIBED AND TAKEN

The amount of ONS prescribed daily varied considerably in the studies reviewed (from 254 kcal in orthopaedic patients (Delmi *et al.*, 1990; Tkatch *et al.*, 1992) to 1175 kcal in patients with liver disease (Mendenhall *et al.*, 1993)). However, ONS intake was documented in only 46% (*n* 24) of trials reviewed. Mean intakes ranged from 251 kcal (in the elderly (Volkert *et al.*, 1996)) to > 1000 kcal (in patients with alcoholic hepatitis (Mendenhall *et al.*, 1993)) in the RCT, and from 151 kcal (in surgical patients (Eneroth *et al.*, 1997)) to > 2000 kcal (in patients with alcoholic hepatitis (Mendenhall *et al.*, 1985)) in the NRT. The amounts of ONS prescribed and taken in individual trials, where reported, have been documented in the tables in Appendix 3.

Table 6.7. Summary of the energy density of oral nutritional supplements used in trials of hospital patients, according to patient group. Range of energy densities of ONS used in trials in each patient group, where information recorded.

Randomized controlled trials		Non-randomized trials/data	
Patient group	Energy density (kcal ml^{-1})	Patient group	Energy density (kcal ml^{-1})
Chronic obstructive pulmonary disease	1.0–2.1	Burns	–
Elderly	1.0–1.5	Elderly	0.45–2.0
Liver disease	0.97–1.5	HIV/AIDS	–
General medical	1.5	Liver disease	–
Neurology	1.0	Malignancy	1.0–1.3
Orthopaedic	1.0–1.2	Orthopaedic	1.0–1.5
Oral/maxillofacial surgery	1.5	Surgery	0.64–1.0
Surgery	1.25–1.5		
Range	0.97–2.1	Range	0.45–2.0

–, no data.

DURATION OF ORAL NUTRITIONAL SUPPLEMENTATION
The duration of ONS use ranged from 7 days in surgical patients (Rana *et al.*, 1992) to 26 weeks in elderly long-term care patients (Larsson *et al.*, 1990) (see Table 6.8). The duration of ONS use differed depending on the patient group, the nutritional status of patients, the location/ward setting of patients and whether ONS were used after discharge from hospital in the community.

Dietary counselling in hospital supplementation trials

Although details about the use of dietary counselling or modified foods/diets to increase energy and protein intakes were not provided in most trials, it is likely that these methods were often used, either alongside ONS or prior to the use of ONS. A few trials (*n* 11) specified that dietary counselling or food modification was used

Table 6.8. Summary of the duration of oral nutritional supplementation in hospital trials. Minimum average duration taken from the trial with the shortest duration of ONS and the maximum average duration from the trial with the longest duration of ONS within each disease/patient group.

Disease/patient group	Minimum average duration (days)	Maximum average duration
Chronic obstructive pulmonary disease	14 (Saudny-Unterberger *et al.*, 1997)	> 57 days (Schols *et al.*, 1995)
Elderly	< 14 (Reilly, J.J. *et al.*, 1995)	26 weeks (Larsson *et al.*, 1990)
Liver disease	20 (Bunout *et al.*, 1989)	77 days (Le Cornu *et al.*, 2000)
General medical	28 (McWhirter and Pennington, 1996)	(1 trial only)
Neurology	10 (Gariballa *et al.*, 1998a)	(1 trial only)
Orthopaedic	10 (Stableforth, 1986)	38 days (Tkatch *et al.*, 1992)
Oral/maxillofacial surgery	42 (Kendell *et al.*, 1982)	10 weeks (Olejko and Fonseca, 1984)
Surgery	7 (Rana *et al.*, 1992)	10 weeks (Beattie *et al.*, 2000)
Range (overall)	7 (Rana *et al.*, 1992)	26 weeks (Larsson *et al.*, 1990)

alongside ONS (COPD (Schols *et al.*, 1995; Saudny-Unterberger *et al.*, 1997); liver disease (Bunout *et al.*, 1989; Le Cornu *et al.*, 2000); oral surgery (Kendell *et al.*, 1982; Olejko and Fonseca, 1984; Antila *et al.*, 1993); burns (Demling and DeSanti, 1998); cancer (Haffejee and Angorn, 1977; Rickard *et al.*, 1979; Cohn *et al.*, 1982)) in hospital patients. In some of these trials, encouragement was given to increase food intake (Cohn *et al.*, 1982; Schols *et al.*, 1995) and, in others, patients received verbal and/or written instructions about improving nutrient intake (energy and protein) (Kendell *et al.*, 1982; Olejko and Fonseca, 1984; Antila *et al.*, 1993). High-energy food snacks or a high-energy and protein diet was occasionally provided for patients (Cohn *et al.*, 1982; Saudny-Unterberger *et al.*, 1997). In specific patient groups, advice was given about texture modification (to orthognathic patients (Antila *et al.*, 1993) and intubated oesophageal-cancer patients (Haffejee and Angorn, 1977)) or reducing protein intakes (in cases of encephalopathy (Bunout *et al.*, 1989)). In two trials, dietary advice was given, presumably to help patients to increase their dietary intakes, but no details were provided (Rickard *et al.*, 1979; Le Cornu *et al.*, 2000).

Main findings of the hospital ONS review

A summary of the key findings from the evidence base for ONS in the hospital setting is presented in Box 6.1. The results of all of the studies reviewed, according to each of the four main questions, have also been summarized in Table 6.9, arranged by body mass index (BMI) and patient group. An indication of the number and proportion of studies that assessed and showed improvement in these four measures is provided in Fig. 6.3 and each is discussed in more detail below. For more specific information about the efficacy of ONS in different patient groups, refer to Appendix 3.

(I) What effect do ONS have on the voluntary food intake and total energy intake of patients in hospital?

ALL PATIENT GROUPS COMBINED

ONS are an effective means of improving total energy and protein intakes in a variety of patient groups in the hospital setting, including patients with COPD, fractured neck of femur, neurological disease, liver disease and cancer, the elderly and surgical patients. A number of studies also indicate that ONS can improve micronutrient intakes in hospital patients (Banerjee *et al.*, 1978, 1981; Kendell *et al.*, 1982; Olejko and Fonseca, 1984; Delmi *et al.*, 1990; Hankey *et al.*, 1993; Volkert *et al.*, 1996) (three NRT (Katakity *et al.*, 1983; Elmstahl and Steen, 1987; Antila *et al.*, 1993)).

In total, 42 trials (72% of all trials) reported the total energy and/or nutrient intake (Table 6.9). In 93% of studies (*n* 39), ONS were associated with improvements in nutritional intake, which were significant in 72% (*n* 28) (see Fig. 6.3). Of those RCT that assessed nutritional intake with ONS (*n* 25, 74% of total RCT), all showed improvements in the total intake of energy and/or nutrients (protein, micronutrients). These improvements were described as statistically significant in 17 trials (68%; only protein/micronutrients in four trials). Similarly, the majority (*n* 14, 82%) of NRT that assessed nutritional intake (*n* 17, 71% of total NRT) indicated that ONS resulted in improvements in total energy and/or nutrient intakes (significant in 11 trials, 79%; only protein/micronutrients in two trials).

The use of ONS, primarily liquid in consistency, appeared not to substantially reduce the voluntary food intake of patients in the hospital setting. The proportion of ONS energy that was additive to food intake was greater than half (50–100%) (assessed in seven RCT), suggesting that ONS did not substantially reduce patients' intake of food. On the contrary, in the majority of studies (*n* 6) (Delmi *et al.*, 1990; Rana *et al.*, 1992; Mendenhall

Table 6.9. Changes in nutrient intake, body weight, function and clinical outcome following oral nutritional supplementation (versus no nutritional support) in the hospital setting related to patients' nutritional status. Trials arranged according to disease group and in alphabetical order.

Supplementation trial	Improved energy and/or nutrient intake	Improved nutritional status	Improved function	Improved clinical outcome
BMI < 20 kg m^{-2}/IBW < 90%				
Randomized, controlled trials				
Schols *et al.* (1995) (i) COPD	√ (v)	√ (v)	√ (t)	n/a
Carver and Dobson (1985) Elderly	n/a	√ (?sig)	n/a	n/a
Larsson *et al.* (1990) (i) Elderly[†∞]	n/a	√ (ns)	√ (t)	√ (ns)
McEvoy and James (1982) Elderly	n/a	√ (v)	n/a	n/a
Potter *et al.* (2001) (i) Elderly[†]	√ (v)	√ (v)	√ (v)	√ (v)
Unosson *et al.* (1992) Elderly[∞]	√ (t)	n/a	√ (v)*	√ (v)
Volkert *et al.* (1996) Elderly	√ N	√ (?sig)	√ (v)	n/a
Brown and Seabrook (1992) A Orthopaedic	√ (?sig)	√ (ns)		√ (?sig)
Beattie *et al.* (2000) Surgical	n/a	√ (v)	√ (v)	√ (ns)
Non-randomized trials/data				
Wanke *et al.* (1996) HIV	n/a	√ (ns)	√ (t)	n/a
Barber *et al.* (1999) Malignancy	√ (t)	√ (t)	√ (t)	n/a
Cohn *et al.* (1982) Malignancy	√ (?sig)	√ (?sig)	n/a	n/a
BMI > 20 kg m^{-2}/IBW > 90%				
Randomized, controlled trials				
Saudny-Unterberger *et al.* (1997) COPD	√ (v)	√ (ns)	√ (v)	n/a
Schols *et al.* (1995) (ii) COPD	√ (v)	√ (v)	√ (t)	n/a
Larsson *et al.* (1990) (ii) Elderly[†]	n/a	√ (v)	√ (t)	√ (v)
Potter *et al.* (2001) (iii) Elderly[†]	√ (v)	√ (?sig)		√ (v)
Bunout *et al.* (1989) Liver disease[††]	√ (v)			√ (ns)
Antila *et al.* (1993) Oral/MF surgery	√ (v)	√ (?sig)		n/a
Kendell *et al.* (1982) Oral/MF surgery	√ (v)	√ (ns)	n/a	n/a
Okejko and Fonseca (1984) Oral/MF surgery	√ (?sig)	√ (v)	n/a	n/a
Schurch *et al.* (1998) Orthopaedic	n/a	n/a	√ (v)	√ (v)
Elbers *et al.* (1997) Surgical	n/a		√ (v)	
Keele *et al.* (1997) Surgical	√ (v)	√ (v)	√ (?sig)	√ (v)
MacFie *et al.* (2000) Surgical	√ (ns)	√ (ns)		
Rana *et al.* (1992) Surgical	√ (v)	√ (ns)	√ (v)	√ (v)
Non-randomized trials/data				
Bos *et al.* (2000) Elderly	√ (t)	√ (v)‡	n/a	n/a
Christie *et al.* (1985) Liver disease	√ N[(t)]	n/a	√ (t)**	n/a
Mendenhall *et al.* (1985) Liver disease[††]	√ (v)	√ (v)	√ (t)	√ (ns)
Lawson *et al.* (2000) Orthopaedic	√ (v)	n/a	n/a	n/a
BMI unknown				
Randomized, controlled trials				
Banerjee *et al.* (1978) Elderly[∞∞]	√ N[(v)]	√ (v)‡		n/a
Banerjee *et al.* (1981) Elderly[∞∞]	√ N[(v)]	√ (v)‡		n/a
Ek *et al.* (1991) Elderly[∞]	n/a	n/a	√ (ns)	n/a
Hankey *et al.* (1993) Elderly	√ (t)			n/a
Hubsch *et al.* (1994) Elderly	√ (?sig)	√ (ns)	√ (ns)	n/a
Reilly, J.J. *et al.* (1995) Elderly	√ (ns)	√ (ns)	n/a	n/a

Continued

Table 6.9. *Continued.*

Supplementation trial	Improved energy and/or nutrient intake	Improved nutritional status	Improved function	Improved clinical outcome
Potter *et al.* (2001) (ii) Elderly	√(v)	√ (?sig)		√(ns)
Le Cornu *et al.* (2000) Liver transplant††	√(ns)	√ (?sig)‡	√(?sig)	√(ns)
Mendenhall *et al.* (1993) Liver disease††	√(v)	√ (v)‡	√(v)*	√(v)*
Gariballa *et al.* (1998a) Neurology	√(?sig)	√ (ns)	√(ns)	√(ns)
McWhirter and Pennington (1996)				
General medical	√ (?sig)	√ (v)	n/a	n/a
Delmi *et al.* (1990) Orthopaedic	√ (?sig)	n/a		√ (v)
Moller-Madsen *et al.* (1988) Orthopaedic	√ (v)		n/a	n/a
Stableforth (1986) Orthopaedic	√ N(t)		n/a	n/a
Tkatch *et al.* (1992) Orthopaedic	n/a	n/a	√ (v)	√ (v)
Murchan *et al.* (1995) A Surgical	n/a	√ (v)		√ (v)
Non-randomized trials/data				
Demling and DeSanti (1998) Burns		√ (?sig)	√ (?sig)	√ (ns)**
Solem *et al.* (1979) Burns	n/a	n/a	√ (ns)	n/a
Bourdel-Marchasson *et al.* (2000) Elderly	√ (v)	n/a	√ (?sig)	
Elmstahl and Steen (1987) Elderly	√ N(t)	√ (t)	n/a	n/a
Katakity *et al.* (1983) Elderly	n/a	n/a	√ (t)	n/a
Ovesen and Allingstrup (1992) Elderly	√ (t)	n/a	n/a	n/a
Craig *et al.* (1994) HIV			√ (t)**	n/a
Okita *et al.* (1985) Liver disease	√ (t)	n/a	√ (t)	n/a
Roselle *et al.* (1988) Liver disease	n/a	n/a	√ (t)	n/a
Bounous *et al.* (1971) Malignancy	√ (ns)	√ (ns)	√ (t)	n/a
Haffejee and Angorn (1977) Malignancy	n/a	√ (?sig)	n/a	n/a
Rickard *et al.* (1983) Malignancy	n/a		n/a	n/a
Doshi *et al.* (1998) A Orthopaedic	√ (v)	n/a	n/a	√ (v)
Williams *et al.* (1989) Orthopaedic	n/a	√ (?sig)	√ (ns)	√ (ns)
Eneroth *et al.* (1997)** Surgical	√ (?sig)	n/a	√ (v)	√ (ns)
Moiniche *et al.* (1995) Surgical			n/a	n/a
Wara and Hessov (1985) Surgical	√ (v)	√ (v)	n/a	n/a

√	Indicates an improvement or less deterioration compared with a control group or compared with baseline measurements.
(v)	Significant compared with a control group receiving no ONS or a placebo.
(t)	Significant change over time/compared with baseline.
ns	Improvement/benefit observed that is not statistically significant.
(?sig)	Improvement/benefit observed but unclear if statistically significant.
n/a	Not assessed in trial.
†	BMI category assumed from information given in paper (no BMI provided).
††	Patients with ascites in whom BMI and/or weight change data may be unreliable.
‡	Nutritional status assessment using only upper-arm anthropometry or markers other than weight.
(i)–(iii)	Specific groups within studies that vary according to initial BMI/nutritional status.
*	Benefits in a specific group of patients only (Mendenhall *et al.* (1993) 'Moderately malnourished' patients; Unosson *et al.* (1992) 'well-nourished group').
**	Significant benefits with one type of ONS relative to another.
***	Some patients may have received ETF and/or PN.
N	Improvement in protein or micronutrient intakes/balance (not energy).
∞	Potentially reports of same patient group.
∞∞	Potentially reports of the same patient group.
A	Abstract.

MF, maxillofacial; IBW, ideal body weight; PN, parenteral nutrition.

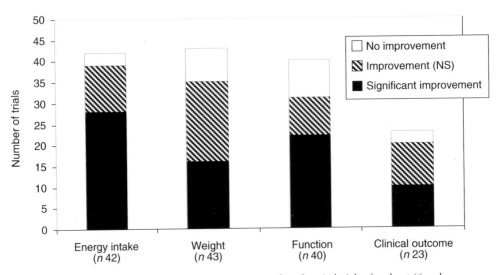

Fig. 6.3. Summary of results for the four outcome measures from hospital trials of oral nutritional supplementation (*n* = total number of trials).

et al., 1993; Reilly, J.J. *et al.*, 1995; Schols *et al.*, 1995; Keele *et al.*, 1997), the food intake of patients receiving ONS was the same (100% of ONS energy additive) or greater than those who were unsupplemented (see Fig. 6.4), irrespective of whether patients were 'underweight' (BMI < 20 kg m^{-2} or < 90% ideal body weight (IBW)) or not (see Fig. 6.5). Whether food intakes are significantly greater in supplemented patients in some trials is difficult to establish due to the lack of individual data. In only one trial was the % of ONS energy additive to food intake calculated as < 50% (31% in liver patients pretransplant (Le Cornu *et al.*, 2000)), although this period of supplementation was undertaken in out-patients prior to admission to hospital, with no apparent checks on compliance with prescribed intakes.

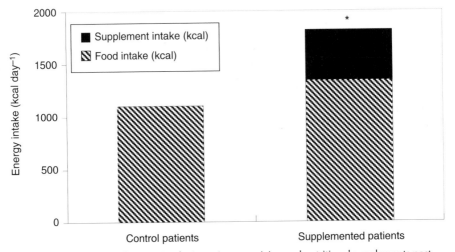

Fig. 6.4. Greater food and total energy intake in patients receiving oral nutritional supplements postsurgery. Data adapted from an RCT (Rana *et al.*, 1992). *Significant increase in total energy intake.

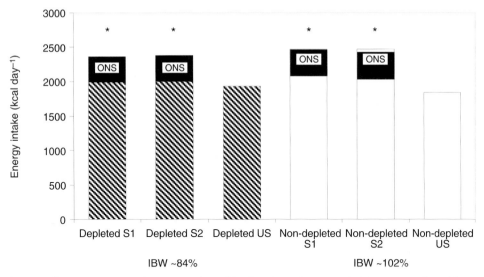

Fig. 6.5. Effect on ONS on total energy intake and food intake in patients with COPD. Data adapted from an RCT (Schols *et al.*, 1995). Supplemented patients not given steroids (S1), given steroids (S2) and unsupplemented patients (US). *Significant increase in total energy intake.

Very few trials (*n* 4) provided an insight into the temporal changes in the intake of food, ONS or total intake over a period of supplementation (Ovesen, 1992; Rana *et al.*, 1992; Keele *et al.*, 1997; Bourdel-Marchasson *et al.*, 2000). All of these trials indicated that the intake of ONS remained relatively constant over time, although the periods of supplementation were relatively short in duration (< 15 days (Ovesen, 1992; Bourdel-Marchasson *et al.*, 2000) and 7 days (Rana *et al.*, 1992; Keele *et al.*, 1997)). In the post-surgical patients (Rana *et al.*, 1992; Keele *et al.*, 1997), voluntary food intake and total energy intake during supplementation improved as patients recovered postoperatively. In sick elderly patients, food intake remained relatively stable or increased during supplementation (Ovesen, 1992; Bourdel-Marchasson *et al.*, 2000).

It is difficult to come to firm conclusions about the impact of ONS on voluntary food intake according to patients' nutritional status. Improvements in total energy intake in patients receiving ONS appeared to occur in trials of patient groups with varying nutritional status. All trials that assessed intake in patients with an average BMI < 20 kg m^{-2} or > 20 kg m^{-2} showed improvements in total energy and/or nutrient intakes (assessed in six trials with BMI < 20 kg m^{-2}; assessed in 11 trials with BMI > 20 kg m^{-2}). However, within these trials, the BMI of individual patients varied considerably. In addition, in the majority of trials (16 RCT, 15 NRT), the average BMI of the patient group was not even documented and could not be calculated from raw data.

INDIVIDUAL PATIENT GROUPS
This analysis suggests that ONS can improve total energy and nutrient intakes across patient groups (COPD, elderly, liver disease, surgery, etc.). In general, there is little or no reduction in food intake with supplementation across disease groups, and appetite and food intake may even improve (see Box 6.3).

(II) What effect do ONS have on the body weight and composition of patients in hospital?

ALL PATIENT GROUPS COMBINED
Use of ONS can improve the nutritional status (body weight, upper-arm anthropometry) of a variety of patients in hospital,

Box 6.3. Effect of oral nutritional supplements on food and total intake in different patient groups (hospital setting). CVA, cerebrovascular accident.

COPD
ONS (1–2 kcal ml^{-1}) can significantly improve energy and protein intakes in patients with acute exacerbations of COPD or stable COPD (two RCT: Schols *et al.*, 1995; Saudny-Unterberger *et al.*, 1997). Total energy intakes were increased by ~350–620 kcal daily in these patients. From the studies reviewed, ONS appears not to suppress voluntary food intake. On the contrary, food intakes may be greater in those given an ONS, whether they are 'underweight' (IBW ~84%) or 'normal weight' (IBW ~102%). Current information suggests that ONS are well tolerated in this patient group.

Elderly
A variety of ONS (1–1.5 kcal ml^{-1}, in prescribed amounts of 265–652 kcal) have been demonstrated to increase total nutrient intake in elderly hospitalized patients with a number of diagnoses. Increases in energy, protein, vitamin and mineral intakes can occur (significant increases reported in five RCT (Banerjee *et al.*, 1978; Unosson *et al.*, 1992; Hankey *et al.*, 1993; Volkert *et al.*, 1996; Potter *et al.*, 2001)). Voluntary food intakes appear to be similar in supplemented and unsupplemented patients, thereby facilitating the increase in total intake with supplementation.

Liver disease
In all the RCT reviewed (*n* 3), ONS (1–1.5 kcal ml^{-1}, intake of > 600 kcal) have been shown to increase total energy and protein intakes in patients with liver disease (alcoholic liver disease and pre-liver transplantation) but not significantly so in those supplemented pre-transplant. Improvements have been observed alongside the use of dietary advice (Le Cornu *et al.*, 2000) and steroid use (Mendenhall *et al.*, 1993). The % of ONS energy additive to food intake ranges from ~30% (pre-transplant) (Le Cornu *et al.*, 2000) to 100% (implying greater food intakes with supplementation in mildly undernourished alcoholic liver-disease patients) (Mendenhall *et al.*, 1993).

Neurology/general medical
ONS (1–1.5 kcal ml^{-1}) in CVA patients (who are able to swallow) and in a group of adult patients with a variety of diagnoses can increase energy and protein intakes (McWhirter and Pennington, 1996; Garibadda *et al.*, 1998a). Using ONS of ~600–700 kcal (for 10 days to 4 weeks) in RCT did not significantly reduce food intake, relative to unsupplemented patients. There were no problems with toleration in these patients, although compliance over a 4-week period in CVA patients was observed in only 50% of patients. The impact of ONS in CVA patients with dysphagia and in patients with other neurological diseases remains to be elucidated in the hospital setting.

Oral/maxillofacial surgery
In all the reviewed trials in mandibular fracture and orthognathic surgical patients (Kendell *et al.*, 1982; Olejko and Fonseca, 1984; Antila *et al.*, 1993), ONS (1.5 kcal ml^{-1}, intake unknown) improved intake. Intakes of energy, a number of vitamins, zinc, copper, selenium and iron were increased, although preoperative supplementation was less effective (Olejko and Fonseca, 1984).

Orthopaedics
ONS (1–1.2 kcal ml^{-1} or 3.85 kcal g^{-1}; prescribed intakes ~250–300 kcal) can increase the energy, protein and calcium intakes of patients hospitalized with a fractured neck of femur (Stableforth, 1986; Moller-Madsen *et al.*, 1988; Delmi *et al.*, 1990; Brown and Seabrook, 1992), significantly so in a couple of RCT (Stableforth, 1986; Moller-Madsen *et al.*, 1988). The information available suggests that food intake is not suppressed substantially by ONS (Delmi *et al.*, 1990). Even with the use of ONS, total intakes may not meet estimated nutritional requirements. Except for large volumes of ONS, which were poorly tolerated, ONS had no major side-effects.

Surgery (gastrointestinal and vascular)
ONS (1–1.5 kcal ml^{-1}), used postoperatively in GI and vascular surgical patients, can improve energy and protein intakes. Even with supplementation, nutritional requirements may not be met in the short term postoperatively. However, ONS use is associated with increases in voluntary food intake (Rana *et al.*, 1992; Keele *et al.*, 1997). It may be that the delivery of a single nutrient or combinations of nutrients or a minimal level of energy intake at a critical time point during recovery may stimulate appetite and intake in some way, perhaps through improvements in well-being (Rana *et al.*, 1992).

including those with COPD, neurological disease and cancer and elderly, surgical and general medical patients.

Overall, 43 trials (74% of all trials) reported changes in body weight/anthropometry following ONS in hospital patients (Table 6.9). Eighty-one per cent of these trials (n 35) showed improvements, either compared with a control group and/or longitudinally, of which 46% (n 16) were statistically significant (Fig. 6.3). Although changes in nutritional status were usually assessed by changes in body weight, in a few trials measurements of upper-arm anthropometry or a combination of anthropometric and biochemical markers were used (indicated by ‡ in Table 6.9). Very few studies recorded the presence or absence of oedema in patients, despite the potential confounding effect on measurements of body weight. In patients with liver disease and ascites, BMI and weight-change data may also be unreliable.

Of the 29 RCT that assessed body weight/anthropometry (85% of all RCT), 83% (n 24) reported improvements (or less deterioration) in supplemented patients compared with unsupplemented patients, and these were statistically significant differences in 46% of trials (n 11). The mean difference in weight change between supplemented and unsupplemented patients was +1.38 kg (calculated using data from 13 RCT; supplemented +0.05 kg; unsupplemented −1.33 kg). Per cent weight-change data from 17 RCT (weighted for sample size, n 1646) across patient groups also suggested less weight loss in supplemented (−1%) than unsupplemented (−4%) patients in the hospital setting (P < 0.03, independent t test). Of the 14 NRT that assessed body weight (58% of total), 11 (79%) showed that improvements occurred and these were significant, either longitudinally or compared with a control group, in five of the trials (36%) (see Table 6.9). The mean weight change in supplemented patients was +0.67 kg (data from seven NRT) and −2.16 kg in unsupplemented patients (data from three NRT).

Weight change according to nutritional status. The difference in weight change between supplemented and unsupplemented groups (COPD, elderly, liver disease and post-surgery) was similar in RCT conducted in patients with a mean BMI < 20 kg m^{-2} (+2.4%; data from five studies) or > 20 kg m^{-2} (+2.6%; data from ten studies) (not significant) (see Fig. 6.6). However, the longitudinal change in supplemented patients was significantly different (P < 0.004, independent t test; +0.7% (BMI < 20 kg m^{-2}) versus −3.1% (BMI > 20 kg m^{-2}) (see Fig. 6.6)).

It was also possible to assess changes in body weight according to the nutritional status of subgroups of patients within some trials. It appeared that improvements in body weight/nutritional status (compared with a control group) occurred following ONS in hospitalized patients who were ‘undernourished’ (BMI < 20 kg m^{-2}) (Brown and Seabrook, 1992; Carver and Dobson, 1995; Schols et al., 1995; McWhirter and Pennington, 1996; Beattie et al., 2000; Potter et al., 2001, group (i)) or ‘well nourished’ (BMI > 20 kg m^{-2}) (Larsson et al., 1990; Rana et al., 1992; Keele et al., 1997; Potter et al., 2001, group (ii)) at the start of supplementation. Indeed, improvements in body weight (greater gain or less loss than in unsupplemented patients) occurred in a similar frequency in studies undertaken in patients with an average BMI < 20 kg m^{-2} or > 20 kg m^{-2} (see Table 6.9). In contrast, in community patients with stable, chronic conditions, improvements in body weight and lean and fat mass were more likely to be observed in those studies in which patients had an average BMI < 20 kg m^{-2} than in those with average BMI > 20 kg m^{-2} (discussed later in this chapter). A clear consensus about the relationship between the initial nutritional status of hospitalized patients and the subsequent efficacy of ONS in improving body weight could not be gained from the existing information. For instance, within the trials reviewed, the BMI of individual patients varied considerably and it is possible that subgroups of patients may have benefited more from

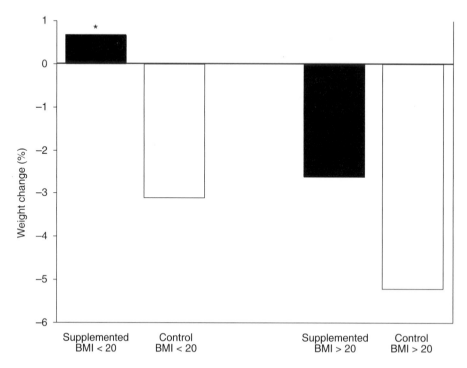

Fig. 6.6. Per cent weight change in supplemented versus control patients from hospital trials (17 RCT; 1646 patients, weighted mean, according to BMI).
*Significantly different longitudinal weight change in supplemented patients ($P < 0.04$) in BMI < 20 kg m^{-2} than in BMI > 20 kg m^{-2} group.

supplementation, in terms of body-weight gain. However, the lack of data for individual patients and the failure of the majority of studies to document the initial nutritional status of patients prevent firm conclusions from being established without further research.

Meta-analysis of % weight change with ONS. The % change in weight in supplemented versus unsupplemented patients was compared using meta-analysis. Meta-analysis of % weight-change data (ten RCT (14 data sets), n 1187) indicated a mean effect size of 0.65 (95% confidence interval (CI) 0.52–0.79), with significant heterogeneity between the studies of a variety of patient groups (surgery, liver disease, COPD, elderly). A larger effect size was found in studies in patients with an average BMI < 20 kg m^{-2} than in those with BMI > 20 kg m^{-2} (BMI < 20 kg m^{-2} mean effect size 1.41 (95% CI 1.06–1.75), five studies; BMI > 20 kg m^{-2} mean effect size 0.44 (95% CI 0.25–0.63); eight studies). An earlier meta-analysis of the effects of nutritional support in adult patients also indicated that routine nutritional supplementation led to consistent improvements in body weight (weighted mean difference 2.06%; 95% CI 1.63–2.49) and upper-arm anthropometry (weighted mean difference 3.16%; 95% CI 2.43–3.89) compared with controls (27 trials) (Potter *et al.*, 1998). However, there were a number of limitations to this analysis, including: (i) the inclusion of trials that used different nutritional interventions (ETF, food supplements and ONS); (ii) the inclusion of trials in a variety of settings; and (iii) the inclusion of only some of the trials that had been published at the time.

INDIVIDUAL PATIENT GROUPS

Figure 6.7 shows that the effect of ONS on % weight change varied with the patient group studied. Combined analysis (weighted for sample size) of each patient group showed % weight gain was greater (or % weight loss less) in supplemented than in unsupplemented patients (by 2–4%). Due to the confounding effects of ascites, liver disease was the one disease category in which % weight loss was greater in supplemented than in control patients (data from one trial only (Bunout et al., 1989)).

The impact of ONS across different patient groups is summarized in Box 6.4. Typically ONS can improve body weight or attenuate weight loss across patient and diagnostic groups.

BODY COMPOSITION

Twelve trials suggested that increments (or attenuated losses) in body fat or lean body mass occurred following ONS in hospital patients. Eight were RCT (in COPD (Schols et al., 1995), elderly (McEvoy and James, 1982; Hankey et al., 1993; Hubsch et al.,

1994; Carver and Dobson, 1995; Potter et al., 2001), oral surgery (Antila et al., 1993) and general medical patients (McWhirter and Pennington, 1996)) and four were NRT (in the elderly (Bos et al., 2000) and in patients with cancer (Cohn et al., 1982; Barber et al., 1999b) and liver disease (Mendenhall et al., 1985)). However, most of these trials used measurements of upper-arm anthropometry as an indication of the changes in fat and fat-free mass accompanying ONS and in some trials the changes were not significant (e.g. Potter et al., 2001). More in-depth study of changes in body composition with ONS is needed.

(III) What effect do ONS have on the body function of patients in hospital?

ALL PATIENT GROUPS COMBINED

This analysis suggests that functional benefits frequently occur following the use of ONS in patients in hospital. The type of functional benefit may vary, depending on the diagnosis or condition of the patient. Reported functional benefits include improvements in muscle strength, walking

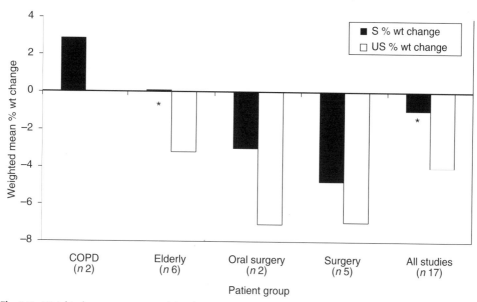

Fig. 6.7. Weighted mean per cent weight change in supplemented (S) compared with control (US) patients according to patient group (data from 17 RCT in the hospital setting, 1646 patients; *n* = number of trials in each patient group). *Significant difference, *P* < 0.04.

Box 6.4. Effect of oral nutritional supplements on body weight, composition and growth in different patient groups (hospital setting).

COPD
Use of ONS can lead to weight gain in COPD patients with stable or acute disease, although the changes may be small (weighted mean % weight change +3% in supplemented patients relative to controls) (Schols *et al.*, 1995; Saudny-Unterberger *et al.*, 1997). Non-response to ONS (smaller weight change) is more likely in older patients with a systemic inflammatory response (Creutzberg *et al.*, 2000).

Elderly
ONS can improve body weight or reduce weight loss in elderly patients, although the changes in weight across trials are variable. This may be due to the efficacy of ONS varying with the age, disease type and status of patients or with the type, quantity and duration of supplementation. Overall, changes in weight are small (weighted mean % change in supplemented patients +3.4% relative to controls) (Larsson *et al.*, 1990; Hankey *et al.*, 1993; Hubsch *et al.*, 1994; Carver and Dobson, 1995; Potter *et al.*, 2001) but are evident in normal weight and underweight (BMI < 20 kg m^{-2}) patients. Although only small changes in weight may occur in the hospital, greater change may be seen after discharge (Volkert *et al.*, 1996). Muscle mass may also be improved with ONS (Hankey *et al.*, 1993; Hubsch *et al.*, 1994).

Liver disease
ONS may improve nutritional status (including muscle mass) (Mendenhall *et al.*, 1993; Le Cornu *et al.*, 2000) but changes in body weight are unreliable in this patient group.

Neurology/general medical
ONS can significantly increase weight and muscle mass in general medical patients (McWhirter and Pennington, 1996) and attenuate weight loss in CVA patients (Gariballa *et al.*, 1998a).

Oral/maxillofacial surgery
ONS can attenuate the weight loss (by ~ 4%) that is typically observed in this patient group postoperatively (Kendell *et al.*, 1982; Antila *et al.*, 1993).

Orthopaedics
Insufficient information prevented any quantitative assessment of the effects of ONS on body weight and composition in this patient group. It appears that weight loss is reduced by the use of ONS (Brown and Seabrook, 1992).

Surgery (gastrointestinal and vascular)
ONS can attenuate the loss of body weight associated with surgery (weighted % weight change +3% relative to controls) (Rana *et al.*, 1992; Elbers *et al.*, 1997; Keele *et al.*, 1997; Beattie *et al.*, 2000; MacFie *et al.*, 2000). Losses of fat and lean tissue can also be reduced (Elbers *et al.*, 1997; Beattie *et al.*, 2000).

distance, well-being, physical and mental health and activity levels (see Table 6.10). Most studies that assessed body function (*n* 31/40, 78%) showed improvements following ONS (see Table 6.9), 71% (*n* 22) of which were significant (Fig. 6.3). Specific functional changes for particular patient groups have been documented in the tables in Appendix 3. The majority of RCT (*n* 17/26, 65%) that assessed patients' function showed improvements with ONS, 71% (*n* 12) of which were significant. All

RCT that documented an improvement in function also reported improvements in body weight and energy/nutrient intake, when these parameters were assessed (see Table 6.9). No trials reported any significant functional detriments associated with the use of ONS.

All of the NRT that reported assessments of function (*n* 14, 58% of total) indicated improvements, 71% (*n* 10) of which were significant. None of these trials showed any functional detriment with ONS.

Table 6.10. Summary of significant improvements in functional and clinical outcomes following ONS in hospital patients (significant changes relative to a control group from randomized controlled trials only). For more information on all functional changes, refer to Appendix 3.

Patient group	Functional/clinical outcome
COPD	Improved ventilatory capacity (Saudny-Unterberger *et al.*, 1997)
Elderly	Lower mortality (Larsson *et al.*, 1990; Unosson *et al.*, 1992; Potter *et al.*, 2001) Improved functional status (Potter *et al.*, 2001) Increased activity (Unosson *et al.*, 1992) and activities of daily living (Volkert *et al.*, 1996) levels Shorter hospital stays (Potter *et al.*, 2001)
Liver disease	Lower mortality (Mendenhall *et al.*, 1993) Improved markers of liver function (Mendenhall *et al.*, 1993)
Orthopaedics	Improved clinical course (lower complication and death rate) (Delmi *et al.*, 1990; Tkatch *et al.*, 1992) Shorter hospital stays (Delmi *et al.*, 1990; Tkatch *et al.*, 1992; Schurch *et al.*, 1998) Retention of bone mineral density in femoral shaft (Tkatch *et al.*, 1992; Schurch *et al.*, 1998)
Surgery[a]	Lower rate of postoperative complications (Rana *et al.*, 1992; Keele *et al.*, 1997) Retention of skeletal (hand-grip) muscle strength (Rana *et al.*, 1992; Beattie *et al.*, 2000) Improved physical and mental health/quality of life (Elbers *et al.*, 1997; Beattie *et al.*, 2000)

[a] Use of a carbohydrate-only ONS in elective surgical patients given preoperatively up until 2 h prior to anaesthesia may reduce postoperative insulin resistance and improve well-being before and after surgery (Ljungqvist *et al.*, 2001; see Appendix 3). Trials of single-macronutrient ONS are not included in the main review.

Functional benefits related to changes in weight or nutritional status. In trials in which a significant functional benefit was observed, the difference in % weight change between supplemented and un-supplemented patients was 3.9%, with supplemented patients losing less weight (−0.9%) than unsupplemented patients (−4.8%; patients with COPD and elderly and surgical patients; 4/9 trials BMI < 20 kg m^{-2}). In trials in which no significant functional benefits were observed, the difference in % weight change between supplemented and control patients was much less (1.3%; patients with liver disease and elderly, neurology and post-surgical patients; 0/10 trials BMI < 20 kg m^{-2}). Although average ONS intakes were similar between these two groups (468 kcal versus 442 kcal daily), the average duration of supplementation was greater in those trials in which significant functional changes were observed (67 days versus 21

days). From a meta-analysis of ten RCT (14 data sets, *n* 1187), the mean effect size for % weight change was greater in studies in which significant functional benefits were observed (0.71 (95% CI 0.52–0.89) versus 0.46 (95% CI 0.16–0.76)), but there was significant heterogeneity between studies.

Functional benefits following ONS were evident in patient groups with an average BMI < 20 kg m^{-2} (six reports (Larsson *et al.*, 1990; Unosson *et al.*, 1992; Schols *et al.*, 1995; Volkert *et al.*, 1996; Beattie *et al.*, 2000; Potter *et al.*, 2001)) or >20 kg m^{-2} (six trials (Larsson *et al.*, 1990; Rana *et al.*, 1992; Schols *et al.*, 1995; Elbers *et al.*, 1997; Saudny-Unterberger *et al.*, 1997; Schurch *et al.*, 1998)) (see Table 6.9). Data available from these trials suggest similar differences in % weight change between supplemented and unsupplemented patients, irrespective of BMI (< or > 20 kg m^{-2}). In some trials, benefits were only seen in 'well-nourished' (as opposed to the 'malnourished' (Unosson et al., 1992)), 'moderately malnourished' (as opposed to the 'severely malnourished' (Mendenhall et al., 1993)) or 'undernourished' (as opposed to the 'well-nourished' (Potter et al., 2001)) patient groups. However, in one study, patients with advanced liver disease who were 'severely malnourished' were less likely to benefit functionally (and clinically (see next question)) from ONS than the 'moderately malnourished' (for criteria, see section on liver disease) (Mendenhall et al., 1993), despite energy and protein intakes increasing significantly with ONS. One of the most likely reasons for this is a greater severity of illness in the more severely malnourished patients.

As the nutritional status/BMI of patients was undocumented in the majority of studies, it was difficult to come to any firm conclusions about the relationship between functional changes and patients' nutritional status. Further research is required in specific groups of patients with similar conditions, stratified according to nutritional status.

INDIVIDUAL PATIENT GROUPS

A variety of different functional benefits are observed across different patient groups. Significant functional changes can

be seen in Table 6.10 (results of RCT only). For more detailed information on the range of functional benefits observed in specific patient groups, refer to Appendix 3.

(IV) What effect do ONS have on the clinical and financial outcome of patients in hospital?

ALL PATIENT GROUPS COMBINED

This analysis suggests that ONS can lead to significant improvements in clinical outcome in a variety of different patient groups in the hospital setting, including the elderly, those with liver disease and surgical and orthopaedic patients. The improvements in outcome include lower mortality rates (Fig. 6.8), lower complication rates (Fig. 6.9) and shorter hospital stays (Fig. 6.10).

Improvements in clinical outcome were seen in 87% (n 20) of all trials that assessed such parameters, 50% (n 10) of which were significant (see Table 6.9). Eighty-eight per cent (n 15/17) of RCT also indicated improvements, which were significant in 60% (n 9).

Mortality. Mortality rates were significantly lower in supplemented (19%, n 181) than unsupplemented (25%, n 248) patients

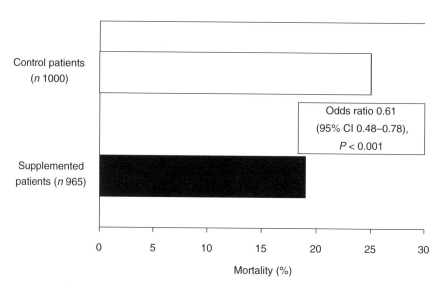

Fig. 6.8. Lower mortality rate with supplementation in hospital patients (11 RCT, 1965 patients).

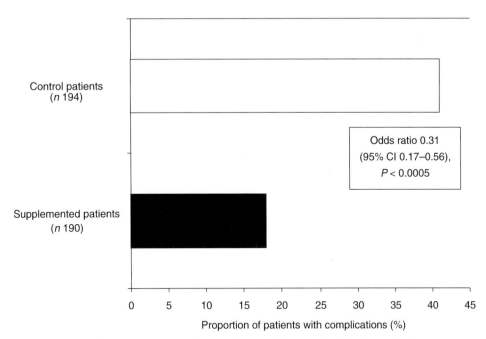

Odds ratio 0.31
(95% CI 0.17–0.56),
P < 0.0005

Fig. 6.9. Lower complication rates in supplemented patients in hospital (7 RCT, 384 patients).

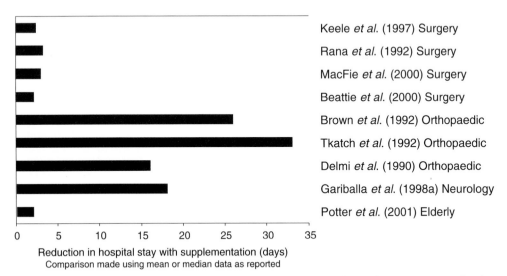

Reduction in hospital stay with supplementation (days)
Comparison made using mean or median data as reported

Fig. 6.10. Reduction in hospital stay with oral nutritional supplements in hospital patients (compared with the length of stay of control patients; 9 RCT).

across diagnostic groups (summary of results from 11 RCT in elderly, liver disease, neurology, surgical and orthopaedic patients; Fig. 6.8).

Meta-analysis. **All trials**. Meta-analysis of mortality data from RCT (11 trials, *n* 1965 (Bunout *et al.*, 1989; Delmi *et al.*, 1990; Larsson *et al.*, 1990; Tkatch *et al.*, 1992;

Unosson *et al.*, 1992; Volkert *et al.*, 1992; Mendenhall *et al.*, 1993; Gariballa *et al.*, 1998a; Le Cornu *et al.*, 2000; MacFie *et al.*, 2000; Potter *et al.*, 2001)) indicated significantly lower mortality in patients receiving ONS (*n* 181/965; odds ratio 0.61 (95% CI 0.48–0.78)) compared with control, unsupplemented patients (*n* 248/1000), with no significant heterogeneity between studies and adequate Rosenthal fail-safe scores.[1]

According to weight change and BMI. Per cent weight change was greater in trials in which significant reductions in mortality were observed (+4.7%) than in trials in which significant differences were not found (+1%; data available from only two RCT in which significant reductions in mortality were observed in patients who were or were not underweight (BMI < 20 kg m^{-2}) (Larsson *et al.*, 1990; Potter *et al.*, 2001)). However, overall, the reduction in mortality rates was most marked in those trials (Larsson *et al.*, 1990; Unosson *et al.*, 1992; Volkert *et al.*, 1996; Potter *et al.*, 2001) in which the average BMI was < 20 kg m^{-2} (17% in supplemented patients versus 26% in control patients, odds ratio 0.57 (95% CI 0.31–1.03), Fig. 6.11). There was little apparent reduction in those trials (Bunout *et al.*, 1989; Larsson *et al.*, 1990; MacFie *et al.*, 2000; Potter *et al.*, 2001) in which patient groups had an average BMI > 20 kg m^{-2}

(19% versus 20%, odds ratio 0.61 (95% CI 0.30–1.27)). For those studies in which the average BMI was unknown (Delmi *et al.*, 1990; Tkatch *et al.*, 1992; Gariballa *et al.*, 1998a; Le Cornu *et al.*, 2000), mortality was lower in supplemented (21%) than in unsupplemented (28%) patients (odds ratio 0.66 (95% CI 0.41–1.05)). (Where studies provided separate data for subgroups of patients according to nutritional status, data were analysed accordingly.)

According to patient group. Meta-analysis of hospital trials in some patient groups indicated that mortality was significantly reduced with ONS compared with routine care in elderly patients (odds ratio 0.58 (95% CI 0.40–0.83); four RCT) and may be reduced in patients with liver disease (odds ratio 0.74 (95% CI 0.29–1.92); three RCT), although larger trials are needed. Figures 6.12 and 6.13 show the lower mortality rates with ONS in trials in the elderly and in patients with liver disease. Figure 6.12 also suggests that reductions in mortality may be greater in elderly patients who are underweight (BMI < 20 kg m^{-2}). However, patients who are 'severely malnourished', and are potentially the sickest patients, may not benefit (Fig. 6.13).

For analysis according to duration and intake of ONS, see 'Combined analysis of ONS studies'.

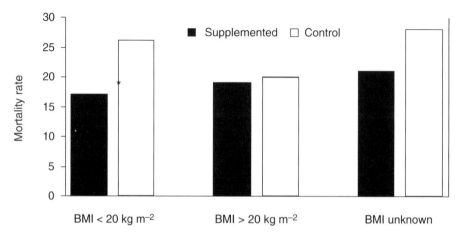

Fig. 6.11. Mortality rate in supplemented versus control hospitalized patients according to BMI (11 RCT; 1965 patients). *Odds ratio 0.57 (95% CI 0.31–1.03).

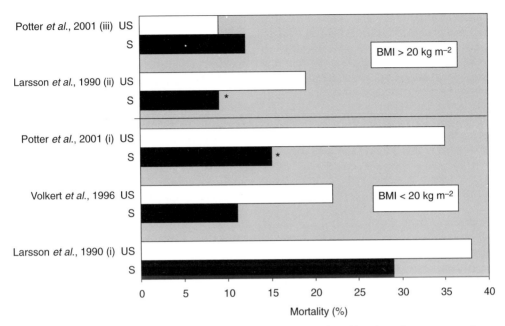

Fig. 6.12. Mortality rates in hospitalized elderly patients receiving oral nutritional supplements, according to BMI. S, supplemented; US, unsupplemented. *Significant reduction in mortality in supplemented patients. (i), (ii) and (iii) indicate patient subgroups according to BMI within trials.

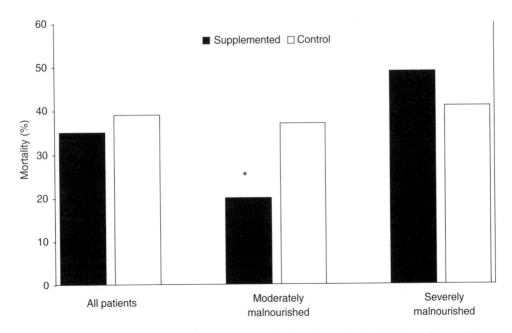

Fig. 6.13. Effect of oral nutritional supplements on mortality in patients with alcoholic liver disease. Data adapted from Mendenhall *et al.* (1993), 273 patients, also given anabolic steroids. * Significant reduction in mortality.

Complication rates. The average rate of complications (infective and others (GI perforation, pressure ulcers, anaemia, cardiac complications)) was significantly lower in supplemented (18%) than in unsupplemented (41%) patients (summary of results from seven RCT, Fig. 6.9).

Meta-analysis. **All trials.** A meta-analysis of RCT in GI and vascular surgical, orthopaedic and stroke patients (*n* 384) (Delmi *et al.*, 1990; Rana *et al.*, 1992; Tkatch *et al.*, 1992; Keele *et al.*, 1997; Gariballa *et al.*, 1998a; Beattie *et al.*, 2000; MacFie *et al.*, 2000) indicated lower complication rates in patients receiving ONS (*n* 35/190) compared with control, unsupplemented patients (*n* 80/194; odds ratio 0.31 (95% CI 0.17–0.56, *P* < 0.0005)), with no significant heterogeneity between studies and an adequate Rosenthal's fail-safe score.

According to weight change and BMI. Complication rates were lower to a similar degree in supplemented patients in trials in which the average BMI was > 20 kg m^{-2} (12% versus 27%; odds ratio 0.38 (95% CI 0.07–1.97), *n* 178, three trials (Rana *et al.*, 1992; Keele *et al.*, 1997; MacFie *et al.*,

2000)) or < 20 kg m^{-2} (12% versus 27%, one trial only (Beattie *et al.*, 2000)). Similarly, complication rates were lower in supplemented patients in those trials in which the BMI was unknown (38% versus 75%, odds ratio 0.21 (95% CI 0.04–1.18), *n* 105, three trials (Delmi *et al.*, 1990; Tkatch *et al.*, 1992; Gariballa *et al.*, 1998a)). Figure 6.14 provides an example of the lower complication rates observed in supplemented orthopaedic patients. Per cent weight change in these trials was small, with the average difference between supplemented and unsupplemented patients ranging from < 1% to 5%.

For analysis according to duration and intake of ONS, see 'Combined analysis of ONS studies'.

Length of hospital stay. Length of hospital stay was shorter in supplemented compared with control patients in all trials reviewed that provided relevant data (*n* 9/9, *P* < 0.004 two-tailed binomial test) (see Fig. 6.10). Average reductions ranged from 2 days (in surgical studies (Keele *et al.*, 1997; Beattie *et al.*, 2000)) to 33 days (in orthopaedics (Tkatch *et al.*, 1992)),

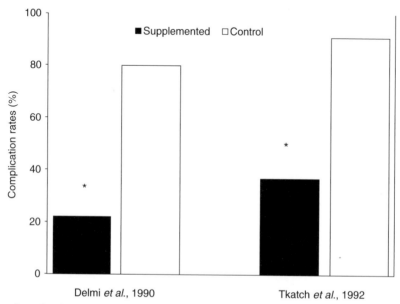

Fig. 6.14. Effect of oral nutritional supplements on complication rates in hospitalized orthopaedic patients. Data from Delmi *et al.*, 1990 (59 patients) and Tkatch *et al.*, 1992 (62 patients). *Supplemented patients significantly better clinical course (including lower complication rates).

depending on the patient group. For example, hospital LOS was significantly shortened and to a greater extent in trials in orthopaedic patients (Delmi *et al.*, 1990; Brown and Seabrook, 1992; Tkatch *et al.*, 1992), for whom total LOS was longer, than in surgical patients, where reductions in hospital days were smaller and average LOS shorter. A meta-analysis of four trials that recorded mean (standard deviation (SD)) of LOS in orthopaedic (Brown and Seabrook, 1992) and surgical (Rana *et al.*, 1992; Keele *et al.*, 1997; Beattie *et al.*, 2000) patients indicated that ONS use was associated with a reduced LOS relative to control patients (effect size −0.80 days (95% CI −1.24 to −0.36)), although there was significant heterogeneity between the studies. Per cent weight change in these studies was small, with an average difference between supplemented and unsupplemented patients of < 1% to 5%. The reduction in LOS with supplementation was greater in trials in which the average BMI was < 20 kg m^{-2} (by 9 days; 19 vs. 28 days) (Brown and Seabrook, 1992; Beattie *et al.*, 2000; Potter *et al.*, 2001) than when it was > 20 kg m^{-2} (by 4 days; 12 vs. 16 days) (Rana *et al.*, 1992; Keele *et al.*, 1997; MacFie *et al.*, 2000; Potter *et al.*, 2001). Statistical analysis of all LOS data was not possible because of the various ways in which data were presented (means, medians, with or without an indication of variability).

Clinical benefits related to changes in weight or nutritional status. The use of ONS may improve clinical outcome in both undernourished (Unosson *et al.*, 1992; Potter *et al.*, 2001) and well-nourished patients (Larsson *et al.*, 1990; Potter *et al.*, 2001). Individually, Larsson *et al.* (1990) were only able to demonstrate significantly lower mortality rates in 'well-nourished' (and not 'malnourished') elderly supplemented patients, while some trials showed significant benefits in patient groups described as 'undernourished' (e.g. Mendenhall *et al.*, 1993; Potter *et al.*, 2001). One further trial indicated that ONS may be less effective at improving the clinical outcome of patients who are 'severely

malnourished' (Mendenhall *et al.*, 1993), but more research is required to address these hypotheses.

Combined analyses of studies of ONS compared with routine clinical care (detailed above) suggest the following:

- Reduction in mortality with ONS maybe more likely:
  (i) in patient groups in which the average BMI is < 20 kg m^{-2} (9% reduction (17% vs. 26%)) than > 20 kg m^{-2} (1% reduction (19% vs. 20%));
  (ii) when there is a greater % weight change (e.g. difference of +4.7% with ETF vs. routine care in trials in which there are benefits, compared with +1.1% when there are not).
- Complication rates are similarly reduced in patient groups with a BMI < 20 kg m^{-2} (15% reduction (12% vs. 27%); one trial) or > 20 kg m^{-2} (15% reduction (12% vs. 27%) three trials).
- LOS is reduced to a greater extent in patient groups with a BMI < 20 kg m^{-2} (19 vs. 28 days) than those with a BMI > 20 kg m^{-2} (12 vs. 16 days).

INDIVIDUAL PATIENT GROUPS
Improvements in clinical outcome have been observed in a number of different patient groups. Significant changes in clinical outcome observed with ONS in different patient groups in RCT can be seen in Table 6.10 (results of RCT only). For more detailed information on the changes in clinical outcome observed in specific patient groups with ONS, refer to Appendix 3 (hospital studies).

NON-RANDOMIZED DATA
Improvements in clinical outcome were also observed in 5/6 NRT that made such an assessment (one significant improvement). None of the trials showed any significant detrimental effects on outcome following ONS. In one trial of elderly patients, there were three more deaths in those receiving an ONS than in a non-randomized control group, but this difference was not significant (Bourdel-Marchasson *et al.*, 2000).

FINANCIAL OUTCOME

None of the trials presented financial data related to the outcome of patients receiving ONS in hospital. Therefore, a retrospective cost analysis was undertaken of nine RCT (see Table 6.11, cost assumptions outlined). This demonstrated mean cost savings of between £352 and £8179 per patient in surgical, orthopaedic, elderly and cerebrovascular accident (CVA) patients. Indeed, the potential cost savings associated with a reduction in length of hospital stay and reduced expenditure on the treatment of complications following appropriate intervention with ONS are significant (Lennard-Jones, 1992; Nutrition Screening Initiative, 1996; Tucker, 1996; Green, 1999). Generally, it was calculated that savings to the National Health Service in the UK of > £266 million annually would be made if appropriate nutritional support was given to malnourished patients (conservative

Table 6.11. Additional mean cost per patient with and without use of oral nutritional supplements (hospital trials).

Trial	Group	Mean cost per patient of additional length of stay (£)	Mean cost per patient of treating complication (£)	Mean cost per patient for ONS (£)	Mean total cost per patient (£)	Mean total saving per patient as a result of nutritional support (£)
Potter et al. (2001) Elderly	Supplemented	0	–	48	48	452
	Control	500	–	0	500	
Gariballa et al. (1998a) Neurology	Supplemented	0	36	84	120	4424
	Control	4500	44	0	4544	
Delmi et al. (1990) Orthopaedic	Supplemented	0	18	96	222	3842
	Control	4000	64[a]	0	4064	
Brown and Seabrook (1992) Orthopaedic	Supplemented	0	–	63	63	6437
	Control	6500	–	0	6500	
Tkatch et al. (1992) Orthopaedic	Supplemented	0	30	114	144	8179
	Control	8250	73[a]	0	8323	
Rana et al. (1992) Surgery	Supplemented	0	12	21	33	832
	Control	825	40	0	865	
Keele et al. (1997) Surgery	Supplemented	0	4	17	21	601
	Control	600	22	0	622	
Beattie et al. (2000) Surgery	Supplemented	0	9	210	219	352
	Control	550	21	0	571	
MacFie et al. (2000) Surgery	Supplemented	0	12	24	36	720
	Control	750	6	0	756	

Assumptions: hospital (hotel) costs: £250 day^{-1}; treatment costs, £80 per complication; ONS £3 day^{-1}.
[a] Complication rates for recovery hospital.

estimate based on nutritional intervention reducing hospital stay by 5 days in 10% of hospital patients at 1992 prices) (Lennard-Jones, 1992). More specifically, a number of other retrospective cost analyses of some of the trials reviewed have demonstrated that cost savings are possible if ONS are used appropriately (Ofman and Koretz, 1997; Green, 1999). Prospective cost evaluations are needed to confirm these observations.

Evidence Base for ONS in the Community Setting

For this review, in addition to the main four questions, the timing of supplementation (additional to question (I)) and the effects of stopping ONS (question V) were also considered.

Summary characteristics of community trials in the ONS review

Study design

One hundred and eight trials (3747 patients) investigating the effects of ONS compared with no nutritional support in patients in the community were systematically reviewed. Forty-four (41%, *n* 2194 patients) were RCT and 64 (59%, *n* 1553 patients) were NRT (see Table 6.12). All trials were reviewed in patient-specific groups and Table 6.12 shows a summary of the number of trials and patients categorized accordingly. The RCT were graded for methodology using Jadad's (Jadad *et al.*, 1996) criteria and a summary of overall scores is shown in Table 6.13. For information about the Jadad scoring system, refer to Chapter 5. For the Jadad scores for

Table 6.12. Summary of trials of oral nutritional supplement use in community patients.

Disease category	Number of trials			Number of patients		
	Randomized	Non-randomized	Total	Randomized	Non-randomized	Total
COPD	9	6	15	171	99	270
Crohn's disease	3	7	10	76	131	207
Cystic fibrosis	3	10	13	39	234	273
Elderly	10	7	17	570	197	767
HIV/AIDS	3	15	18	650	494	1144
Liver disease	2	0	2	61	0	61
Malignancy	9	8	17	392	202	594
Renal disease	2	10	12	40	192	232
Other diseases	3	1	4	195	4	199
Total	44	64	108	2194	1553	3747

Table 6.13. Summary of the Jadad scores for community randomized controlled trials (Jadad *et al.*, 1996). Individual codes relating to the design of each study can be seen in the summaries in Appendix 4. For an explanation of the Jadad scoring system, refer to Chapter 5.

Jadad score	Number of trials (%)	Patient group (number of trials)
1	12 (27%)	COPD (4), cystic fibrosis (1), elderly (2), malignancy (4), renal (1)
2	23 (52%)	COPD (3), Crohn's disease (3), cystic fibrosis (2), elderly (4), HIV (2), liver disease (2), malignancy (4), renal (1), other (2)
3	7 (16%)	COPD (1), elderly (3), HIV (1), malignancy (1), other (1)
4	2 (5%)	COPD (1), elderly (1)
5	0	–

–, no data.

individual trials, refer to Appendix 4. Sixty-four trials were non-randomized and were coded according to whether they had a non-random control group (given no nutritional support) (B) or not (C). Eighty per cent of NRT were simply longitudinal observations of patients undertaken before and after a period of ONS (51 trials coded C; COPD six; Crohn's disease seven; cystic fibrosis seven; elderly three; HIV 14; malignancy four; renal disease nine; other one) and the rest had a control group (13 trials coded B; cystic fibrosis three; elderly four; HIV one; malignancy four; renal disease one). RCT comparing groups of patients receiving two or more different types of ONS were also reviewed as non-randomized data and coded C.

For some diseases, no studies in the community setting were reviewed (e.g. neurological diseases).

Community settings

Most studies (> 80%) were conducted in patients living at home, including those who had started ONS in hospital and were being followed up as out-patients (e.g. Woo *et al.*, 1994; Keele *et al.*, 1997) and those who were receiving ONS prior to hospital admission (e.g. McCarter *et al.*, 1998). Fewer than 20% of studies were undertaken in patients in nursing or residential homes or in a research centre.

ONS used in community trials

CONSISTENCY, TYPE AND COMPOSITION OF ONS
Liquid ONS (either commercial sip feeds or powders reconstituted to form a liquid supplement) were used in more than 80% of the studies reviewed. A minority of studies reported using bars, puddings, powders added to normal food and drink or home-made (non-commercial) ONS. In six studies (Chandra and Puri, 1985; Stauffer *et al.*, 1986; Flynn and Leightty, 1987; Donahoe *et al.*, 1989; Dowling *et al.*, 1990; Hayes *et al.*, 1995), neither the name nor the type of ONS used was documented. The energy density of ONS varied considerably (from 0.6 to 3.8 kcal ml^{-1}), as did their composition (protein hydrolysate, ele-

mental, medium-chain triglyceride-enriched, branched-chain amino acid-enriched and formulas with extra arginine, omega-3 fatty acids and nucleic acids). Standard formulas containing a mix of macronutrients (e.g. ~15% energy as protein, 35% energy as fat, 50% energy as carbohydrate) and micronutrients were also commonly used. Further details of the ONS used in individual studies can be found in Appendix 4.

AMOUNT OF ONS PRESCRIBED AND TAKEN
The amount of ONS prescribed daily (recorded in 78% of trials, *n* 84) ranged from 200 kcal to 2661 kcal (when used as a sole source of nutrition). ONS intake (reported in 48% of trials, *n* 52) also varied, ranging from 47 kcal to 3000 kcal. The amount of ONS prescribed and taken in individual studies, where reported, is summarized in Appendix 4. Table 6.14 contains a summary according to patient group.

DURATION OF ORAL NUTRITIONAL SUPPLEMENTATION
The duration of supplementation ranged from less than 2 weeks (Flynn and Leightty, 1987; McCarter *et al.*, 1998) to over 2 years (Allan *et al.*, 1973).

Dietary counselling in community supplementation trials

Although information about the use of dietary counselling or modified foods/diets to increase energy and protein intakes was not provided in most trials, it is likely that these methods were often used, prior to or alongside the use of ONS. Nearly one-third (31%, *n* 33) of the studies reviewed reported the use of dietary counselling/advice in patients given ONS (COPD five trials; elderly three trials; cystic fibrosis four; renal disease three; malignancy eight; HIV/AIDS eight; other two). In some cases, dietary counselling had been used unsuccessfully before the trial, and ONS were being used as the next therapeutic option (Smathers *et al.*, 1992; Burger *et al.*, 1994; Tolia, 1995). However, the dietary counselling varied across specialities and over the years that studies had been undertaken.

Table 6.14. Range of documented prescribed amounts of ONS and ONS intakes from community trials.

Patient group (total number of trials)	Range of prescribed ONS (number of trials)	Range of ONS intake (number of trials)
COPD (15)	400–1080 kcal (9)	347–1080 kcal (7)
Crohn's disease (10)	600–2661 kcal[a] (7)	550–3000 kcal (4)
Cystic fibrosis (13)	500–1200 kcal (11)	462–1413 kcal (6)
Elderly (17)	200–1080 kcal (14)	200–815 kcal (9)
HIV/AIDS (18)	480–1500 kcal (14)	310–695 kcal (11)
Liver disease (2)	1000–2400 kcal[a] (2)	889–1800 kcal (2)
Malignancy (17)	500–2400 kcal[a] (13)	167–2500 kcal[a] (7)
Renal disease (12)	200–800 kcal (11)	321–2375 kcal (3)
Other diseases (4)	750 kcal (3)	47–570 kcal (3)

[a] When prescribed as a sole source of nutrition.

Advice ranged from general encouragement to increase energy/food intakes (Parsons *et al.*, 1983) to specific advice in relation to modifying textures of foods to maximize intake in cancer patients (Arnold and Richter, 1989), individualized counselling to increase vitamin and calcium intakes in COPD patients (Ganzoni *et al.*, 1994), aspects of hygiene and dealing with GI symptoms (e.g. diarrhoea, vomiting) in HIV/AIDS patients (Berneis *et al.*, 2000) and reductions in fibre intakes during abdominal radiotherapy (Brown *et al.*, 1980; Foster *et al.*, 1980). In older trials, the dietary recommendations given were often unlike current recommendations (e.g. advice on how to consume a low-fat diet in patients with cystic fibrosis (Berry *et al.*, 1975)). Where indicated, the health professional providing the counselling was usually a dietitian (e.g. Openbrier *et al.*, 1984; Ovesen and Allingstrup, 1992; Chlebowski *et al.*, 1993; Pichard *et al.*, 1998; Berneis *et al.*, 2000). In some cases, dietary counselling was specifically not given, either because patients were on ONS alone (e.g. studies in Crohn's disease) or because the trial aimed to investigate the effects of ONS *per se* on dietary intake.

Main findings of the community ONS review

A summary of the key findings from the evidence base for ONS in the community setting is presented in Box 6.2. The results

of all of the studies reviewed, according to each of the four main questions, have also been summarized in Table 6.15, arranged by BMI and patient group. An indication of the number and proportion of studies that assessed and showed improvement in these four measures is provided in Fig. 6.15 and each is discussed in more detail below. For more specific information about the efficacy of ONS in different patient groups, refer to Appendix 4.

(I) What effect do ONS have on the voluntary food intake and total energy of patients in the community?

ALL PATIENT GROUPS COMBINED
Total energy and nutrient intake. This analysis suggests that ONS increase total energy intake in a variety of patient groups (COPD, cystic fibrosis, Crohn's disease, HIV, elderly, surgery, liver disease). Most (84%, *n* 52) studies that assessed energy intake showed an increase, which was significant in 65% (*n* 34) (see Table 6.15). The effect of ONS versus no nutritional support on total energy intake was assessed in 32 RCT. In 91% of these studies (29/32), an increase in total energy intake with supplementation was demonstrated and this was statistically significant in 72% (*n* 21; in 12 trials versus a control group, in nine trials over time; the others were either not statistically evaluated or not statistically significant (Fig. 6.15)). In addition, 77% of NRT (*n* 23/30) that made assessments demonstrated an

Table 6.15. Changes in nutrient intake, body weight, function and clinical outcome following oral nutritional supplementation (versus no nutritional support) in the community setting related to patient's nutritional status.

Supplementation trial	Improved energy and/or nutrient intake	Improved nutritional status	Improved function	Improved clinical outcome
BMI < 20 kg m^{-2}/IBW < 90%				
Randomized, controlled trials				
Donahoe *et al.* (1989) A COPD	√ (?sig)	√ (t)	√ (t)	n/a
Efthimiou *et al.* (1988) COPD	√ (t)	√ (t)	√ (t)	n/a
Fuenzalida *et al.* (1990) COPD	√ (t)	√ (t)	√ (t)	n/a
Knowles *et al.* (1988) COPD	√ (t)	√ (t)	√ (t)	n/a
Lewis *et al.* (1987) COPD	√ (v)	n/a	√ (ns)	n/a
Norregaard *et al.* (1987) A COPD	√ (t)	√ (t)	√ (?sig)	n/a
Otte *et al.* (1989) COPD	√ (?sig)	√ (v)		n/a
Rogers *et al.* (1992) COPD	√ (v)	√ (v)	√ (v)	n/a
Harries *et al.* (1983) Crohn's	√ (v)	√ (v)	√ (ns)	n/a
Kalnins *et al.* (1996) Cystic fibrosis (P)		√ (ns)		n/a
Steinkamp *et al.* (2000) Cystic fibrosis (P)	√ (t)	√ (t)	√ (?sig)	n/a
Gray-Donald *et al.* (1995) Elderly	√ (ns)	√ (v)	√ (v)	n/a
Lauque *et al.* (2000) (i) Elderly	√ (t)	√ (?sig)		n/a
Persson *et al.* (2000b) A Elderly	n/a	√ (v)	√ (t)	n/a
Volkert *et al.* (1996) Elderly	n/a	√ (t)	√ (v) **	n/a
Woo *et al.* (1994) Elderly	√ (v)	√ (t)	√ (v)	n/a
Non-randomized trials/data				
Pardy *et al.* (1986) COPD	√ (?sig)	√ (ns)		n/a
Sridhar *et al.* (1994) COPD	n/a	√ (ns)		n/a
Stauffer *et al.* (1986) COPD	√ (t)	√ (ns)	n/a	n/a
Wilson *et al.* (1964) COPD	√ (t)	n/a	n/a	n/a
Wilson *et al.* (1986) COPD	n/a	√ (t)	√ (t)	n/a
Harries *et al.* (1984) Crohn's	√ (?sig)	√ (t)	√ (t)	n/a
Logan *et al.* (1981) Crohn's	n/a	√ (ns)	√ (t)	
Allan *et al.* (1973) Cystic fibrosis (P)	n/a	√ (t)	√ (?sig)	n/a
Barclay and Shannon (1975) Cystic fibrosis (P)	n/a		√ (ns)	n/a
Berry *et al.* (1975) Cystic fibrosis (P)	n/a	√ (t)	√ (t)	n/a
Kashirskaja *et al.* (1996) Cystic fibrosis (P)	n/a	√ (?sig)	√ (t)	√ (t)
Parsons *et al.* (1983) Cystic fibrosis (P)	√ (t)	√ (t)	√ (ns)	n/a
Rettammel *et al.* (1995) Cystic fibrosis (P)			n/a	n/a
Shepherd *et al.* (1983) Cystic fibrosis (P)	√ (?sig)	√ (t)	√ (t)	n/a
Skypala *et al.* (1998) Cystic fibrosis (P)	√ (t)	√ (t)	n/a	n/a
Yassa *et al.* (1978) Cystic fibrosis (P)	n/a	√ (t)	√ (t)	n/a
Cederholm and Hellström (1995) Elderly	n/a	√ (v)	√ (t)	n/a
Gray-Donald *et al.* (1994) Elderly	√ (t)	√ (t)	√ (t)	n/a
Lipschitz *et al.* (1985) Elderly	√ (?sig)	√ (?sig)		n/a
Welch *et al.* (1991) Elderly	√ (t)	√ (t)	n/a	n/a
Fogaca *et al.* (2000) HIV		√ (ns)		n/a
Cuppari *et al.* (1994) Renal	√ (t)	√ (t)	n/a	n/a
BMI > 20 kg m^{-2}/IBW > 90%				
Randomized, controlled trials				
Fiatarone *et al.* (1994) Elderly	√ (t)**	√ (t)		n/a
Fiatarone Singh *et al.* (2000) Elderly	√ (ns)	√ (v)	√ (t)	n/a
Krondl *et al.* (1999) Elderly	√ N (v)	n/a		n/a
Lauque *et al.* (2000) (ii) Elderly	√ (t)	√ (?sig)		n/a

Continued

Table 6.15. *Continued.*

Supplementation trial	Improved energy and/or nutrient intake	Improved nutritional status	Improved function	Improved clinical outcome
Meredith *et al.* (1992) Elderly	√ (t)	√ (v)		n/a
Berneis *et al.* (2000) HIV	√ (ns)	√ (ns)		n/a
Gibert *et al.* (1999) HIV	√ (v)	√ (ns)	n/a	n/a
Rabeneck *et al.* (1998) HIV	n/a		√ (t)	n/a
Foster *et al.* (1980) Malignancy	n/a	√ (ns)	n/a	n/a
Jensen and Hessov (1997) GI surgery	√ (v)	√ (v)	n/a	n/a
Keele *et al.* (1997) GI surgery	√ (v)	√ (ns)		n/a
Broqvist *et al.* (1994) Cardiac	√ (v)	√ (?sig)		n/a
Non-randomized trials/data				
Geerling *et al.* (2000b) Crohn's	n/a	n/a	√ (t)**	n/a
Breslow *et al.* (1993) Elderly	√ (t)	n/a	√ (t)	n/a
Yamaguchi *et al.* (1998) Elderly	√ (t)	√ (v)	n/a	n/a
Chlebowski *et al.* (1993) HIV	√ (?sig)		n/a	n/a*
Dowling *et al.* (1990) HIV		√ (ns)	n/a	n/a
Hoh *et al.* (1998) HIV	√ (t)			n/a
Pichard *et al.* (1998) HIV	√ (? sig)**	√ (ns)	√ (?sig)	n/a
Stack *et al.* (1996) HIV	n/a	√ (?sig)	n/a	n/a
Süttman *et al.* (1996) HIV	√ (ns)	√ (v)**	√ (t)**	n/a
McCarter *et al.* (1998) Malignancy	n/a	n/a		
Wallner *et al.* (1990) Malignancy	n/a	√ (v)	n/a	n/a
Patel and Raftery (1997) Renal	√ (v)	n/a	n/a	n/a
Patel *et al.* (2000) Renal	√ (t)	√ (ns)	n/a	n/a
BMI unknown				
Randomized, controlled trials				
Ganzoni *et al.* (1994) COPD	√ (ns)	√ (t)		n/a
Lindor *et al.* (1992) Crohn's	n/a	n/a		
O'Morain *et al.* (1984) Crohn's	n/a	√ (t)	√ (t)	√ (t)
Sondel *et al.* (1987) Cystic fibrosis (P)	√ (v)		n/a	
Chandra and Puri (1985) Elderly	n/a	√ (t)	√ (v)	n/a
Simko (1983) Liver disease	√ (v)			n/a
Hirsch *et al.* (1993) Liver disease	√ (v)	√ (t)	√ (t)	√ (v)
Arnold and Richter (1989) Malignancy	√ (v)	√ (ns)	n/a	
Bounous *et al.* (1975) Malignancy		√ (v)	√ (v)	n/a
Brown *et al.* (1980) Malignancy	n/a	√ (ns)	n/a	n/a
Douglass *et al.* (1978) Malignancy	√ (?sig)		√ (ns)	
Elkort *et al.* (1981) Malignancy	n/a	√ (?sig)		
Evans *et al.* (1987) Malignancy	√ (t)	√ (ns lung)		
Flynn and Leightty (1987) Malignancy	n/a	n/a	n/a	√ (?sig)
Nayel *et al.* (1992) Malignancy	n/a	√ (v)	n/a	√ (ns)
Kuhlmann *et al.* (1997) A Renal	√ (?sig)	√ (?sig)	n/a	n/a
Wilson *et al.* (2001) Renal	n/a	n/a	n/a	√ (ns)
Non-randomized trials/data				
Openbrier *et al.* (1984) COPD	n/a	√ (t)	n/a	n/a
Akobeng *et al.* (2000) Crohn's P	n/a	√ (?sig)	√ (?sig)	n/a
Fell *et al.* (2000) Crohn's P	n/a	√ (?sig)	√ (t)	n/a
Kirschner *et al.* (1981) Crohn's (P)	√ (?sig)	√ (?sig) g	n/a	n/a
Raouf *et al.* (1991) Crohn's	n/a	n/a	√ (?sig)	n/a
Hayes *et al.* (1995) A Cystic fibrosis (P)	n/a	n/a	n/a	n/a
Bunker *et al.* (1994) Elderly	n/a	n/a		n/a
Burger *et al.* (1994) HIV	n/a		n/a	

Continued

Table 6.15. *Continued.*

Supplementation trial	Improved energy and/or nutrient intake	Improved nutritional status	Improved function	Improved clinical outcome
Chan *et al.* (1994) HIV	n/a	✓ (?sig)	✓ (t)	
Chlebowski *et al.* (1992) A HIV	n/a	✓ (t**)	✓ (?sig)	
Gaare *et al.* (1991) A HIV			n/a	n/a
Hellerstein *et al.* (1994) A HIV	n/a	n/a	✓ (t)	n/a*
Richards *et al.* (1996) A HIV	✓ (?sig)		n/a*	n/a
Singer *et al.* (1992) A HIV	n/a	✓ (?sig)	n/a*	n/a
Wandall *et al.* (1992) HIV	n/a	✓ (t)	n/a	n/a
Baker *et al.* (1977) A Malignancy	n/a	n/a	n/a	n/a
Barber *et al.* (1999a) Malignancy	n/a	✓ (?sig)	n/a	n/a
Barber *et al.* (2000) Malignancy	n/a	✓ (t)	n/a	n/a
Bounous *et al.* (1973) A Malignancy	n/a	n/a	n/a	n/a
Crossland and Higgins (1977) A Malignancy	n/a	n/a	✓ (?sig)	n/a
Ovesen and Allingstrup (1992) Malignancy	✓ (t)**	✓ (t)**	n/a	n/a
Cockram *et al.* (1998) Renal	n/a	n/a	n/a	n/a
Lynch *et al.* (1983) Renal			n/a	n/a
Mareckova *et al.* (1995) A Renal		n/a	n/a	n/a
Ortiz *et al.* (1992) Renal			n/a	n/a
Smathers *et al.* (1992) Renal	n/a	n/a	n/a	n/a
Young *et al.* (1978) Renal	n/a	n/a	n/a	n/a
Yulo *et al.* (1997) A Renal	n/a	n/a	n/a	n/a
Tolia (1995) Other (P)	✓ (t)	✓ (? sig) g	n/a	n/a

✓	Indicates an improvement or less deterioration compared with a control group or over time.
(v)	Significant compared with a control group receiving no ONS or a placebo.
(t)	Significant change over time.
(?sig)	Improvement/benefit observed but unclear if statistically significant.
(ns)	Improvement/benefit observed that is not statistically significant.
n/a	Not assessed in trial.
A	Abstract.
(P)	Includes paediatrics.
g	Growth.
*	Significant benefits to outcome with one type of ONS relative to another.
**	Improvement observed only in a specific supplemented group (Geerling *et al.*, 1998c).
N	Improvement in protein or micronutrient intakes (not energy).

increase in total energy intake, which was significant in 13 (57%).

ONS appear to increase energy intakes in patient groups with an average BMI < 20 and > 20 kg m^{-2}. Improvements in total energy intake were documented in 93% of RCT in which the mean BMI of patients was < 20 kg m^{-2} (13/14; significant in ten (77%)) and in 90% of those with a mean BMI > 20 kg m^{-2} (9/10; significant in seven (77%)). However, improvement in intake occurred to a greater extent in studies of underweight patients (mean BMI < 20 kg m^{-2}) (see section on spontaneous food intake).

The use of exercise alongside ONS may further stimulate appetite and food intake. For example, in one trial in elderly residential care patients, total energy intake was only significantly increased in those patients given resistance exercise in addition to supplementation (Fiatarone *et al.*, 1994).

A number of trials in a variety of different patient groups provided information that suggested that protein and micronutrient intakes were significantly increased with ONS. Trials indicating significant improvements in protein intakes included those in

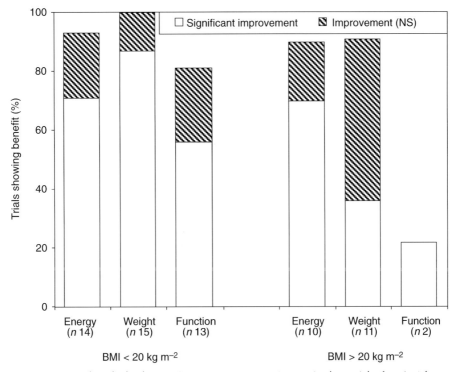

Fig. 6.15. Summary of results for three main outcome measures (energy intake, weight, function) from community trials of ONS according to BMI (*n* = total number of trials).

COPD patients (Lewis *et al.*, 1987; Norregaard *et al.*, 1987), patients with liver (Hirsch *et al.*, 1993) or renal disease (Cuppari *et al.*, 1994; Mareckova *et al.*, 1995; Patel and Raftery, 1997; Patel *et al.*, 2000), the elderly (Welch *et al.*, 1991; Gray-Donald *et al.*, 1994; Woo *et al.*, 1994; Yamaguchi *et al.*, 1998; Krondl *et al.*, 1999; Lauque *et al.*, 2000), those with cancer (Arnold and Richter, 1989), post-surgery (Jensen and Hessov, 1997) or with congestive heart failure (Broqvist *et al.*, 1994). Improvements in micronutrient intakes with ONS were also documented in a range of patient groups, including HIV patients (Hoh *et al.*, 1998) and the elderly (free-living, in nursing homes or receiving meals on wheels (Welch *et al.*, 1991; Woo *et al.*, 1994; Yamaguchi *et al.*, 1998; Krondl *et al.*, 1999)), with improvements in vitamin status also being reported in studies in elderly patients (Lipschitz *et al.*, 1985) and in patients with Crohn's disease (Geerling *et al.*, 2000b).

Although ONS may increase total energy intake, a reduction in food intake and/or ONS intake may occur over time, particularly if ONS are used for long periods of time in chronically ill patients. The change in food intake and total energy intake during the period of supplementation was assessed in only eight trials (cancer (Arnold and Richter, 1989; Ovesen and Allingstrup, 1992), COPD (Lewis *et al.*, 1987; Knowles *et al.*, 1988; Fiatarone Singh *et al.*, 2000), elderly (Lipschitz *et al.*, 1985; Yamaguchi *et al.*, 1998), HIV (Pichard *et al.*, 1998)). These suggested that, with longer-term ONS, a reduction in food intake and total energy intake may occur over time (Yamaguchi *et al.*, 1998), often returning close to baseline levels. In one trial the increase in total energy intake was transient, lasting for only 1–2 months out of a total of 6 months of supplementation (Pichard *et al.*, 1988).

There appeared to be no clear relationship between reported ONS intake and significant increases in total energy intake from the studies reviewed. Significant increases in total energy intake were reported with ONS intakes ranging from 347 kcal (Knowles *et al.*, 1988) to 1080 kcal (Fuenzalida *et al.*, 1990). Failure to increase total energy intake substantially was also documented in trials in which the ONS intake was purported to be < 238 kcal (Dowling *et al.*, 1990) or up to 1413 kcal (Rettamel *et al.*, 1995). This may be because checks on compliance were limited or inadequate in the trials reviewed. Also, it is likely that the duration, type (composition or consistency), time and frequency of ONS consumption and the disease of patients may affect the ability of ONS to improve energy and nutrient intake. Combining ONS with other therapies (e.g. exercise) may have a 'synergistic' effect in increasing total energy intake (Fiatarone *et al.*, 1994), although this requires further investigation.

Spontaneous food intake. This analysis suggests that ONS provide largely additional energy to that taken as food in patients in the community. The extent to which supplemental energy intake replaced or added to the energy taken from food could be assessed in 25 trials (for methodology, refer to Chapter 5). On average, the increment in total energy intake during supplementation was equivalent to 69% of the energy consumed as a supplement, but this varied widely across studies from 0% to > 100% (Fig. 6.16). Indeed, in some studies, voluntary food intake actually increased during the period of ONS (as indicated by > 100% of ONS energy additive) (e.g. RCT in post-surgical patients (Jensen and Hessov, 1997); cross-over trial in Crohn's disease (Harries *et al.*, 1983); NRT in patients on haemodialysis (Cuppari *et al.*, 1994)), a phenomenon also observed in some trials in the hospital setting (Rana *et al.*, 1992). This could be due to the stimulation of appetite with supplementation. However, the lack of information about the methods used to assess intake and the variability in patients' responses make it difficult to assess whether the apparent increases in food intake are statistically significant or whether they are due to differences in the methodology used in various trials.

The % of supplement energy additional to food intake was greater in studies (n 11) in which the patients had a mean BMI < 20 kg m^{-2} (83%, range 43–135%), than in those (n 10) with a mean BMI > 20 kg m^{-2} (45%, range 0–93%) (Fig. 6.16). Indeed, the frequency with which more than 50% of the ONS energy was additive to food intake was significantly greater in studies of patients with an average BMI < 20 kg m^{-2} than in those with BMI > 20 kg m^{-2} ($P < 0.024$; Fisher's exact test) (Fig. 6.17).

Appetite. Remarkably little is known about the impact of ONS on appetite in patients in the community with chronic disease. No studies formally assessed the effect of ONS on appetite sensations (hunger, fullness and desire to eat). Anecdotal observations during supplementation included fullness (early satiety), often associated with abdominal bloating, which was reported to occur more frequently in patients receiving the high energy density supplements or large volumes of unpalatable formulas. A study in adults reported that reducing the volume and increasing the frequency of ONS intake relieved bloating (Rettamel *et al.*, 1995). In children with cystic fibrosis, one study (Sondel *et al.*, 1987) reported that 25% of patients lost their appetite after taking the supplement during the day, whereas another reported no loss of appetite when the supplement was given during the night (Hayes *et al.*, 1995). In adults, anecdotal reports suggested that ONS improved anorexia in patients with HIV, at least temporarily, but this was not supported by long-term measurements of total energy intake (Pichard *et al.*, 1998). Other studies in cancer patients reported loss of appetite over time, irrespective of whether or not an ONS was consumed (Nayel *et al.*, 1992).

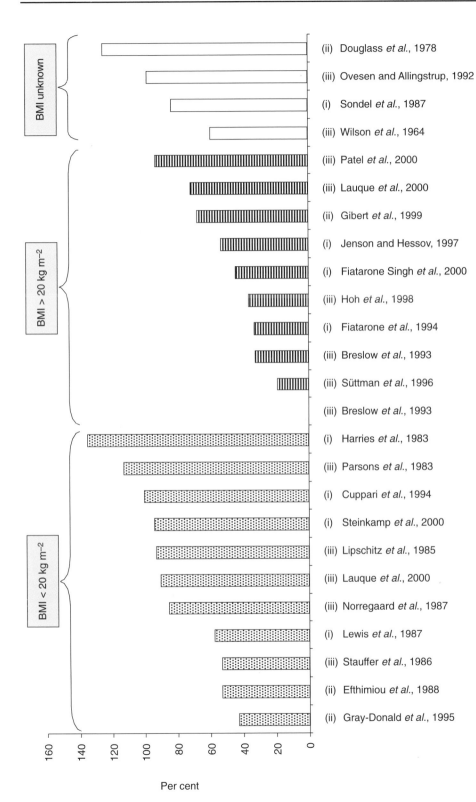

Fig. 6.16. Increment in total energy intake as a proprtion (%) of the energy consumed as a supplement (data from community ONS studies according to BMI, see Chapter 5 for calculation methods (i), (ii) and (iii)).

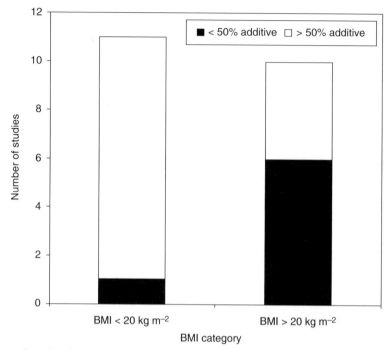

Fig. 6.17. Number of studies in which more than or less than 50% of supplement energy is additive to food intake (according to BMI, $P < 0.024$).

The composition (including energy density) and the consistency of the ONS may be factors that determine the impact ONS have on appetite and subsequent food intake. On the basis of the limited and often anecdotal and conflicting information from patient studies in the community, no firm conclusions were reached about the effects of the composition and energy density of the ONS or the timing of ONS consumption on appetite and total intake. Further research is required.

INDIVIDUAL PATIENT GROUPS

ONS consistently improve total energy intake across different patient groups. In most groups (including COPD and surgery), supplemental energy intake is largely additional to food intake (see Box 6.5).

(Ia) Is the timing of supplementation important in community patients?

The time of day and the frequency with which ONS are consumed is likely to have

an important effect on appetite and food intake. This in turn may determine whether structural and functional measures are altered. However, no firm conclusions have been reached about the optimal frequency and timing of ONS consumption from the current evidence base.

Twenty-three studies (elderly (n 10), malignancy (n 4), cystic fibrosis (n 4), Crohn's disease (n 1), COPD (n 1), postoperative (n 1), congestive heart failure (n 1), renal disease (n 1)) indicated when ONS should be consumed, but patients' compliance with this timing was not verified.

The 'recommendations' about timing of supplementation varied widely and included the following:

- Between meals (Douglass *et al.*, 1978; Lipschitz *et al.*, 1985; Stauffer *et al.*, 1986; Ovesen and Allingstrup, 1992; Smathers *et al.*, 1992; Broqvist *et al.*, 1994; Woo *et al.*, 1994; Volkert *et al.*, 1996; Keele *et al.*, 1997).

Box 6.5. Effect of ONS on food and total intake in different patient groups (community setting).

COPD
ONS (1–2 kcal ml^{-1}) can increase total energy intakes in patients with COPD in the community. Studies suggest that > 50% of the energy is additive to food intake (Lewis *et al.*, 1987; Norregaard *et al.*, 1987; Efthimiou *et al.*, 1988). Large volumes of supplementation or energy dense feeds (2 kcal ml^{-1}) may lead to bloating (Lewis *et al.*, 1987; Fuenzalida *et al.*, 1990). Otherwise no adverse effects were reported.

Crohn's disease
When used as a supplement to food intake, ONS (0.8–1.5 kcal ml^{-1}) can increase total energy intake without substantially reducing food intake (Harries *et al.*, 1983). ONS may also be used as a sole source of nutrition in those with acute exacerbations (adults and children).

Cystic fibrosis
In adult and paediatric cystic fibrosis patients, ONS (1–2 kcal ml^{-1}) can increase total energy intake without reducing food intake substantially. In the studies reviewed, the majority of energy (> 80%) (Parsons *et al.*, 1983; Sondel *et al.*, 1987; Steinkamp *et al.*, 2000) was additive to food intake, although large volumes of unpalatable feeds may suppress appetite (Yassa *et al.*, 1978).

Elderly
ONS (0.6–2 kcal ml^{-1}) can increase total energy and nutrient intakes in healthy free-living elderly and in those with disease living at home or in institutions. If used for long periods of time, food and total intake can decrease (Fiatarone Singh *et al.*, 2000). The provision of a variety of ONS types (Lauque *et al.*, 2000) or the use of other treatments (e.g. exercise therapy) alongside ONS may be beneficial (Fiatarone *et al.*, 1994).

HIV/AIDS
A variety of different types of ONS (bars, sweet and savoury drinks) may be more effective at increasing total energy intakes in HIV/AIDS patients than one type of ONS used for long periods of time. Increasing variety may prevent the suppression of food intake observed over time in some patients (Pichard *et al.*, 1998). ONS can increase vitamin and mineral intakes (Hoh *et al.*, 1998).

Liver disease
ONS (1 kcal ml^{-1}) can significantly improve both energy and protein intakes. The impact of supplementation on appetite and food intake has not been investigated in the trials reviewed.

Malignancy
Improvements in total energy intake (Evans *et al.*, 1987; Arnold and Richter, 1989) and in food intake may occur with use of ONS (0.8–1.3 kcal ml^{-1}) in cancer patients, although these increments may not be sustained over time (Arnold and Richter, 1989).

Renal disease
ONS (1–2 kcal ml^{-1}) can improve energy and protein intakes and may not substantially reduce food intake in those with chronic renal disease (including patients on haemodialysis (HD) and continuous ambulatory peritoneal dialysis (CAPD)) but RCT are needed.

Surgery (gastrointestinal)
ONS used in surgical patients discharged from hospital can increase total energy and protein intakes. Food intake appears not to be suppressed and may even be increased during ONS (Jensen and Hessov, 1997; Keele *et al.*, 1997).

- Small sips throughout the day (Berry *et al.*, 1975; Bounous *et al.*, 1975; Yassa *et al.*, 1978; Lindor *et al.*, 1992).
- With the main meal (Breslow *et al.*, 1993).
- Early morning (Meredith *et al.*, 1992; Cederholm and Hellström, 1995).
- Afternoon/evening (Sondel *et al.*, 1987; Meredith *et al.*, 1992; Fiatarone *et al.*, 1994; Cederholm and Hellström, 1995).

- Night (Hayes *et al.*, 1995). One study involved waking up children in the middle of the night so that they could consume a supplement.
- Spread throughout the week (no specific times of day given) (Krondl *et al.*, 1999).

These 'recommendations' were mostly based on the belief that total energy intake would be increased maximally, with minimal suppression of appetite.

No formal comparisons between the effects of these different schedules (i.e. times of supplement consumption) on appetite and food intake were made in the different disease groups and there was insufficient evidence from the trials reviewed to make any conclusions regarding the recommended times for ONS consumption and subsequent outcome measures (total energy intake, structural or functional/clinical outcomes). Further investigations are needed.

(II) What effect do ONS have on the body weight and composition of patients in the community?

ALL PATIENT GROUPS COMBINED

ONS can improve body weight and muscle mass in a variety of community-based patient groups with chronic diseases (including the elderly and those with COPD, cystic fibrosis, Crohn's disease, renal disease and cancer). Improvements in body weight were documented in 85% (*n* 72) of all trials that reported assessments, with 60% (*n* 43) showing a statistically significant increase (see Table 6.15).

More than 90% of RCT (*n* 36) that assessed changes (*n* 39) in body weight showed an increase or less loss of weight with ONS, of which 64% were statistically significant (*n* 23). In ten studies, weight gain was significantly greater or weight loss was significantly less than in a control group who were unsupplemented and, in 13 studies, the changes were analysed as significant compared with the baseline.

Per cent weight change in supplemented relative to unsupplemented patients could be calculated from 30 RCT (*n* 1452 patients;

COPD, elderly, HIV, liver disease, cancer, surgery). The mean % weight change (weighted for sample size) in supplemented patients was 2.58% and in unsupplemented patients 0.71% (mean difference 1.87%; $P < 0.001$; independent t test).

Meta-analysis of % weight change from supplemented and unsupplemented groups of patients in 13 sets of randomized, controlled data (*n* 509, with complete data for mean and SD of % weight change) suggested a small, non-significant cumulative effect size of 0.51 (95% CI 0.30–0.71), with considerable heterogeneity between studies.

Improvements in body weight with ONS were observed in 78% (*n* 38) of the NRT that made such assessments and significant improvements over time were noted in 41%. The average longitudinal increase in body weight in NRT (data from 24 trials) was 1.2 kg.

Greater reported or prescribed intakes of ONS did not necessarily relate to greater weight gain. There appeared to be no level of reported ONS intake above which significant weight gain was always observed across the trials reviewed. For example, no significant changes in weight were found in studies in which ONS intake was either 497 kcal (Lewis *et al.*, 1987) or 1045 kcal (Stauffer *et al.*, 1986). In other studies, significant weight changes were reported when ONS intakes ranged from 329 kcal (Gray-Donald *et al.*, 1995) to 1080 kcal (Fuenzalida *et al.*, 1990). Assuming that reported ONS intakes are accurate (which may be in doubt if compliance was not checked), it is likely that a combination of factors (e.g. duration of ONS, disease condition, ONS composition and volume) may also be important determinants of the effects of ONS on weight changes.

Weight change according to BMI. This analysis suggests that improvements in body weight are more likely in patient groups with an average BMI < 20 kg m^{-2} (or IBW $< 90\%$ or equivalent). For example, all of the RCT in which patients had a mean BMI < 20 kg m^{-2} showed a greater increase or a smaller decrease in weight in supplemented than in unsupplemented patients (*n* 15 data sets), with significant increases in 87% of trials (13/15 trials; eight observed over time, five compared with a control group) (Fig. 6.15). In contrast, significant improvements in weight were only observed in 36% (4/11) of trials in patients with an average BMI > 20 kg m^{-2}.

Longitudinal % weight change in patients receiving ONS was greater (*P* < 0.054; independent *t* test) in RCT of patients with a mean BMI < 20 kg m^{-2} (+4.6%, *n* 12 trials) than in those > 20 kg m^{-2} (+1.74%, *n* 11 RCT) (see Fig. 6.18; all trials +2.6%). The difference in % weight change between supplemented and unsupplemented patients was also greater (BMI < 20 kg m^{-2} +3.1% versus BMI > 20 kg m^{-2} +1.3%; *P* < 0.09; independent *t* test). Meta-analysis of % weight change data from trials of patients with a mean BMI < 20 kg m^{-2} (three trials, duration 6–13 weeks, ONS 329–1080 kcal, *n* 125) (Otte *et al.*, 1989; Fuenzalida *et al.*, 1990; Gray-Donald, 1995) showed a greater effect size (0.84 (95% CI −0.31 to 1.83)) than trials in patients with a mean BMI > 20 kg m^{-2} (four trials, duration 6–16 weeks, 40–358 kcal, *n* 314; effect size 0.52 (95% CI −0.21 to 0.83)) (Fiatarone *et al.*, 1994; Keele *et al.*, 1997; Rabeneck *et al.*, 1998; Fiatarone Singh *et al.*, 2000), with

no significant heterogeneity between studies. However, very few studies were available for this analysis and the findings in each group were not significant.

Improvements in weight and/or growth (in children) were also more likely in NRT in which patients were at risk of malnutrition (BMI < 20 kg m^{-2}; IBW < 90% or weight-for-height < 90%). In NRT in which the average BMI was < 20 kg m^{-2} (or equivalent), 90% showed improvements in body weight over time and 57% were statistically significant. Increases in body weight/growth were found in fewer trials in which the average BMI was > 20 kg m^{-2} (64%, significant changes in only 27% of trials). Quantitatively, however, the average weight change was similar in NRT in which the average BMI of patients was < 20 kg m^{-2} (+1.75 kg) or > 20 kg m^{-2} (+1.13 kg).

INDIVIDUAL PATIENT GROUPS

The impact of ONS on body weight varies according to the condition of the patients. In all diagnostic categories except liver disease, supplemented patients show more weight gain (or less weight loss) than the unsupplemented, control patients. Figure 6.19 summarizes the effects of ONS on % weight change according to disease/condition (weighted

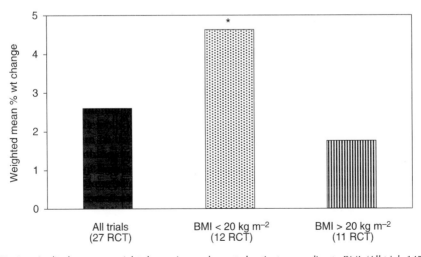

Fig. 6.18. Longitudinal per cent weight change in supplemented patients according to BMI. (All trials 1452 patients; BMI < 20 kg m^{-2} 363 patients; BMI > 20 kg m^{-2} 869 patients.) *Difference according to BMI *P* < 0.054.

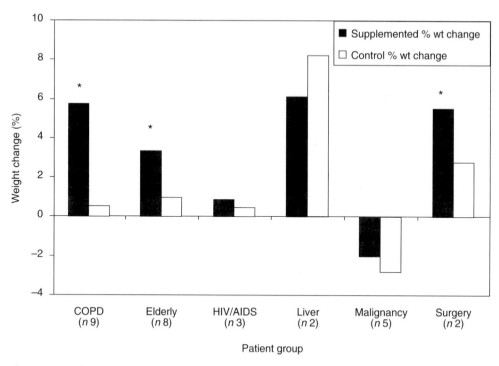

Fig. 6.19. Weighted mean per cent weight change in supplemented compared with control patients according to disease/patient group (results of 29 RCT (1364 patients) in the community setting, see text for details). *Supplemented versus control group; $P < 0.05$.

for the number of subjects in each category). The greatest difference in weight change between the supplemented and unsupplemented patients (5.2% of body weight; $P < 0.002$; independent t test) was in those with COPD, who received ONS for between 1 and 4 months. In this group of patients, BMI (or % IBW) was consistently lower than in the other disease categories. For a summary of changes in body weight according to diagnosis, see Box 6.6. For more details, refer to Appendix 4.

GROWTH

This review suggests that ONS can improve growth in growth-retarded children. The effects of ONS on growth in growth-retarded children (aged 4 months to 19 years) could be assessed in 14 studies. These lasted between 2 months and 5 years and involved patients with cystic fibrosis (11 studies (Allan et al., 1973; Barclay and Shannon, 1975; Berry et al., 1975; Yassa et al., 1978; Parsons et al., 1983; Shepherd et al., 1983; Rettamel et al., 1995; Kalnins et al., 1996; Kashirskaja et al., 1996; Skypala et al., 1998; Steinkamp et al., 2000)), Crohn's disease (two studies (Kirschner et al., 1981; Fell et al., 2000)), and failure to thrive due to multiple causes (one study (Tolia, 1995)). All showed an improvement in growth (seven significant improvements in weight or height centiles, two non-significant changes, five not statistically evaluated). Only two of these studies incorporated a randomized, controlled design and both were in children with cystic fibrosis (Kalnins et al., 1996; Steinkamp et al., 2000). Nine trials had no unsupplemented control group and, in a further three trials that involved a control group, it was non-randomly selected and/or not appropriately matched for disease severity with the supplemented patients.

Box 6.6. Effect of ONS on body weight, composition and growth in different patient groups (community setting).

COPD
Weight gains follow ONS use in COPD patients. On average, gain in weight (weighted mean) was 5% greater in ONS patients than in controls (results from nine RCT). Increases in muscle and fat mass may follow ONS.

Crohn's disease
ONS may increase body weight and muscle mass in adults and can improve growth in growth-retarded children. Well-designed trials are needed.

Cystic fibrosis
Information predominantly from NRT suggests that ONS improve body weight and typically increase growth in growth-retarded children.

Elderly
ONS can improve body weight in elderly patients living at home or in nursing or residential homes, and in those who do or do not have active disease. Per cent weight gain in supplemented patients was 2% greater than in controls (weighted analysis of eight RCT). However, weight gain was greater in trials of underweight (average difference +5%) (BMI < 20 kg m^{-2}) than in 'normal' weight (BMI > 20 kg m^{-2}; +1.8%) patients. ONS may increase muscle mass (Cederholm and Hellström, 1995).

HIV/AIDS
From the studies reviewed, ONS appear to have little effect on body weight in HIV/AIDS patients within the ideal weight range (BMI 20–25 kg m^{-2}).

Liver disease
Body weight is an unreliable indicator of nutritional status in patients with ascites (present in the trials reviewed). Other measures (upper-arm anthropometry) suggest that there may be improvements in muscle mass (Simko, 1983; Hirsch *et al.*, 1993), although these techniques may also be confounded by fluid shifts.

Malignancy
From the trials reviewed, it appears that the impact of ONS on body weight is variable and that there may be little difference between supplemented and control groups. Few changes in body composition have been documented either. Findings are confounded by the heterogeneity of the patients and the likelihood of oedema.

Renal disease
Due to a lack of RCT, there is insufficient information to assess whether ONS increase body weight or improve body composition in those with renal disease.

Surgery (gastrointestinal)
ONS used postoperatively in GI surgical patients before and after discharge from hospital can improve body weight and muscle mass.

BODY COMPOSITION

The use of ONS in community patients (with a variety of conditions: cancer, Crohn's disease, cystic fibrosis, COPD, HIV/AIDS, the elderly) may lead to increases in muscle and fat mass.

Only 44 (41% of total) studies (cancer six, Crohn's disease three, cystic fibrosis four, elderly six, COPD ten, HIV/AIDS ten, liver two, other three) assessed the effects of ONS on body composition. Twenty-five studies (56%) suggested increases in muscle and/or fat tissue (evaluated as statistically significant in 20). The majority of trials that reported positive changes in body composition with ONS occurred in patient groups who were at risk of malnutrition (BMI < 20 kg m^{-2} or equivalent). Significant improvements in indices of body composition (fat and/or fat-free mass) occurred in 12 trials in which mean BMI was < 20 kg m^{-2} (COPD (Stauffer *et al.*, 1986; Wilson *et al.*, 1986; Norregaard *et al.*, 1987; Efthimiou *et al.*, 1988; Fuenzalida *et al.*, 1990), Crohn's disease (Harries *et al.*, 1983, 1984), cystic fibrosis (Shepherd *et al.*, 1983; Skypala *et al.*, 1998), HIV (Fogaca *et al.*, 2000), elderly (Cederholm and Hellström, 1992; Woo *et al.*, 1994)) and in only two trials in which BMI was > 20 kg m^{-2} (significant increases in fat (Broqvist *et al.*, 1994; Jensen and Hessov, 1997) and muscle mass (Jensen and Hessov, 1997)). The majority of trials used measurements of upper-arm anthropometry as indicators of changes in fat mass and lean body mass. Overall, there is insufficient information to come to firm conclusions about the effect of ONS on the body composition of community-based patients suffering with a range of different conditions. Further research is needed.

(III) What effect do ONS have on the body function and clinical outcome of patients in the community?

BODY FUNCTION – ALL PATIENT GROUPS COMBINED
The present analysis indicates that ONS can improve a variety of body functions in community patients. These include respiratory muscle function, hand-grip strength and walking distances in COPD patients (Rogers *et al.*, 1992), and immunological

benefits (Chandra and Puri, 1985), a reduction in falls (Gray-Donald *et al.*, 1995) and increased activities of daily living (Volkert *et al.*, 1992; Woo *et al.*, 1994) in the elderly (see Tables 6.16 and 6.17). Functional improvements were also noted in growth-retarded children with cystic fibrosis, Crohn's disease and other conditions. These included significant improvements in growth (z scores for weight, height, bone), clinical scores (general activity, pulmonary, nutrition) and a variety of anecdotal improvements in psychological and behavioural functions (see sections on Crohn's disease and cystic fibrosis).

Functional outcome measures have been summarized according to disease category (see Tables 6.16 and 6.17). The clinical importance of some of the laboratory measurements and biochemical changes is uncertain. No significant functional detriments were associated with the use of ONS.

Nearly two-thirds (63%) of RCT (n 22) that assessed tissue/body function (total 35) showed improvements, 45% (n 10) of which were significant over time and 27% (n 6) statistically significant compared with a control group (see Table 6.15). Most (74%) NRT showed improvements in function (23/31 that made assessments), 65% of which were significant changes over time (Fig. 6.15).

Table 6.16. Summary of significant functional and clinical outcome improvements following ONS in community patients (significant changes relative to a control group from randomized controlled trials only).

Patient group	Functional/clinical outcome
COPD	Improved respiratory muscle function (Rogers *et al.*, 1992) Improved hand-grip strength (Rogers *et al.*, 1992) Walking distances (Rogers *et al.*, 1992)
Elderly	Immunological benefits (Chandra and Puri, 1985) Reduced number of falls (Gray-Donald *et al.*, 1995) Increased activities of daily living (Volkert *et al.*, 1992; Woo *et al.*, 1994)
HIV/AIDS	Improved cognitive function (Rabeneck *et al.*, 1998)
Liver disease	Lower incidence of severe infections (Hirsch *et al.*, 1993) Lower frequency of hospitalization (Hirsch *et al.*, 1993)
Malignancy	Immunological benefits (Bounous *et al.*, 1975)

Table 6.17. Summary of the effects of oral nutritional supplements on body function and clinical outcome in community patients.

Disease	Change in function/outcome – mean BMI < 20 kg m⁻²	Change in function/outcome – mean BMI > 20 kg m⁻²	Change in function/outcome – mean BMI unknown
COPD	**Donahoe *et al.*, 1989**: Improved respiratory muscle strength, hand-grip strength, 12 min walking distance (all sig. vs. baseline) **Efthimiou *et al.*, 1988**: Less breathlessness, lower oxygen cost of breathing, improved well-being (?). Sig. increased 6 min walking distance, respiratory muscle strength and hand-grip strength (all sig. vs. baseline). No change in FEV, FVC or blood gases **Fuenzalida *et al.*, 1990**: Respiratory muscle function during exercise, duration of exercise and immunological status improved (sig. vs. baseline) **Knowles *et al.*, 1988**: Respiratory muscle strength increased only in those with an increase in total energy intake > 30% (sig. vs. baseline). No change in respiratory muscle function **Lewis *et al.*, 1987**: NS change in respiratory muscle function **Norregaard *et al.*, 1987**: Improved respiratory function (? sig. vs. baseline) **Otte *et al.*, 1989**: No difference in pulmonary function, immunological function, well-being or walking distance **Pardy *et al.*, 1986**: No change in respiratory muscle function (vs. baseline) **Rogers *et al.*, 1992**: Improved respiratory muscle function (expiratory), hand-grip strength, 12 min walking distance (all sig. vs. control). No change in quality of life or dyspnoea **Sridhar *et al.*, 1994**: No change in FEV, respiratory muscle strength or *VO₂* max. (vs. baseline)		**Ganzoni *et al.*, 1994**: No change in walking distances or ventilatory parameters

Continued

Table 6.17. *Continued.*

Disease	Change in function/outcome – mean BMI < 20 kg m^{-2}	Change in function/outcome – mean BMI > 20 kg m^{-2}	Change in function /outcome – mean BMI unknown
	Wilson *et al.*, 1986: Increased hand-grip strength, respiratory function (sig.) and sense of well-being (?sig. vs. baseline). No change in FEV, FVC, lung volume		
Crohn's disease	**Harries *et al.*, 1983**: Decrease in CDAI (NS) and improved well-being (NS vs. baseline) **Harries *et al.*, 1984**: Reduction in serum orosomucoids (sig. vs. baseline) indicative of decreased disease activity **Logan *et al.*, 1981**: Decrease in gastro-intestinal protein loss (sig. vs. baseline), increased energy and sense of well-being (?sig.)		**Geerling *et al.*, 1998b,c/2000b** (abstracts): Reduction in CDAI score and improved muscle strength with enriched feed (sig. vs. baseline). No change in quality of life **O'Morain *et al.*, 1984**: Reduction in clinical scores at 1 week and 3 months (sig. vs. baseline) **Raouf *et al.*, 1991**: 9/11 patients (whole-protein feed) (?sig.) and 9/13 patients (amino acid feed) (?sig.) reach remission
Malignancy		**McCarter *et al.*, 1998**: No effect on immunological function (vs. baseline)	**Arnold and Richter, 1989**: No difference in tumour response rate, survival rate, side-effects and treatment interruptions (vs. control) **Bounous *et al.*, 1975**: Less radiation-induced diarrhoea (?sig.). Less reduction of total lymphocyte count (sig. vs. control) **Crossland and Higgins, 1977**: Increased sense of well-being (?sig. vs. baseline) **Douglass *et al.*, 1978**: Improved DCH (NS vs. baseline) **Elkort *et al.*, 1981**: No difference in response to treatment (recurrence rate) or treatment toxicity (vs. control). Association between gain or loss of weight with an increased risk of recurrences in one group **Evans *et al.*, 1987**: No difference in tumour response rate, survival times or treatment toxicity (vs. control)

Group		
Elderly	Breslow *et al.*, 1993: Decrease in truncal pressure-ulcer surface area and stage IV ulcers (sig. vs. baseline). Cederholm and Hellström, 1995: Increased hand-grip strength (sig. vs. baseline). No change in peak expiratory flow or DCH Gray-Donald *et al.*, 1994: General well-being and total lymphocyte count (sig. vs. baseline). Increased hand-grip strength (NS vs. baseline) Gray-Donald *et al.*, 1995: Lower number of falls (0%) in S than US patients (21%) (sig.). No change in hand-grip strength, well-being or self-perceived health Lipschitz *et al.*, 1985: No change in immunological parameters Persson *et al.*, 2000b: Improved ADL (sig. vs. baseline). Volkert *et al.*, 1996: More independent patients (ADL) in good 'compliers' (sig. vs. control) Woo *et al.*, 1994: Greater ADL score 2 months after ONS stopped (sig. vs. control), mental test score improved after 1 month and life satisfaction after 2 months (NS vs. control)	Fiatarone *et al.*, 1994: No effect on mobility or muscle strength. Fiatarone Singh *et al.*, 2000: Improved ADL (sig. vs. baseline). No changes in habitual physical activity, depression, cognitive function, muscle strength or number of medications Krondl *et al.*, 1999: No changes in quality of life (SF-36) or general well-being questionnaire (NS vs. baseline) but sig. increases in some components (sig. vs. baseline) Lauque *et al.*, 2000: No changes in hand-grip strength (NS vs. control) Meredith *et al.*, 1992: No effect on dynamic muscle strength	Flynn and Leightty, 1987: Fewer complications, shorter length of stay by 3 days (?, vs. control). No difference in rate of sig. complications Nayel *et al.*, 1992: Less treatment delay, with a lower incidence of severe mucosal reactions (NS vs. control). Bunker *et al.*, 1994: No change in immunological parameters Chandra and Puri, 1985: Higher rate of seroconversion and a higher mean antibody titre (sig. vs. control) following influenza-virus vaccination
HIV/AIDS	Fogaca *et al.*, 2000: No changes in immunological parameters, intestinal morphometry stable	Berneis *et al.*, 2000: No changes in lymphocyte CD4 count or cytokine receptor concentrations or quality of life	Chan *et al.*, 1994: Reduced stool weight and stool fat (sig. vs. baseline) Chlebowski *et al.*, 1992: Subjective:

Continued

Table 6.17. *Continued.*

Disease	Change in function/outcome – mean BMI < 20 kg m^{-2}	Change in function/outcome – mean BMI > 20 kg m^{-2}	Change in function/outcome – mean BMI unknown
		Chlebowski *et al.*, 1993: Lower hospitalization rate in those taking an enriched ONS relative to a standard ONS (sig.) **Pichard *et al.*, 1998**: Improvement in anorexia and GI symptoms (?sig. vs. baseline) **Rabeneck *et al.*, 1998**: Cognitive function: short-term recall and long-term storage improved (sig. vs. baseline). No change in quality of life. Increase in hand-grip strength (NS vs. control) **Süttman *et al.*, 1996**: Increased serum concentration of soluble tumour necrosis factor receptor proteins in those taking an enriched ONS (sig. vs. baseline)	increased well-being and energy levels in ~30% (?sig. vs. baseline) **Hellerstein *et al.*, 1994**: Higher % lymphocyte count, reduced stool frequency, fewer hospitalizations (all sig. vs. baseline in those taking enriched ONS) **Hoh *et al.*, 1998**: No change in quality of life or lymphocyte counts (NS vs. baseline) **Richards *et al.*, 1996**: 7.4 times greater risk of > 50% drop in CD4 count in those taking an enriched ONS compared with a standard ONS (sig.) **Singer *et al.*, 1992**: Improved IgA (sig.) and β_2 microglobulin (NS) in those taking an enriched ONS compared with the standard ONS **Simko, 1983**: No deterioration in grade of encephalopathy **Hirsch *et al.*, 1993**: Lower incidence of severe infections resulting in a lower frequency of hospitalization (sig. vs. control). No difference in mortality or number of hospital days **Wilson *et al.*, 2001**: Shorter stays in hospital (NS vs. control)
Liver			
Renal		**Keele *et al.*, 1997**: No change in fatigue, well-being or hand-grip strength **Broqvist *et al.*, 1994**: No change in maximal work capacity or respiratory gases, or muscle concentrations of ATP, creatine or glycogen	
Other			

sig., significant; ?sig., unclear whether statistically significant. FEV, forced expiratory volume; VO_2 max., maximum oxygen consumption; S, supplemented; US, unsupplemented; DCH, delayed cutaneous hypersensitivity; ADL, activities of daily living; NS, not significant; IgA, immunoglobulin A; FVC, forced ventilatory capacity; CDAI, Crohn's disease activity index.

Functional changes related to BMI and per cent weight change. In general, significant improvements in body function were more likely to occur in patient groups with a BMI < 20 kg m^{-2} than a BMI > 20 kg m^{-2}. Functional benefits were observed in 81% (13/16) of RCT in which the mean BMI was < 20 kg m^{-2} and in only 22% (2/9 trials) of those with a mean BMI > 20 kg m^{-2} ($P < 0.009$; Fishers exact test). The findings were similar in NRT, with significant improvements in function more likely in trials in which patients had an average BMI < 20 kg m^{-2} (improvements in 75% of trials (12/16 trials), of which 75% were significant (n 9)).

Improvements in function across patient groups did not appear to be related to longitudinal weight change, which was similar for RCT that showed significant benefit (weighted mean +3.73%, n 11) compared with those that did not (weighted mean

+3.25%, n 12 studies, 14 data sets). However, in underweight patients with COPD and in elderly patients, significant functional benefits were only demonstrated in trials in which 2 kg or more of weight gain was achieved (see Fig. 6.20).

BODY FUNCTION – INDIVIDUAL PATIENT GROUPS
ONS can improve different functions across patient groups. Tables 6.14 and 6.15 indicate the specific functional changes according to patient group. For more information, refer to Appendix 4.

CLINICAL OUTCOME
This analysis suggests that ONS can improve the clinical outcome of some groups of community patients (see Table 6.15). Although very few studies (17 in total) assessed the effects of ONS on clinical outcome, benefits included reduced hospitalizations (Hirsch *et al.*, 1993),

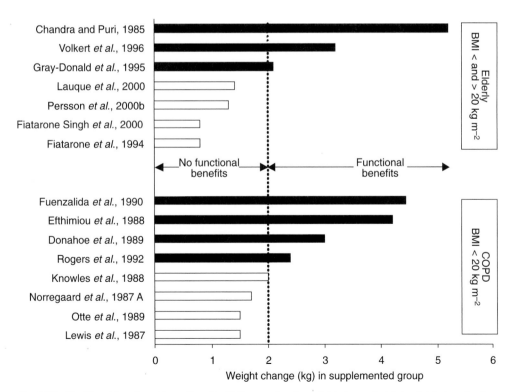

Fig. 6.20. Significant functional benefits with ONS according to weight change in trials of elderly patients and underweight COPD patients (black bars represent significant functional benefit; weight gain of 2 kg or more associated with significant functional benefit). A, abstract.

shorter lengths of hospital stay (Wilson *et al.*, 2001) and fewer infections/complications (Flynn and Leightty, 1987; Hirsch *et al.*, 1993) (see Table 6.16). Some studies, particularly those in cancer patients, did not find improvements in responses to treatment or survival (Douglass *et al.*, 1978; Elkort *et al.*, 1981), although these studies were typically too small to assess such outcomes. Detriments may also occur when certain types of ONS are used inappropriately in weight-stable overweight patients with certain diseases (e.g. cancer patients (Evans *et al.*, 1987)).

Mortality. Meta-analysis of only three RCT in patients with liver cirrhosis or malignant disease suggested an odds ratio of 0.78 (95% CI 0.10–6.32) with supplementation compared with routine care (Douglass *et al.*, 1978; Arnold and Richter, 1989; Hirsch *et al.*, 1993). However, there was significant heterogeneity within the analysis and only small numbers of patients and trials were included. Therefore, this is unlikely to be a reliable estimate of the effect of ONS on mortality and further investigation is required.

Complication rates. Complication rates, including infections, may be reduced by the use of ONS in community patients. Meta-analysis of only three RCT in patients with liver cirrhosis or malignancy suggested an odds ratio of 0.24 (95% CI 0.04–1.65; no significant heterogeneity) with supplementation compared with routine care (Flynn and Leightty, 1987; Nayel *et al.*, 1992; Hirsch *et al.*, 1993). More trials are needed.

There appeared to be no relationship between the reported intake of ONS and the occurrence of significant improvements in functional or clinical outcomes. In addition to the need to ascertain ONS compliance, other factors, such as the duration of ONS and the disease activity of the patient group, also need to be considered. For more information about changes in clinical outcome with ONS in patient-specific groups and in individual trials, refer to Appendix 4.

COST EFFICACY

None of the studies reviewed made any assessments of the cost-effectiveness of using ONS in the community setting. Therefore prospective evaluation of the financial consequences of using ONS in the community is required.

(V) What are the effects of stopping ONS in patients in the community?

Although some of the benefits of ONS may be lost once patients stop consuming them, some improvements in body weight and function are retained.

The effects of stopping ONS were assessed in only nine trials, between 8 days and > 6 months after their withdrawal, in patients with COPD, Crohn's disease, cystic fibrosis, cancer, renal disease and other conditions. The increment in energy intake accompanying ONS was often not sustained once ONS were stopped, with energy intake typically returning close to baseline values (Table 6.18). Weight gain persisted following cessation of ONS in five trials (Bounous *et al.*, 1975; Yassa *et al.*, 1978; O'Morain *et al.*, 1984; Woo *et al.*, 1994; Patel *et al.*, 2000), although this was not a consistent finding (Efthimiou *et al.*, 1988; Knowles *et al.*, 1988). When functional benefits were reported, there was a general loss of that function after ONS were stopped, although in many studies a degree of functional benefit was maintained above baseline values during follow-ups of varying periods (see Table 6.18).

Combined Analysis of ONS Studies in Hospital and Community Patients

In following our multilayer approach to assessing the evidence (see Chapter 5), combined analysis was undertaken of RCT of ONS in hospital and community patients for a number of outcome measures: % weight change, mortality rates, complication rates and length of hospital stay.

Table 6.18. Summary of the effects of stopping oral nutritional supplements in community patients.

Authors, trial design and condition	Effect of supplement	Effect of stopping supplement	When assessed
Efthimiou *et al.*, 1988 Randomized COPD	Weight gain (sig.) Increase in TEI (sig.) Functional benefits (sig.)	30% of gained weight lost TEI returns to baseline Deterioration in some functions to baseline, others remain significantly above baseline	3 months
Knowles *et al.*, 1988 Randomized COPD	Weight gain (sig.) Increase in TEI (sig.) Functional benefits in some patients (sig.)	Weight returns close to baseline TEI returns to baseline Functional benefits not assessed	1 month
O'Morain *et al.*, 1984 Randomized Crohn's disease	Weight gain (sig.) TEI not assessed Reduction in Crohn's disease activity (sig.) (longitudinal)	Weight gain persisted TEI not assessed Reduction in Crohn's disease activity persists (effect of spontaneous remission not assessed)	2 months
Yassa *et al.*, 1978 Non-randomized cystic fibrosis	Improved height and weight *z* scores and bone age (all sig.) TEI not assessed	Slower increase in height and weight (sig.), bone age continues to improve TEI not assessed	6 months and 1 year
Woo *et al.*, 1994 Randomized Elderly	Weight gain (sig.) Increase in TEI (sig.) Function not assessed	Similar weight gain in S and US Greater gain in muscle (NS) and fat (sig.) in S vs. US TEI not assessed Functional benefits	2 months
Arnold and Richter, 1989 Randomized Malignancy	Similar weight loss in S and US (?sig.) Increase in TEI (NS) Function not assessed	Similar weight loss in S and US TEI not assessed No functional benefits	3 months
Bounous *et al.*, 1975 Non-randomized Malignancy	Weight gain (NS) Increase in TEI (NS) Functional benefits (?sig.)	Weight gain persisted TEI not assessed Functional benefits persisted	8 days
Patel *et al.*, 2000 Non-randomized Renal disease	Increase in TEI (sig.) Weight gain (?sig.) Function not assessed (increase in PCR)	Food intake unchanged (TEI reduced) Weight gain (sig.) No functional assessments (PCR returned to baseline)	6 months
Tolia, 1995 Non-randomized Other	Weight gain/growth (?sig.) Increase in TEI (sig.)	Weight loss (?sig.) TEI not assessed	Not clear

NS, not significant; PCR, protein catabolic rate; sig., significant; S, supplemented; ?sig., unclear if statistically significant; TEI, total energy intake; US, unsupplemented.

Per cent weight change

- Mean change in weight was +2.4% in supplemented relative to unsupplemented patients (ONS +0.64%, unsupplemented −1.78%; $P < 0.001$; results of 46 RCT (57 data sets, data weighted for sample size)), from across patient groups (general, neurology, elderly, surgery, malignancy,

COPD, liver disease, HIV/AIDS) (see Fig. 6.21).

- When weighted analysis was performed according to BMI, gain in weight with ONS was evident for trials of patients with a mean BMI < 20 kg m^{-2} (+2.6% longitudinal change; +3.33% compared with control group; 17 RCT in COPD, elderly, cystic fibrosis and surgical patients). In studies where mean BMI was > 20 kg m^{-2}, there was an attenua-

tion of % weight loss (−0.46% longitudinal change; +2.11% compared with unsupplemented group; 22 RCT in COPD, HIV/AIDS, elderly, liver disease, malignancy, surgical patients) (refer to Fig. 6.22). Longitudinal % weight change in supplemented patients in trials with a mean BMI < 20 kg m^{-2} was significantly greater than in those with a BMI > 20 kg m^{-2} ($P < 0.004$; independent t test). The difference in % weight

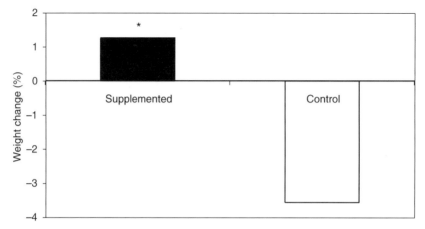

Fig. 6.21. Per cent weight change in supplemented versus control patients from hospital and community trials (weighted mean, data from 57 sets of randomized data, 3098 patients; *$P < 0.001$).

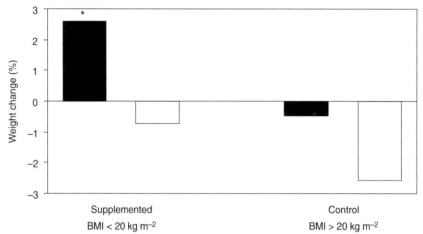

Fig. 6.22. Per cent weight change in supplemented versus control patients from hospital and community trials (weighted mean, according to BMI). BMI < 20 kg m^{-2} 18 sets of RCT (732 patients); BMI > 20 kg m^{-2} 28 sets of RCT (1806 patients). *Longitudinal weight change in supplemented patients and difference in per cent weight change between supplemented and control patients significantly greater for BMI < 20 kg m^{-2} than > 20 kg m^{-2} ($P < 0.01$).

change between supplemented and control patients was also significantly greater in trials in which mean BMI was < 20 kg m^{-2} than in those with BMI > 20 kg m^{-2} ($P < 0.01$, independent t test).

- Meta-analysis of % weight change from 22 RCT (27 data sets) suggested a mean effect size of 0.61 (95% CI 0.50–0.71), with significant heterogeneity between the studies, which were undertaken in diverse patient groups and in both hospital and community settings. Even if studies in which unusual weight changes could have occurred were excluded (studies in liver disease), the mean effect size was 0.59 (95% CI 0.48–0.70).

- Meta-analysis of RCT according to BMI indicated a greater mean effect size in studies with a mean BMI < 20 kg m^{-2} (1.28 (95% CI 1.02–1.54), eight data sets) than with a mean BMI > 20 kg m^{-2} (0.47 (95% CI 0.32–0.61), 14 data sets). There was significant heterogeneity between studies in the analysis.

Mortality

- Mortality was found to be lower in supplemented (19%) than in unsupplemented (25%) patients (see Fig. 6.23). Meta-analysis of the results of 17 data sets (from 14 trials, three community and 11 hospital, n 2096) suggested an odds ratio for mortality of 0.62 (95% CI 0.49–0.78) with ONS. There was no significant heterogeneity between studies undertaken in various patient groups (e.g. elderly, liver disease, neurology, orthopaedics and malignancy) and Rosenthal's fail-safe score was 83 (scores > 87 adequate).

- If results from only one of the trials considered a potential duplication of data was included in this analysis ((Larsson *et al.*, 1990) included and (Unosson *et al.*, 1992) excluded), the odds ratio was similar (0.63 (95% CI 0.48–0.81)).

- Due to a lack of BMI results in community studies that reported mortality, it was not possible to undertake a combined analysis of hospital and community trials.

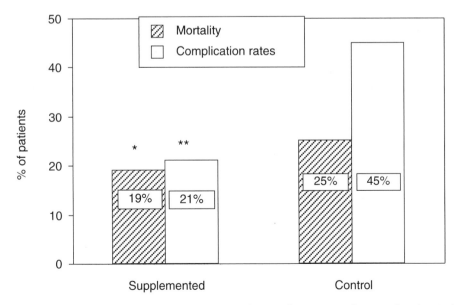

Fig. 6.23. Lower mortality and complication rates in supplemented versus control patients from hospital and community studies. *Mortality 14 RCT, n 2096; odds ratio 0.62 (95% CI 0.49–0.78). **Complication rates 10 RCT, n 494; odds ratio 0.29 (95% CI 0.18–0.47).

- The reduction in mortality rates appeared to be similar for trials in which ONS were given for ≤ 1 month (odds ratio 0.57 (95% CI 0.35–0.92); eight RCT) or > 1 month (odds ratio 0.64 (95% CI 0.47–0.87); nine RCT; no significant heterogeneity). When analysed according to intake, mortality was significantly reduced in trials in which ONS intake was < 600 kcal (odds ratio 0.58 (95% CI 0.43–0.78); 11 RCT). The reduction in mortality did not reach significance in the few trials in which intake was > 600 kcal (odds ratio 0.75 (95% CI 0.42–1.36); five RCT).

Complication rates

- Complication rates in supplemented patients (21%; 52/246) were found to be lower than in unsupplemented patients (45%; 111/248) (see Fig. 6.23). Complications included postoperative complications, infectious complications and post-radiotherapy complications (mucositis – objective mucosal reaction).
- Meta-analysis of ten trials (n 494) indicated an odds ratio for all complication rates of 0.29 (95% CI 0.18–0.47) with supplementation, with no significant heterogeneity between studies and a high Rosenthal's fail-safe score.
- The reduction in complication rates was significant whether ONS were given for ≤ 1 month (odds ratio 0.42 (95% CI 0.19–0.95); five RCT) or for more than 1 month (odds ratio 0.19 (95% CI 0.08–0.45); no significant heterogeneity). When analysed according to intake, complication rates were significantly reduced in trials in which ONS intake was < 600 kcal (odds ratio 0.27 (95% CI 0.14–0.53); six RCT) but insufficient trials in which intakes exceeded 600 kcal prevented any further analysis.

Length of hospital stay

- All 11 RCT, primarily from the hospital setting (community n 1) showed a consistent reduction in mean or median LOS with ONS (27 vs. 40 days; 11/11 RCT; two-tailed binomial test $P < 0.001$; reduction of 13 days, ranging from 2 to 36 days). As data were variously reported as mean (sometimes with SD) or medians, meta-analysis has not been undertaken.

Other Methods for Increasing Dietary Intake

It may be possible to improve clinical outcome to a similar extent to ONS simply by increasing nutritional intake by other means. This could be by dietary manipulation involving the provision of more food, by increasing the nutrient density of the diets provided (dietary fortification) or by counselling patients to increase their intake. Box 6.7 provides a summary of the key findings about the efficacy of different dietary strategies, which are considered individually below.

Dietary fortification with energy and protein

Food is incontrovertibly the best vehicle for nutrient consumption . . . Food and the act of eating provide biochemical, physiological and psychological benefits that supplements do not.

(Tripp, 1997)

As the above quote suggests, some workers have preferentially emphasized the value of food.

Dietary fortification or enrichment of foods in the treatment of DRM is undertaken with the aim of increasing the energy and protein density of a food or diet. This is often undertaken by adding ingredients to foods that are rich in energy and/or protein (e.g. cream, milk, skimmed-milk powder, oil, butter, sugar) (Odlund-Olin et al., 1996), which can lead to marked changes in the taste and mouth-feel of food items. These may or may not be desirable changes. Commercial single-macronutrient supplements, in liquid or powder form, can also be used; these are typically easy and convenient to use and

> **Box 6.7.** Key findings from the evidence base for dietary counselling and fortification.
>
> Nutritional intake
> Dietary manipulation using a combination of dietary counselling or fortification of the diet (using energy- and protein-rich foods, food ingredients (e.g. cream, skimmed-milk powder) or supplements) can be effective at improving intakes of energy and, to a lesser extent, protein, particularly in institutionalized patients (e.g. hospitals, nursing homes). Consideration should also be given to improving the micronutrient intakes of those with low dietary intake and at risk of DRM.
>
> Body weight, function and outcome
> Improvements in body structure may occur with dietary manipulation but the impact of these methods on functional- and clinical outcome measures has not been widely studied. Research with RCT is needed across patient groups and health-care settings.
>
> Comparison with ONS
> Dietary manipulation may not be as effective as ONS at improving nutritional (macro- and micronutrient) intake or body structure, at least in some patient groups. Comparative studies of functional and clinical outcome are lacking.

are relatively tasteless additions for fortifying a wide range of foods (Table 6.1). They include energy ONS (carbohydrate and/or fat ONS) and protein ONS. Alternatively, energy- or protein-rich foods/snacks can be added to the diet (Hanning *et al.*, 1993; Nielsen *et al.*, 1995; Turic *et al.*, 1998). The provision of such foods as part of the menus provided in hospitals, nursing and residential homes has been recommended as a low cost initiative to prevent or treat DRM (Odlund-Olin *et al.*, 1996; Allison, 1998). As the findings of research in healthy subjects, lean and obese adults and undernourished children suggest (Booth *et al.*, 1970; Geliebter, 1979; Rolls *et al.*, 1988; Barkeling *et al.*, 1990; de Graaf *et al.*, 1992; Sanchez-Grinan *et al.*, 1992; Blundell *et al.*, 1993; Brown *et al.*, 1995; Stubbs *et al.*, 1995, 1998; Poppit and Prentice, 1996; Bell and Rolls, 2001), changing the energy density or the macronutrient composition of food may influence hunger and satiety and total food intake. Similarly, longitudinal observational trials in patients at risk of DRM in the clinical setting have also suggested that changing the energy or protein density of diets may improve intake (see Box 6.8). These studies have predominantly been undertaken in elderly subjects in institutions (Odlund-Olin *et al.*, 1996; Gall

et al., 1998b; Lorefalt *et al.*, 1998; Barton *et al.*, 2000b). RCT assessing the impact of dietary fortification on clinical outcome, compared with routine clinical care, are lacking. Improving the nutrient density of the diet (in terms of vitamins, minerals and trace elements), as well as increasing the energy and protein content, may also be important for the functional and clinical recovery of the patient with DRM, particularly as deficiency states and/or insufficient intakes of a plethora of vitamins, minerals and trace elements occur (e.g. in the elderly (Finch *et al.*, 1998)). In the community, it is likely that the provision of foods, either as part of meals on wheels (Krassie *et al.*, 2000), as fortified food products (de Jong *et al.*, 1999) or as ONS, may be a more effective strategy than dietary counselling alone, although comparative studies are needed. Other strategies, such as modifying the organoleptic/sensory qualities of foods (Schiffman and Warwick, 1993; Blundell and Stubbs, 1999), altering the timing and frequency of food consumption (Brown *et al.*, 1995) or the provision of a variety of different foods (varying in taste, texture, mouth feel, etc.) (Rolls *et al.*, 1981), may also be effective ways to increase nutritional intake in different patient groups, but further investigation is warranted.

Box 6.8. The effectiveness of dietary fortification in different patient groups.

- In elderly in-patients (Odlund-Olin *et al.*, 1996), increasing the energy content of a hospital diet from 7.0 MJ (1670 kcal) to 10.5 MJ (2520 kcal) daily (using oil, cream, sour cream, butter and milk, no weight or volume given to calculate energy density) significantly increased energy intakes (to 25 kcal kg^{-1} day^{-1}) and body weight after 3 weeks but no changes in function were observed. The costs of this initiative were very low (an increase of 4% compared with the normal cost of hospital food).

- In a crossover trial in elderly hospitalized patients, increasing the energy density of the foods provided (with butter, cream, cheese, glucose polymers, increasing total energy provision by 14% or 200 kcal), whilst reducing portion sizes (by ~20%), increased energy intakes (from 1425 kcal to 1711 kcal) and reduced wastage (Barton *et al.*, 2000b). As in other studies, this type of fortification did not improve protein intakes (Gall *et al.*, 1998b).

- Energy and protein intakes and protein retention were improved in liver cirrhosis patients after the consumption of energy- and protein-enriched foodstuffs for 38 days (Nielsen *et al.*, 1995). Strict dietary restrictions (e.g. low sodium, low potassium, low lactose) that accompany some types of liver and renal disease may limit the efficacy of food fortification in this patient group.

- In elderly long-term-care patients, food snacks facilitated increases in energy intakes of ~30%, whilst also improving the intake of protein and a number of micronutrients. Functional and clinical outcome measures were not reported in this study (Turic *et al.*, 1998).

- In community-based cystic fibrosis patients, the provision of additional food snacks (milk shakes, tinned puddings, breakfast drink) was able to elevate patients' energy intakes (by ~445 kcal daily), but changes in respiratory function, muscle strength and growth did not occur (Hanning *et al.*, 1993).

- An RCT of free-living elderly (BMI ~24 kg m^{-2}) suggested that the provision of nutrient-dense foods (fruit and dairy products fortified with micronutrients, given twice daily) corrected deficiencies of some micronutrients (e.g. vitamins B_2, B_{12} and D) and significantly improved the intakes of a number of vitamins (B_1, B_2, B_6, B_{12}, C, D, E, A) compared with a control group (*n* 34) (de Jong *et al.*, 1999).

Dietary counselling

In routine practice, dietary counselling to improve the nutritional intakes of malnourished patients is often recommended as the first line of nutritional intervention, prior to using ONS or in combination with ONS. The effectiveness of such a strategy will depend on a number of factors (outlined in Box 6.9) and has been little studied in the clinical setting (see Box 6.10 for some examples of trials (Macia *et al.*, 1991; Bories and Campillo; 1994, Schwenk *et al.*, 1994; Chlebowski *et al.*, 1995)). Most of the trials neglect to report information about the person giving the dietary counselling, the advice given, the counselling methods used or patients' compliance and understanding of the advice, and RCT are mostly lacking.

Ultimately, there is a need for RCT to gain greater insights into the effects of providing a diet rich in energy, protein and other nutrients and the impact of dietary counselling on total food/nutrient intake and outcome measures in distinct patient groups in both hospital and community settings.

There is also a need for comparative research of dietary fortification or counselling with the other main form of intervention discussed in this chapter, ONS.

A Comparison of Dietary Manipulation with ONS

There is currently very little evidence with which to assess the relative efficacy of ONS and dietary manipulation. The current

---

Box 6.9. Components affecting the efficacy of dietary counselling.

- The person giving the counselling. Motivational, counselling skills, good nutritional/dietetic knowledge and the ability to convey knowledge in educating the patient are all important (see Thomas, 1994).

- The methods of counselling and the information or advice provided. It is assumed that oral and written dietary instructions to increase energy and protein intakes, given at regular intervals, are most appropriate, although the evidence base for using this approach in the treatment of DRM is lacking. The advice given as part of counselling to help malnourished patients increase energy and nutrient intakes is important (i.e. what to have, when and how to have it) and yet there appear to be few evidence-based guidelines in existence to define the best and most effective practices. This is an area for further research.

- The patient. As with any other form of treatment, the effectiveness of dietary counselling will vary depending on the patient, with factors such as age, education, disease state, culture and psychological status being important.

Box 6.10. The effectiveness of dietary counselling in different patient groups. MAMC, mid-arm muscle circumference; TSF, triceps skin-fold thickness.

- Simple encouragement to improve food intake (diet provided 40 kcal kg^{-1} day^{-1}) for 1 month in hospitalized alcoholic cirrhosis patients significantly increased energy and protein intakes, despite patients reportedly having adequate intakes at the start of the study. Some significant improvements in nutritional status (e.g. MAMC, TSF) were recorded, as were some changes in liver function tests, but the lack of a control group limits the interpretation of these findings (Bories and Campillo, 1994).

- In free-living individuals with HIV, dietary counselling (with ONS if needed) was able to maintain patients' energy intakes at baseline levels. Attempts were also made to address specific nutritional deficiencies. Nevertheless, counselling was unable to prevent body weight progressively decreasing during the 6-month study period (Chlebowski *et al.*, 1995).

- In HIV-infected patients with low spontaneous intake (< 31.5 kcal kg^{-1}), dietary counselling was of limited value due to anorexia (present in 69% of patients), dysphagia, nausea and altered taste sensations (Schwenk *et al.*, 1994).

- In an RCT of cancer patients undergoing radiotherapy, dietary counselling (oral and written instructions about the most appropriate foods to have during treatment, mistakes in eating habits to be avoided and tips on diet preparation for each individual) led to smaller reductions in anthropometric parameters and intake after a 2-year period. Fewer side-effects of treatment (dysphagia, anorexia, diarrhoea) in those given counselling than in the control group were also noted, but no statistical comparisons between the groups were presented (Macia *et al.*, 1991).

---

evidence base suggests that ONS (with or without dietary counselling) may be more effective than dietary counselling alone or the provision of food snacks (Baldwin *et al.*, 2002). Meta-analysis of four trials comparing dietary manipulation (counselling or fortification) with ONS suggests that, after 3 months, those receiving ONS have significantly greater weight gain and energy intakes. Three examples of individual studies from different health-care settings can be found in Box 6.11 (Murphy *et al.*, 1992; Turic *et al.*, 1998; Schwenk *et al.*, 1999b). It is likely that ONS, particularly liquid ones, will have different effects on appetite and total dietary intake from those of fortifying

---

Box 6.11. Comparison of oral nutritional supplements with dietary manipulation in different patient groups.

Institutionalized community patients
- In an RCT in elderly patients in long-term care (BMI ~20 kg m^{-2}), a 6-week trial comparing ONS with food snacks suggested that both forms of intervention could improve energy and protein intakes. However, the ONS group had significantly higher intakes of energy and all nutrients (protein, vitamins and minerals) than the food-snack group (although body weight gain was greater in the food-snack group) (Turic et al., 1998).

Free-living community patients
- In a free-living patient group with HIV infection and weight loss (BMI ~20 kg m^{-2}), those patients randomized to receive an ONS had significantly greater total energy intakes than controls for the first 4 of 8 weeks only and changes in body cell mass and weight gain over the study period were no different between groups (Schwenk et al., 1999b). The authors suggested that the use of ONS may be more practical in some groups of free-living patients. For example, those in the control group of Schwenk's trial found the preparation of energy-dense meals difficult and many favoured the use of ONS. Typically, these patients were men from non-traditional or single households with no carers to help with meal provision (Schwenk et al., 1999b).
- A comparative study (non-randomized) in HIV patients (16 weeks) suggested that both dietary counselling and ONS use significantly increased energy intakes (Murphy et al., 1992). However, the observation that dietary counselling was more effective at improving protein intakes and body weight than ONS may simply have been because the supplemented group had higher baseline protein intakes (94 g vs. 71 g) and body weight (Murphy et al., 1992).

Hospital patients
- No trials – comparative RCT are needed.

---

the diet with energy- and protein-rich snacks, due in part to the differences in consistency/texture and gastric emptying rates (Pliner, 1973; Kissileff, 1985; Hulshof et al., 1993; Guinard and Brun, 1998). In the absence of a consensus from the current evidence, it seems pragmatic to give consideration to the likely efficacy of dietary counselling/fortification in the individual patient, considering their social circumstances, their disease status and their preferences, in addition to the types of ONS available for use (flavours, volumes, consistencies). Overall, short- and long-term evaluations (> 3 months) of the efficacy of dietary manipulation and ONS in both hospital and community settings are needed, including their impact on functional and clinical outcomes. Therefore, despite the widespread practice of recommending dietary counselling as a first-line treatment to improve nutritional intakes in patients who are malnourished or at risk of malnutrition, the evidence base is currently inadequate and research in this area is warranted.

While the efficacy of ONS is considered (as earlier in this chapter), the concomitant use of dietary counselling also has to be addressed. For example, dietary counselling (encouragement to eat and other forms of counselling, often not well defined) was sometimes used alongside ONS (Kendell et al., 1982; Olejko and Fonseca, 1984; Antila et al., 1993; Schols et al., 1995; Le Cornu et al., 2000) and, in other studies, a high-energy and protein diet or food snacks, in combination with ONS, were provided (Cohn et al., 1982; Demling and DeSanti, 1998). In other studies, it is likely that counselling or fortified diets were given alongside supplementation but not reported. Alternatively, assistance with meals to facilitate intake, as reported in one trial of ONS (Bourdel-Marchasson et al., 2000), may have been given. In such cases, it is difficult to disentangle the effects of the different strategies used to improve nutrient intake. These issues highlight a need for carefully controlled trials and explicit reporting of treatments used within individual trials.

There may be other strategies (flavour/odour enhancement (Schiffman, 1983; Schiffman and Warwick, 1993), environmental (Association of Community Health Councils for England and Wales, 1997), behavioural (Stark *et al.*, 1990, 1996)) for increasing the nutritional intake of patients at risk of DRM and some of these have been summarized in Box 6.12. However, the strategies adopted to improve nutritional intake (dietary or other means) may vary, depending on the patient group, including the type and state (acute or chronic) of disease and the age of patients. For example, in elderly nursing-home residents, it has been suggested that non-liquid ways of improving nutritional intake in the elderly may be more successful than liquid feeds. The suggestions included non-liquid supplementation (especially in the incontinent and in light of the reductions in thirst perception in elderly individuals), attention to the aesthetic and hedonic properties of food, such as taste, presentation, aroma and seasoning, or altering the nutrient density and the diversity of the habitual diet itself. In contrast, in younger patients, behavioural strategies or easy-to-use liquid sip feeds may be more effective (Fiatarone Singh *et al.*, 2000). Before conclusions can be made, further research is needed.

Discussion

This systematic review of 166 trials (*n* 7630 subjects) has highlighted the fact that ONS given to some patient groups can produce marked reductions in mortality and complication rates and shorten hospital stays. Unlike previous analyses, the present one not only has provided an overall combined analysis of different groups of patients across hospital and community settings, but has also assessed the effects of ONS in different health-care settings, in different groups of patients and according to nutritional status. In addition, it has attempted to provide insights into the possible mechanisms by which ONS may influence outcome. For example, the extent to which ONS suppress food intake and increase total energy intake (question I) and the changes in weight and lean tissue mass (question II) accompanying supplementation have been considered, as has the importance of chronic protein-energy status.

Box 6.12. Other potential strategies for increasing nutrient intake in patients at risk of malnutrition.

Flavour and odour enhancement
Flavour enhancement of nutrient-dense foods (using roast beef, ham, natural bacon, prime beef, maple and cheese flavours) has been shown to increase food consumption in elderly patients in a residential home over a 3-week period. Significant improvements in immune function (total lymphocyte count, total B- and total T-cell counts) and in grip strength accompanied the increase in food intake (Schiffman and Warwick, 1993). This may be a particularly effective strategy in the elderly in whom changes in taste and odour sensations occur with ageing and with disease (Schiffman, 1983).

Environmental changes
The ways in which food are provided and the environment for dining may be important in maximizing patients' dietary intakes and the dining expectations of residents of long-term-care facilities have been summarized elsewhere (Case *et al.*, 1997). These include providing a pleasant atmosphere for dining (e.g. use of tablecloths), having staff in the dining-room to help with eating and providing meals that are social occasions for all residents. The reports *Hungry in Hospital* (Association of Community Health Councils for England and Wales, 1997) and *Hospital Food as Treatment* (Allison, 1999) have also highlighted many problems with food provision in the hospital environment and have provided recommendations to help maximize patients' nutritional intakes.

Behavioural therapy
Child behaviour-management training may assist parents in helping their child meet their energy (and other nutrient) requirements (Stark *et al.*, 1990, 1996).

The main functional and clinical outcome parameters (questions III and IV) were often dramatically improved, effects unlikely to be reproduced by many other treatments (e.g. pharmacological interventions) in clinical practice:

- The overall reduction in mortality in supplemented compared with unsupplemented patients was 24% (19% versus 25% mortality; $P < 0.001$; Fig. 6.23). Meta-analysis of 17 RCT (three from the community setting; total n 2096) of a variety of patient groups suggested an odds ratio of 0.62 (95% CI 0.49–0.78).
- The greatest reduction in mortality was in patient groups who were underweight (BMI < 20 kg m^{-2}).
- Complications, including postoperative and infective complications and those following radiotherapy, were reduced twofold with ONS compared with routine care (from 45% to 21%, $P < 0.001$; Fig. 6.23), across a number of patient groups, particularly in the hospital setting (Table 6.10). Meta-analysis of ten RCT (n 494) across a number of patient groups (orthopaedics, surgery, cancer, liver disease) in both hospital and community settings indicated an odds ratio with ONS of 0.29 (95% CI 0.18–0.47), irrespective of the BMI of the patient groups.
- Hospital LOS was reduced with ONS in all the reviewed trials providing data (estimated average reduction 13 days; range 2–36 days).
- Financial savings may accompany ONS. Retrospective calculations from hospital studies of ONS (see Table 6.11) suggested savings of between £352 and £8179 per patient on the basis of reduced complications and shorter hospital stays.
- A wide range of functional improvements, often disease-specific, accompanied ONS that were not seen in unsupplemented patients receiving routine clinical care (see Tables 6.10, 6.16 and 6.17). No significant functional detriments with ONS were found.
- In the community, functional benefits were more likely in underweight patients (BMI < 20 kg m^{-2}). There was

no clear relationship between functional improvements with ONS and chronic protein-energy status in hospital patients.

Before examining the possible mechanisms or explanations for these improvements, it is necessary to briefly consider a couple of general issues that place the findings in perspective. First, the overall mortality of the hospitalized patients was high (25% in unsupplemented patients). This is considerably greater than the overall mortality of patients in hospital, which was about 3% in National Health Service trusts in England between 1991 and 1997. Even in those aged 75 years and over, the mortality was only about 9.5% (Department of Health, 1998). The high mortality rate indicated by the meta-analysis presented in this chapter reflects the types of patients who were selected and included in some of the trials. In some cases, trials involved acutely ill elderly patients or severely ill patients with liver disease at high risk of dying (e.g. ~38% mortality rate (Larsson *et al.*, 1990; Mendenhall *et al.*, 1993)). In other trials, mortality was much lower (< 10%). Secondly, Fig. 6.1 can be used to illustrate the types of patients included in trials of ONS and subsequently in the meta-analysis. Patients who are well nourished and have an adequate intake (right side of distribution curve) do not require ONS and are not generally included in clinical trials. In contrast, those who are at high risk of undernutrition and are not eating well, usually as a result of severe acute or chronic disease, are more likely to be included in such trials (left side of distribution curve in Fig. 6.1). It is these patients that are most likely to benefit from ONS.

Although it is difficult to provide a single explanation for the beneficial effects of ONS on functional and clinical outcomes, a number of possible mechanisms exist. Such mechanisms may depend on the type and the severity of the disease and the effectiveness of ONS at increasing total energy and nutrient intake. It is possible that the functional and clinical benefits result from an increase in body weight and fat-free body mass, which is mainly composed of muscle. Since loss of body mass, particularly lean body mass, is associated with functional impairments (see Chapters 1 and 4), gain of body mass and lean tissue would be expected to improve tissue function and clinical outcome, especially in those with a low BMI (chronic protein-energy malnutrition). Insights into these possibilities are obtained by examining the relationship between functional and clinical outcomes, BMI and changes in body mass (and lean body mass) from the trials reviewed.

In community studies in which ONS produced significant functional benefits, the difference in mean % weight change between supplemented and control patients was +3.7%, only slightly greater than in those trials in which ONS produced no functional benefits (+3.25%). However, when the findings were analysed according to the mean BMI of patients, ONS were more likely to produce benefits when the BMI was < 20 kg m^{-2} (81% of trials showing benefit) than when it was > 20 kg m^{-2} (22% of trials; $P < 0.009$). Furthermore, ONS largely added to food intake (Fig. 6.16) and produced a greater weight gain (Fig. 6.18) when the mean BMI of patients was < 20 kg m^{-2}. In contrast, in those trials in which the mean BMI was > 20 kg m^{-2}, there was typically greater suppression of food intake with ONS and less weight gain. Since impaired body function is more likely to exist in individuals with a BMI < 20 kg m^{-2}, improvements in function are also more likely to occur when nutritional intervention is given to such patients. Similarly, when there has been no loss of function, no improvements in function with ONS can be expected. A general implication of these findings in the community setting is that there is a stronger indication for prescribing ONS to those with a BMI < 20 kg m^{-2} than to those with BMI > 20 kg m^{-2}. Of course, this review of trials has major limitations, in that it was based on the mean results of a group of patients. Trials in which the mean BMI of patients was < 20 kg m^{-2} may have included some individuals with a BMI > 20

kg m^{-2}, but it was not possible to undertake subgroup analysis to assess the effectiveness of ONS according to the BMI of individual patients.

In the trials in which ONS produced functional benefits in the hospital setting, % weight change in supplemented patients (−0.9%) was greater than in control patients (−4.8%) by 3.9%. In trials that did not demonstrate significant functional benefits, the mean difference was only 1.3% of body weight, possibly because the duration of ONS was threefold shorter. (The patient groups in trials showing functional benefits (COPD, elderly and surgical patients) were similar to those in trials not showing benefits.) Another difference between hospital and community studies is that ONS in the hospital setting were equally likely to produce functional benefits when the mean BMI of patients was < 20 kg m^{-2} (six trials) or > 20 kg m^{-2} (six trials), whereas in the community the benefits were predominantly in those who were underweight (BMI < 20 kg m^{-2}). However, in the hospital setting, the major reduction in mortality produced by administering ONS was largely due to benefits in those with a BMI < 20 kg m^{-2} (17% vs. 26%) rather than those with a BMI > 20 kg m^{-2} (19% vs. 20%).

One interpretation of these observations is that ONS provided during critical periods of an illness can influence body function and improve clinical outcome independently of chronic protein-energy status (assessed using BMI). ONS may lead to beneficial effects on outcome by improving the function of tissues and cells involved in the inflammatory and immune responses (see Chapter 1). This may be due to the supply by ONS of one or more macronutrients or micronutrients (e.g. one or a mix of nutrients) at a critical time and in sufficient amounts. Perhaps deficiency of one or more essential nutrients is corrected. As the deficiency of a number of micronutrients can lead to loss of appetite or fatigue, corrections of such deficiencies with ONS may further improve appetite and food intake (see Chapter 1). (It is difficult to assess the role of other nutrients (e.g. micronutrients) in the current review, partly because micronutrient status was virtually never assessed and partly as studies including supplements containing only micronutrients were not included in this review.) This theory is consistent with a number of individual trials that showed benefits (both to function and clinical outcome), despite small changes in body weight or fat-free mass with ONS (Rana *et al.*, 1992; Keele *et al.*, 1997; Saudny-Unterberger *et al.*, 1997; Potter *et al.*, 2001, group (ii)). One must also consider the limitations of using body weight as an indicator of chronic protein-energy status in some patient groups, particularly in the acutely ill. Indeed, in many investigations, changes in fluid balance and the presence of oedema may have confounded measurement of weight (but were often not recorded). The extent that body weight is improved may vary, depending on the prescribed ONS intake, the duration of supplementation or patients' tolerance of the ONS and their actual intake. Alternatively, it could be that different ONS affect hunger and satiety to different degrees, depending on the composition, the consistency or the time of administration, all of which may determine the extent to which total energy intake and body mass are increased. Indeed, increases in nutritional intake with supplementation are important, whatever the way in which ONS improve function and outcome. The findings of this review suggest that ONS add to rather than replace food intake when used in addition to diet. Both the hospital and the community reviews have consistently indicated significant improvements in total energy intakes among many patient groups given ONS. Protein, vitamin, mineral and trace element intakes may also improve. One of the potential reasons for the marked improvements in patients' total intakes is that ONS appear not to suppress appetite and voluntary food intake substantially in most patient groups. Typically, they provide largely additional energy and nutrients to those obtained in the diet. The reasons for this still require exploration, but the consistency (usually liquid), the composition of

the feeds or the time they are given may be factors. The findings of this review suggest that, in trials of patients with chronic disease in the community, the majority of ONS energy (on average ~70%) is additive to food intake, with the greatest amount additive (and least suppression of appetite and food intake) in underweight patients (BMI < 20 kg m^{-2}). In many other cases, in hospital and community trials, food intake is greater in those randomized to supplementation than in a control group. Whether these are significant increases is difficult to establish, due to the lack of individual data. Such an increase may occur because the additional energy or nutrients, supplied at a critical stage in disease or recovery, improve appetite through greater physical or psychological well-being. Could similar effects be achieved simply by the provision of extra food or by counselling patients to increase the energy and protein contents of their diet at such times? As discussed earlier in this chapter, there are very few data on the impact of increasing the availability of food or of dietary manipulation on clinical or functional outcomes. Furthermore, there have been very few comparative studies addressing the efficacy of one form of oral nutritional intervention compared with another (e.g. ONS versus counselling).

A further explanation for the positive effects of ONS observed in this review may relate to publication bias or poorly designed studies. It is well established that studies that show no effect of an intervention on an outcome measure are less likely to be published (publication bias) (Dickersin *et al.*, 1994). Therefore, as part of this analysis, an indication of the potential effect of a publication bias, assessed by funnel plots and Rosenthal's fail-safe scores, has been given. For analyses of mortality and complication rates with ONS compared with routine clinical care, adequate fail-safe scores suggested that the publication of a relatively large number of additional trials showing a negative effect would be needed to lose the significant results obtained. Although these statistics suggest that publication bias is unlikely, it does not entirely exclude it. In addition, both positive and negative results observed in individual trials may relate to the quality of the study design and execution. Although this chapter has presented the findings of systematic reviews and meta-analyses (often regarded as the highest level of evidence), the results are only as good as the individual studies that have been included. Wherever possible, the main findings of the four review questions (I–IV) have been based on RCT (47% of total trials reviewed). However, in some patient groups (e.g. children with cystic fibrosis or other diseases causing severe growth failure) NRT can still provide valuable and sometimes the only information available. This is often the case in patient groups for whom it is considered unacceptable ethically to recruit to a control group within an RCT in which no nutritional intervention is given.

Other methodological considerations could have some impact on the outcome of individual trials and the findings of this review as a whole. For RCT, the use of blinding and placebos, the ways used to randomize patients and the extent of follow-up of patients reported in trials are important. To assess these aspects of study design and the likelihood of bias, Jadad scoring (Jadad *et al.*, 1996) was used and, as Fig. 6.24 illustrates, > 50% of trials had low methodological scores (less than a total score of 2, range from 0 (weakest design) to 5 (strongest design)). In most trials, this was due to the failure to blind both patients and investigators (double blind) to the intervention by using an appropriate placebo feed. Indeed, very few trials, mostly in elderly patients, reported the use of a placebo ONS and whether these were effective is unclear (Otte *et al.*, 1989; Whittaker *et al.*, 1990; Tkatch *et al.*, 1992; Fiatarone *et al.*, 1994; Carver and Dobson, 1995; Fiatarone

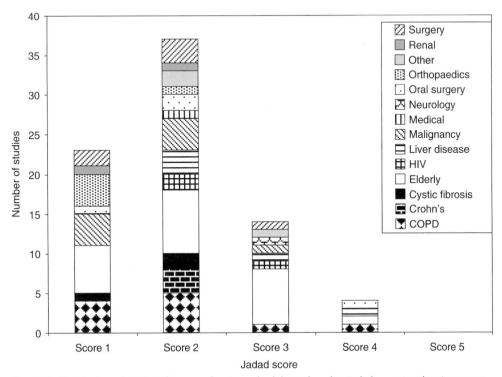

Fig. 6.24. Distribution of ONS studies according to methodological quality (Jadad scores) and patient group.

Singh *et al.*, 2000). Practically, there may be difficulties in providing non-nutritional placebos that have a similar appearance and consistency to feeds (as opposed to watered-down feeds), which is necessary for complete blinding (see Chapter 10). The extent to which the main findings of the analysis have been confounded by the failure to provide placebos in the trials reviewed probably depends on the outcomes being assessed. It is likely that knowledge about which patients are part of the intervention arm of an RCT will influence some outcomes (e.g. functional assessments, particularly those with a subjective element), but other 'harder' outcomes (e.g. mortality) may be more difficult to influence (Schultz and Grimes, 2002b). Nevertheless, the use of effective placebos in future RCT should be considered in order that any potential bias will be reduced.

Another methodological consideration that may have some implications for the findings of the review relate to the power of individual trials to detect significant changes in outcome measures (see Chapter 10 for more details). Although 12 trials included > 100 subjects (see Fig. 6.25), 57% included ≤ 30. Therefore, it is likely that sample size in many cases was insufficient to detect significant changes in functional or clinical outcomes (type II error). Of the trials reviewed, very few reported the use of power statistics to determine the necessary sample size prior to undertaking the study (e.g. Evans *et al.*, 1987; Chlebowski *et al.*, 1993; Keele *et al.*, 1997; Saudny-Unterberger *et al.*, 1997; Gariballa *et al.*, 1998a; MacFie *et al.*, 2000; see Chapter 10), despite mortality rates and complication rates being the main endpoints of many of the trials included in this analysis. Therefore, we have provided a guide (see Table 6.19, Figs 6.26 and 6.27) to

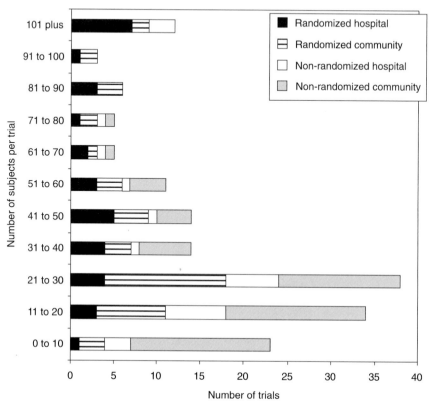

Fig. 6.25. Distribution of the number of subjects in individual ONS trials.

Table 6.19. Total number of subjects in an individual trial required to detect difference in proportions with 80% power (significance *P* < 0.05), assuming equal-sized groups. Reduction in mortality (25% vs. 19%) requires 748 per group (total 1496); reduction in complication rates (41% vs. 18%) requires 61 per group (total 122).

Proportion in supplemented group	Proportion in unsupplemented group											
	35%	32.5%	30%	27.5%	25%	22.5%	20%	17.5%	15%	12.5%	10%	7.5%
40%	2,942	1,288	712	448	304	218	164	126	98	78	64	52
35%	–	11,230	2,754	1,198	658	410	276	198	146	110	86	68
30%	2,754	10,790	–	10,228	2,502	1,080	588	362	242	170	124	94
25%	658	1,142	2,502	9,724	–	9,096	2,188	932	500	300	200	138
20%	276	388	588	1,010	2,188	8,404	–	7,652	1,812	758	398	236
15%	146	184	242	334	500	848	1,812	6,834	–	5,956	1,372	556

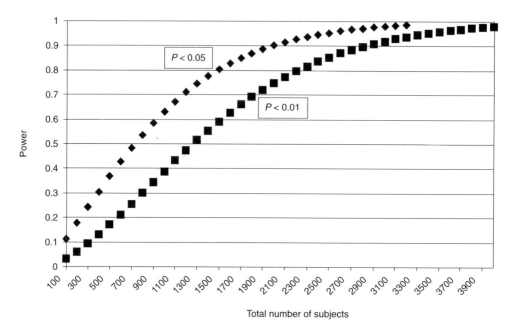

Fig. 6.26. Sample size required to observe a difference in mortality (25% and 19%) in two equally sized groups, according to power and significance level ($P < 0.05$ and $P < 0.01$. Generated using SPSS SamplePower 2 software for PC).

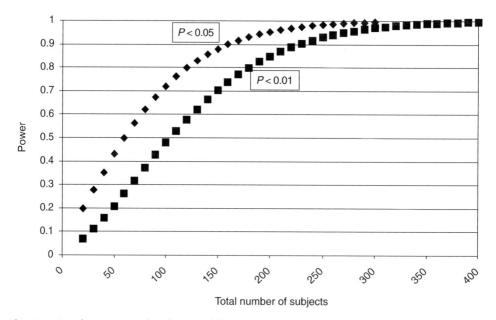

Fig. 6.27. Sample size required to observe a difference in complication rates (41% and 18%) in two equally sized groups, according to power and significance level ($P < 0.05$ and $P < 0.01$. Generated using SPSS SamplePower 2 software for PC).

the total number of subjects required in trials to detect differences in the proportions of patients with a certain outcome (e.g. mortality, complication rates) with an 80% power (significant at $P < 0.05$ level, assuming equal numbers of patients in both groups), using power statistics. These calculations suggest that, to detect a difference in mortality rate of 25% and 19% (difference between unsupplemented and supplemented patients using combined analysis in this chapter), 748 patients per group (total patient n 1496) would be needed in an individual trial. Similarly, to detect a difference in complication rates of 40% (controls) and 20% (approximate reduction achieved with supplementation shown in this review), 164 patients in total (82 per group) would be needed. These calculations are based on 80% power at the $P < 0.05$ level. Figures 6.26 (mortality) and 6.27 (complication rates) show that, to detect a similar magnitude of difference with increased power and significance level ($P < 0.05$ to $P < 0.01$), larger sample sizes are required. In this systematic review, a few small trials showed significant improvements in outcome (e.g. mortality and complication rates) because the observed differences between treatment and control groups were large. Other trials showed smaller differences that were not significant, possibly because of the small sample size (type II error). Therefore, by combining the results obtained by different trials, sample size and power are increased. This may explain why some of the effects of ONS (e.g. on mortality) were significant in the meta-analysis but not in the individual (constituent) trials.

Apart from the need for better-designed trials (see Chapter 10), future research should investigate the cellular, molecular and tissue mechanisms that may explain the impact of ONS on functional and clinical outcomes. Investigations should also be undertaken to assess the effects of different types of ONS (in terms of nutrient composition and consistency) that are available. The impact of the timing of administration, both in terms of the time of day or night and the time of intervention during a period of treatment (e.g. provision of ONS

during a critical period of recovery), should also be assessed across patient groups. One specific example of the importance of providing an ONS at a critical time is the provision of carbohydrate-containing ONS prior to surgery. These have been shown to improve preoperative well-being, reduce postoperative insulin resistance and shorten length of hospital stay (Ljungqvist *et al.*, 2001).

Conclusion

This chapter has highlighted the current evidence base (166 trials, 7630 patients) of ONS efficacy in patients across disease groups and health-care settings. In summary, marked improvements in clinical outcome (mortality, complication rates and reduced length of stay) appear likely when ONS are used in certain patient groups at risk of DRM, particularly in the hospital setting. A wide range of functional benefits have also been documented following the use of ONS in patients with both acute and chronic diseases. The mechanisms by which these improvements occur may be through increases in energy and nutrient intake, body weight and muscle mass. Alternatively, it may be that the supply of one or a mix of nutrients at a critical time in the treatment of a patient's disease can influence body function, independently of effects on gross body structure. Ultimately, further research is required to ascertain the benefits to outcome of this simple means of nutritional intervention across patient groups in both hospital and community settings. Although there may also be benefits associated with increasing the dietary intake of patients by fortification or counselling, there is little evidence at present to suggest that improvements in function or clinical outcome are forthcoming. Well-designed trials that investigate different strategies (e.g. dietary fortification, additional food snacks, flavour or odour enhancement, changes to food consistency, dining environment, etc.) of dietary manipulation are needed across patients in both hospital and community settings.

For some patient groups at high risk of DRM, provision of nutrients via the oral route may not be possible. This could be because of obstructive conditions or neurological injury making swallowing and eating difficult or unsafe. Otherwise, it could be that poor appetite limits total nutrient intake. In such cases, bypassing the oral route, by supplying nutrients by tube, may be safer and more effective than either dietary manipulation or ONS. The efficacy of this form of nutritional therapy is discussed in the next chapter of this book.

Additional Studies Obtained Since Completion of Data Collection (December 2001 onwards)

Vlaming *et al.* (2001) indicated that the administration of ONS to 'thin' hospital patients (mixed group, unintentional 5–10% weight loss or BMI of 18–22 kg m^{-2}) did not affect hospital stay, with average length of stay 2.8 days greater for supplemented relative to control patients (95% CI −0.8 to +6.3).

Faxén Irving *et al.* (2002) found in an NRT that the use of ONS in demented elderly patients (*n* 22) improved body weight significantly (+3.4 kg) over 6 months. No functional improvements were observed (e.g. cognitive function, activities of daily living (ADL)).

Wouters-Wesseling *et al.* (2002) found in an RCT of elderly nursing-home patients (*n* 42) that ONS (135 kcal) for up to 12 weeks significantly improved the intakes of a number of micronutrients (e.g. vitamin B_6, B_{12}, D and folate). No functional improvements (e.g. Barthel scores) were noted.

Note

[1]Removal of potentially duplicated data (Unosson *et al.*, 1992) from analysis has little effect on the result (odds ratio for mortality with ONS 0.61 (95% CI 0.47–0.81), adequate fail-safe scores).

7
Evidence Base for Enteral Tube Feeding

Systematic Review of Enteral Tube Feeding

This chapter provides the evidence base for enteral tube feeding (ETF) for a wide variety of patients in hospital and community settings. The systematic review and meta-analysis presented in this chapter suggest that ETF can significantly improve clinical outcome, reducing mortality and complication rates. A number of functional benefits are also observed. These improvements in outcome, which are associated with the marked increases in total energy and nutrient intakes provided by ETF, may be due to the attenuation of loss of body mass and function or to the supply of one or a mix of nutrients at a critical time in recovery. A summary of the key findings of the reviews of ETF in hospital and community settings can be found in Boxes 7.1 and 7.2.

The previous chapter of this book has highlighted that, in some patients at risk of disease-related malnutrition (DRM), oral nutritional supplements (ONS) or dietary manipulation may be the optimal ways to increase nutrient intake. In cases where oral nutritional support is either unable to increase total nutrient intake sufficiently (e.g. in a patient with a poor appetite) or is contraindicated (e.g. cerebrovascular accident (CVA) patient with dysphagia and risk of

aspiration), then ETF may be the most appropriate way to increase nutritional intake.

An Introduction to ETF

Indications for ETF and ETF techniques

The general indications and contraindications of ETF are summarized in Table 7.1. The feed can be delivered through a variety of routes using different tubes, depending on the patient group (e.g. whether there is abnormal upper gastrointestinal (GI) anatomy or risk of aspiration) and the duration of treatment (short- or long-term). There are fine-bore nasoenteral tubes (nasogastric, nasoduodenal, nasojejunal), gastrostomy tubes (surgical, percutaneous endoscopic or fluoroscopic) and jejunostomy tubes (surgical, percutaneous endoscopic). Many of these ETF routes have been used in the trials included in the systematic review presented later in this chapter (for details, see Appendices 5 and 6). Most ETF involves the use of a pump to deliver continuous infusions of feed over many hours, during the day, night or both. Sometimes boluses of feed are given (200–400 ml over 20–60 min), often by syringe, at intervals during the day. The timing and rate of ETF will vary depending on the site of feeding (e.g. gastric or jejunal), GI function and

Box 7.1. Key findings from the evidence base for enteral tube feeding in the hospital setting (74 trials (*n* 2769); 33 RCT (*n* 1358)). RCT, randomized controlled trials; CI, confidence interval; COPD, chronic obstructive pulmonary disease; BMI, body mass index.

ETF can substantially increase nutritional intake
Ninety-eight per cent of trials (and all RCT) assessing intake with ETF showed improvements in total energy intake (of which 62% were significant). On average, ETF increased energy intake by ~1000 kcal day^{-1} compared with routine care in the RCT reviewed. ETF does not substantially suppress food intake.

ETF typically attenuates loss of body weight and lean tissue
In 81% of RCT in patients with burns, critical illness, cystic fibrosis, liver disease and those post-surgery, ETF produced weight gain or attenuated weight loss relative to a control group (of which 53% were significant). The effect on weight appears to involve improvements or better retention of lean and fat tissue mass. Meta-analysis of % weight change suggests a mean effect size with ETF of 1.41 (95% CI 0.66–2.16) compared with routine care, but with significant heterogeneity between studies.

ETF can improve functional outcomes
ETF was found to produce functional benefits in 67% of RCT in patients with COPD, cystic fibrosis, liver disease, cancer and those post-surgery. These included significant improvements in respiratory function, liver function, bowel function, wound healing, well-being and immune function, depending on the patient group. Such benefits were typically accompanied by substantial improvements in weight (~6% difference between ETF and control patients).

ETF can improve clinical outcome and may be cost-effective
Mortality and complication rates were significantly reduced by ETF compared with routine care in some patient groups:

● Mortality was significantly lower with ETF (11% vs. 22%), with meta-analysis suggesting an odds ratio of 0.48 (95% CI 0.30–0.78). The reduction in mortality occurred to a similar extent in trials with a mean BMI < 20 kg m^{-2} or > 20 kg m^{-2}. Weight change (+6–8% difference between ETF and control patients) was associated with improvements in mortality but there was no clear relationship with the duration of ETF.
● Complication rates, including sepsis, wound and urinary infections and pneumonia, were significantly lower with ETF than with routine care (33% vs. 48%), with meta-analysis suggesting an odds ratio of 0.50 (95% CI 0.35–0.70). Significant reductions in infective complications were also noted (odds ratio 0.26 (95% CI 0.15–0.44)). Weight change may be associated with the improvements in complications.
● Small reductions in hospital stay may accompany ETF.
● Cost savings are likely to occur when complication rates are markedly reduced.

Methodology
Only 46% of trials were randomized and poor study designs (low Jadad scores, small sample sizes) were some of the limitations of the data set. Therefore larger RCT to assess the clinical and cost-effectiveness of ETF are required.

patient's tolerance of ETF. Social factors should also be considered in the patient on home ETF. All of these different ways of ETF have been used in the studies reviewed later in this chapter. For more details on ETF techniques, refer to ASPEN (2002). Information about the complications associated with ETF can be found in the *Oxford Textbook of Medicine* (Elia, 1996a).

Types of feeds

A variety of nutritionally complete tube feeds are available for use in adults and children (Tables 7.2 and 7.3). Some are powder based, such as Nutrison Powder (Nutricia), but most are liquid. These liquid formulas typically have similar nutritional compositions, although the energy densities (0.5–2 kcal ml^{-1}), protein contents and

---

Box 7.2. Key findings from the evidence base for enteral tube feeding in the community setting (47 trials (*n* 1321), three RCT (*n* 52)). RCT, randomized controlled trials; COPD, chronic obstructive pulmonary disease; HIV, human immunodeficiency virus; NRT, non-randomized trials.

The findings, predominantly from non-randomized trials suggest that:

ETF can improve or maintain nutritional intake
All trials that assessed total energy intake indicated that it was improved by ETF (*n* 14). When used as a supplement to food intake, ETF did not suppress appetite and dietary intake substantially. ETF was also used effectively as a sole source of nutrition for prolonged periods of time (e.g. stroke patients, patients with inflammatory bowel disease).

ETF can improve body weight, lean tissue mass and growth in children
ETF increased or maintained weight over variable periods of time in all trials that made assessments (significant improvement in all three RCT). In trials that assessed body composition, 88% indicated improvements in fat mass and/or muscle mass in a variety of patient groups, such as COPD, cystic fibrosis, HIV and renal disease. ETF improved growth in infants and children with cancer, cystic fibrosis, HIV and gastrointestinal disease.

ETF can improve functional and clinical outcomes
Eighty-eight per cent of trials reported improvements in function with ETF. These varied with the patient group and included improved well-being/quality of life and pulmonary function and reductions in pressure-ulcer surface area. Some trials suggested improvements in clinical outcome, such as fewer and shorter hospitalizations, lower mortality rates and reduced use of medication in certain patient groups.

ETF in the community can be cost-effective
The increasing use of ETF at home provides substantial cost saving to the hospital, but places greater demands on carers in the community, who are often family members.

Methodology
The majority of trials reviewed were small NRT, partly due to the ethical difficulties of withholding or withdrawing ETF in patients with severe chronic disease, for whom ETF is usually the sole or predominant source of nutrition.

---

sources may vary, and some do not include fibre. There is also an extensive range of specialized tube feeds available that vary in composition for use in specific patient groups. These include:

- peptide and medium-chain triglyceride-based feeds, e.g. Peptisorb (Nutricia) and Perative (Abbott) that may be used in patients with malabsorption;
- low sodium/low electrolyte feeds, e.g. Nutrison Low Sodium (Nutricia), Nepro (Abbott) that may be used in patients with liver or renal disease;
- feeds with altered fat and carbohydrate proportions for patients with diabetes, e.g. Nutrison Diabetes (Nutricia);
- feeds enriched with specific nutrients (e.g. glutamine, arginine, omega-3 fatty acids) for use in critically ill patients,

e.g. Stresson Multi Fibre (Nutricia), Impact (Novartis);
- feeds which are complete in micronutrients in one litre for patients with low energy requirements, e.g. Nutrison Vitaplus Multi Fibre (Nutricia), Jevity Plus (Abbott).

The choice of feed and the quantity of feed prescribed will depend on the patients' general clinical condition, GI function and estimated nutritional requirements (energy requirements can be calculated using the Schofield equation (Schofield *et al.*, 1985)). The amount of tube feed given will also depend on whether ETF is used as the sole source of nutrition (e.g. in patients who are unable to swallow food due to a neurological condition or an obstructive cancer) or in addition to food intake (e.g. in patients who

Table 7.1. Guidelines for the use of enteral tube feeding in the adult patient (Elia, 1996a).

1 Conditions where ETF should be a part of routine care
   (a) Protein-energy malnutrition (greater than 10% weight loss) with little or no oral intake for the previous 5 days
   (b) Less than 50% of the required oral nutrient intake for the previous 7–10 days
   (c) Severe dysphagia or swallowing-related difficulties, e.g. head injury, strokes, motor neurone disease
   (d) Major, full-thickness burns
   (e) Massive small-bowel resection (in patients with 50–90% small-bowel resection, ETF is given to hasten gut
       regeneration and return to oral intake, often in combination with parenteral nutrition)
   (f) Low-output enterocutaneous fistulae (< 500 ml day^{-1})[a] (elemental diets may hasten closure of fistula)

2 Conditions where ETF would normally be helpful
   (a) Major trauma (see 1a and 1b)
   (b) Radiation therapy (see 1a and1b)
   (c) Mild chemotherapy (see 1a and 1b)

3 Conditions where ETF is of limited or undetermined value
   (a) Immediate postoperative period or post-stress period if an adequate oral intake will be resumed within 5–7 days
   (b) Acute enteritis
   (c) Less than 10% of the small intestine remaining (parenteral nutrition is usually indicated)

4 Conditions/situations in which ETF should not be used
   (a) Complete mechanical intestinal obstruction
   (b) Ileus or intestinal hypomotility
   (c) Severe uncontrollable diarrhoea
   (d) High-output fistulas
   (e) Severe acute pancreatitis
   (f) Shock
   (g) Aggressive nutritional support not desired by the patient or legal guardian, in accordance with hospital policy
       and existing law
   (h) Prognosis not warranting aggressive nutritional support

[a]If the fistula is proximal, the feeding should be distal. If the fistula is distal, sufficient proximal length must be present to allow sufficient absorption.
Fistulas due to malignancy, radiation and distal obstruction are unlikely to close spontaneously.

have a poor appetite due to cystic fibrosis, chronic obstructive pulmonary disease (COPD), infections or cancer).

The availability of tube feeds in terms of types of products varies from country to country. Tube feeds should always be used under medical supervision, with the appropriate medical devices for administration. Reimbursement of tube feeds for use in the community also varies between countries.

Evidence Base for ETF

As discussed briefly in Chapter 5, the use of ETF in developed countries such as Britain is increasing, particularly in the community setting. In 2000, it was estimated that the point prevalence of patients on home ETF in Britain was 20,000.

Annual growth rates for home ETF have been between 15 and 20% since 1996 (Elia *et al.*, 2001b). In both hospital and community settings, ETF is used in patients with a wide variety of conditions and ages (from paediatrics to the elderly) in the short (days to weeks, as in acute disease) or long term (months, years, as in chronic disease) either to prevent or to treat DRM. ETF can be used to provide nutritional support in a number of ways:

1. As a sole source of nutrition (e.g. in the early postoperative period, in patients unable to swallow safely).
2. As a supplement to food intake (e.g. in those unable to take sufficient orally due to eating difficulties, anorexia).
3. In combination with parenteral nutrition (PN).

Table 7.2. Examples of 'nutritionally complete', whole protein tube feeds for adults.

Enteral tube feed	Presentation of tube feed	Energy content (kcal 100 ml^{-1})	Protein content (g 100 ml^{-1})
Nutrison Multi Fibre[a] (Nutricia)	Nutrison Pack (500 ml, 1000 ml, 1500 ml) Bottle (500 ml)	100	4
Nutrison Energy Multi Fibre[a] (Nutricia)	Nutrison Pack (500 ml, 1000 ml, 1500 ml) Bottle (500 ml)	150	6
Isosource Fibre[a] (Novartis)	Flexibag (500 ml, 1000 ml, 1500 ml) Bottle (500 ml)	100	3.8
Isosource Energy Fibre[a] (Novartis)	Flexibag (500 ml) Bottle (500 ml)	150	4.9
Sondalis Fibre[a] (Nestle)	Dripac-flex (500 ml, 1000 ml) Bottle (500 ml) Can (375 ml)	100	3.8
Sondalis 1.5[b] (Nestle)	Dripac-flex (500 ml, 1000 ml)	150	5.6
Fresubin Original Fibre[a] (Fresenius)	Easybag (500 ml, 1000 ml) Bottle (500 ml)	100	5.5
Fresubin Energy Fibre[a] (Fresenius)	Easybag (500 ml,1000 ml) Bottle (500 ml)	150	5.6
Jevity[a] (Abbott)	Ready-to-hang rigid container (500 ml, 1000 ml, 1500 ml) Cans (8 fl.oz and 32 fl.oz)	105	4.0
Enrich Plus[a] (Abbott)	Ready-to-hang rigid container (500 ml)	153	6.25

[a]Similar feeds also available without fibre; [b]does not contain fibre.
This table was compiled based on information available to the authors at the time of writing (July 2002). This is not a complete overview of all products available on the market, but is intended to give examples of the main products. Not all products/presentations are available in all countries. Furthermore, product names, presentations and compositions may vary between countries, and may be subject to change. For more accurate information, contact individual manufacturers.

Can ETF be safely and effectively used in different patient groups that vary according to age and disease? Previous reviews and meta-analyses that have attempted to address this question have provided only partial answers. One of the reasons for this is that some analyses have combined trials of ETF and other nutritional interventions (e.g. ONS) together, to compare their efficacy with routine clinical care. In these types of analyses, it is difficult to separate out the benefits due to the individual treatment modalities (Potter *et al.*, 1998; Ferreira *et al.*, 2000; Lewis *et al.*, 2001). Other meta-analyses and reviews have focused on the efficacy of ETF in specific conditions (e.g. COPD (Ferreira *et al.*, 2000), postoperative GI surgical (Lewis *et al.*, 2001), chronic non-malignant disorders (Aker, 1979)), and some at particular stages of a condition (Lewis *et al.*, 2001), which makes it difficult to generalize the findings to other stages of a condition or to other diseases. A number of meta-analyses have also compared the efficacy of ETF using feeds differing in composition (e.g. 'standard' feed versus enriched 'immunomodulatory' feeds (Heyland *et al.*, 2001b)) or compared with another nutritional intervention, particularly PN (e.g. Braunschweig *et al.*, 2001), discussed in great detail in Chapter 9. Despite these previous meta-analyses, there is no comprehensive review that summarizes the available information of the effectiveness of ETF according to specific diseases, combinations of diseases and stages of disease (e.g. acute or chronic stages of a condition) in different settings (hospital and community). Also, few reviews have related the functional and clinical effects of ETF with changes in body weight and initial nutritional status.

Table 7.3. Examples of 'nutritionally complete' tube feeds for paediatrics.

Enteral tube feed	Target age group/ body weight	Presentation of tube feed	Energy content (kcal 100 ml^{-1})	Protein content (g 100 ml^{-1})
Infatrini[b] (Nutricia)	Infants 0–12 months/ up to 8 kg body weight	Bottle (100 ml)	100	2.6
Nutrini Multi Fibre[a] (Nutricia)	Children aged 1–6 years/ 8–20 kg body weight	Pack (500 ml) Bottle (200 ml)	100	2.8
Nutrini Energy Multi Fibre[a] (Nutricia)	Children aged 1–6 years/ 8–20 kg body weight	Pack (500 ml) Bottle (200 ml)	150	4.1
Tentrini Multi Fibre[a] (Nutricia)	Children aged 7–12 years/ 21–45 kg body weight	Pack (500 ml) Bottle (500 ml)	100	3.3
Tentrini Energy Multi Fibre[a] (Nutricia)	Children aged 7–12 years/ 21–45 kg body weight	Pack (500 ml) Bottle (500 ml)	150	4.9
Novasource Junior (Novartis)	Children aged 1–6 years/ 8–20 kg body weight	Flexibag (500 ml) Bottle (250 ml)	100	N/A
Isosource Junior[b] (Novartis)	Children aged 1–6 years/ 8–20 kg body weight	Flexibag (500 ml) Bottle (250 ml)	122	2.7
Sondalis Junior[b] (Nestle)	Children aged 1–6 years	Dripac-flex (500 ml)	100	3.0
Frebini (Fresenius)	Children aged 1–12 years	Bottle (500 ml)	100	2.5
Paediasure Fibre[a] (Abbott)	Children aged 1–6 years/ > 8 kg body weight	Ready-to-hang rigid container (500 ml) Can (250 ml, 8 fl.oz)	101	2.8
Paediasure Plus Fibre[a] (Abbott)	Children aged 1–6 years/ > 8 kg body weight	Ready-to-hang rigid container (500 ml)	150	4.2

[a]Similar feeds also available without fibre; [b]Does not contain fibre; N/A: data not available
This table was compiled based on information available to the authors at the time of writing (July 2002). This is not a complete overview of all products available on the market, but is intended to give examples of the main products. Not all products/presentations are available in all countries. Furthermore, product names, presentations and compositions may vary between countries, and may be subject to change. For more accurate information, contact individual manufacturers.

From a clinical perspective, it is clear that ETF is indicated for particular conditions (Fig. 7.1). There is often little doubt about the value of ETF in patients who are likely to recover from prolonged unconsciousness or in those with swallowing difficulties who otherwise have good health or quality of life (left side of distribution curve, Fig. 7.1). In several such situations, it would be unethical to withhold ETF (and a randomized controlled trial (RCT) could not be undertaken). In contrast, ETF is not generally indicated in patients who are able to take sufficient orally to meet their nutritional requirements (right side of distribution curve, Fig. 7.1). The controversy exists in the intermediate group of patients (see Fig. 7.1) who are unable either to eat or to tolerate the required amount of food

orally. This may be due to severe dietary inadequacy for a short period of time or less severe dietary inadequacy over a more prolonged period of time. In general, reductions in intake in such patients will be greater than in those considered for ONS (and included in ONS trials). Intake may be reduced because of anorexia or poor tolerance of, or complications associated with, oral intake. In such patients, continuous or intermittent ETF over prolonged periods of time may lead to better tolerance and greater nutritional intake. The section that follows primarily examines the use of ETF in this intermediate group of patients in an attempt to clarify some of the controversial issues and provide an evidence-based approach to treatment. It addresses the use of ETF either as a sole source of

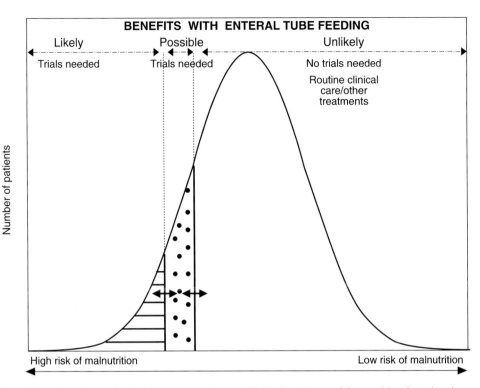

Fig. 7.1. Benefits of enteral tube feeding according to risk of malnutrition and the need for clinical trials.

nutrition or as a supplement to food intake. As stated in Chapter 5, the systematic review has addressed four main questions:

(I) What effect does ETF have on the voluntary food intake (in those patients able to eat) and total energy intake of patients?
(II) What effect does ETF have on the body weight and composition of patients?
(III) What effect does ETF have on the function of patients?
(IV) What effect does ETF have on the clinical and financial outcome of patients in hospital and community settings?

Where possible, evidence has been drawn from RCT. The efficacy of ETF has been addressed by taking a multilayer approach to assessing the evidence. This has embraced individual RCT and non-randomized trials (NRT) and summaries for patient-specific groups according to setting (see Appendices 5 and 6). This chapter provides a summary of the main findings of effectiveness of ETF overall and according to health-care setting

(hospital/community) and patient group (age/disease). It also attempts to analyse the effect of the intake and duration of ETF.

Summary of the Study Design of Trials Reviewed

Hospital setting

Randomized and non-randomized trials according to patient group

Seventy-four trials (2769 patients) of ETF in the hospital setting were reviewed. Thirty-three were RCT (1358 patients) comparing ETF with no nutritional support in a variety of patient groups. Forty-one were NRT (1411 patients). All trials were reviewed in patient-specific groups, defined by condition (e.g. COPD) or age (e.g. elderly, paediatrics). Tables 7.4 and 7.5 give a summary of the numbers of trials and patients categorized according to patient group.

Table 7.4. Summary of randomized controlled trials of enteral tube feeding in hospital patients. For some diseases/conditions, no trials of ETF were reviewed (e.g. renal disease, HIV/AIDS).

Disease/patient group	Number of randomized controlled trials reviewed	Total number of patients in trials reviewed
Burns	2	100
Chronic obstructive pulmonary disease	1	10
Critical illness/injury	6	258
Gastroenterology	1	60
General medical	1	51
Liver disease	6	228
Malignancy	2	11
Orthopaedics	2	140
Paediatrics (cystic fibrosis)	1	22
Surgery	11	478
Total	33 (45% of total)	1358

Table 7.5. Summary of non-randomized trials of enteral tube feeding in hospital patients. For some diseases/conditions, no trials of ETF in hospital patients were reviewed (e.g. renal disease, HIV/AIDS).

Disease/patient group	Number of non-randomized trials reviewed	Total number of patients in trials reviewed
Burns	1	46
Chronic obstructive pulmonary disease	1	16
Critical illness/injury	4	101
Elderly	2	237
Gastroenterology	6	115
General medical	8	304
Liver disease	3	23
Malignancy	4	109
Neurology	2	70
Paediatrics	7	158
Surgery	3	232
Total	41 (55% of total)	1411

Methodological issues

All the trials reviewed were categorized and coded according to study design. RCT were coded for methodology using the Jadad scoring system (Jadad *et al.*, 1996) and a summary of total scores is given in Table 7.6 (see Chapter 5 for methodology). The higher the score, the better the study design (highest score 5). The components of these scores for each individual RCT can be seen in Appendices 5 and 6.

Community setting

Randomized and non-randomized trials according to disease group

Forty-seven trials (1321 patients) of ETF in the community setting were reviewed. Only three were a randomized, controlled design (52 patients) comparing ETF with no nutritional support in adult patients with COPD or cancer and in paediatrics. Forty-four trials were a non-randomized

Table 7.6. Summary of randomized trial Jadad scores (Jadad *et al.*, 1996). See Chapter 5 for an explanation of Jadad scoring and see Appendix 5 for scores for individual studies.

Total Jadad score	Number of studies (%)	Patient group
0	1 (3%)	Paediatrics (1)
1	5 (15%)	Burns (1); liver disease (2); surgery (2)
2	20 (61%)	Burns (1); critic illness/injury (4); GI (1); general medical (1); liver disease (4); malignancy (2); orthopaedic (2); surgery (5)
3	5 (15%)	Critically ill (2); surgery (3)
4	2 (6%)	COPD (1); surgery (1)
5	0 (0%)	–

design (1269 patients). All trials were reviewed in disease-specific or age-specific (e.g. paediatrics, elderly) groups. Tables 7.7 and 7.8 give a summary of the numbers of trials and patients categorized according to patient group.

Methodological issues

All the RCT trials reviewed were categorized and coded according to study design. The Jadad scores of the three RCT were 1 (Donahoe *et al.*, 1994), 2 (Hearne *et al.*,

Table 7.7. Summary of randomized controlled trials of enteral tube feeding in community patients.

Disease/patient group	Number of randomized controlled trials reviewed	Total number of patients in trials reviewed
Chronic obstructive pulmonary disease	1	11
Malignancy	1	31
Paediatrics	1	10
Total	3 (6% of total)	52

Table 7.8. Summary of non-randomized trials of enteral tube feeding in community patients. For some diseases/conditions, no trials of ETF in this setting were reviewed (e.g. liver disease).

Disease/patient group	Number of non-randomized trials reviewed	Total number of patients in trials reviewed
Chronic obstructive pulmonary disease	1	4
Cystic fibrosis	10	147
Elderly	2	40
Gastroenterology	1	44
General medical/mixed	8	353
HIV/AIDS	5	135
Malignancy	3	259
Neurology	1	30
Paediatrics[a]	12	249
HIV	1	18
Gastroenterology	5	69
General/mixed diagnoses	3	89
Malignancy	3	73
Renal	1	8
Total	44 (94% of total)	1269

[a]Excluding cystic fibrosis – separate category.

1985) and 2 (Patrick *et al.*, 1986). The components of these scores can be seen in the tables in Appendix 6. The higher the score, the better the design (highest score 5).

Summary of ETF Used in the Trials Reviewed

Routes of ETF

A variety of tubes and routes were used for ETF in the studies reviewed. These included nasogastric, duodenal and jejunal tubes, typically fine-bore in size. Gastrostomy and jejunostomy tubes were also used, particularly in the community (~50% of studies used a gastrostomy tube).

The way in which ETF was administered varied depending on the patient group and included giving ETF continuously for 24 h, nocturnally, diurnally or as boluses.

Composition of enteral tube feeds

The studies reviewed used a variety of different formulas. In hospital and community studies, formulations were mostly commercially produced (where reported), with only six studies using hospital-made formulations (de Vries *et al.*, 1982; Seri and Aquilio, 1984; Shukla *et al.*, 1984; Tandon *et al.*, 1984; Chiarelli *et al.*, 1990; Singh *et al.*, 1998). The tube feeds used in the studies reviewed were mostly mixed macronutrient (protein, fat, carbohydrate) polymeric formulations that were nutritionally 'complete'. In some studies peptide or elemental feeds, feeds enriched with medium-chain triglycerides or branched-chain amino acids or low in sodium were used. The energy density of feeds, where reported, ranged from 0.9 kcal ml^{-1} to 4 kcal ml^{-1} (hospital-made feed), although most feeds ranged between 1 kcal ml^{-1} and 1.5 kcal ml^{-1}. In many studies, a variety of tube feeds were used, often in combination with other feeds or modular supplements (protein or carbohydrate) in order that the nutrient and fluid requirements of patients in different disease groups could be met.

Prescription and duration of ETF

The amount of tube feed prescribed varied according to the patient group and the indications for using ETF (sole source of nutrition vs. supplement to food intake or PN). Typically ETF was prescribed either as the sole form of nutrition or in combination with oral food intake, in order to meet energy/nutritional requirements. Available data comparing prescribed and provided amounts of ETF are summarized in the tables in Appendices 5 and 6 (where such data were provided).

The duration of ETF also depended on the patient group and the reason for using this method of nutritional support. For hospital-based trials, the duration of ETF ranged from ~5 to ~50 days, with ETF continuing for up to 3 months in patients subsequently discharged home with tube feeding. The duration of ETF in community-based trials ranged from less than 1 month to 5 years.

Summary of Main Findings from Hospital and Community Trials

Due to the lack of RCT of ETF in community patients, community- and hospital-based trials have been addressed separately in the section below. The four main review questions (I–IV) are addressed systematically below, and a summary of the outcomes can be seen in Tables 7.9 (hospital) and 7.10 (community). An indication of the number and proportions of trials that did or did not show improvements in the main outcome parameters (energy intake, body weight and body function) is given in Figs 7.2 (hospital) and 7.3 (community).

(I) What effect does ETF have on the voluntary food intake (in those patients able to eat) and total energy intake in patients in hospital and community settings?

In the studies reviewed, ETF was found to be a relatively safe and effective way of improving total energy and/or nutrient intakes in patients in both hospital and community settings.

Table 7.9. Changes in nutrient intake, nutritional status, function and clinical outcome following enteral tube feeding (versus no nutritional support) in hospital (trials arranged according to body mass index (BMI) and patient group).

ETF trial	Improved energy and/or nutrient intake	Improved nutritional status	Improved function	Improved clinical outcome
BMI < 20 kg m^{-2}/IBW < 90%/growth retardation				
Randomized, controlled trials				
Whittaker *et al.* (1990) COPD	✓ (t)	✓ (v)	✓ (v)	n/a
Cabre *et al.* (1990) Liver disease †	✓ (v)		✓ (v)	✓ (v)
Bastow *et al.* (1983) Orthopaedics †	✓ (? sig)	✓ (v)	n/a	✓ (v)
Shepherd *et al.* (1988) Paediatrics (CF)	✓ (? sig)	✓ (t)	✓ (t)	n/a¶
Non-randomized trials/data				
Goldstein *et al.* (1988) COPD	✓ (v)		✓ (t)	n/a
Afdhal *et al.* (1989) GI	n/a	✓ (t)	✓ (t)	n/a
Rigaud *et al.* (1991) GI	n/a	✓ (t)	✓ (t)	n/a
Bastow *et al.* (1985) GI	✓ (? sig)	✓ (? sig)	n/a	n/a
Bennegard *et al.* (1983) General	✓ (t)	✓ (t)	n/a	n/a
Gentile *et al.* (2000) General	n/a	✓ (t)	n/a	n/a
Hebuterne *et al.* (1995) General †	✓ (t)	✓ (t)	n/a	n/a
Schneider *et al.* (1996) General	✓ (t)	✓ (t)	✓ (t)	n/a
Winter *et al.* (2000) General	n/a	✓ (? sig)	✓ (? sig)	n/a
Daniels *et al.* (1989) Paediatrics (CF)	✓ (t)	✓ (t)	n/a	n/a
Morin *et al.* (1980) Paediatrics (GI)	✓ (? sig)	✓ (t)	✓ (? sig)	n/a
BMI > 20 kg m^{-2}/IBW > 90%				
Randomized, controlled trials				
De Ledinghen *et al.* (1997) Liver disease	✓ (? sig)	✓ (ns)		
Kearns *et al.* (1992) Liver disease ††	✓ (v)	✓ (? sig)	✓ (v)	✓ (ns)
Sullivan *et al.* (1998) Orthopaedics	✓ (v)	n/a		✓ (ns)
Beier-Holgersen and Boesby (1996) Surgery	✓ (? sig)	n/a	✓ (v)	✓ (v) £
Carr *et al.* (1996) Surgery	✓ (v)	✓ (? sig)	✓ (v)	✓ (ns)
Ryan *et al.* (1981) Surgery †	✓ (v)	✓ (v)	n/a	✓ (v)
Singh *et al.* (1998) Surgery	✓ (v)	n/a	n/a	✓ (v)
Watters *et al.* (1997) Surgery	n/a			
Non-randomized trials/data				
Mowatt-Larssen *et al.* (1992) Critically ill/injury	✓ (? sig)		n/a	n/a
Smith *et al.* (1982) Liver disease	✓ (? sig)	✓ ‡(? sig)	✓ (? sig)	n/a
Bruning *et al.* (1988) Malignancy	n/a			n/a
Yeung *et al.* (1979b) Surgery	✓ (v)	✓ (? sig)	n/a	
BMI unknown				
Randomized, controlled trials				
Chiarelli *et al.* (1990) Burns	n/a	✓ (ns)	n/a	✓ (ns)
Jenkins *et al.* (1994) Burns	✓ (v)	n/a	n/a	✓ (v)
Chuntrasakul *et al.* (1996) Critically ill/injury	✓ (v)	✓ (v)	n/a	✓ (ns)
Kompan *et al.* (1999) Critically ill/injury	✓ (v)	n/a	✓ (? sig)	✓ (v)
Minard *et al.* (2000) Critically ill/injury	✓ (v)	n/a	n/a	✓ (ns)
Moore and Jones (1986) Critically ill/injury	✓ (? sig)	✓ (? sig)	✓ (t)	✓ (v)
Seri and Aquilio (1984) Critically ill/injury	n/a			✓ (ns)
Taylor *et al.* (1999) Critically ill/injury	✓ (v)	n/a	n/a	✓ (v)
Pupelis *et al.* (2001) GI	✓ (v)	n/a	✓ (v)	✓ (v)
McWhirter and Pennington (1996) General	✓ (? sig)	✓ (v)	n/a	n/a
Calvey *et al.* (1984) Liver disease	n/a	n/a	n/a	
Foschi *et al.* (1986) Liver disease	n/a		n/a	✓ (v)
Hasse *et al.* (1985) Liver disease	✓ (v)	n/a	n/a	✓ (v)
Tandon *et al.* (1984) Malignancy	n/a	✓ (t)	✓ (t)	✓ (? sig)

Continued

Table 7.9. *Continued.*

ETF trial	Improved energy and/or nutrient intake	Improved nutritional status	Improved function	Improved clinical outcome
Van Bokhorst (2000, 2001) Malignancy	✓ (v)	✓ (ns)	✓ (v)	✓ (ns)
Elmore *et al.* (1989) Surgery	n/a	n/a	n/a	
Frankel and Horowitz (1989) Surgery	n/a	n/a		
Hoover *et al.* (1980) Surgery	✓ (v)	✓ (v)	n/a	n/a
Sagar *et al.* (1979) Surgery	✓ (? sig)	✓ (v)		✓ (v)
Schroeder *et al.* (1991) Surgery	✓ (v)	✓ (ns)	✓ (v)	✓ (ns)
Smith *et al.* (1985) Surgery	n/a	✓ (ns)	n/a	
Non-randomized trials / data				
Hansbrough and Hansbrough (1993) Burns	✓ (? sig)	n/a	n/a	n/a
Clifton *et al.* (1985) Critically ill/injury	n/a		n/a	n/a
Grahm *et al.* (1989) Critically ill/injury	✓ (v)	✓ (? sig)	n/a	✓ (v)
Kirby *et al.* (1991) Critically ill/injury	✓ (? sig)	n/a	n/a	n/a
Lipschitz and Mitchell (1982) Elderly	✓ (? sig)	✓ (t)	✓ (t)	n/a
Treber and Harris (1996) Elderly	n/a	n/a	n/a	✓ (v)
Abad-Lacruz *et al.* (1988) GI	n/a		✓ (t)	n/a
Kudsk *et al.* (1990) GI	n/a	n/a	✓ (? sig)	n/a
Royall *et al.* (1994) A GI	n/a	✓ (? sig)	✓ (t)	n/a
Yeung *et al.* (1979b) GI			n/a	n/a
Dresler *et al.* (1987) General	n/a	✓ (ns)	n/a	n/a
Taylor (1993) General	n/a	n/a	n/a	n/a
Keohane *et al.* (1983) Liver disease	n/a		✓ (t)	n/a
Soberon *et al.* (1987) Liver disease	✓ (t)	n/a		n/a
De Vries *et al.* (1982) Malignancy	n/a	✓ (v)	n/a	
Haffejee and Angorn (1979) Malignancy	✓ (? sig)	✓ (? sig)	✓ (t)	n/a
Lipschitz and Mitchell (1980) Malignancy	n/a	n/a	✓ (v)	n/a
Norton *et al.* (1996) Neurology	n/a	✓ (? sig)*	n/a	n/a
Park *et al.* (1992) Neurology	✓ (? sig)	✓ (? sig)	n/a	n/a
Chellis *et al.* (1996) Paediatrics (ICU)	✓ (? sig)	n/a	n/a	n/a £
Finch and Lawson (1993) Paediatrics (mixed)**	n/a	✓ (? sig)	n/a	n/a
Leite and Fantozzi (1998) Paediatrics (neuro)**	✓ N(t)	n/a	n/a	n/a
Smith *et al.* (1986) Paediatrics (GI)	n/a	n/a	n/a	✓ (ns) £
Yahav *et al.* (1985) Paediatrics (cardiac)**	✓ (t)	✓ (? sig)	n/a	n/a
Moncure *et al.* (1999) Surgery	✓ (v)	n/a	n/a	
Shukla *et al.* (1984) Surgery	n/a	✓ (v)	✓ (v)	✓ (? sig)

✓   Indicates an improvement or less deterioration compared with a control group or over time.
(v)   Significant compared with a control group receiving no ETF or a placebo.
(t)   Significant change over time.
(? sig) Improvement/benefit observed but unclear if statistically significant.
(ns)   Improvement/benefit observed that is not statistically significant.
n/a   Not assessed in trial.
A   Abstract.
‡   Assessment using only upper-arm anthropometry or other markers (not weight).
*   Improvement in those given PEG feeding only.
**   Improvement observed only in a sub-group of ETF patients.
N   Improvement in protein or micronutrient intake/balance (not energy).
†   BMI category assumed from information on nutritional status given in paper (no BMI provided).
††   Measurement of nutritional status and changes in body weight could be confounded by ascites.
¶   Significant improvement in 'very thin' patients only.
£   Financial savings calculated.
GI   Gastrointestinal disease; CF, cystic fibrosis; ICU, intensive care unit; IBW, ideal body weight; PEG, percutaneous endoscopic gastrostomy; BMI, body mass index.

Table 7.10. Changes in nutrient intake, nutritional status, function and clinical outcome following enteral tube feeding (versus no nutritional support) in the community (trials arranged according to body mass index and patient group).

ETF trial	Improved energy and/or nutrient intake	Improved nutritional status	Improved function	Improved clinical outcome
BMI < 20 kg m^{-2}/IBW < 90%/growth retardation				
Randomized, controlled trials				
Donahoe *et al.* (1994) A COPD	n/a	✓ (t)	n/a	n/a
Hearne *et al.* (1985) Malignancy	✓ (? sig)	✓ (v) †	n/a	
Patrick *et al.* (1986) Paediatrics (CP)	✓ (? sig)	✓ (v)	n/a	n/a
Non-randomized trials/data				
Irwin and Openbrier (1985) A COPD	n/a	✓ (? sig)	✓ (? sig)	✓ (? sig)
Bertrand *et al.* (1984) Cystic fibrosis (P)	✓ (t)	✓ (t)		n/a
Boland *et al.* (1986) Cystic fibrosis (P)	n/a	✓ (? sig)	✓ (ns) *	n/a
Dalzell *et al.* (1992) Cystic fibrosis (P)	n/a	✓ (v)	✓ (v)	✓ (ns)
Levy *et al.* (1985) Cystic fibrosis (P)	n/a	✓ (t)	✓ (? sig)	n/a
Moore *et al.* (1986) Cystic fibrosis (P)	✓ (t)	✓ (t)	✓ (t)	n/a
O'Loughlin *et al.* (1986) Cystic fibrosis (P)	✓ (t)	✓ (t)	✓ (? sig) *	n/a
Shepherd *et al.* (1983) Cystic fibrosis (P)	✓ (? sig)	✓ (t)	✓ (t)	n/a
Shepherd *et al.* (1986) Cystic fibrosis (P)	n/a	✓ (v)	✓ (v)	n/a
Smith, D.L. *et al.* (1994) Cystic fibrosis (P)	n/a	✓ (t)	✓ (ns)	n/a
Steinkamp and von der Hardt (1994) Cystic fibrosis (P)	n/a	✓ (t)	✓ (t)	n/a
Bastow *et al.* (1985) General	✓ (? sig)	✓ (? sig)	✓ (ns)	n/a
Schneider *et al.* (2000b) General	n/a	✓ (? sig)	n/a	n/a
Kotler *et al.* (1991) HIV/AIDS	n/a	✓ (? sig)	✓ (? sig)	n/a
Süttmann *et al.* (1993) HIV/AIDS	n/a	✓ (t)	n/a	n/a
Aiges *et al.* (1989) Paediatrics (GI)	✓ (? sig)	✓ (t)	✓ (t)	n/a
Belli *et al.* (1988) Paediatrics (GI)	✓ (t)	✓ (v)	✓ (v)	n/a
Chin *et al.* (1990) Paediatrics (GI)	n/a	✓ (v) **	n/a	
Cosgrove and Jenkins (1997) Paediatrics (GI)	n/a	✓ (t)	n/a	✓ (t)
Duche *et al.* (1999) Paediatrics (GI)	✓ (? sig)	✓ (? sig)	n/a	n/a
Papadopoulou *et al.* (1995) Paediatrics (mixed)	n/a	✓ (t)	n/a	n/a
Henderson *et al.* (1994) Paediatrics (mixed)	n/a	✓ (t)	n/a	n/a
Aquino *et al.* (1995) Paediatrics (malignancy)	n/a	✓ (? sig)	n/a	n/a
Den Broeder *et al.* (2000) Paediatrics (malignancy)	n/a	✓ (t)	n/a	n/a
Den Broeder *et al.* (1998) Paediatrics (malignancy)	n/a	✓ (v)		
Sayce *et al.* (2000) Renal	n/a	✓ (t)	n/a	✓ (? sig)
BMI > 20 kg m^{-2}/IBW > 90%				
Randomized, controlled trials				
None				
Non-randomized trials/data				
Breslow *et al.* (1993) Elderly	✓ (ns)	✓ (ns)	✓ (t)**	n/a
Mansfield *et al.* (1995) GI	n/a	✓ (? sig)	✓ (? sig)	n/a
BMI Unknown				
Randomized, controlled trials				
None				
Non-randomized trials/data				
Chernoff *et al.* (1990) Elderly	n/a	n/a	✓ (? sig)	n/a
Bannerman *et al.* (1999) A General	n/a	n/a		n/a
Edington *et al.* (1994) General	✓ (? sig)	✓ (ns)	n/a	
Jager-Wittenaar *et al.* (2000) General	n/a	n/a	n/a	✓ (? sig)
Pareira *et al.* (1954) General	✓ (? sig)	✓ (? sig)	n/a	n/a
Schneider *et al.* (2000a) A General	n/a	n/a	✓ (t)	n/a
Von Herz *et al.* (2000) General	n/a	n/a	✓ (t)	n/a

Continued

Table 7.10. *Continued.*

ETF trial	Improved energy and/or nutrient intake	Improved nutritional status	Improved function	Improved clinical outcome
Brantsma *et al.* (1991) HIV/AIDS	n/a	✓ (? sig)	✓ (ns) ***	n/a
Cappell and Grodil (1993) HIV/AIDS (P)	n/a	✓ (ns)	n/a	✓ (? sig)
Ockenga *et al.* (1994) HIV/AIDS	n/a	n/a	n/a	n/a
Fietkau *et al.* (1991) Malignancy	n/a	✓ (? sig)	✓ (? sig)	n/a
Roberge *et al.* (2000) Malignancy	n/a	n/a	✓ (t)	n/a
Shike *et al.* (1989) Malignancy	n/a	✓ (? sig)	n/a	n/a
Wicks *et al.* (1992) Neurology	✓ (? sig)	✓ (? sig)	n/a	n/a
Balfe *et al.* (1990) Paediatrics (mixed)	n/a	✓ (ns)	n/a	n/a
Greene *et al.* (1981) Paediatrics (mixed)	n/a	✓ (? sig)	n/a	n/a

✓   Indicates an improvement or less deterioration compared with a control group or over time.
(v)   Significant compared with a control group receiving no ETF or a placebo.
(t)   Significant change over time.
(? sig) Improvement/benefit observed but unclear if statistically significant.
(ns)   Improvement/benefit observed that is not statistically significant.
n/a   Not assessed in trial.
A   Abstract.
(P)   Includes paediatrics.
*   No improvements in pulmonary parameters (FEF, FEV_1, FVC), benefits in subjective ratings only.
**   Benefits in one group of ETF patients only.
***   Observational improvement.
†   Excludes nasopharyngeal cancers.
HIV, human immunodeficiency virus; AIDS, acquired immune deficiency syndrome; BMI, body mass index; CP, cerebral palsy; IBW, ideal body weight; FEV_1, forced expiratory volume in 1 s; FVC, forced ventilatory capacity; FEF, forced expiratory flow.

Nutritional intake in hospital patients

Ninety-eight per cent (45/46) of studies that assessed changes in total energy intake with ETF in hospital patients showed improvements. Of these, 62% (*n* 28) were significant, relative to a control group (*n* 20, 16 RCT) or to the baseline period in the same group (*n* 8, one RCT). All the RCT that assessed the impact of ETF on total energy intake (*n* 24) showed improvements. Of these, 71% were significant either when compared with a control group given no ETF (with or without voluntary food intake) (67%, *n* 16) or over time (4%, *n* 1) (see Fig. 7.2). These trials were undertaken in patients with burns (Jenkins *et al.*, 1994), COPD (Whittaker *et al.*, 1990), cystic fibrosis (Shepherd *et al.*, 1988), critical illness/trauma (Moore and Jones, 1986; Kompan *et al.*, 1999; Taylor *et al.*, 1999; Minard *et al.*, 2000), GI disorders (Pupelis *et al.*, 2001), general medical conditions (McWhirter and Pennington, 1996), liver disease (Cabre *et al.*, 1990; Kearns *et al.*, 1992; Hasse *et al.*, 1995), cancer (Tandon *et al.*, 1984) or following surgery (GI or orthopaedic) (Sagar *et al.*, 1979; Hoover *et al.*, 1980; Ryan *et al.*, 1981; Bastow *et al.*, 1983; Schroeder *et al.*, 1991; Beier-Holgersen and Boesby, 1996; Carr *et al.*, 1996).

Ninety-five per cent (21/22) of NRT that assessed energy intakes showed improvements in total energy intake with ETF, of which > 50% were significant over time (*n* 7) or compared with a non-random control group (*n* 4). These were trials undertaken in patients with burns (Hansbrough and Hansbrough, 1993), COPD (Goldstein *et al.*, 1988), head injury (Grahm *et al.*, 1989), the elderly (Lipschitz and Mitchell, 1982), general medical conditions (Bennegard *et al.*, 1983; Bastow *et al.*, 1985; Hebuterne *et al.*, 1995; Schneider *et al.*, 1996), liver disease (Soberon *et al.*, 1987; Smith *et al.*, 1992), cancer (Haffejee and Angorn, 1979) or cystic fibrosis (Daniels *et al.*, 1989) or in those post-surgery (Yeung *et al.*, 1979b; Moncure *et al.*, 1999).

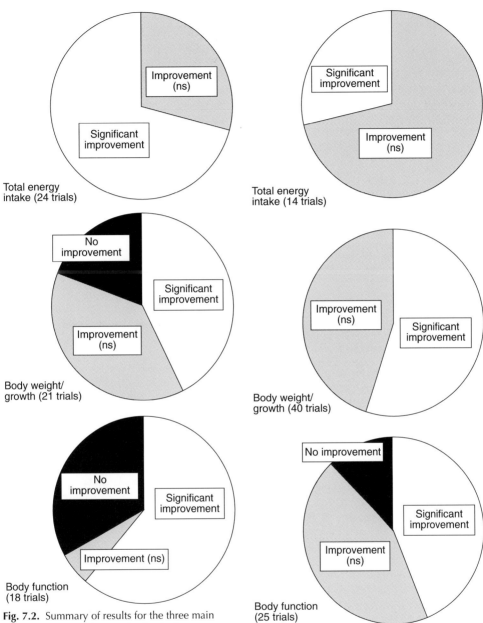

Fig. 7.2. Summary of results for the three main outcome measures (energy intake, body weight/growth, body function) from hospital trials of enteral tube feeding (RCT and NRT *n* 24 trials).

Fig. 7.3. Summary of results for the three main outcome measures (energy intake, body weight/growth, body function) from community trials of enteral tube feeding (RCT and NRT *n* 40 trials).

Nutritional intake in community patients

Fourteen trials in the community made assessments of the changes in total energy intake with ETF. All of these reported improvements either compared with a con-

trol group (RCT in cancer patients (Hearne *et al.*, 1985) and paediatrics (Patrick *et al.*, 1986)) or compared with pre-ETF intakes (a variety of trials in general medicine, paediatric and elderly patients) (Shepherd *et al.*, 1983; Bertrand *et al.*, 1984; Moore *et al.*, 1986; O'Loughlin *et al.*, 1986; Belli *et al.*, 1988; Breslow *et al.*, 1993; Duche *et al.*, 1999) (see Fig. 7.3). In 29% of these trials, the improvements were statistically significant (Bertrand *et al.*, 1984; Moore *et al.*, 1986; O'Loughlin *et al.*, 1986; Belli *et al.*, 1988). The improvements in total energy intake with ETF appeared not to be sustained once the artificial nutrition was stopped (Moore *et al.*, 1986).

These findings highlight the efficacy of using ETF to maintain or improve nutritional intake in two different ways: as a sole source of nutrition in patients in whom food intake is contraindicated or as a supplement to food intake in patients able to eat. The use of ETF for these purposes is discussed below.

Use of ETF as a sole source of nutrition in hospital and community patients

In patients who are physically unable to eat or in whom food intake is contraindicated, ETF appears to be the most effective and physiological way of providing nutrition to meet macro- and micronutrient requirements. As ETF is relatively safe and easy to administer and generally widely tolerated by patients with a wide range of diagnoses, it has increasingly been used as a sole source of nutrition in both hospital and community patients:

● The surveys and studies reviewed have highlighted the ease of use and effectiveness of ETF as a sole source of nutrition in those patient groups with chronic disease in whom food intake is contraindicated (e.g. stroke patients and those with other dysphagic conditions, patients with inflammatory bowel disease (IBD)) (Elia *et al.*, 2000a, 2001a). ETF is commonly used in this way in patients in both the community and hospital settings. For example, ETF as a sole source of nutrition may promote remission in both adults and children with Crohn's disease, in community and hospital settings (Afdhal *et al.*, 1989; Rigaud *et al.*, 1991; Royall *et al.*,

1994; Mansfield *et al.*, 1995). More specifically, home ETF is most commonly used as a sole source of nutrition in patients with neurological conditions (CVA, persistent vegetative state (PVS), multiple sclerosis (MS), etc.) (Wicks *et al.*, 1992; Howard *et al.*, 1995; Elia *et al.*, 2000a, 2001a,b). Indeed, national surveys suggest that in the community there has been marked growth in the use of ETF as a sole source of nutrition in adults with chronic diseases, particularly those with CVA or obstructive cancers that prevent oral intake (Howard *et al.*, 1995; Elia *et al.*, 2001b). Before the development of ETF, these patients would have become progressively malnourished, often remaining in hospital for prolonged periods of time, some ultimately dying from dehydration or starvation or the complications of the underlying disease. ETF allows patients to be discharged home or to long-term care while an adequate nutrient intake is maintained.

● Hospital-based studies suggest that ETF can be used to maintain energy and nutrient balance to a significantly greater extent than routine clinical care or delaying the use of ETF, particularly at critical times when oral nutrition would not be feasible or recommended. These include the early post-burn period (two RCT), critical illness and injury (six RCT), in the early postoperative period (seven RCT), in pancreatitis (one RCT) and following an oesophageal variceal bleed (one RCT). In these studies ETF into the duodenum or jejunum has particularly been used to maximize the nutritional intake of such patients. If ETF is not used, the nutritional supply to these patient groups would be low at a time when some of the nutritional requirements are increased (e.g. burns). The alternative parenteral route is substantially more expensive and should be reserved for those patients in whom the GI tract is not functioning (see Chapter 9). In some cases, a combination of ETF and PN may be appropriate (e.g. postoperative GI surgical patient with moderate–severe intestinal failure).

- Specific feeds may be used as the sole source of nutrition in a number of patient groups. These include modified formulations for diabetic patients to aid glycaemic control (Craig *et al.*, 1998) and specific feeds for use in critically ill and post-surgical cancer patients. These are not considered in any depth in this review.
- Distressing appetite sensations may occur in patients fed solely by tube. A small survey of tube-fed patients in hospital and community settings indicated that between 20 and 50% experienced hunger and as many as 83% had a desire to eat. One-third of patients on long-term home ETF were distressed by hunger (Stratton, 1999). A couple of studies (in head and neck cancer patients who were nil by mouth and solely fed by tube their estimated requirements) have also suggested that ETF may not be as satiating as oral intake. During 21 days of ETF, 50% of cancer patients were thirsty and > 50% felt deprived of the act of eating, even after just 7 days (Bruning *et al.*, 1988). In a similar patient group, 46% were moderately hungry while receiving ETF (Roberge *et al.*, 2000). Strategies to prevent distressing appetite sensations in those in whom food intake is contraindicated need investigation. Similarly, manipulation of ETF so that it has a minimal effect on the appetite of patients who are trying to increase their oral intake would be desirable (Stratton, 1999).

In summary, ETF as a sole source of nutrition has become an indispensable treatment for patients who are unable to eat due to acute or chronic disease, in both the short and long term.

Use of ETF as a supplement to food intake in hospital and community patients

ETF can be used as an effective way of increasing the nutritional intake of patients who are able to eat (see Fig. 7.4). The studies reviewed have highlighted the efficacy of using ETF as a supplement to food intake in patients across age-groups (paediatrics to elderly), settings (hospitals, community) and diagnostic groups (neurology, cancer, COPD, cystic fibrosis, GI and liver disease, human immunodeficiency virus (HIV) and in those recovering from surgery and other medical procedures).

Only a few studies in hospitalized patients (*n* 9: Sagar *et al.*, 1979; Ryan *et al.*, 1981; Lipschitz and Mitchell, 1982; Bastow *et al.*, 1983; Bennegard *et al.*, 1983; Tandon *et al.*, 1984; Smith *et al.*, 1992; Hebuterne *et al.*, 1995; McWhirter and Pennington, 1996) reported the impact of ETF on voluntary food intake. The findings suggested that the energy provided by ETF in patients with

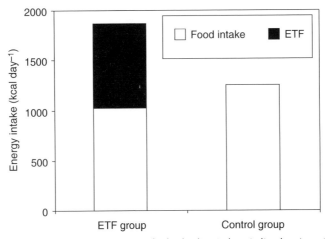

Fig. 7.4. Increase in total energy intake with enteral tube feeding in hospitalized patients (data adapted from McWhirter and Pennington, 1996; 51 patients).

various conditions was largely additive to food intake, because it had little effect on oral intake (Fig. 7.4). On the contrary, some studies indicated that ETF might help to stimulate appetite and improve voluntary food intake in previously anorectic/under-nourished patients during their recovery (Sagar *et al.*, 1979; Ryan *et al.*, 1981; Lipschitz and Mitchell, 1982; Bennegard *et al.*, 1983; Tandon *et al.*, 1984; Smith *et al.*, 1992; Hebuterne *et al.*, 1995). The findings from the community studies are similar. Information from five community-based trials (Pareira *et al.*, 1954; Greene *et al.*, 1981; Bastow *et al.*, 1985; O'Loughlin *et al.*, 1986; Süttman *et al.*, 1993) suggested that ETF had little suppressive effect on appetite/food intake. In addition, it appears that stimulation of appetite and food intake had occurred when weight gain followed ETF, although these observations were longitudinal and there was no control group (Greene *et al.*, 1981; Bastow *et al.*, 1985). Furthermore, controlled investigations in healthy subjects have suggested that the energy provided by ETF is largely additional to that taken orally and has little suppressive effect on appetite (Stratton *et al.*, 1998; Stratton and Elia, 1999b).

Effects of ETF on intake according to patient group

The efficacy of ETF at increasing nutritional intake when used as a sole source of nutrition or as a supplement to food intake varies across different patient groups, as indicated in Box 7.3. ETF can be an effective supplement to improve the total nutritional intake of a variety of patients when used in combination with the oral route. In patients unable to eat sufficient food to meet their energy requirements, ETF has little effect in suppressing their oral intake. The benefits to body function and clinical outcome of using ETF as a sole source of nutrition or as a supplement to food intake are subsequently discussed.

For more details about the individual studies, including references within patient-specific groups, see Appendices 5 and 6.

(II) What effect does ETF have on the body weight and composition of patients in hospital and community settings?

ETF can be used to improve body weight and nutritional status or to prevent loss of weight (including fat and muscle mass) in a variety of diagnostic groups across hospital and community settings.

Body weight changes in hospital patients

ETF may improve body weight or reduce weight loss compared with routine care in hospital patients. Most trials (78%, 40/51) assessing body weight found that ETF produced greater increments in body weight (or smaller losses in weight), of which 50% were significant (9 (23%) versus a control group; 11 (28%) versus baseline)). These included studies of patients receiving ETF as a sole source of nutrition or as a supplement to food intake. A similar proportion (81%) of RCT showed improvements in body weight (17/21), 53% (*n* 9) of which were significant compared with a control group (*n* 7) or over time (*n* 2) (see Fig. 7.2). These included trials undertaken in patients with burns (Chiarelli *et al.*, 1990), COPD (Whittaker *et al.*, 1990), cystic fibrosis (Shepherd *et al.*, 1988), critical illness (Moore and Jones, 1986), general medical conditions (McWhirter and Pennington, 1996), cancer (Tandon *et al.*, 1984) and liver disease (de Ledinghen *et al.*, 1997) and in orthopaedic (Bastow *et al.*, 1983) and other surgical patients (Sagar *et al.*, 1979; Hoover *et al.*, 1980; Ryan *et al.*, 1981; Smith *et al.*, 1985; Schroeder *et al.*, 1991; Carr *et al.*, 1996). Combined analysis of % weight change (weighted for sample size) from nine RCT in adults (*n* 312) indicated an attenuation of weight loss (−1.12%) in patients receiving ETF versus controls (−6.62%) (see Fig. 7.5) (Ryan *et al.*, 1981; Tandon *et al.*, 1984; Moore and Jones, 1986; Chiarelli *et al.*, 1990; Whittaker *et al.*, 1990; Schroeder *et al.*, 1991; Chuntrasakul *et al.*, 1996; McWhirter and Pennington, 1996; de Ledinghen *et al.*, 1997). Meta-analysis of four trials (*n* 129)

Box 7.3. Effect of ETF on food and total intake in different patient groups (hospital and community settings).

Burns (hospital only)
ETF in patients with acute burns injury, who are often unable to take nutrition orally, may facilitate a substantial energy, nitrogen and micronutrient intake throughout the recovery period.

COPD (hospital only)
Total energy intakes can be significantly improved when ETF is used as a supplement to food intake in patients with COPD in hospital.

Critical injury/illness (hospital only)
ETF (particularly duodenal/jejunal feeding) can be valuable as the sole source of nutrition in such patients in that total energy and protein intakes can be greatly increased (relative to no nutritional support). There is increasing interest in using modified/enriched enteral feeds to improve the intake of a number of nutrients (omega-3 fatty acids, arginine, glutamine, β-carotene) during critical illness.

Cystic fibrosis
ETF, typically as a supplement to food intake, has been shown to improve energy and nutrient intakes in patients with cystic fibrosis in the community and the hospital. A high-energy diet given orally may be as effective as ETF within the hospital setting.

Elderly (NRT only)
ETF can increase total nutritional intake and may lead to improvements in food intake in elderly patients in hospital and community settings.

Gastrointestinal disease
ETF can be used as a sole source of nutrition in patients with various GI diseases (e.g. acute pancreatitis, Crohn's disease) and post-GI-surgery to maintain nutritional supply when patients are otherwise nil by mouth as food intake is contraindicated.

General medical/mixed patient groups
ETF can be a useful way of increasing the energy and nutrient intakes of a variety of hospitalized and community patients who are unable to consume sufficient oral diet. ETF appears not to substantially reduce food intake, which may even improve. ETF is also a valuable means of maintaining nutritional intake in those in whom food intake is contraindicated, both for short periods of time in hospital and for long periods of time in the community.

HIV/AIDS (community NRT only)
Very limited data suggest that ETF may improve energy intakes without affecting oral intake.

Liver disease
ETF as a supplement to food intake can increase energy and nutrient intakes substantially in patients with liver disease (cirrhosis, alcoholic liver disease) and in patients post-liver-transplant. The impact of ETF on food intake requires exploration.

Malignancy
ETF as a supplement to diet may improve appetite and food intake and increase total nutritional intake in some patients with cancer. In those patients with severe anorexia and undergoing cancer treatments, ETF may be preferred by patients and be more effective than the oral route as a way of providing nutritional support in both hospital and community settings.

Neurology (NRT only)
ETF, particularly via gastrostomy, is a valuable means of providing a sole source of nutrition to CVA patients and others who are dysphagic and in whom food intake is contraindicated.

Orthopaedics (hospital only)
Overnight ETF in fractured neck of femur patients can significantly improve total intake, without substantially reducing food intake.

Paediatrics
In both hospital and community settings, ETF can be used as a way of increasing the nutritional intake of children with a variety of conditions, either when used in addition to food or as a sole source of nutrition (conditions include congenital heart disease, critical illness, Crohn's disease and other GI diseases, cerebral palsy, cancer, HIV/AIDS, cystic fibrosis).

Renal disease (community NRT only)
No data on intake.

Surgery (hospital only)
ETF in the early postoperative period and beyond can significantly increase intake compared with standard management. In patients given ETF, food intake may be similar to or greater than in those on diet alone (controls).

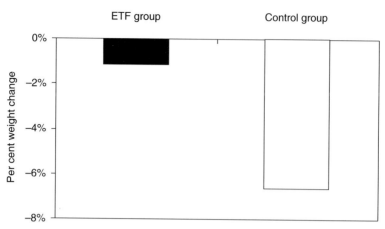

Fig. 7.5. Attenuation of weight loss with enteral tube feeding in the hospital setting (results of nine RCT, 312 patients; weighted mean analysis).

that presented appropriate data (mean and standard deviation (SD) of % weight change) (Ryan *et al.*, 1981; Chiarelli *et al.*, 1990; Schroeder *et al.*, 1991; Chuntrasakul *et al.*, 1996) suggested a mean effect size of 1.41 (95% confident interval (CI) 0.66–2.16), with significant heterogeneity between study results (fixed-effects model).

As most studies failed to document the body mass index (BMI), it is difficult to establish conclusions about changes in weight in relation to initial nutritional status. For example, % weight change following ETF was greater in one trial in which patients were initially underweight (difference of +6%) (Whittaker *et al.*, 1990) than when average BMI was > 20 kg m^{-2} (+3%) (Ryan *et al.*, 1981). In children with cystic fibrosis, the relationship of weight gain to initial nutritional status was explored, with a significant correlation between the extent of initial underweight and subsequent weight gain (Shepherd *et al.*, 1988). In another trial, weight gain was only observed when ETF was 'successful' (well tolerated by patients and prescribed volumes received by patient) (Smith *et al.*, 1985).

Twenty-three NRT (77%, 23/30) that assessed changes in body weight with ETF also showed weight gain over time or greater weight gain/less weight loss than a control group (of which 48% were signifi-

cant, *n* 11). These trials included patients in paediatric (Daniels *et al.*, 1989; Finch and Lawson, 1993) and elderly groups (Lipschitz and Mitchell, 1982) and in various diagnostic groups, including COPD (Goldstein *et al.*, 1988), critical illness/ injury (Grahm *et al.*, 1989), GI disease (Afdhal *et al.*, 1989; Rigaud *et al.*, 1991; Royall *et al.*, 1994), general medical conditions (Bennegard *et al.*, 1983; Bastow *et al.*, 1985; Dresler *et al.*, 1987; Hebuterne *et al.*, 1995; Schneider *et al.*, 1996; Gentile *et al.*, 2000; Winter *et al.*, 2000), cancer (Haffejee and Angorn, 1979; de Vries *et al.*, 1982), neurological disease (Park *et al.*, 1992; Norton *et al.*, 1996) and those post-surgery (Yeung *et al.*, 1979b; Shukla *et al.*, 1984). In those with neurological conditions (CVA), using a percutaneous endoscopic gastrostomy (PEG) for ETF appeared to be more effective at improving nutritional status than nasogastric (NG) feeding (Park *et al.*, 1992; Norton *et al.*, 1996). Overall, the average longitudinal weight change from 19 NRT of ETF across diagnostic groups was +2.15 (4.73) kg.

Body weight changes in community patients

In community patients, ETF may improve or maintain body weight and nutritional status. All studies that assessed changes in body weight (*n* 40) showed some benefit (weight gain or less weight loss) (see Fig. 7.3). Some studies suggested that ETF was an effective way of stabilizing weight and nutritional status (Chernoff *et al.*, 1990; Breslow *et al.*, 1993; Von Herz *et al.*, 2000), but the majority of trials (*n* 36) indicated that ETF could lead to weight gain in community patients. Significant improvements in body weight were reported in the three RCT that involved COPD (Donahoe *et al.*, 1994), cancer (Hearne *et al.*, 1985) and paediatric patients (Patrick *et al.*, 1986). From these RCT, the difference in % weight change between ETF and control patients ranged from +39% (paediatrics) (Patrick *et al.*, 1986) to +7.5% in adult cancer patients (Hearne *et al.*, 1985). Meta-analysis of these data could not be undertaken because the standard deviation of % weight change was not reported. Similarly, 19 NRT (51%) showed significant improvements in weight, compared either with a non-random control group (*n* 5) or with baseline values (*n* 14) obtained in trials of patients with cystic fibrosis, HIV/AIDS and renal disease and in paediatric and adult patients with a variety of disorders. In all of these trials, average BMI was < 20 kg m^{-2}.

Changes in body weight with ETF according to patient group

The effectiveness of ETF at increasing body weight or attenuating weight loss varied substantially across different patient groups, as shown in Box 7.4. Lean tissue mass also appears to be maintained to a greater degree with ETF, compared with routine clinical care. For more details, see Appendices 5 and 6, although information is lacking for some patient groups in some care settings.

Body composition changes in hospital and community patients

There is limited information from the studies reviewed about the changes in body composition following ETF in the hospital setting. Ten RCT and 14 NRT in critically ill, injured, general medical, orthopaedic and surgical patients and in those with COPD, liver disease, cancer and cystic fibrosis made some assessment of body composition, principally by using upper-arm anthropometry. Two RCT (Bastow *et al.*, 1983; McWhirter and Pennington, 1996) and 11 NRT indicated improvements in such anthropometric parameters, of which nine (two RCT) were significant, typically over time. These showed increases in fat and/or muscle mass or an attenuation of loss. Other trials, including those in patients with liver disease (Foschi *et al.*, 1986; Cabre *et al.*, 1990) and cancer (Van Bokhorst-de van der Schueren *et al.*, 2001) and those post-surgery (Schroeder *et al.*, 1991; Carr *et al.*, 1996), found no benefits (total of *n* 11, eight RCT and three NRT). Very few trials assessed the presence of oedema, which may confound measurements of body weight and other anthropometric parameters, including the presence of ascites in those with liver disease.

In the community, 16 trials made assessments of body composition following a period of ETF. Eighty-eight per cent of these studies (*n* 14) indicated improvements in fat and/or muscle mass with ETF in patients with COPD (Irwin and Openbrier, 1985; Donahoe *et al.*, 1994), cystic fibrosis (Shepherd *et al.*, 1983; Bertrand *et al.*, 1984; Levy *et al.*, 1985; Boland *et al.*, 1986; O'Loughlin *et al.*, 1986; Steinkamp and von der Hardt, 1994), HIV/AIDS (Brantsma *et al.*, 1991; Süttmann *et al.*, 1993), cancer (Fietkau *et al.*, 1991; den Broeder *et al.*, 2000) and renal disease (Sayce *et al.*, 2000) and in mixed groups of general medical patients (Bastow *et al.*, 1985). In only two trials were the changes not statistically significant (Bastow *et al.*, 1985; Irwin and Openbrier, 1985). In one trial in children with cystic fibrosis, no improvements were observed (Moore *et al.*, 1986) and, in a group of elderly patients, measurements of mid-arm muscle area improved in 46% and deteriorated in 54% of patients (Bannerman *et al.*, 1999).

Box 7.4. Effect of ETF on body weight, composition and growth in different patient groups (hospital and community settings).

Burns (hospital only)
ETF may reduce the weight loss typically seen in those with burn injury.

COPD (hospital only)
ETF can significantly increase body weight compared with a control group and may improve muscle mass.

Critical injury/illness (hospital only)
ETF can attenuate some of the weight loss that accompanies critical illness and injury, compared with routine clinical care.

Cystic fibrosis
ETF may facilitate increases in body weight or improvements in growth in growth-retarded children with cystic fibrosis, in hospital and community settings. Muscle mass may also be improved.

Elderly (NRT only)
ETF in elderly patients in both hospital and community settings may lead to weight stabilization or weight gain.

Gastrointestinal disease (NRT only)
The use of ETF in patients with GI disease (Crohn's disease) may increase body weight and body fat.

General medical/mixed patient groups
ETF can improve body weight and indices of muscle mass in patients with acute and chronic diseases in hospital, compared with controls. In the community, ETF may also be used as a means of maintaining nutritional status in patients who are unable to eat (e.g. CVA patients).

HIV/AIDS (community NRT only)
In underweight patients with HIV and AIDS, ETF may lead to improvements in body weight and lean tissue.

Liver disease (hospital only)
Gain in body weight or less loss of weight compared with routine care has been found in this patient group, but the confounding effects of ascites need to be considered. Assessment of body composition may be more reliable as an indicator of the effects of this intervention on nutritional status.

Malignancy
ETF can significantly reduce weight loss or lead to weight gain in patients with cancer, including those receiving chemotherapy. In some groups (e.g. nasopharyngeal cancer), gastrostomy feeding may be more effective at improving nutritional status than nasogastric feeding.

Neurology (NRT only)
ETF is one of the main ways of maintaining or improving the nutritional status of patients with neurological disease who are unable to eat (in whom food intake is contraindicated). The impact on body weight and composition when used as a supplement to intake requires study.

Orthopaedics (hospital only)
ETF can improve body weight and fat mass when used in hospitalized fractured neck of femur patients. It may be most effective in the most undernourished patients.

Paediatrics
ETF can improve growth in growth-retarded children with a variety of conditions (cerebral palsy, liver disease, HIV/AIDS, cancer, renal disease, congenital heart disease, cystic fibrosis (see above)).

Renal disease (community NRT only)
ETF may increase body weight, fat and muscle mass in haemodialysis patients.

Surgery (hospital only)
ETF can significantly attenuate the weight loss that typically occurs postoperatively when compared with control patients.

ETF and growth of children in hospital and community settings

This review suggests that ETF in infants and children with growth failure may improve growth (weight-for-age, weight-for-height and height-for-age). For example, two NRT in the hospital setting indicated improvements in the growth of children with Crohn's disease (significant) (Morin *et al.*, 1980) or a variety of diagnoses (Finch and Lawson, 1993).

In the community setting, improvements in growth (including weight-for-age, weight-for-height and height-for-age) were recorded in 21 trials (one RCT: Patrick *et al.*, 1986) in growth-retarded children with conditions that included cystic fibrosis (Shepherd *et al.*, 1983, 1986; Bertrand *et al.*, 1984; Levy *et al.*, 1985; Boland *et al.*, 1986; Moore *et al.*, 1986; O'Loughlin *et al.*, 1986; Dalzell *et al.*, 1992; Steinkamp and von der Hardt, 1994; see Fig. 7.6), HIV (Henderson *et al.*, 1994), GI disease (Belli *et al.*, 1988; Aiges *et al.*, 1989; Chin *et al.*, 1990; Cosgrove and Jenkins, 1997; Duche *et al.*, 1999), cancer (Aquino *et al.*, 1995; den Broeder *et al.*, 1998, 2000) and a mixed diagnostic group (Greene *et al.*, 1981; Patrick *et al.*, 1986; Papadopoulou *et al.*, 1995). These improvements were assessed as significant in all but four trials (Greene *et al.*, 1981; Aquino *et al.*, 1995; Papadopoulou *et al.*, 1995; Duche *et al.*, 1999).

(III) What effect does ETF have on the body function of patients in hospital and community settings?

ETF can lead to a variety of functional benefits compared with the use of routine clinical care in the hospital or community setting (see Tables 7.9 and 7.10). The type of functional benefit varies depending on the diagnostic group of the patient. Functional benefits within different disease groups are summarized in Tables 7.11 and 7.12 and in Appendices 5 and 6.

Functional outcomes in hospital patients

Functional benefits may follow the use of ETF in a variety of patient groups in the hospital setting. Of those trials that assessed body function (*n* 35), 77% showed functional benefits (*n* 27), of which 22 (81%) were significant (see Table 7.9 and Fig. 7.2). Sixty-seven per cent of RCT that assessed function (12/18) suggested that ETF produced benefits in patients with COPD (Whittaker *et al.*, 1990), cystic fibrosis (Shepherd *et al.*, 1988), critical illness/injury (Moore and Jones, 1986; Kompan *et al.*, 1999), GI disease (Pupelis *et al.*, 2001), liver disease (Cabre *et al.*, 1990; Kearns *et al.*, 1992) and cancer (Tandon *et al.*,

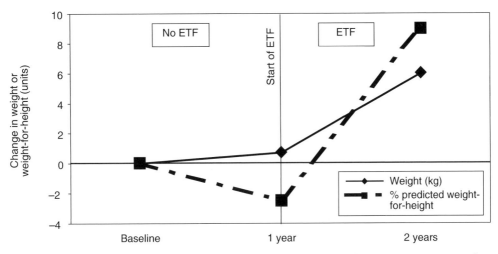

Fig. 7.6. Improved growth following enteral tube feeding in community paediatric patients in an NRT (data adapted from Steinkamp and von der Hardt, 1994; *n* 14).

Table 7.11. Summary of significant functional outcome benefits from RCT (compared with control group) according to patient group following enteral tube feeding in the hospital setting (significant changes over time from RCT and NRT in parentheses).

Disease/patient group	Improvements in functional outcome following ETF in hospital patients
COPD	Improved maximal expiratory pressure and sustained inspiratory pressure (endurance) (Whittaker *et al.*, 1990)
	(Improved maximal inspiratory and expiratory pressures, hamstring strength and endurance (Goldstein *et al.*, 1988))
Cystic fibrosis	(Improved forced expiratory volume (Shepherd *et al.*, 1988))
Critically ill/injury	Prevention of increases in intestinal permeability seen in those not given ETF (Kompan *et al.*, 1999), improved immune function (Moore and Jones, 1986)
Elderly	(Improved immune function (Lipschitz and Mitchell, 1982))
Gastroenterology	Earlier return of GI function (Pupelis *et al.*, 2001)
	(Improvements in Crohn's disease activity/inflammatory markers (Abad-Lacruz *et al.*, 1988; Afdhal *et al.*, 1989; Rigaud *et al.*, 1991; Royall *et al.*, 1994))
	(Improved vitamin status (Abad-Lacruz *et al.*, 1988))
General medical	(Improved immunological parameters (Schneider *et al.*, 1996))
	(Improved intestinal absorption and GI function (Winter *et al.*, 2000))
Liver disease	Improved liver function (Cabre *et al.*, 1990; Kearns *et al.*, 1992)
Malignancy	Improved physical and emotional functioning and dyspnoea symptoms (Van Bokhorst-de von der Schueren *et al.*, 2000b, 2001)
	(Immunological improvements (Haffejee and Angorn, 1979; Lipschitz and Mitchell, 1980; Tandon *et al.*, 1984))
Surgery	Earlier return of bowel function (Beier-Holgersen and Boesby, 1996),
	Significant attenuation of increases in gut permeability (Carr *et al.*, 1996)
	Greater wound-healing rate (Schroeder *et al.*, 1991)
	(Immunological benefits (Shukla *et al.*, 1984))

Table 7.12. Summary of improvements in functional and clinical outcome according to patient group following enteral tube feeding in the community setting from NRT only (non-significant trends in parentheses). This table contains information from non-randomized trials only – none of the RCT made assessments of function.

Disease/patient group	Improvements in functional and clinical outcome following ETF in community patients
COPD	(Improved maximal inspiratory and expiratory pressures, less breathlessness (Irwin and Openbrier, 1985))
	(Frequency and duration of hospital stays reduced (Irwin and Openbrier, 1985))
Cystic fibrosis	Improved well-being (O'Loughlin *et al.*, 1986)
	Less deterioration or improvements in pulmonary function (Shepherd *et al.*, 1986; Steinkamp and von der Hardt, 1994)
	Improved clinical scores (Shepherd *et al.*, 1983; Moore *et al.*, 1986)
	Fewer episodes of pneumonia (O'Loughlin *et al.*, 1986)
	(Increased daily activities (Levy *et al.*, 1985; Boland *et al.*, 1986))
	(Lower mortality and hospital admissions (Dalzell *et al.*, 1992))
Elderly	Reduction in pressure ulcer surface area (Breslow *et al.*, 1993)
GI/liver disease	Reduction in Crohn's disease activity[a] (Belli *et al.*, 1988; Mansfield *et al.*, 1995)
(adults and paediatrics)	Improved clinical scores (Aiges *et al.*, 1989)
	Reduction in medication (Cosgrove and Jenkins, 1997)
General medical	Improved quality of life (Schneider *et al.*, 2000a)
	(Shorter hospital stay (Jagar-Wittenear *et al.*, 2000))
HIV/AIDS	Immunological benefits (Kotler *et al.*, 1991) (Improved quality of life (Brantsma *et al.*, 1991))
Malignancy	(Improved quality of life (Roberge *et al.*, 2000))
Renal disease	(Shorter hospital stay (Sayce *et al.*, 2000))

[a]Significant in paediatrics only.

1984;Van Bokhorst-de van der Schueren *et al.*, 2000b) and in surgical patients in the postoperative period (Schroeder *et al.*, 1991; Beier-Holgersen and Boesby, 1996; Carr *et al.*, 1996). In all but one of these trials (Kompan *et al.*, 1999), the functional benefits were statistically significant. Similarly, 88% (15/17) of NRT in patients with a variety of conditions (including COPD (Goldstein *et al.*, 1988), GI disease (Abad-Lacruz *et al.*, 1988; Afdhal *et al.*, 1989; Kudsk *et al.*, 1990; Rigaud *et al.*, 1991; Royall *et al.*, 1994), general medical conditions (Schneider *et al.*, 1996; Winter *et al.*, 2000), liver disease (Smith *et al.*, 1982; Keohane *et al.*, 1983) and cancer (Haffejee and Angorn, 1979; Lipschitz and Mitchell, 1980) and in post-surgical (Shukla *et al.*, 1984) and elderly (Lipschitz and Mitchell, 1982) patients) indicated improvements in functional measures with ETF, of which 73% (*n* 11) were significant. From the findings of the RCT and the NRT reviewed, the functional outcomes found to improve with ETF in specific patient groups are shown in Table 7.11.

Average % weight change in studies documenting significant functional changes with ETF was 6% greater than in controls ((−0.46 vs. −6.36) data from four studies (*n* 167) in adults (Tandon *et al.*, 1984; Moore and Jones, 1986; Whittaker *et al.*, 1990; Schroeder *et al.*, 1991)). There was insufficient data to assess the changes in weight in trials that did not show functional benefits. However, functional benefits were more likely in trials in which patients were underweight. All RCT and NRT in patient groups with an average BMI < 20 kg m^{-2} showed functional benefits (where assessed), compared with 50% of trials in patients with an average BMI > 20 kg m^{-2} (see Table 7.9). As the number of trials that documented BMI was small (see Table 7.9), further studies are needed to confirm this observation.

Of the 35 trials that assessed function, only eight found no positive effect of ETF (see Fig. 7.2), and these were typically small trials. In one small trial of patients post-GI surgery (Watters *et al.*, 1997), those fed enterally had a lower vital capacity (a measure of respiratory function) and physical activity levels in the postoperative period than the control group. The majority of trials reviewed (53% of all trials, *n* 39) did not make any assessments of functional outcomes following ETF. Therefore, future investigations in this area are required (refer to Chapter 10 for guidance on designing studies).

Functional outcomes in community patients

The appropriate use of ETF in patients in the community can also lead to improvements in some functional outcome measures. Eighty-eight per cent of trials that formally assessed function (*n* 22/25) reported improvements (see Table 7.10 and Fig. 7.3) and all were NRT. In 11 trials, the changes were significant over time (*n* 8) or compared with a control group (*n* 3). The type of functional benefit varied, depending on the diagnostic group, but a variety of improvements were seen in patients with COPD (Irwin and Openbrier, 1985), cystic fibrosis (Shepherd *et al.*, 1983, 1986; Levy *et al.*, 1985; Boland *et al.*, 1986; Moore *et al.*, 1986; O'Loughlin *et al.*, 1986; Dalzell *et al.*, 1992; Steinkamp and von der Hardt, 1994), GI disease (Mansfield *et al.*, 1995), HIV (Brantsma *et al.*, 1991; Kotler *et al.*, 1991) and cancer (Fietkau *et al.*, 1991; Roberge *et al.*, 2000) and in paediatric (Greene *et al.*, 1981; Belli *et al.*, 1988; Aiges *et al.*, 1989), elderly (with pressure ulcers) (Chernoff *et al.*, 1990; Breslow *et al.*, 1993) and mixed groups of adult patients (Schneider *et al.*, 2000c; Von Herz *et al.*, 2000). These are summarized in Table 7.12.

In some NRT, anecdotal information suggested that patients' activity levels increased following ETF (Pareira *et al.*, 1954; Bastow *et al.*, 1985). Some studies (both hospital- and community-based) indicated improvements in some biochemical markers (Greene *et al.*, 1981; Seri and Aquilio, 1984; Fietkau *et al.*, 1991; Süttmann *et al.*, 1993; Edington *et al.*, 1994; Watters *et al.*, 1997), although these were not consistently reported (Chuntrasakul *et al.*, 1996; den Broeder *et al.*, 2000).

Functional benefits according to patient group

The functional changes following ETF for each specific patient group have been summarized in Tables 7.11 (hospital) and 7.12 (community), for conditions for which data exists. For detailed information on the functional outcomes for each of the patient groups from individual studies, refer to Appendices 5 and 6.

(IV) What effect does ETF have on the clinical and financial outcome of patients in hospital and community settings?

Clinical outcome can be improved by the use of ETF instead of routine clinical care in a variety of patient groups in both hospital and community settings. Reductions in mortality rates, complication rates, and hospital stays can occur.

Clinical outcome in hospital patients

Thirty-six hospital trials reported assessments of clinical outcome following ETF and the majority (75%, n 27) showed some improvements. Specifically, 79% (23/29) of RCT suggested some clinical benefit following ETF, of which 57% (n 13) were assessed as statistically significant compared with a control group (see Table 7.9). These trials were undertaken in patients with various diseases or conditions, including burns (Chiarelli et al., 1990; Jenkins et al., 1994), critical illness/injury (Moore and Jones, 1986; Kompan et al., 1999; Taylor et al., 1999; Minard et al., 2000), GI disease (Pupelis et al., 2001), liver disease (Foschi et al., 1986; Cabre et al., 1990; Kearns et al., 1992; Hasse et al., 1995), cancer (Tandon et al., 1984) and in orthopaedic (Bastow et al., 1983) and other surgical patients (Sagar et al., 1979; Ryan et al., 1981; Schroeder et al., 1991; Beier-Holgersen and Boesby, 1996; Carr et al., 1996). Significant improvements in clinical outcome are shown in Table 7.13.

Difference in % weight change (weighted for sample size) was greater

(+10.2%, n 77 (Ryan et al., 1981; Moore and Jones, 1986)) in those trials in which clinical outcome improved significantly, compared with those trials in which such improvements were not documented (+5.3%, n 152 (Tandon et al., 1984; Chiarelli et al., 1990; Schroeder et al., 1991; Chuntrasakul et al., 1996)). Attenuation of weight loss was more likely with ETF than weight gain within these studies. However, interpretation of these findings is limited because of the small number of studies available for such analysis.

It is difficult to ascertain from the current available evidence whether changes in clinical outcome were more likely in trials in which patients had a BMI < 20 kg m^{-2} or > 20 kg m^{-2}. All the trials that assessed clinical outcome with patient groups that were underweight showed significant improvements (n 2/2), compared with only 50% of those in patients with an average BMI > 20 kg m^{-2} (3/6). Due to the small number of these studies, definitive conclusions cannot be made.

Of the NRT, 57% (4/7) reported improvements in clinical outcome following a period of ETF or compared with a control group in head injury (Grahm et al., 1989), general medical (Taylor, 1993), elderly (Treber and Harris, 1996), surgical (Shukla et al., 1984) and paediatric (Smith et al., 1986) patients (see Tables 7.9 and 7.13).

Although nine trials found no improvements in clinical outcome with ETF (Yeung et al., 1979b; de Vries et al., 1982; Calvey et al., 1984; Smith et al., 1985; Elmore et al., 1989; Frankel and Horowitz, 1989; de Ledinghen et al., 1997; Watters et al., 1997; Moncure et al., 1999), half of the trials (38, 51%) reviewed did not report changes in clinical outcome following ETF. Many of the trials that did assess outcome had insufficient sample sizes to adequately detect changes in such measures (see Figs 6.26 and 6.27 and the discussion in Chapter 6).

The impact of ETF on the three main clinical outcome measures in hospital patients is discussed separately below.

Table 7.13. Summary of improved clinical outcomes according to disease group following enteral tube feeding in hospital patients (significant changes from randomized controlled trials, with non-significant trends and non-randomized data in parentheses).

Disease/condition	Improvements in clinical outcome following ETF
Burns	(Shorter hospital stays (Chiarelli *et al.*, 1990))
	Fewer wound infections (Jenkins *et al.*, 1994)
Critical illness/injury	Lower number of infective complications (Moore and Jones 1986; Taylor *et al.*, 1999)
	(Lower mortality (Chuntrasakul *et al.*, 1996; Minard *et al.*, 2000))
	(Better neurological outcome (Taylor *et al.*, 1999))
Elderly	(Shorter length of hospital stay (Treber and Harris, 1996))
Gastrointestinal disease	Lower rate of reoperation (Pupelis *et al.*, 2001)
	(Lower rate of other complications (Pupelis *et al.*, 2001))
	Lower mortality (Pupelis *et al.*, 2001)
General medical	(Lower mortality rate with earlier introduction of ETF (Taylor, 1993))
Liver disease	Lower mortality rate (Cabre *et al.*, 1990)
	Lower complication rate (Foschi *et al.*, 1986), including viral complications (Hasse *et al.*, 1995)
Malignancy	(Lower mortality (Tandon *et al.*, 1984))
Orthopaedics	Shorter rehabilitation time (Bastow *et al.*, 1983)
	Shorter length of hospital stay[a] (Bastow *et al.*, 1983)
	(Lower mortality (Bastow *et al.*, 1983))
Paediatrics	(Shorter length of hospital stay (Smith *et al.*, 1986))
	(Reduced PN use (Smith *et al.*, 1986))
Surgery	Lower rate of postoperative complications, including infective complications (Beier-Holgersen and Boesby, 1996; Singh *et al.*, 1998)
	Shorter length of hospital stay (Sagar *et al.*, 1979)
	(Slightly lower mortality (Beier-Holgersen and Boesby, 1996))
	Less PN use after ETF (Beier-Holgersen and Boesby, 1996) and shorter requirement for i.v. catheter (Ryan *et al.*, 1981)

[a]'Very thin' patients only.
i.v., intravenous.

MORTALITY

This analysis suggests that the use of ETF in hospital patients can reduce mortality. Twelve trials (13 sets of data) provided information on mortality rates following ETF in a variety of patients groups: burns (Jenkins *et al.*, 1994); critical illness/injury (Chuntrasakul *et al.*, 1996; Minard *et al.*, 2000); GI/liver diseases (Cabre *et al.*, 1990; Kearns *et al.*, 1992; de Ledinghen *et al.*, 1997; Pupelis *et al.*, 2001); cancer (Tandon *et al.*, 1984); orthopaedics (Bastow *et al.*, 1983; Sullivan *et al.*, 1998); and surgery (Beier-Holgersen and Boesby, 1996; Singh *et al.*, 1998). Most (69%, 9/13) trials showed a reduction in mortality with ETF, with two trials showing significant reductions (Cabre *et al.*, 1990; Pupelis *et al.*, 2001). A combined analysis of these trials indicated that mortality rates were significantly lower in

patients receiving ETF (11%, 34/299) than controls (22%, 66/301; data from 12 RCT, *n* 600; $P < 0.001$; see Fig. 7.7). Similar differences in mortality rates were observed in trials of patients with a BMI < 20 kg m^{-2} (11% vs. 23%; two studies, *n* 184 (Bastow *et al.*, 1983; Cabre *et al.*, 1990)), BMI > 20 kg m^{-2} (13% vs. 19%; five studies, *n* 176 (Kearns *et al.*, 1992; Beier-Holgersen and Boesby, 1996; de Ledinghen *et al.*, 1997; Singh *et al.*, 1998; Sullivan *et al.*, 1998)) or in which BMI was unknown (11% vs. 23%; five studies, *n* 267 (Tandon *et al.*, 1984; Jenkins *et al.*, 1994; Chuntrasakul *et al.*, 1996; Minard *et al.*, 2000; Pupelis *et al.*, 2001)).

Meta-analysis

All trials. Meta-analysis of these trials revealed an odds ratio in favour of ETF of

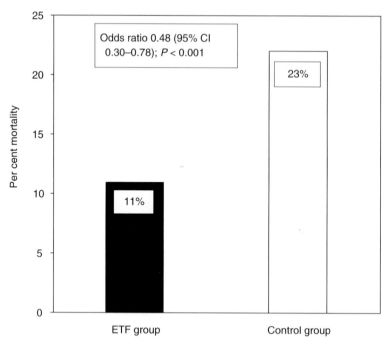

Fig. 7.7. Lower mortality rates with enteral tube feeding compared with routine clinical care (12 RCT, 600 patients).

0.48 (95% CI 0.30–0.78), with no significant heterogeneity between studies. However, preliminary statistics (Rosenthal's fail-safe score, quartile plots) suggest that larger numbers of trials/patients are needed to assess the impact of ETF on mortality, if publication bias or differences in responses between patient populations are to be excluded. Within the trials included in the meta-analysis, there was variation in the mortality response associated with ETF. Nine RCT showed a reduction in mortality, of which two were significant, and four trials showed increases, none of which were significant. The lack of significance in some of these individual trials probably represents a type 2 error due to small sample sizes (see Fig. 6.26, Chapter 6). In those trials that showed non-significant reductions in mortality (n 7), the difference in % weight change between ETF and control groups was 6–8%. (There were no data on differences in % weight change in the trials in which significant reductions in mortality were documented and in trials in which small increases in mortality were found.)

According to BMI. For studies in which the mean BMI of patients was < 20 kg m^{-2}, the odds ratio for mortality with ETF was lower (0.44 (95% CI 0.07–2.81), n 157, two trials (Bastow *et al.*, 1983; Cabre *et al.*, 1990)), compared with those with a BMI > 20 kg m^{-2} (odds ratio 0.62 (95% CI 0.2–1.94), n 176, five trials (Kearns *et al.*, 1992; Beier-Holgersen and Boesby, 1996; de Ledinghen *et al.*, 1997; Singh *et al.*, 1998; Sullivan *et al.*, 1998)), although in neither group were the reductions significant, possibly due to the small numbers included in the analysis.

According to patient group. Meta-analysis of studies in some patient groups also indicated that mortality may be reduced, but not significantly so, and the small numbers of studies limit conclusions: critical illness/injury (three studies, odds ratio 0.23 (95% CI 0.03–2.16)); liver disease (three studies, odds ratio 0.42 (95% CI 0.05–3.44)) and orthopaedics (three studies, odds ratio 0.52 (95% CI 0.06–4.28)).

According to duration of ETF. The duration of ETF in the trials included in the meta-analysis ranged from 5 days in surgical patients (Beier-Holgersen and Boesby, 1996) to 4 weeks in those with liver disease (Kearns *et al.*, 1992). Meta-analysis suggested that significant reductions in mortality were observed with feeding for 1 month or less (odds ratio 0.53 (95% CI 0.32–0.87); 12 RCT, no significant heterogeneity), but insufficient trials in which ETF was given for < 2 weeks or for > 1 month prevented further analysis.

According to intake of ETF. In the trials included in the meta-analysis, the energy intake of ETF ranged from < 1000 kcal (Sullivan *et al.*, 1998) to > 3000 kcal (Jenkins *et al.*, 1994). Meta-analysis suggested significant reductions in mortality when > 1000 kcal of ETF were given (odds ratio 0.47 (95% CI 0.26–0.86); nine RCT, no significant heterogeneity), but there was an insufficient number of trials using smaller quantities of feed to proceed any further with the analysis.

There is a need for further RCT to assess the effects of ETF on mortality across different patient groups. In particular, assessments of clinical outcome following ETF are lacking in patients with neurological disease, COPD and GI disease and in paediatric and elderly patients. Larger sample sizes are also required to ensure sufficient statistical power to detect changes in mortality (see Chapter 6). From the current data set, the average sample size of trials showing reduced mortality was 42, compared with 55 for those showing no significant differences.

COMPLICATION RATES

ETF may reduce the rate of complications, particularly infective/septic complications. Nineteen trials assessed rates of complications with ETF, 17 of which provided data that could be used for analysis. Complications recorded varied according to the diagnoses or treatments (e.g. surgery) of patients and included sepsis, wound, uri-

nary and other infections, pneumonia, pulmonary failure, acute myocardial infarction, anastomotic leaks, wound dehiscence and bowel obstructions. Most studies (76%, *n* 13) indicated that complication rates were lower in tube-fed patients than in controls. Seven trials indicated significant reductions in complication rates with ETF (Foschi *et al.*, 1986; Moore and Jones, 1986; Jenkins *et al.*, 1994; Beier-Holgersen and Boesby, 1996; Singh *et al.*, 1998; Taylor *et al.*, 1999; Pupelis *et al.*, 2001). In three of these trials, the observations related to septic/infective complications only (Moore and Jones, 1986; Jenkins *et al.*, 1994; Singh *et al.*, 1998).

Combined analysis of these trials (17 RCT, *n* 749) suggested that total complication rates in tube-fed patients were significantly lower (33%) than in controls (48%, *P* < 0.001; see Fig. 7.8).

ETF may be more effective at reducing infective/septic complications than routine care in the groups of patients studied. Combined analysis suggested that 23% of tube-fed patients (*n* 51/219) experienced such complications compared with 47% of controls (*n* 104/223, *P* < 0.001; see Fig. 7.8).

Trials that did not provide detailed data on complication rates reported that with ETF the rates were similar to (Smith *et al.*, 1985) or less than (Chuntrasakul *et al.*, 1996) the controls.

Meta-analysis of complication rates. Meta-analysis of the results of 17 RCT (*n* 749) that had recorded total complication rates indicated an odds ratio of 0.50 (95% CI 0.35–0.70), with no significant heterogeneity between studies. Funnel plots and Rosenthal's fail-safe score suggested that reporting bias may be a problem.

According to BMI and weight change. Analysis of complication rates according to BMI was limited, as 5/6 of the trials in which mean BMI was documented were in those with a mean BMI > 20 kg m^{-2} (odds ratio 0.36 (95% CI 0.14–0.92)). Similarly it was not possible to relate changes in complication rates with changes in body weight due to a lack of data. From the two trials that provided data, it was only possible to high-

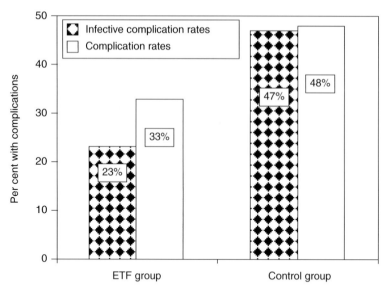

Fig. 7.8. Lower complication rates, including infective complications, with enteral tube feeding compared with routine clinical care (hospital RCT). Complications: odds ratio 0.50 (95% CI 0.35–0.70), $P < 0.001$; 17 RCT; 749 patients. Infective complications: odds ratio 0.26 (95% CI 0.15–0.44), $P < 0.001$; 9 RCT; 442 patients.

light that the difference in % weight change between ETF and control patients was greater in the trial in which complication rates were significantly reduced (+5.2% with ETF (Moore and Jones, 1986)) than not (+1.8% (Schroeder *et al.*, 1991)).

According to patient group. Meta-analysis of studies in some patient groups indicated that complication rates may be reduced, although small numbers and heterogeneity limit conclusions (critical illness/injury, liver disease and surgery; see Appendix 5 for details).

According to duration of ETF. The duration of ETF in the trials in the meta-analysis ranged from 5 days in surgical patients (Beier-Holgersen and Boesby, 1996) to 4 weeks in those with burns (Jenkins *et al.*, 1994). Meta-analysis suggested that significant reductions in complications were observed with feeding for 1 month or less (odds ratio 0.54 (95% CI 0.37–0.78); 15 RCT, no significant heterogeneity). None of the trials included in the analysis involved ETF for > 1 month. In trials in which ETF was given for only 1 week or less (seven RCT), meta-analysis suggested that compli-

cation rates were significantly reduced (odds ratio 0.36 (95% CI 0.17–0.77)).

According to intake of ETF. The energy intake in the trials included in the meta-analysis ranged from < 1000 kcal (Sullivan *et al.*, 1998) to > 3000 kcal (Jenkins *et al.*, 1994). Meta-analysis suggested significant reductions in complication rates when > 1000 kcal of ETF were given (odds ratio 0.53 (95% CI 0.35–0.81); 12 RCT, no significant heterogeneity), but there was an insufficient number of trials using smaller quantities of feed to proceed further with analysis.

Meta-analysis of infective complication rates. When infective/septic complications were analysed separately in a meta-analysis (results from nine trials, n 442), an odds ratio of 0.26 (95% CI 0.15–0.44) was found, with no significant heterogeneity between studies and no indication of a publication bias.

LENGTH OF STAY (LOS) IN HOSPITAL
Nineteen RCT assessed LOS as an outcome measure following ETF. Of these, 53% (n 10) indicated shorter stays with ETF, two of which were significant reductions (Sagar *et al.*, 1979; Bastow *et al.*, 1983). No trials indi-

cated significantly longer hospital stays with ETF. As LOS data were presented as means (with or without SD) or medians, a meta-analysis was not undertaken. Simple calculations averaging the results of all trials indicated that LOS was shorter by 1 day (ETF 23 days, control 24 days). In the two trials in which hospital stay was significantly reduced, stays were shortened on average by 9 days ('very thin' orthopaedic patients (Bastow *et al.*, 1983)) and 5 days (surgical patients (Sagar *et al.*, 1979)). The greatest reduction was in one trial in burns patients, in which hospital stay was reduced by an average of 20 days (Chiarelli *et al.*, 1990). Length of hospital stay may not be a good indicator of outcome as there are many factors, often social, that determine the time of discharge. Indeed, one study was able to show that the postoperative day on which all the clinical discharge criteria were met (as distinct from organizational or social criteria) was earliest in those on ETF (Elmore *et al.*, 1989), but actual days of discharge for all groups were later (Elmore *et al.*, 1989).

Other reviews of outcome in hospital patients

A meta-analysis assessing the use of enteral nutrition (ONS or ETF) early rather than later in a range of hospitalized patients with acute illness (burns, postoperative, head injured, trauma) suggests that the incidence of infections and hospital stay may be significantly reduced, although considerable heterogeneity existed between studies (Marik and Zaloga, 2001).

Clinical outcome in community patients

Only 11 trials made a comparison of patients' clinical outcome after ETF in the community (one RCT (Hearne *et al.*, 1985) and ten NRT (Irwin and Openbrier, 1985; Chin *et al.*, 1990; Dalzell *et al.*, 1992; Cappell and Godil, 1993; Edington *et al.*, 1994; Ockenga *et al.*, 1994; Cosgrove and Jenkins, 1997; den Broeder *et al.*, 1998; Jager-Wittenaar *et al.*, 2000; Sayce *et al.*, 2000)). Of these, 55% (*n* 6/11) suggested benefits to clinical outcome following ETF, but all were NRT (Irwin and Openbrier,

1985; Dalzell *et al.*, 1992; Cappell and Godil, 1993; Cosgrove and Jenkins, 1997; Jager-Wittenaar *et al.*, 2000; Sayce *et al.*, 2000). Many of these clinical outcomes were anecdotally or subjectively recorded, with no quantitative data provided, and the lack of control groups meant changes in disease activity (e.g. Crohn's disease, COPD) and the effects of other confounding variables (e.g. medication) could not be excluded. In summary, the possible benefits to clinical outcome included the following:

- COPD: A marked reduction in the 'frequency, duration and intensity of pulmonary-related hospital stays', from 83 days during the 6 months before ETF to 12 days during the 6 months after ETF (Irwin and Openbrier, 1985).
- Pregnancy: Shorter hospital stays when ETF was used as part of the treatment regimen for hyperemesis gravidarum, compared with an earlier period when no nutritional support was given (Jager-Wittenaar *et al.*, 2000) (duration not quantified).
- Crohn's disease: Significant reductions in steroid doses during ETF in children with Crohn's disease, with 60% no longer requiring medication (Cosgrove and Jenkins, 1997).
- Renal failure: A 40% lower than average number of days in hospital for patients receiving haemodialysis and ETF compared with a typical patient not given nutritional support (Sayce *et al.*, 2000).
- Cystic fibrosis: Lower hospital admission rates and lower mortality rates in growth-retarded patients with cystic fibrosis given ETF compared with a non-random control group receiving conventional treatment (no ETF) (Dalzell *et al.*, 1992).

A meta-analysis was not carried out because there were no suitable data from RCT.

None of the trials reviewed suggested significant detriments to clinical outcome from using ETF. A number of studies (Kotler *et al.*, 1991; Henderson *et al.*, 1994; Bannerman *et al.*, 1999; Duche *et al.*, 1999; Schneider *et al.*, 2000a) reported general information about the outcome of patients on ETF at home (% mortality, % returning to oral intake), but the lack of control groups limited the full interpretation of these data (see Appendix 6 for more details). In HIV/AIDS patients, two trials were able to suggest that the clinical outcome of PEG feeding in this patient group was associated with either similar (Ockenga et al., 1994) or better (Cappell and Godil, 1993) mortality rates than among non-HIV patients receiving PEG feeding.

The use of disease-specific enteral formulations in some patient groups in the community may also lead to improvements in outcome compared with the use of standard feeds. For example, the use of a modified feed for diabetics led to fewer fevers, pneumonia and urinary-tract infections (non-significant) than a standard enteral feed (Craig et al., 1998). Similarly, other disease-specific formulas have been developed for use in patients with pressure ulcers and in cancer patients, although their efficacy in community patients with chronic illness has not been investigated in this review.

Clinical outcome according to patient group

Improvements in clinical outcome (mortality, complication rates and reduced LOS) have been found in a number of different patient groups following ETF, particularly in the hospital setting. A summary of these can be seen in Tables 7.12 and 7.13 (where data exist). For detailed information on changes in clinical outcome in specific studies in different patient groups, refer to Appendices 5 and 6.

Cost efficacy

Since ETF can produce improvements in clinical outcome, it is also likely to be cost-effective in both hospital and community settings. Although only a few trials included prospective calculations of cost (see below), a number of trials included estimates or retrospective calculations. Indeed, a small number of studies reviewed (n 7) in the hospital setting made some estimates of the financial benefits of using ETF in hospitalized patients. Specifically, using data gathered prospec-

tively, it was estimated that huge cost savings could be made if head-injured patients were given early ETF in the UK (with the associated reduction in complication rates and hospital stays that ensued following ETF) (Taylor et al., 1999; see Appendix 5). An earlier study by the same author in a group of general medical patients also predicted that savings of > £4519 (1993 UK prices) per patient could be made if ETF were introduced early in a patient's hospital stay thus preventing prolonged periods of starvation (Taylor, 1993).

Four trials undertook prospective assessment of costs during ETF (Smith et al., 1986; Hasse et al., 1995; Beier-Holgersen and Boesby, 1996; Chellis et al., 1996). In two studies of ETF in paediatric patients, cost savings were highlighted (Smith et al., 1986; Chellis et al., 1996). In critically ill children, the use of ETF instead of PN led to savings of US$2701 per patient (Chellis et al., 1996). Similarly, the introduction of a protocol to encourage the appropriate use of ETF in children with intractable diarrhoea led to cost savings of US$14,750 per patient, as hospital stays and the use of PN were reduced (Smith et al., 1986). Furthermore, in adults undergoing surgery, investigators suggested that 'postoperative enteral feeding may reduce the need for TPN [total PN] and reduce expenditure' (Carr et al., 1996), although no financial estimates were given in this study (Carr et al., 1996) (refer to Chapter 9 for more information on cost comparisons between ETF and PN). However, another study in adult surgical patients confirmed that the use of ETF in the early postoperative period did reduce hospital costs (~£1000 per patient) compared with a control group (~£2000 per patient) given a placebo (Beier-Holgersen and Boesby, 1996). In contrast, in patients undergoing liver transplant, those receiving ETF did not have different hospital costs from control patients receiving intravenous (i.v.) fluids (Hasse et al., 1995).

The use of disease-specific enteral formulations may also be cost-effective if clinical outcome is improved. Indeed, two meta-analyses of studies in critically ill and surgical patients in the hospital setting, using feeds enriched with nutrients that may modulate immune and inflammatory markers, have indicated the cost efficacy of ETF, with significant improvements in outcome and reductions in resource use (i.e. reduced hospital stays), although this is not a consistent observation (Heyland *et al.*, 2001b). In the community, the use of diabetic feeds for diabetes (Craig *et al.*, 1998) could also lead to financial savings with reduced health-care resource use, as clinical outcome is improved (e.g. reduced infection rates and fewer pressure ulcers).

In the community, the use of home nutritional support, as opposed to the hospitalization of such patients, has been predicted to save substantial amounts of money each year (estimates in 1995 of > £90 million annually for the UK for ETF and PN (Elia, 1995)). Although patients on home ETF are occasionally hospitalized, surveys have suggested that < 1% of patients at any one time are in hospital (Elia *et al.*, 2001b). Therefore the savings to the health-care system are likely to be substantial. Indeed, the improvements in clinical outcome seen in some studies of community patients, such as reduced hospital stays (Irwin and Openbrier, 1985; Dalzell *et al.*, 1992; Jager-Wittenaar *et al.*, 2000; Sayce *et al.*, 2000), will lead to cost savings and increased availability of health-care resources (e.g. hospital beds). However, although the increasing use of home artificial nutritional support will undoubtedly lead to cost savings for health-care systems, there are likely to be implications for other individuals (e.g. carers) in terms of cost, financial as well as physical and emotional. These implications have yet to be assessed or quantified.

Unfortunately, very few studies of ETF in hospital or community settings have made formal financial assessments. Indeed, in 1995, a review of the literature found that < 20% of studies (1980–1994) of home enteral nutrition included information about cost efficacy (Pironi and Tognoni, 1995). However, it seems likely, if functional outcomes and complications of disease can be significantly improved by ETF, that cost savings will result, particularly as ETF is a relatively cheap and complication-free therapy.

An American evidence-based review of the clinical and cost-effectiveness of enteral feeding (Nutrition Screening Initiative, 1996), including both ONS and ETF, concluded that these forms of nutritional support were highly cost-effective, as the extracts below illustrate:

> The regular and appropriate administration of medical foods [ONS and ETF] in the treatment of a wide range of conditions . . . improves health outcomes resulting in lower costs to the nation's healthcare system.

> The savings result from a number of factors including reduced medical complications, reduced length of hospital stay, reduced hospital re-admissions, improved wound healing, enhanced immune function and increased use of enteral versus parenteral routes of administrations.

> These savings more than offset the cost of additional patients receiving medical foods.
> (Nutrition Screening Initiative, 1996)

This report also calculated that:

> consistent and appropriate use of medical nutrition therapy . . . would have saved the nation's health care system over $150 million in 1994, and would result in a projected seven-year savings of $1.3 billion between the years 1996 and 2002.
> (Nutrition Screening Initiative, 1996)

For a discussion of the cost efficacy of ETF compared with PN, refer to Chapter 9.

Combined analysis of ETF trials in hospital and community patients

Combined analysis of studies from the hospital and the community setting was carried out for % weight change data (no RCT data on mortality or complication rates from community ETF studies). Meta-analysis of the results of five studies (*n* 146) (Ryan *et al.*, 1981; Hearne *et al.*, 1985; Chiarelli *et al.*, 1990; Schroeder *et al.*, 1991; Chuntrasakul *et al.*, 1996) indicated a mean effect size of 1.41 (95% CI 0.81–2.01). However, there was significant heterogeneity between the study results, as one might expect from the variety of diagnostic groups involved (COPD, surgery, critical illness, cancer).

Discussion

Reductions in mortality rates (from 23% to 11%; $P < 0.001$) and complication rates (48% to 33%; $P < 0.001$) and a range of functional improvements with ETF compared with routine care have been highlighted by this systematic review of 121 trials (4090 patients). Functional benefits with ETF, often specific to the diagnostic category of patients, have been observed across patient groups in hospital and community settings. These include improved muscle strength, increased walking distances, better quality of life and improved immune function. Similarly, improvements in clinical outcome have been observed across a number of patient groups in the hospital setting, including surgical patients, critically ill patients and those with liver disease. Meta-analysis suggests significant reductions in mortality (odds ratio 0.48 (95% CI 0.30–0.78)) and complication rates (odds ratio 0.50 (95% CI 0.35–0.70)), particularly infective/septic complications (odds ratio 0.26 (95% CI 0.15–0.44)), with ETF across patient groups. The high incidence of mortality (23%) observed in these patients provides an indication that those selected for trials of ETF are often severely ill and at high risk of malnutrition (towards the left of Fig. 7.1). Indeed, the mortality observed in this group was considerably higher than the mortality of patients in hospital in general (about 3% in National Health Service (NHS) trusts in England between 1991 and 1997 (Department of Health, 1998)). For example, in one trial of elderly fractured neck of femur patients, mortality was 30% (Sullivan *et al.*, 1998), while, in patients with severe liver disease, mortality was as high as 47% (Cabre *et al.*, 1990). It is likely that, in less sick patients who are at lower risk of DRM, such marked differences in clinical outcome may not be observed with ETF (towards the right of Fig. 7.1).

These improvements in functional and clinical outcomes have been established through systematically reviewing the literature and undertaking meta-analyses. Although systematic reviews and meta-analyses are regarded as the highest level of evidence, the design and the quality of the individual studies included in such analyses are also important. For the present analysis, in addressing the evidence base using a multilayer approach, both RCT and NRT were included for completeness. The main findings and the combined analysis of efficacy of ETF were based on the results of RCT wherever possible (45% of hospital trials and 6% of community trials). However, considering the findings of NRT is also important in some groups of patients, in whom RCT comparing ETF with no nutritional support might not be possible, clinically or ethically. This is often the case for patients with chronic disease in the community (hence the low proportion of RCT in this setting). Examples where RCT comparing ETF with no nutritional support would not be undertaken include CVA patients in whom food intake is contraindicated and ETF is the only means of providing nutrition via the GI tract. Also, in children with severe growth failure associated with disease (e.g. cystic fibrosis or Crohn's disease), it may be difficult ethically to withhold ETF in a group randomized to routine clinical care.

In interpreting the results of the studies used in the systematic review, it is necessary to consider their quality. In the present analysis, the methodology of RCT was assessed using Jadad's criteria (Jadad *et al.*, 1996). This system scores studies according to the methods of randomization used, the use of placebos and blinding and the reporting of patient follow-up through the trial. Although composite Jadad scores for all RCT of ETF have been summarized in the tables in Appendices 5 and 6, Fig. 7.9 indicates the distribution of total Jadad scores for the hospital and community ETF trials reviewed (from 0 weakest design to 5 strongest design: see Chapter 5). Most of the RCT reviewed had a score of 2 or less (80%). In most cases, this was due to the failure of studies to blind patients and investigators with the use of placebo tube feeding. Only two trials used a placebo feed in the control arm of the studies (Whittaker *et al.*, 1990;

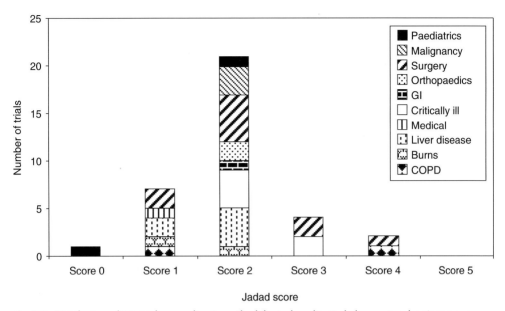

Fig. 7.9. Distribution of ETF trials according to methodological quality (Jadad scores) and patient group.

Beier-Holgersen and Boesby, 1996) and a similar approach has been undertaken successfully in controlled studies of ETF in healthy subjects (Stratton, 1998, 1999). However, in the clinical setting, apart from the problems associated with the practicalities of formulating a placebo feed that has a similar appearance and consistency to a nutritional feed (to ensure complete blinding of both patients and investigators: see Chapter 10), there is also an ethical dilemma. Is it ethically appropriate to place a tube in a patient to allow infusion of a non-nutritious placebo? Specifically, there are the potential risks associated with the placement of certain types of feeding tubes (e.g. PEG tubes) and the potential complications (e.g. infections at the PEG site) to consider. Even with the use of an NG tube, the insertion of which is less invasive, there may be a degree of discomfort for the patients involved. Therefore, although it is generally recommended that use of double-blinding (and hence placebo) is desirable in attaining the perfect study design, this is not always possible clinically/practically and, for studies of ETF, may be considered unethical.

Does this affect the interpretation of the findings of such studies and of this review? For some parameters, failure to blind can potentially bias some outcome measures (e.g. records of intake or feed tolerance, quality of life). For other 'harder' outcomes (e.g. mortality), it is unlikely that bias can substantially alter them (Schultz and Grimes, 2002b). Even for some clear-cut major complication rates (e.g. pressure ulcers, acute myocardial infarction), the impact of bias on outcome may be limited.

When considering the impact of the methodology of the individual trials on the findings of this review, the total number of patients in trials must also be assessed. As highlighted in Chapter 6, large trials are required if they are to have sufficient power to detect significant changes in clinical outcome measures, such as mortality and complication rates, with nutritional intervention. If trials are small, there is the likelihood that differences in clinical outcome that do exist are not detected (type II error). As Fig. 7.10 illustrates, sample sizes in individual trials (both RCT and NRT) were typically small and with insufficient power to detect changes to outcome (only 17% had > 50 subjects in total). Furthermore, very few trials

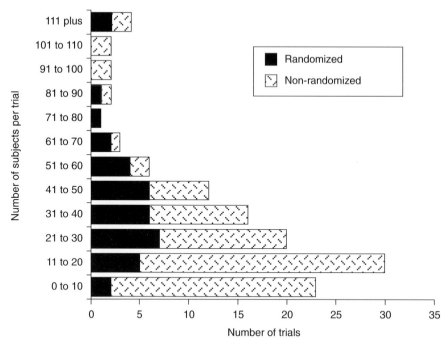

Fig. 7.10. Distribution of the number of subjects in each of the ETF trials reviewed.

(< 5%) reported power calculations at the start of the investigations. For greater power, the results of these individual studies have been combined in a meta-analysis (e.g. 600 patients included in the meta-analysis of mortality).

The findings of this systematic review and the meta-analyses are predominantly based on studies that have been published and are therefore easily accessible for reviewing. It is possible that studies that show no effect of an intervention (e.g. ETF) on an outcome measure are less likely to be published (publication bias) (Dickersin *et al.*, 1994) and hence less likely to be reviewed. Therefore, as part of this analysis, an indication of the potential effect of a publication bias, assessed by funnel plots and fail-safe scores, was given. For analyses of both mortality and complication rates with ETF compared with routine clinical care, low fail-safe scores suggested that the publication of a small number of additional trials showing a negative effect would be needed to lose the significant results obtained. Therefore, larger RCT are

needed in disease-specific groups to confirm the reductions in mortality and complication rates observed in this review.

Let us now consider some pathophysiological explanations for the marked improvements in clinical outcome observed with ETF, compared with routine care. In the patient groups studied, total dietary intake was markedly increased by ETF (by a mean of ~1000 kcal day^{-1} compared with control patients) (see Fig. 7.11). This effect was observed particularly in those in whom food intake was contraindicated (e.g. critically ill, early postoperative period in GI surgical patients, CVA patients with dysphagia). In those who were unable to consume enough orally, the use of ETF as a supplement to food also substantially increased total intake. In such cases, ETF does not appear to markedly reduce intake from the diet, so that the intake from ETF and food are largely additive. Controlled studies in healthy subjects have also indicated that appetite and food intake are largely unaffected by continuous infusions of feed by tube, at least in the short term (Stratton,

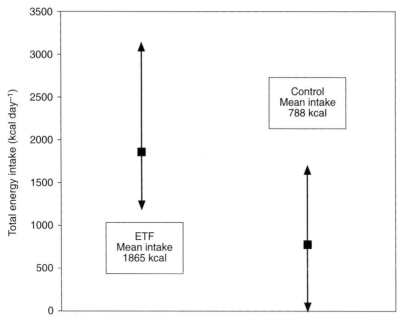

Fig. 7.11. Substantially greater energy intakes with ETF compared with routine clinical care (findings from all RCT providing data).

1998, 1999). This may be because feed is infused at a slow rate, usually continuously over many hours and often overnight during sleep. The delivery of feed also bypasses the upper GI tract and the associated cephalic-phase response. In addition to these factors, the liquid consistency or the composition of the tube feed may explain why appetite and food intake are not substantially suppressed with ETF, although further study is required in this area.

Since dietary intake was considerably greater in the ETF groups compared with control groups (Fig. 7.11), it is not surprising that the increases in weight and lean body mass (when measured) were also greater in the ETF group. This is a plausible mechanism, particularly if we consider that the differences in % weight change between ETF and control patients in RCT that showed significant benefits to clinical outcome was much greater (10%) than in trials in which improvements were not found (5%) (see Fig. 7.12). Similarly, in individual trials demonstrating improvements in mortality, differences in % weight change between intervention and control

groups were ~6–8%. Greater weight change in ETF patients compared with control patients was also found when complication rates were significantly reduced (5%, one trial) than when they were not (1.8%, one trial), although only two trials provided such data (Moore and Jones, 1986; Schroeder *et al.*, 1991). The greater difference in weight change between ETF and control patients in certain trials is likely to be due to a greater total energy intake as a result of either higher prescribed amounts and better tolerance to feeding a longer duration of feeding and possibly the composition of the feed used. However, limitations in the data provided regarding these aspects of intervention make it difficult to establish conclusions.

Since dietary lack, which produces loss of weight, leads to loss of body function, while increased intake improves body function (see Chapter 1) in malnourished individuals without disease, it is reasonable to suggest that similar effects occur in the presence of disease. The mechanisms may involve multiple processes that produce the following manifestations:

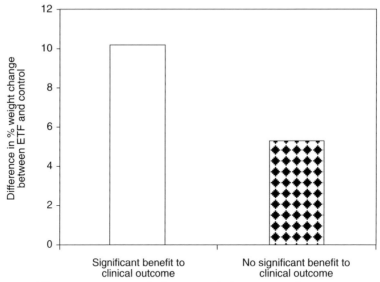

Fig. 7.12. Greater difference in per cent weight change in trials showing a significant improvement in clinical outcome (mortality or complications) with enteral tube feeding. Data from RCT included in meta-analyses.

- Improvement in the muscle mass, including diaphragmatic muscle mass, resulting in increased muscle strength, increased cough pressure and a reduction in the risk of chest infections.
- Improved sensitivity of the respiratory centre to oxygen, which may reduce the need for artificial ventilation in critically ill patients.
- Increased physical activity, which reduces the risk of developing pressure ulcers and thromboembolism.
- Improvement in immune function, reducing the risk of infection.
- Improvement in psychological function and well-being, which favours recovery.

It is possible for nutrients to improve the function of tissues independently of tissue mass. Many of the patients included in reviewed trials are likely to have had individual nutrient deficiencies that detrimentally affected the function of many tissues. Improving the status of these nutrients could have contributed to the positive effects of ETF. However, available information does not allow us to examine whether the benefits were the result of improving the status of individual nutrients or a combination of nutrients.

Formulations used for ETF are usually nutritionally complete, containing energy (carbohydrate and fat), protein, vitamins, minerals and trace elements. Therefore, improvements in complication rates and mortality could be a result of the supply of one or more specific nutrients at a critical time influencing one or more body systems (e.g. immune function). This is a concept that needs further exploration. For a fuller understanding of the impact of ETF on both functional and clinical outcomes, further study of the metabolic changes accompanying feeding are needed in larger RCT in specific patient groups.

In conclusion, the currently available evidence suggests that ETF is superior to routine clinical care in a number of patient groups at high risk of malnutrition (to the left of Fig. 7.1). For some patient groups, the use of ETF as a means of supplying a sole source of nutrition is undisputed (e.g. chronic CVA patients in whom food intake is contraindicated). For other groups of patients for whom there may be uncertainty about the benefits of ETF relative to routine clinical care (intermediate part of Fig. 7.1), greater improvements in body function and in clinical outcome with ETF have been demonstrated. However, larger trials are needed to confirm these observations in such groups. Exploration of the mechanisms by which such improvements in outcome occur should also be undertaken, in particular focusing on the impact of increased energy and nutrient intakes and relative improvements in body weight that have been observed with ETF in this review. For patients who are less sick and at lower risk of malnutrition (to the right of Fig. 7.1), other means of nutritional support may be effective (see Chapter 6 for a discussion of the efficacy of ONS and dietary manipulation). In contrast, at the other end of the spectrum, in patients at high risk of malnutrition and in whom intestinal failure is observed to some degree, PN may be indicated either as a sole source of nutrition or in combination with ETF, and this is discussed in Chapter 9.

This chapter has addressed the available evidence of the efficacy of ETF across all patient groups in hospital and community settings ('generalizable' findings: see Fig. 5.6, Chapter 5). This is complemented by a more detailed account of the evidence base for ETF in specific conditions and patient groups in Appendix 5 and 6 (for specificity). For greater 'generalizability', it could also be argued that the evidence of the efficacy of ETF should be considered together with the other form of enteral nutrition support, ONS, across patient groups. The aim of both these prescribed treatments is to increase nutritional intake in patients at risk of malnutrition. Therefore, a combined analysis of ONS and ETF as compared with routine clinical care is presented in the next chapter of this book (Chapter 8).

8
Combined Analysis of the Effects of Oral Nutritional Supplements and Enteral Tube Feeding

The previous two chapters of this book (Chapters 6 and 7) have addressed the impact of oral nutritional supplements (ONS) and enteral tube feeding (ETF) compared with routine clinical care on a number of physiological and clinical outcome measures. Individually, ONS and ETF have been shown to improve clinically relevant outcome measures (e.g. mortality, complication rates, hospital stay) and a number of functional measures (e.g. muscle strength, immune function) across a wide variety of hospital and community patients.

Previous meta-analyses have combined studies involving a range of interventions (ONS, ETF, dietary interventions) in different health-care settings, to assess their impact on outcome (typically body weight and mortality) (Potter *et al.*, 1998; Ferreira *et al.*, 2000). This approach has been criticized on the basis of the heterogeneity of the component data sets, which are of little value to the practising clinician interested in treating individual patients. However, it can be justified on the basis that inadequate intake produces adverse effects (malnutrition) (see Chapters 3 and 4) and that improving the intake, by whatever means, will prevent such detriments and improve outcome. Therefore, meta-analysis involving a combination of trials of ONS and ETF has been undertaken for three reasons:

- It provides 'generalizable' results obtained with a larger number of trials and patients.
- It updates previous meta-analyses.
- It establishes the multilayer approach for establishing the evidence base, the components of which can be found in Chapters 6 and 7 (ONS and ETF meta-analyses) and in Appendices 3–6 (individual studies).

Undertaking Combined Analysis of Studies of ONS and ETF

Randomized controlled trials (RCT) of ONS and ETF retrieved in the systematic review process (see Chapters 6 and 7), with relevant data on the following outcomes:

- mortality,
- complication rates,
- length of hospital stay,
- body weight,

were combined and analysed. Throughout this analysis the term 'ONS and ETF' is used. The trials involved in this review assessed the effects of one or other form of intervention, and not both combined. For details of the methodology used for systematic reviewing and meta-analysis, see Chapter 5. All studies were scored according to their design using the Jadad criteria

(Jadad *et al.*, 1996) and scores for individual trials can be seen in Appendices 3–6. The trials included were undertaken in a range of patients, including those with burns, critical illness/injury, liver disease, cancer and neurological disease and in elderly and post-surgical patients.

Findings of Combined Analysis of Trials of ONS and ETF

Combined analysis of a total of 30 sets of randomized controlled data suggests that mortality rates and complication rates (postoperative, post-radiotherapy, infective) are significantly reduced and length of hospital stay is shortened (by an average of 13 days) with ONS and ETF compared with routine clinical care. The changes in weight that accompany intervention with ONS and ETF are generally small and are greatest in trials of patients who are underweight (body mass index (BMI) < 20 kg m^{-2}) (see Box 8.1).

The impact of ONS and ETF on the three clinically relevant outcome measures is discussed in more detail below.

Mortality

Mortality is significantly lower in patients given ONS and ETF (17%) than in control patients given routine clinical care (24%, P < 0.001; see Fig. 8.1). This analysis was undertaken with data from 3258 patients from a number of different patient groups (elderly, liver disease, neurology, orthopaedics, cancer, surgery, critical illness/injury and burns). Meta-analysis of these trials (30 sets of data from RCT) suggested an odds ratio (OR) with ONS and ETF of 0.59 (95% confidence interval (CI) 0.48–0.72), with no significant heterogeneity between studies and an adequate Rosenthal's fail-safe score. Although this statistic suggests that publication bias is unlikely, it cannot be excluded. Figure 8.2

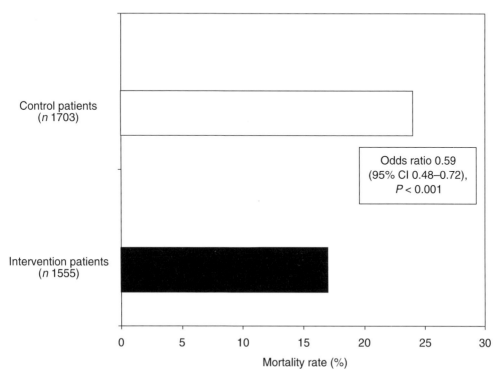

Control patients (*n* 1703)

Intervention patients (*n* 1555)

Odds ratio 0.59 (95% CI 0.48–0.72), P < 0.001

Mortality rate (%)

Fig. 8.1. Lower mortality rates following intervention with oral nutritional supplements and enteral tube feeding (30 sets of RCT data, *n* 3258).

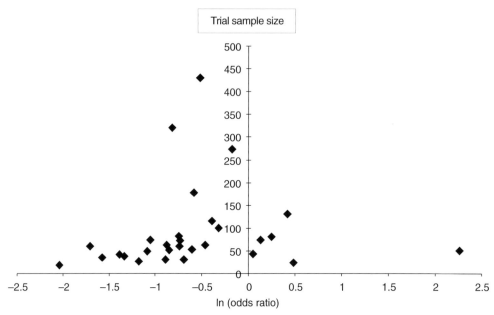

Grand mean for ln odds ratio −0.53 (95% CI −0.73 to −0.32)

Fig. 8.2. Odds ratio (natural log (ln)) for the risk of mortality with ONS and ETF compared with routine care in individual studies according to trial sample size.

provides a visual indication of the ORs (shown as natural log (ln) for the purposes of visual presentation) obtained in individual trials, according to trial sample size (funnel plot). This plot indicates that most trials showed a lower risk of mortality with ONS and ETF than with routine care (ln (odds ratio) less than 0 or OR less than 1), including the largest trials. However, some of the largest effects (both positive and neg-

ative) were observed in the smallest trials (refer to Chapters 6 and 10 for a discussion of the importance of sufficiently large sample sizes to detect true significant improvements in clinical outcomes).

Table 8.1 provides a summary of the results of meta-analysis of mortality rates from all trials, of hospital and community trials individually, and according to BMI (< or > 20 kg m^{-2}). As Table 8.1 shows,

Table 8.1. Meta-analysis results for mortality from RCT of ONS and ETF (30 data sets from 26 RCT, n 3258).

Groups of RCT	Number of data sets	Model	Odds ratio	95% CI	Significant heterogeneity
All hospital and community trials	30	Fixed	0.59	0.48–0.72	No
Community trials only	3	Fixed	0.78	0.10–6.32	Yes
		Random[a]	1.02	0.03–37.9	Yes
Hospital trials only	27	Fixed	0.58	0.47–0.72	No
Trials with average BMI < 20 kg m^{-2} (hospital and community)	7	Fixed	0.54	0.36–0.83	No
Trials with average BMI > 20 kg m^{-2} (hospital and community)	15	Fixed	0.61	0.39–0.97	No

[a]The more conservative random-effects model was used when there was significant heterogeneity with a fixed-effect model.

significant reductions in mortality were seen in trials in which the average BMI of patients was < 20 kg m^{-2} and > 20 kg m^{-2}. As most of the trials in the analysis were undertaken in the hospital setting, it is not surprising that significant reductions in mortality are not seen in the community trials alone. Table 8.2 provides data from the individual trials included in the meta-analysis. Analysis excluding potential duplicate information from Unosson *et al.* (1992) does not alter the findings of this meta-analysis (OR 0.59 (95% CI 0.47–0.73), no significant heterogeneity, high fail-safe score).

The impact of the duration of ONS and ETF on mortality was analysed. A significant reduction in mortality was observed when the duration of ONS and ETF exceeded 2 weeks (OR 0.59 (95% CI 0.48–0.74); 23 sets of RCT data, no significant heterogeneity, adequate Rosenthal's fail-safe score). Significant reductions in mortality were not seen with shorter interventions (less than 2 weeks), probably due to the smaller data set (OR 0.67 (95% CI 0.30–1.46), six sets of data from RCT). No consistent pattern was observed as the duration of interventions increased up to and exceeding 6 months. When the intake of ONS and ETF was considered in the analysis, significant reductions in mortality were observed in trials in which intake was 600 kcal or less (OR 0.58 (95% CI 0.43–0.78), 11 sets of data) or greater than 600 kcal (OR 0.61 (95% CI 0.44–0.85), 17 sets of data). However, more trials are needed before firm conclusions can be made about the impact of either the duration or the intake of ONS and ETF on mortality.

Complication rates

Complication rates are significantly lower in patients given ONS and ETF (28%) than in those given routine care (46%, *P* < 0.001) (see Fig. 8.3). This includes the rate of a wide range of complications (infective and non-infective), including those following surgery or radiotherapy. Meta-analysis of 27 sets of randomized controlled data in 1710 patients suggested an OR of 0.41 (95% CI 0.31–0.53), with no significant heterogeneity between trials and a high Rosenthal's fail-safe score (Table 8.3). Figure 8.4 shows that, in the majority of studies, there was a lower risk of complications with ONS and ETF than with routine care (ln OR less than 0, equivalent to an OR < 1). This is observed in some of the larger trials. However, some of the largest effects (both positive and negative) were observed in the smallest trials (refer to Chapters 6 and 10 for a discussion of the importance of sufficiently large sample sizes to detect true significant improvements in clinical outcomes). Data from the individual trials can be seen in Table 8.4. Significant reductions in complication rates were observed in hospital-based trials (see Table 8.3) and there was a trend towards improvements in community trials too, but data are lacking. There were also insufficient data to examine whether the nutritional status (BMI) of patients has an effect on the incidence of complications (see Table 8.3).

The impact of the duration of ONS and ETF on complication rates was analysed. Similar significant reductions in complication rates were observed when the duration of ONS and ETF was 2 weeks or less (OR 0.43 (95% CI 0.29–0.66); 13 sets of RCT data, no significant heterogeneity) or more than 2 weeks (OR 0.42 (95% CI 0.28–0.63); 12 sets of RCT data, no significant heterogeneity, adequate Rosenthal's fail-safe score). However, there was no consistent relationship between length of feeding and reduction in risk, with individual trials showing significant reductions with feeding lasting less than 1 week or between 1 and 2 months. When the intake of ONS and ETF was considered in the analysis, significant reductions in complication rates were observed in trials in which intake was 600 kcal or less (OR 0.52 (95% CI 0.36–0.75), 15 sets of data) or greater than 600 kcal (OR 0.27 (95% CI 0.14–0.53), six sets of data). Individual trials also demonstrated reductions in complication rates with intakes of ONS and ETF less than 500 kcal. There is a

Table 8.2. Mortality rates from RCT of ONS and ETF in hospital (H) and community (C) patients for combined analysis.

Trial	Setting	Intervention	Condition	BMI category	Intervention dead	Intervention alive	Control dead	Control alive
Larsson et al., 1990 (i)	H	ONS	Elderly	<20	17	42	21	35
Larsson et al., 1990 (ii)	H	ONS	Elderly	>20	12	126	34	148
Potter et al., 2001 (i)	H	ONS	Elderly	<20	5	29	14	26
Potter et al., 2001 (ii)	H	ONS	Elderly	Unknown	8	82	13	74
Potter et al., 2001 (iii)	H	ONS	Elderly	>20	8	54	6	62
Unosson et al., 1992[a]	H	ONS	Elderly	<20	28	169	51	182
Volkert et al., 1996	H	ONS	Elderly	<20	4	31	8	29
Bunout et al., 1989	H	ONS	Elderly	>20	2	15	5	14
Le Cornu et al., 2000	H	ONS	Liver	>20	5	37	9	31
Mendenhall et al., 1993	H	ONS	Liver	Unknown	48	89	53	83
Gariballa et al., 1998a	H	ONS	Neurology	Unknown	2	19	7	14
Tkatch et al., 1992	H	ONS	Orthopaedics	Unknown	3	30	4	25
Delmi et al., 1990	H	ONS	Orthopaedics	Unknown	6	19	10	17
MacFie et al., 2000	H	ONS	Surgery	>20	33	42	13	12
Hirsch et al., 1993	C	ONS	Liver	Unknown	3	23	6	19
Douglass et al., 1978	C	ONS	Malignancy	Unknown	8	5	13	4
Arnold and Richter, 1989	C	ONS	Malignancy	Unknown	3	20	0	27
Jenkins et al., 1994	H	ETF	Burns	Unknown	5	35	4	36
Chuntrasakul et al., 1996	H	ETF	Critical illness/injury	Unknown	1	20	3	14
Minard et al., 2000	H	ETF	Critical illness/injury	Unknown	1	11	4	11
Pupelis et al., 2001	H	ETF	GI	Unknown	1	29	7	23
Cabre et al., 1990	H	ETF	Liver	<20	2	14	9	10
De Ledinghen et al., 1997	H	ETF	Liver	>20	3	9	2	10
Kearns et al., 1992	H	ETF	Liver	>20	2	14	4	11
Tandon et al., 1984	H	ETF	Malignancy	Unknown	6	23	13	20
Bastow et al., 1983 (i)	H	ETF	Orthopaedics	<20	2	23	5	18
Bastow et al., 1983 (ii)	H	ETF	Orthopaedics	<20	5	34	4	31
Sullivan et al., 1998	H	ETF	Orthopaedics	>20	0	8	3	7
Beier-Holgersen and Boesby, 1996	H	ETF	Surgery	>20	2	28	4	26
Singh et al., 1998	H	ETF	Surgery	>20	4	17	4	18

[a]Unosson et al. (1992) possibly duplicate data from Larsson et al. (1990), analysis undertaken with and without this trial.
GI, gastrointestinal. (i), (ii) and (iii) patient subgroups according to BMI category within trials.

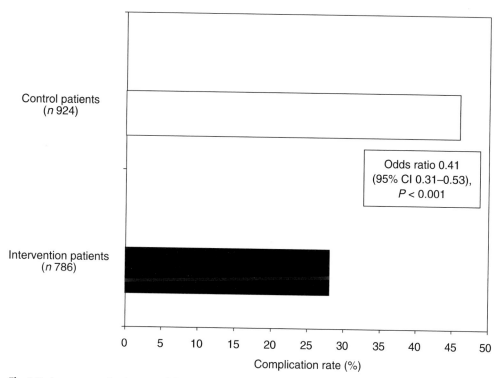

Fig. 8.3. Lower complication rates following intervention with oral nutritional supplements and enteral tube feeding (27 RCT, *n* 1710).

Table 8.3. Meta-analysis results for complication rates from RCT of ONS and ETF (27 RCT, *n* 1710).

Groups of RCT	Number of data sets	Model	Odds ratio	95% CI	Significant heterogeneity
All complications					
All hospital and community trials	27	Fixed	0.41	0.31–0.53	No
Community trials only	3	Fixed	0.24	0.03–1.65	No
Hospital trials only	24	Fixed	0.42	0.32–0.57	No
Trials with average BMI < 20 kg m^{-2} (hospital and community)	Insufficient data				
Trials with average BMI > 20 kg m^{-2} (hospital and community)	8	Fixed	0.37	0.20–0.67	No
Infective complications					
All hospital and community trials	10	Fixed	0.34	0.21–0.55	No

need for more trials before firm conclusions can be made about the effect the duration or the intake of ONS and ETF has on the rate of complications.

A separate analysis (Table 8.3) highlights that the incidence of infective complication rates was significantly lower in patients receiving ONS and ETF (24%) than those given routine care (44%, *P* < 0.001). Meta-analysis suggested that the OR for infective complications with ONS and ETF was 0.34 (95% CI 0.21–0.55), with no significant heterogeneity between studies and a high fail-safe score.

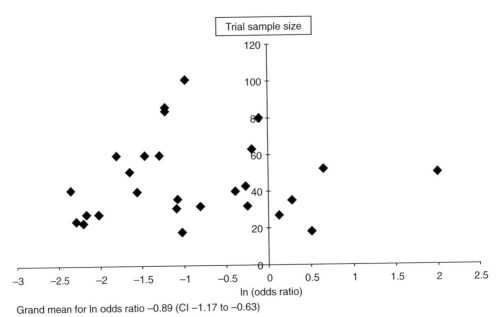

Grand mean for ln odds ratio −0.89 (CI −1.17 to −0.63)

Fig. 8.4. Odds ratio (natural log (ln)) for risk of complications with ONS and ETF from individual studies according to trial sample size.

Length of hospital stay

Most studies (70%, *n* 21) showed reductions in the length of hospital stay with ONS and ETF, relative to a control group given routine clinical care (see Table 8.5). Reductions in individual trials ranged from 1 day to 36 days (mean change −6 days compared with controls) across patient groups (elderly, orthopaedics, surgery, neurology, liver disease, critical illness/injury and cancer). As data from individual trials were presented as means or medians, with or without an indication of the variability of results, a meta-analysis was not undertaken.

Body weight

Improvements in body weight occur with ONS and ETF, with either greater % weight gain or less % weight loss than in patients given routine clinical care. Weighted analysis of mean % weight change indicated a greater improvement (+2.85%) in patients

on ONS and ETF relative to controls (ONS and ETF −0.28%; controls −3.12%). Analysis showed that the changes in % weight were relatively small across the various patient groups (surgery, elderly, cancer, chronic obstructive pulmonary disease (COPD), human immunodeficiency virus (HIV), critical illness/injury, burns) (see Table 8.6 for data from individual trials). Meta-analysis of all RCT providing appropriate data (mean and standard deviation (SD) of % weight change in intervention and control groups) suggested a mean effect size of 0.65 (95% CI 0.55–0.75, fixed-effects model), with considerable heterogeneity between studies (32 sets of randomized controlled data). Using the more conservative random-effects model, the effect size was 0.94 (95% CI 0.60–1.28) (see Table 8.7 for a summary of the analysis). Of interest was the greater effect size (1.28 (95% CI 1.03–1.53)) for % weight change with ONS and ETF in trials undertaken in patients with a BMI < 20 kg m^{-2} than in those with BMI > 20 kg m^{-2}, shown in Table 8.7.

Table 8.4. Complication rates from RCT of ONS and ETF in hospital (H) and community (C) patients for combined analysis.

Trial	Setting	Intervention	Condition	BMI category	Intervention Comp.	Intervention No comp.	Control Comp.	Control No comp.	Type of complications
Jenkins *et al.*, 1994	H	ETF	Burns	Unknown	21	19	22	18	All
Minard *et al.*, 2000	H	ETF	Critical illness/injury	Unknown	6	6	7	8	All
Moore and Jones, 1986	H	ETF	Critical illness/injury	Unknown	14	18	15	16	All
Seri and Aquilio, 1984	H	ETF	Critical illness/injury	Unknown	1	9	2	6	Infective
Taylor *et al.*, 1999	H	ETF	Critical illness/injury	Unknown	26	16	36	6	Infective
Pupelis *et al.*, 2001	H	ETF	GI	Unknown	1	29	8	22	Infective
Cabre *et al.*, 1990	H	ETF	Liver	< 20	7	9	7	12	Infective
Foschi *et al.*, 1986	H	ETF	Liver	Unknown	5	23	15	17	All
Hasse *et al.*, 1995	H	ETF	Liver	Unknown	3	11	8	9	Infective
Van Bokhorst-de van der Schueren *et al.*, 2001	H	ETF	Malignancy	Unknown	7	8	9	8	All
Sullivan *et al.*, 1998	H	ETF	Orthopaedic	> 20	7	1	8	2	All
Beier-Holgersen and Boesby, 1996	H	ETF	Surgery	> 20	8	22	19	11	All
Carr *et al.*, 1996	H	ETF	Surgery	> 20	0	14	3	11	Infective
Frankel and Horowitz, 1989	H	ETF	Surgery	Unknown	1	24	0	25	All
Schroeder *et al.*, 1991	H	ETF	Surgery	Unknown	4	12	7	9	All
Singh *et al.*, 1998	H	ETF	Surgery	> 20	11	10	13	9	All
Watters *et al.*, 1997	H	ETF	Surgery	> 20	0	13	3	12	All
Hirsch *et al.*, 1993	C	ONS	Liver	Unknown	2	24	9	16	Infective
Flynn and Leightty, 1987	C	ONS	Malignancy	Unknown	6	13	10	7	All
Nayel *et al.*, 1992	C	ONS	Malignancy	Unknown	9	2	12	0	Mucositis
Gariballa *et al.*, 1998a	H	ONS	Neurology	Unknown	9	11	11	9	Infective
Delmi *et al.*, 1990	H	ONS	Orthopaedic	Unknown	2	7	12	3	All
Tkatch *et al.*, 1992	H	ONS	Orthopaedic	Unknown	7	12	20	2	All
Beattie *et al.*, 2000	H	ONS	Surgery	< 20	6	46	13	36	Infective
MacFie *et al.*, 2000	H	ONS	Surgery	> 20	4	23	2	23	All
Keele *et al.*, 1997	H	ONS	Surgery	> 20	4	39	12	31	All
Rana *et al.*, 1992	H	ONS	Surgery	> 20	3	17	10	10	Infective

Comp., complications; No comp., no complications; GI, gastrointestinal.

Box 8.1. Key findings from the evidence base for ONS and ETF.

Combined meta-analysis of studies of ONS and ETF across patient groups and health-care settings suggested the following:

Mortality
Significant reductions in mortality (17% vs. 25% $P < 0.001$; odds ratio 0.59 (95% CI 0.48–0.72), n 3258) occur with ONS and ETF in patient groups who are or are not underweight (BMI < 20 kg m^{-2}) but are more likely if ONS and ETF are given for more than 2 weeks.

Complication rates
Significant reductions in complication rates (28% vs. 46%, $P < 0.001$; odds ratio 0.41 (95% CI 0.32–0.53), n 1710), particularly infective complications (25% vs 44%, $P < 0.001$; odds ratio 0.34 (95% CI 0.21–0.55)), occur with ONS and ETF. The effect of initial nutritional status (BMI) and the duration and intake of ONS and ETF require further study.

Length of hospital stay
Reduction in length of hospital stay occurs in most trials (70%) with ONS and ETF, with an average difference of –6 days compared with controls.

Body weight
Small improvements in body weight occur with ONS and ETF, particularly in patient groups who are initially underweight (BMI < 20 kg m^{-2}).

Discussion

The combined analysis of ONS and ETF trials demonstrated significantly and clinically relevant effects compared with routine clinical care (see Box 8.1) on mortality, complications and length of stay.

The quality and limitations of the trials and the possible mechanism by which the benefits are produced have been discussed in Chapters 6 and 7. They may involve an increase in body weight and lean tissue mass and an improvement in the function of the existing tissues or cells, including immune and inflammatory cells. It is uncertain whether these benefits are produced by specific nutrients or by a combination of nutrients. Nevertheless, such changes to outcome have potentially important financial implications.

This chapter has focused on the benefits to outcome of using ONS and ETF to improve nutritional intake in patients at risk of disease-related malnutrition (DRM). However, in some patient groups, the use of ONS and ETF may not be an effective way to increase nutrient intake. This is usually because patients have some degree of intestinal failure, and feeding that bypasses the GI tract is required (e.g. parenteral nutrition). The use and efficacy of parenteral nutrition are considered in the next chapter of this book.

Table 8.5. Hospital length of stay from RCT of ONS and ETF in hospital (H) and community (C) patients for combined analysis. Average length-of-stay data include means and medians (see Appendices 3, 4 and 5 for details).

Trial	Patient group	Setting	Type of nutritional intervention	Nutritional intervention group average length of stay (days)	Control group average length of stay (days)	Difference in averages (days)
Potter et al., 2001[a]	Elderly	H	ONS	16	18	−2
Gariballa et al., 1998	Neurology	H	ONS	24	42	−18
Delmi et al., 1990a	Orthopaedics	H	ONS	24	40	−16
Tkatch et al., 1992	Orthopaedics	H	ONS	69	102	−33
Brown and Seabrook, 1992	Orthopaedics	H	ONS	21	47	−26
Beattie et al., 2000	Surgery	H	ONS	18	21	−3
MacFie et al., 2000	Surgery	H	ONS	10	13	−3
Rana et al., 1992	Surgery	H	ONS	13	16	−3
Keele et al., 1997	Surgery	H	ONS	11	13	−2
Flynn and Leightty, 1987	Malignancy	C	ONS	18	21	−3
Wilson et al., 2001	Renal	C	ONS	71	107	−36
Chiarelli et al., 1990	Burns	H	ETF	69	89	−20
Jenkins et al., 1994	Burns	H	ETF	34	33	1
Minard et al., 2000	Critical illness/injury	H	ETF	30	21	9
Moore and Jones, 1986	Critical illness/injury	H	ETF	25	30	−5
Pupelis et al., 2001	GI	H	ETF	35	36	−1
De Ledinghen et al., 1997	Liver	H	ETF	15	13	2
Hasse et al., 1995	Liver	H	ETF	16	18	−2
Kearns et al., 1992	Liver	H	ETF	11	12	−1
Van Bokhorst et al., 2001[b]	Malignancy	H	ETF	31	41	−10
Bastow et al., 1983[b]	Orthopaedics	H	ETF	29	38	−9
Sullivan et al., 1998	Orthopaedics	H	ETF	38	24	14
Beier-Holgersen and Boesby, 1996	Surgery	H	ETF	8	12	−4
Carr et al., 1996	Surgery	H	ETF	10	9	1
Elmore et al., 1989	Surgery	H	ETF	4	4	0
Frankel and Horowitz, 1989	Surgery	H	ETF	2	2	0
Sagar et al., 1979	Surgery	H	ETF	14	19	−5
Schroeder et al., 1991	Surgery	H	ETF	10	15	−5
Singh et al., 1998	Surgery	H	ETF	14	13	1
Watters et al., 1997	Surgery	H	ETF	17	16	1
Estimated average				24	30	−6

[a] Subgroups within this study (see Appendix 3 for details).
[b] Data for one intervention group only (see Appendix 5 for details).

Table 8.6. Per cent weight change from RCT of ONS and ETF in hospital (H) and community (C) patients for combined analysis.

Trial	Setting	Intervention	Condition	BMI category	Intervention			Control		
					x % weight	SD % weight	No.	x % weight	SD % weight	No.
Simko, 1983	C	ONS	Liver	Unknown	5.6	13.2	7	1.9	5.9	3
Keele et al., 1997 (H & C ONS)	C	ONS	Other – surgery	>20	7.58	12.3	15	4.7	3.87	15
Elkort et al., 1981	C	ONS	Malignancy	Unknown	1.57	7.9	12	2.1	9.4	14
Larsson et al., 1990 (ii)	H	ONS	Elderly	>20	-1.8	6.46	138	-6.5	20.2	182
Keele et al., 1997	C	ONS	Other – surgery	>20	5.89	6.3	16	3.35	8.76	19
Potter et al., 2001 (i)	H	ONS	Elderly	<20	3.4	6	22	-1.3	7.6	27
Potter et al., 2001 (ii)	H	ONS	Elderly	Unknown	0.3	5.9	78	-0.8	6.2	67
Arnold and Richter, 1989	C	ONS	Malignancy	Unknown	-6	5.5	23	-5	4	27
Gray-Donald et al., 1995	C	ONS	Elderly	>20	4	4.8	24	1.2	3.3	24
Potter et al., 2001 (iii)	H	ONS	Elderly	>20	1	4.6	42	-1.2	5.2	57
Carver and Dobson, 1995	H	ONS	Elderly	<20	7.51	3.86	20	1.32	3.75	20
Nayel et al., 1992	C	ONS	Malignancy	Unknown	6.3	3.5	11	-1.1	3.7	12
Flatarone et al., 1994 (no ex)	C	ONS	Elderly	>20	1.5	3.4	24	-0.8	3.1	26
Schols et al., 1995 (ii)	H	ONS	COPD	>20	1.56	3.4	33	-0.54	3.26	38
Otte et al., 1989	C	ONS	COPD	<20	3.29	3	13	0.4	2	15
Flatarone et al., 1994 (ex)	C	ONS	Elderly	>20	1.8	3	25	0.4	3	25
Antila et al., 1993	H	ONS	Oral surgery	>20	-3.8	2.7	8	-6	3.8	9
Fuenzalida et al., 1990	C	ONS	COPD	<20	7.54	2.3	5	4.6	2.7	4
Bunout et al., 1989	H	ONS	Liver	>20	-8.82	2.1	17	-6.23	2.41	19
Keele et al., 1997	H	ONS	Surgery	>20	-3.33	1.52	43	-6.03	1.15	43
Schols et al., 1995 (i)	H	ONS	COPD	<20	5	1.11	39	0.92	0.74	25
Beattie et al., 2000	H	ONS	Surgery	<20	-5.6	1	52	-9.8	2	49
Saudny-Unterberger et al., 1997	H	ONS	COPD	>20	0.29	0.93	14	-0.13	0.32	10
Elbers et al., 1997	H	ONS	Surgery	>20	-8.41	0.93	10	-8.18	0.76	10
Lauque et al., 2000	C	ONS	Elderly	>20	1.44	0.86	24	-1.37	0.82	26
Larsson et al., 1990 (i)	H	ONS	Elderly	<20	0	0.77	59	-1.5	3.74	56
Rabeneck et al., 1998	C	ONS	HIV	>20	-0.15	0.63	49	-0.15	0.5	50
Chiarelli et al., 1990	H	ETF	Burns	Unknown	-2.9	2.7	10	-5.4	3.3	10
Chuntrasakul et al., 1996	H	ETF	Critical illness	Unknown	-9.81	1.5	21	-16.6	2.2	17
Ryan et al., 1981	H	ETF	Surgery	>20	-2.8	1.16	7	-6.1	1.35	7
Schroeder et al., 1991	H	ETF	Surgery	Unknown	-4.26	4.1	16	-6.14	3.22	16
Hearne et al., 1985	C	ETF	Malignancy[a]	<20	0.2	5.9	9	-7.3	4.2	8

[a]Not nasopharyngeal cancer.
x % weight, mean per cent weight change; SD, standard deviation; H & C ONS group given ONS in hospital and community, ex, resistance training also given; no ex, no resistance training given; (i), (ii) and (iii) patient subgroups according to BMI category within trials.

Table 8.7. Meta-analysis results for per cent weight change from RCT of ONS and ETF (32 data sets from 25 RCT).

Groups of RCT	Number of data sets	Model	Effect size	95% CI	Significant heterogeneity
All hospital and community trials	32	Fixed	0.65	0.55–0.75	Yes
		Random[a]	0.94	0.60–1.28	Yes
Community trials only	14	Fixed	0.53	0.33–0.73	Yes
		Random[a]	0.76	0.27–1.25	No
Hospital trials only	18	Fixed	0.7	0.57–0.83	Yes
		Random[a]	1.08	0.57–1.58	Yes
Trials with average BMI < 20 kg m^{-2} (hospital and community)	15	Fixed	1.28	1.03–1.53	Yes
		Random[a]	1.52	0.65–2.40	No
Trials with average BMI > 20 kg m^{-2} (hospital and community)	15	Fixed	0.48	0.34–0.62	Yes
		Random[a]	0.65	0.21–1.10	Yes

[a]The more conservative random-effects model was used when there was significant heterogeneity with a fixed-effects model.

9
Parenteral Nutrition: a Comparison with Enteral Tube Feeding

The previous two chapters have focused on the use of enteral nutritional support as a means of sustaining or improving nutritional intake with the aim of preventing or treating disease-related malnutrition (DRM). In particular, the efficacy of dietary counselling and fortification, oral nutritional supplements (ONS) and enteral tube feeding (ETF) compared with routine clinical care has been discussed. However, in some patients at risk of DRM, parenteral nutrition (PN) is the most appropriate method of feeding (Fig. 9.1). The main indications for use of PN include prolonged gastrointestinal (GI) failure in the form of ileus, peritonitis, severe and recurrent pancreatitis, high intestinal fistulas, short-bowel syndrome and severe inflammatory disease of the intestine (e.g. severe mucositis following cytotoxic therapy or Crohn's disease complicated by fistulas). PN may also be used in the perioperative period. For further discussion on the indications and complications associated with PN, refer to Elia (1996a). It is recognized that for these conditions there is often little alternative but to feed parenterally (e.g. severe intestinal failure, especially when it is likely to be prolonged; left-hand side of Fig. 9.1). However, in other instances, the use of PN is more controversial and has led to a large number of clinical trials and meta-analyses being carried out. These generally fall into two main categories: those in which PN is compared with routine clinical care and those in which PN is compared with ETF. These are considered separately below, with a review of published trials and meta-analyses.

Parenteral Nutrition Compared with Routine Clinical Care

In studies in which PN has been compared with routine clinical care, the form of nutrition provided as part of routine care has varied, sometimes including oral feeding and ETF or combinations. Therefore, it is not surprising that variable results have been obtained from meta-analyses of these studies. Here are some examples:

- PN is compared with routine clinical care in the surgical patient (Heyland *et al.*, 2001a). Meta-analysis of 27 randomized controlled trials (RCT) (*n* 2907), predominantly in adult GI surgical patients, suggests no effect of PN on mortality and a non-significant reduction in complication rates (relative risk 0.81 (95% confidence interval (CI) 0.65–1.01)) in the group as a whole. In studies of 'malnourished patients', complication rates are significantly reduced (relative risk 0.52 (95% CI 0.30–0.91)).

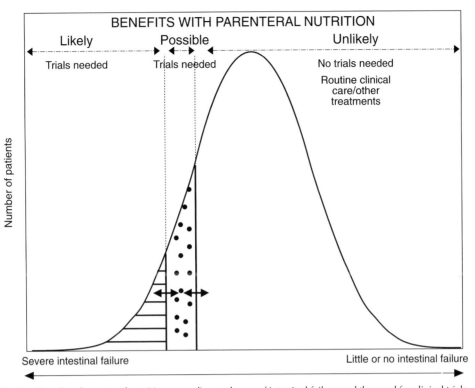

Fig. 9.1. Benefits of parenteral nutrition according to degree of intestinal failure and the need for clinical trials.

- PN is compared with routine care in the perioperative period (Detsky *et al.*, 1987). Meta-analysis of 11 RCT suggests PN has no effect on the risk of complications or fatalities following major surgery.
- PN is compared with routine care (may have included use of enteral nutrition) in critically ill patients (Heyland *et al.*, 1998). Meta-analysis of 26 RCT suggests that the use of PN in this patient group might be associated with increased morbidity and mortality.
- PN is compared with routine clinical care in cancer patients undergoing chemotherapy (McGeer *et al.*, 1990). Meta-analysis of 12 RCT in patients with various types of cancer (lung, GI, acute leukaemia) undergoing chemotherapy suggests that PN might be detrimental. PN use is associated with a significant increase in infectious complications and a trend towards decreased survival and poorer tumour response (Kaminski *et al.*,

1990). (In many of these trials, patients were well nourished and it has been suggested that methodological flaws and poor PN techniques were a problem.)
- PN is compared with routine clinical care across patients with a range of diagnoses (Koretz *et al.*, 2001). Meta-analysis of 82 RCT suggests that PN does not influence mortality or total complication rates but significantly increases infectious complication rates (one additional infection for every 20 patients treated, effect mostly in cancer patients receiving therapy). Meta-analyses of these trials were also undertaken in the following subgroups of patients:
  - Surgical patients in the perioperative period: meta-analysis of 41 RCT suggests no effect of PN used pre- and/or postoperatively on postoperative mortality or complications (tendency for a reduction with PN) or length of hospital stay (Koretz *et al.*, 2001).
  - Cancer patients undergoing therapy:

meta-analysis of 19 RCT in cancer patients receiving chemotherapy (three RCT in those being treated with radiation (with or without chemotherapy) and four RCT in bone marrow transplant (BMT) patients) suggests no effect of PN on survival (although patients in one RCT with end-stage malignancy lived significantly longer with PN than controls), increases in total complication rates and infectious complication rates and an adverse effect on tumour response rates (Koretz *et al.*, 2001).

- Low birth weight infants: meta-analysis of five RCT suggests that PN has no significant effect on survival and does not affect total or infectious complication rates or length of hospital stay (Koretz *et al.*, 2001).

The results of these analyses need to be carefully considered, for at least four reasons. First, severely malnourished patients have often been excluded from studies of PN (e.g. Von Meyenfeldt *et al.*, 1992; Fan *et al.*, 1994), even though they are likely to respond to this form of nutritional support (Heyland *et al.*, 1998). Secondly, the adverse effects of PN compared with routine care observed in some studies may be attributable to hyperglycaemia and other metabolic abnormalities associated with overfeeding (e.g. prescribed intakes of PN up to 40 kcal kg^{-1} body weight (Kinsella *et al.*, 1981) or 3000–5000 kcal daily (Bower *et al.*, 1986; Veterans Affairs TPN Cooperative Study Group, 1991)). However, overfeeding is practised much less commonly now than when these studies were undertaken and so the extent to which the findings of the earlier studies are relevant to current practice is not entirely clear. Thirdly, there are issues in individual trials in relation to differences in the composition of PN formulations used (e.g. with or without lipids), the variety of different types of patients involved, the duration of PN and the hygienic techniques used. Fourthly, it could be argued that trials

that have randomized patients to receiving PN or an oral diet are of limited clinical value as intravenously feeding patients who are able to tolerate intake orally could be considered inappropriate. A detailed review of the efficacy of PN relative to routine care is beyond the scope of this book and for more information the reader is referred to other publications – Klein *et al.* (1997), Heyland *et al.* (1998) and Koretz *et al.* (2001).

Parenteral Nutrition: a Comparison with Enteral Tube Feeding

PN is a very specialized nutritional intervention typically used for patients at high risk of DRM who have intestinal failure. Usually, whenever the gut is available, oral or enteral nutrition should be used, as it is simpler, more physiological and cheaper than PN (see below).

However, controversy about the value of PN relative to ETF or an oral diet exists when the intake by the enteral route is limited, often because of poor tolerance to feeding or the potential complications associated with feeding by this route. For example, there is the risk of aspiration pneumonia in patients with gastro-oesophageal reflux or neurological swallowing difficulties, or the possibility of precipitation of attacks of pancreatitis in patients who have already had recurrent, acute episodes. It should be stressed that there is often no conflict between the use of PN and ETF (see Fig. 9.2), since there are clear-cut indications for each mode of feeding (e.g. PN for prolonged intestinal failure and ETF in patients unable to swallow but with a functioning gut). In other situations, it is appropriate to use both ETF and PN (Fig. 9.2) (e.g. in the patient who has undergone severe GI surgery (MacFie, 2000a) and is being weaned from PN to ETF). Therefore, the following section, which compares PN with ETF, only applies to certain patient groups for whom there is uncertainty about the relative benefits of PN and ETF (Fig. 9.2).

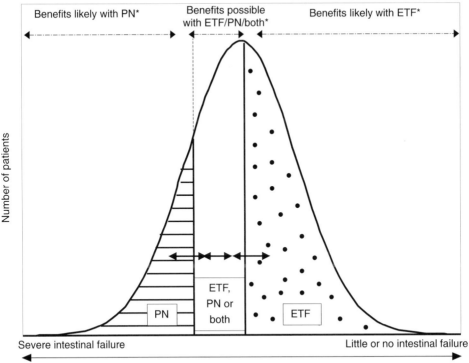

Fig. 9.2. Benefits with enteral tube feeding or parenteral nutrition and the need for clinical trials in some patient groups * (patient population at high risk of malnutrition).

Use of parenteral nutrition and enteral tube feeding in clinical practice

In the large majority of cases, if the GI tract is functioning and accessible, ETF is the method of choice for artificial nutritional support, according to standards set by the American Society of Parenteral and Enteral Nutrition (ASPEN) (1995, 2002). Table 7.1 in Chapter 7 has provided a summary of guidelines for the use of ETF and for PN the indications are mentioned earlier in this chapter. Ideally, the route selected for nutritional support must be appropriate for meeting the nutritional requirements of the patient and for meeting the goals of treatment (in terms of improved nutrient intake, anthropometric, functional or clinical outcome measures). The method chosen should also be the safest and most cost-effective (ASPEN, 1988). Therefore, ETF is used considerably more as a method of nutritional support than PN in both hospi-

tal and community settings. Data from the British Artificial Nutrition Survey (BANS) indicate that, in Britain, ETF is practised ~tenfold more frequently than PN (data from 1999, hospital and community settings) (Elia *et al.*, 2000a). At the end of 1999, it was estimated that ~500 people received home PN, compared with ≥ 15,000 on home ETF. In the hospital setting, PN is also practised significantly less frequently than ETF (by about four times: estimated 0.7 patients (PN) versus 2.9 patients (ETF) per 100 hospital beds in 1999) (Elia *et al.*, 2000a). Whilst recent years have seen marked growth in the use of ETF, particularly at home, the use of PN in hospital and community settings has grown less (Elia *et al.*, 2000a). Estimates from France and Italy suggest a similar prevalence of PN use in the home setting to Britain of around two to four patients per million of population, whereas the figures for the USA are much higher (~80 per million) (Pironi and

Tognoni, 1995). As in the UK, the prevalence of home ETF is much greater than that
of home PN in these countries, accounting
for 80–90% of all home artificial nutritional
support (HANS) (Pironi and Tognoni, 1995)
(for more information on UK and US surveys, refer to Chapter 7 (for home ETF) or
the following publications (for home ETF
and PN): Howard *et al.* (1995) and Elia *et al.*
(2000a, 2001b)). For many of these patients
who typically have chronic disease, the use
of PN or ETF is clear-cut (as discussed
above and illustrated in Fig. 9.2). However,
for those conditions in which ETF or PN
could be used, there are a number of considerations to be made when assessing the relative efficacy of these methods.

Physiology

ETF is undoubtedly more physiological
than intravenous feeding in that the GI
tract is utilized for the digestion (depending on the feed composition) and absorption of nutrients, as with a normal diet
consumed orally. This may be important
for the control of appetite and energy balance (Stratton and Elia, 1999b) and for the
function and integrity of the GI tract.
Indeed, it is hypothesized that the sole use
of PN and the failure to provide any nutrients enterally, particularly in the long term,
may have detrimental effects on the morphology and function of the intestine.
Although some studies have suggested
adverse effects of PN on intestinal function
(Guedon *et al.*, 1986), comparative studies
in humans are few and relatively short-
term (Wicks *et al.*, 1994; Suchner *et al.*,
1996; Reynolds *et al.*, 1997). Therefore, at
present, there is insufficient evidence to
suggest that ETF is superior to PN in this
respect (Lipman, 1998; Green, 1999), and
so further studies are needed.

It is suggested that one of the consequences of intestinal morphological
changes that may follow prolonged periods
of gut rest (e.g. with intravenous feeding) is
bacterial translocation. This can be defined
as the passage of viable indigenous bacteria
or bacterial products from the GI tract to
the mesenteric lymph nodes and other

organs. The enteral delivery of nutrients by
ETF may prevent this process. However, at
the present time, there is no clinical evidence to suggest that PN promotes bacterial
translocation or that ETF can prevent it in
a clinically relevant manner (Lipman,
1995, 1998; Green, 1999; MacFie, 2000b).
Therefore, the clinical significance of this
process remains to be established.

Safety

It is widely believed that ETF is safer than
PN, although few studies have fully compared the safety and the rates of complications of these two methods of nutritional
support (Lipman, 1998). It has been
hypothesized that PN may predispose
patients to having more infections and so
any clinical advantages that arise from the
use of PN must overcome this disadvantage
(Koretz, 1994). Indeed, in postoperative
oesophagogastric patients, there were more
life-threatening complications with PN
than with jejunostomy feeding (Baigire *et
al.*, 1996) and in laryngectomy patients,
ETF-related complications were clinically
less significant than those associated with
PN (Iovinelli *et al.*, 1993). A meta-analysis
of eight studies comparing the efficacy of
early ETF with PN, in a variety of surgical
patients, found that fewer of the enterally
fed patients developed septic complications (Moore *et al.*, 1992). Other trials have
suggested no differences (Von Meyenfeldt
et al., 1992; Woodcock *et al.*, 2001). In
addition, care is needed when interpreting
the findings of older studies in which overfeeding, leading to hyperglycaemia,
occurred with PN, which may have contributed to these morbidities.

Clearly, both PN and ETF are associated
with complications (mechanical, infectious, metabolic), although the majority can
be avoided if correct clinical practices are
observed in hospital and community settings (Lipman, 1998). National and international expert committees on the use of
artificial nutritional support have published recommended standards for patients
receiving these methods of feeding, either
in hospital or in the home environment,

which can be referred to for practical guidance (ASPEN, 1988, 1995; Elia *et al.*, 1994; Sizer, 1996).

Comparison of clinical efficacy of PN and ETF in specific patient groups

Although the following review of individual studies and meta-analyses shows variable results when the clinical efficacy of ETF and PN is compared, in specific groups of patients, during particular phases of disease, it generally shows that ETF has similar or superior effects to PN. However, in interpreting the results obtained in specific groups of patients, the following general issues should be kept in mind:

- The results apply to groups of patients at a particular phase of disease or injury with variable degrees of intestinal failure. During different phases of the same condition, when intestinal failure is less of a problem, PN is not likely to be required and so comparisons between PN and ETF are less valuable.
- The macro- and micronutrient composition of the feeds given intravenously or enterally generally vary. For example, the amino acid composition of parenteral and enteral feeds is invariably different. PN typically lacks specific amino acids, such as glutamine, at least in the studies evaluated.
- The quantity of energy and protein provided by PN is often greater than that from ETF because poor tolerance to enteral feeding restricts intake (due either to gastric stasis, as in the early postoperative period, or to GI side-effects, as in patients receiving BMT or certain types of chemotherapy). The provision of greater intakes intravenously than enterally may theoretically have positive effects relative to ETF (e.g. when the amount of ETF provided is extremely low) or negative effects (e.g. when intake by ETF is adequate or near adequate and PN is in excess of requirements, with the potential for adverse effects associated with overfeeding).

- Each modality of treatment can produce a range of potentially beneficial effects and a range of complications. A comparison between two modalities of treatment (ETF versus PN) represents the balance between the benefit and detriment associated with each therapy. For example, although PN can provide adequate amounts of nutrients, even when there is GI failure, an important complication is catheter-related sepsis. The incidence of this complication is increased in patients who are immunosuppressed and those who are hyperglycaemic as a result of overfeeding or glucose intolerance. The complications of PN, including catheter-related sepsis may explain why PN has not been found to be more effective than ETF, at least in some patient groups, and why in some circumstances it may be inferior to ETF. This means that, in comparing PN and ETF, there are nutritional and non-nutritional considerations. For example, poor hygienic technique is a major cause of catheter-related sepsis (non-nutritional), but poor control of glucose concentrations in critically ill patients, who typically receive PN (nutritional), increases a wide range of complications, including mortality (Van den Berghe *et al.*, 2001; see Chapter 1).
- Severely malnourished patients are often excluded from trials, even though they are likely to respond to nutritional support (e.g. Iovinelli *et al.*, 1993).

Bone marrow transplantation

BMT is used for the treatment of patients with severe aplastic anaemia, leukaemia and some other malignancies. As there are many adverse sequelae (anorexia, nausea, vomiting, diarrhoea and mucositis) associated with such a procedure, an adequate oral diet is usually unachievable and artificial nutritional support is required. Traditionally, PN has been the chosen method for the nutritional support of patients undergoing BMT. Indeed, in one trial, patients given PN were found to have significantly improved survival and increased disease-free survival, with longer times to relapse, than patients given no nutritional support (Weisdorf *et al.*, 1987). However, a comparative study has found little difference in efficacy between using PN and ETF (Szeluga *et al.*, 1987), with nutrition-related costs being two to three times greater in parenterally fed patients. Furthermore, another study suggests that ETF may be more effective clinically as well as financially in this patient group (Todd, A.J. *et al.*, 2000). This preliminary report indicated that episodes of pyrexia and diarrhoea were significantly fewer in patients fed via ETF (nasogastric (NG) tube and oral intake). There was also a trend towards a reduction in the number of episodes of nausea and vomiting and a shorter length of hospital stay by an average of 5 days (Todd, A.J. *et al.*, 2000). Therefore, in BMT patients, while both PN and ETF are clinically effective, recent preliminary findings suggest that ETF may be more effective clinically while being a cheaper treatment to administer. The findings of a larger RCT are awaited.

Critical illness/injury (including head injury)

Increasingly, ETF is being used in critically ill or severely injured patients instead of PN, and Chapter 7 includes a review of studies of ETF in this patient group. Although some studies and meta-analyses have shown no significant differences in outcome in enterally and parenterally fed patients with critical illness/injury (Adams *et al.*, 1986; Hadley *et al.*, 1986; Cerra *et al.*, 1988; Moore *et al.*, 1992) and severe head injury (Hadley *et al.*, 1986; Young *et al.*, 1987), others suggest that ETF, typically into the jejunum, may be superior to PN in this patient group. Here are some examples:

- In a study of 24 critically ill patients (with complications following surgery or respiratory failure), those randomized to ETF had better GI-tract mucosal permeability compared with the PN group (Hadfield *et al.*, 1995).

- In a study of patients with multisystem trauma (*n* 63 with abdominal trauma index > 15), the nitrogen balance was similar in the ETF (jejunal) and PN groups, but there was significantly less septic morbidity in those fed enterally (Moore and Moore, 1991).

- Meta-analysis concluded that septic morbidity rates in high-risk surgical patients were reduced in those given ETF compared with those given PN (Moore *et al.*, 1992), although this may relate to differences in intake between groups (see above).

- Patients with blunt and penetrating trauma (abdominal trauma index >15) who were randomized to be fed enterally (jejunal) sustained significantly fewer pneumonias, intra-abdominal abscesses and episodes of line sepsis than parenterally fed patients (Kudsk *et al.*, 1992). The ETF group also had significantly fewer infections per patient and significantly fewer infections per infected patient (Kudsk *et al.*, 1992).

- Patients with head injury fed by ETF exhibited significant improvements in the Glasgow coma scale (suggesting improved neurological outcome), compared with stable scores in the PN group (Suchner *et al.*, 1996), although similar benefits were not observed in another study (trend towards better neurological outcome in the PN group (Young *et al.*, 1987)).

Larger, well-designed RCT that assess both clinical and cost outcomes are required in these patient groups. The importance of the time of intervention during treatment and the benefits of using specialized, disease-specific formulations also require exploration.

GI disease

GI disease frequently limits nutritional intake and the digestion and absorption of food. Therefore, nutritional support is often required in this patient group. Unless there is intestinal failure or the need for complete bowel rest, ETF is typically used in preference to PN. Studies indicate that the use of PN during bowel rest is less effective than ETF or a regular diet at inducing remission (McIntyre *et al.*, 1986; Gonzalez-Huix *et al.*, 1993). For patients with severe inflammatory bowel disease, ETF (using elemental, peptide or whole-protein feeds) is most commonly used, either alone or in combination with steroid therapy, to induce remission (Zachos *et al.*, 2001). Furthermore, in children, the use of ETF may be preferable to steroid treatment, in order to maintain growth (Heuschkel *et al.*, 2000) (growth and development can be hindered by steroids). Also, in children with severe intractable diarrhoea, ETF and PN have been shown to have similar effects on body weight, although ETF was associated with faster resolution of malabsorption and diarrhoea than PN (small RCT, *n* 13) (Orenstein, 1986). A discussion of the use of ETF and PN in patients undergoing GI surgery can be found below.

Liver transplantation

Two trials comparing the use of ETF and PN in liver-transplant patients have supported the use of ETF in this patient group (Mehta *et al.*, 1994; Wicks *et al.*, 1994). In one retrospective trial, patients fed enterally (*n* 55) started on an oral diet sooner, reached an adequate oral intake significantly earlier and had a lower frequency of postoperative ileus than the parenterally fed patients (*n* 20) (Mehta *et al.*, 1994). Patients not meeting their nutritional requirements orally were sent home on ETF, allowing quicker discharge from hospital (Mehta *et al.*, 1994). In a small prospective RCT (*n* 24), ETF was found to be of comparable efficacy to PN. The recovery of an oral diet, the maintenance of arm anthropometric values and changes in GI absorptive capacity were similar in the two groups of patients but the costs of ETF compared with PN were much lower (Wicks *et al.*, 1994). The specific use of branched-chain amino acids in the treatment of hepatic encephalopathy is not considered here.

Malignancy

There is a high prevalence of malnutrition in cancer patients in hospital and community settings (see Chapter 2), which may impair patients' quality of life and patients' response to treatments. Therefore, some form of nutritional support is often recommended as an integral part of the treatment of patients with cancer. Both ETF and PN are commonly used to provide nutritional support for patients with cancer, although it is generally recommended that ETF should be the method of choice in cancer patients who have a functioning GI tract (Bozzetti, 1992). Comparisons of the effectiveness of ETF and PN in this patient group are limited but evidence suggests that both methods improve nutritional indices (body weight, fat mass, nitrogen balance) and visceral protein status, and that ETF improves indices of immune function (Bozzetti, 1992). More recent trials, particularly in cancer patients undergoing surgery (Bozzetti *et al.*, 2001; Braga *et al.*, 2001), suggest that, although patients receiving ETF experience more GI symptoms (e.g. diarrhoea, abdominal distension), their outcome is significantly better than those fed parenterally (see below). In addition to surgery, ETF and PN are often used alongside chemotherapy and/or radiotherapy in the treatment of cancer patients.

CHEMOTHERAPY

In patients receiving chemotherapy for a variety of cancers, ETF may be preferable to PN (Koretz, 1994). Meta-analyses in patients receiving PN during chemotherapy suggest that survival may be reduced, the response to chemotherapy poorer and the infection rates higher (Klein *et al.*, 1986; Koretz *et al.*, 2001). However, there are methodological criticisms of the studies used in the analysis that make it difficult to draw firm conclusions (e.g. exclusion of severely undernourished patients). Therefore, it seems pragmatic to suggest that ETF is the preferred method of support during chemotherapy until well-designed RCT in cancer-specific groups show otherwise.

Studies in irradiated patients with a variety of cancers suggest that ETF and PN have similar metabolic effects (see Donaldson, 1984, for a review), but their effects on outcome have not been compared (quality of life, complication rates, etc.). Although individual studies of either ETF or PN have suggested beneficial effects of their use during radiation to patients with head, neck, oesophagus and abdominal/pelvic cancers (Donaldson, 1984), well-designed comparative trials in patients at risk of DRM are lacking. RCT are required if the efficacy of ETF versus PN in patients with different types of cancer undergoing radiation and other treatments (e.g. surgery) (Donaldson, 1984; Jensen, 1985) is to be ascertained.

SURGERY
In cancer patients undergoing surgery (often for head and neck or GI cancer), PN and ETF are used perioperatively. The clinical benefits of using these two methods before surgery have been discussed elsewhere (Jensen, 1985) (studies undertaken in mixed groups of surgical patients are discussed below). However, here are some examples of specific studies comparing these two forms of therapy. In an RCT of 257 patients with cancer of the stomach, pancreas or oesophagus, no significant differences were found in nutritional, immunological or inflammatory variables between patients given PN (n 131) or ETF (n 126) postoperatively. Infectious and non-infectious complication rates, length of hospital stay and mortality rates also did not differ between groups. However, intestinal oxygenation recovered significantly faster in enterally fed patients and ETF was four times less expensive than PN (Braga et al., 2001). A more recent report from the same group, comparing ETF (n 159) with PN (n 158) in malnourished GI surgical patients, found significantly lower complication rates and significantly shorter postoperative stays in those enterally fed. However, the incidence of 'adverse events' was significantly greater

in the ETF group (mild GI symptoms) (Bozzetti et al., 2001).

Although both methods of nutritional support can improve nutritional parameters and may reduce postoperative morbidity and mortality, RCT are required to compare the clinical and cost efficacy of ETF and PN in perioperative cancer patients. The effectiveness of using disease-specific enteral formulas compared with PN in cancer patients, including those formulated with the aim of modulating immune and inflammatory parameters, also requires investigation.

TERMINAL CARE
Ideally, PN should be a treatment that is reserved for cancer patients who cannot be fed via the GI tract (Tchekmedyian, 1995) and so its use in the feeding of advanced cancer and acquired immune deficiency syndrome (AIDS) patients, particularly in the home setting in some countries (Howard et al., 1995; Pironi and Tognoni, 1995), is controversial. Furthermore, the use of PN is not recommended as an adjunct to cancer therapy because of the limited benefits and the high risks and expenses of using this mode of support (Tchekmedyian, 1995). It is unclear whether any significant prolongation of life with improved quality of life can be gained from using intravenous feeding in terminal cancer patients. Therefore, ETF in most cases (if the GI tract is functioning and enteral access is feasible) is preferable if nutritional support is warranted.

In cancer patients, there is generally a lack of evidence supporting the use of one type of nutritional support over another. Therefore, it is pragmatic to encourage the use of ETF as a largely safer, cheaper and more physiological treatment than PN. Indeed, a recent review of evidence-based medicine concluded that, for specialized nutritional support, ETF rather than PN should typically be used, being a potentially safer and more physiological method (Ashley and Howard, 2000). The benefits of using enteral nutrition (ONS and ETF) in cancer patients in hospital and community settings is discussed in Chapters 6 and 7. Ultimately, the provision of optimal nutritional care for cancer patients and other patient groups requires a multidisciplinary approach, with doctors, dietitians, nurses and pharmacists (Shils, 1979) working as a team. Deciding what method of nutritional support to use for each individual patient requires primarily clinical judgement (Lipman, 1998), while the evidence-based information is lacking, although the availability of resources may also influence decisions about treatment (see Chapter 5).

Acute pancreatitis

In the past, PN has typically been the favoured means of nutritional support in the treatment of patients with acute pancreatitis. However, RCT of patients with severe acute pancreatitis report that the resolution of the disease is similar whether enteral (into the jejunum) or parenteral feeding is used, although complications tend to be fewer with ETF (small trial (*n* 15) (Abou-Assi *et al.*, 2000). Other RCT suggest that ETF is safe and may be more effective than PN in this patient group (Kalfarentzos *et al.*, 1997; McClave *et al.*, 1997; Windsor *et al.*, 1998). In these trials, jejunal ETF is typically well tolerated without adverse effect on the course of the disease. In one trial, enterally fed patients (nasoenteric tube, elemental diet, *n* 18) experienced fewer total complications and were at lower risk of developing septic complications than the parenterally fed individuals (*n* 20) (Kalfarentzos *et al.*, 1997). In another trial (*n* 34) (Windsor *et al.*, 1998), total ETF attenuated the acute-phase response and improved disease severity. Systemic inflammatory response syndrome (SIRS), sepsis, organ failure and intensive-care unit (ICU) stay were also globally improved in the enterally fed patients, but similar improvements were not seen in the parenterally fed group (Windsor *et al.*, 1998). Therefore, several authors favour the use of ETF above PN in patients with severe acute pancreatitis.

Surgery

The studies reviewed suggest that, in some groups of patients undergoing major surgery, those receiving ETF (typically into the duodenum and jejunum) have a number of outcome advantages over those fed parenterally in the postoperative period. These include the following:

- Significantly shorter lengths of hospital stay (by an average of 8 days in patients undergoing total laryngectomy (Iovinelli *et al.*, 1993)).
- Lower infective complication rates (nonsignificantly lower in patients undergoing major hepatic resection (Shirabe *et al.*, 1997)).
- Quicker return of bowel movements postoperatively (Feilhauer *et al.*, 2000).
- Fewer life-threatening complications (in postoperative oesophagogastric patients (Baigire *et al.*, 1996)).
- Fewer septic complications (in a variety of surgical patients, meta-analysis of trials (Moore *et al.*, 1992)).

Other perioperative studies have found no differences in outcome between enterally and parenterally fed patients (e.g. GI surgical cancer patients (Von Meyenfeldt *et al.*, 1992; Pacelli *et al.*, 2001) and upper GI surgical patients (Reynolds *et al.*, 1997)), although the small size of some of these trials may mean that a type II error is likely (i.e. significant differences exist but are not detected due to insufficient power). Other authors have shown that, in some patient groups (including GI surgical and vascular surgical patients in whom GI function is uncertain), PN may be superior to ETF (Woodcock *et al.*, 2001). These differences in results are likely to be due to the inclusion of different types of patients in these clinical trials (see Fig. 9.2 for the relationship of severity of intestinal failure and potential efficacy of ETF or PN).

ETF may also be as effective at improving nutritional status and visceral protein status as PN, if not more effective, in a variety of surgical groups (major abdominal surgery (Heylen *et al.*, 1987; Hamaoui *et* al., 1990) and neurosurgery (Suchner et al., 1996)). In one trial, it appeared that PN patients had slightly reduced absorptive function (not significant) and that ETF patients maintained better absorption of vitamin A (Suchner et al., 1996). However, both nutritional support methods have been shown to be effective ways of ensuring a greater nutritional intake in the pre-operative (Von Meyenfeldt et al., 1992) and early postoperative period than would be possible without nutritional support (nil by mouth and intravenous fluids), typically with similar efficacy (although not always) (Bower et al., 1986; Fletcher and Little, 1986; Heylen et al., 1987; Hamaoui et al., 1990; Iovinelli et al., 1993; Suchner et al., 1996; Reynolds et al., 1997). Studies in surgical patients also indicate that ETF can be more cost-efficient than PN (Bower et al., 1986; Hamaoui et al., 1990).

In general, authors have found that ETF is preferable to PN as a means of nutritional support in specific groups of surgical patients due to clinical and/or cost benefits, as the following quotations reflect:

> The efficacy and safety of enteral nutrition, combined with its decreased cost, make it an attractive alternative to PN in properly selected patients. Increased use of enteral nutrition under these circumstances may allow for reduced costs of nutritional support without sacrificing quality of therapy.
> (Bower et al., 1986)

> Enteral nutrition is well tolerated after major upper GI surgery and is considerably less expensive than TPN... on this basis, it [ETF] can be recommended.
> (Reynolds et al., 1997)

However, these conclusions are not shared universally (Woodcock et al., 2001) and some would argue that a combination of ETF and PN might be most effective (MacFie, 2000a), depending on the patient group in question (Fig. 9.2).

Other diseases

Prospective RCT are needed in other patient groups in whom there is uncertainty about the efficacy of ETF versus PN (including liver and renal disease).

Narrative reviews by experts in these specialist areas suggest that ETF should be used where feasible instead of PN.

LIVER DISEASE

ETF is recommended as a safe alternative to PN for the nutritional replenishment of patients with chronic liver disease (Cabre and Gassull, 1993), even in those with oesophageal varices. Indeed, a number of studies of ETF have documented outcome benefits with the use of ETF in patients with liver disease (see Chapter 7) and specialized formulas have been developed particularly for use in patients with chronic liver disease. In contrast, the use of PN can have a number of disadvantages. These include the high incidence of catheter-related complications in advanced cirrhotics and problems with large volumes of parenteral fluid delivery leading to water retention (Cabre and Gassull, 1993).

RENAL DISEASE

It has been suggested that ETF should provide at least some of the nutritional needs of a patient with acute renal failure (Druml, 1993). Furthermore, commercial enteral feeds have been specifically formulated in order that the nutritional and fluid requirements of such patients can be met. In some patients, especially those with acute renal failure, it may be difficult to meet the specific requirements from ETF alone and supplementary PN may be useful (Druml, 1993). However, because tolerance to fluid/volume load is limited, electrolyte and fluid derangements can quickly develop. Therefore, regular monitoring in this patient group is recommended to avoid any metabolic complications resulting from artificial nutritional support.

In many of the above trials, the small sample sizes and the potential for a type II error need to be considered (see Chapter 10). Ultimately, larger trials in disease-specific groups are needed where there is controversy about which method of feeding to use (ETF versus PN). These should be preceded by power calculations that have estimated the sample size of patients required to assess differences in outcome between enterally and parenterally fed patients.

Financial issues

Not enough is known about the cost-effectiveness of either ETF or PN as individual methods of nutritional support (Twomey and Patching, 1985; Green, 1999) and so comparison of the financial efficacy of these two treatments is difficult. Analyses of the cost–benefit and the cost-effectiveness of nutritional support in hospital and community settings need to be undertaken prospectively as part of large, well-designed RCT in specific patient groups (for a discussion, see Twomey and Patching, 1985; Green, 2001a). However, it is clear that PN is a substantially more expensive treatment than ETF, in both hospital and home settings. For example, the average cost of PN in hospital patients in the USA was estimated to be ~US$500 compared with < US$30 for ETF in 1985 (Twomey and Patching, 1985) (excluding costs of hospital stay). A full breakdown of the costs for PN was also highlighted in this review (Twomey and Patching, 1985) and included costs for pharmacy and supplies (PN solutions, tubing, pump, dressings and medications), laboratory and professional monitoring and the treatment of complications. The costs of some of the more common complications of intravenous therapy, including systemic sepsis, pneumothorax and subclavian vein thrombosis, were also highlighted (Twomey and Patching, 1985), although their relative infrequency contributed only ~$13 to the estimated daily costs. Other minor complications of PN (e.g. hyperglycaemia, catheter migration, arterial injury) were estimated to have little effect on cost, but the cost implications of life-threatening complications (e.g. massive air embolus) were difficult to calculate.

In contrast to PN, the costs for ETF are known to be markedly lower, with the cost of feeds, equipment and monitoring being significantly less. In the community setting in the UK, some of the costs for ETF equipment (e.g. pumps) and monitoring are increasingly being met by commercial companies. Most hospitals in the UK now use a commercial company to provide a service for patients discharged on home ETF (Elia *et al.*, 2001b) and this service includes supply of feed and equipment to patients and a telephone helpline. The funding for feeds/equipment may be from a hospital or community budget (see Howard and Bowen, 2001, for more information) and the general practitioner is mostly responsible for prescribing. However, practices differ across Europe due to differences in health-care systems. In the UK, there are proposals to change the way home ETF is funded to reduce the costs of this treatment even further. This involves providing feeds from the hospital setting at cheaper 'contract' prices instead of by prescription in the community. Although this may produce cost savings in the short term, it is anticipated that such changes in funding may detrimentally affect the clinical care of patients receiving this type of treatment, which will eventually have cost implications. For a review of these issues, see Howard and Bowen (2001).

The cost-effectiveness of ETF and PN and the systems that support these treatments needs to be evaluated in the short and long term and should not simply focus on the costs of feeding and personnel (including carers in the community) *per se*, without a consideration of the effects of these methods of feeding on patients' clinical outcome. Indeed, a full cost-effectiveness analysis must take into account the savings associated with the benefits of a treatment offset against its costs and any complications. However, it can be difficult to 'cost' many of the benefits of nutritional support, such as improvements in muscle strength, walking distance and quality of life and reduced mortality rates. It is likely that cost savings associated with the improvements in outcome observed following the use of ETF (e.g. reduced complication rates, reduced ICU/hospital stays, quicker recovery times) will far exceed the relatively small costs of feeding (Green, 1999). This may be less likely with

PN because of the greater expense of this therapy and the costs of treating the complications associated with intravenous feeding. As this quote simply states, 'in patients with functioning GI tracts the adage "If the gut works use it" reflects both good physiology and good economics' (Twomey and Patching, 1985). Indeed, unlike ETF, which has relatively low costs, the high costs of PN mean that, if clinical outcome is not demonstrably improved, it is unlikely to be cost-effective. Therefore, with PN and, to a lesser extent, ETF, identification of those patients who will benefit from nutritional support before initiation of treatment is ideal (Twomey and Patching, 1985).

For cost savings to be apportioned to either ETF or PN, clinical trials are needed to assess clinical outcomes and associated costs with sufficient power to detect differences in these parameters. Of the studies reviewed in this book and by other workers (ETF and PN) (Koretz, 1994), sample sizes and study designs are frequently insufficient and inadequate to detect meaningful changes in outcome and hence cost parameters. Most of the existing financial data comparing ETF and PN have been provided by studies from America, some of which have been summarized in the very thorough review by Lipman (1998), who concluded that enteral nutrition is less expensive than parenteral nutrition. Table 9.1 summarizes both prospective and retrospective calculations and estimates of the costs of ETF compared with PN in a number of different patient groups (listed in alphabetical order according to first author). Although this table highlights a plethora of different cost estimates (average per patient, daily, monthly and annual figures) for patients with a variety of different conditions, it consistently shows that ETF is cheaper than PN. This supports the findings of a detailed review (Lipman, 1998). ETF has been shown by prospective and retrospective estimates and calculations to be cheaper in many patient groups. These include BMT or liver transplantation patients, those post-trauma/post-surgery

and those with mild pancreatitis. It has also been shown to be cheaper in both community and hospital settings. The total cost of home ETF has been estimated to be ~10% of that of home PN. Other estimates suggest that the use of ETF and PN in the community setting accounts for savings of ~75% and 60–76% on hospital costs for ETF and PN, respectively (Pironi and Tognoni, 1995).

Conclusions

For some patients, PN provides the only and the most effective way of increasing nutritional intake to prevent or treat DRM (e.g. in patients with severe intestinal failure). In clinical practice, this is likely to include a minority (< 5%) of patients. This is because, in most patients with a functioning GI tract, ETF is the method of choice if artificial nutritional support is required. However, there are conditions for which there is uncertainty about whether ETF, PN or a combination of both methods is the most effective way to provide nutritional support (see Fig. 9.2). In such situations, consideration should be given to the physiology and the safety of the respective methods and the current evidence base discussed in this chapter (i.e. the clinical efficacy). From the analysis in which PN was compared to ETF in specific patient groups, at particular stages of their illness, ETF was generally found to be as effective as PN, if not more effective, at lower cost. However, in some situations when GI function is inadequate, PN has been shown to be superior to ETF (Woodcock *et al.*, 2001). Nevertheless, it is hoped that the overview presented in this chapter will help to reduce at least some of the controversy surrounding the use of ETF versus PN in particular patient groups. Ultimately, the decision to use one or other or both means of artificial nutrition may depend on clinical judgement, the resources available to fund nutritional support and the acceptability and tolerance of each specific mode of nutritional support.

Table 9.1. Costs of parenteral nutrition versus enteral tube feeding in various patient groups.[a]

Author/study	Type of cost/patient group	Parenteral nutrition	Enteral tube feeding (as a % of PN cost)
Adams et al., 1986	Daily cost for feeding following laparotomy post-trauma (USA)	$153	24
Allison, 1995	Average weekly cost of feeding hospital patients (UK)	£350–£500	14–20
Bower et al., 1986	Average patient charge for feeding postoperatively (USA) (upper GI and pancreaticobiliary surgery)	$2,313	37[b]
Braga et al., 2001	Average daily per-patient cost of feeding (Italy)	$91	27
Cerra et al., 1988	Total feeding cost for septic patients (USA)	$330,661	69[b]
Hamaoui et al., 1990	Average daily cost for feeding major abdominal surgical patients (USA)	$102	43[b]
Howard et al., 1995	Average daily charge for home-fed patients (USA)	$280	12
Kalfarentzos et al., 1997	Average daily per-patient feeding cost during severe acute pancreatitis (UK)	£100 (feed, not complications)	30
McClave et al., 1997	Mean per-patient charge for feeding (mild acute pancreatitis) (USA)	$3,294	53[b]
Reynolds et al., 1997	Average per-patient cost for feeding postoperatively (upper-GI surgery, USA)	$200	10
Szeluga et al., 1987	Cost of 28-day feeding programme for a bone-marrow transplant patient (USA)	$2,575	44
Tchekmedyian, 1995	Average monthly charges for home cancer patients (USA)	$8,400 ($7,140–11,700)	12
Twomey and Patching, 1985	Average hospital cost for feeding per patient (USA)	$503	<6
Wicks et al., 1994	Average daily per-patient feeding cost for patients undergoing liver transplant (UK)	£75–85 (feed plus complications)	8 (feed only)
Windsor et al., 1998	Average daily per-patient feeding cost during severe acute pancreatitis (UK)	£75 (not including disposables)	7

[a]The absolute costs associated with different studies are not comparable since they include different components and are taken from studies in different countries undertaken at different times over a 15-year period.
[b]Difference evaluated to be statistically significant (most studies/reviews did not report statistics).

10
Undertaking Clinical Nutrition Intervention Trials

Introduction

In Chapters 6 and 7 we assessed the quality of many clinical nutrition trials and found frequent inadequacies in study design, as well as in the analysis and reporting of results. Amongst the most common identifiable problems were selection and allocation of patients to the control and treatment groups, inadequate sample sizes (lack of power statistics) and inadequate analysis of some of the results. Flawed or inadequate study designs may be considered to be unethical because they may expose patients to unnecessary risk or inconvenience, use financial and other resources that could be used more beneficially elsewhere and stimulate unnecessary further research to examine the claims made. The brief sections that follow provide practical guidelines that aim to prevent these problems from arising. A fuller analysis of the issues can be found elsewhere (Pockock, 1983, 1985). Here we begin by considering some of the basic principles and purposes of clinical trials.

Principles and Purposes of Clinical Trials

Science aims to understand variability in nature, statistics provides methods to assess this variability, and study design controls and reduces variability to make assessment more reliable and valid. One of the most important contributions of statistics to medicine and nutritional science is study design. This has three purposes:

- To reduce or eliminate bias from a treatment effect, e.g. to reduce systematic error by ensuring that each patient has an equal chance of receiving the treatment or placebo (or alternative treatment) (see glossary for various types of bias).
- To control and reduce error so that confounding variability that is not of interest to the experiment is removed.
- To allow hypotheses to be examined with acceptable statistical power, i.e. by reducing bias and error, treatment effects can be estimated with greater reliability and confidence.

When the outcome measure is highly variable, large samples are needed to obtain reliable results. A reduction in variability implies that the study has more power (see Glossary). This means that a smaller sample size can be used to achieve the same power as a study with greater outcome variability.

There are two types of methods for controlling and reducing variability due to experimental error. The first is an indirect statistical method, which is carried out after the results become available, e.g.

analysis of covariance (ANCOVA) can be used to control for continuous variables that are not evenly matched between the groups. The second is a direct experimental method (study design), in which subjects are selected and allocated into homogeneous and comparable experimental groups and subjected to treatments under standardized experimental conditions. Study design is concerned with the second, more direct method of controlling and reducing variability (Winer *et al.*, 1991).

Study designs can be divided into observational (descriptive) and interventional (experimental) designs. They can also be divided into prospective or retrospective studies, and longitudinal or cross-sectional studies, but these are not mutually exclusive. For example, interventional studies can also be prospective and longitudinal. Interventional studies are in principle more powerful, in respect of inferences and causality, than observational studies, which are descriptive in nature. When observational studies are used to make comparisons between groups, significant differences do not necessarily prove that the variable under consideration is the cause. For example, several observational studies have shown that undernourished patients have more postoperative complications than normally nourished individuals (Chapter 4), but this does not prove that undernutrition is responsible for the increased complications. It is possible that complications are caused by the underlying disease, which coincidentally also causes malnutrition. If malnutrition is involved in the causal pathway, then it should be possible to demonstrate through an intervention study that appropriate nutritional treatment reduces the number of complications. Therefore, in this book a clear distinction is made between observational (descriptive) studies and interventional (experimental) studies.

This chapter focuses on the design of clinical trials, which can be defined as planned experimental human studies that aim to assess the effects of one or more interventions or treatments. Clinical trials are often categorized into one of four phases, according to their experimental status (Everitt and Pickles, 1999):

Phase I trial: clinical pharmacology and toxicity investigations.
Phase II trial: initial clinical investigations for treatment effects.
Phase III trial: full-scale evaluation of treatment.
Phase IV: post-marketing evaluation (e.g. for long-term adverse effects).

Clinical trials correspond to phase III trials. The conclusions that emerge from such trials obviously depend on the methodology used. Use of poor methodology, either in assessing the outcome variables or in designing the study, can provide misleading results, which at worst may ultimately harm the patient.

It is essential to clarify thoughts in advance of starting the study, not only to prevent misunderstanding from occurring between those involved in planning and executing the trial, but also to consider and clarify ethical and statistical issues. These are achieved by writing a protocol, which can be regarded as a formal statement of the scientific basis, aims and planned procedures associated with the trial and its analysis. The key items of protocols are given in Table 10.1. Several of them are discussed in more detail in the two main sections that follow: 'Designing Clinical Trials' and 'Analysing Results of Clinical Trials'.

Designing Clinical Trials

Define a hypothesis, treatment groups and appropriate outcome variables

One of the first steps in undertaking a clinical trial is to define a hypothesis and identify key outcome measures, in the light of existing knowledge (see Annex 10.1, which provides aids to establishing such knowledge). For example, a hypothesis might be that perioperative nutritional support decreases postoperative fatigue. The outcome variables may be either subjective (e.g. those obtained on visual analogue scales) or objective measures of fatigue.

Table 10.1. Key features of protocols for clinical trials.

Background of the area, identifying deficiencies in knowledge that are amenable to investigation
Objectives and/or hypothesis to be examined
Treatments, including a comparison group
Primary (± secondary or intermediate) outcome variables
Methods for assessing outcome variables
Study design
Sample size calculations
Patient selection and allocation
Ethical issues, including patient consent and anonymity, data protection
Practical issues: administration, recording progress of study, including protocol violations, establishment of database
Statistical analysis
Writing up the study, authorship and dissemination of results

The objective measures of fatigue may involve voluntary tests (e.g. grip strength) or involuntary tests (e.g. electrical stimulation tests). In any case, the hypothesis and outcome variables should be established before the study is begun.

It is usual to first identify a primary outcome variable, which is subjected to the main analysis, but additional intermediary (or secondary) variable(s) may also be included, which will be subjected to additional analyses. For example, if muscle biopsies are taken in a study on fatigue, they may be used to establish intermediary outcome measures, such as the histological appearance or concentration of metabolites implicated in causing muscle fatigue. They may provide plausible mechanisms responsible for any positive primary outcome measures. There may be more than one primary and intermediary outcome variable. Indeed, several outcome variables are often included in clinical trials (Roland and Torgerson, 1998) so that an overall balance can be obtained about the benefits of the intervention, which may include pathophysiological (e.g. effect on disease process), psychological (e.g. well-being) or economic end-points. Therefore, it is not surprising that nutritional intervention trials often include both specific and general outcome variables. However, the trial usually requires more subjects when several outcome variables are being assessed, because the likelihood of a positive chance finding is increased.

The following issues are relevant to outcome variables:

1. Each sample size calculation is based on a single variable. When more than one outcome variable is used, it may be necessary to undertake more than one sample-size calculation (see below).
2. The use of multiple statistical tests will increase the likelihood that a significant result will occur by chance. This needs to be taken into account at both the planning and the analytical stage (see below).
3. The choice of outcome variable depends on the study. A list of some of the variables used in clinical trials involving nutritional interventions is given in Table 10.2. Some of these are specific to the disease, such as encephalopathy in liver disease, respiratory function in chronic obstructive pulmonary disease and cytotoxicity or radiation-induced damage in cancer patients. Others are non-specific, such as muscle strength, well-being and weight change. Functional measurements, such as the number of falls in older subjects, quality of life and walking distance, are generally of greater clinical relevance than isolated measurements of changes in body weight or circulating concentrations of metabolites, which may or may not relate to the functional outcome measures.
4. Appropriate methodology, with known specificity and reproducibility, should be available. In multicentre studies, it is particularly important to ensure consistency in procedures and in the equipment used, so that variability and bias can be reduced.

Table 10.2. Some specific and general outcome variables used to assess the effectiveness of nutritional support in different groups of patients (see Chapters 6 and 7 and Appendices 3–6).

Disease	Outcome variable
Chronic obstructive pulmonary disease	Respiratory muscle strength
	Pulmonary function tests
	Walking distance
	Hand-grip strength
	Well-being/quality of life
	Weight change
Crohn's disease	Gastrointestinal function
	Inflammatory status
	Sense of energy and well-being
	Muscle strength
Malignancy	Disease recurrence
	Survival time
	Cytotoxicity (e.g. mucositis)
	Radiation-induced diarrhoea
	Immune function tests
	Well-being/quality of life
	Weight change
Elderly	Number of falls
	Pressure ulcer surface area
	Mental tests
	Immune function tests
	Activities of daily living
	Grip strength
	Well-being/quality of life
	Self-perceived health
	Mortality
	Length of hospital stay
HIV/AIDS	Immune function tests
	Gastrointestinal symptoms and function
	Cognitive function
	Well-being/quality of life
Liver disease	Grade of encephalopathy
	Mortality
	Rate of hospitalization
	Incidence of infections

Obviously, in designing studies to assess the effect of a nutritional intervention, it is necessary to decide on the type of treatment (if any) to be given to the control group. Some possibilities are given below:

- A new enteral formula or oral supplement is compared with an established formula or supplement, e.g. an immunonutrition formula is compared with a standard formula (Braga *et al.*, 1999; Senkal *et al.*, 1999).
- A formula is compared with a 'placebo' feed containing virtually no nutrients

(Whittaker *et al.*, 1990; Carver and Dobson, 1995), as in experimental studies on appetite regulation (Stratton, 1999).

- A formula is compared with no formula (Keele *et al.*, 1997).
- A formula is compared with routine therapy, which may include the use of other nutritional therapy in some patients (Pupelis *et al.*, 2001).
- Enteral tube feeding is compared with parenteral nutrition (Bozzetti *et al.*, 2001).
- A formula taken orally is compared with dietetic counselling (Turic *et al.*, 1998)

or other nutritional therapy, such as tube feeding (McWhirter and Pennington, 1996), or with drug therapy, such as steroids in Crohn's disease (O'Morain *et al.*, 1984).

Some of the advantages and disadvantages of these are shown in Table 10.3. Only the first two are amenable to blinding, whereby the patient and/or observer is unaware of the 'treatment' allocation, i.e. whether the patient has been allocated to the treatment or control group. A double-blind trial refers to a study where neither the patient nor the observer is aware of the treatment allocation, whereas a single-blind study refers to a study where only the patient is unaware of the allocation. Most clinical trials cited

Table 10.3. Advantages and disadvantages of using different types of control groups in clinical nutrition trials.

Type of comparison	Advantages	Disadvantages
New formula versus standard formula	Can be double-blind Can demonstrate superiority of one product over another	Since differences are often small, large sample sizes may be necessary to demonstrate an effect Multicentre trials may be necessary The nutrients responsible for any observed differences may be difficult to identify, since composition of products often differ in multiple ways[a]
New liquid formula versus watery placebo (placebo)	More likely to demonstrate a significant effect than when another feed is used as the control	Watery placebo may not have the same taste, texture or appearance as formula Watery placebo may be unethical in undernourished patients in need of nutritional support
New formula versus routine care	No placebo effect Benefit more likely to be demonstrated when routine care is inadequate	Not possible to fully blind (can be partially overcome if independent observers 'blind' to the interventions make objective judgements) Results depend on the quality of routine care, which may vary considerably from one health-care setting to another The routine care may include use of the new formula The trial may alter routine care
Tube feeding versus parenteral nutrition		Not possible to blind Ethical difficulties in randomizing certain types of patients (e.g. those with intestinal failure who require parenteral nutrition) The feeds may differ in multiple ways[a]
Formula versus dietary counselling		Not possible to blind May alter practice in an unacceptable manner (counselling is normally provided when a supplement is started)
Formula versus drug or tube feeding or parenteral nutrition		Not possible to blind May alter practice Unethical for certain types of patients (e.g. those with swallowing difficulty or intestinal failure)

[a]Attempts may be made to establish isonitrogenous and isocaloric delivery of feeds, but even these may differ in the proportion of energy derived from fat and carbohydrate.

in this book are not blinded studies (described as open studies) for either the observer or the patient. This means that for most trials there is potential for a variable amount of bias, which may partly explain the variable results obtained for similar groups of patients (see Chapters 6 and 7). Wherever possible, attempts should be made to design double-blind studies, but the composition of the control formula may need to be considered very carefully (Table 10.3). Unblinding should be carried out after the trial has been completed. If it is deemed necessary to unblind the study before it is complete so as to assess whether it is ethically justifiable to continue (i.e. if a marked and statistically significant difference is shown in the interim analysis, it may be unethical to continue the study), it should be carried out by a third party who is not involved with those performing the study. The interim analysis can also provide information on the variability in response, which can be used to establish or review the appropriate sample size, with advice from a statistician.

Sample size

Sample size should not be subjectively and arbitrarily decided. This is partly because a small sample size may fail to demonstrate a statistically significant effect when one really exists (type 2 error), and partly because it may lead to little confidence in a positive result in situations where there is really no significant effect. Therefore, sample size should be based on procedures that produce a high probability of detecting a significant effect if one truly exists, and reasonable certainty that no effect exists if it is not demonstrated by the trial. In calculating sample size, it is necessary to consider three variables.

1. Significance (P value): the specified probability of observing by chance an effect of a given magnitude (or greater than this magnitude) when in reality no effect exists (true null hypothesis). For example, suppose that a nutritional supplement does not alter cognitive function. However, when the conventional value of $P < 0.05$ is used to indicate a significant result, there is a 5% chance of such a result when in reality there is no actual change in cognitive function (type I error). If a value of $P < 0.01$ is used as the criterion for significance, there is only a 1% chance of observing a significant change in cognitive function; therefore the chances of obtaining a type 1 error can be reduced by choosing a smaller P value, although this increases the probability of a type 2 error (see below).

2. Power: the certainty or probability that a study of a given sample size will yield a statistically significant result when a real effect of a given magnitude exists. A study in which a significant result is obtained with 80% power indicates that there is only 80% certainty in the result being correct. In 20% of samples a significant result will be obtained when in reality there is no effect (20% chance of a type 2 error).

3. Effect size index: the magnitude of the effect (effect size) is the extent to which the null hypothesis is false, i.e. the extent to which the outcome variables differ between control and treatment groups. For Student's *t* tests and tests of two proportions, the difference between the groups is typically expressed as a fraction of the standard deviation (standardized difference or effect size index), so that calculations of sample size can be generic, e.g. an effect size expressed in centimetres is 100 times greater than when expressed in metres, but the two are exactly the same when expressed as fractions of the standard deviation.

For two independent samples, the effect size index is:

$$m_a - m_b/\sigma$$

where $m_a - m_b$ = expected difference between group means expressed in original measurement units, and σ = standard deviation of either population, since they are assumed to be equal.

For comparison of two proportions, the effect size index is:

$$p_a - p_b/\sigma$$

where $p_a - p_b$ = expected difference in proportions between groups, σ = standard deviation of the groups, corresponding to $\sqrt{p(1 - p)}$, where $p = p_a + p_b/2$ (assuming that the two groups are of equal size). For example, if the incidence of postoperative complications was 20% ($p_a = 0.2$) and the hypothesis is that the complications could be reduced to 10% ($p_b = 0.1$) by providing nutritional support, the effect size index can be calculated to be $0.2 - 0.1/\sqrt{0.15 \times 0.85}$, or 0.28.

The same result can be obtained by using percentage values throughout instead of proportions ($20 - 10/\sqrt{15 \times 85} = 0.28$).

It should be clear that significance, power, effect size and sample size cannot be viewed in isolation. When three of the four variables are specified, the fourth can be calculated. Here, the variables are used to calculate sample size. It should also be clear that large sample sizes are needed when:

1. The P value is small (less likelihood that the statistically significant result has occurred by chance);
2. The power is great (more power implies more certainty in a significant result);
3. The effect size index is small (it is easier to detect a larger effect than a smaller and less obvious effect).

A common procedure for calculating sample sizes is to use a significance value of 5% ($P = <0.05$ or a 5% chance of obtaining a significant result when there is no effect or a 5% chance of a type 1 error) and a power of 80% (20% chance of finding no significant effect when one really exists – type 2 error). This procedure implies that a type 1 error is four times more harmful than a type 2 error (the ratio of 20% and 5%). However, these criteria may be inappropriate for specific situations, i.e. they need to be considered according to the issue or hypothesis being addressed. For example, if the aim of an investigation (not necessarily a clinical trial) is to identify drugs or pharmaconutrients for more detailed subsequent investigations, it may be reasonable to use high power (e.g. 95%) and a high P value (e.g. 0.15 or even 0.2),

so that potentially useful products are not missed. In contrast, if there is concern that a new feed with unusual constituents might cause side-effects, then it might be reasonable to maintain a high power (e.g. 95% or more) but to reduce the P value to 0.01 or lower, so that any side-effects will be detected with considerable certainty.

The effect size index should represent a clinically significant effect. If an estimate of the standard deviation (variability in outcome variable) is not available to calculate an effect size index, a pilot study can be undertaken to establish it. It may also be possible to start the trial and use the early part of the trial to estimate the standard deviation. Although it is sometimes assumed that sample size calculations cannot be undertaken without pilot data or prior estimate of the true effect, this is not true. It is possible to undertake calculations based on estimates of clinically or theoretically important effects, e.g. if 10% reduction in feed-related complications (from 25% to 15%) is considered to be clinically important, the effect size index is 0.25. Cohen (1988) has proposed small, medium and large effect size indices for the social sciences, and they have become widely adopted. These conventions have also been adopted by some computer software packages (e.g. Statistical Package for Social Sciences (SPSS) SamplePower 2.0). For the independent t test and differences between two independent proportions, a small effect size index corresponds to 0.20, medium to 0.50 and large to 0.80. When these are used to calculate sample sizes necessary to achieve a significant result with 80% power, the values correspond to 393, 64 and 26 per group, respectively. When possible, it is better to use clinically relevant criteria than these conventions. Nevertheless, the conventions can act as a sort of 'reality check'.

It would be advantageous to plan any clinical trial with a low P value, high power and small effect size indices so that small differences in clinically important measures are assessed with high confidence, irrespective of whether the result is significant, but this would require more subjects, more work and more expense, which in some cases may be unrealistic. Therefore, it is necessary to consider all these issues in sample size calculations. If the required sample size of the study is so high as to require an unrealistic amount of resources, then it is probably best not to undertake the study.

Sample size calculations can be undertaken using the following:

1. Published sample size tables (provided by Machin and Campbell, 1987; Cohen, 1988). Table 10.4 shows sample sizes needed to demonstrate different effect sizes with $P < 0.05$ and 80% power.
2. Nomograms (e.g. Altman, 1995).
3. Formulas; e.g. when the outcome variables are to be compared using Student's two-sample t test or the test for two proportions, sample size can be calculated approximately using the following formula ($P < 0.05$ and 80% power):

Number of subjects per group = 16/(effect size index)^2

For an effect size index of 0.5, the number per group is 64 (16/0.25).

4. Computer packages, e.g. SPSS SamplePower 2.0 or Samplesize V2.0 (see Annex 10.2).
5. Advice of a statistician. Advice is generally recommended when there is uncertainty about the principles and procedures. It is also generally recommended when the outcome variable is survival time or when the study is complex and involves multiple centres.

Two examples of statistical power analysis are given below to illustrate the procedures for calculating sample sizes involving differences between proportions (example 1) and differences between means (example 2), using a published sample size table (Table 10.4).

Example 1

Fifty per cent of a population of elderly subjects has been reported to have falls over a 6-month period. Since a recent survey of this population showed frequent deficiency of thiamine, an investigator considered the possibility that thiamine deficiency may cause confusion and be responsible for the high incidence of falls

Table 10.4. Number of subjects per group needed to detect the stated values of effect size indices (0.1–1.4), with significance ($P < 0.05$ and < 0.01; two-tailed for both) and power (0.70–0.99)[a] (based on Cohen 1988).

Power	0.1	0.2	0.3	0.4	0.5	0.6	0.7	0.8	1.0	1.2	1.4
$P < 0.05$											
0.70	1235	310	138	78	50	35	26	20	13	10	7
0.80	1571	393	175	99	64	45	33	26	17	12	9
0.85	1797	450	201	113	73	51	38	28	19	14	10
0.90	2102	526	234	132	85	59	44	34	22	16	12
0.95	2600	651	290	163	105	73	54	42	27	19	14
0.99	3675	920	409	231	148	103	76	58	38	27	20
$P < 0.01$											
0.70	1924	482	215	122	79	55	41	32	21	15	12
0.80	2338	586	259	148	95	67	49	38	25	18	14
0.85	2611	654	292	165	106	74	55	43	28	20	15
0.90	2978	746	332	188	120	84	62	48	31	22	17
0.95	3564	892	398	224	144	101	74	57	37	26	20
0.99	4808	1203	536	302	194	136	100	77	50	35	26

Header spanning columns 0.1–1.4: Effect size index

[a]The table is suitable for comparison of means (independent sample t test) and comparison of two proportions (independent two-proportion test) assuming equal-sized groups.

within this population (50% over 6 months). Therefore she planned to undertake a randomized placebo-controlled clinical trial to assess if thiamine administration reduced the number of falls. She felt that, if there was a reduction in the proportion that fell from 50% to 25%, this would represent a clinically relevant change, with important health and economic consequences. The specifications are as follows:

- $P < 0.01$ (2-tailed);
- power, 90%;
- effect size index, 0.52 (50 − 25/√37.5 × 62.5).

She turned to Table 10.4 (lower half) and found that, for an effect size index of 0.5, 120 subjects per group are required and, for an effect size index of 0.6, 84 subjects per group are required. By linear interpolation between these two values, she calculated that, for an effect size index of 0.52, 115 subjects per group are required. However, she did not have access to 230 subjects, but she was willing to relax the stringency of the specifications. These were now set as follows:

- $P < 0.05$
- power, 80%
- effect size index, 0.52 (as before)

By a similar procedure as above and with the use of Table 10.4 (upper half), she calculated that the required sample size was 62 per group (124 in total). She now found that a study of this size was within her resources and she proceeded with the next part of the trial.

Example 2

A clinician was concerned about the high prevalence of undernutrition and poor quality of life of patients in residential homes. She became aware that malnutrition can adversely affect psychological and social function and decided to examine the hypothesis that nutritional support will produce a change in the quality of life. A validated visual analogue scale was administered to the residents (0 = worst imagin-

able quality of life and 100 = best imaginable quality of life). She found that the mean score was 60 (standard deviation 20). Increasing the score to 75 would be clinically important. She therefore set the following criteria for sample size calculations:

- $P < 0.05$;
- power 80%; and
- effect size index 0.75 (75 − 60/20).

By reference to Table 10.4 (upper half) and extrapolation to a mid-point value between an effect size index of 0.7 (33 subjects) and 0.8 (26 subjects), she calculated that about 30 subjects per group were required.

Clinical trials often compare changes in outcome variables. A trial sets out to test the hypothesis that nutritional supplements produce changes in the quality of life that are greater in magnitude than those that occur in the control group. Here, the standard deviation of the change is used in the calculations, although this information is frequently not available. Another modification concerns sample size calculations when the allocation ratio is not 1:1, which is assumed by Table 10.4. If for logistic reasons it is necessary to allocate three patients to a control group for every patient allocated to a treatment group, the allocation ratio is 3:1. This will affect the way the sample size is calculated. One way to do this (Cohen, 1988) is to adjust the value shown in Table 10.4, which can be considered as the harmonic mean (n):

$$n = 2n_a n_b / n_a + n_b$$

Thus, if three times more subjects are allocated to group n_a than to group n_b, then by substitution into the above equation $3n_b$ for $1n_a$ ($3n$ in group $b = 1n$ in group a) it can be shown that $n = 1.5n_b$ ($2 \times 3n_b \times n_b/4n_b$). Conversely, $n_b = 0.67n$ and $n_a = 3n_b$ or $2n$. Thus, the total sample size ($n_a + n_b = 4n_b$) is $2.67n$ (not $2n$, which is the value for equal-sized groups).

Although other procedures are required for certain tests, such as the odds ratio and time to event, the studies reported in this book have generally not used these methods, and therefore the relevant power calculations are not discussed here.

Pilot studies

Pilot studies are often undertaken before the start of a clinical trial so that the practicalities, including compliance with the intervention, can be assessed. For example, patients may experience discomfort associated with specific procedures or unhappiness due to the multiple tests that they are subjected to. It may be possible to address both of these issues before the clinical trial begins. These may also provide logistic information about the feasibility and practicality of undertaking certain procedures, the time taken to obtain some measurements and the suitability of the forms used to record the data. Pilot studies can also provide some information about the effect size index and the variability of the outcome variables, which are of value in calculations of sample sizes.

Selection of patients

In order to be able to make inferences about the treatment effect from the sample of subjects investigated to the overall population of interest (external validity), it is desirable to aim for random selection and random allocation of subjects to the control and treatment groups. In practice, random selection from the population of interest is frequently not achieved for practical reasons. Therefore, it is important to clarify and report on the selection procedure used. For example, since there is so much variability in the characteristics of patients admitted to intensive care units, the entry criteria for a clinical trial might be restricted to only those that are likely to affect outcome, such as age and disease severity. The study might exclude patients with multiorgan failure in an attempt to reduce variability further. Alternatively, the study may wish to consider a more homogeneous group of patients, such as only those with burns. However, even here it may be appropriate to select patients according to age and extent of burn. One of the disadvantages of using a large number of exclusion criteria (restrictive entry characteristics) is that the results will be less 'generalizable'. In the case of a clinical trial on burned patients, it would be inappropriate to extrapolate the results to other groups of patients. As another example, consider a clinical trial that aims to assess the effect of a nutrition screening tool, which is linked to a care plan, on clinically relevant outcome variables, such as length of hospital stay or complications. Results obtained from patients with a single diagnosis are likely to be of limited value to a hospital that manages patients with a wide range of diagnoses. It may be necessary to undertake a study with 'all comers' or much less restrictive entry criteria, but such a study will require large numbers of patients to combat the wide variability in expected results. Planned subgroup analyses may be necessary because different patient groups are known to have very different lengths of hospital stay, e.g. patients undergoing cardiac surgery compared with hernia repair. Patient selection may also be affected by ethical considerations. For example, just as it is unethical to withhold antihypertensive treatment in patients with high blood pressure (Elwood, 1982), it is unethical to withhold nutritional treatment in patients with a very low body mass index (BMI) who are severely undernourished (Fig. 10.1). All these issues should be considered at the planning stage in conjunction with the proposed hypothesis.

Allocation of patients

Whatever selection criteria are used, it is essential to use an appropriate procedure to allocate patients to a treatment or control group. Sometimes studies may allocate patients to several groups, but this chapter will focus on only two groups, so that the principles and procedures involved can be illustrated more easily. The allocation can be based on randomization or minimization, which is probably the only generally accepted non-random allocation procedure. Both aim to reduce bias by ensuring that the two groups are very similar to each other, although there is no absolute guarantee that this will be achieved.

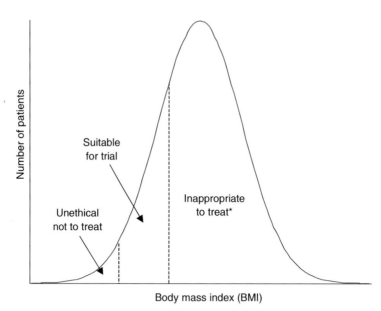

Fig. 10.1. Suitability of a population of weight-stable subjects for participation in a nutritional interventional trial, with weight and body function as outcome measures. (*In weight-losing patients, it may be appropriate to treat or include in a trial.)

Random allocation

Described below are three general randomization procedures that aim to ensure that individual subjects have the same chance of being placed in the treatment and the control groups (Altman, 1995; Schultz and Grimes, 2002a). Apart from reducing bias (except that which occurs by chance), random allocation of the population sampled ensures that statistical tests based on probability theory are valid. The allocation procedure is normally carried out by an individual who does not interact with the patients and who conceals the identity of the treatment and control group, e.g. by providing the allocation in sealed opaque envelopes or conveying the information by telephone through a third party. Although randomized allocation can be achieved using results obtained by tossing a coin, this procedure may not allow a retrospective check of the allocating process (audit tracking). For this reason, random numbers generated by a computer or random numbers published in tables can be used to allocate patients to the treatment groups. (The patients may be aware of the random

number allocated to them, but not the code for the treatment category.) It is also possible to use software packages and on-line computer web-sites to obtain randomization sequences and allocations (e.g. www.sghms.ac.uk/phs/staff/jmb/jmb.htm). A table of two-digit random numbers generated from EXCEL is shown in Annex 10.1.

RANDOMIZED SIMPLE ALLOCATION
Table 10.5 shows a sequence of 50 two-digit numbers that can be used to categorize patients into group A or B depending on whether the random numbers are even (group A) or odd (group B). Thus, the allocation sequence for the first ten patients is as follows:

Random number:
24 23 36 44 14 10 15 02 79 78
Allocation to group:
A B A A A A B A B A

Seven of the first ten patients (70%) are allocated to group A and the remaining three to group B (30%). This uneven allocation is simply the result of chance. When all 50 numbers in this random sequence are allocated (Table 10.5), 24 of the patients

Table 10.5. A sequence of 50 randomly generated two-digit numbers.

24	23	36	44	14	10	15	02	79	78
27	07	91	84	89	26	03	75	66	39
39	87	30	20	41	78	19	39	76	16
99	68	54	58	91	69	32	72	02	41
75	18	53	77	83	85	46	03	68	08

end up in group A (48%) and 26 in group B (52%). If subjects are randomly allocated into groups A and B, according to whether the numbers in the above sequence were less than 50 (group A) or 50 or more (group B), eight out of the first ten patients are allocated to group A and the remaining two to group B. By the time all 50 patients are allocated, 27 (54%) end up in group A and 23 (46%) in group B. These examples are used to illustrate that uneven random allocation can adversely affect small studies. This is because studies are most powerful when the subjects are equally divided between groups (see below). Randomized block allocation can be used to overcome this problem.

RANDOMIZED BLOCK ALLOCATION

This procedure allows numbers in the two groups to be very close to each other throughout the allocation process. For example, if there are two groups, A and B, it is possible to allocate subjects in blocks of two (two at a time). There are only two permutations containing both A and B (AB and BA). These permutations can be allocated randomly, e.g. even numbers in a random sequence might be chosen to represent AB and odd numbers BA. It is clear that groups cannot differ by more than one at any stage during the allocation process. One of the problems with this procedure is that the operator could correctly guess every second allocation. Therefore, it may be desirable to use larger blocks. For example, if we consider blocks of four, each containing two As and two Bs, there are six possible permutations: 1, AABB; 2, ABAB; 3, ABBA; 4, BBAA; 5, BABA; 6, BAAB. Blocks can be chosen at random to create an allocation sequence, e.g. using numbers 1–6 generated randomly or using only the

numbers beginning with 1–6 in a random sequence of numbers, such as that shown in Annex 10.1. Using this allocation procedure, the two groups will not differ by more than two at any stage. However, it is possible to deduce the allocation of every fourth patient. This problem may be overcome by allocating patients using a combination of blocks, e.g. blocks of 2, 4 and 6. Obviously, guessing is much more difficult if the type of allocation used is concealed from those that interact with the patient. Occasionally, large studies allocate patients in large blocks of 10–20, making it virtually impossible to guess the allocation.

RANDOMIZED STRATIFIED ALLOCATION

Although randomized simple allocation aims to remove bias, it commonly does not do this for characteristics such as age and severity or stage of disease that strongly affect outcome of disease. This problem is likely to arise in small studies that include several prognostic characteristics. Although the uneven allocation of characteristics to the groups will have arisen by chance, the effect is to bias the study. A procedure for achieving reasonable balance between the strongly prognostic characteristics is stratified randomization. Separate block randomization procedures are used for each prognostic characteristic, which is treated as a subgroup (stratum). If, for example, it is felt that a clinical trial should stratify patients according to the presence and absence of lymph nodes, two separate lists of random numbers are prepared so that patients with and without lymph nodes can be separately allocated to the treatment and control groups. In multicentre studies, it is usual to include centre as a subgroup and to randomize patients within each centre. Stratification may involve several factors, but the number of independent randomizations can rapidly become large. For example, when there are two levels (e.g. with or without lymph nodes) for each of three variables, the required number of separate randomizations rises to 12 ($2 \times 3 \times 2 = 12$). Critics of the randomized stratified procedure (Meier, 1981) argue that this increased complexity increases the risk of errors. Therefore, if there is uncertainty about whether a particular characteristic affects outcome, it is reasonable to exclude it from the stratification procedure (Pockock, 1983). In practice, it is not common to include more than two strata.

Non-random allocation: minimization

Minimization aims to minimize imbalance between subgroups of prognostic factors at each stage of the trial (Altman, 1995). It achieves an overall balance of prognostic factors, even in small studies, although not necessarily for each combination. An example will help to illustrate the use of minimization. Suppose that ten patients with chronic obstructive pulmonary disease have already been allocated to receive treatment A and another nine to receive treatment B. The distribution of three prognostic characteristics (age, BMI, other diseases), each with two subgroups, is shown in Table 10.6, while the imbalance is shown in Table 10.7. The next patient to be allocated is less than 65 years old, has a BMI of less than 20 kg m^{-2} and also suffers from heart disease. Since the aim is to establish two groups as similar as possible, it would be advantageous to allocate the patient to the treatment with the smaller overall score, which is treatment B (Table 10.7). In this way the overall imbalance is reduced without the use of a random component. However, this procedure may introduce a small bias because each allocation depends on the characteristics of the previously allocated patients. Therefore, this procedure may be modified by including a randomized component, whereby the allocation is weighted in favour of the group with the smaller overall score (e.g. 3 or 4 to 1 in favour of allocating the 20th patient to treatment B).

Table 10.6. Distribution of characteristics in the first 19 patients with chronic obstructive pulmonary disease involved in a clinical trial involving allocation by minimization.

		Treatment A (*n* 10)	Treatment B (*n* 9)
Age	< 65 years	6	5
	≥ 65 years	4	4
Body mass index	< 20 kg m^{-2}	7	6
	≥ 20 kg m^{-2}	3	3
Other diseases	Yes	7	7
	No	3	2

Table 10.7. Imbalance of the three characteristics, shown for the purpose of allocating the 20th patient (< 65 years, body mass index < 20 kg m^{-2} and other diseases) using minimization.[a]

		Treatment A (*n* 10)	Treatment B (*n* 9)
Age	< 65 years	6	5
Body mass index	< 20 kg m^{-2}	7	6
Other diseases	Yes	7	7
	Overall score	20	18

[a]The 20th patient is allocated to treatment B.

Concealment

Whichever allocating procedure is used (Schulz and Grimes, 2002b), it is better if those interacting with the patients do not know how the randomization sequence was established. A common procedure for concealing treatment allocation in randomized trials is to use a central telephone randomization system. This system, which is particularly useful for large randomized trials, involves supplying details to a 'third party', so that the eligibility criteria can be checked and the patient assigned to a particular treatment group. Another system is for a third party to allocate in sealed, nontransparent envelopes, ensuring that key information is not transferred on pressure-sensitive paper or carbon paper inside the envelope (Altman and Schulz, 2001).

Analysing Results of Clinical Trials

Summarize entry characteristics

With appropriate allocation procedures, there should be little imbalance in entry characteristics between treatment and control groups. If there is substantial imbalance in entry characteristics that are suspected of being of prognostic importance, they can be adjusted statistically (see below).

Main analysis

This is the most important analysis of the trial, which involves a comparison of the main prespecified outcome variable between control and treatment groups. It can usually be carried out using standard statistical tests. In studies involving independent groups and continuous outcome variables (e.g. muscle strength or quality of life on a visual analogue scale), use can be made of the unpaired Student's *t* test (two samples), analysis of variance (more than two samples), Mann–Whitney U test (two groups) and Kruskal–Wallis test (more than two groups). For studies involving categorical outcome variables, use is made of the chi-square test. For paired or matched samples, use can be made of the paired Student's *t* test, the Wilcoxon paired *t* test and the sign test. There are special statistical procedures for analysing crossover trials (Altman, 1995), in which the treatment given to each group is switched so that each group receives both treatments, often with an intervening 'wash-out' period.

Multiple comparisons: analysis of multiple outcome variables, several subgroups and several time points

Some trials include several secondary or intermediate variables. The more variables that are used in the analysis, the greater the likelihood of obtaining a significant result by chance when in reality there is no difference (type 1 error). It is therefore prudent to restrict the number of outcome variables at the outset, but, if there are several important outcome variables that must be included, then it is necessary to correct for the risk of a type 1 error. One way of doing this is to use the Bonferroni correction, where the critical value for significance ($P < 0.05$) is divided by the number of tests. For example, if four outcome variables are examined, then the corrected significance level is 0.0125 (0.05/4). Many computer programs provide corrected values using the Bonferroni or other tests. Details of this and other tests are found in standard textbooks on statistics (e.g. Howell, 1997).

The same issues apply to multiple analyses of subgroups or different time points. The chances of obtaining a significant result when there is no effect is increased by undertaking more tests. Again a correction is necessary. There may be so many combinations of characteristics that, if the data are analysed in different ways in the hope that some result will be significant, the chances are that a significant result will occur. Therefore, if subgroup analysis is deemed to be important, this should be specified at the outset, before the study begins. Deviations from this procedure should be reported.

Changes over time

Many studies undertake measurements of the outcome variable at baseline and again at the end of the treatment period. It is possible to undertake a Student's *t* test to assess if there has been a significant change in each group. However, the primary aim of the trial is to assess if there are different responses between the groups. Therefore, it is far better (although unfortunately it has often not been considered in the trials reported in this book) to calculate the changes from baseline for each patient and compare the differences between groups using an unpaired *t* test. Other statistical tests, such as a mixed/split plot analysis can achieve the same result. ANCOVA can offer some advantages in special circumstances (Vickers and Altman, 2001). For serial measurements over time (time-series analyses), expert statistical advice should be sought.

Statistical adjustment of variables (indirect method for controlling and reducing variability)

As indicated above, an appropriate study design is the direct way of controlling and reducing variability, but there may still be substantial imbalances between the entry characteristics of the groups, especially in small trials (e.g. age, severity of disease, BMI). Adjustment can be made using ANCOVA or multiple regression (Huitema, 1980; Howell, 1997). Statistical advice should be sought when necessary.

Incomplete data sets and protocol violations

If the data sets are incomplete, the underlying reasons should be examined and reported. Were the entries inadvertently omitted? Were the measurements not made? Did the patients drop out of the study because of complications? Did the patients drop out because they moved to another area or had an incidental problem? If the drop-outs were due to causes not directly related to the study, it is reasonable to exclude them

from the analysis, especially if they account for only a small proportion of the total number of patients and are approximately equally divided between the groups. It would be unreasonable to exclude or ignore from the analysis patients who withdrew or were suspected of having withdrawn as a direct result of the treatment, especially if the withdrawals were unequally divided between the groups. One approach is to analyse the results after assigning both the most optimistic and the most pessimistic to the drop-outs and report both sets of results together with the assumptions used. There will be confidence in the overall results of the study if both types of analyses come to similar conclusions.

For individuals who remain in the study but do not comply with the protocol, either intentionally or unintentionally (non-compliers), it is generally recommended that they remain in the analysis, which is termed intention-to-treat analysis. It is also possible to undertake analysis only on those that received the product or on everyone who received a certain preset intake of feed (compliance analysis), but the results may be biased. Nevertheless, some confidence emerges if similar results are obtained with each type of analysis.

Writing Up Results and Assessing the Quality of Clinical Trials

The check-list in Table 10.8 provides some insight into important issues that need to be considered in writing up papers. Such a list is not only useful for increasing the chances of acceptance of papers by journals, but also for assessing the quality of papers after they have been published, e.g. for meta-analysis. Therefore, a judgement on the quality and validity of the work will be made according to the way the paper is written up. The validity of a trial has two components (see Glossary): internal validity, which is the extent to which systematic error or bias (selection, performance, detection and attrition bias; see Glossary) has been minimized; and external validity, which is the extent to which the results of a trial can be safely

Table 10.8. Check-list of items to include when reporting a randomized trial.[a]

Paper section and topic	Item	Description
Title and abstract	1	How participants were allocated to interventions (e.g. 'random allocation', 'randomized' or 'randomly assigned')
Introduction Background	2	Scientific background and explanation of rationale
Methods Participants	3	Eligibility criteria for participants and the settings and locations where the data were collected
Interventions	4	Precise details of the interventions intended for each group and how and when they were actually administered
Objectives	5	Specific objectives and hypotheses
Outcomes	6	Clearly defined primary and secondary outcome measures and, when applicable, any methods used to enhance the quality of measurements (e.g. multiple observations, training of assessors)
Sample size	7	How sample size was determined and, when applicable, explanation of any interim analyses and stopping rules
Randomization – sequence generation	8	Method used to generate the random allocation sequence, including details of any restriction (e.g. blocking, stratification)
Randomization – allocation concealment	9	Method used to implement the random allocation sequence (e.g. numbered containers or central telephone), clarifying whether the sequence was concealed until interventions were assigned
Randomization – implementation	10	Who generated the allocation sequence, who enrolled participants and who assigned participants to their groups
Blinding (masking)	11	Whether or not participants, those administering the interventions and those assessing the outcomes were blinded to group assignment. When relevant, how the success of blinding was evaluated
Statistical methods	12	Statistical methods used to compare groups for primary outcome(s). Methods for additional analyses, such as subgroup analyses and adjusted analyses
Results Participant flow	13	Flow of participants through each stage (a diagram is strongly recommended). Specifically, for each group report the numbers of participants randomly assigned, receiving intended treatment, completing the study protocol and analysed for the primary outcome. Describe protocol deviations from study as planned, together with reasons
Recruitment	14	Dates defining the periods of recruitment and follow-up
Baseline data	15	Baseline demographic and clinical characteristics of each group
Numbers analysed	16	Number of participants (denominator) in each group included in each analysis and whether the analysis was by 'intention-to-treat'. State the results in absolute numbers when feasible (e.g. 10/20, not 50%)
Outcomes and estimation	17	For each primary and secondary outcome, a summary of results for each group, and the estimated effect size and its precision (e.g. 95% confidence interval)
Ancillary analyses	18	Address multiplicity by reporting any other analyses performed, including subgroup analyses and adjusted analyses, indicating those prespecified and those exploratory
Adverse events	19	All important adverse events or side-effects in each intervention group
Discussion Interpretation	20	Interpretation of the results, taking into account study hypotheses, sources of potential bias or imprecision and the dangers associated with multiplicity of analyses and outcomes
Generalizability	21	Generalizability (external validity) of the trial findings
Overall evidence	22	General interpretation of the results in the context of current evidence

[a]Further details of all of these items can be found on www.consort-statement.org.

extrapolated to other circumstances. Since external validity is often a matter of judgement, it is not surprising that much emphasis has been placed on internal validity. A large number of quality assessment scales have been produced to assess the quality of various components of trials, so that a single score can be ultimately achieved (composite scales). As many as 25 different scales were identified by Moher *et al.* in 1995 and 1996 and another 14 by Juni *et al.* in 1999. The results obtained by different scales do not agree, because they do not always incorporate the same items or attribute the same weighting to the items. Some scales include a wide range of items, including the use of sample calculations before and after the study, side-effects and data presentation, including statistical tests and confidence intervals. One of the simplest scales, the Jadad quality assessment scale (Jadad *et al.*, 1996) (used in the analysis of trials in this book), incorporates only three items, which are common to most other scales: randomization; blinding; and patient attrition. There is a need to report not only whether these were features of the trial but also the procedures used to ensure that the issues were adequately addressed. The Consort recommendations for attrition are illustrated as a flow diagram (Fig. 10.2). It has been increasingly used as a framework for reporting attrition in clinical trials, and included in papers submitted to various peer-reviewed journals.

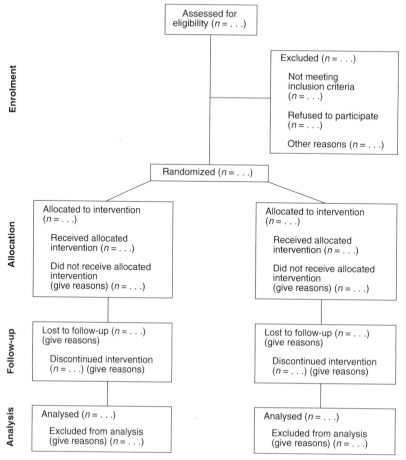

Fig. 10.2. Diagram showing the flow of participants through each stage of a randomized trial (based on the revised Consort diagram: www.consort-statement.org).

This short introduction to some of the main issues involved in clinical trials is not a substitute for discussions and advice from those with experience in randomized trials, including statisticians. It is far better to seek advice about study design and analysis before the study has begun rather than ending up with results that are difficult or impossible to interpret. The following quotation by the famous statistician Sir Ronald Fisher emphasizes this sentiment:

> To call in a statistician after the experiment is done may be no more than asking him to perform a post-mortem examination: he may be able to say what the experiment died of.

Annex 10.1: Table of Random Numbers between 0 and 99

64	36	59	20	46	9	9	39	81	30	10	62	44	77	27	31	16	31	78	51
21	99	90	45	69	2	44	66	20	18	80	97	12	51	79	9	81	74	55	12
57	70	25	96	10	7	0	62	51	24	31	71	3	64	97	55	5	6	96	87
85	60	34	57	61	31	23	7	19	81	60	55	55	62	23	78	77	60	86	52
73	28	64	1	81	19	34	37	67	25	11	19	98	93	94	6	16	43	4	8
40	49	86	56	91	30	20	80	2	67	97	18	33	86	10	83	50	30	37	81
17	3	20	25	64	13	61	31	26	76	61	2	84	26	9	74	82	7	22	13
34	63	81	88	9	55	94	78	93	11	5	81	44	71	58	92	89	13	4	79
78	96	65	8	27	33	44	65	88	96	89	53	62	65	65	1	85	84	98	36
59	63	22	93	71	52	64	49	74	64	84	38	42	62	12	64	38	17	2	5
66	83	60	50	24	4	35	43	89	79	50	91	59	73	36	59	6	68	40	31
36	61	8	34	18	28	19	88	89	4	29	67	91	2	77	43	50	8	0	31
2	54	63	15	45	41	58	21	64	13	92	68	78	70	66	36	98	11	14	24
64	54	22	73	92	42	29	4	36	28	60	11	97	7	94	12	50	7	97	51
35	80	90	48	97	51	85	99	93	52	67	4	46	89	52	7	87	66	18	77
70	23	27	29	87	62	61	30	39	46	2	75	15	30	29	37	11	46	97	9
95	6	49	65	17	35	10	83	19	57	38	81	39	26	7	72	42	79	98	90
65	91	30	15	47	73	47	72	84	86	91	47	16	14	31	41	33	5	29	3
22	97	34	25	93	74	35	37	49	44	88	18	82	94	48	91	67	51	26	68
52	33	8	18	22	64	87	74	29	72	7	31	10	21	11	15	16	79	42	79
39	11	61	26	56	79	81	96	94	45	53	59	15	95	28	16	85	58	83	46
94	39	83	44	66	58	97	3	47	54	61	18	22	25	54	0	51	77	5	34
85	94	85	68	14	80	26	65	86	14	96	17	75	47	83	30	64	64	44	96
81	95	22	16	54	92	43	64	8	23	1	62	3	31	40	97	46	38	46	91
16	18	3	35	53	93	84	37	88	83	75	16	22	30	11	48	34	65	59	64
43	76	83	16	70	82	86	61	84	31	71	99	37	40	32	81	98	2	36	8
9	60	3	90	51	51	33	92	54	97	29	34	19	49	46	30	61	53	46	69
60	97	76	32	45	53	47	54	92	42	24	45	34	1	12	54	68	48	10	32
45	41	49	75	72	40	17	74	2	77	18	51	53	96	61	61	70	23	68	16
47	81	21	96	80	49	32	31	76	69	9	25	55	79	7	91	90	22	53	29
78	45	62	65	15	16	52	65	67	79	37	12	84	56	93	52	6	34	14	17
98	6	68	77	77	2	7	96	1	41	63	80	33	61	37	23	42	1	10	10
4	46	59	46	45	3	18	77	22	70	40	66	86	4	8	59	73	16	35	52
77	72	28	88	65	94	55	71	61	7	39	85	77	6	67	69	42	67	18	94
15	35	40	14	17	26	65	44	49	9	18	57	82	58	8	63	13	90	98	62
96	97	45	65	69	8	34	96	51	32	99	23	55	10	93	61	66	76	16	37
44	60	63	11	96	61	62	93	25	1	72	35	15	72	56	30	14	27	58	86
13	87	10	1	68	90	3	84	56	14	13	88	1	15	43	80	49	75	60	16
32	47	25	55	40	27	43	99	8	65	86	89	55	64	12	12	1	98	69	48
19	34	64	5	44	94	68	99	21	41	53	43	64	13	13	65	56	93	85	87
1	3	24	42	72	31	58	69	49	86	83	37	27	96	2	76	24	76	54	72
87	58	35	73	83	73	79	20	4	93	86	79	28	20	50	34	60	97	53	33
42	51	34	90	37	58	38	28	40	80	81	47	26	3	44	5	98	89	53	88
61	49	20	28	89	98	33	7	18	82	60	74	76	15	89	12	13	19	91	29
10	79	33	77	86	2	35	59	42	68	1	96	88	24	1	43	46	45	38	83

59	8	66	70	60	15	85	26	85	38	62	90	3	17	76	44	60	38	52	69
50	95	96	59	34	6	20	63	28	41	71	70	39	78	91	72	43	71	58	31
22	11	12	44	49	33	23	78	53	26	23	21	39	36	54	97	21	72	16	14
74	50	39	52	2	58	56	58	67	68	93	3	61	12	75	10	44	73	66	31
80	83	78	11	32	12	61	46	89	99	64	97	55	2	52	66	97	45	97	71
51	53	11	29	10	54	62	71	99	46	95	49	6	79	61	93	57	4	42	66
7	74	28	78	22	86	77	12	27	8	56	52	22	11	49	50	6	72	37	8
29	71	56	78	90	32	70	18	34	51	58	58	47	61	87	35	21	0	77	83
90	50	8	88	66	3	39	77	79	60	73	99	94	65	5	43	20	15	52	81
73	16	93	22	33	34	14	58	14	32	85	67	25	32	44	76	95	14	71	3
88	86	43	58	95	24	25	79	5	68	93	59	35	11	28	31	77	79	60	32
43	60	2	6	8	83	68	76	46	8	46	23	22	33	32	21	3	68	67	74
15	29	28	42	91	60	73	18	37	42	19	92	41	14	35	77	75	12	73	54
11	40	62	23	26	47	85	87	42	65	85	35	4	89	76	92	65	80	75	42
64	51	40	51	97	80	34	12	44	78	45	90	17	29	5	14	31	47	13	49
46	60	88	3	40	38	47	19	92	32	24	95	44	9	58	62	17	72	41	69
38	24	37	44	43	86	82	53	15	15	60	80	36	81	43	26	40	96	55	3
34	45	36	91	11	39	88	46	71	85	60	91	7	2	63	62	77	86	95	66
69	37	0	60	4	31	45	75	52	54	19	64	88	37	41	69	80	8	88	80
95	65	74	67	16	49	46	68	7	31	22	33	16	14	67	85	47	41	40	2
4	36	59	23	61	38	93	70	13	10	86	64	25	24	1	76	35	2	41	54
28	45	98	32	38	16	4	57	24	87	61	12	87	56	51	57	36	72	71	10
94	62	5	29	72	87	82	45	68	53	14	12	83	88	18	0	76	6	43	97
85	60	96	61	80	75	43	10	29	98	12	45	77	90	63	97	5	1	51	3
82	77	98	96	95	99	58	47	0	80	75	44	38	38	32	64	46	73	34	46
0	96	20	70	90	9	45	2	40	16	72	8	72	75	59	82	12	46	19	16
94	30	76	59	68	24	83	83	11	9	68	40	1	4	33	38	41	36	33	89
54	23	25	21	4	21	36	41	19	65	35	93	11	40	83	38	47	86	35	49
58	10	30	33	27	81	27	20	44	35	53	12	38	97	10	70	11	5	92	95
93	34	98	0	80	35	7	86	36	1	42	43	11	47	27	51	3	95	8	78

Annex 10.2: Aids to Undertaking a Clinical Trial

Literature on randomized clinical trials

Before undertaking a clinical trial, it is important to be aware of what has already been or is being carried out to prevent unnecessary duplication. The following strategy, which is largely based on Lefevre and Clarke (2001), includes useful addresses/web-sites for identifying individual trials and multiple trials (meta-analyses). All may be useful but none provides a complete picture of the literature. Therefore, it is often necessary to combine different sources of information.

Major databases

- Cochrane library: The largest source of randomized controlled trials, which includes a collection of databases, among which are the Cochrane Controlled Trials Register and Cochrane Database of Systematic Reviews. Available from: Update Software, Summertown Pavilion, Middle Way, Summertown, Oxford OX2 7LG or http://www.medlib.com and http://www. hcn.net.au. A list of registers of clinical trials can help identify unpublished and/or ongoing trials (appendix in the Cochrane Reviewer's Handbook – http://www.cochrane.org/cochrane/hbo ok.htm). A list of journals searched by the Cochrane Collaboration can be found at http://cochrane.org/srch.htm.
- Other databases: Although clinical trials appearing in Pubmed – MEDLINE http://www.nbci.nlm.nih.gov./PubMed and EMBASE http://www.embase.com/ otherdb – are included in the Cochrane library, not all of the clinical trials are identified. Furthermore, many nutrition articles do not appear in MEDLINE or other commonly available databases (Avenell *et al.*, 2001). Further databases may also be considered, such as Allied and Alternative Medicine (AMED), biological abstracts (BIOSIS), CAB Health and Cumulative Index to Nursing and Allied Health Literature (CINAHL).

Journals

A wide range of journals publish papers on undertaking clinical trials.

Reference lists and cross-referencing

Reference lists at the end of journal articles can identify previously published clinical nutrition trials that are not included on electronic databases. Cross-referencing of articles appearing on one list/database and another list/database can also identify published clinical nutrition trials.

Conference proceedings

The British Library web-site http://www. bl.uk contained information on over 350,000 conferences worldwide in 2001.

Ongoing and/or unpublished studies

- UK National Research Register http:// www.doh.gov.uk/research/nrr.htm: ongoing health research in the UK together with ongoing systematic reviews.
- Clinical Trials Gov (USA) http://www. clinicaltrials.gov: clinical trials in the USA.
- Computer Retrieval of Information on Scientific Projects in the USA (CRISP) http://www-commons.cot.nih.gov/crisp: controlled trials supported by the US Department of Health and Human Services.
- Glaxo Wellcome register http://ctr. glaxowellcome.co.uk: Glaxo Wellcome register of clinical trials.
- Meta-register of controlled trials http:// www.controlled-trials.com: integration of several registers of controlled trials – organized by the publisher of *Current Science*.
- Registers of specific disease categories: e.g. cancer-specific registers of controlled trials in the UK http:// www.ctu.mrc.ac.uk/ukccr and the USA http://cancernet.nci.nih.gov.

Contacting experts in the field

Building a network is another useful way of identifying published articles on clinical trials, especially if the network is international. Contacts through national and international nutrition societies may be valuable.

Randomization software and services

A useful directory for a randomization directory has been produced by Martin Bland (http://www.sghms.ac.uk/Department/ phs/guide/randser.htm) at St George's Medical School (see modified summary below).

Randomization programs

- Clinstat (St George's Hospital Medical School, London, England): This free program, developed by Martin Bland, is suitable for small-scale trials. It provides blocked and unblocked allocations and random sampling. Randomization is found under main menu option 8. It prints simple lists of random allocations. For stratified randomization, a blocked randomization list is printed separately for each stratum.
- www.randomization.com: Free online randomization while you wait. It prints simple lists of random allocations.
- Experimental Design Generator and Randomizer (EDGAR) http://www.jic. bbsrc.ac.uk/services/statistics/edgar.htm (John Innes Centre, Norwich, England): EDGAR is a free online randomization program. This is designed for agriculture and does Latin squares and split plots as well as simple randomization. It randomizes while you wait and prints lists of random allocations.
- Stata UK branch – http://www.timber-lake.com.uk/software/stata/stata.htm – Timberlake Consultants. Stata is a commercial general statistical analysis program, with an add-on called 'ralloc', which does simple randomization, stratified randomization and blocked randomization.

- EaSt 2000 USA – http://www.cytel.com/ new.pages/EAST.2.html: a commercial program for sequential trials, aimed at the pharmaceutical industry.
- PARADIGM Registration–Randomization Software http://telescan.nki/paradigm. html (Netherlands/UK): A free web-based package produced by the Netherlands Cancer Institute and the UK Medical Research Council Cancer Trials Office. Operates interactively during your study.
- KEYFINDER http://lib.sat.cmu.edu/ designs/: A free interactive program useful for statisticians. It produces factorial designs, including blocked and/or fractional–replicate designs with user-specified confounding and aliasing properties.

Randomization services

Some of these services emerged from academic research, while others are purely commercial. These services are not free and not cheap. Telephone randomization may be provided during normal working hours or 24 h per day, sometimes by a voice-activated computer or by a person next to a telephone.

- Health Services Research Trial Support Unit Department of Health Sciences and Clinical Evaluation (University of York, England – http://www.york.ac.uk/ Departments/hsce/trials1): collaboration with researchers on various aspects of trial design and analysis, including telephone randomization.
- Birmingham Clinical Trials Unit (Birmingham, England – http://www.bctu. bham.ac.uk): customized minimization randomization programs and a telephone service.
- MRC/ICRF/BHF (Medical Research Council/Cancer Research UK/British Heart Foundation) Clinical Trial Service Unit and Epidemiological Studies Unit (University of Oxford, England – http://www.ctsu.ox.ac.uk/): collaborates on trials, especially large-scale trials.
- The Nottingham Clinical Research Group Research Organization (Nottingham, England – http://www.ncrl.ac.uk): offers

telephone randomization, statistical analysis and writing up of reports, primarily to the pharmaceutical industry.

- The Northern and Yorkshire Clinical Trials and Research Unit (NYCTRU) (University of Leeds, England – http://www.leeds.ac.uk/medicine/res_school/epid_hsr/nyctru.htmlat): offers a wide range of collaborative trial services, including medical statistics, computer programming, trial coordination, data management, e.g. in psychosocial medicine, oncology, research ethics and pharmaceutical work. Support is offered from the grant-application stage through to publication.
- Clinical Trials Research Unit (CTRU) (University of Auckland, New Zealand, http://www.ctru.auckland.ac.nz/services/randomisation.html): offers 24 h randomization.
- The NHMRC (National Health and Medical Research Council) (Clinical Trials Centre of the University of Sydney, Australia, http://www.ctc.usyd.edu.au/7randcentre/randcent.shtml): provides a randomization service, 6 a.m. to 8 p.m. daily (24 h a day for acute cardiovascular trials).
- Duke Clinical Research Institute (DCRI) (Duke University Medical Center, USA, http://www.dcri.duke.edu/services/randomization.html): a 24 h on-site, staffed randomization service with interactive voice-response system technology and emergency unblinding.
- Rho, Inc. North Carolina, USA (http://www.rhoworld.com/services/services_ivrs.htm): randomization systems and services offer an interactive voice-response system for managing patient randomization during clinical trials, 24 h per day. It also offers biostatistics, clinical management, medical writing and statistical programming.
- Covance InterActive Trial Management Systems, Princeton (New Jersey, USA – http://www.covance.com/itms/index.html): offers randomization by an interactive voice-response system, mainly for the pharmaceutical industry.

- The Sealed Envelope (London – http://www.thesealedenvelope.com/default.htm): Offers internet online random allocation system 24 h a day.
- ClinPhone (http://www.clinphone.com/cp_1.html Nottingham, Brussels, New Jersey, Chicago): Offers a service orientated towards the pharmaceutical industry, including data collection and telephone randomization.
- Clinical Data Care http://www.clinicaldatacare.com/ Lund, Sweden, with international offices: offers many trials services including telephone randomization.
- ASCOPHARM http://www.ascopharm.com/randomisationtext.html: a variety of central randomization systems orientated to the pharmaceutical industry. Other services include biostatics and data management.

Software programs for power statistics, including sample size calculations

Several software packages are available for undertaking power statistics. Some examples are indicated below:

- SPSS SamplePower 2.0, international with central offices in Chicago, USA – http://www.spss.com: offers power statistics using a wide range of tests, including ANCOVA, multiple regression and survival analysis. It can display results graphically and as formal reports.
- SamplesizeV2.0, Blackwell Science Ltd UK – 1987–1997 M. Machin, M.J. Campbell, P.M. Fayers, A.P.Y. Pinol: user-friendly power statistics package with a wide range of tests.
- nQuery Advisor Version 2.0, http://www.statsol.ie, Statistical Solutions Ltd, Cork, Ireland: user-friendly statistical package for sample size calculations for many types of design, including standard designs, crossover designs, survival analysis, regression and non-parametric tests.
- Stata, http://www.timberlake.com.uk/software/stata/stata.htm, UK branch – Timberlake Consultants: stata is a gen-

eral statistical package orientated towards statisticians. It includes sample size and power statistics

Reporting clinical trials

The CONSORT statement www.consort-statement.org is an important research tool that takes an evidence-based approach to improving the quality of reports of randomized trials. The statement is available in six languages and has been endorsed by prominent medical journals, such as *The Lancet, Annals of Internal Medicine* and the *Journal of the American Medical Association*. Its critical value to researchers, health-care providers, peer reviewers, journal editors and health policy makers is that

it increases confidence in the integrity of the reported results of research.

CONSORT comprises a check-list (see Table 10.8) and flow diagram (Fig. 10.2) to help improve the quality of reports of randomized controlled trials. It offers a standard way for researchers to report trials. The check-list includes items based on evidence that need to be addressed in the report; the flow diagram provides readers with a clear picture of the progress of all participants in the trial, from the time they are randomized until the end of their involvement. The intention is to make the experimental process more clear, so that the data can be evaluated in a more appropriate way. This is an extensive and useful web-site with explanations and definitions of terms and cross-referencing makes this a useful web-site.

11

An Overview and Some Future Directions

Current Evidence Base for Clinical Nutrition

In the last decade the practice of medicine has continued to change as new investigative techniques and new modalities of treatment have been introduced. This has coincided with a scrutinization and reassessment of traditional practices, in the light of evidence-based medicine, which has received increasing attention by regulatory bodies that focus on the cost–benefit and cost-effectiveness of treatments. Much of this emphasis has concerned specific forms of treatments for particular conditions, such as the use of interferon in multiple sclerosis, new anti-diabetic drugs for type 2 diabetes, and the efficacy of statins for improving the circulating profile of lipoproteins and reducing the risk of cardiovascular disease. The establishment of an adequate evidence-base for nutritional support is more challenging, not only because it can be provided in a wide variety of ways, but also because it is given to patients with variable nutritional status suffering from a wide range of clinical conditions. Furthermore, since nutritional support can affect every system of the body, it has a role in every medical discipline, from paediatrics to geriatrics, and in every health-care setting. This means that the evidence base for the treatment of disease-related malnutrition must take into account an enormous number of disease–nutrient interactions, which may express themselves in both obvious and not so obvious ways. For example, although nutritional support may improve muscle strength as a result of increasing muscle mass, it may also produce functional and subtle psychological changes that are not related to measurable changes in body composition. Establishing such an evidence base is of the utmost importance as disease-related malnutrition is a global public health problem. It is particularly widespread across health-care settings affecting individuals with a whole variety of diseases and conditions (see Chapter 2). In addition, the spectrum of adverse consequences of disease-related malnutrition has serious implications both clinically and financially for individuals and society. Not only are physical and psychological functions, quality of life and recovery from illness and injury impaired by disease-related malnutrition, but mortality, stays in hospital and the utilization of other health-care resources (care homes, medical consultations, prescriptions) are increased, with great cost to individuals and to health-care providers. However, as a prerequisite to the effective treatment of disease-related malnutrition, improved methods of detection (see Chapter 1), and greater awareness of the causes and consequences of this condition (see Chapters 3 and 4) are essential.

After establishing a structured, multi-layered evidence base, the current state of knowledge for the detection and treatment of disease-related malnutrition has been examined in different ways, according to disease categories, acute and chronic conditions, health-care setting, nutritional status, and the effectiveness of different types of nutritional support (Chapters 5–9). In particular, the focus has been on the areas of current uncertainty. For example, it is known that clinically malnourished individuals usually benefit from nutritional support, while well nourished individuals with no history of weight loss do not normally require nutritional support. However, between these extremes there is an intermediate group of patients, for whom the value of nutritional support is less apparent (see Fig. 5.2, Chapter 5), and in whom the evidence base for the role of nutritional support needs particular attention. The efficacy of ONS and ETF was addressed by a systematic review of a total of 287 trials (11,720 patients). Figures 11.1 and 11.2 provide an overview of findings from randomized controlled trials (RCT; *n* 114) of the impact of oral nutritional supplements (ONS) and enteral tube feeding (ETF) on the two main clinical outcomes, mortality and complication rates. These figures are portrayed in a way that illustrates our multi-layered approach to establishing the evidence base. The results are presented according to the type of treatment (ONS and ETF) and the health-care setting (hospitals, mostly with acute conditions, and community, mostly with chronic conditions). The spectrum of evidence is displayed vertically, from the 'generizable' at the top (combined treatments across a mix of patient groups and settings) to the more specific at the bottom (specific treatments, specific patient groups, specific RCT). Details of the analyses and of individual trials are available in Chapters 6, 7 and 8 and in the accompanying appendices. The organization of information in this way established a useful platform for examining clinical outcome.

Clinical and functional outcome

Mortality and complication rates

It appears that for the two major clinical outcomes (mortality and complication rates) the evidence is stronger at the generic than at the specific level. At a generic level, ETF and ONS result in a considerable reduction in mortality in the hospital setting, with ONS producing a 32% reduction and ETF a 50% reduction. Despite publication of trials of variable quality, some of which may have been selected for publication on the basis of positive results, it is difficult to ignore hard end points such as mortality, especially since the extent of improvements produced by nutritional support cannot easily be produced by other treatments. The mortality in the control groups may seem high[1], but this reflects the frailty and disease severity of the patient groups studied, which often included elderly patients in hospital.

There were virtually no data on the effects of ONS on mortality in community-based patients. Since the mortality of patients in the community is much lower than in hospital, community-based studies addressing this issue would require large numbers of subjects and lengthy follow-up. Mortality statistics for home ETF are available from a few countries only, but the largest set of results has emerged from the British Artificial Nutrition Survey (BANS). Table 11.1 shows the status of all adult patients after 1 year of starting home ETF, as well as the status of patients with specific diagnoses. Mortality varies with the condition, but it generally slows down with time so that most patients receiving artificial nutrition in the UK survive for considerably longer than a year. The majority of these patients, who have swallowing difficulties, would die quickly from aspiration pneumonia if they did not receive ETF. For obvious ethical reasons, randomized controlled trials have not been undertaken in such patients to compare the effects of ETF with no ETF on mortality. Similarly, most patients with chronic intestinal failure, especially those with

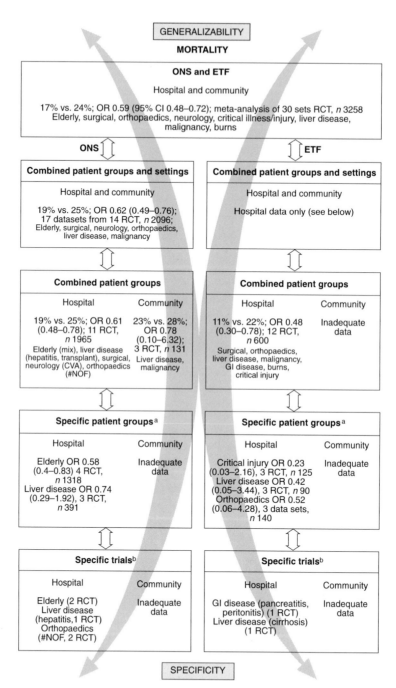

Fig. 11.1. A multi-layer summary of the evidence base for the effects of oral nutritional supplements (ONS) and enteral tube feeding (ETF) on mortality in hospital and community settings. [a]Data from meta-analysis of three or more randomized controlled trials (RCT) in one disease/patient group; [b]randomized controlled trials demonstrating a significant reduction in mortality. OR, odds ratio; 95% CI, 95% confidence interval; n, number of patients; #NOF, fractured neck of femur; CVA, cerebrovascular accident; GI, gastrointestinal. Odds ratios relate to the results of nutrition relative to routine care. Percentages (where provided) indicate the incidence in the nutrition group (ONS or ETF) vs. the control group.

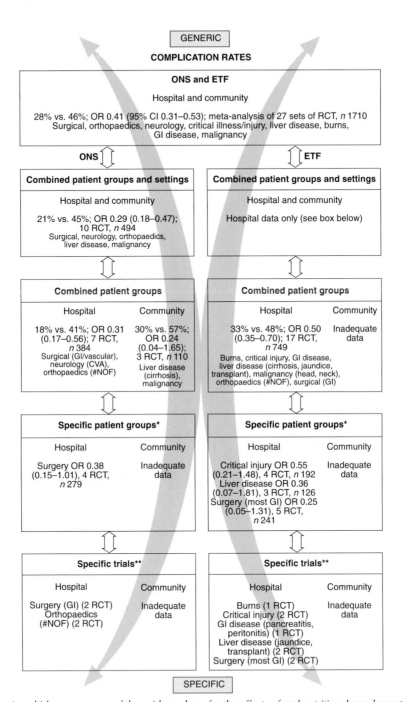

Fig. 11.2. A multi-layer summary of the evidence base for the effects of oral nutritional supplements (ONS) and enteral tube feeding (ETF) on complication rates in hospital and community settings. *Data from meta-analysis of three or more randomized controlled trials in one disease/patient group; ** randomized controlled trials demonstrating a significant reduction in complication rates; OR, odds ratio; 95% CI, 95% confidence interval; *n*, number of patients; #NOF, fractured neck of femur; CVA, cerebrovascular accident; GI, gastrointestinal. Odds ratios relate to the results of nutrition relative to routine care. Percentages (where provided) indicate the incidence in the nutrition group (ONS or ETF) vs. the control group.

Table 11.1. Status of selected adult patient groups and all patient groups combined at 12 months after starting home enteral tube feeding (HETF) and home parenteral nutrition (HPN) in the UK (Elia *et al.*, 2001).

	Number of patients (n)	Continuing (%)	Died (%)	Returned to oral (%)	Other[a] (%)
HETF					
Cerebrovascular disease	6,044	52.5	33.1	12.9	1.5
Motor neurone disease	925	34.8	62.9	1.3	0.9
Multiple sclerosis	911	80.6	14.2	3.6	1.6
Parkinson's disease	423	50.6	41.1	5.4	2.9
All diagnoses	16,247	49.9	33.8	14.3	2.0
HPN					
Crohn's disease	188	76.1	3.7	16.5	3.7
Pseudo-obstruction/ motility disorders	38	89.5	0.0	10.5	0.0
Radiation enteritis	26	84.6	7.7	7.7	0.0
Vascular disease: ischaemic	33	90.9	0.0	9.1	0.0
Vascular disease: thrombotic	20	90.0	5.0	5.0	0.0
All diagnoses	467	74.2	8.1	15.1	2.6

[a]In hospital, refused treatment and withdrawn.

intestinal motility problems and short-bowel syndrome (mainly due to Crohn's disease and vascular disease of the small intestine), would die if not given home parenteral nutrition (PN), although some could linger on in a very malnourished state. It is clear that home PN prolongs survival in these patients and that clinical trials to compare home PN with no intervention would also be unethical. Trials that have attempted to ascertain the relative merits of ETF over PN in a number of patient groups have also been controversial (Chapter 9). In addition, the results of such trials need to be interpreted cautiously since differences in outcome between the two forms of treatment may be due not only to the route of feeding but also the composition and volume of feeds infused, as well as to specific complications associated with each form of treatment (e.g. catheter-related sepsis in patients receiving PN).

At a more specific level, significant effects of nutritional support in reducing mortality were found in individual trials and particular patient groups (e.g. ONS in hospitalized elderly). In these smaller analyses, the effects of intervention on mortality had to be substantial so that a significant difference could be detected (the

demonstration of smaller changes in mortality would require a larger sample size). For example, power calculations suggested that a reduction in mortality from 25% to 19% (the average difference in mortality produced by ONS in hospital) would require a total sample size of 1496 patients or 748 per group (for 80% power and $P < 0.05$ (two-tailed)), which is considerably more than that of any individual study or combination of studies for a particular patient group. However, collaboration between centres may allow such studies to be undertaken in the future.

Statistical evidence of the effects of ONS and ETF in reducing complication rates, especially infective complications, also appeared to be stronger at the generic than the specific level, although individual trials suggested improvements in a number of patient groups (see Fig. 11.2). Since death occurs less frequently than other disease complications, a study with a given sample size can assess complication rates with more confidence than mortality. This may explain why, at the more specific level, there is greater information about the effects of nutritional intervention on complication rates than on mortality. The database of RCT assessing complication rates was more extensive for ETF than ONS (more trials, larger patient numbers) in the hospital setting, and more extensive for ONS than ETF in the community setting. The overall reduction in complications (ETF and ONS in hospital and the community) is again impressive (64% reduction from 46% to 28%), but the lack of double-blind, placebo-controlled trials makes it difficult to assess the exact magnitude of the true effect. For example, most trials of ETF did not give a placebo feed via an enteral tube to the control group, and most ONS trials did not include a placebo supplement. However, it is recognized that blinded placebo-controlled trials are practically and often ethically more difficult when nutritional rather than pharmaceutical interventions are involved (e.g. insertion of tubes/intravenous catheters for placebo feeding) (see Chapter 10).

Functional outcomes

A wide variety of functional benefits have been observed in RCT of ONS and ETF in different patient groups, as highlighted in Chapters 6 and 7. Benefits have been observed in both hospital and community settings for ONS, but for ETF, the majority of evidence is in hospital patients. Functional benefits that have been reported from RCT include the following: improved respiratory function and muscle strength in patients with COPD; immunological benefits in a wide range of patient groups; improved liver function in those with liver disease; better wound healing, quality of life, muscle strength and gastrointestinal function in surgical patients; improved physical and emotional functioning in patients with malignancy; improved activities of daily living and fewer falls in the elderly; and greater retention of bone mineral density in orthopaedic fractured neck of femur patients. However, the issues raised above about the appropriate blinding of trials are again relevant here. In addition, a surprising number of trials failed to assess body function, leaving gaps in the current evidence base. In particular, there is a need to obtain greater insights into the patient's perspective, with more attention given to

the effects of nutritional intervention on quality of life. Trials are also required to assess the longer-term effects of intervention, on both functional and clinical outcomes, especially during the transition from hospital to community settings.

Length of hospital stay

The combination of reduced complication rates and improved body function may explain why many trials reported a reduction in length of hospital stay. However, the different ways in which length of hospital stay was reported (e.g. mean or median, with or without a standard deviation or range) makes it difficult to undertake detailed statistical analysis. Nevertheless, 11 out of 11 trials of ONS reported reduced length of hospital stay ($P < 0.001$; two-tailed binomial test, see Chapter 6), although we are aware of a study published since our analysis was undertaken that showed a small increase in the length of hospital stay in the group given ONS (Vlaming *et al.*, 2001). If this study was included in the analysis the binomial test would still remain significant. ETF had a less consistent effect on hospital stay (reduction in 53% (*n* 10) of RCT (*n* 19) that assessed hospital stay, significant reduction in two trials), possibly because of the variability in length of stay, the small numbers of patients involved in the analyses and the effect of ETF on mortality. For example, since death in hospital may reduce length of hospital stay, a higher mortality rate in the control group compared to the ETF group would tend to shorten length of hospital stay. The majority of trials did not indicate that this was taken into account, in which case the effect of ETF in reducing length of hospital stay would have been underestimated.

Possible mechanisms by which nutritional support influences outcome

The present work raises at least two major issues about the mechanisms by which nutritional support might produce benefits.

The first concerns the effects of ONS and ETF on appetite, food and total energy intake. In hospital and community trials, supplemental energy largely added to food intake. In community trials, the reduction in food intake corresponded on average to about a third of the energy content of the feed, with total energy intake increasing by an amount equivalent to about two-thirds of supplemental energy. The reduction in food intake with supplementation was less in trials in which the mean body mass index (BMI) was < 20 kg m^{-2} than in those in which mean BMI was > 20 kg m^{-2}. In addition, studies in both patients and healthy volunteers suggest that ETF can produce marked increases in total energy intake, often without substantially suppressing food intake (Stratton and Elia, 1999). It is intriguing that some hospital trials suggest that food intake is not suppressed by ONS or ETF, at least over a period of days, and that in some instances it may actually be stimulated. Although it may be difficult to adequately control for the effects of disease and to accurately measure intake in the clinical setting, the possibility of disinhibition of appetite deserves further study. Overall, the mechanisms by which ONS and ETF can provide largely additional energy are unknown. The liquid consistency, composition and texture of feeds, continuous administration (in the case of ETF) and the timing of feeding, may all be factors. Information on the effects of different methods of nutritional support on appetite in patients with disease is mostly lacking, especially when the delivery of feed totally (PN) or partially (ETF) bypasses the gastrointestinal tract. A summary of this area of research is provided by Stratton and Elia (1999). It is also unclear whether dietary counselling and the provision of additional or fortified food items can produce similar increments in nutritional intake and similar functional and clinical benefits as ONS. Although dietary counselling is often recommended as the first step in dealing with patients with poor nutritional intake, the evidence base for its effectiveness is surprisingly poor in comparison with that for ONS (see Chapter 6, Fig. 6.3 for a summary).

The second issue concerns the putative mechanisms by which ONS and ETF improve clinical outcome and body function. The increased energy and nutrient intakes resulting from the intervention could produce an increase in the mass of body tissues, such as muscle. This may explain the increase in muscle strength that was observed in some studies. In trials of ETF, in which the increases in total energy intake and body weight were considerably greater than the control group, it is reasonable to link the clinical and functional benefits to the increase in lean body mass and body weight. Furthermore, in community patients given ONS, the increase in body weight and functional benefits were more likely to occur in underweight individuals with a BMI < 20 kg m^{-2} than in those with a BMI > 20 kg m^{-2}, who presumably had less functional deficit. For elderly patients and those with COPD, functional benefits were generally only observed when body weight increased by more than 2 kg. However, in other trials that reported improvements in outcome, weight change was often very small compared with the control group. Our analysis was also limited by the presentation of study average values for BMI and weight change rather than individual patient values. Nevertheless, the available information raises the possibility that nutrients provided during key periods of an illness influence the function of tissues, especially those of the inflammatory and immune system, affecting the incidence of infections. One of the main effects of nutritional support in surgical patients was to reduce infective complications (mainly wound infections), which were among the most common postoperative complications. Since wound infections are likely to be due to seeding of bacteria during the operation, and since the time of recognition of infections is often only a few days after the operation, it is reasonable to suggest that nutrients provided over the short perioperative period could enhance bacterial killing and prevent wound infections from developing. Such effects may not be unique to nutrients. For example, animal and human studies have shown that intraoperative hypothermia increases the risk of postoperative infections, and that prevention of this mild hypothermia reduces the incidence of wound infections, improves wound healing and sepsis scores, and shortens hospital stay (see Chapter 4). In one recent study (Melling *et al.*, 2001) as little as 30 min whole body or local warming in the preoperative period produced a marked reduction in wound infection rates. Similarly, the effects of preoperative carbohydrate in surgical patients and strict blood glucose control using pharmacological doses of insulin in critically ill patients have been found to have remarkable effects on clinical outcome, as discussed in Chapter 1, including a significant reduction in mortality in intensive care patients (Van den Berghe *et al.*, 2001). Taken together, these observations suggest that there are windows of opportunity for introducing physical, nutritional and/or other metabolic interventions that can potentially improve clinical outcome. The detailed mechanisms require investigation. The supply of nutrients during critical periods of the development of disease can be regarded as part of a spectrum of other programming effects that may also be important in apparently healthy subjects. These include the effects of folic acid administration during the first few weeks of pregnancy in preventing neural tube defects in the offspring (MRC, 1991) and programming of the immune system, cardiovascular risk and hypertension during fetal and early postnatal life (Chapter 1). Whether common mechanisms are involved in producing these long-term manifestations, which take decades to appear, and the short-term clinical manifestations, which take only a few days to appear, is unclear.

Limitations of the Current Evidence Base

As anticipated at the outset of this project, given the large number of medical conditions in which nutritional support may be required, it is clear that the database for specific patient categories is substantially incomplete. Such areas, which can be surmised from Figs 11.1 and 11.2, are also indicated in individual Chapters 6 (ONS and dietary manipulation), 7 (ETF) and 9 (PN). In view of this, clinicians may have little or no information about the role of nutritional support in certain types of patients. In this case, they have no option but to base their judgement on past experience, and the evidence associated with the more general effects of nutritional support.

There are a number of general limitations to systematic reviews and meta-analyses, which also apply to those reported in this book. Publication bias, or the preferential publication of studies with significant results, is one of them. Although funnel plots (e.g. see Figs 8.2 and 8.4 in Chapter 8) and formal statistical tests did not typically suggest publication bias at a generic level (analysis of all studies combined), these techniques do not necessarily exclude the possibility. Furthermore, some of the more specific analyses of individual interventions (ONS or ETF) on specific patient groups indicated that publication bias could be a problem. Failure to double-blind trials is another potential problem that has already been mentioned. This is likely to have more effect on subjective measurements or events, rather than on objective, unambiguous outcomes such as mortality. Another limitation concerns the use of certain summary statistics for subgroup analysis. In assessing the effect of chronic protein-energy status, reliance was placed on the mean BMI. Mortality, complication rates and functional outcomes were assessed according to whether the mean BMI of each study group was below or above 20 kg m^{-2}. This is far from ideal since a study of patients with a mean BMI < 20 kg m^{-2} may include a substantial proportion with a BMI > 20 kg m^{-2} and vice versa. From the available data it was not possible to assess if the mortality or the complication rates in each group predominantly involved subjects with a BMI < 20 kg m^{-2}, > 20 kg m^{-2} or whether subjects were evenly distributed below and above this cut-off point.

Some Future Directions

New information

It is obviously necessary to consider new information about the efficacy of different methods of nutritional support, which is constantly emerging, and to update and intermittently re-analyse relevant data-bases. Since information on individual patients would add another dimension to databases, attempts should be made through collaborative effort to consolidate such information. National organizations or a network of individuals involved in nutritional support are encouraged to con-sider organizing such activities. They are also encouraged to consider organizing high quality multi-centre trials to address outstanding issues, such as the effective-ness of nutritional support in aiding recov-ery during the transition from hospital to the community, and the potential mecha-nisms of action, in particular patient groups. The conceptual framework will also change and evolve as advances in mol-ecular biology and genetics emerge. For example, genetic polymorphisms of cytokines appear to predispose to and affect the outcome of a variety of acute and chronic diseases. Consequently, it is possi-ble that particular types of nutritional sup-port may benefit some patients and not others with the same disease, depending on genotypes that influence the handling and actions of nutrients, immune responses, catabolic responses and other clinically rel-evant body functions. If this is the case, a new conceptual framework that takes into account the new evidence as it emerges will be needed. Scientific investigation into the mechanisms that link metabolic demand to clinical outcome may also provide new conceptual frameworks for considering the efficacy of nutritional support.

Patient journey and continuity of care

The role of nutritional support throughout the patient journey, from the community, into hospital and back into the community, needs greater consideration. Figure 11.3 provides an example of a patient's journey. Weight typically decreases before admis-sion to hospital, continues to deteriorate in hospital, and may even continue to do so after discharge from hospital. Recovery from moderate to severe illness may take weeks or months, but detailed information about recovery of various bodily functions following acute diseases of varying severity is lacking. However, it is believed that the ability to undertake a full day's work is one of the last functions to return to normal in adults. Critically ill patients may take more than 6 months to fully recover, especially if they are elderly.

Information on the longer-term effects of nutritional support during the transition from one health-care setting to another is also scanty. This may be partly due to inad-equacies in the continuity of care for the detection and management of disease-related malnutrition for patients who are transferred from one health-care setting to another. One of the problems is that differ-ent malnutrition screening tools are used to assess both the risk of malnutrition and the effects of nutritional intervention across patient groups and health-care settings. Since the criteria for malnutrition vary, this will influence the identification and treat-ment of malnourished patients, as well as the results of meta-analyses. Furthermore, even when different tools are applied to the same group of patients they may iden-tify different patients as being malnour-ished, even when the total proportion of malnourished patients identified by each tool is similar. An example concerns a group of 75 patients who were screened using two screening tools (M. Elia, R.J. Stratton and D. Longmore, unpublished). One tool identified 29% (n 22) of patients in a medical ward as being at risk of mal-nutrition and the other 32% (n 25). The chance corrected measure of agreement was reasonably good (kappa = 0.66, where a kappa of 0.00 corresponds to no agree-ment and 1.00 to perfect agreement), but even so, 11 patients were categorized as malnourished by one of the two tools and not the other.

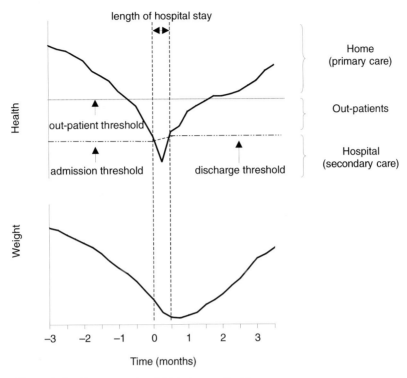

length of hospital stay

Health

out-patient threshold

admission threshold

discharge threshold

Home
(primary care)

Out-patients

Hospital
(secondary care)

Weight

−3   −2   −1   0   1   2   3

Time (months)

Fig. 11.3. Change in health status and weight during a patient journey.

Agreement between other screening tools has been found to be even poorer than in the above example, mainly because they rely on a different number and type of criteria. Some of these are subjective and others objective. Furthermore, some include only indices of chronic protein-energy status (BMI or arm anthropometry), others only indices of acute protein-energy status such as recent weight loss), while others use combinations of the two. The most common indicator for nutritional status in the studies that were reviewed in this book was a weight-for-height index, such as BMI. This was used in our analysis, although it is recognized that it provides a crude and inadequate characterization of nutritional status (see Chapter 1). The situation would be improved if information was also available for weight loss, and if different research groups used common criteria to identify individuals at risk of malnutrition. Unfortunately, national and international agencies have not agreed on cut-off points

for significant unintentional weight loss or growth failure, although some professional organizations have attempted to do so.

Conclusion

The current evidence base outlined in this book suggests that nutritional intervention can be effectively used in the treatment of disease-related malnutrition. However, malnutrition remains a substantial, costly problem that is often unrecognized and consequently untreated in our society. Even the most fundamental measurements of weight and height are often not routinely undertaken in clinical practice and there is currently no universally agreed screening method to detect disease-related malnutrition. There is a definite need to increase awareness about treatable malnutrition and to ensure that nutritional screening is routinely undertaken and appropriate nutritional support provided throughout the health-care system, from hospital patients to groups of patients in the community. Without detection of disease-related malnutrition, appropriate nutritional assessment and support will not be forthcoming, to the detriment of individuals and society.

Note

[1]National statistics in England suggest that the average mortality of patients over 75 years during their hospital stay is 9% (Department of Health, 1998).

Appendix 1
Prevalence of Disease-related Malnutrition

CRITERIA COMMONLY USED TO DEFINE MALNUTRITION

Body Mass Index

Body mass index (BMI) is a simple tool that provides an indication of an individual's chronic protein-energy status.

$$BMI = \frac{Weight\ (kg)}{Height\ (m)^2}$$

Cut-off values for BMI for indicating risk of chronic protein-energy malnutrition typically range from 18.5 to 20 kg m^{-2} (see Chapter 1).

Percentage Ideal Body Weight (Weight Index)

Frame size is estimated or determined from measurements of height and wrist circumference or elbow breadth. For example, elbow breadth is measured using a calliper and entered into the following equation:

$$Frame\ index\ 2 = \frac{Elbow\ breadth\ (mm)}{Height\ (cm)} \times 100$$

The derived frame index 2 is then compared with reference values for small, medium and large frames, as defined for the appropriate age and gender of the subject (Howell, 1998).

Percentage ideal body weight (IBW) (sometimes know as weight index (WI)) can then be calculated by comparison with standard tables for ideal or desirable weight for a given height, gender and frame size. Several reference tables are available, e.g. the 1983 Metropolitan Life Height and Weight Insurance Tables, tables from the National Health and Nutrition Examination Survey (NHANES) nutrition surveys in the USA and Frisancho anthropometric standards (Matarese and Gottschlich, 1998; Shopbell et al., 2001). Ideal weight (or reference weight (RW)) may also be calculated according to regression equations (e.g. Warnold and Lundholm, 1984):

$$RW\ (women) = 0.65 \times height - 40.4$$
$$RW\ (men) = 0.80 \times height - 6.20$$

Percentage IBW is then calculated according to the following equation:

$$\%\ IBW = \frac{Actual\ weight\ (kg)}{IBW} \times 100$$

The following gradings are often used (Shopbell et al., 2001):

80–90% IBW: mild malnutrition
70–79% IBW: moderate malnutrition
$\leq$ 69% IBW: severe malnutrition

Percentage Weight Loss

In adults, unintentional weight loss of more than 10% of body weight over 3–6 months is considered to be physiologically and clinically significant. As the normal intra-individual variation in weight is about ±5%, unintentional weight loss between 5 and 10% over 3–6 months has been recommended as an indication of the risk of malnutrition developing. However, in the studies reviewed, unquantified weight loss (in terms of the amount of weight lost and over what time span) is sometimes used as one of the criteria to define malnutrition. For further details, refer to Chapter 1 and Elia (2000b).

Subjective Global Assessment

As part of the subjective global assessment (SGA) (Detsky et al., 1987), five features of a patient's history are elicited:

1. Weight loss in 6 months: < 5% small, 5–10% potentially significant, > 10% definitely significant. The rate and pattern of weight loss are considered.
2. Dietary intake in relation to a patient's usual pattern – normal or abnormal. The duration and degree of abnormal intake are noted.
3. Presence of significant gastrointestinal (GI) symptoms (anorexia, nausea, vomiting, diarrhoea) – persisting on a daily basis for a period longer than 2 weeks.
4. Functional capacity or energy level (bedridden to full capacity).
5. Metabolic demands of the underlying disease state (low to high stress).

Four features of a physical examination are noted as normal, mild, moderate or severe. These are:

1. Loss of subcutaneous fat in triceps region and mid-axillary line at the level of the lower ribs.
2. Muscle wasting in the quadriceps and deltoids.
3. Presence of oedema in the ankles and the sacral region.
4. Presence of ascites.

On the basis of these features of history and physical examination, the clinician subjectively identifies a rank to indicate a patient's nutritional status as follows:

SGA A: well nourished
SGA B: moderate or suspected malnutrition
SGA C: severe malnutrition.

Mini Nutritional Assessment

The Mini Nutritional Assessment (MNA) is a screening tool to evaluate an individual's risk of malnutrition (Guigoz et al., 1994). It includes 18 items, involving anthropometry, general assessments, dietary assessments and subjective assessment. A total score categorizes patients as follows:

Score $\geqslant$ 24 points: well nourished
Score 17–23.5 points: at risk of malnutrition
Score < 17 points: malnourished

Maastricht Index

The Maastricht index (MI) was developed in Maastricht, The Netherlands, to determine patients with malnutrition (de Jong et al., 1985). It was based on a survey of 18 objective nutritional measurements in a group of 50 patients requiring total parenteral nutrition on the basis of clinical judgement and 38 control patients admitted for elective minor surgical procedures. Discriminant analysis was performed and the following equation was developed:

MI = 20.68 − (0.24 × albumin, g l^{-1}) − (19.21 × prealbumin, g l^{-1}) − (1.86 × TLC, 10^9 l^{-1}) − (0.04 × % IBW)

Patients with a score > 0 are considered malnourished (Naber et al., 1997; Huang et al., 2000).

Nutritional Index

The nutritional index (NI) is a modification of the Maastricht index (Von Meyenfeldt et al., 1992):

NI = (0.14 × albumin, g l^{-1}) + (0.03 × % IBW) + (0.73 × TLC, 10^9 l^{-1}) − 8.90

Values less than 1.31 are considered to reflect abnormal nutritional status.

Nutrition Risk Index

The nutrition risk index (NRI) as described by the TPN Cooperative Study Group, (Veterans Affairs, 1991) is derived from serum albumin and the ratio of actual to usual body weight according to the following equation:

NRI = (1.519 × albumin, g l^{-1}) + (0.417 × $\frac{\text{(current weight)}}{\text{(usual weight)}}$ × 100

NRI score > 97.5: borderline malnourished
NRI score 83.5–97.5: mildly malnourished
NRI score < 83.5: severely malnourished

Prognostic Nutritional Index

The prognostic nutritional index (PNI) was described by Dempsey *et al.* (1988). It was developed as a means of trying to identify those patients undergoing major surgery at most risk of developing complications or death, using the following equation:

PNI (% risk) = 158 − 16.6 (albumin, g dl^{-1}) − 0.78 (triceps skin-fold thickness (TSF), mm) − 0.2 (transferrin, mg dl^{-1}) − 5.8 (delayed hypersensitivity (DH), graded 0–2)

PNI < 40%: low risk
PNI 40–50%: intermediate risk
PNI > 50%: high risk

Other Indices

A variety of other anthropometric indices have been used as criteria to define malnutrition (e.g. TSF, mid-arm muscle circumference), either in combination with other anthropometry or in combination with a variety of biochemical (e.g. albumin, prealbumin, transferrin) or immunological (e.g. total lymphocyte count) parameters. The cut-off values used to define risk of malnutrition also vary.

Children

The criteria to assess malnutrition in children are different from those used in adults and include assessment of weight-for-height, weight-for-age and height-for-age.

Acute nutritional status in children is most commonly measured using weight-for-height, according to the following equation:

Acute nutritional status =

$$\frac{\text{actual weight (kg)}}{50^{\text{th}} \text{ percentile weight for current height}} \times 100$$

Chronic nutritional status in children is most commonly measured using height-for-age, according to the following equation:

Chronic nutritional status =

$$\frac{\text{actual height (cm)}}{50^{\text{th}} \text{ percentile height for current age}} \times 100$$

Various classifications have been used to quantify nutritional status, the most common being the Waterlow classification (Waterlow, 1972), as shown in Table A1.1.

Table A1.1. The Waterlow classification of nutritional status.

Nutritional status	Acute malnutrition (wasting) (weight-for-height in %)	Chronic malnutrition (stunting) (height-for-age in %)
Grade 0 (normal)	> 90%	> 95%
Grade 1 (mild)	80–90%	90–95%
Grade 2 (moderate)	70–80%	85–90%
Grade 3 (severe)	< 70%	< 85%

EXPLANATION OF STUDY SUMMARY TABLES

In the following tables, details of all studies referred to in Chapter 2 have been summarized. The studies are arranged in alphabetical order (based on the name of the first author) within each section. Where logical, they have been further subdivided into subgroups, e.g. types of surgery, treatment for cancer, community versus hospital. Where data or information has not been reported in the paper/abstract reviewed, a dash '–' has been used in tables to indicate the lack of data.

Table A1.2. Prevalence of malnutrition in hospitalized patients (mixed diagnoses)[a].

Study	Time of assessment	Patients (n)	Diagnosis	Prevalence of malnutrition (% of patients)	Criteria for definition	Mean BMI (SD) of group (kg m^{-2})	BMI < 20 kg m^{-2} (%)	Change in nutritional status over time
Arnold et al., 2001, UK Abstract	Retrospective. Included in analysis if data in medical or nursing notes (only 36% of cases had data in 1999 review)	83	–	14%	BMI ≤ 20	–	14	48% lost wt (mean 3.6%) according to review of notes and 52% gained wt (mean 2.7%) (H stay ≥ 7 days)
Audivert et al., 2000, Spain Abstract	Admission	300	–	33% 41.6%	BMI < 20 and TSF or MAMC < 15th percentile SGA	–	–	–
Braunschweig et al., 2000, USA	Admission	404	Mixed H stay ≥ 7 days	31% 23%	SGA B SGA C	SGA B 25.5 SGA C 23.5	– –	59% undernourished at discharge (total n 404). 31% had decline in nutr. status during H stay
Cederholm et al., 1993, Sweden	Admission	205	Acute admissions, including CV, N, R, Rh	20% 36% MOF 33% R 20% CHF 13% Rh 0% CV, N	3 or more of: WI < 80%, TSF or MAMC < 10th percentile, low albumin, low DH	–	–	–
Chima et al., 1997, USA	Admission	173 (TH)	Mixed	32% at risk High at-risk groups were: GI 59% Infectious disease 59% Pneumonia/TB 42%	Risk defined as one or more of: < 75% IBW, low albumin, ≥ 10% wt loss in 1 month	–	–	–

Reference	Timing	n (setting)	Patient group	Prevalence	Criteria		Prevalence	Comments
Comi *et al.*, 1998, Italy Abstract	On admission and after 15 (± 2) days	705 (10 H)	Mixed GM and GS	19.1%	BMI < 20 and TSF < 10 mm (M) < 15 mm (F)	–	19.1%	Nutritional status (incl. lymphocytes, albumin and prealbumin) worsened in 60.2% and improved in 24.4%
Corish *et al.*, 2000a, Ireland	Admission	594 (2 TH)	Mixed, including GM, R, E, GS, O	11%	BMI < 20 and TSF or MAMC < 15th percentile	–	13.5%	Wt loss in 43% of 'underweight', 66% of 'normal weight' and 65% in 'overweight' and 'obese' (total *n* 202, median LOS 12 days)
Dechelotte *et al.*, France Abstract	–	1230 (UH)	Mixed GM and GS	28.6% 13.3%	SGA B SGA C	–	–	–
Edington *et al.*, 2000, UK	Admission	850 (2 TH, 2 DGH)	Mixed, including GS, O, GM, E, CV, N, GI, ON	20% 22.4% TH 16.5% DGH	BMI < 20 and TSF or MAMC < 15th percentile, or wt loss ≥ 10% in 6 months and BMI < or > 20, or BMI < 20 and wt loss < 10% in 6 months	–	–	–
Kamath *et al.*, 1986, USA	Admission	3047 (33 H)	All admissions	58%	Deficient in 1 or more of: albumin, Hb or TLC, W/H < 10th percentile	–	–	–
Kelly *et al.*, 2000, UK	Admission	219 (TH)	GM and GS, acute	16.2% 13%	BMI < 18.5 or BMI 18.5–20.0 and wt loss > 3 kg in 3 months	–	18%	–

Table A1.2. *Continued.*

Study	Time of assessment	Patients (n)	Diagnosis	Prevalence of malnutrition (% of patients)	Criteria for definition	Mean BMI (SD) of group (kg m^{-2})	BMI < 20 kg m^{-2} (%)	Change in nutritional status over time
Kyle et al., 2001, Switzerland	Admission	995 (UH)	Mixed GM and GS	17.3% 31%	BMI < 20 < 10th percentile for FFM (BIA)	24.1 (3.9)	17.3%	–
Landi et al., 2000, Italy	Admission, daily updates	9170 (M) 9145 (F) (79 H)	Mixed	3.8% (M) 15% (M) 7.3% (F) 20% (F)	BMI < 18.5 BMI 18.5–21.7 BMI < 18.5 BMI 18.5–21.7	24.9 (3.9) (M) 24.9 (5.0) (F)	–	–
Larsson et al., 1994b, Sweden (Swedish)	–	382 (4 H)	Mixed	20% 7%	SGA B SGA C	SGA B 20.8 SGA C 17.5	–	Negative energy and nitrogen balance observed
McWhirter and Pennington, 1994, UK	Admission	500 (TH)	Mixed: GS (n 100) GM (n 100) R (n 100) O (n 100) E (n 100)	40% 27% 46% 45% 39% 43%	BMI < 20 and TSF or MAMC < 15th percentile	–	37.4%	64% lost wt (total n 112), including 75% of 'undernourished' (n 55) Mean wt loss 5.4% (n 112)
Middleton et al., 2001, Australia	–	819 (2 TH)	Mixed	30% 6%	SGA B SGA C	–	–	–
Naber et al., 1997, The Netherlands	Admission	155 (UH)	Mixed, non-GS	45% 57% 62%	SGA NRI MI			Sig. improvement in nutr. status during admission (n 90) if MI used (? LOS unclear)

Study		n	Type of patients	Prevalence	Method			
Peake et al., 2000, UK Abstract	0–2 days (16.5%) 3–7 days (25.3%) 8–14 days (21%) 15–30 days (18%) 30+ days (19%)	553	Mixed	29% 35% at risk	NAT including diagnosis, age, recent oral intake, BMI, % wt loss, nausea, vomiting, pain	—	—	—
Perman et al., 2001, Argentina Abstract	—	1000 (38 H)	—	36.2% 11.2%	SGA B SGA C	—	—	—
Planas et al., 2001, Spain Abstract	Admission	404 (UH)	Mixed, non-trauma	46%	SGA	—	—	—
Reilly et al., 1988, USA	Admission, retrospective review	771 (1 UH, 1 DGH)	GM and GS	55% total 59% medical IBD 55% Pneumonia 63% Fractures 45% Surgical 48% Bowel 60% Orthopaedic 44% Abdominal 46%	LOM – any one of: low albumin, TLC, % IBW < 80%, subjective rating or appearance, 15% wt loss in 3 months	—	—	—
Reilly, H.M. et al., 1995, UK	Admission	153	Mixed, including P	24% moderate 26% high risk	NRS for adults and children: includes appetite, ability to eat, stress factor, % wt loss and BMI or W/L (P)	—	—	—
Strain et al., 1999, UK Abstract	Admission	326 (TH)	Mixed (expected stay ≥ 7 days)	24% 30%	BMI < 20 and TSF or MAMC < 10th percentile and/or wt loss BAPEN recommendation of wt, ht and wt loss	—	—	Wt loss in 68%, wt gain in 23%, 8% wt stable (total n 95)

Table A1.2. *Continued.*

Study	Time of assessment	Patients (n)	Diagnosis	Prevalence of malnutrition (% of patients)	Criteria for definition	Mean BMI (SD) of group (kg m⁻²)	BMI < 20 kg m⁻² (%)	Change in nutritional status over time
Thorsdottir et al., 1999, Iceland	Admission	82 (UH)	GM and GS	21%	3 or more of: BMI < 20, low albumin, TLC, prealbumin, Hb, TSF and MAMC < 10th percentile, wt loss 5–10% in 1–6 months	–	5%	–
Vlaming et al., 1999, UK Abstract	Admission	423 (TH)	Acute admissions to GM, GS, O (< 65 years)	15% (M) 18% (F)	BMI < 20	25.2 (M) 25.4 (F)	15% (M) 18% (F)	–
Waitzberg et al., 2001, Brazil	1st 48 h (22.1%) 3–7 days (27.9%) 8–15 days (23.3%) > 16 days (26.7%)	4000 (25 H)	Mixed GM and GS	48.1% 12.6%	SGA B + C SGA C (severe)	–	–	–

[a] Patients who were too ill or unable to give consent, or who were bedridden and could not be weighed were often excluded (Weekes, 1999; Edington et al., 2000). Surrogate measures for height, including arm span (Coats et al., 1993; Edington et al., 2000) and knee height (McWhirter and Pennington, 1994; Corish et al., 2000a), and for weight (Corish et al., 2000a) were used in some studies. Very few studies recorded excluding patients with gross fluid retention (Weekes, 1999; Corish et al., 2000a). One study reported including oedematous patients and fluid retention was not corrected for in calculations of BMI or weight loss (Strain et al., 1999). Very few studies included paediatrics and, in those which did, results were not presented separately (Reilly, H.M. et al., 1995).

CHF, congestive heart failure; CV, cardiovascular; E, elderly; GI, gastrointestinal; GM, general medicine; GS, general surgery; IBD, inflammatory bowel disease; MOF, multiple organ failure; O, orthopaedics; ON, oncology; N, neurology; P, paediatrics; R, respiratory medicine; Rh, rheumatology; DGH, district general hospital; H, hospital; TH, teaching hospital; UH, university hospital; BIA, bioelectrical impedance; DH, delayed hypersensitivity; FFM, fat-free mass; Hb, haemoglobin; incl., including; LOM, 'likelihood of malnutrition'; MI, Maastricht index; NAT, nutritional assessment tool; NRI, nutrition risk index; NRS, nutrition risk score; nutr, nutritional; TLC, total lymphocyte count; W/H, weight-for-height; W/L, weight-for-length; WI, weight index; SD, standard deviation; MAMC, mid-arm muscle circumference; TB, tuberculosis; LOS, length of stay; BAPEN, British Association for Parenteral and Enteral Nutrition.

Table A1.3. Summary of the prevalence of malnutrition using a variety of criteria in general medical patients admitted to hospital, according to country.

Country	Number of subjects	Prevalence of malnutrition (risk) % [a]	BMI < 20 kg m^{-2} (%)	Reference
Germany	100	21	–	Pirlich *et al.*, 2000 Abstract
Lebanon	82	35	–	Aoun *et al.*, 1993
UK	186	9	22	Weekes, 1999 Abstract
		22		
		31		
USA	135	34	–	Anderson *et al.*, 1985
USA	228	38	–	Coats *et al.*, 1993
USA	100	56	–	Robinson *et al.*, 1987
USA	134	48	–	Weinsier *et al.*, 1979

[a] When more than one result is provided for a given study (unless specifically explained), the results have been obtained by applying different criteria to the same group of patients.

Table A1.4. Prevalence of malnutrition in hospitalized medical patients.

Study	Time of assessment	Patients (n)	Prevalence of malnutrition (% of patients)	Criteria for definition	Mean BMI (SD) of group (kg m^{-2})	BMI < 20 kg m^{-2} (%)	Change in nutritional status over time
Agradi et al., 1984, Italy	Admission	100	45%	General nutritional index (combination of anthropometric indices)	–	–	Worsening of most parameters of nutritional status during hospitalization
Anderson et al., 1985, USA	Admission	135	34% 46%	Recent wt loss > 4.5 kg Inability to eat for 1 week	–	–	–
Aoun et al., 1992, Lebanon	–	82 (UH)	35%	At least 4 abnormal of: albumin, transferrin, CHI, TLC, % wt loss, MAMC, TSF	–	–	–
Coats et al., 1993, USA	Admission and 14th day of hospital stay	228 (UH)	38%	LOM score, includes < 90% IBW, low TSF, MAMC, TLC, plasma albumin, folate, ascorbate, haematocrit	–	–	By day 14, 46% had a high LOM score
Pirlich et al., 2000, Germany Abstract	Admission	100 (UH)	21%	SGA B + C	–	–	–
Robinson et al., 1987, USA	Admission	100 (UH)	40% 16% (borderline)	Wt loss > 10% or, if history unknown, global assessment	–	–	–
Weekes, 1999, UK Abstract	After admission (77% within 3 days)	186 (TH)	9% 31%	BMI < 18 MAMC < 15th percentile	23.7 (14.2–43.3)	22%	–
Weinsier et al., 1979, USA	Admission	134 (TH)	48%	LOM score (see Coats et al., 1993)	–	–	–

CHI, creatinine–height index; LOM, likelihood of malnutrition; MAMC, mid-arm muscle circumference; SD, standard deviation; TH, teaching hospital; TLC, total lymphocyte count; UH, university hospital.

Table A1.5. Prevalence of malnutrition in general medical patients in the community.

Study	Patients (*n*)	Diagnosis	Prevalence of malnutrition (% of patients)	Criteria for definition	Mean BMI (SD) of group (kg m^{-2})	BMI < 20 kg m^{-2} (%)	Change in nutritional status over time
Edington *et al.*, 1996, UK	441	Mixed, chronic diseases, including R, GI (52%) and ON (48%)	> 8%	BMI < 20 and TSF or MAMC < 15th percentile	–	–	–
Edington *et al.*, 1999, UK	10,317	ON 55%[a] CV 45%	7.7% (ON) 5.3% (CV)	BMI < 20	– –	7.7% (ON) 5.3% (CV)	– –
Martyn *et al.*, 1998, UK	11,357	Mixed, including R, GI, N	12.5%	BMI < 20	–	12.5%	–

[a]Also reported separately in section on malignancy.
CV, cardiovascular; GI, gastrointestinal; MAMC, mid-arm muscle circumference; N, neurology; ON, oncology; R, respiratory medicine; SD, standard deviation.

Causes and Consequences of Disease-related Malnutrition in Patients with Mixed Diagnoses

Factors associated with weight loss and the development of malnutrition in general hospital patients are numerous, some of which have been outlined in Table A1.6. In those who are hospitalized or living in institutions, the provision of food or patients intake of food is commonly inadequate (see Chapter 3 for more details) and low nutrient intake has been linked to adverse clinical outcome, particularly in the elderly (Hall *et al.*, 2000). Furthermore, disease-related malnutrition has many deleterious conse-quences for patients in the hospital and community setting. Both functional and clinical outcomes are worse for patients who are undernourished. In addition, greater use of health care resources in hospital and community settings translates into greater financial costs for undernourished patients.

From the data available, it is not possible to separate the effects of malnutrition and the impact of the disease severity on outcome. It is likely that those patients who are more undernourished are also sicker individuals. In some instances, it is likely that the consequences of weight loss/malnutrition may perpetuate further weight loss and deterioration in nutritional status.

Table A1.6. Potential causes and possible consequences of disease-related malnutrition in patients with mixed diagnoses.

Causes/factors	Consequences
Poor food intake (Browne and Moloney, 1998; Gall *et al.*, 1998; Shirley and Moloney, 2000; Valla *et al.*, 2000) for a variety of reasons (see Chapter 2)	Lower muscle strength (HGS) (Cederholm *et al.*, 1993), lower peak expiratory flow (Cederholm *et al.*, 1993), reduced functional ability (Naber *et al.*, 1997), and lower time ambulant (Cederholm *et al.*, 1993)
Severe anorexia (Agradi *et al.*, 1984)	Lower mood (women only) (Cederholm *et al.*, 1993)
Increasing disease severity (Edington *et al.*, 2000)	Higher complication and infection rates (Reilly *et al.*, 1988; Larsson *et al.*, 1994b; Naber *et al.*, 1997; Braunschweig *et al.*, 2000; Edington *et al.*, 2000)
Infections (Edington *et al.*, 2000)	Increased nosocomial infection (Dechelotte *et al.*, 2001)
Greater medication use (Naber *et al.*, 1997)	Longer hospital stay (Weinsier *et al.*, 1979; Anderson *et al.*, 1985; Robinson *et al.*, 1987; Reilly *et al.*, 1988; Coats *et al.*, 1993; Larsson *et al.*, 1994b; Chima *et al.*, 1997; Naber *et al.*, 1997; Audivert *et al.*, 2000; Braunschweig *et al.*, 2000; Edington *et al.*, 2000; Middleton *et al.*, 2001; Perman *et al.*, 2001; Planas *et al.*, 2001; Waitzberg *et al.*, 2001)
Disease duration > 2 years (Cederholm *et al.*, 1993)	
Old age (Cederholm *et al.*, 1993)	
Multiple organ failure (Cederholm *et al.*, 1993)	Higher hospital charges and costs (Robinson *et al.*, 1987; Reilly *et al.*, 1988; Chima *et al.*, 1997; Braunschweig *et al.*, 2000)
Failure to assess the nutritional status of the majority (> 50%) of admission patients (Kamath *et al.*, 1986; Vlaming *et al.*, 1999)	Higher mortality (Weinsier *et al.*, 1979; Reilly *et al.*, 1988; Coats *et al.*, 1993; Martyn *et al.*, 1998; Edington *et al.*, 1999; Corish *et al.*, 2000a; Landi *et al.*, 2000; Middleton *et al.*, 2001)
Failure to refer undernourished patients to a dietitian (Roubenoff *et al.*, 1987; Reilly, H.M. *et al.*, 1995; Kelly *et al.*, 2000; Peake *et al.*, 2000; Tessier *et al.*, 2000; Kruizenga *et al.*, 2001; Waitzberg *et al.*, 2001)	Higher rates of readmission to hospital (Planas *et al.*, 2001)
	Greater number of new drug prescriptions (Naber *et al.*, 1997; Martyn *et al.*, 1998; Edington *et al.*, 1999; Edington *et al.*, 2000)
Failure to document nutritional information in the medical notes (McWhirter and Pennington, 1994; Kelly *et al.*, 2000; Peake *et al.*, 2000; Perman *et al.*, 2001; Waitzberg *et al.*, 2001)	Less likelihood of discharge home with self-care and greater likelihood of using home health-care services (Chima *et al.*, 1997)
	Higher rates of hospital admission (community patients) (Martyn *et al.*, 1998)
Failure to provide nutritional support (Robinson *et al.*, 1987)	Higher GP consultation rates (community patients) (Martyn *et al.*, 1998; Edington *et al.*, 1999)

GP, general practitioner; HGS, hand-grip strength.

Table A1.7. Summary of the prevalence of malnutrition using a variety of criteria in elderly patients admitted to hospital and in different community settings, according to country.

Country	Number of subjects	Prevalence of malnutrition (risk) (%)[a]	BMI < 20 kg m^{-2} (%)	IBW < 90% (%)	Sector	Reference
Hospital, mixed diagnoses						
Belgium	151	6.5 – 85	17	–	Mixed	Joosten *et al.*, 1999
Canada	152	59.2	–	–	Mixed	Azad *et al.*, 1999
France	918	24.5 (acute)	–	–	Mixed	Compan *et al.*, 1999
		32.5 (subacute)				
		24.7 (long-term)				
Germany	300	22	–	–	Mixed acute	Volkert *et al.*, 1992
Ireland	218	16	16	–	Mixed	Corish *et al.*, 2000b Abstract
		10				
		28				
Italy	286	27	–	–	Mixed	Incalzi *et al.*, 1996
Norway	121	55	–	55	Mixed	Mowé and Bøhmer, 1991
Norway	311	57	–	–	Mixed acute	Mowé *et al.*, 1994
Sweden	78	30	30	–	Mixed acute	Andersson *et al.*, 2001 Abstract
Sweden	96	55	–	–	Mixed acute	Cederholm and Hellström, 1992
Sweden	337	36	36	–	Mixed	Flodin *et al.*, 2000
Sweden	501	29	–	–	Long-term care	Larsson *et al.*, 1990
Sweden	18	33	–	61	Long-term care	Sidenvall and Ek, 1993
Switzerland	219	35.9	–	–	Mixed acute	Mühlethaler *et al.*, 1995
		30.3				
		13.7				
Switzerland	1145	78.6	–	–	Mixed	Van Nes *et al.*, 2001
UK	20	35	35	–	Mixed acute	Klipstein-Grobusch *et al.*, 1995
UK	65	26	29	–	Mixed	Watson, 1999 Abstract
USA	250	39	–	–	Mixed	Sullivan *et al.*, 1989

Continued

Table A1.7. Summary of the prevalence of malnutrition using a variety of criteria in elderly patients admitted to hospital and in different community settings, according to country.

Country	Number of subjects	Prevalence of malnutrition (risk) (%)[a]	BMI < 20 kg m^{-2} (%)	IBW < 90% (%)	Sector	Reference
Hospital, general medical						
France	324	45.6 (M)/62.4 (F)	–	–	Medical	Constans *et al.*, 1992
Ireland	49	83.7	–	–	Medical acute	Charles *et al.*, 1999
Ireland	24	21	21	–	Medical	Corish *et al.*, 2000b Abstract
		17				
		33				
Scandinavia	56	28.5	–	–	Medical	Sandström *et al.*, 1985
Sweden	205	20	–	–	Medical acute	Cederholm *et al.*, 1995
UK	69	22	–	–	Medical acute	Potter *et al.*, 1995
USA	369	21 (M)/27 (F)	–	–	Medical	Covinsky *et al.*, 1999
		40.7				
Hospital, ICU						
France	116	8	–	–	ICU, mainly medical, > 24 h ventilation	Dardaine *et al.*, 2001
		29 (M)/16 (F)				
		20 (M)/12 (F)				
Home (out-patients)						
Denmark	61	38	23	–	Contact via GP	Beck *et al.*, 2001a
Norway	106	14	–	–	No acute illness	Mowé *et al.*, 1994
Sweden	80	64.5	34	–	Mixed, nursed at home	Saletti *et al.*, 1999
Sweden	70	49	–	–	Leg and foot ulcers	Wissing and Unosson, 1999
Sheltered accommodation/community resident home						
Sweden	261	33	–	–	Mixed	Christensson *et al.*, 1999
Sweden	28	40	0	–	–	Faxén Irving *et al.*, 1999
		0				
		18				

					Reference
Sweden	872	70 (SF) 90 (OPH) 90 (GLD) 100 (NH)	18 (SF) 25 (OPH) 19 (GLD) 33 (NH)	–	Mixed	Saletti et al., 2000
Nursing home					
Sweden	192	50	–	–	–	Nordenram et al., 2001
USA	2811	11.8	–	–	Mixed	Abbasi and Rudman, 1993
USA	156	19	–	–	Mixed	Morley and Kraenzle, 1994
USA	232	59	–	–	Mixed	Pinchcofsky-Devin and Kaminski, 1986
USA	53	69.8	–	–	Mixed	Sacks et al., 2000
USA	115	85	–	42	–	Shaver et al., 1980
USA	130	69	–	–	Mixed	Silver et al., 1988
USA	50	54	–	–	Mixed	Thomas et al., 1991

[a] When more than one result is provided for a given study (unless specifically explained) the results have been obtained by applying different criteria to the same group of patients. For more details, refer to Tables A1.8–A1.10.

GLD, group living for the demented; GP, general practitioner; ICU, intensive care unit; NH, nursing home; OPH, old people's home; SF, service flats (sheltered accommodation).

Table A1.8. Prevalence of malnutrition in hospitalized elderly patients (mixed diagnoses).[a]

Study	Time of assessment	Patients (*n*)	Diagnoses	Prevalence of malnutrition (% of patients)	Criteria for definition	Mean BMI (SD) of group (kg m^{-2})	BMI < 20 kg m^{-2} (%)	Change in nutritional status over time
Andersson *et al.*, 2001, Sweden Abstract	–	78	Mixed acute admissions (mean 83, SD 7 years, sex N/R)	30%	BMI < 20	–	30%	–
Azad *et al.*, 1999, Canada	Admission	152	Mixed including GM, O, GS, N (66 M, 86 F, mean 79, range 65–93 years)	44.1% moderate risk 15.1% malnourished	Detailed nutritional assessment including anthropometry, TLC, serum albumin, cholesterol, and risk factors for malnutrition	–	–	–
Cederholm and Hellström 1992, Sweden	Admission	96	Acute, mixed including CV, R, N, ON (31 M, 65 F, mean 80, SD 1 year)	55% CV 32% R 36% N 18% ON 56% Multiple 67% 28%	At least 2 (including 1 anthro.) of: DH, WI, TSF, albumin < 10th percentile of matched controls WI < 80%	–	–	–
Compan *et al.*, 1999, France	Admission and discharge (except long-term care)	918	AC (*n* 299) SAC (*n* 196) LTC (*n* 423) (303 M, 615 F, mean 83, range 55–103 years)	26% 24.5% (AC) 32.5% (SAC) 24.7% (LTC)	MNA	24.1 (3.4) 24.0 (4.7) 24.6 (5.4)	–	Nutritional status tended to improve with the duration of hospitalization in the acute-care group
Corish *et al.*, 2000b, Ireland Abstract	–	218	Mixed (age, sex N/R)	16% 10% 28%	BMI < 20 BMI < 20 + MAMC/TSF < 15th percentile BMI + MAMC/TSF < 15th percentile	–	16%	–

Reference	Setting	N	Population	Prevalence	Criteria	BMI	%	Comments
Flodin *et al.*, 2000, Sweden	Admission, retrospective	337	Mixed, including CV, ON, N, O, R, GI (70% acute) (128 M, 249 F, mean 81.4, SD 8 years)	36%	BMI < 20	22.2 (4.3) Lowest in COPD and ON and highest in diabetics	36%	—
Incalzi *et al.*, 1996, Italy	Admission and discharge	286	Mixed, including CV, R, ON, N, GM (143 M, 163 F, mean 79, range 79–99 years)	27%	BMI < 21	—	—	Depletion in 27% of patients from admission to discharge (depletion = MAC decreased by 3.6% or more)
Joosten *et al.*, 1999, Belgium	Admission	151	Mixed, including CHF, ON, CVA, ID, MOD (49 M, 102 F, mean 82.8 range 70–99 years)	30% 62% 10% 18% 85% 6.5% 62% 52% 26%	MAC < P10 + alb < 35 g l^{-1} Low BMI, TSF, MAMC or alb CAMA < 16/16.9 cm^2 BMI < P5 Low MAMC, TSF or alb BMI < 18 and TSF or MAMC < P5 Low BMI, MAC or TSF MNA 17–23.5 MNA < 17	23.7 (2.7) (M) 24.1 (5.4) (F)	17%	—
Klipstein-Grobusch *et al.*, 1995, UK	Admission from patient's own home	20	Acutely ill, mixed including CV, N, O, ON, R (8 M, 12 F, mean 82, SD 5 years)	35% 30% 62%	BMI < 20 MAC < P10 + alb < 35 g l^{-1} Low BMI, etc.	21.4 (4.7)	35%	Small loss of weight (−0.2 kg) and MAMC (−0.4 mm sig.) during hospitalization

Continued

Table A1.8. *Continued*

Study	Time of assessment	Patients (n)	Diagnoses	Prevalence of malnutrition (% of patients)	Criteria for definition	Mean BMI (sd) of group (kg m⁻²)	BMI < 20 kg m⁻² (%)	Change in nutritional status over time
Larsson *et al.*, 1990, Sweden	On admission, 8 and 26 weeks	501	Long-term care admissions, mixed	29% 32% (F) 23% (M)	3 or more of: (i) IBW < 80%, low TSF, MAMC; (ii) low albumin, prealbumin; (iii) low DH (at least 1 from each group)	Approx. 88% IBW	–	Decreased anthro. measures in malnourished up to 26 weeks (% IBW was unchanged); 26% of well-nourished pt were undernourished by 26 weeks (control arm of intervention study)
Mowé and Bøhmer, 1991, Norway	Admission	121	Non-critically ill, mixed (50 M, 71 F, mean 78.2, range 70–98 years)	55%	IBW < 90%	24.6 (M) 25.9 (F)	55% (< 90 % IBW)	–
Mowé *et al.*, 1994, Norway	Admission	311	Acutely ill, mixed diagnoses (140 M, 171 F, range 70–91 years)	57% 53% (M) 61% (F)	At least one of: BMI < 20; TSF ≤ 5 mm, MAMC ≤ 20 cm; alb ≤ 35 g l⁻¹ (M) BMI < 19.2; TSF ≤ 9mm; MAMC ≤ 19 cm; alb. ≤ 35 g l⁻¹ (F)	22.1 (M) 21.7 (F)	–	–
Mühlethaler *et al.*, 1995, Switzerland	Admission	219	Mixed (69 M, 150 F, mean 81.6, range 66–95 years)	35.9% 30.3% 13.7%	MAMA < 5th percentile TSF < 5th percentile BW < 80% of age and sex average	–	–	–

Reference	Timing	n	Population	Prevalence	Criteria			
Sidenvall and Ek, 1993, Sweden	Admission 3 and 6 weeks	18	Long-term care (> 3 weeks), mixed (5 M, 13 F, mean 81.4, SD 7.7 years)	33%	3 or more of: IBW < 90%, albumin, prealbumin, Hb below reference values	93 (16)% IBW	61% (IBW < 90%)	−1.44% (2.7%) IBW
Sullivan et al., 1989, USA	Admission to discharge	250	Mixed, including GM and GS	39%	At risk: albumin < 30 g l⁻¹, TLC < 1.5 cells mm⁻³ or history of wt loss or < 5th percentile for BMI	–	–	–
Van Nes et al., 2001, Switzerland	Admission	1319 (1145 analysed)	Mixed (396 M, 923 F, mean 84.2 years)	60% 18.6%	MNA 17–23.5 (at risk) MNA < 17 (malnourished)	–	–	–
Volkert et al., 1992, Germany	Admission	300	Acute, mixed (73 M, 227 F, mean 82.3, range 75–97 years)	22%	Graded by physician – clinical impression (reduced subcutaneous fat, low MAC)	M: BMI 23.0 (14.4–30.5) F: BMI 23.4 (11.9–39.1) n = 215	–	–
Watson, 1999, UK Abstract	Admission	65	Mixed, no details (M : F 2 : 3, mean 80.3 years)	26%	BMI < 20 + TSF or MAMC < 10th percentile	–	29%	–

[a] Patients were typically excluded from studies if they suffered severe cognitive impairment, if they were unable to give informed consent/answer questions (Sidenvall and Ek, 1993; Klipstein-Grobusch et al., 1995) or if they had cancer (Klipstein-Grobusch et al., 1995). Small numbers in same disease groups (due to heterogeneity of patients in studies) means data likely to be unreliable estimate of incidence of malnutrition (Cederholm and Hellström, 1992).

alb, albumin; anthro., anthropometric; CHF, congestive heart failure; CV, cardiovascular; GI, gastrointestinal; GM, general medicine; GS, general surgery; ID, infectious disease; MOD, multi-organ dysfunction; O, orthopaedics; ON, oncology; N, neurology; R, respiratory medicine; AC, acute care; SAC, sub-acute care; LTC, long-term care; alb, albumin; BW, body weight; CAMA, corrected arm muscle area; DH, delayed hypersensitivity; Hb, haemoglobin; P, percentile; TLC, total lymphocyte count; WI, weight index; SD, standard deviation; N/R, not recorded; MAMC, mid-arm muscle circumference; MAC, mid-arm circumference; COPD, chronic obstructive pulmonary disease.

Table A1.9. Prevalence of malnutrition in hospitalized elderly medical and ICU patients.

Study	Time of assessment	Patients (n)	Diagnoses	Prevalence of malnutrition (% of patients)	Criteria for definition	Mean BMI (SD) of group (kg m^{-2})	BMI < 20 kg m^{-2} (%)	Change in nutritional status over time
Cederholm et al., 1995, Sweden	Admission, follow-up at 9 months	205	Acute medical admissions (84 M, 121 F, mean 75, SD 1 years)	20%	Subnormal values for at least 3 of 5 variables: WI, TSF, MAMC, albumin and DH	–	–	125 of 158 survivors underwent follow-up. Of 19 who were malnourished at admission, nine had improved nutritional status and ten remained malnourished
Charles et al., 1999, Ireland	Admission	49	Acute medical admissions (21 M, 28 F, mean approx. 80 years)	4.1% (mild) 18.4% (mod.) 61.2% (severe)	Risk (1–3) based on indices of weight, anthropometry, nutritional intake and albumin	19.2 (3.7)	–	Nutritional status deteriorated in 29% of patients originally classed as well nourished. Improvement or maintenance of indices with nutritional intervention was seen in 75% of those classed as at risk
Constans et al., 1992, France	Admission, follow-up on 15th day	324	Medical care unit (128 M, 196 F, > 70 years)	30% (M, mod.) 41% (F, mod.) 15.6% (M, severe) 21.4% (F, severe)	Moderate: MAC < 10th percentile or albumin < 35 g l^{-1} Severe: MAC < 10th percentile and albumin < 35 g l^{-1}	–	–	53 patients had follow-up measurements made. MAC and albumin decreased over time
Corish et al., 2000b, Ireland Abstract	–	24	Medicine for the elderly (age, sex N/R)	21% 17% 33%	BMI < 20 BMI < 20 + MAMC/TSF < 15th percentile BMI + MAMC or TSF < 15th percentile	–	21%	–
Covinsky et al., 1999, USA	Admission	369	General medical (140 M, 229 F, mean 80.3 years)	24.4% 16.3%	SGA B SGA C	–	–	–

Reference	Measurement timing	n	Subjects	Prevalence	Definition	BMI (SD)			Comments
Dardaine *et al.*, 2001, France	Admission to ICU	116	Acute admissions to ICU (mainly medical), ventilation for min. 24 h (65 M, 51 F, mean 76.5, range 70–91 years)	8% 29% (M) 16% (F) 20% (M) 12% (F)	BMI < 21 MAC < 10th percentile MAC < 10th percentile Severe: MAC < 10th percentile + albumin < 35 g l^{-1}	27 (6.0)	—	—	—
Potter *et al.*, 1995, UK	Admission follow-up until discharge	69	Acute medical admissions (24 M, 45 F, mean 82.2, range 69–96 years)	22% 21% (M) 27% (F)	BMI < 5th percentile CAMA < 16 cm^2 (M) CAMA < 16.9 cm^2 (F)	21.9 (4.8) 21.6 (5.0) (M) 22 (4.6) (F)	—	—	41 patients had two or more data sets collected. MAMC decreased significantly between admission and discharge
Sandström *et al.*, 1985, Sweden, Norway, Finland	Admission	56	General medical (25 M, 31 F, mean 70, SD 9 years)	28.5%	Three or more abnormal parameters (WI, MAMC, TSF, albumin, TIBC, haemoglobin, iron)	—	—	—	Likelihood of developing malnutrition as result of energy intake falling below 21 kcal kg^{-1} body wt was seen in 36%

CAMA, corrected arm muscle area; DH, delayed hypersensitivity; ICU, intensive care unit; MAC, mid-arm circumference; MAMC, mid-arm muscle circumference; min., minimum; mod., moderate; N/R, not recorded; SD, standard deviation; TIBC, total iron binding capacity; WI, weight index.

Table A1.10. Prevalence of malnutrition in elderly patients in the community.

Study	Location	Time of assessment	Patients (*n*)	Diagnoses	Prevalence of malnutrition (% of patients)	Criteria for definition	Mean BMI (SD) of group (kg m^{-2})	BMI < 20 kg m^{-2} (%)	Change in nutritional status over time
Home									
Beck *et al.*, 2001a, Denmark	Home	After contact with GP, follow-up after 6 months	61	No acute illness, contact via GP (18 M, 43 F, mean 75, range 71–81 years)	38%	MNA 17–23.5	20.7 (MNA < 23) 24.7 (MNA > 23)	23%	56% were followed up. Median MNA score was similar to baseline. Trend towards higher rate of acute disease, hospitalization and need for home care in those with MNA ≤ 23 at baseline
Mowé *et al.*, 1994, Norway	Home	Age- and sex-matched controls for a hospital study	106	No acute illness (54 M, 52 F, range 70–91 years)	14% 13% (M) 15% (F)	One or more of the following: BMI < 20; TSF ≤ 5 mm; MAMC ≤ 20 cm; albumin ≤ 35 g l^{-1} (M) BMI < 19.2; TSF ≤ 9 mm; MAMC ≤ 19 cm; albumin ≤ 35 g l^{-1} (F)	24.4 (M) 25.4 (F)	–	–
Saletti *et al.*, 1999, Sweden	Nursing care at home	–	80	Mixed, including CHF, COPD and diabetes (11 M, 69 F, mean 84, SD 6 years)	62% 2.5%	MNA 17–23.5 (at risk) MNA < 17 (malnourished)	22.7 (5)	34%	–
Wissing and Unosson, 1999, Sweden	Home	–	70	Leg or foot ulcers (20 M, 50 F, mean 79.2, SD 6.5 years)	46% 3%	MNA 17–23.5 (at risk) MNA < 17 (malnourished)	At risk: 23.1 (4.1) (M) 26 (6.2) (F) Malnourished: 16.5 (0.4) (F)	–	–

Sheltered accommodation/community resident home

Reference	Setting	Study design	n	Subjects	Prevalence	Criteria	BMI	% low BMI	Comments
Christensson *et al.*, 1999, Sweden	Community resident home	Within 2 weeks of admission	261	Mixed (*n* 133 from own home, *n* 61 from hospital, *n* 67 from other care home) (113 M, 148 F, mean approx. 83 years)	33% 29% (home) 43% (hospital) 33% (other care home)	2 or more subnormal nutritional variables (WI, TSF, MAMC, prealbumin, albumin)	—	—	—
Faxén Irving *et al.*, 1999, Sweden	Sheltered housing	Recruitment and 6-month follow-up	28	7 M, 21 F, mean 81, SD 7 years	40% 0% 11% 7%	Wt loss > 10% since age 60 years BMI < 20 SGA B SGA C	26.6 (3.1) (M) 25.6 (3.2) (F)	0%	No deterioration in nutritional status at 6-month follow-up
Saletti *et al.*, 2000, Sweden	Assisted accommodation		872	Mixed (270 M, 602 F, mean 85, SD 8 years)	48% 36% 49%/21% (SF) 57%/33% (OPH) 51%/39% (GLD) 29%/71% (NH)	MNA 17–23.5 (at risk) MNA < 17 17–23.5/ < 17 per group	23.6 (4.5) 24.2 (5) (SF) 23.6 (5) (OPH) 23.9 (4) (GLD) 22.3 (4) (NH)	23% 18% (SF) 25% (OPH) 19% (GLD) 33% (NH)	—

Nursing home

Reference	Setting	Study design	n	Subjects	Prevalence	Criteria	BMI	% low BMI	Comments
Abbasi and Rudman, 1993, USA	26 nursing homes	Last recorded info for all residents, retrospective	2811	Mixed (age/sex N/R)	11.8%	IBW < 80%	—	—	—
Morley and Kraenzle, 1994, USA	Nursing home	All residents in nursing home for > 3 months	156	Chronically ill, mixed including R, N, ON	19% 15% short stayers (3–6 months) 21% in long stayers (> 6 months)	Weight loss of ≥ 2.3 kg during nursing home stay	—	—	Criteria used to define risk of malnutrition relates to weight loss during stay in nursing home

Continued

Table A1.10. *Continued.*

Study	Location	Time of assessment	Patients (n)	Diagnoses	Prevalence of malnutrition (% of patients)	Criteria for definition	Mean BMI (SD) of group (kg m^{-2})	BMI < 20 kg m^{-2} (%)	Change in nutritional status over time
Nordenram et al., 2001, Sweden	Nursing home	–	192	–	25% at risk 25% PEM	Nutrition score 0–1: non-PEM 1–2: at risk 3–7: PEM	–	–	–
Pinchcofsky-Devin and Kaminski, 1986, USA	Nursing home	–	232	Mixed (104 M, 128 F, mean 72.9, SD 12 years)	59% 100% in patients with PU	Graded mild, moderate or severe on basis of anthropometric and biochemical parameters	–	–	–
Sacks et al., 2000, USA	Long-term care	<2 weeks after admission	53	Mixed (11 M, 42 F, mean 83.2, SD 5.8 years)	52.8% 17%	SGA B (mild/mod.) SGA C (severe)	25.7 (2.6) (A) 21.4 (3.7) (B) 17.7 (3.8) (C)	–	–
Shaver et al., 1980, USA	Nursing home	Survey of all residents	115	21 M, 94 F, mean approx. 80, range 48–101 years	85%	Moderate/severe depletion of ≥ 1 somatic protein parameter and ≥ 1 visceral protein	23.0 (M) 21.2 (F)	42% (< 90% IBW)	–
Silver et al., 1988, USA	Academic nursing home	Survey of residents present for > 6 months	130	Mixed, n 87 elderly (sex N/R, mean 78 years)	46% 23%	10% below ABW 20% below ABW	–	–	24% had lost 4.5–8.6 kg and 45% had lost > 9.1 kg during their nursing-home stay
Thomas et al., 1991, USA	Nursing home	Admission, 8–10-week follow-up	50	Mixed (22 M, 28 F, mean 76, SD 13 years)	54%	Index ≥ 4, based on anthropometric and biochemical indices	25.5 (11.7) (index < 3; n 24) 19 (4.1) (index > 4; n 26)	–	27 patients remained at end of follow-up. Improvement of score occurred in 63% (10/16) of those with original score ≥ 4. 1/11 with original score < 4 became malnourished. 6/16 remained malnourished.

GP, general practitioner; SF, service flats (sheltered accommodation); OPH, old people's home; GLD, group living for the demented; NH, nursing home; ABW, average body weight; CHF, congestive heart failure; PEM, protein-energy malnutrition; PU, pressure ulcers; SD, standard deviation; COPD, chronic obstructive pulmonary disease; info, information; MAMC, mid-arm muscle circumference; N/R, not recorded; R, respiratory medicine; N, neurology; ON, oncology.

Causes and Consequences of Disease-related Malnutrition in the Elderly

There are many causes of malnutrition in the elderly (Goodwin, 1989; Fischer and Johnson, 1990; Lipschitz, 1991; Morley and Kraenzle, 1994; Morley, 1996), most of which have been highlighted in Chapter 3. Robbins (1989) described the 'nine d's' of weight loss in the elderly: dentition, dysgeusia, dysphagia, diarrhoea, disease, depression, dementia, dysfunction and drugs. Although alone each of these may represent a rather minor problem, these factors frequently coexist. However, the relative emphasis of each may vary according to the location of patients. For example, eating dependency is a particular problem in institutionalized elderly patients (estimates of between 32% and 50% of nursing home residents in the USA (Siebens *et al.*, 1986)). This has been associated with an increased 6-month mortality and multiple other impairments (absence of teeth, difficulty in swallowing, impaired cognition) (Siebens *et al.*, 1986). Many studies in elderly patients, particularly those in hospitals and nursing homes, have consistently shown extremely poor nutritional intakes (MacLennan *et al.*, 1975; Vir and Love, 1979; Morgan *et al.*, 1986; Thomas *et al.*, 1986; Elmstahl and Steen, 1987; Stratton, 1994; Elmstahl *et al.*, 1997). Furthermore, an official review of the care of older people in general hospitals in the UK has revealed concerns about the non-availability and poor quality of food and drink (Health Advisory Service, 1998). Reports of lack of help from staff to feed patients who need assistance with reaching or eating their food are also documented (Health Advisory Service, 1998). In addition, a high frequency of nutritional deficiencies, including micronutrient deficiencies (Vir and Love, 1979; Greer *et al.*, 1986; Burns *et al.*, 1989; Finch *et al.*, 1998) has been reported, particularly in elderly people in hospitals and nursing homes.

Importantly, weight loss and malnutrition are associated with adverse functional and clinical outcomes in elderly patients (summarized in Table A1.11). A large retrospective review of 8428 hospital admissions indicated that the deleterious effects of extremes of body weight take on increasing importance with increasing age, with a low weight being a more important predictor of mortality than overweight in older hospitalized subjects (Potter *et al.*, 1988).

From the data available it is not possible to separate the effects of malnutrition and the impact of the disease severity on outcome. For example, patients may be more severely undernourished because disease severity is greater. More information on the causes and consequences of malnutrition can be gathered from Chapters 2 and 3.

Table A1.11. Possible causes and potential consequences of disease-related malnutrition in elderly patients.

Causes/factors	Consequences
Poor food intake in hospitals (Sandström et al., 1985; Elmstahl, 1987; Jones et al., 1988; Mowé et al., 1994; Klipstein-Grobusch et al., 1995; McCargar et al., 1995; Incalzi et al., 1996; Elmstahl et al., 1997; Sullivan et al., 1999; Barton et al., 2000a), nursing homes (Van der Wielen et al., 1996; Persson et al., 2000; Eastwood et al., 2001; Hollis and Henry, 2001; Lengyel et al., 2001) and at home (Lewis et al., 1993) for a variety of reasons (see Chapter 3)	Lower ADL (Incalzi et al., 1996; Covinsky et al., 1999; Flodin et al., 2000)
	Lower TLC (Incalzi et al., 1996)
	Pressure ulcers (Pinchcofsky-Devin and Kaminski, 1986)
	Greater use of medications (Incalzi et al., 1996)
	Increased falls (Vellas et al., 1992)
	Increased complications (Sullivan et al., 1990; Sacks et al., 2000)
	Increased risk of sepsis (Potter et al., 1995)
Anorexia (Incalzi et al., 1996)	Longer hospital stay (Incalzi et al., 1996; Sullivan et al., 1989; Van Nes et al., 2001)
Dental problems (Sidenvall and Ek, 1993; Sheiham et al., 2001)	Higher mortality (Sullivan et al., 1990, 1991; Thomas et al., 1991; Constans et al., 1992; Volkert et al., 1992; Cederholm et al., 1995; Mühlethaler et al., 1995; Covinsky et al., 1999; Flodin et al., 2000; Mowé and Bøhmer, 2000; Sacks et al., 2000; Dardaine et al., 2001; Van Nes et al., 2001)
Depression (Morley and Kraenzle, 1994)	
Poor mental state (Incalzi et al., 1996)	
Use of many medications (Incalzi et al., 1996)	Greater dependence on mobility aids (Wissing and Unosson, 1999)
Motor dysfunction (Sidenvall and Ek, 1993)	Greater dependence on home-help services (Wissing and Unosson, 1999)
Lack of identification/recognition of malnutrition (Mowé and Bøhmer, 1991)	
Lack of dietetic referral for at-risk patients (Sullivan et al., 1989)	Reduced likelihood of discharge from nursing home (Thomas et al., 1991)
Failure to provide nutritional support for at-risk patients (Sullivan et al., 1989; Mowé and Bøhmer, 1991)	Increased need for nursing home care following hospital discharge (Covinsky et al., 1999)
	Increased risk of non-elective hospital readmission (Friedmann et al., 1997)
	Increased risk of institutionalization (Payette et al., 2000)

ADL, activities of daily living; TLC, total lymphocyte count.

Table A1.12. Summary of the prevalence of malnutrition using a variety of criteria in patients with COPD in the community and in hospital, arranged according to country.

Country	n	Prevalence of malnutrition (%)[a]	IBW < 90% (%)	BMI < 20 kg m^{-2} (%)	Reference
COPD: community					
Brazil	32	19 (normoxaemic) 25 (hypoxaemic)	19 (normoxaemic) 25 (hypoxaemic)	–	Godoy et al., 2000
Canada	135	24	24	–	Gray-Donald et al., 1989
Denmark	2132	5 (M) / 16 (F)	–	5 (M) / 16 (F)	Landbo et al., 1999
Netherlands	86	49 (E) / 26 (CB)	–	–	Baarends et al., 1997 Abstract
Netherlands	72	21	–	–	Engelen et al., 1994
Netherlands	99	49 (E) / 22 (CB) 37 (E) / 12 (CB)	–	–	Engelen et al., 1999
Netherlands	83	25 42 33	25	–	Schols et al., 1989
Netherlands	253	34	34	–	Schols et al., 1993
Netherlands	42	52 (E) / 40 (CB)	–	–	Schols et al., 1999
USA	60	27 33 5 0	–	–	Braun et al., 1984b
USA	126	23	–	23	Sahebjami et al., 1993
USA	779	24	24	–	Wilson et al., 1989
COPD: hospital					
France	50	60	34	–	Laaban et al., 1993
Iceland	34	38	–	24	Thorsdottir et al., 2001
Iceland	10	30	–	30	Thorsdottir and Gunnarsdottir, 2002

CB, chronic bronchitis; COPD, chronic obstructive pulmonary disease; E, emphysema.
[a]When more than one result is provided for a given study (unless specifically explained), the results have been obtained by applying different criteria to the same group of patients. For more details, refer to Table A1.13.

Table A1.13. Prevalence of malnutrition in chronic obstructive pulmonary disease (COPD).

Study	Time of assessment	Patients (*n*)	Diagnosis	Prevalence of malnutrition (% of patients)	Criteria for definition	Mean BMI (SD) of group (kg m^{-2})	BMI < 20 kg m^{-2} (%)	Change in nutritional status over time
Community								
Baarends *et al.*, 1997, Abstract NL	–	86	COPD (E, 32 M, 11 F; CB, 37 M, 6 F) Age N/R	49% (E) 26% (CB) (*P* < 0.05)	Weight loss	–	–	–
Braun *et al.*, 1984b, USA	Admission to a rehabilitation programme	60	COPD (42 M, 18 F, mean 62, SE 1.3 years)	27% 33% 5% 0%	Weight loss > 5% in 12 months TSF < 60% of standard IBW < 60% MAMC < 60% of standard	–	–	–
Engelen *et al.*, 1994, NL	First presentation for routine lung function tests	72	COPD, stable (55 M, 17 F, mean 62, SD 13 years)	21%	IBW < 90% and/or FFM IBW < 67 (F)/ < 69 (M)%	–	–	–
Engelen *et al.*, 1999, NL	Admission to a pulmonary rehabilitation center	99	COPD, moderate to severe, 49 E, 50 CB (77 M, 22 F; mean 64 years)	49% (E) 22% (CB) (*P* < 0.05) 37% (E) 12% (CB)	Recent involuntary weight loss Lean mass depletion	24.5 (4.3) 22.6 (3.2) (E) 26.3 (4.3) (CB) (*P* < 0.001 E vs. CB)	–	–
Godoy *et al.*, 2000, Brazil	Admission to rehabilitation or oxygen therapy programmes	32	Normoxaemic (12 M, 4 F; mean 63.6, SD 7.0 years) Hypoxaemic (10 M, 6 F; mean 65.2, SD 10.8 years)	19% (norm.) 25% (hypox.)	IBW < 90%	23 (M, norm.) 23.8 (F, norm.) 23.5 (M, hypox.) 23.4 (F, hypox.)	19% (norm.) 25% (hypox.) < 90% IBW	–

Continued

Reference	Setting	n	Patients	Prevalence	Criteria	BMI	Prevalence	
Gray-Donald et al., 1989, Canada	—	135	COPD, severe (100 M, 35 F, mean 63.6 years)	24.4% / 14%	IBW <90% / IBW <90% and TSF <60% normal	—	24% (<90% IBW)	—
Landbo et al., 1999, Denmark	—	2132	COPD (1218 M, mean 57.7, SD 11.0 years; 914 F, mean 55, SD 10.8 years)	5% (M) / 16% (F)	BMI <20	22.5 (3.8) (M) / 24.1 (4.6) (F)	5% (M) / 16% (F)	—
Sahebjami et al., 1993, USA	Attendance at chest clinic	126	COPD, stable (M, mean approx. 64 years)	23%	BMI <20	—	23%	—
Schols et al., 1989, NL	Admitted to a pulmonary rehabilitation centre	83	COPD, stable (71 M, 12 F, mean 62, SD 8 years)	25% / 42% / 33%	IBW <90% / CHI <60% and/or IBW <90% / Wt loss ≥ 10% of UBW	—	25% (<90% IBW)	—
Schols et al., 1993, NL	1 week after admission to rehabilitation programme	253	COPD, stable (203 M, 52 F, mean age 65, SD 8 (M), 62 SD 9.0 (F))	34%	IBW <90%	—	34% (<90% IBW)	—
Schols et al., 1999, NL	Admitted to a pulmonary rehabilitation centre	42	COPD, severe lung function impairment (27 E, mean 67, SD 8 years; 15 CB, mean 67, SD 5 years)	52% (E) / 40% (CB)	Recent involuntary weight loss	21.6 (3.0) (E) / 25.1 (3.3) (CB) ($P < 0.001$)	—	—
Wilson et al., 1989, USA	Data from IPPB trial	779	COPD (M, age N/R)	24%	IBW <90%	—	24% (<90% IBW)	—

Table A1.13. *Continued*

Study	Time of assessment	Patients (*n*)	Diagnosis	Prevalence of malnutrition (% of patients)	Criteria for definition	Mean BMI (SD) of group (kg m^{-2})	BMI < 20 kg m^{-2}	Change in nutritional status over time
Hospital Laaban *et al.*, 1993, France	Admission	50	COPD, acute respiratory failure, 27 MV (38 M, 12 F, mean 65, SD 13 years)	60% 34%	Multiparameter nutritional index IBW < 90%	–	34% (< 90% IBW)	–
Pouw *et al.*, 2000, NL (Retrospective case control study)	Admission and discharge (mean LOS 12 days) Cases: readmitted within 14 days Controls: not readmitted	28 (14 cases)	COPD, acute exacerbation (16 M, 12 F, mean approx. 70 years)	–	–	21.3 (3.1) (cases) 22.4 (5.9) (controls)	–	BMI of cases decreased significantly during hospital stay to 20.7 (3.0) (*P* < 0.01) and remained low at readmission (20.3, SD 3.2). BMI did not change in controls
Thorsdottir *et al.*, 2001, Iceland	–	34	COPD, acute exacerbation (15 M, 19 F, mean 73 years)	38%	≥ 3 of 7 measures below reference values: BMI <20, TSF, MAMC/ MAMA <5th percentile, albumin <38 g l^{-1}, prealbumin <180 mg l^{-1}, TLC < 1.82 × 10^9 l^{-1}, wt loss > 5% in previous months	28.2 (5.7) (WN; *n* 21) 20.8 (4.2) (MN; *n* 13)	24%	–
Thorsdottir and Gunnarsdottir 2002, Iceland	Admission and after 7–10 days	10	COPD, acute exacerbation (4 M, 6 F, mean 72, range 62–89 years)	30%	≥ 3 of 7 measures below reference values (see above)	23.8 (4.9)	30%	No significant change in nutritional status over time

CB, chronic bronchitis; E, emphysema; IPPB, intermittent positive pressure breathing; MN, malnourished; MV, mechanical ventilation; TLC, total lymphocyte count; WN, well nourished; SD, standard deviation; NL, Netherlands; SE, standard error; MAMC, mid-arm muscle circumference; FFM, fat-free mass; LOS, length of stay; N/R, not recorded; CHI, creatinine–height index; UBW, usual body weight; MAMA, mid-arm muscle area.

Causes and Consequences of Disease-related Malnutrition in Chronic Obstructive Pulmonary Disease (COPD)

The proposed causes and possible consequences of malnutrition in COPD are summarized in Table A1.14. As in other diseases, the causes of malnutrition are probably multifactorial. Few studies have actually measured food intake, and of those that have looked at intake in stable patients, intake does not appear to be dramatically reduced (Baarends *et al.*, 1997; Schols *et al.*, 1999). However, as with other diseases, such as acquired immune deficiency syndrome (AIDS), acute exacerbations of the disease may compromise food intake. Only one study has examined this (Thorsdottir and Gunnarsdottir, 2002), and showed that food intake was insufficient to improve nutritional status. Others have also shown a significant negative energy balance due to insufficient intake in COPD patients in a rehabilitation programme (Tang *et al.*, 2002). Other reasons for reduced intake have also been proposed, as well as other possible explanations.

Several studies have highlighted the relationship between weight loss/malnutrition and adverse outcome. As with other diseases, it is not possible to separate the effects of malnutrition and the impact of disease severity on outcome. Studies of nutritional intervention in COPD are examined in Chapters 6–8.

Table A1.14. Possible causes and potential consequences of disease-related malnutrition in COPD.

Causes/factors	Consequences
Reduced food intake, possibly due to the following: • Dyspnoea due to irregular breathing while eating or reduced functional residual capacity during gastric filling (Congleton, 1999)[a] • Arterial oxygen desaturation due to altered breathing patterns during chewing and swallowing (Schols et al., 1991) • Hypoxia-related appetite suppression (Congleton, 1999) • Acute exacerbations (Vermeeren et al., 1997; Creutzberg et al., 2000) • Raised plasma TNF-α levels (Schols, 1999)	Reduced lung function and dyspnoea (Openbrier et al., 1983; Braun et al., 1984b; Keim et al., 1986; Wilson et al., 1989; Sahebjami et al., 1993, 2000; Braulio et al., 2001) Reduced maximal oxygen consumption (VO_2 max.) (Gray-Donald et al., 1989) Decreased peripheral muscle function (Engelen et al., 1994)[b] Decreased exercise performance (Schols et al., 1989, 1993; Yoshikawa et al., 1999; Kobayashi et al., 2000)[c]
Increased REE (Donahoe et al., 1989; Wilson et al., 1990; Schols et al., 1991; Hugli et al., 1996; Vermeeren et al., 1997; Nguyen et al., 1999)	Decreased QOL (Mostert et al., 2000)[c]
Increased energy requirement for augmenting ventilation (Donahoe et al., 1989; Mannix et al., 1999)	Increased need for hospitalization (Braun et al., 1984a)
Increased TEE due to non-resting component (Baarends et al., 1997)[d]	Increased postoperative complications during lung volume reduction surgery (Nezu et al., 2001)
Imbalance between energy intake and energy requirements during acute exacerbations (Vermeeren et al., 1997; Creutzberg et al., 2000)	Increased mortality (Wilson et al., 1989; Connors et al., 1996; Gray-Donald et al., 1996; Incalzi et al., 2001)
Elevated systemic inflammatory response (Schols, 1999; Schols et al., 1999; Creutzberg et al., 2000)	
Raised plasma TNF-α levels (Nguyen et al., 1999)	
Altered metabolic handling of nutrients (Goldstein et al., 1988; Green and Muers, 1991)	
Theophylline treatment (Nguyen et al., 1999)	

[a]Others suggest that dyspnoea during mealtimes is unlikely to reduce intake (Gray-Donald et al., 1998).
[b]Deficit in skeletal muscle function is also likely to be caused by chronic inactivity and muscle deconditioning (Bernard et al., 1998; Clark et al., 2000).
[c]Not in all studies (Gray-Donald et al., 1989).
[d]Raised TEE not shown in all studies (Hugli et al., 1996; Tang et al., 2002).
TNF-α, tumour necrosis factor alpha; REE, resting energy expenditure; TEE, total energy expenditure; QOL, quality of life.

Table A1.15. Summary of the prevalence of malnutrition using a variety of criteria in patients with gastrointestinal or liver disease in the hospital and the community, arranged according to country.

Country	Patients (*n*)	Prevalence of malnutrition (%)[a]	BMI < 20 kg m⁻² (%)	IBW < 90% (%)	Reference
Gastrointestinal disease: hospital					
Chile	175	54	–	–	Hirsch *et al.*, 1991
Germany	100	38	–	–	McWhirter *et al.*, 1994b Abstract
UK	100	27	–	–	Pirlich *et al.*, 1994b Abstract
Gastrointestinal disease: community					
UK	100	16	–	–	McWhirter *et al.*, 1994b Abstract
Liver disease: hospital					
Denmark	37	78	–	–	Nielsen *et al.*, 1993
Germany	92	41	–	–	Koch *et al.*, 2001 Abstract
Italy	212	54	–	–	Alberino *et al.*, 2001
USA	284	47.2 (mild disease)	–	–	Mendenhall *et al.*, 1984b
		61.5 (moderate disease)			
		77.8 (severe disease)			
Liver disease: community					
Thailand	60	13.3	–	13.3	Roongpisuthipong *et al.*, 2001
		11.7			
		38			
		35			
UK	80	33	–	–	Wicks *et al.*, 1995
USA	132	3	–	–	Thuluvath and Triger, 1994
		19			
		35			
Liver disease: location unclear					
Germany	45	100	–	–	Plauth *et al.*, 1998 Abstract
		51			
Italy	1053	35	–	–	Merli *et al.*, 1996

Continued

Table A1.15. *Continued*

Country	Patients (*n*)	Prevalence of malnutrition (%)[a]	BMI < 20 kg m^{-2} (%)	IBW < 90% (%)	Reference
Liver disease: awaiting liver transplant					
UK	65	54	–	–	Davidson *et al.*, 1999
UK	102	79	–	–	Harrison *et al.*, 1997
		28			
UK	41	39	7	–	Jackson *et al.*, 1996 Abstract
		7			
UK	164	54	–	–	Madden *et al.*, 1994 Abstract
		23			
		71			
USA	20	85	0	–	Hasse *et al.*, 1993
USA	99	99	–	–	Stephenson *et al.*, 2001

[a]When more than one result is provided for a given study (unless specifically explained) the results have been obtained by applying different criteria to the same group of patients. For more details, refer to Table A1.16.

Table A1.16. Prevalence of malnutrition in patients with gastrointestinal and liver disease[a].

Study	Time of assessment	Patients (n)	Diagnosis	Prevalence of malnutrition (% of patients)	Criteria for definition	Mean BMI (SD) of group (kg m^{-2})	BMI < 20 kg m^{-2} (%)	Change in nutritional status over time
Gastrointestinal disease: hospital								
Hirsch et al., 1991, Chile	Admission	175	GI disease, benign and malignant (age/sex N/R)	38% 16%	SGA B SGA C	–	–	–
McWhirter et al., 1994b, UK Abstract	Admission	100	GI disease (no details given)	38%	BMI < 20 and TSF and/or MAMC < 15th percentile	–	–	–
Pirlich et al., 2000, Germany Abstract	Admission	100	GI disease (no details given)	27%	SGA B + C	–	–	–
Gastrointestinal disease: community								
Geerling et al., 2000a, Netherlands	Within 6 months of diagnosis	69	CD (n 23) UC (n 46)	–	Body composition Dietary intake Biochemistry Muscle strength	22.2 (2.7) 23.1 (3.0)	–	–
Geerling et al., 1998a, Netherlands	Long-standing CD (> 10 years)	32	CD in remission	–	Body composition Dietary intake Biochemistry Muscle strength	23.2 (3.7)	–	–
McWhirter et al., 1994b UK Abstract	First clinic visit	100	GI disease (no details given)	16%	BMI < 20 and TSF and/or MAMC < 15th percentile	–	–	–

Continued

Table A1.16. *Continued*

Study	Time of assessment	Patients (n)	Diagnosis	Prevalence of malnutrition (% of patients)	Criteria for definition	Mean BMI (SD) of group (kg m^{-2})	BMI < 20 kg m^{-2} (%)	Change in nutritional status over time
Liver disease: hospital								
Alberino *et al.,* 2001, Italy	Admission	212	Liver cirrhosis (A and NA) Child A, B and C (143 M, 69 F, mean 57.4, SD 10.4 years)	54%	MAMC and/or TSF < 10th percentile	26.2 (4.2) (CA) 25.0 (4.3) (CB) 26.0 (4.0) (CC)	–	–
Koch *et al.,* 2001, Germany Abstract	Admission?	92	Child A liver cirrhosis (53 M, 39 F, age N/R)	41%	BCM < 2 SD of control Lymphocytes < 1000 μl^{-1}, and/or albumin < 35 g l^{-1}	26.8 (M) 26.6 (F)	–	–
Mendenhall *et al.,* 1984b, USA	Between 5 and 10 days after admission	284	Alcoholic hepatitis (mean 50.2, SE 0.47 years, sex N/R)	47.2% (mild) 61.5% (moderate) 77.8% (severe)	All of: low % IBW (no value given), decreased LBM (CHI), failure to react to skin tests	22.7 (mild) 21.4 (moderate) 20.6 (severe)	–	–
Nielsen *et al.,* 1993, Denmark	Median 11 (range 2–38) days after admission	37	Alcoholic liver cirrhosis (26 M, 11 F, med. 46, range 31–82 years)	35% (mild) 43% (moderate)	Clinical judgement	20.2 (calculated from med. wt and ht)	–	–
Liver disease: community								
Roongpisuthipong *et al.,* 2001, Thailand	Clinic visit	60	Liver cirrhosis (A and NA) Child A, B and C (33 M, 27 F, mean approx. 56 years)	13.3% 11.7% 38% 30% 5%	IBW < 90% BMI < 18.5 TSF < 10th percentile SGA B SGA C	22.0 (3.9) (A) 24.5 (3.4) (NA)	13.3% < 90% IBW	–

Reference	Setting	n	Patient group	Prevalence	Criteria				
Thuluvath and Triger, 1994, USA	Clinic visit	132	Chronic liver disease (A and NA) (49 M, 83 F, mean approx. 50 years)	3% 19% 35%	IBW < 80th percentile MAFA < 5th percentile MAMA < 5th percentile	—	—		—
Wicks et al., 1995, UK	Clinic visit	80	Primary biliary cirrhosis (6 M, 74 F, mean 55, range 29–75 years)	33%	MAC and/or TSF < 5th percentile	—	—		—
Liver disease: location unclear									
Merli et al., 1996, Italy	—	1053	Liver cirrhosis (A and NA) (635 M, 400 F, age N/R)	35%	MAMA and/or MAFA < 5th percentile	—	—		—
Plauth et al., 1998, Germany Abstract	—	45	Liver cirrhosis (A and NA) Child A, B and C (age/sex N/R)	100% 51%	MAMA < 5th percentile BCM < 35% of IBW	—	—		—
Liver disease: awaiting liver transplant									
Davidson et al., 1999, UK	Consideration for liver transplant	65	Liver cirrhosis, hepatocellular (n 31; A and NA) and biliary (n 34) (25 M, 40 F, mean 54.6, SE 2.2 years)	54%	BMI, wt loss as % actual body weight, TSF, and/or MAMC < 80% of reference	24.1 (SE 0.8)	—		—
Harrison et al., 1997, UK	On liver transplant waiting list (med 8, range 1–59 weeks pre-transplant)	102	Cholestatic liver disease (n 58) and parenchyma cirrhosis (n 44) (range 17–69 years, sex N/R)	79% 28%	MAC and TSF < 25th percentile MAC and TSF < 5th percentile	—	—		—
Hasse et al., 1993, USA	Evaluation for liver transplant	20	Mixed liver diseases[b] (7 M, 13 F, mean 44.3, range 17–61 years)	70% 15%	SGA B SGA C	—	0%		—

Continued

Table A1.16. Continued

Study	Time of assessment	Patients (n)	Diagnosis	Prevalence of malnutrition (% of patients)	Criteria for definition	Mean BMI (SD) of group (kg m^{-2})	BMI < 20 kg m^{-2} (%)	Change in nutritional status over time
Jackson et al., 1996, UK Abstract	Acceptance on to liver transplant list	41	Chronic liver disease (20 M, 21 F, mean 51, range 17–69 years)	39% 7%	TSF and/or MAMC < 5th percentile BMI < 20	–	7%	–
Madden et al., 1994, UK Abstract	Prior to liver transplant	164	Details N/R Age/sex N/R	54% 23% 71% 34% (mild) 25% (mod.) 12% (severe)	MAMC < 5th percentile TSF < 5th percentile Nutritional assessment based on intake, anthropometry and wt loss	–	–	–
Müller et al., 1994, Germany	On liver transplant waiting-list and mean 432 (103–1022) days post transplant	26	Mixed liver diseases[b] (14 M, 12 F, range 23–65 years)	–	–	101% IBW	–	+4.9% IBW (−17 to +33%) NS reduction in BCM and increase in fat mass
Richardson et al., 2001, UK	Awaiting liver transplant and three 3-month intervals afterwards	23	PBC (n 13); HC (n 10) (10 M, 13 F, mean 53.9, SD 1.9 years)	–	BMI Pre-illness weight loss TSF MAMC BIA	24.9 (SE 0.9)	–	Mean BMI increased to 27.8 (SE 0.87) by 9 months post transplant (P < 0.0001). TSF and fat mass also increased significantly
Stephenson et al., 2001, USA	Admission for liver transplant	99	Mixed liver diseases (60 M, 39 F, mean 47, SD 2.3 years)	35% 32% 32%	SGA ranking: Mild Moderate Severe	–	–	–

[a] Documentation of the presence or absence of ascites is needed in studies of patients with liver disease. Body weight measurements were corrected for ascites in one study (Mendenhall et al., 1984b).

[b] Including a few patients with hepatocellular carcinoma.

A, alcoholic; BCM, body cell mass; BIA, bioelectrical impedance analysis; CD, Crohn's disease; CHI, creatinine–height index; HC, hepatocellular; LBM, lean body mass; MAFA, mid-arm fat area; MAMA, mid-arm muscle area; NA, non-alcoholic; PBC, primary biliary cirrhosis; UC, ulcerative colitis; N/R, not recorded; MAMC, mid-arm muscle circumference; SD, standard deviation; SE, standard error; MAC, mid-arm circumference; NS, not significant; med., median; CA, CB, CC, child A, B, C.

Causes and Consequences of Disease-related Malnutrition in Patients with GI and Liver Disease

There are many causes of malnutrition in patients with GI and liver disease. These have been summarized in Table A1.17. Although malabsorption might be expected to be a major factor in these patients, surprisingly little information could be found to substantiate this assertion. As in other patient populations, reduced food intake again appears to play a pivotal role in poor nutritional status. Even though energy intakes may not appear to be low relative to recommended intakes for healthy populations, they may be low relative to needs for individual patients (Rigaud *et al.*, 1994).

Although resting energy expenditure (REE) has been shown to be raised in liver cirrhosis (Plauth *et al.*, 1998) and Crohn's disease (Al-Jaouni *et al.*, 2000), total energy expenditure (TEE) may in fact not be increased. Normal TEE has been shown in patients (*n* 13) with active Crohn's disease requiring nutritional support by assessment of energy intake and changes in body energy stores using a combined body-scan technique (Stokes and Hill, 1993). As in other diseases, any increase in REE may be more than compensated for by a decrease in physical activity. Extent of disease activity may influence ability to handle nutrients. For example, patients with Crohn's disease have been shown to have increased fat oxidation which correlates with disease activity (Al-Jaouni *et al.*, 2000).

The consequences of poor nutritional status have mainly been examined in relation to outcome after liver transplant. As in other diseases, it is not possible to separate the effects of malnutrition and the impact of disease severity on outcome.

More information on the causes and consequences of malnutrition can be gathered from Chapters 3 and 4.

Table A1.17. Possible causes and potential consequences of disease-related malnutrition in patients with gastrointestinal and liver disease.

Causes/factors	Consequences
Poor food intake (Nielsen *et al.*, 1993; Rigaud *et al.*, 1994; Davidson *et al.*, 1999; McCollum, 2000; Richardson *et al.*, 2001) due to:	Lower hamstring muscle strength in men with long-standing Crohn's disease (Geerling *et al.*, 1998a)
• Anorexia, nausea, vomiting, abdominal discomfort, encephalopathy, presence of ascites and/or early satiety (Rigaud *et al.*, 1994; Wicks *et al.*, 1995; Jackson *et al.*, 1996; Bannerman *et al.*, 2001)	Lower survival rate/increased mortality in cirrhosis (Alberino *et al.*, 2001)
• Altered taste (Madden *et al.*, 1997)	Increased intraoperative transfusion requirements during liver transplant (Stephenson *et al.*, 2001)
• Medical advice/diet restrictions, e.g. low fat, low sodium (Rigaud *et al.*, 1994; Wicks *et al.*, 1995)	
• Depression (Rigaud *et al.*, 1994)	Increased complications post-liver transplant (Harrison *et al.*, 1997)
• Less pleasure associated with eating (Rigaud *et al.*, 1994)	Increased LOS post-liver transplant (Stephenson *et al.*, 2001)
• Alcohol intake (Thuluvath and Triger, 1994)	
	Lower survival rate/increased mortality post-liver transplant (Madden *et al.*, 1994)
Modified metabolism (Plauth *et al.*, 1998; Al-Jaouni *et al.*, 2000)	
Hormonal alterations (Alberino *et al.*, 2001)	
Malabsorption (Stokes, 1992; Rigaud *et al.*, 1994)	

LOS, length of stay.

Table A1.18. Summary of the prevalence of malnutrition using a variety of criteria in patients with HIV infection and AIDS in the community and in hospital, arranged according to country.

Country	Number of subjects (n)	Prevalence of malnutrition (%) [a]	Some degree of weight loss (%)	BMI < 20 kg m^{-2} (%)	Reference
HIV infection and AIDS: community					
Canada	37	46	46	–	Parisien et al., 1993
France	2376	11	–	–	Malvy et al., 2001
		10			
		32			
France	124	38	38	–	Niyongabo et al., 1997
Germany	65	30	–	–	Ockenga et al., 1997 Abstract
Germany	53	87	–	–	Süttmann et al., 1991
		53			
		68			
		25			
UK	162	12.6	–	12.6	Hodgson et al., 2001 Abstract
USA	43	38 (HIV)/50 (ARC)/	38 (HIV)/50 (ARC)/	–	Dworkin et al., 1990
		78 (AIDS)	78 (AIDS)		
USA	77	73	73	–	Guenter et al., 1993
USA	633	8	14	8	Kim et al., 2001
		14			
USA	56	55	55	–	Luder et al., 1995
		30			
HIV infection and AIDS: hospital					
Sweden	25	> 50	–	–	Karlsson and Nordstrom, 2001
USA	71	98	98	–	Chlebowski et al., 1989
USA	48	64	–	–	Trujillo et al., 1992
		29			

[a]When more than one result is provided for a given study (unless specifically explained) the results have been obtained by applying different criteria to the same group of patients. For more details, refer to Table A1.19.
ARC, AIDS-related complex; HIV, human immunodeficiency virus.

Table A1.19. Prevalence of malnutrition in patients with HIV infection and AIDS in the community.

Study	Patients (n)	Diagnosis	Prevalence of malnutrition (% of patients)	Criteria for definition	Mean BMI (SD) of group (kg m^{-2})	BMI < 20 kg m^{-2} (%)	Change in nutritional status over time
Dworkin et al., 1990, USA	43	Clinically stable HIV infection[a] (9 M, 4 F, mean 34.5, SD 7.5 years), ARC (6 M, 6 F, mean 36.3, SD 10 years), AIDS (14 M, 4 F, mean 34.2, SD 5.7 years)	38% (HIV) 50% (ARC) 78% (AIDS)	History of wt loss	–	–	–
Guenter et al., 1993, USA	77	HIV infection (74 M, 3 F), mean 38.7 years (range 23–67)	42% 22% 9%	UBW 90–100% UBW 80–90% UBW < 80%	–	–	–
Hodgson et al., 2001, UK Abstract	162	HIV infection (95 M, 67 F), 134 on HAART, age N/R	5.6% 7%	BMI <18.5 BMI 18.5–20	Med. 23.7	12.6%	–
Kim et al., 2001, USA	633	HIV infection (44%) and AIDS (56%) (463 M, mean 39, SD 7.6 years; 61% AIDS; 170 F, mean 37, SD 7 years, 44% AIDS) 71% using protease inhibitors or antiretrovirals	8% (all) 14% (all) 16% (M) 7% (F)	BMI < 20 Involuntary wt loss of > 10% of initial body weight or sustained loss of > 5% in previous 6 months (HIV wasting syndrome)	–	8% 7% (M) 10% (F)	–
Luder et al., 1995, USA	56	HIV infection (n 16), ARC (n 23) and AIDS (n 17) (47 M, 9 F, mean age approx. 40 years)	55% 30%	Wt loss Involuntary wt loss > 10% of pre-illness weight (HIV wasting syndrome)	25.5 (5.2) (stable wt) 21.2 (2.4) (wt loss) P = 0.0001	–	–

Study	n	Population	Prevalence	Criteria	BMI (SD) / baseline	Notes
Malvy et al., 2001, France	2376	All stages of HIV infection[b] (1738 M, 638 F, median 31 (range 18–78) years; 675 (28.4%) developed AIDS during follow-up 77% using antiretrovirals)	10% 32% (of n 1570)	History of invol. wt loss > 10% During follow-up: BMI < 18.5 at least once	Median at baseline: 21.5 (range 14–37.9) –	66.5% experienced weight loss (median 6% of baseline, range 0.4–42%)
Niyongabo et al., 1997 France	124	HIV infection (CDC A, n 47; CDC B, n 22) and AIDS (CDC C, n 55), M : F ratio 3.3 : 1, mean 36.3, SD 7 years	13% 17% 8%	Wt loss vs. UBW: 5–10% 10–20% > 20%	21.4 (3.7)	–
Ockenga et al., 1997, Germany Abstract	65	Clinically stable asymptomatic HIV infection (CDC I: n 26; II: n 14; III: n 30), mean 38, SD 10 years, sex N/R	30% I: 10% II: 21% III: 50%	IBW < 80%, BMI < 18 and/or BCM ratio > 1.0	20 (3)	–
Parisien et al., 1993, Canada	37	Asymptomatic (11 M, mean 34.2, SD 6.4 years) and symptomatic (n 9, mean 35.6, SD 8.6 years) HIV infection and clinically stable AIDS (n 17, mean 32.1, SD 5.2 years)	46% 18% (AS) 44% (S) 65% (AIDS) 11% 9% (AS) 0% (S) 18% (AIDS)	Wt loss Wt loss > 10% UBW	23.1 (3.5) (AS) 22.8 (2.5) (S) 21.5 (2.4) (AIDS) –	–

Continued

Table A1.19. Continued

Study	Patients (n)	Diagnosis	Prevalence of malnutrition (% of patients)	Criteria for definition	Mean BMI (SD) of group (kg m^{-2})	BMI < 20 kg m^{-2} (%)	Change in nutritional status over time
Süttmann et al., 1991, Germany	53	HIV infection without OI, WR-1 (2 M), WR-2 (9 M, 2 F), WR-3 (3 M), WR-4 (5 M), WR-6 (21 M, 1 F), age 20–67 years	87% 53% 68% 25%	Clinical signs IBW < 90% FM < 20% BW BCM < 30% BW and ECM > 50% BW	22.3 (WR-1) 23.5 (WR-2) 19.9 (WR-3) 20.9 (WR-4) 20.2 (WR-5) 21.4 (WR-6)	–	–

[a] All out-patients except seven AIDS patients.
[b] In- and out-patients. Follow-up for median 43.1 (range 0.7–148) months.

ARC, AIDS-related complex (a general term covering those with symptomatology indicative of AIDS, but without having an indicator disease for AIDS); AS, asymptomatic; BCM, body cell mass; BW, body weight; CDC, centres for disease control classification (higher class indicates more advanced disease); ECM, extracellular mass; FM, fat mass; S, symptomatic; UBW, usual body weight; WR, Walter Reed classification (higher class indicates more advanced disease); HIV, human immunodeficiency virus; HAART, highly active antiretroviral therapy; N/R, not recorded; OI, opportunistic infection; SD, standard deviation; med., median.

Table A1.20. Prevalence of malnutrition in patients admitted to hospital with HIV infection and AIDS.

Study	Time of assessment	Patients (*n*)	Diagnosis	Prevalence of malnutrition (% of patients)	Criteria for definition	Mean (SD) BMI of group (kg m⁻²)	BMI < 20 kg m⁻² (%)	Change in nutritional status over time
Chlebowski *et al.*, 1989, USA	At diagnosis of AIDS	71	AIDS (68 M, 3 F, mean 32, SD 2 years)	98% 32% 41% 25%	Wt loss vs. UBW < 10% 10–20% > 20%	–	–	–
Karlsson and Nordstrom 2001, Sweden	Admission	25	HIV positive	> 50%	SGA B + C	–	–	–
Trujillo *et al.*, 1992, USA	Admission	48	AIDS (mean 35.7, SE 1.0 years, sex N/R)	64% 29%	Wt loss > 10% UBW Wt loss > 20% UBW	20.4 (SE 0.4)	–	–

HIV, human immunodeficiency virus; N/R, not recorded; SD, standard deviation; SE, standard error; UBW, usual body weight.

Causes and Consequences of Malnutrition in Human Immunodeficiency Virus (HIV) Infection and AIDS

Quite a number of studies have measured food intake in patients with HIV infection and AIDS and, surprisingly, not many of these demonstrated significant impairments (see Chapter 3 and Appendix A2) compared with normal healthy controls and public health recommendations. Despite this, it is generally considered that a reduction in food intake is a primary reason for the loss of weight frequently seen (Macallan *et al.*, 1995; Beaugerie *et al.*, 1998; Melchior *et al.*, 1999; Sheehan and Macallan, 2000). The probable explanation for this is that the majority of studies examined food intake in clinically stable patients without ongoing opportunistic infections. In contrast, those with ongoing infections have a dramatic decrease in food intake (Grunfeld *et al.*, 1992). In longitudinal studies of weight change, Macallan *et al.* (1993) demonstrated that acute weight loss episodes were associated with systemic infections and, in turn, with reduced intake.

Increased REE has been reported by a number of groups, even in the absence of opportunistic infections (Hommes *et al.*, 1990; Grunfeld *et al.*, 1992; Melchior *et al.*, 1993, 1999; Slusarczyk, 1994). However, increased REE is not associated with ongoing weight loss (Schwenk *et al.*, 1996), and increases may be explained by a relative increase in the fraction of visceral tissue comprising body cell mass (BCM) in wasted individuals (Macallan, 1996; Schwenk *et al.*, 1996). Furthermore, TEE is reduced during weight loss (Macallan *et al.*, 1995). Therefore it is thought that a raised REE alone is unlikely to be responsible for weight loss in HIV infection. However, other metabolic factors are likely to contribute to wasting. The proposed causes and possible consequences of malnutrition in HIV infection and AIDS are summarized in Table A1.21. As with other diseases, it is not possible to make causal inferences from these reports. Potential benefits of nutritional support in HIV infection and AIDS are discussed in Chapters 6–8.

Table A1.21. Possible causes and potential consequences of disease-related malnutrition in HIV infection and AIDS.

Causes/factors	Consequences
Reduced food intake (Macallan *et al.*, 1995; Beaugerie *et al.*, 1998; Melchior *et al.*, 1999; Sheehan and Macallan, 2000) due to: • Oral lesions (Migliorati and Migliorati, 1997) • Taste and smell dysfunction (due to oral pathology such as candidiasis, medications, central nervous system lesions, cranial nerve abnormalities and sinusitis) (Heald and Schiffman, 1997) • Reduced appetite, nausea, vomiting (Kim *et al.*, 2001) • Opportunistic infections (Grunfeld *et al.*, 1992; Macallan *et al.*, 1993; Summerbell *et al.*, 1993) • Diarrhoea (food intake may be voluntarily restricted or appetite may be suppressed due to unabsorbed nutrients in the lower intestine) (Castetbon *et al.*, 1997; Sheehan and Macallan, 2000; Kim *et al.*, 2001) • Lack of assistance with food shopping and/or preparation (Kim *et al.*, 2001) • Deliberate efforts to lose weight (Kim *et al.*, 2001) • Unavailability of protease inhibitors or antiretroviral drugs (Kim *et al.*, 2001) or voluntary cessation of drug therapy (Summerbell *et al.*, 1993) • Allergic drug reactions (Summerbell *et al.*, 1993) • Sociodemographic factors (low educational status, low household income, injection drug use, not living with an adult care giver, living with children) (Kim *et al.*, 2001) • Major psychiatric disorders (Summerbell *et al.*, 1993) • Stress due to bereavement, loss of home or job (Summerbell *et al.*, 1993) Opportunistic infections (Summerbell *et al.*, 1993; Melchior *et al.*, 1999) Hypermetabolism due to opportunistic infections (Grunfeld, 1992; Macallan *et al.*, 1993; Melchior *et al.*, 1993) Altered metabolism, including increased fat oxidation, increased *de novo* lipogenesis, increased protein turnover and increased insulin sensitivity (Hommes *et al.*, 1991a,b,c; Heyligenberg *et al.*, 1993; Macallan *et al.*, 1995, 1998; Salas-Salvadó and Garcia-Lorda, 2001) Diarrhoea (Summerbell *et al.*, 1993; Melchior *et al.*, 1999) Malabsorption (Kotler *et al.*, 1990; Keating *et al.*, 1995; Koch *et al.*, 1996; Jimenez-Expositio *et al.*, 1998) due to mucosal abnormalities (Gillin *et al.*, 1985; Miller *et al.*, 1988; Ullrich *et al.*, 1989) and/or gastrointestinal disease (Kapembwa *et al.*, 1990; Macallan *et al.*, 1993; Blanchard *et al.*, 1996)	Faster progression from HIV to AIDS (Malvy *et al.*, 2001) Increased LOS in in-patients (Mijàn *et al.*, 1998) Increased mortality (Kotler *et al.*, 1985; Chlebowski *et al.*, 1989; Guenter *et al.*, 1993; Ott *et al.*, 1995; Palenicek *et al.*, 1995; Mijàn *et al.*, 1997; Melchior *et al.*, 1999; Kim *et al.*, 2001)

LOS, length of stay.

Table A1.22. Standardized incidence rate of cancer in Eur-15 countries per 100,000 males and females in 1995 (standard world population). EU-15 population on 1 January 1995: 181,332,400 (males); 190,257,100 (females). Adapted from European Commission (2001). See this report for cancer rates in individual European countries.

Type of cancer	Men	Women
All sites but skin	278.7	202.6
Bronchus/lung	54.1	11.0
Colon/rectum	34.0	23.2
Female breast	–	65.1
Prostate	34.1	–
Stomach	15.4	7.2
Oesophagus	6.6	1.4
Bladder	21.9	4.3
Larynx	8.3	0.6
Testis	5.5	–
Cervix uteri	–	9.9
Ovary	–	10.1
Corpus uteri	–	10.9
Leukaemia	8.1	5.0
Liver	6.7	2.1
Non-Hodgkin's lymphoma	9.9	6.2
Hodgkin's disease	2.1	1.6
Pancreas	6.8	4.4
Lip, oral cavity, pharynx	15.1	2.7
Kidney	9.5	4.2
Skin melanoma	5.3	6.2
Multiple myeloma	2.8	1.9
Brain, nervous system	6.9	4.9
Thyroid	1.5	3.1

Table A1.23. Summary of the prevalence of malnutrition using a variety of criteria in patients with malignancy in the community and in hospital, arranged according to country.

Country	Number of subjects (*n*)	Prevalence of malnutrition (%) [a]	Some degree of weight loss (%)	BMI < 20 kg m^{-2} (%)	Reference
Hospital: prior to surgery					
Colombia	40	62.5	–	–	Rey-Ferro *et al.*, 1997
Netherlands	64	31	–	–	Van Bokhorst-de van der
		23			Schueren *et al.*, 1997
		67			
Sweden	75	5	–	–	Ulander *et al.*, 1998
UK	39	46	–	–	Bashir *et al.*, 1990
		36			
UK	84	56	–	–	Brookes, 1982
UK	59	76	75	6	Corish *et al.*, 1998 Abstract
		6			
		75			
		37			
UK	60	13.3	–	13.3	Jagoe *et al.*, 2001a
		25			
		23			
		5			
USA	101	33	–	–	Meguid *et al.*, 1986
USA	143	58	–	–	Martin *et al.*, 1999 Abstract
Hospital: various therapies					
Sweden	48	51	–	–	Hammerlid *et al.*, 1998
USA	5044	57.3	57.3	–	Daly *et al.*, 2000
Radiotherapy					
UK	61	13	26	13	Collins *et al.*, 1999
		26			
UK	100	57	57	–	Lees, 1999
USA	249	48	–	–	Beaver *et al.*, 2001

Continued

Table A1.23. *Continued*

Country	Number of subjects (n)	Prevalence of malnutrition (%)[a]	Some degree of weight loss (%)	BMI < 20 kg m^{-2} (%)	Reference
Chemotherapy					
Denmark	104	46	–	–	Ovesen et al., 1993
Germany	40	15	–	15	Wolf et al., 2001 Abstract
UK	1555	51 (M) / 44 (F)	–	–	Andreyev et al., 1998
USA	3047	32	–	–	DeWys et al., 1980
Bone marrow transplantation					
Turkey	74	75 12 26	–	–	Gungor et al., 2001 Abstract
USA	1662	11	–	–	Deeg et al., 1995
Untreatable cancer					
UK	20	85 35	85	35	Wigmore et al., 1997
Community: various cancers/ treatments					
Sweden	297	67 10	–	–	Bosaeus et al., 2001
Sweden	87	80 (GI)/33 (Ur) 52 (GI)/9 (Ur)	80 (GI)/33 (Ur)	–	Persson et al., 1999
UK	5074	7.7	–	7.7	Edington et al., 1999

[a]When more than one result is provided for a given study (unless specifically explained) the results have been obtained by applying different criteria to the same group of patients. For more details, refer to Table A1.24.
GI, gastrointestinal; Ur, urological.

Table A1.24. Prevalence of malnutrition in patients with malignancy in hospital prior to surgery/various therapies.

Study	Patients (n)	Diagnosis	Prevalence of malnutrition (% of patients)	Criteria for definition	Mean (SD) BMI of group (kg m⁻²)	BMI < 20 kg m⁻² (%)	Change in nutritional status over time
Hospital: prior to surgery							
Bashir *et al.*, 1990, UK	39	Thoracotomy for bronchial cancer (mean 61.9 years, sex N/R)	46% 21% 15%	BMI + TSF + SSF < 25th percentile IBW 80–90% IBW < 80%	–	36% < 90% IBW	–
Brookes 1982, UK	84	Untreated primary SCC of head and neck (age/sex N/R)	39% (deficit) 15% (malnut.) 2% (severe malnut.)	General nutritional status assessment (based on anthropometry, biochemistry and N excretion)	–	–	–
Corish *et al.*, 1998, Ireland Abstract	59	Lung (*n* 16) H and N (*n* 13) Bowel (*n* 12) Oes. (*n* 10) Ovary (*n* 4) Gastric (*n* 2) Panc-duo (*n* 2) (37 M, 22 F, mean 66, range 31–90 years)	63% (at risk) 13% (severe) 6% 75% 37%	NRI (at risk) NRI (severe) BMI ≤ 20 Wt loss (mean 11.2%) Wt loss > 10%/6 months	15.2 24.9 25.3 21.6 24.8 27.6 28.4	6%	76% lost weight in hospital (mean 5.6% of admission weight). Following discharge, 70% lost weight within 3 months (mean 5.9% body weight)
Jagoe *et al.*, 2001a, UK	60	Lung cancer (43 M, 17 F, mean 63.5, range 36–80 years)	13% 25% 23% 5%	BMI ≤ 20 IBW ≤ 90% Wt loss > 5% Wt loss > 10%	25.4 (4.7)	13.3%	–
Martin *et al.*, 1999, USA Abstract	143	Oesophagogastrectomy for cancer (124 M, 19 F, med. 60 years)	58%	Wt loss (preop.)	–	–	87% had postop. wt loss, of which 21% had wt loss > 10% of immediate preop. wt. Postop. wt loss was greater in those who had lost less wt preop.

Continued

Table A1.24. *Continued*

Study	Patients (n)	Diagnosis	Prevalence of malnutrition (% of patients)	Criteria for definition	Mean (SD) BMI of group (kg m^{-2})	BMI <20 kg m^{-2} (%)	Change in nutritional status over time
Meguid et al., 1986, USA	101	Colorectal cancer (mean 66 years, range 32–85)	33%	Albumin < 35 g l^{-1} and 2 other abnormal values: recent wt loss > 10%, W/H, MAMC or TSF < 10th percentile	–	–	–
Rey-Ferro et al., 1997, Colombia	40	Gastric adenocarcinoma (22 M, 18 F, mean 54, SD 14 years)	5% (mild) 42.5% (mod.) 15% (severe)	NRI > 97.5 NRI 83.5–97.5 NRI < 83.5	–	–	–
Ulander et al., 1998, Sweden	75	Colorectal surgery for cancer (38 M, 37 F, mean 71.4, range 41–90 years)	5%	SGA B and C[a]	–	–	39% wt loss ≥ 5% during hospital stay. Mean % wt loss 4.7 (4.4)%, greatest in M (6.1%)
Van Bokhorst-de van der Schueren et al., 1997, NL	64	Advanced head and neck cancer (mean 61, SD 10 years, sex N/R)	31% 17% (mild) 3% (mod.) 3% (severe) 67%	Wt loss > 10%/6 months 80–90% IBW 70–79% IBW < 69% IBW NI < 1.31	–	23% < 90% IBW	–
Hospital: various therapies							
Daly et al., 2000, USA	5044	Oesophageal cancer (3 : 1 M : F, mean 67.3 years)[b]	57%	Weight loss	–	–	–
Hammerlid et al., 1998, Sweden	48	Head and neck cancer (36 M, 12 F, mean 67, range 40–88 years)	51%	2 or more abnormal values: – > 5% wt loss, MAMC and TSF < reference, WI < 0.80, BMI < 20, albumin < 33 g l^{-1}	–	–	–

[a] Day before surgery and on discharge.
[b] n 828 hospitals included.
NI, nutrition index; NRI, nutrition risk index; Oes, oesophageal; Panc-duo, pancreatoduodenal; SSF, subscapular skin-fold thickness; W/H, weight-for-height; WI, weight index; SD, standard deviation; N/R, not recorded; MAMC, mid-arm muscle circumference; NL, The Netherlands; malnut., malnutrition; mod., moderate; preop., preoperative; postop., postoperative; SCC, squamous cell carcinomas.

Table A1.25. Prevalence of malnutrition in patients with malignancy prior to and during radiotherapy and chemotherapy, untreatable cancer and patients in the community.

Study	Location	Time of assessment	Patients (n)	Diagnosis	Prevalence of malnutrition (% of patients)	Criteria for definition	Mean (SD) BMI of group (kg m^{-2})	BMI <20 kg m^{-2} (%)	Change in nutritional status over time
Radiotherapy									
Beaver et al., 2001, USA	Hospital	Prior to and during radiotherapy	249	Head and neck cancer (187 M, 62 F; mean 58 years)	48%	Wt loss > 10% UBW in 6 months, 5% in 1 month, or > 7% BMI lost in 6 months	–	–	33% had severe weight loss during chemotherapy, most pronounced in those who had already lost weight
Collins et al., 1999, UK	Hospital	Prior to and after radiotherapy – retrospective	61	Early laryngeal squamous-cell cancer (51 M, 10 F, age N/R)	40% 13% 26%	BMI < 25 BMI < 20 Wt loss (mean 5.4%)	25	13%	BMI at end of treatment was significantly lower than at start (23.5)
Lees, 1999, UK	Regional oncology centre	Prior to radiotherapy	100	Head and neck cancer	57%	Wt loss (mean 10%)	–	–	–
Chemotherapy and bone marrow transplantation									
Andreyev et al., 1998, UK	–	Prior to chemotherapy	1555	Mix of solid tumours (1030 M, 525 F, med. 61, range 16–84 years)	51% (M) 44% (F)	Wt loss	–	–	–
Deeg et al., 1995, USA	–	Prior to BMT	1662	Haematological cancers (952 M, 710 F, mean age N/R)	9% 2%	IBW 85–95% IBW < 85%	–	–	–

Continued

Table A1.25. *Continued*

Study	Location	Time of assessment	Patients (n)	Diagnosis	Prevalence of malnutrition (% of patients)	Criteria for definition	Mean (SD) BMI of group (kg m^{-2})	BMI <20 kg m^{-2} (%)	Change in nutritional status over time
DeWys et al., 1980, USA	Out-patients from many centres	Prior to chemotherapy –retrospective	3047	Mix of cancers (age/sex N/R)	32% (all) breast 14% (n 289) sarcoma 18% (n 189) colon 28% (n 307) lung small-cell 34% (n 436) lung non-small-cell 36% (n 590) pancreas 54% (n 111) gastric ~65% (n 317)	Wt loss > 5% in 6 months	–	–	–
Gungor et al., 2001, Turkey Abstract	Hospital	Prior to high-dose chemotherapy for BMT	74	Haematological cancer? (age/sex N/R)	75% 12% 26%	NRI < 97.5 BMI < 18.5 SGA B + C	–	–	–
Ovesen et al., 1993, Denmark	Out-patients	Newly diagnosed, prior to chemotherapy	104	Small cell lung, breast and ovarian cancer (24 M, 80 F, mean approx. 59, range 22–77 years)	46%	Wt loss > 5% in 3 months (self-report)	22.3 (3.3) (wt loss) 25.7 (3.6) (wt stable)	–	–
Wolf et al., 2001, Germany Abstract	–	Prior to chemotherapy	40	Gynaecological cancer: ovary (n 22) or breast (n 18) (F, age N/R)	15%	BMI < 20	–	15%	–

Study	Setting	Timing/duration	n	Patients	Prevalence	Criteria	BMI	%	Comments
Untreatable cancer									
Wigmore et al., 1997, UK	Out-patients	At diagnosis and monthly intervals until death	20	Unresectable pancreatic cancer (12 M, 8 F, median 60 years)	85% / 35%	Wt loss / BMI < 20	20.7 (19.5–23.6)	35%	All patients had lost weight at time of death. BMI was < 20 in 65% at time of death
Community: various cancers/treatments									
Bosaeus et al., 2001, Sweden	Out-patients	–	297	Unselected cancer patients, solid tumours (160 M, 137 F, mean age 67 years, range 30–90)	43% / 24% / 10%	Wt loss > 10% / Wt loss 5–10% / BMI < 18.5	23.4 (3.8) (M) / 22.5 (3.7) (F)	–	–
Edington et al., 1999, UK	Community	–	5074	Cancer	7.7%	BMI < 20	–	7.7%	–
Persson et al., 1999, Sweden	Out-patients	Median duration of disease since diagnosis 6 (range 1–145) months	87	GI (n 54) and Ur (n 33) cancers (61 M, 26 F, med. 65, range 21–80 years)	80% (GI) 33% (Ur) / 52% (GI) 9% (Ur)	Wt loss in previous 12 months / SGA B + C	–	–	–

BMT, bone marrow transplantation; GI, gastrointestinal; N/R, not recorded; NRI, nutrition risk index; SD, standard deviation; Ur, urological; UBW, usual body weight.

Causes and Consequences of Disease-related Malnutrition in Cancer

The causes of weight loss and malnutrition in cancer patients are multifactorial (Strain, 1979; Von Meyenfeldt *et al.*, 1988), some of which are shown in Table A1.26. Lipman (1991) summarized the causes as:

1. Inadequate intake due to primary tumour-induced anorexia and/or obstructing lesions.
2. Toxicity from chemotherapy or radiotherapy producing anorexia, nausea, vomiting or malabsorption.
3. The primary catabolic effects of the tumour.
4. The abnormal metabolism of nutrients.

In addition, many of the studies reviewed have highlighted the relationship of weight loss and malnutrition to adverse outcome. In particular, for many tumour types, an inverse relationship between the degree of weight loss and median survival and performance status have been documented (DeWys *et al.*, 1980; DeWys, 1986). However, the role of disease severity must also be considered. From the data available, it is not possible to separate the effects of malnutrition and the impact of the disease severity on outcome. It is likely that those patients who are more undernourished are also sicker individuals. It is also likely that the consequences of weight loss/malnutrition may perpetuate further weight loss and deterioration in nutritional status.

Ultimately, effective nutritional support using oral nutritional supplements (ONS) or enteral tube feeding (ETF) is required in the prevention or treatment of cancer-related malnutrition (Shils, 1979; Bozzetti, 1992), where appropriate (depending on the patient's condition, extent of palliative care, etc.). For a review of the efficacy of these modes of nutritional support, see Chapters 6–8.

Table A1.26. Possible causes and potential consequences of disease-related malnutrition in patients with malignancy.

Causes/factors	Consequences
Reduced food intake (Holmes and Dickerson, 1991; Ovesen *et al.*, 1991; Levine and Morgan, 1994; Choileain *et al.*, 1995; Pattison *et al.*, 1997a; Persson *et al.*, 1999; Bosaeus *et al.*, 2001) due to:	Reduced muscle function (Zeiderman and McMahon, 1989)
• Deterioriation in taste, smell and appetite (anorexia) due to the tumour and/or therapy (Macqueen and Frost, 1998; Wu *et al.*, 1998; Mutlu and Mobarhan, 2000; Nitenberg and Raynard, 2000; Broadhead *et al.*, 2001b)	Reduced performance status after chemotherapy (DeWys *et al.*, 1980; Andreyev *et al.*, 1998)
• Altered food preferences/food avoidance/food aversion (Holmes, 1993; Broadhead *et al.*, 2000b; Schuetz *et al.*, 2000)	Lower quality of life: lower general health, lower social functioning, lower outlook/happiness (Ovesen *et al.*, 1993; Andreyev *et al.*, 1998)
• Problems with eating (Persson *et al.*, 1999)	Tendency for greater depression, anxiety, insomnia in weight-losing patients (NS) (Ovesen *et al.*, 1993)
• Dysphagia, odynophagia or partial/total GI obstruction (Nitenberg and Raynard, 2000)	
• Early satiety, nausea and vomiting (Wu *et al.*, 1998; Nitenberg and Raynard, 2000)	Higher prescription rates and consultation rates (Edington *et al.*, 1999)
• Soreness, dry mouth, sticky saliva, painful throat and problems opening mouth during radiotherapy (Broadhead *et al.*, 2001b)	Increased complications after surgery (Meguid *et al.*, 1986; Van Bokhorst-de van der Schueren *et al.*, 1997)
• Oral lesions and oesophagitis (Nitenberg and Raynard, 2000)	
• Mucositis due to chemo- or radiotherapy (Raber-Durchaler, 1999)	Increased need for reventilation after surgery for lung cancer (Jagoe *et al.*, 2001b)
• Gastrointestinal problems due to immunosuppression (Agarwal *et al.*, 1998)	
• Acute and/or chronic radiation enteritis during/after radiotherapy (Yeoh *et al.*, 1993; Sekhon, 2000)	Lower chemotherapy response rates (DeWys *et al.*, 1980; Andreyev *et al.*, 1998)
• Depression, anxiety (Mutlu and Mobarhan, 2000)	Increased risk of chemotherapy-induced toxicity (Andreyev *et al.*, 1998)
• Cancer-related pain (Mutlu and Mobarhan, 2000)	
• Hypercalcaemia (Mutlu and Mobarhan, 2000)	Shorter duration of remission after chemotherapy (Rickard *et al.*, 1983)
Malabsorption due to atrophy of the small bowel mucosa, chemotherapy or radiotherapy (Nitenberg and Raynard, 2000)	Increased mortality, especially in GI cancer patients (Persson *et al.*, 1999), after surgery (Meguid *et al.*, 1986; Rey-Ferro *et al.*, 1997; Van Bokhorst-de van der Schueren *et al.*, 2000b; Jagoe *et al.*, 2001b), after BMT (Deeg *et al.*, 1995; Dickson *et al.*, 1999) and after chemotherapy (Andreyev *et al.*, 1998)
Metabolic disturbances (Mutlu and Mobarhan, 2000; Nitenberg and Raynard, 2000)	
Humoral and inflammatory responses (e.g. increased or abnormal cytokine activity/production, abnormal eicosanoid production, excessive monocyte and macrophage activation, altered lymphocyte function, cancer-specific cachectic factors) (Mutlu and Mobarhan, 2000; Nitenberg and Raynard, 2000)	Shorter survival (Gogos *et al.*, 1998; Hammerlid *et al.*, 1998), also after surgery (Corish, 1998; Van Bokhorst-de van der Schueren *et al.*, 1999), after chemotherapy (De Wys *et al.*, 1980) and in non-small-cell lung cancer (Palomares *et al.*, 1996)

BMT, bone marrow transplant; GI, gastrointestinal; NS, not significant.

Table A1.27. Summary of the prevalence of malnutrition using a variety of criteria in patients with neurological disease (stroke and non-stroke) in hospital and the community, arranged according to country.[a]

Country	Number (*n*)	Prevalence of malnutrition (%)	BMI < 20 kg m^{-2} (%)	Reference
Stroke: hospital				
Canada	49	4	–	Finestone *et al.*, 1995
Spain	104	16.3	–	Davalos *et al.*, 1996
Sweden	100	16	–	Axelsson *et al.*, 1988
Sweden	50	8	–	Unosson *et al.*, 1994
UK	201	31	31	Gariballa *et al.*, 1998b
UK	130	66	–	Murray *et al.*, 2000 Abstract
Non-stroke: community				
France	55	16.4	–	Desport *et al.*, 1999
UK	318 (H) 99 (C)	> 60	> 60	Kennedy *et al.*, 1997
UK	43	56	–	Thomson *et al.*, 2001 Abstract

[a]For more details, refer to Tables A1.28 and A1.29.
C, community; H, hospital.

Table A1.28. Prevalence of malnutrition in patients with neurological disease – cerebrovascular accident (stroke).

Study	Time of assessment	Patients (*n*)	Diagnosis	Prevalence of malnutrition (%)	Criteria for definition	Mean BMI (SD) of group (kg m^{-2})	BMI < 20 kg m^{-2} (%)	Change in nutritional status over time
Axelsson *et al.*, 1988, Sweden	Admission and weekly until discharge	100	Acute stroke (64 M, 36 F, mean 71.4, range 51–90 years)	16%	2 or more of IBW < 80%, low TSF, low MAMC, low albumin, prealbumin, transferrin	101% IBW (M) 103% IBW (F)	–	At discharge, 22% 'undernourished' (total *n* 78, average stay 13 days)
Davalos *et al.*, 1996, Spain	Admission and after 1 week	104	Acute stroke (67 M, 37 F, mean 66, SD 10 years)	16.3%	Serum albumin < 35 g l^{-1} or TSF or MAMC < 10th percentile	–	–	Increased 'malnutrition': 26.4% after 1 week (*n* 91 pt in total) and 35% after 2 weeks (*n* 43 pt in total)
Finestone *et al.*, 1995, Canada	Admission	49	Rehab. for acute stroke (32 M, 17 F, mean approx. 61, range 20–78 years)	49%	2 or more of: BMI < 20/ < 90% IBW or sig. wt loss (> 7.5% in 3 months); low sum of skin-folds; low MAMC; low albumin; low TLC; low transferrin	–	–	Incidence of 'malnutrition' decreased to 34% at 1 month, 22% at 2 months, 19% at follow-up to 4 months later
Garibaldi *et al.*, 1998b,[b] UK	Admission, after 2 and 4 weeks	201	Acute stroke (81 M, 120 F, mean 77.9, IQR 72–84 years)	31%	BMI < 20	22.2 (3.9) (M) 22.9 (5) (F)	31%	Most who remained in hospital showed marked and sig. deterioration in all measures of nutritional status within 4 weeks of admission. Within 14 days of admission, 64% of pt who survived (*n* 96) lost wt, with 45% losing wt in the next 14 days (total *n* 52). Similar wt loss in M and F

Continued

Table A1.28. *Continued*

Study	Time of assessment	Patients (n)	Diagnosis	Prevalence of malnutrition (%)	Criteria for definition	Mean BMI (SD) of group (kg m⁻²)	BMI < 20 kg m⁻² (%)	Change in nutritional status over time
Murray et al., 2000, UK Abstract	Admission and discharge	130	Acute stroke (58 M, 72 F, mean 78.4, SD 10.8 years)	13% (mod. risk) 53% (high risk)	Nutrition risk score based on wt loss, BMI, appetite and food intake, stress factors	–	–	32% died during admission. Mean LOS was 41 (SD 41) days.14% were mod. risk and 22% high risk at discharge
Unosson et al., 1994[b], Sweden	Admission and after 2 and 9 weeks	50	Acute stroke (23 M, 27 F, mean approx. 79, SD 4.4 years)	8%	3 or more of: (i) IBW < 80%, low TSF, MAMC (ii) low albumin, prealbumin (iii) low DH (at least 1 from each group)	93% IBW (M) 99% IBW (F)	–	Slight deterioration in nutr. status at 9 weeks, with small losses of wt, TSF, body fat and body cell mass.

[a]Patients with other diseases or receiving ongoing medication excluded (n 90), of which 16.7% assessed as 'undernourished' using the same criteria (Davalos *et al.*, 1996).
[b]Use of surrogate measures for height (e.g. arm span) (Garibaldi *et al.*, 1998b) or supine height (Unosson *et al.*, 1994).
DH, delayed hypersensitivity; rehab, rehabilitation; TLC, total lymphocyte count; SD, standard deviation; IQR, interquartile range; mod, moderate; nutr, nutritional; sig, significant; MAMC, mid-arm muscle circumference; LOS, length of stay.

Table A1.29. Prevalence of malnutrition in patients with neurological disease/disorders – non-stroke.

Study	Location	Time of assessment	Patients (n)	Diagnosis	Prevalence of malnutrition (%)	Criteria for definition	Mean (SD) BMI of group (kg m⁻²)	BMI < 20 kg m⁻² (%)	Change in nutritional status
Desport et al., 1999, France	Referral neurology practice	Mean 29 (SD 25) months after onset of disease	55	Amyotrophic lateral sclerosis (mean 63.2 SD 11.2 years, sex N/R)	16.4%	BMI < 18.5	23.0 (5.1)	–	–
Kennedy et al., 1997, UK	Community (C) Hospital (H)	–	99 (C) 318 (H)	Intellectual and neurological disability (a) feed independently (b) partial assistance (c) dependence (C: 58 M, 41 F, H: 173 M, 145 F, age N/R)	> 60%	BMI < 20	C (a) 26.4 M 28.0 F (b) 19.9 M 22.4 F (c) 18.8 M 20.9 F H (a) 23.7 M 27.5 F (b) 20.5 M 24.4 F (c) 19.8 M 18.4 F	> 60%	–
Thomson et al., 2001, UK Abstract	Rehabilitation unit	Admission (approx. 29 days after injury), during rehab. and discharge	43	TBI (28 M, 5 F) and ABI (5 M, 5 F). Age between 16 and 64 years	56% (total) Mild: 26% (n 11) Moderate: 23% (n 10) Severe: 7% (n 3)	Mild: BMI < 20 + MAMC or TSF < 15th percentile Moderate: BMI < 18 + TSF or MAMC < 5th percentile Severe: BMI < 16 + TSF or MAMC < 5th percentile	20.7	–	Mean wt loss of 12.6% since injury in those given no nutrition and 5% wt loss in those given nutritional support

[a] Values presented as median BMI, includes paediatrics and adults.
ABI, anoxic brain injury, e.g. due to ischaemia, anaemia; MAMC, mid-arm circumference; N/R, not recorded; rehab., rehabilitation; SD, standard deviation; TBI, traumatic brain injury, e.g. due to falls, assaults, road-traffic accidents.

Causes and Consequences of Disease-related Malnutrition in Stroke Patients

Some of the causes and consequences of disease-related malnutrition in stroke patients have been summarized in Table A1.30. There are many causes of malnutrition in patients with neurological disease, although one of the main factors is likely to be difficulty with eating. Video recording of a group of patients with Parkinson's disease has highlighted problems with handling food on a plate, transporting food to the mouth, manipulating food in the mouth and swallowing (Athlin *et al.*, 1989). One of the factors typically associated with the development of malnutrition in stroke patients is the inability to swallow (Axelsson *et al.*, 1984; Davalos *et al.*, 1996). Approximately 30% of patients with semi-hemisphere cerebrovascular accident (CVA) may have difficulty swallowing (Barer, 1989) and such impairment has been significantly inversely related to functional ability 1 and 6 months post-CVA (Barer, 1989). Davalos *et al.* (1996) found that after 1 week in hospital, 48% of patients with swallowing incapacity were undernourished versus 14% of those with a normal swallow. Many other eating problems have been documented in stroke patients (Axelsson *et al.*, 1984, 1989), including chewing problems, hoarding of food in the mouth, leakage of food from the mouth and anorexia (Axelsson *et al.*, 1984). The presence of such eating disturbances has been strongly correlated with a long stay or death in the stroke unit (Axelsson *et al.*, 1984). Similarly, patients who are undernourished clearly have a poorer clinical outcome than those who are well nourished, although the confounding effects of disease severity have to be considered. From the data available, it is not possible to separate the effects of malnutrition and the impact of the disease severity on outcome. For example, patients may be more severely undernourished because disease severity is greater.

Table A1.30. Possible causes and potential consequences of disease-related malnutrition in stroke patients.

Causes/factors	Consequences
Poor food intake (Brynes *et al.*, 1998; Gariballa *et al.*, 1998b) due to feeding problems/dysphagia (Axelsson *et al.*, 1984; Davalos *et al.*, 1996; Finestone *et al.*, 1995)	Lower functional capacity (Davalos *et al.*, 1996)
	Pressure ulcers (Davalos *et al.*, 1996)
Old age (Axelsson *et al.*, 1988; Finestone *et al.*, 1995)	Greater incidence of urinary- and respiratory-tract infections (Davalos *et al.*, 1996)
Previous CVA (Finestone *et al.*, 1995)	Longer hospital stay (Davalos *et al.*, 1996)
Lack of community care at follow-up (Finestone *et al.*, 1995)	Higher mortality (Davalos *et al.*, 1996)
	Greater likelihood of dying or not being discharged from hospital (Axelsson *et al.*, 1988; Gariballa *et al.*, 1998b)

Table A1.31. Summary of the prevalence of malnutrition using a variety of criteria in patients with fractured neck of femur in hospital, arranged according to country.

Country	Number (*n*)	Prevalence of malnutrition (%) [a]	BMI < 20 kg m^{-2} (%)	Reference
France	40	33	–	Paillaud *et al.*, 2000
New Zealand	66	42.4	–	Hanger *et al.*, 1999
Sweden	88	25.5	25.5	Bachrach-Lindström *et al.*, 2001
		37.5		
Sweden	42	50	36	Ponzer *et al.*, 1999
Sweden	50	38	–	Unosson *et al.*, 1995
Switzerland	20	50	50	Jallut *et al.*, 1990
UK	23	43.5	–	Brown and Seabrook, 1992 Abstract
UK	32	41	–	Lumbers *et al.*, 1996
UK	75	13	–	Lumbers *et al.*, 2001
		46		
UK	49	63	–	Murphy *et al.*, 2000
UK	119	31	–	Maffulli *et al.*, 1999

[a]When more than one result is provided for a given study (unless specifically explained) the results have been obtained by applying different criteria to the same group of patients. For more details, refer to Table A1.32.

Table A1.32. Prevalence of malnutrition in fractured neck of femur patients.

Study	Time of assessment	Patients (n)	Prevalence of malnutrition (% of patients)	Criteria for definition	Mean (SD) BMI of group (20 kg m⁻²)	BMI < 20 kg m⁻² (%)	Change in nutritional status over time
Bachrach-Lindström et al., 2001, Sweden	4–6 days after surgery and 1 and 3 months afterwards	88 (F, mean 84.2, SD 5 years)	28% (C)/23% (I); 38% (C)/37% (I)	BMI < 20; BMI < 20 and/or TSF and/or MAMC < 10th percentile plus albumin < 36 g l⁻¹	21.7 (3.) (C); 23.6 (4) (I)	28% (C)/23% (I)	Body weight and BMI deteriorated over the 3 month follow-up
Brown and Seabrook, 1992, UK Abstract	–	23 (F, age N/R)	43.5%	Low W/H, TSF and MAC	22 (2) (WN); 17 (1) (UN)	–	Mean body weight and upper arm anthropometry decreased in all patients, especially in those not receiving supplements
Hanger et al., 1999, New Zealand	Admission – acute	66 (15 M, 51 F, mean 81.5, SD 7.6 years)	42.4%	Low result in at least 2 of: TSF, MAMA, prealbumin	–	–	–
Jallut et al., 1990ᵇ, Switzerland	Admission	20 (F, mean 81, SD 4 years)	50%	BMI < 20	20.7 (3.1)	50%	−0.84 (2.1) kg over 5–6 days (n 15)
Lumbers et al., 1996ᶜ, UK	Admission and discharge and up to 26 weeks after	60 (F) THR (n 28, mean 75.2 years) FNF (n 32, mean 81.3 years)	4% THR; 41% FNF	3 or more of: low body wt (< 48 kg), TSF, MAMC, albumin and haemoglobin < 5th percentile	–	–	–
Lumbers et al., 2001, UK	Admission – acute	75 (F, mean 80.5, range 61–103 years)	46%; 13%; 65%; 46%	Mindex < 50th percentile; Mindex < 10th percentile; MAMC < 50th percentile; MAMC < 10th percentile	24.1 (4.7)	–	–
Maffulli et al., 1999, UK	Admission and on 5th postop day	119 (91 F, 28 M, mean approx. 80 years)	31%	BMI < 18 (MAC if unable to be weighed)	24.3 (5.3) M, IT; 23.6 (4.5) M, IC; 21.9 (4.4) F, IT; 19.1 (2.9) F, IC	–; –; –; –	Feasibility of weighing patients on the 5th postop day was the most important prognostic indicator for complications

Murphy et al., 2000, UK	Admission – acute (n 7 elective THR)	49 (F, mean 80, range 61–103 years)	47% (at risk) 16%	MNA 17–23.5 (at risk) MNA <17 (malnutrition)	23.7 (4.3)	–	–
Paillaud et al., 2000, France	Admission to rehab. unit (20 days after hip fracture surgery)	40 (35 F, 5 M, mean 84, range 70–91 years)	33% (all F)	MAC <23 cm TSF <10 mm (F), <6 mm (M)	–	–	−2.7 kg after 30 days (n 20; NS) −0.7 kg after 60 days (n 20; NS)
Ponzer et al., 1999, Sweden	Admission – acute	42 (F, mean 80, SD 7 years)	50%	BMI ≤ 20 and reduced IGF-1 and IGFBP-1 levels	22 (4.3)	36%	–
Unosson et al., 1995[c], Sweden	Admission	50 (42 F, 8 M, mean approx. 84 years)	38%	2 or more of: wt index < 80%, low TSF, MAMC, prealbumin, albumin	74% IBW (UN) 91% IBW (WN)	–	At discharge (approx 30 days after admission), 52% 'undernourished' Reduction in wt (3% of pt), TSF (16% of pt.) and body fat (14% of pt.)

[a]All studies include only FNF patients unless otherwise stated, and all in hospital unless otherwise stated.
[b]Estimations of body weight common in this patient group (Jallut et al., 1990).
[c]Exclusion of patients with other diseases (renal, hepatic, malignant disease) (Unosson et al., 1995), including dementia (Lumbers et al., 1996).
THR, total hip replacement (elective); FNF, fractured neck of femur (emergency); IGF-1, insulin-like growth factor 1; IGFBP-1, insulin-like growth factor binding protein 1; IT, intertrochanteric; IC, intracapsular; Mindex, weight/demispan; NS, not significant; UN, undernourished; WN, well nourished; SD, standard deviation; N/R, not recorded; MAMA, mid-arm muscle area.

Causes and Consequences of Disease-related Malnutrition in Patients with Fractured Neck of Femur (FNF)

There are many causes of weight loss and malnutrition in this group of patients, many of whom are elderly. In particular, patients' dietary intakes (both macro- and micronutrients) may be insufficient to meet nutritional requirements (Older *et al.*, 1980; Gegerie *et al.*, 1986; Jallut *et al.*, 1990; Lumbers *et al.*, 1998, 2001; Murphy *et al.*, 2000; Paillaud *et al.*, 2000), due to a poor appetite, physical difficulties with eating or other factors (Ponzer *et al.*, 1999). Some of these factors are highlighted in Table A1.33. As the quote below highlights, malnutrition is associated with adverse functional and clinical outcomes in patients with FNF:

> Deficiency in both micronutrients and macronutrients appears to be strongly implicated in the pathogenesis and the consequences of hip fracture in osteoporotic elderly. Such deficiencies can accelerate age-dependent bone loss, increase the propensity to fall by impairing movement coordination, and affect protective mechanisms that reduce the impact of falling.
>
> (Bonjour *et al.*, 1996)

As in other diseases, from the data available it is not possible to separate the effects of malnutrition and the impact of the disease severity on outcome. For example, patients may be more severely undernourished because disease severity is greater. Prevention and treatment of disease-related malnutrition in orthopaedic patients are both clinically and financially warranted, if patients' outcome can be improved. As Chapters 6–8 highlight, the appropriate use of ONS and ETF in undernourished patients with FNF can lead to significant improvements in clinical outcome.

More information on the causes and consequences of malnutrition can be gathered from Chapters 3 and 4.

Table A1.33. Causes and consequences of disease-related malnutrition in patients with fractured neck of femur.

Causes/factors	Consequences
Poor food intake (Older *et al.*, 1980; Gegerie *et al.*, 1986; Jallut *et al.*, 1990; Doshi *et al.*, 1998; Lumbers *et al.*, 1998, 2001; Barton *et al.*, 2000a; Murphy *et al.*, 2000; Paillaud *et al.*, 2000; Bachrach-Lindström *et al.*, 2001) due to:	Lower mobility (Lumbers *et al.*, 1996)
	Lower mental function (Lumbers *et al.*, 1996)
	Lower quality of life (Ponzer *et al.*, 1999) [a]
• Anorexia (Ponzer *et al.*, 1999)	Low mood (Ponzer *et al.*, 1999) [a]
• Dental problems (Ponzer *et al.*, 1999)	
• Depression (Ponzer *et al.*, 1999) [a]	Depression (Ponzer *et al.*, 1999) [a]
• Low mood (Ponzer *et al.*, 1999) [a]	
• Poor quality of life (Ponzer *et al.*, 1999) [a]	Reduced hand-grip strength (Lumbers *et al.*, 1996; Ponzer *et al.*, 1999)
• Low cognitive scores (Ponzer *et al.*, 1999) [a]	
	Higher complication rate (Patterson *et al.*, 1992; Paillaud *et al.*, 2000)
	Longer time in convalescence/health care (Bastow *et al.*, 1983; Patterson *et al.*, 1992; Lumbers *et al.*, 1996)
	Higher mortality (Bastow *et al.*, 1983; Patterson *et al.*, 1992; Lumbers *et al.*, 1996)

[a]Associated with patients identified as undernourished (could be a cause and/or a consequence).

Table A1.34. Summary of the prevalence of malnutrition using a variety of criteria in patients with renal disease in the community and in hospital, arranged according to country.

Country	Number (n)	Prevalence of malnutrition (%)[a]	BMI < 20 kg m^{-2} (%)	Reference
Renal disease: predialysis				
Australia	50	28	–	Lawson *et al.*, 2001
Sweden	115	48	–	Heimburger *et al.*, 2000
Renal disease: haemodialysis				
Australia	64	36	–	Laws *et al.*, 2000
France	7123	24	24	Aparicio *et al.*, 1999
		22		
		62		
France	20	40 (> 25 years)	–	Chazot *et al.*, 2001
		10 (shorter term)		
South Africa	37	59	–	Herselman *et al.*, 2000
UK	57	33	33	Engel *et al.*, 1995
		17		
		56		
USA	58	72	25.9	Thunberg *et al.*, 1981
		25.9		
Renal disease: continuous ambulatory peritoneal dialysis				
Europe and USA	224	41	–	Young *et al.*, 1991
UK	147	48	–	Harty *et al.*, 1993
Renal disease: dialysis (mixed)				
Denmark	48	54	–	Marckmann, 1988
Italy	487	51 (> 65 years)	–	Cianciaruso *et al.*, 1995
		31 (41–64 years)		
		27 (18–40 years)		
Netherlands	250	16	16	Jager *et al.*, 2001
Renal disease: hospital				
UK	20	50	–	Hartley *et al.*, 1997

[a] When more than one result is provided for a given study (unless specifically explained) the results have been obtained by applying different criteria to the same group of patients. For more details, refer to Table A1.35.

Table A1.35. Prevalence of malnutrition in patients with renal disease.[a]

Study	Time of assessment	Patients (n)	Treatment	Prevalence of malnutrition (% of patients)	Criteria for definition	Mean (SD) BMI of group (20 kg m⁻²)	BMI < 20 kg m⁻²	Change in nutritional status over time
Community								
Aparicio et al., 1999, France	Cross-sectional study on 1 day	7123	HD (4108 M, 3015 F, mean 62.2, SD 15.9 years)	24% 22% 62% 36%	BMI < 20 IBW < 90% Ob/ex LBM < 90% Serum prealbumin < 300 mg l⁻¹	23.3 (4.6)	24%	–
Chazot et al., 2001, France	HD for mean 304 months HD for mean 51 months	10 10	HD, 2 groups matched (12 M, 8 F, mean approx. 59 years)	40% 10%	BMI < 18.5 BMI < 18.5	19.3 (2.6) 21.4 (2.8)	– –	– –
Cianciaruso et al., 1995, Italy	CAPD for mean 2.1 years or HD for mean 3.6 years	487	CAPD or HD (n 62 aged 18–40; n 239 aged 41–64; n 183 aged 65–91 years)	51% > 65 years 31% 41–64 years 27% 18–40 years	SGA (? B + C, not described)	% IBW 93% > 65 years 97% 41–64 years 88% 18–40 years	–	–
Engel et al., 1995, UK	Long-term HD, follow-up within 7 months	57	HD (41 M, 16 F, med. 64, range 27–81 years)	33% 30% 21% 17% 56%	BMI < 20 PI < 0.8 g kg⁻¹ IBW Albumin < 35 g l⁻¹ Wt loss > 5% in 6 months At least 1 of above	–	33%	47 patients underwent follow-up. Risk-factor profile showed some improvement: 36% had at least 1 risk factor (21% had low BMI, 19% had low PI, 6% had low albumin, 8.5% had wt loss > 5% since first review)
Harty et al., 1993, UK	CAPD for mean 22, range 3–113 months	147	CAPD (85 M, 62F, mean 51, range 19–79 years)	28–32% (moderate) 13–16% (severe)	Composite nutritional index based on anthropometry, biochemistry and SGA	24.2 (4.3)	–	–

Reference	n	Setting	Population	Prevalence	Criteria	Mean value	%	Comments
Heimburger *et al.*, 2000, Sweden	115	Prior to dialysis	ESRD, prior to dialysis (69 M, 46 F, mean 52, range 23–69 years)	37% (mild) 9% (mod.) 2% (severe)	SGA 2 SGA 3 SGA 4	24.4 (4.5)	—	—
Herselman *et al.*, 2000, S. Africa	37	Long-term HD, follow-up for 26, range 12–33 months	HD (25 M, 11 F, mean 40, range 20–65 years)	59%	Composite scoring system, including BMI < 18.5, MAMA < 15th percentile, low FM and FFM, low albumin	OP 22.9 (4.1) (20.4 (2.6) in pt hospitalized for infection)	—	Deterioration in the nutritional status of patients followed up for 24 months (*n* 15; NS)
Jager *et al.*, 2001, NL	250	3 months after start dialysis, 2 year follow-up	HD (*n* 132) PD (*n* 118)	16% (all) 14% (HD) 19% (PD)	BMI < 20	23.9 (4.1) (all) 24.5 (4.4) (HD) 23.1 (3.5) (PD)	16% (all) 14% (HD) 19% (PD)	BMI increased in both groups. Body fat increased in PD, but no change in LBM
Laws *et al.*, 2000, Australia	64	HD > 1 month (range 1–200 months)	HD (31 M, 33 F, mean approx. 65, range 37–85 years)	23% (mod.) 13% (severe)	SGA B SGA C	—	—	—
Lawson *et al.*, 2001, Australia	50	Prior to dialysis	CRF (predialysis)	20% 8%	SGA B	29 (5.0) (WN) 22.7 (2.9) (MN)	—	—
Marckmann, 1988, Denmark	48	Dialysis (mean 39, range 3–188 months), follow-up at 2 years	HD (22 M, 10 F, med. 42, range 21–68 years); CAPD (9 M, 7 F, med. 59, range 29–73 years)	54% 25% slight 29% severe 53% HD 56% CAPD	Score based on TSF, MAMC, transferrin, relative body wt (score 3–4: slight; 5–8: severe)	—	—	19% died within 2 years, all of whom had a score of 4 or more
Thunberg *et al.*, 1981, USA	58	HD (mean 30.8, range 2–102 months)	HD (30 M, 28 F, mean 48.2, SD 17 years)	72% 25.9%	TSF < 90% of ideal BMI < 20	Approx. 22.5	25.9%	10 M and 8 F were followed up at 6 and 18 months. Little change in nutritional status seen
Young *et al.*, 1991, Europe and USA	224	CAPD > 3 months (mean 32.2, SD 26.7 months)	CAPD (132 M, 92 F, mean 53.35, range 14–87 years)	41% 33% mild–moderate 8% severe	Modification of SGA	24.3	—	—

Continued

Table A1.35. *Continued*

Study	Time of assessment	Patients (*n*)	Treatment	Prevalence of malnutrition (% of patients)	Criteria for definition	Mean (SD) BMI of group (20 kg m⁻²)	BMI < 20 kg m⁻²	Change in nutritional status over time
Hospital								
Hartley *et al.*, 1997, UK Abstract	Admission to nephrology ward	20	HD (*n* 10) CRF (*n* 4) ARF (*n* 1) Others (*n* 5) (11 M, 9 F, mean 64, range 40–84 years)	50% (mild/moderate)	SGA B	24.3 (WN) 20.8 (UN)	–	–

[a]Oedema-free weight used, although the time anthropometric measurements were undertaken in relation to dialysis was not always described (Cianciaruso *et al.*, 1995). CRF, chronic renal failure; ESRD, end-stage renal disease; ARF, acute renal failure; HD, haemodialysis; CAPD, continuous ambulatory peritoneal dialysis; ob/ex, observed/expected; OP, out-patients; PD, peritoneal dialysis; PI, protein intake; UN, undernourished; WN, well nourished; SD, standard deviation; LBM, lead body mass; NL, The Netherlands; FFM, fat-free mass; MAMC, mid-arm muscle circumference; MN, malnourished; NS, not significant; MAMA, mid-arm muscle area; FM, fat mass.

Causes and Consequences of Disease-related Malnutrition in Patients with Chronic Renal Failure

The causes of weight loss and malnutrition in patients with chronic renal failure and end-stage renal disease (ESRD) are numerous (Bergstrom, 1995; Toigo *et al.*, 2000), as summarized in Table A1.36.

Table A1.36. Possible causes and potential consequences of disease-related malnutrition in patients with chronic renal failure.

Causes/factors	Consequences
Inadequate energy and protein intakes relative to requirements (Thunberg *et al.*, 1981; Cooper and Beaven, 1993; Lorenzo *et al.*, 1995; Fraser *et al.*, 1999; Herselman *et al.*, 2000) due to:	Reduced grip strength in predialysis patients (Heimburger *et al.*, 2000)
• Iatrogenic restriction of protein in predialysis patients (Hartley, 2001)[a]	Increased likelihood of acute hospitalization in predialysis patients (Lawson *et al.*, 2001)
• Severe anorexia (Young *et al.*, 1991; Bergstrom, 1999)	Reduced physical activity (Johansen *et al.*, 2000)
• Impaired taste sensitivity (Middleton and Allman-Farinelli, 1999)	
• Impaired smell (Griep *et al.*, 1997)	Increased morbidity (e.g. number of hospitalizations, number of days in hospital per patient and
• Nausea and vomiting (Bergstrom, 1999; Stenvinkel *et al.*, 2000)	infection-related morbidity) in HD or CAPD (Acchiardo *et al.*, 1983; Engel *et al.*, 1995; Ikizler *et al.*,
Duration on dialysis (Young *et al.*, 1991; Chazot *et al.*, 2001)	1999; Kopple *et al.*, 1999; Herselman *et al.*, 2000)[b]
Inadequacy of dialysis (Bergstrom, 1995)	Increased mortality in predialysis patients (Lawson *et al.*, 2001)
Losses of nutrients in dialysate (Bergstrom, 1995)	
Lower residual renal function (Young *et al.*, 1991)	Increased mortality in patients receiving dialysis (Marckmann, 1989; Kopple *et al.*, 1999)
Delayed gastric emptying (Stenvinkel *et al.*, 2000)	
Hormonal derangements (Stenvinkel *et al.*, 2000)	
Inadequate control of acidosis (Stenvinkel *et al.*, 2000), although this is controversial (Dumler *et al.*, 1999)	
Inflammation (Bistrian and Khaodhiar, 1999; Kaysen, 1999; Stenvinkel *et al.*, 2000)	
Presence of other diseases (e.g. diabetes; Young *et al.*, 1991; Stenvinkel *et al.*, 2000)	

[a] Low-protein diets (0.6 g protein kg^{-1} body weight day^{-1} or less) have traditionally been used in the predialysis period to correct uraemic symptoms, slow the progression of renal failure and delay the initiation of dialysis (Maroni, 1998; Aparicio *et al.*, 2001; Hartley, 2001). However, their use is now contentious, with fears that this may induce malnutrition (Hartley, 2001). Others argue that, in carefully selected patients, their use may prevent rather than induce malnutrition (Aparicio *et al.*, 2001).
[b] Magnitude of inflammatory response is also an independent predictor of hospitalization in patients receiving HD (Ikizler *et al.*, 1999). Furthermore, the extent of renal failure is likely to be an important factor (Acchiardo *et al.*, 1983; Young *et al.*, 1991).
CAPD, chronic ambulatory peritoneal dialysis; HD, haemodialysis.

Table A1.37. Number of operations performed in The Netherlands in 1992, categorized by type of surgery. Adapted from Ministry of Health, Welfare and Sports, 1995 (Statistics Netherlands, 1995).

Type of main operation[a]	Number of operated patients (*n*)	Number of operated patients per 100,000 average population
Musculoskeletal system	152,406	1,004
Digestive system	112,722	742
Obstetrics	57,918	755 (per 100,000 women)
Eyes	57,093	376
Gynaecology	49,485	645 (per 100,000 women)
Male genital organs	29,863	398 (per 100,000 men)
Breast	25,894	337 (per 100,000 women)
Urinary system	27,665	182
Circulatory system	27,533	181
Nose and nasal sinuses	25,766	170
Skin and subcutaneous tissue	23,903	157
Throat	23,339	154
Heart	18,342	121
Nervous system	15,852	104
Ears	13,751	91
Mouth	5,994	39
Lungs and bronchi	4,772	31
Blood and lymph system	4,297	28
Endocrine glands	3,345	22
Total	679,940	4,478

[a] Does not include repeat or further operations during a single hospital stay.

Table A1.38. Summary of the prevalence of malnutrition using a variety of criteria in surgical and ICU patients in hospital and the community arranged according to country.

Country	Number of subjects (n)	Prevalence of malnutrition (%)[a]	BMI < 20 kg m^{-2} (%)	IBW < 90% (%)	Reference
Surgery, mixed (benign and malignant, general): hospital					
France	408	32.4	–	–	Cohendy et al., 1999
Lebanon	94	23	–	23	Aoun et al., 1993
		23			
		53			
Norway	244	39	21	–	Bruun et al., 1999
		43			
Sweden	199	35	–	–	Larsson et al., 1994a
UK	808	6	6	–	Harrison, 1997 Abstract
UK	105	87	–	–	Hill et al., 1977
UK	46	35	–	–	Senapati et al., 1990
		65			
Surgery, mixed (benign and malignant, general): community					
UK	123	10.5	–	–	Edington et al., 1997
Surgery, mixed (benign and malignant, gastrointestinal): hospital					
Canada	202	31	–	–	Detsky et al., 1987
Canada	50	0	–	–	McLeod et al., 1995
New Zealand	66	45	–	–	Haydock and Hill, 1986
New Zealand	102	17	–	–	Windsor and Hill, 1988
		41			
Sweden	112	28	–	–	Symreng et al., 1983
UK	244	14	–	–	Brown et al., 1982
		82			
UK	150	6 (M)/13 (F)	6% (M)/13% (F)	–	Fettes et al., 2001a Abstract
UK	175	5 (M)/13 (F)	5% (M)/13% (F)	–	Fettes et al., 2001b Abstract
USA	100	62	–	–	Buzby et al., 1980
USA	245	50	–	–	Shaw-Stiffel et al., 1993
Surgery, mixed (benign and malignant, gynaecological and urological): hospital					
USA	74	11	–	–	Anderson et al., 1984

Continued

Table A1.38. *Continued*

Country	Number of subjects (n)	Prevalence of malnutrition (%) [a]	BMI < 20 kg m^{-2} (%)	IBW < 90% (%)	Reference
Surgery, benign, non-transplant					
Denmark	47	72	–	–	Pedersen and Pedersen, 1992
Japan	23	78	–	78	Nezu et al., 2001
South Africa	52	21	13	–	Dannhauser et al., 1995a,b
		13			
		38			
Sweden	215	12	–	–	Warnold and Lundholm, 1984
USA	51	53	–	–	Mazolewski et al., 1999
Surgery, benign, prior to transplant					
Canada	229	37	37	–	Madill et al., 2001
France	74	55	49	–	Schwebel et al., 2000
		49			
		72			
UK	65	54	–	–	Davidson et al., 1999
UK	102	28	–	–	Harrison et al., 1997
UK	164	54	–	–	Madden et al., 1994 Abstract
		23			
		71			
USA	20	85	–	–	Hasse et al., 1993
USA	99	99	–	–	Stephenson et al., 2001
Surgery, malignancy: hospital					
Colombia	40	62.5	–	–	Rey-Ferro et al., 1997
Netherlands	64	31	–	23	Van Bokhorst-de van der
		23			Schueren et al., 1997
		67			
Sweden	75	5	–	–	Ulander et al., 1998
UK	39	46	–	36	Bashir et al., 1990
		36			
UK	84	56	–	–	Brookes, 1982
UK	59	76	6	–	Corish et al., 1998 Abstract
		6			
		75			

Table A1.38. *Continued*

Country	Number of subjects (n)	Prevalence of malnutrition (%)[a]	BMI < 20 kg m^{-2} (%)	IBW < 90% (%)	Reference
UK	60	13.3 25 23	13.3	25	Jagoe et al., 2001a
USA	143	58	–	–	Martin et al., 1999 Abstract
USA	101	33	–	–	Meguid et al., 1986
Intensive care unit					
Portugal	44	6.8 16	6.8	16	Ravasco et al., 2002
Taiwan	49	100	–	–	Huang et al., 2000
USA	4301	59	–	–	Galanos et al., 1997
USA	129	43	–	–	Giner et al., 1996
Brain injury during rehabilitation					
UK	33	0 10 0 26	0	–	French and Merriman, 1999
UK	43	100 56	–	–	Thomson et al., 2001 Abstract

[a] When more than one result is provided for a given study (unless specifically explained) the results have been obtained by applying different criteria to the same group of patients. For more details, refer to Table A1.39.
ICU, intensive care unit.

Table A1.39. Prevalence of malnutrition in surgical patients.[a]

Study	Time of assessment	Patients (n)	Procedure	Prevalence of malnutrition (% of patients)	Criteria for definition	Mean (SD) BMI (kg m^{-2})	BMI < 20 kg m^{-2} (%)	Change in nutritional status over time
Surgery, mixed (benign and malignant, general): hospital								
Aoun et al., 1993, Lebanon	Admission	94	Mixed surgery (62 M, 32 F, mean 47.1, SD 18.7 years)	23 18 5 53	Wt loss IBW 80–90% IBW < 80% At least 3 abnormal measures (wt loss, TSF + SSF, MAMC, CHI, albumin, transferrin)	–	23 < 90 IBW	–
Bruun et al., 1999, Norway	After 1 week of hospital stay (includes patients on nutrition support)	244	GI (cancer, IBD, 77 M, 101 F, mean 67.5, range 22–92 years) and O (FNF and other fractures, 18 M, 48 F, mean 76, range 39–91 years) surgery	39 43 (GI) 27 (O) 28 33 (GI) 14 (O) 15 17 (GI) 8 (O)	BMI < 20 and > 5% wt loss in 3 months Wt loss > 5% UBW Wt loss > 10% UBW	–	21 21 (GI) 20 (O)	Of n 64: 17% wt-stable or gained wt, 50% lost up to 5% wt, 25% lost 5–10% wt and 8% lost 10–15% wt (wt loss may be due to loss of oedema in n 14)
Cohendy et al., 1999, France	Admission	408	Mixed elective surgery (50% M, mean 72, range 60–98 years)	25.5 6.9	MNA 17–23.5 MNA < 17	25.2	–	–
Harrison, 1997, UK Abstract	Admission	808	Elective surgery[b] (485 M, 323 F, med. 61, range 18–81 years)	6 4 1 1	BMI < 20 BMI < 20 + (TSF or MAMC < 15th percentile) BMI < 18 + (TSF or MAMC < 5th percentile) BMI < 16 + (TSF or MAMC < 5th percentile)	–	6	–
Hill et al., 1977,	Various time points in the	105	Mixed minor and major surgery,	87	Wt loss	–	–	Frequency of abnormal values for wt loss,

Reference	Timing	N	Population	Prevalence	Criteria					Comments
UK	course of hospital stay		benign and malignant (55 M, 50F, mean 53.8, range 17–85 years)			–	–	–	–	MAMC, albumin, transferrin, haemoglobin and vitamin stores (>50%) was highest in those patients assessed more than 1 week after major surgery
Larsson *et al.*, 1994a, Sweden	Admission	199	Mixed surgery, GI (malignant or benign), endocrine and vascular disease (110 M, 89 F, mean 59, range 22–83 years)	35% (39% of patients with malignant GI disease)	3 or more of: wt loss >10%, IBW < 80%, abnormal TSF, MAMC, prealbumin, albumin	–	–	–	–	–
Senapati *et al.*, 1990, UK	Presurgery	46	Mixed surgery (27 M, 19 F, mean 59.6, range 24–84 years)	35% / 65%	<100% BW/IBW × 100 / <100% BW/UBW × 100	–	–	–	–	–
Surgery, mixed (benign and malignant, general): community										
Edington *et al.*, 1997, UK	Within 6 weeks of surgery, post-discharge	123	Mixed major surgery, benign and malignant (74 M, 49 F, mean 64, range 23–90 years)	8.1% / 0% / 2.4%	BMI < 20 + (TSF or MAMC < 15th percentile) / BMI < 18 + (TSF or MAMC < 5th percentile) / BMI < 16 + (TSF or MAMC < 5th percentile)	–	–	–	–	Measurements were made post-discharge, within 6 weeks of surgery
Surgery, mixed (benign and malignant, gastrointestinal): hospital										
Brown *et al.*, 1982, UK	Prior to surgery	244	Major surgery for malignant and benign GI disease (med. 57, range 16–84 years, sex N/R)	14% / 82%	IBW < 80% / MAMC > 2 SD below normal range	–	–	–	–	–
Buzby *et al.*, 1980, USA	Admission	100	Mixed GI surgery (44 M, 56 F, mean 58, SE 1.8 years)	23% (mod. risk) / 39% (high risk)	PNI (based on albumin, transferrin, TSF and delayed hypersensitivity)	–	–	–	–	–

Continued

Table A1.39. Continued

Study	Time of assessment	Patients (n)	Procedure	Prevalence of malnutrition (% of patients)	Criteria for definition	Mean (SD) BMI (kg m^{-2})	BMI < 20 kg m^{-2} (%)	Change in nutritional status over time
Detsky et al., 1987, Canada	Presurgery	202	Major GI surgery (mean 52.7, SD 17.7 years, sex N/R)	21% 10%	SGA B SGA C	–	–	–
Fettes et al., 2001a, UK Abstract	Admission and on starting oral diet (+7 days after surgery)	150	Elective moderate/ major GI surgery[b] (range 18–80 years, sex N/R)	9% 6% (M) 13% (F)	BMI < 20	26.8 (M) 24.6 (F)	9% 6% (M) 13% (F)	52 M, 61 F reassessed. Wt loss was more common (90% vs. 59%, $P < 0.001$) and greater (4.1% vs. 1.6%; $P < 0.01$) in M than F. 34% of patients lost > 5% body wt. Sig. reduction of TSF, MAMC (greater in M) and hand grip strength (greater in F)
Fettes et al., 2001b, UK Abstract	Admission and on starting oral diet	175	Elective major GI surgery[b] (age/sex N/R)	5% (M) 13% (F)	BMI < 20	–	5% (M) 13% (F)	Postop. wt loss was more common (88% vs. 57%; $P < 0.001$) and greater (4% vs. 13%; $P \leq 0.001$) in M than F. M had greater loss of MAMC, but F showed a greater decrease in grip strength
Haydock and Hill, 1986, NZ	Presurgery	66	Elective GI surgery	45% 32% (mild) 14% (mod./ severe)	Mild: wt ≥ 5% of 'well' wt and reduced dietary intake Mod./severe: wt > 10% below 'well' wt and < 3rd percentile for BMI	24.1 (4.3) (mild) 18.1 (2.2) (mod./severe)	–	–
McLeod et al., 1995, Canada	–	(i) 25 (ii) 25	(i) Whipple procedure[c] (benign or malignant) (13 M, 12 F,	0%	SGA B and C	(i) 26.1 (4.9) (ii) 28.2 (4.4)	–	–

Continued

Reference	Timing	n	Patient group	Prevalence	Criteria			
			mean 57.7, SD 14.6 years) (ii) cholecystectomy (13 M, 12 F, mean 58, SD 11.1 years)					
Shaw-Stiffel et al., 1993, USA	Retrospective analysis	245	Major GI surgery (colorectal, small bowel, benign or malignant, mean 68, SD 15.4 years)	50%	Low albumin and prealbumin, wt loss > 10% in 6 months, or history of poor oral intake	—	—	—
Symreng et al., 1983, Sweden	Admission	112	Elective GI surgery (68 M, 44 F, mean 55, range 16–86 years)	28%	3 or more of: WI < 80%, low TSF, MAMC, albumin, prealbumin transferrin, cholinesterase, fibronectin, DH	—	—	—
Windsor and Hill 1988, NZ	Day before surgery	102	Major GI surgery, mixed (mean approx. 65 years, sex N/R)	17% / 41%	Wt loss > 10% UBW in 3 months / Wt loss > 10% with evidence of physiological impairment (dysfunction ≥ 2 organ systems)	—	—	—
Surgery, mixed (benign and malignant, gynaecological and urological): hospital								
Anderson et al., 1984, USA	Admission	74	Gynaecological and urological surgery, 26% malignant (21 M, 53 F, mean age approx. 53 years)	11%	Wt loss > 10%	—	—	—
Surgery, benign, non-transplant								
Dannhauser et al., 1995a, S. Africa	Within 36 h of admission	52	Benign GI (n 27) or cardiovascular (n 25) surgery (33 M, 19 F, mean 59 years)	21% / 21% / 13%	Wt loss > 10% in 6 months / IBW < 90 % / BMI < 20 (M); < 19 (F)	—	13% (< 19 in F)	—
Dannhauser et al., 1995b, S. Africa	Within 36 h of admission	52	Benign GI (n 27) or cardiovascular (n 25) surgery (33 M, 19 F, mean 59 years)	38% / 11% (mild) / 27% (mod.)	≥ 2 criteria present: appetite loss > 5 days, inadequate oral intake, high-risk diagnosis, wt loss > 10% in 6 months	—	—	—

Table A1.39. *Continued*

Study	Time of assessment	Patients (n)	Procedure	Prevalence of malnutrition (% of patients)	Criteria for definition	Mean (SD) BMI (kg m^{-2})	BMI <20 kg m^{-2} (%)	Change in nutritional status over time
Mazolewski et al., 1999, USA	Presurgery	51	LVR for end-stage emphysema (37 M, 14 F, mean 70 years)	53%	'Low' BMI (mean 20.9 SD 2.05)	–	–	–
Nezu et al., 2001, Japan	Presurgery	23	Bilateral LVR for COPD (M, mean 65.4, SD 7.8 years)	78%	IBW < 90%	18.6 (1.9)	78% < 90% IBW	–
Pedersen and Pedersen, 1992, Denmark	Presurgery	47	Amputations for lower extremity ischaemia	Poor 34% Reduced 38%	Graded reduced or poor nutr. status: wt loss, TSF, MAMC, albumin, prealbumin	–	–	–
Warnold and Lundholm, 1984, Sweden	Admission	215	Major vascular (52 M, 25 F, mean 61.6 years), minor vascular (32 M, 24 F, mean 55.3 years), abdominal (40 M, 32 F, mean 55.7 years), other (5 M, 3 F, mean 65.1 years) (non-cancer)	12% 18% (major vascular) 4% (minor vascular) 13% (abdominal)	2 or more of: WI < 0.8, low MAMC, low albumin or wt loss ≥ 5%	–	–	–
Surgery, benign, prior to transplant								
Davidson et al., 1999, UK	Consideration for liver transplant	65	Liver cirrhosis Hepatocellular (n 31; alcoholic and non-alcoholic) and biliary (n 34) (25 M, 40 F, mean 54.6, SE 2.2 years)	54%	BMI, weight loss as % actual body weight, TSF, and/or MAMC < 80% of reference	24.1 (SE 0.8)	–	–
Harrison et al., 1997, UK	On liver transplant waiting list (med. 8, range	102	Cholestatic liver disease (n 58) and parenchyma cirrhosis (n 44) (range	79% 28%	MAMC and TSF < 25th percentile MAMC and TSF < 5th percentile	–	–	–

Reference	n	Subjects	Prevalence	Criteria			Comments
Hasse et al., 1993, USA Evaluation for liver transplant 1–59 weeks pretransplant	20	17–69 years, sex N/R; Mixed liver diseases[d] (7 M, 13 F, mean 44.3, range 17–61 years)	70% 15%	SGA B SGA C	–	0%	–
Jackson et al., 1996, UK Abstract Acceptance on to liver transplant list	41	Chronic liver disease (20 M, 21 F, mean 51, range 17–69 years)	39% 7%	TSF and/or MAMC <5th percentile BMI < 20	–	7%	–
Madden et al., 1994, UK Abstract Prior to liver transplant	164	Age/sex N/R	54% 23% 71% 34% (mild) 25% (mod) 12% (severe)	MAMC < 5th percentile TSF < 5th percentile Nutritional assessment based on intake, anthropometry and wt loss	–	–	–
Madill et al., 2001, Canada Prior to lung transplant (retro review)	229	CF (24%), emphysema (33%), IPF (17%), PPH (7%), other (19%) (125 M, mean 42.1, SD 12.8 years; 104 F, mean 43.6, SD 13.2 years)	27% 10%	BMI 17–20 BMI < 17	–	37%	–
Müller et al., 1994, Germany On liver transplant waiting list and mean 432 (103–1022) days post-transplant	26	Mixed liver diseases[d] (14 M, 12 F, range 23–65 years)	–	–	101% IBW	–	+4.9% IBW (−17 to +33%) NS reduction in body cell mass and increase in fat mass
Richardson et al., 2001, UK Awaiting liver transplant and three × 3 months intervals afterwards	23	PBC (n 13); HC (n 10) (10 M, 13 F, mean 53.9, SD 1.9 years)	–	BMI Pre-illness weight loss TSF MAMC BIA	24.9 (SE 0.9)	–	Mean BMI increased to 27.8 (SE 0.87) by 9 months post-transplant ($P < 0.0001$). TSF and fat mass also increased significantly

Continued

Table A1.39. *Continued*

Study	Time of assessment	Patients (n)	Procedure	Prevalence of malnutrition (% of patients)	Criteria for definition	Mean (SD) BMI (kg m^{-2})	BMI < 20 kg m^{-2} (%)	Change in nutritional status over time
Schwebel et al., 2000, France	Candidates for lung transplant	74	Bronchiectasis or CF (38%), emphysema (33%), IPF (20%), PPH (8%) (24 M, 54 F, mean 42.3, SD 14.4 years)	55% 49% 72%	IBW < 90% BMI < 20 BMI < 20 or LBM (CHI) < 60% of predicted	20.4 (4.3)	49%	–
Stephenson et al., 2001, USA	Admission for liver transplant	99	Mixed liver diseases (60 M, 39 F, mean 47, SD 2.3 years)	99% 35% (mild) 32% (mod.) 32% (severe)	SGA	–	–	–
Surgery, malignancy: hospital (all assessments made preoperatively unless otherwise stated)								
Bashir et al., 1990, UK		39	Thoracotomy for bronchial cancer (mean 61.9 years, sex N/R)	46% 21% 15%	BMI + TSF + SSF < 25th percentile 80–90% IBW < 80% IBW	–	36% (< 90% IBW)	–
Brookes, 1982, UK		84	Untreated primary SCC of head and neck (age/sex N/R)	39% (deficit) 15% (malnut.) 2% (severe malnut.)	General nutritional status assessment (based on anthropometry, biochemistry and N excretion)	–	–	–
Corish et al., 1998, Ireland Abstract		59	Lung (n 16), H and N (n 13), Bowel (n 12), Oes. (n 10), Ovary (n 4), Gastric (n 2), Panc-duo (n 2) (37 M, 22 F, mean 66, range 31–90 years)	63% (at risk) 13% (severe) 6% 75% 37%	NRI NRI BMI < 20 Wt loss (mean 11.2%) Wt loss > 10% in 6 months	15.2 24.9 25.3 21.6 24.8 27.6 28.4	6%	76% lost weight in hospital (mean 5.6% of admission weight). Following discharge, 70% lost weight within 3 months (mean 5.9% body weight)
Jagoe et al., 2001a, UK		60	Lung cancer (43 M, 17 F, mean	13% 25%	BMI < 20 IBW < 90%	25.4 (4.7)	13.3%	–

Reference	N	Patient group	Prevalence	Criteria			Comments
Martin et al., 1999, USA Abstract	143	Oesophagogastrectomy for cancer (124 M, 19 F, med 60 years)[e]	23%, 5%, 58%	Wt loss > 5%, Wt loss > 10%, Wt loss (preop.)	–	–	87% had postop. wt loss, of which 21% had wt loss > 10% of immediate preop. wt.
Meguid et al., 1986, USA	101	Colorectal cancer (mean 66 years, range 32–85)	33%	Albumin < 35 g l⁻¹ and 2 other abnormal values: recent wt loss > 10%, W/H, MAMC or TSF < 10th percentile	–	–	–
Rey-Ferro et al., 1997, Colombia	40	Gastric adenocarcinoma (22 M, 18 F, mean 54, SD 14 years)	5% (mild), 42.5% (mod.), 15% (severe)	NRI > 97.5, NRI 83.5–97.5, NRI < 83.5	–	–	–
Ulander et al., 1998, Sweden	75	Colorectal surgery for cancer[f] (38 M, 37 F, mean 71.4, range 41–90 years)	5%	SGA B and C	–	–	39% wt loss ≥5% during hospital stay. Mean % wt loss 4.7 (4.4)%, greatest in M (6.1%)
Van Bokhorst-de van der Schueren et al., 1997, NL	64	Advanced head and neck cancer (mean 61, SD 10 years, sex N/R)	31%, 17% (mild), 3% (mod.), 3% (severe), 67%	Wt loss > 10% in 6 months, IBW 80–90%, IBW 70–79%, IBW < 69%, NI < 1.31	–	23% (< 90% IBW)	–

$Albumin < 35$ g l^{-1}

[a]Confounding factors were rarely noted in any of these studies (e.g. oedema; Bruun et al., 1999).
[b]No details on types of patients or types of GI surgery.
[c]Whipple procedure consists of a cholecystectomy and a pancreaticoduodenectomy.
[d]Including a few patients with hepatocellular carcinoma.
[e]Pre- and post-surgery, retrospective review.

IBD, inflammatory bowel disease; IPF, idiopathic pulmonary fibrosis; LVR, lung volume reduction surgery; NI, nutrition index; NRI, nutrition risk index; O, orthopaedic; PNI, prognostic nutritional index; PPH, primary pulmonary hypertension; SSF, subscapular skin-fold thickness; W/H, weight-for-height ratio; MAMC, mid-arm muscle circumference; CHI, creatinine–height index; BIA, bioelectrical impedance analysis; HC, hepatocellular cirrhosis; PBC, primary biliary cirrhosis; UBW, usual body weight; MNA, Mini Nutritional Assessment; N/R, not recorded; SE, standard error; BW, body weight; NL, The Netherlands; NS, not significant; CF, cystic fibrosis; H and N, head and neck; Oes., oesophageal; Panc-duo, pancreatoduodenal; IBW, ideal body weight; med., median; mod., moderate; postop, postoperative; retro, retrospective; SCC, squamous cell carcinoma.

Causes and Consequences of Disease-related Malnutrition in Surgical Patients

A number of studies have documented adverse sequelae associated with changes in weight in surgical patients (see Table A1.40). In addition to the adverse effects of weight loss on outcome, other studies have highlighted the fact that patients who are undernourished during their hospital admission have a poorer outcome, both clinically and functionally, than the well nourished. These include increased length of stay (LOS), reduced well-being, impaired wound healing and increases in morbidity and mortality. As in other patient groups, it is not possible from the data available to separate the effects of malnutrition and the impact of the disease severity on outcome. It is likely that those patients who are more undernourished are also sicker individuals. It is also likely that the consequences of weight loss/malnutrition may perpetuate further weight loss and deterioration in nutritional status.

Despite clear indications that disease-related malnutrition adversely affects outcome, a number of the studies reviewed have highlighted the problems of lack of recognition and lack of treatment of malnutrition in the hospital setting in surgical patients (Bruun *et al.*, 1999).

Table A1.40. Possible causes and potential consequences of disease-related malnutrition in surgical patients

Causes/factors	Consequences
Poor food intake (Rana *et al.*, 1992; Jensen and Hessov, 1997; Keele *et al.*, 1997; Maskell *et al.*, 1999; Barton *et al.*, 2000a) due to various reasons including:	Fatigue (Christensen and Kehlet, 1984)
• Reduced appetite, vomiting, diarrhoea, swallowing difficulties (Corish *et al.*, 1998)	Abnormal wound healing (Haydock and Hill, 1986) and greater frequency of impaired wound healing (Pedersen and Pedersen, 1992)
• (Perceived) reduced gastrointestinal motility (Bengmark, 1998) • Presence of inflammatory or malignant disease	Low well-being ratings (lower mood, endurance, attitude to others and future orientation, greater anxiety and loneliness)/impaired quality of life (Larsson *et al.*, 1994a)
Altered metabolism as a result of inflammatory or malignant disease (Heslin and Brennan, 2000)	Increased complication rates (Buzby *et al.*, 1980; Symreng *et al.*, 1983; Warnold and Lundholm, 1984; Meguid *et al.*, 1986; Mughal and Meguid, 1987; Windsor and Hill, 1988; Pedersen and Pedersen, 1992; Sagar and Macfie, 1994; Dannhauser *et al.*, 1995a,b; Gianotti *et al.*, 1995; Harrison *et al.*, 1997; Van Bokhorst-de van der Schueren *et al.*, 1997; Martin *et al.*, 1999; Mazolewski *et al.*, 1999; Schwebel *et al.*, 2000; Desseigne *et al.*, 2001; Jagoe *et al.*, 2001b; Nezu *et al.*, 2001; Stephenson *et al.*, 2001)
Altered metabolism and catabolism as a response to surgical stress (proportional to the magnitude of surgical stress) (Heslin and Brennan, 2000; Maxfield *et al.*, 2001)	Longer hospital stay (Warnold and Lundholm, 1984; Windsor and Hill, 1988; Pedersen and Pedersen, 1992; Shaw-Stiffel *et al.*, 1993; Ulander *et al.*, 1998; Mazolewski *et al.*, 1999; Stephenson *et al.*, 2001)
Failure to screen or assess the nutritional status of patients and their risk of malnutrition, e.g. records of weight in only 59% of medical notes and records of height in only 51% of notes (Bruun *et al.*, 1999)	Longer rehabilitation period (following orthopaedic surgery) (Bastow *et al.*, 1983; Patterson *et al.*, 1992; Lumbers *et al.*, 1996)
Failure to treat malnutrition with nutritional support, e.g. nutritional support given to only 23% of all patients (Bruun *et al.*, 1999)	Increased mortality (Buzby *et al.*, 1980; Brown *et al.*, 1982; Meguid *et al.*, 1986; Mughal and Meguid, 1987; Madden *et al.*, 1994; Sagar and Macfie, 1994; Van Bokhorst-de van der Schueren *et al.*, 1997, 2000; Corish *et al.*, 1998; Schwebel *et al.*, 2000; Jagoe *et al.*, 2001b; Madill *et al.*, 2001)

Table A1.41. Typical case mix on general intensive care units (adapted from Hill *et al.*, 1995).

Primary problem	Patients (*n*)
Respiratory	
Pneumonia	17
Asthma	2
COPD	8
Others	8
Total respiratory	35 (12.4%)
Cardiovascular	
Post-cardiac surgery	16
Cardiac medical	8
Post-cardiac arrest	7
Pulmonary	1
Total cardiovascular	32 (11.3%)
Neurological	
ICH/CVA	7
Guillain–Barré syndrome	5
Encephalitis/meningitis	3
Status epilepticus	2
Post-neurosurgery	2
Others	5
Total neurological	24 (8.5%)
Renal	
Acute renal failure	5 (1.8%)
Surgical	
Multiple trauma	37
Upper GI	47
Lower GI	28
Major vascular	26
Pancreatitis	10
Liver transplant	4
Other surgery	10
Total surgical	162 (57%)
Others	
Overdose/poisoning	6
Haematological	5
Metabolic	6
MOF	2
Miscellaneous	6
Total others	25 (8.8%)

CVA, cerebrovascular accident; ICH, intracerebral haemorrhage; MOF, multiple organ failure.

Table A1.42. Prevalence of malnutrition in patients in intensive care units (ICU)

Study	Time of assessment	Patients (n)	Diagnosis	Prevalence of malnutrition (% of patients)	Criteria for definition	Mean (SD) BMI of group (kg m^{-2})	BMI < 20 kg m^{-2}	Change in nutritional status over time
Galanos et al., 1997	Admission	4301	Serious illness (43% ARF/MOSF, 34% COPD/CHF/cirrhosis, 17% cancer, 6% coma) (2451 M,1850 F, mean 62, SD 15.5 years)	59%	Wt loss	24.7 (7.2)	–	–
Giner et al., 1996, USA	Admission to medical/ surgical ICU	129	Mixed (TISS on admission approx. 27) (71 M, 58 F, median age approx. 58, range 17–88 years)	43%	Albumin < 35 g l^{-1} and W/H ratio < 100%	–	–	–
Huang et al., 2000, Taiwan	Admission to ICU and 14th day	49	Mixed. 3 groups according to feeding: ETF (16 M, 6 F), PN (7 M, 2 F), ETF + PN (10 M, 8 F), mean age 67, 55 and 64 years for each group	100%	MI (includes prealbumin, albumin, TLC and % IBW, score > 0 indicates risk)	21.8 (ETF n 22) 26.4 (PN n 9) 24.5 (ETF + PN n 18)	–	MI sig. lower by day 14, although only 3 pt classified as 'not undernourished' with a score < 0. No sig. changes in wt or arm anthropometry
Ravasco et al., 2002, Portugal	Admission	44	Medical conditions, respiratory failure requiring MV (24 M, 20 F, mean 55, range 17–83 years)	6.8% 16%	BMI < 20 IBW < 90%	–	6.8%	–

ARF, acute respiratory failure; CHF, congestive heart failure; MI, Maastricht index; MOSF, multiple organ system failure; MV, mechanical ventilation; TISS, therapeutic intervention scoring system; < 20, minimal to moderate severity of illness; > 20, severe illness; TLC, total lymphocyte count; W/H, weight-for-height; SD, standard deviation; PN, parenteral nutrition; ETF, enteral tube feeding.

Table A1.43. Prevalence of malnutrition in brain-injured patients during rehabilitation.

Study	Time of assessment	Patients (n)	Diagnosis	Prevalence of malnutrition (% of patients)	Criteria for definition	Mean (SD) BMI of group (kg m^{-2})	% BMI < 20 kg m^{-2}	Change in nutritional status over time
French and Merriman, 1999, UK	Several years after injury	33	Brain injury requiring long-term treatment for acquired behavioural problems (31 M, 2 F, mean 33, range 16–63 years)	0% 10% 0% 26%	BMI < 19.9 MAC < 5th percentile TSF < 5th percentile MAMC < 5th percentile	–	0%	–
Thomson et al., 2001, UK Abstract	Admission (median time from injury to admission: 29 (7–328) days) and discharge	43	TBI (28 M, 5 F) and ABI (5 M, 5 F). Age between 16–64 years	100% 26% 23% 7%	Wt loss since injury (mean 12.6% UBW) BMI < 20 + (TSF or MAMC < 15th percentile) BMI < 18 + (TSF or MAMC < 5th percentile) BMI < 16 + (TSF or MAMC < 5th percentile)	–	–	Mean duration rehab. (including nutritional support where indicated) was 61 (range 1.9–52.5) days. Mean weight gain during rehab. was 4.9 kg. Mean % wt loss from time of injury was 5% at discharge. 23% remained nutritionally depleted

ABI, anoxic brain injury, e.g. due to ischaemia, anaemia; TBI, traumatic brain injury, e.g. due to falls, assaults, road traffic accidents; SD, standard deviation; MAC, mid-arm circumference; MAMC, mid-arm muscle circumference; UBW, usual body weight; rehab., rehabilitation.

Table A1.44. Prevalence of malnutrition in children with disease. W/H: low values indicate wasting (acute malnutrition). W/A, BMI/A and BMI also indicate wasting. H/A: low values indicate stunting (chronic malnutrition).

Study	Location	Time of assessment	Patients (n)	Diagnosis	Prevalence of malnutrition (% of patients)	Criteria for definition	% W/H of group	W/H < 90% (%)	Change in nutritional status over time
General/mixed diagnoses									
Hankard et al., 2001, France (French)	Hospital	> 48 h after admission	58	Mixed: GM, GS and PS (> 6 months, age/sex N/R)	21% 12%	BMI < −2 SDS BMI < −2 SDS (excl. AN, n6)	—	—	—
Hendricks et al., 1995, USA	Tertiary care facility	All in-patients	268	Mixed (50% M, 50% F, age 0–18 years)	24.5% (35% in < 2 years) 17.4% 5.8% 1.3% 27.3% (46% in < 2 years) 14.5% 7.7% 5.1%	Acute: W/H < 90% 81–90% mild 70–80% moderate <70% severe Chronic: H/A < 95% 90–95% mild 85–89% moderate < 85% severe	—	24.5%	—
Hendrikse et al., 1997, UK	Children's hospital and out-patients	Admission or clinic visit	226	Mixed: GM, GS and OP (140 M, 86 F, 7 months–16 years)	8% (wasted) 16% 15% (stunted) 16%	W/H < 80% W/A < 5th percentile H/A < 5th percentile W/A and H/A −1 SDS to −2 SDS	—	—	—
McCarthy and McIvor, 2001, UK Abstract	Children's hospital	Admission	31	– Age, sex N/R	13% 0% 16% 10% 10% 13% 16% 0%	W/H 80–90% (Waterlow) W/H < 80% (Waterlow) W/H 80–90% (Hendrikse) W/H < 80% (Hendrikse) W/A −1.0 to −2.0 SDS W/A −2.0 SDS BMI/A 80–90% BMI/A < 80%	—	13–26% (depending on reference)	—
Moy et al., 1990, UK	Children's hospital	Representative sample	255	Mixed: acute GM, GS and elective GS (sex N/R, age 3 months–18 years)	19% at risk 14% severely wasted 22% at risk 16% severely stunted	W/H −1 to −2 SDS W/H < −2 SDS H/A −1 to −2 SDS H/A < −2 SDS	Acute/elective −0.25 (1.33) Chronic −0.24 (1.06)	—	—

Continued

Table A1.44. *Continued*

Study	Location	Time of assessment	Patients (n)	Diagnosis	Prevalence of malnutrition (% of patients)	Criteria for definition	% W/H of group	W/H < 90% (%)	Change in nutritional status over time
Sermet-Gaudelus et al., 2000, France	Children's hospital	Admission	296	– >1 month old	26% 7% 5% 14%	Acute: W/A < 85% 80–84% (mild) 75–79% (moderate) <75% (severe)	–	37.5% (<90% IBW)	65% lost wt during stay and 45% lost >2% of admission wt. 'Malnutrition' did not increase the risk of nutritional depletion during hospital stay
Cardiology									
Cameron et al., 1995, USA	Tertiary referral teaching hospital	Admission (retrospective)	160	Cardiac (medical and surgical) (90 M, 60 F, newborn–24 years)	33% 18% 12% 3% 64% 21% 31% 12% 6%	Acute: W/H < 90% 80–89% (mild) 70–79% (moderate) <70% (severe) Chronic: H/A < 95% 91–94% (mild) 86–90% (moderate) <86% (severe) Acute and chronic	–	33%	–
Venugopalan et al., 2001, Oman	Out-patients	–	152	Congenital heart defects (78 M, 74 F, mean 3.3, SD 3.6 years)	27% 24%	Acute: W/A < 3rd percentile and H/A > 3rd percentile Chronic: W/A and H/A < 3rd percentile	–	–	–
Cerebral palsy									
Dahl and Gebre-Medhin, 1993, Sweden	Rehabilitation centre	Admission	44	Cerebral palsy (n 30) and myelomeningocoele (n 14)	38%[a] 30%[a]	W/A < –2 SDS H/A < –2 SDS	–	–	–
Dahl et al., 1997, Sweden	Home	– (parental interviews, records and measurements)	35	Cerebral palsy, moderate to severe (23 M, 12 F, med. 8 years)	49% 43%	W/H or TSF <2.5th percentile (wasting) H/A or lower-leg length <2.5th percentile (stunting)	–	–	–

Study	Setting	Age	n	Patient group	Prevalence	Criteria			
Kong et al., 1999, Hong Kong	Disability unit	–	62	Cerebral palsy (35 M, 27 F, mean 7.1, range 2.3–14 years)	68%	Bone age delay of >1 year	–	–	–
Stallings et al., 1993, USA	Home	–	154	Cerebral palsy (85 M, 69 F, mean 7.3, range 2–17.4 years)	28% 29% 23%	TSF <15th percentile W/A <5th percentile Height by upper-arm length <5th percentile (stunted)	–	–	–
Sullivan et al., 2000, UK	Home (questionnaire)	–	240	Cerebral palsy (153 M, 118 F, mean 8.9, range 4–13 years)	38%	Underweight (parent's view)	–	–	–
Thommessen et al., 1991, Norway	Home (retrospective)	–	42	Cerebral palsy (mean approx. 5.5, range 1–13 years)	15% 48%	W/H <2.5th percentile and/or TSF <5th percentile and/or EI <70% RDA H/A <2.5th percentile	–	–	–
Chronic obstructive pulmonary disease									
Viola et al., 2000, France Abstract	–	Mean 11.4 (3.2) years	50	Stable COPD (sex N/R)	28%	W/H <90%	–	28%	–
Cystic fibrosis (CF)									
Lai et al., 1998, USA[b]	1993 National CF Patient Registry data	–	13,116	Cystic fibrosis (6925 M, 6191 F, age 0–18 years)	46.6% 0–1 years 10.9% wasted 8.3% stunted 27.3% both 22% 1–10 years 3.8% wasted 9.6% stunted 8.5% both 34% 11–18 years 9% wasted 8% stunted 17% both	Stunted and/or wasted W/A < 5th percentile H/A < 5th percentile Both of above As above As above	–	–	–

Continued

Table A1.44. Continued

Study	Location	Time of assessment	Patients (n)	Diagnosis	Prevalence of malnutrition (% of patients)	Criteria for definition	% W/H of group	W/H < 90% (%)	Change in nutritional status over time
McNaughton et al., 2000, Australia	Out-patients	–	226	Cystic fibrosis	7.5% (M) 1.7% (F) 6.8% (M) 8.3% (F) 7.7% (M) 7.3% (F) 30% (M) 22% (F)	W/H < –2.0 SDS W/A < –2.0 SDS H/A < –2.0 SDS < 80% predicted TBK for age	z score –0.07 (1.09) (M) –0.04 (0.93) (F)	–	–
Westwood and Saitowitz, 1999, S. Africa	Out-patients	–	38	Cystic fibrosis (children and adolescents)	47% (> 10 years) 14.3% (< 10 years) 16%	W/H < 90% H/A < 5th percentile	Med. 93 (IQR 84–101)	47% (> 10 years) 14.3% (< 10 years)	–
Wiedemann et al., 2001, Germany	Out-patients (paeds (P) and adults (A))	–	2325 (P) 1110 (A)	Cystic fibrosis	26.8% (< 6 years) 22% (6–12 years) 25% (6–12 years) 31% (> 12 years) 38.3% (adults)	Acute: W/H < 90% BMI < 19	97.2 (11.9)	26.8%	–
Intensive care									
Almeida Santos et al., 1998, Spain (Spanish)	PICU	Admission	65	Respiratory failure (1–158 months)	60% 63% 13%	W/H < 90% W/A < 90% H/A < 90%	–	60%	–
Briassoulis et al., 2001, Greece	PICU	Admission	71	Critical illness, MV (1.29 M:1 F, mean 6 years; 2 months–17 years)	27% 21% (at risk) 6% (severe) 21% 17% (at risk) 4% (severe)	Acute: W/H < 90% W/H 70–89% W/H < 70% Chronic: H/A < 95% H/A 85–95% H/A < 85%	–	27%	–
Hulst et al., 2001, NL Abstract	8 PICUs	All children on 1 day	51	Mixed acute and/or chronic illness (sex N/R, med. age 6 months (8 days–16.5 years)	16% 29% 0 23%	Acute (Waterlow) Acute (SDS) Chronic (Waterlow) Chronic (SDS)	–	–	–

Reference	Setting	Timing	n	Population	Prevalence (%)	Criteria				Comments
Pollack *et al.*, 1981, USA	Medical PICU	Within 48 h of admission	50	Medical admissions (no chronic organ failure or cancer) (sex N/R, age from 0 years)	40% 24% 6% 10% 22% 6% 10% 6%	Acute: W/H < 90% W/H 80–90% W/H 70–79% W/H < 79% Chronic: H/A < 95% H/A 80–95% H/A 85–89% H/A < 85%	–	40%	–	–
Pons Leite *et al.*, 1993, Brazil	PICU	Admission	46	Mixed (22 M, 24 F, med. 22.5, range 3–175 months)	17% 22% 26%	W/H < 80% H/A < 90% Both	–	–	–	–
Malignancy Deeg *et al.*, 1995, USA	–	Prior to BMT	576	Haematological cancers (344 M, 298 F, < 18 years, mean age N/R)	12% 4%	85–95% IBW < 85% IBW	–	–	–	–
Kurugöl *et al.*, 1997, Turkey	Hospital	Remission (*n* 25) Active disease (*n* 20)	45	Leukaemia, bone tumours and other tumours (27 M, 18 F, mean 10.5, SD 5.4 years)	51.1% 11.1% 11.1% 28.9%	Acute: W/H ≤ 95% 90–95% 85–90% < 85%	–	40%	–	–
Pietsch and Ford, 2000, USA	–	Diagnosis (retrospective)	127	Haematological and solid (incl. brain) tumours (sex N/R, age 0–18 years)	47% (of *n* 81) 15% (of *n* 81) 1% (of *n* 81) 11% (of *n* 81) 1% (of *n* 81) 32% (of *n* 127) 14% (of *n* 78) 3% (of *n* 78)	W/H < 50th percentile W/H < 20th percentile W/H < 80% W/H z score < −1 W/H z score < −2 BMI < 16 BMI z score < −1 BMI z score < −2	–	–	–	–
Reilly *et al.*, 1999, UK	–	Diagnosis (retrospective)	1,019	ALL (767 M, 252 F, med. 4.4 range 0.4–14.9 years)	8% (M) 7% (F)	BMI < −2.0 SDS	–	–	–	–
Smith *et al.*, 1990, UK	Children's out-patients	Diagnosis	48	Solid tumours (25 M, 23 F, med. age 4.3, range 0.5–16 years)	7% 26% 30%	H/A < −2.0 SDS and/or W/H < 80% MAC < 5th percentile TSF < −2.0 SDS	100%	–	–	Prevalence of malnutrition increased from 27 to 46% ($P < 0.05$) during therapy, despite 33% of patients receiving nutritional support

Continued

Table A1.44. *Continued*

Study	Location	Time of assessment	Patients (n)	Diagnosis	Prevalence of malnutrition (% of patients)	Criteria for definition	% W/H of group	W/H < 90% (%)	Change in nutritional status over time
Smith et al., 1991, UK	Children's out-patients	Diagnosis	100	Solid and haematological tumours (52 M, 48 F, median 5, range 0.3–16.5 years)	5%[c] 20% 23%	H/A <–2.0 SDS and/or <80% W/H[c] MAC < 5th percentile TSF <–2.0 SDS	100%[c]	–	–
Yaris et al., 2002, Turkey	–	Diagnosis, at 3 months and at end of therapy	47	Lymphoma, brain tumour, soft-tissue and bone sarcoma, other solid tumours	29.8% 19.2% 2.1% 8.5%	Wasted and/or stunted Wasted (Waterlow) Stunted (Waterlow) Wasted and stunted	–	–	After 3 months, overall rate of malnutrition was 38.3%. In those reassessed at end of therapy (n 27), rate was 18.5%
Renal disease									
Pereira et al., 2000, Brazil	Paediatric nephrology clinic	6 times during a 12-month period	30	ESRD 23 PD 4 IPD 19 CAPD 7 HD (12 M, 18 F, mean 9.3, SD 7.4 years)	53% 63% 43%	W/A <–2.0 SDS H/A <–2.0 SDS MAMA/A <–1.65 SDS	Med. 91.5 (IQR 8.7) (1) Med. 92.7 (IQR 11.4) (6)	Approx. 50%	Statistical changes over time not recorded

[a] Includes 14 patients with myelomeningocoele, who tend to be overweight rather than underweight.

[b] This paper also used other methods of defining malnutrition and showed considerable variation depending on which method was applied. Gender-specific information is also given. A further report comparing CF registries in the USA and Canada has also been published (Lai *et al.*, 1999). In the UK, mean weight and height of children with CF have been reported to be 0.5 SD below the norm in the first 10 years of life (Morison *et al.*, 1997).

[c] Authors wary of using weight as an indicator of nutritional status due to the confounding effects of tumour mass in children with cancer (Smith *et al.*, 1991).

AN, anorexia nervosa; ALL, acute lymphoblastic leukaemia; CAPD, continuous ambulatory peritoneal dialysis; ESRD, end-stage renal disease; GM, general medicine; GS, general surgery; HD, haemodialysis; IPD, intermittent peritoneal dialysis; PD, peritoneal dialysis; PICU, paediatric intensive care unit; PS, psychiatry; BMI/A, body mass index for age; H/A, height-for-age; IQR, interquartile range; MAMA/A, mid-arm muscle area for age; med., median; RDA, recommended daily allowance; SDS, standard deviation score; TBK, total body potassium (an indicator of body cell mass); W/A, weight-for-age; W/H, weight-for-height; N/R, not recorded; NL, The Netherlands; MAC, mid-arm circumference; MV, mechanical ventilation; OP, out-patient.

Table A1.45. Main types, forms, incidence and survival rates of childhood cancers in the UK (adapted from Lissauer and Clayden, 1997; Ward, 2001).

Type of cancer	Forms	Incidence in 1998 (UK)	3-year survival rate (1993–1997)
Leukaemias (approx. 30–45% of all childhood cancers)	Acute lymphoblastic leukaemia	113	88%
	Acute myeloid leukaemia	–	–
	Chronic myeloid leukaemia	–	–
Lymphomas (approx. 9–15% of all childhood cancers)	Hodgkin's disease	13	98%
	Non-Hodgkin's lymphoma	17	81%
	Burkitt's lymphoma	–	–
Solid tumours (approx. 40% of all childhood cancers)	Brain tumours (23% of all childhood cancers)	–	–
	Wilms' tumour (6% of all childhood cancers)	23	85%
	Neuroblastoma (6% of all childhood cancers)	25	64%
	Rhabdomyosarcoma (4% of all childhood cancers)	15	72%
	Osteosarcoma (5% of all childhood cancers)	6	64%
	Ewing's sarcoma	6	67%
	Primitive neuroectodermal tumour	17	57%

Causes and Consequences of Disease-related Malnutrition in Paediatrics

There are many factors that are associated with the development of malnutrition in children, many of which will be similar to the reasons seen in adults (see Chapter 3 and disease-specific sections of this appendix). These include food intakes that are inadequate to meet recommended allowances, pain and moderate/severe stress associated with disease (see Table A1.46). The consequences of malnutrition in children are both short- and long-term and can include impairments in growth and in other aspects of development (physical and intellectual) (see Chapter 4). Other consequences for function and outcome have been less well investigated in children than in adults, but findings in adults are likely also to be relevant to children (see relevant sections).

Table A1.46. Possible causes and potential consequences of disease-related malnutrition in children.

Causes	Consequences
Poor food intake (Smith *et al.*, 1991; Chin *et al.*, 1992; Dahl and Gebre-Medhin, 1993; Kurugöl *et al.*, 1997; Norman *et al.*, 2000; Sermet-Gaudelus *et al.*, 2000)	Impaired growth (see Table A1.44)
	Poor cognitive function (Berkman *et al.*, 2002)
Pain and stress associated with disease (Sermet-Gaudelus *et al.*, 2000)	Increased risk of infections (Grantham-McGregor, 2002)
	Reduced duration of remission in neuroblastoma (Rickard *et al.*, 1983)
	Increased mortality in CF (Corey *et al.*, 1988), HIV infection (McKinney *et al.*, 1994; Berhane *et al.*, 1997; Fontana *et al.*, 1999; Amadi *et al.*, 2001), malignancy (Rickard *et al.*, 1983; Deeg *et al.*, 1995; Mejía-Arangure *et al.*, 1999)

Appendix 2
Energy and Protein Intakes in Disease

Table A2.1. Food intake in patients with mixed diagnoses in hospitals.

Investigator	Type of patients/n	Assessment method	Energy intake (kcal day^{-1})	Protein intake (g day^{-1})	Other nutrient intake
Browne and Moloney, 1998, Ireland Abstract	Two public hospitals A (16 M, 10 F) B (13 M, 12 F) Age/BMI N/R	3-day weighed food intake (excluding snacks)	1310 (SD 285) (M, A) 1285 (SD 190) (F, A) 1595 (SD 450) (M, B) 1620 (SD 450) (F, B)	–	Low vitamin C, Fe (F) and Ca intakes (see Shirley and Moloney, 1998)
Gall et al., 1998, UK	Orthopaedic, medical and female elderly patients[a] (27 M, mean 60.5, SE 2.4 years; 54 F, mean 74, SE 1.5 years) BMI N/R	3-day dietary record	1405 (SE 62)	51.2 (SE 2.1) (14.5en%)	–
Shirley and Moloney, 2000, Ireland Abstract	Private hospital[b] (11 M, 19 F, age 19–65 years) BMI N/R	3-day weighed food intake (excluding snacks)	1820 (SD 445)	–	Low Fe intakes (F)
Valla et al., 2000, France Abstract	University hospital[c] Rheumatology/n = 25 Pneumonology/n = 22 Orthopaedics/n = 11 Geriatrics/n = 19 (35 M, 42 F, mean 73, SD 15 years, mean BMI 23.7, SD 5.5	Calculated by difference from food provision and wastage	1125 (SD 530)	–	–

[a]Patients were excluded if they were not eating freely for a minimum of 3 days.
[b]Patients all capable of independent feeding.
[c]Patients with dysphagia, those fasted or needing nutritional support were excluded.
BMI, body mass index (kg m^{-2}); en%, percentage of energy intake from protein; N/R, not recorded; SD, standard deviation; SE, standard error.

Table A2.2. Food intake in general medical patients in hospitals.

Investigator	Type of patients/*n*	Assessment method	Energy intake (kcal day⁻¹)	Protein intake (g day⁻¹)	Other nutrient intake
Barton *et al.*, 2000a, UK	General medical Ward study: daily mean 27 patients Subgroup: 9 M, 13 F, mean 65, range 40–98 years	Calculated by difference from whole ward food provision and wastage over 27 days. Checked against 3-day weighed records in a subgroup	1400 (ward study) 1380 (sᴅ 364) (subgroup)	43.5	–
Sandström *et al.*, 1985, Sweden	General elderly medical (25 M, 31 F, mean 70, sᴅ 9 years)	Dietary history (home) Weighed food intake (hospital)	2380 (sᴅ 550) (M, home) 1690 (sᴅ 310) (M, hosp.) 1860 (sᴅ 405) (F, home) 1570 (sᴅ 335) (F, hosp.)	72 (sᴅ 19) 74 (sᴅ 15) 60 (sᴅ 15) 68 (sᴅ 13)	–

sᴅ, standard deviation.

Table A2.3. Food intake in elderly patients with mixed diagnoses in hospitals.

Investigator	Type of patients/n	Assessment method	Energy intake (kcal day⁻¹)	Protein intake (g day⁻¹)	Other nutrient intake
Barton et al., 2000a, UK	Elderly Ward study: daily mean 22 patients Subgroup: 6 M, 14 F, mean 73, range 52–98 years	Calculated by difference from whole ward food provision and wastage. Checked against 3-day weighed records in a subgroup	1380 (ward study) 1390 (SD 289) (subgroup)	44.6	–
Elmstahl, 1987, Sweden	Long-stay mobile geriatrics (14 M, 16 F, mean 83, range 68–92 years)	4-day weighed food intake	1610 (SD 330) 1745 (M) 1490 (F)	–	–
Elmstahl et al., 1997, Sweden	Long-stay geriatrics/n = 61	9-day dietary record	1360 (SD 310) 1560 (SD 230) (M) 1280 (SD 310) (F)	58 (17en%) 66 (17en%) (M) 54 (17en%) (F)	More than 50% of patients had low intakes of vitamins D, C, B$_{12}$ and Fe
Jones et al., 1988, UK	Long-stay geriatrics/n = 90	Weighed food intake/ vitamin C analysis	745	29	Low intakes of vitamin C and fibre
Klipstein-Grobusch et al., 1995, UK	Elderly patients with acute illness (8 M, 12 F, mean 82, SD 5 years, mean BMI 21.4, SD 4.7	2–3-day weighed food intake 3 times between admission and 28 days	1145 (SD 357)	–	Low intake of various vitamins, especially vitamin C
McCargar et al., 1995, Canada	Chronic-care geriatrics (3 M, 29 F, mean 84 years) in 2 centres	3-day dietary record	1610 (SE 68) (F)	66 (SE 4.4) (F)	Low fibre intake
Sullivan et al., 1999, USA	Elderly patients/n = 497	Patient observations and records	1430 (SD 547)	0.34 g kg⁻¹ IBW (SD 0.18) (low intake; n = 102) 0.92 g kg⁻¹ IBW (SD 0.26) (others: n 395)	–

IBW, ideal body weight. For other abbreviations, see Table A2.1.

Table A2.4. Food intake in the elderly living in the community (residential and nursing homes and receiving nursing care at home).

Investigator	Type of patients/n	Assessment method	Energy intake (kcal day⁻¹)	Protein intake (g day⁻¹)	Other nutrient intake
Eastwood *et al.*, 2001, UK Abstract	Institutionalized elderly (15 M, 27 F, mean 84 years) Free-living controls (21 M, 29 F, mean 74 years) BMI N/R	4-day weighed food intake	1550 (SD 500) 1833 (SD 430)	14.4 en% (SD 2.3) 15.5 en% (SD 3.3)	Low intakes of NSP in institutionalized group
Hollis and Henry, 2001, UK Abstract	Healthy geriatric residents (7 M, 13 F, mean approx. 83 years) in a residential care home, BMI N/R	7-day weighed food intake	1140 (SD 85) (M) 985 (SD 190) (F)	32.6 (SD 8.2) (F) 39.7 (SD 4.3) (M)	Low intakes of vitamins and trace elements
Lasheras *et al.*, 1999, Spain	Nursing home (NH) residents (49 M, 112 F, mean 80.4 years, BMI approx. 25.7) Elderly living at home (85 M, 106 F, mean 72 years, BMI approx. 28.5)	Food-frequency questionnaire	2095 (SD 345) (M, NH) 1895 (SD 335) (M, home) 1900 (SD 290) (F, NH) 1620 (SD 80) (F, home)	67.8 (SD 14.1) (M, NH) 63.5 (SD 13.6) (M, home) 62.2 (SD 9.8) (F, NH) 58.6 (SD 12.9) (F, home)	Low intakes of vitamins A, C and D in many subjects
Lengyel *et al.*, 2001, Canada Abstract	Geriatric residents (17 M, 31 F, mean 88 years, BMI N/R) in 5 long-term care facilities	3-day dietary record	1500	–	Low intakes of Mg, trace elements, vitamins and fibre
Lewis *et al.*, 1993	Elderly with venous leg ulcers in the community (5 M, 15 F, mean 76, range 65–86 years, BMI 29, SD 1.12)	Diet history and 5-day dietary record	1190 (SD 229)	56.1 (SD 4.5) (19 en%)	Mean Zn and vitamin C intakes were low; Fe intake and protein quality of concern
Johnson *et al.*, 1995, USA	Nursing home residents > 65 years (51 F, 31 regular diet, 20 puréed diet), age/BMI N/R	7-day observation of foods consumed	2155 (regular) 1785 (puréed)	88 (regular) 78 (puréed)	Many had low intakes of Fe, Zn, Ca and vitamin D
Persson *et al.*, 2000a, Sweden	Weight-stable geriatric residents (13 M, 18 F, mean 86 years) in 5 nursing homes, BMI N/R	7-day dietary record	1730 (SD 310)	–	–

Continued

Table A2.4. *Continued*

Investigator	Type of patients/*n*	Assessment method	Energy intake (kcal day^{-1})	Protein intake (g day^{-1})	Other nutrient intake
Van der Wielen *et al.*, 1996, Netherlands	Nursing-home residents (40 F, mean 81.5, SD 7.1 years, BMI N/R)	Modified dietary history method	1550 (SD 285)	–	Low intake of vitamins B$_1$, B$_2$, B$_6$ and C in many nursing home residents
	Admission to nursing home (10 M, 11 F, approx. 80 years, BMI N/R)		2095 (SD 525)		
	Sedentary free-living elderly (52 M, 68 F, approx. 77 years, BMI approx. 27)		2095 (SD 595)		
	Active free-living elderly (34 M, 32 F, approx. 76 years, BMI approx. 24.7)		2405 (SD 550)		

NH, nursing home; NSP, non-starch polysaccharide. For other abbreviations, see Table A2.1.

Table A2.5. Food intake in elderly living at home and in sheltered accommodation.

Investigator	Type of patients/*n*	Assessment method	Energy intake (kcal day^{-1})	Protein intake (g day^{-1})	Other nutrient intake
Beck *et al.*, 2001a, Denmark	Elderly at home (GP contact) (18 M, 43 F, age 71–81 years, BMI 18–25.5)	4-day dietary record	1810 (1545–2310) (at risk) 1975 (1645–2285) (WN)	–	–
Caughey *et al.*, 1994b, UK	Elderly in sheltered accommodation (54 M, mean 73, range 65–89 years; 160 F, mean 81, range 66–95 years)	24hr dietary recall	1939 (SD 500) (M) 1570 (SD 550) (F)	68.3 (SD 18.2) 57.6 (SD 18.2)	Low intakes of vitamins D and B$_6$ seen in > 60% of F and >70% of M
Charlton, 1997, UK	Elderly men > 70 years, free-living and sheltered accommodation (*n* 66, mean 78.9, range 70–93 years, BMI 24.4, SD 4.0)	Semi-quantified food-frequency questionnaire	2165 (SD 550)	84.9 (SD 20.7) (15.7en%)	Low intakes of NSP and vitamin D
De Jong *et al.*, 1998, Netherlands Abstract	Frail elderly (35 M, 110 F, age/BMI N/R)	3-day dietary record	2025 (men) 1640 (women)	–	–
Finch *et al.*, 1998, UK	Free-living elderly > 65 years (*n* 1275) and institutionalized elderly (*n* 412)	4-day weighed food intake (National Diet and Nutrition Survey)	1910 (M, FL) 1425 (F, FL) 1655 (I, teeth) 1685 (I, no teeth)	16.1 en% (M, FL) 16.5 en% (F, FL)	Low intakes of vitamins D and K and Mg often reported
Gretebeck and Boileau, 1998, USA	Healthy weight-stable elderly (8 F, mean 68, SD 5 years, 64.9, SD 8.6 kg)	7-day dietary record with daily review by investigator	1600 (SD 136)	–	–
Inelmen *et al.*, 2000, Italy	Healthy elderly aged 70–75 years (97 M, 93 F)	Modified dietary history method	2210 (SD 560) (M) 1740 (SD 525) (F)	71 (SD 20.3) (M) 13 (SD 2.1) en% 59.9 (SD 20.9) (F) 14 (SD 2.4) en%	A high proportion had Ca intakes lower than recommendations. Fe intakes were low in 20% of M and 47% of F. Low intakes of vitamins B$_1$, B$_2$, C and A were reported in a smaller number of subjects

Continued

Table A2.5. *Continued*

Investigator	Type of patients/*n*	Assessment method	Energy intake (kcal day⁻¹)	Protein intake (g day⁻¹)	Other nutrient intake
Klipstein-Grobusch *et al.*, 1999, UK	Healthy elderly (2225 M, mean 67, range 55–93 years; 3029 F, mean 68, range 55–94 years)	Semi-quantitative food-frequency questionnaire	2310 (SD 545) (55–64 years) 2215 (SD 500) (65–74 years) 2120 (SD 405) (75–84 years) 2165 (SD 450) (85–95 years)	93.3 (SD 22.1) 86.2 (SD 18.4) 82 (SD 19.1) 82.4 (SD 17.4)	Men showed a general decline in energy and nutrient intake with age. This trend was not seen in women to the same extent
Lumbers *et al.*, 1998, UK Abstract	Healthy elderly (15 F, age/BMI N/R)	Four 24 h dietary recalls	1610 (SD 286)	67.7 (SD 22.2) (16.8 en%)	Mg, Se and Zn intakes borderline
Mowé *et al.*, 1994, Norway	Elderly > 70 years Hospital (31 M, 45 F) Home (48 M, 47 F) Mean age/BMI N/R	Semi-structured interview of usual intake at home	2475 (SD 835) (M, home) 1810 (SD 525) (M, hosp.) 1740 (SD 430) (F, home) 1690 (SD 570) (F, hosp.)	–	Men in hospital had significantly lower intakes of vitamins A, D, niacin and Fe than home group. No differences seen in F
Nicolas *et al.*, 2000, France	Healthy elderly (2 M, mean 72.6 SD kg; 73 F, mean 60.1, SD 9.3 kg, age > 55 years), 4-year follow-up (18 M, 64 F)	3-day partially weighed food record, checked by dietitian	2140 (SD 250) (M) 1730 (SD 345) (F) 2070 (SD 400) (M) 1735 (SD 350) (F)	17.5 (SD 3.8) en% (M) 18.3 (SD 3.1) en% (F) 17.1 (SD 3.1) en% (M) 17.7 (SD 2.8) en% (F)	Intakes of Ca, Zn, vitamins A, B₁, B₂, B₆ and folate lower than recommendations
Rea *et al.*, 1998, UK Abstract	Elderly > 70 years (including 55 > 90 years), free-living (26 M, 79F, mean age/BMI N/R)	24 h dietary questionnaire	1540	55 (14.3) en%	Poor intake of some micronutrients in some subjects, particularly vitamins D, C, folate and Ca
Saini *et al.*, 1998, UK Abstract	Elderly (11 M, 22 F, mean approx. 75 years)	3-day dietary record	1645 (SD 226) (M) 1475 (SD 179) (F)	64.1 (SD 8) (M) (15.6 en%) 57.8 (SD 10.7) (F) (15.7 en%)	Mean vitamin D and NSP intakes low; Ca borderline

FL, free-living; GP, general practitioner; I, institutionalized; NSP, non-starch polysaccharide; WN, well nourished. For other abbreviations, see Table A2.1

Table A2.6. Food intake in patients with chronic obstructive pulmonary disease (COPD).

Investigator	Type of patients/n	Assessment method	Energy intake (kcal day^{-1})	Protein intake (g day^{-1})	Other nutrient intake
Community					
Baarends *et al.,* 1997, Netherlands Abstract	COPD (emphysema, 32 M, 11 F, age N/R; chronic bronchitis, 37 M, 6 F, age N/R)	Dietary history	1970 (SD 560) (E) 2115 (SD 530) (CB) (NS)	–	–
Schols *et al.,* 1999, Netherlands	COPD, admitted to a pulmonary rehabilitation centre (emphysema, 27 M; 67 SD 8 years; chronic bronchitis, 15 M; 67 SD 5 years)	Cross-checked dietary history	2145 (SD 536) (E) 1805 (SD 533) (CB) (*P* = 0.055)	–	–
Tang *et al.,* 2002, Hong Kong	COPD, admitted to a pulmonary rehabilitation programme (10 F, mean 74, SD 9 years)	Dietary record (period not specified)	1150 (SD 360)	–	–
Hospital					
Thorsdottir and Gunnarsdottir, 2002, Iceland	COPD, admitted to hospital for acute exacerbation (4 M, 6 F, mean 72, range 62–89 years)	4-day weighed food intake from day 4 of admission	Median 1820 (IQR 1560–1995) Median 27 kcal kg^{-1}	Median 90 (IQR 76–98)	–

CB, chronic bronchitis; E, emphysema; IQR, interquartile range; NS, no significant difference. For other abbreviations, see Table A2.1.

Table A2.7. Food intake in patients with gastrointestinal or liver disease.

Investigator	Type of patients/n	Assessment method	Energy intake (kcal day^{-1})	Protein intake (g day^{-1})	Other nutrient intake
Gastrointestinal disease, community					
Geerling *et al.*, 1998a, Netherlands	Long-standing CD with small-bowel involvement (> 10 years) (14 M, 18 F, mean 40, IQR 34.3–54 years, BMI 23.3, SD 3.7) Healthy controls (*n* 32, age- and sex-matched)	Cross-checked dietary history	2665 (SD 835) (CD) 2450 (SD 880) (control)	14.4 (SD 3.0) en% 15.9 (SD 3.3) en%	Poor intake of many nutrients in both CD and controls. Fibre and P intakes significantly lower in CD compared with controls
Geerling *et al.*, 2000a, Netherlands	Recently diagnosed IBD (within 6 months) CD (8 M, 15 F, mean 30.1, SD 10.2 years, BMI 22.2, SD 2.7) UC (25 M, 21 F, mean 37.8, SD 14.7 years, BMI 23.1, SD 3) Healthy controls (*n* 69, age- and sex-matched)	Cross-checked dietary history	2620 (SD 810) (CD) 2570 (SD 835) (control) 2450 (SD 620) (UC) 2450 (SD 835) (control)	14.7 (SD 2.2) en% 14.7 (SD 2.8) en% 14.8 (SD 2.5) en% 16.1 (SD 2.8) en%	Protein, Ca, P and vitamin B$_2$ intakes significantly lower in UC compared with controls
Gastrointestinal disease, community and hospital					
Rigaud *et al.*, 1994, France	CD, no malabsorption Wt loss > 10% in 3 months (13 M, 17 F, mean 32, SD 8 years, BMI 19.1, SD 2) Stable wt (17 M, 16 F, mean 35, SD 10 years, BMI 20.9, SD 3)	Dietary history (intake at home) 7-day weighed food intake (hospital)	Wt loss, home: 2135 (SD 500) Wt loss, hosp.: 1680 (SD 350) Stable, home: 2635 (SD 435) Stable, hosp.: 2220 (SD 540) (WL vs. WS: *P* < 0.01)	71.9 (SD 16) 61.5 (SD 15) 88.6 (SD 18) 79.6 (SD 19) (WL vs. WS: *P* < 0.01)	–
Liver disease, awaiting liver transplant, community					
Davidson *et al.*, 1999, UK	Biliary cirrhosis (3 M, 31 F, mean 57.7, SE 1.6 years) Hepatocellular cirrhosis (22 M, 9 F, mean 51.2, SE 1.7 years) Healthy subjects (9 M, 9 F, mean 50.2, SE 2.7 years)	3-day dietary record	1665 (SD 95) (BC) 1550 (SD 95) (HC) 2145 (SD 120) (control)	–	–

			Energy intake	Protein intake	Comments
Jackson *et al.*, 1996, UK Abstract	Chronic liver disease (20 M, 21 F, mean 51, range 17–65 years)	Dietary history	1745	—	—
McCollum, 2000, UK Abstract	Stable chronic liver disease (CLD) assessed for liver transplant/*n* 7 Healthy subjects/*n* 5 Age/sex/BMI N/R	1 day weighed intake	1700 (SD 350) (CLD) 2660 (SD 265) (control)	—	—
Richardson *et al.*, 2001, UK	Liver transplant waiting-list (PBC 13, HC 10, 10 M, 13 F, mean 53.9, SD 1.9 years)	3-day dietary record	1540 (SE 124)	60.3 (SE 5.6)	—
Liver disease, community					
Thuluvath and Triger, 1994, USA	Stable PBC (11 F) Controls (5 F) Age/BMI N/R	1 week assessment (no details)	1490 (SD 380) 1483 (SD 540)	62 (SD 18) 72 (SD 23)	—
Liver disease, hospital					
Nielsen *et al.*, 1993, Denmark	Stable alcoholic liver cirrhosis (26 M, 11 F, median 46, range 31–82 years)	24 h dietary recall	Median 1690 (1190–3000)	Median 54 (14–101)	Low median intakes of Mg, Zn, vitamins B_1, D, E and folate

BC, biliary cirrhosis; CD, Crohn's disease; CLD, chronic liver disease; HC, hepatocellular cirrhosis; IBD, inflammatory bowel disease; PBC, primary biliary cirrhosis; UC, ulcerative colitis; WL, weight-losing; WS, weight-stable. For other abbreviations, see Table A2.1.

Table A2.8. Food intake in patients with human immunodeficiency virus (HIV) infection and acquired immune deficiency syndrome (AIDS).

Investigator	Type of patients/n	Assessment method	Energy intake (kcal day^{-1})	Protein intake (g day^{-1})	Other nutrient intake
Community					
Beaugerie *et al.*, 1998, France	HIV infection with chronic diarrhoea, median duration of diarrhoea 8 (1–133) months (109 M, 7 F, mean 32, SD 8 years)	2-day dietary record (2 days prior to hospitalization for investigation of chronic diarrhoea)	25.2 (8.1) kcal kg^{-1} UBW (range 9.7–54.7)	61 (22.1) (range 15–165)	–
Dowling *et al.*, 1990, Ireland	Clinically stable HIV infection (CDC II, 15 M, 2 F, median 27 years) and AIDS (CDC IV, 15 M, 2 F, median 29 years)	7-day dietary history Out-patients	2855 (1260) (II) 2475 (1120) (IV)	94 (35) (II) 75 (37) (IV)	Average intakes of micronutrients assessed were adequate
Dworkin *et al.*, 1990, USA	Clinically stable HIV infection (9 M, 4 F, mean 34.5, SD 7.5 years), ARC (6 M, 6 F, mean 36.3, SD 10 years), AIDS (14 M, 4 F, mean 34.2, SD 5.7 years)	3-day dietary record (all out-patients except 7 AIDS patients)	31.9 (17.7) kcal kg^{-1} (HIV) 34.6 (7.8) kcal kg^{-1} (ARC) 39.1 (13.2) (AIDS) kcal kg^{-1} (NS)	1.4 (0.6) g kg^{-1} (HIV) 1.5 (0.5) g kg^{-1} (ARC) 1.9 (1.0) g kg^{-1} (AIDS) (NS)	Almost 90% of all patients had deficient intake of at least one micronutrient
Foskett *et al.*, 1991, UK	Clinically stable HIV infection and AIDS (11 M), CDC classification: II (n 1), III; (n 1), IV (n 9)	7-day weighed food intake	2570 (SE 120)	91.9 (SE 5.5)	–
Hogg *et al.*, 1995, Canada	Clinically stable HIV infection, AIDS-free (139 M, median 38 years)	24 h recall questionnaire	Median 2200	Median 94	–
Keithley *et al.*, 1992, USA	HIV infection and AIDS (33 M, mean 35 years), modified WR staging (I: n 9, II: n 13, III: n 9, IV: n 2)	4-day dietary record	2900 (580) (I) 2370 (990) (II) 2355 (55) (III) 1795 (n 1) (IV)	114 (21) (I) 98 (46) (II) 93 (9) (III) 73 (n 1) (IV)	100% of all subjects had deficient intake of at least one nutrient
Kim *et al.*, 2001, USA	HIV infection (44%) and AIDS (56%) (463 M, mean 39, SD 7.6 years; 61% AIDS; 170 F, mean 37, SD 7 years, 44% AIDS)	3-day dietary record	37.5% failed to meet RDA	11% failed to meet RDA	42% failed to meet RDA for Zn, 52% failed to meet RDA for vitamin A

Continued

Reference	Subjects	Method	Energy intake	Protein intake	Comments
Luder *et al.*, 1995, USA	HIV infection (*n* 16), ARC (*n* 23) and AIDS (*n* 17) (47 M, 9 F, mean age approx. 40 years)	3-day dietary record	1935 (587) (WS) 26 (8) kcal kg⁻¹ 2040 (575) (WL) 32 (10) kcal kg⁻¹ ($P = 0.02$) Mean 74% of RDA	80 (32) (WS) 1.1 (0.4) g kg⁻¹ 83 (29) (WL) 1.3 (0.5) g kg⁻¹ ($P = 0.02$)	Large proportions of patients had intakes of vitamin B₆, Mg, Zn and/or Cu < 90% of RDA. 84% took micronutrient supplements (2–50,000% of RDA)
Ockenga *et al.*, 1997, Germany Abstract	Clinically stable asymptomatic HIV infection (CDC I: *n* 26; II: *n* 14; III: *n* 30), mean 38, SD 10 years, sex N/R	7-day dietary record	2430 (622) 2700 (511) (I) 40 (12) kcal kg⁻¹ (I) 2330 (470) (II) 35 (7) kcal kg⁻¹ (II) 2285 (650) (III) 39 (11) kcal kg⁻¹ (III) (NS)	—	Intake of at least one micronutrient (vitamins A, D, E, C, B₁, B₂, B₆, folate, Se and Zn) was < 50% of RDA in 91% and of at least three micronutrients 50% in 35%
Parisien *et al.*, 1993, Canada	Asymptomatic (11 M, mean 34.2, SD 6.4 years) and symptomatic (9 M, mean 35.6, SD 8.6 years) HIV infection and clinically stable AIDS (17 M, mean 32.1, SD 5.2 years)	7-day dietary record	2500 (330) (AS) 36 kcal kg⁻¹ 2060 (346) (S) 29 kcal kg⁻¹ 2155 (395) (AIDS) 33 kcal kg⁻¹ ($P < 0.05$)	98 (AS) 1.4 (0.2) g kg⁻¹ 85 (S) 1.2 (0.4) g kg⁻¹ 89 (AIDS) 1.4 (0.3) g kg⁻¹	—
Sharkey *et al.*, 1992, Canada	Clinically stable HIV infection and AIDS (28 M), CDC classification II–IV Mean approx. 73 kg, age N/R HIV-negative controls (8 M, mean approx. 79 kg, age N/R)	7-day weighed food record (*n* 21) or food-frequency questionnaire (*n* 6)	2715 (SE 145) (HIV+) 2550 (SE 190) (HIV−)	94 (SE 6) (HIV+) 97 (SE 7) (HIV−)	Average intakes of micronutrients assessed were adequate
Smit *et al.*, 1996, USA	Clinically stable HIV infection (*n* 41) and AIDS (*n* 4) (32 M, 13 F, mean 37.8, SD 4.6 years). All injecting drug users	24 h dietary recall	3305 (1340)	132 (66)	Low intakes of fibre, vitamins A and E, Ca and Zn reported

Table A2.8. *Continued*

Investigator	Type of patients/n	Assessment method	Energy intake (kcal day⁻¹)	Protein intake (g day⁻¹)	Other nutrient intake
Woods *et al.*, 2002, USA	HIV infection (386 M, mean 40, SD 7.6 years; 130 F, mean 38, SD 7.4 years)	3-day dietary record and semi-quantitative food-frequency questionnaire	Median (IQR) CD4 < 200 2935 (2350–3470) (M) 40.3 (33.7–47.9) kcal kg⁻¹ 1880 (1500–2585) (F) 30 (24.3–46) kcal kg⁻¹ CD4 200–499 2835 (2320–3230) (M) 36.9 (29.3–44.7) kcal kg⁻¹ 2135 (1565–2635) (F) 31 (21.8–40) kcal kg⁻¹ CD4 > 500 2815 (2470–3500) (M) 36 (29.5–43.9) kcal kg⁻¹ 2081 (1370–2620) (F) 29.4 (18.1–37.1) kcal kg⁻¹ (*P* = 0.001; M, kcal kg⁻¹)	Median (IQR) M/F CD4 < 200 1.5 (1.1–1.9) kcal kg⁻¹ 1.1 (0.9–1.5) kcal kg⁻¹ CD4 200–499 1.3 (1.1–1.6) kcal kg⁻¹ 1.0 (0.79–1.5) kcal kg⁻¹ CD4 > 500 1.4 (1.1–1.8) kcal kg⁻¹ 1.0 (0.6–1.5) kcal kg⁻¹	Poor intakes (< 75% of DRI) of several micronutrients noted, particularly in women, and especially for folate, vitamins A and C, Fe and Zn
Hospital Trujillo *et al.*, 1992, USA	AIDS (*n* 48; mean 35.7, SE 1.0 years, sex N/R)	Daily food record	1100 (SE 85) (range 455–2020)	53 (SE 4.1) (range 25–100)	

ARC, AIDS-related complex; AS, asymptomatic; CDC II–IV, Centers for Disease Control classification (higher class indicates more advanced disease); DRI, dietary reference intake; HIV+, HIV positive; HIV–, HIV negative; IQR, interquartile range; NS, no significant difference; RDA, recommended daily allowance; S, symptomatic; WL, weight-losing; WR I–IV, Walter Reed classification (higher class indicates more advanced disease); WS, weight-stable; UBW, usual body weight. For other abbreviations, see Table A2.1.

Table A2.9. Food intake in patients with malignancy.

Investigator	Type of patients/*n*	Assessment method	Energy intake (kcal day^{-1})	Protein intake (g day^{-1})	Other nutrient intake
Community Bosaeus *et al.,* 2001, Sweden	Unselected cancer patients, solid tumours (160 M, 137 F, mean age 67 years, range 30–90 years)	4-day dietary record	1715 (627) Range 250–4650 26 (10) kcal kg^{-1} Range 4–77 kcal kg^{-1} 1915 (650) (M) 1480 (515) (F)	66 (24) Range 17–197 0.99 (0.39) g kg^{-1} Range 0.2–3.1 g kg^{-1} 73 (26) (M) 58 (18) (F)	–
Broadhead *et al.,* 2001a, UK Abstract	Oral and pharyngeal cancer prior to/during radiotherapy (14 M, 3 F, mean 63, range 38–89 years)	4-day retrospective food-frequency questionnaire	1900 (pretreatment) 1350 (after 3 weeks) 1435 (after 6 weeks)	75.7 (pretreatment) 50.4 (after 3 weeks) 60.3 (after 6 weeks)	Fibre intake decreased from 13.4 g day^{-1} prior to treatment to 6.5 g day^{-1} after 6 weeks
Choileáin *et al.,* 1995, Ireland Abstract	Head and neck cancer patients undergoing radiotherapy (*n* 38, age/sex/BMI N/R)	7-day dietary history 5 times over 2 months (baseline data presented)	29.5 kcal kg^{-1}	0.91 g kg^{-1}	–
Jagoe *et al.,* 2001a, UK	Lung cancer, prior to admission for surgery (*n* 47, age/sex/BMI N/R)	5-day dietary record	2025 (880–3000) (30% had low energy intake)	74.1 (35.9–143.8) (13% had low protein intake)	62% had reduced vitamin C intake (only micronutrient measured)
Macqueen and Frost, 1998, UK	Newly diagnosed squamous-cell carcinoma prior to and during radiotherapy (larynx, 9 M, 1 F; pharynx, 5 M, 5 F, mean 64, range 48–81 years)	3-day dietary record	2620 (larynx, pre) 2405 (larynx, end) 2255 (pharynx, pre) 875 (pharynx, end)	–	Energy intake reflected the pattern of intake of each nutrient
Ovesen *et al.,* 1991, Denmark	Patients with cancer of ovary, breast or lung before and after 1 and 3 chemotherapy cycles (16 M, 36 F, mean 57, range 22–75 years, mean 67.3, SD 12.5 kg)	3-day weighed food intake	1905 (SD 550) (start) 1975 (SD 570) (1 month) 1930 (SD 595) (3 months)	62 (SD 19) (start) 65 (SD 23) (1 month) 64 (SD 22) (3 months)	–
Pattison *et al.,* 1997a, UK Abstract	Advanced cancer, no active treatment (*n* 22) Age-matched geriatric controls (*n* 16), age/sex/BMI N/R	3-day weighed food intake	845 (SE 85) (cancer) 1405 (SE 93) (control)	16 en% 18 en%	–

Continued

Table A2.9. *Continued*

Investigator	Type of patients/n	Assessment method	Energy intake (kcal day^{-1})	Protein intake (g day^{-1})	Other nutrient intake
Staal-van den Brekel *et al.*, 1994, Netherlands	Newly diagnosed lung cancer (82 M, 18 F, mean 65, SD 9 years, mean 70.2, SD 14.3 kg)	Dietary history	2140 (SD 796) (central tumour) 1950 (SD 550) (peripheral tumour)	–	–
Hospital					
Holmes and Dickerson, 1991, UK	Cancer patients admitted to hospital (12 M, 16 F, age/BMI N/R)	3-day weighed food intake	1345 (SD 470)	46.9 (SD 19.4) (16 en%)	Mean folate and Fe intakes of concern
Levine and Morgan, 1994, UK Abstract	Cancer cachexia patients in hospital (5 M, 5 F, mean 55.3, SD 9.7 years, BMI 19, SD 3 kg m^{-2}) General medical controls (age/sex-matched, BMI 22, SD 2)	Choice of 200 foods; 3-day weighed food intake, chemical analysis	1425 (SD 690) (cancer) 26.2 (SD 1.9) kcal kg^{-1} 2310 (SD 595) (control) 38 (SD 1.9) kcal kg^{-1}	49 (SD 27) (14 en%) 0.9 (SD 0.4) g kg^{-1} 74 (SD 23) (13 en%) 1.2 (SD 0.3)	

For abbreviations, see Table A2.1.

Table A2.10. Food intake in neurology patients (stroke or dysphagia in hospital).

Investigator	Type of patients/*n*	Assessment method	Energy intake (kcal day^{-1})	Protein intake (g day^{-1})	Other nutrient intake
Brynes *et al.*, 1998, UK Abstract	Dysphagia requiring texture modified diet + supplements and/or NG feed (*n* 23, mean 82, range 57–98 years)	24 h weighed food intake	Median 865 (0–1900)	–	–
	Non-dysphagic elderly controls (*n* 27, mean 81, range 69–90 years)		Median 1055 (115–2500)	–	–
Gariballa *et al.*, 1998b, UK	Acute stroke without dysphagia (11 M, 10 F, mean 80, range 63–90 years, mean 57, SD 8.9 kg)	Daily dietary record by nurses/catering composition data	1085 (SD 345)	44.1 (SD 12.8) (16.3 en%)	–

en%, percentage of energy intake from protein; NG, nasogastric; SD, standard deviation.

Table A2.11. Food intake in orthopaedic patients.

Investigator	Type of patients/n	Assessment method	Energy intake (kcal day⁻¹)	Protein intake (g day⁻¹)	Other nutrient intake
Hospital					
Bachrach-Lindström et al., 2001, Sweden	Elderly women, FNF (13 F, mean approx. 84 years)	7-day dietary record 1 month after FNF	1325 (SD 500)	44.4 (SD 14.5)	–
Barton et al., 2000a, UK	Orthopaedics (FNF, THR, FF, hand surgery) Ward study: daily mean 21 patients Subgroup: 10 M, 6 F, mean 53, range 28–85 years	Calculated by difference from whole-ward food provision and wastage. Checked against 3-day weighed records in a subgroup	1450 (ward study) 1465 (SD 395) (subgroup)	43.6	–
Gegerie et al., 1986, Switzerland	Elderly women, FNF (n 16, mean 77 years)	Weighed food intake (total 50 daily balance studies)	1105	35	–
Jallut et al., 1990 Switzerland	Elderly women, FNF (20 F, mean 81, SD 4 years, mean 52.7, SD 7.5 years)	Weighed food intake/dietary record on days 3–8/9	1095 (SD 333)	38.1 (SD 16.6) (13.9 en%)	–
Lawson et al., 2000	Orthopaedic patients (9 M, 19 F, age/BMI N/R)	24 h food intake calculated 1 day every 2 weeks of entire study (mean 12 days after admission, range 3–37 days) by difference from food provision and wastage of meals. Snacks recorded separately	Med. 1290	52.2	–
Lumbers et al., 1998, UK Abstract	Elderly women, FNF (14 F, age/BMI N/R)	Four 24 h dietary recalls	870 (SD 342)	35.3 (SD 10.8) (16.2 en%)	Low intakes of Ca, Mg, Fe, Zn, Se
Lumbers et al., 2001, UK	Elderly women, FNF (75 F, mean 80.5, SD 8.2 years)	3-day 24 h dietary recalls with menu-card prompts	1020 (SD 300)	43 (SD 13)	Low intakes of vitamin B_6, folate Ca, Mg, Se, Zn and NSP
Murphy et al., 2000, UK	Elderly women, FNF (n 7) and THR (n 7) (mean 80, range 61–103 years)	3-day 24 h dietary recalls with menu-card prompts 5 days postop	Med. 1050 (CI 900–1070)	Med. 43 (CI 36–45)	Low median intakes of vitamins B_6, A, D, folate and Ca, Mg, K, Fe, Se, Zn, NSP

Older *et al.*, 1980, UK	Elderly women, FNF (19 F, mean 78 years)	3-day weighed food intake	1010 (day 3) 1040 (day 7) 1100 (day 14)	40.8 (day 3) 36.5 (day 7) 41.5 (day 14)	Low intakes of vitamins D, C, B_1, B_2 and niacin
Rehabilitation Paillaud *et al.*, 2000, France	Elderly, FNF (5 M, 35 F, mean 84, SE 1.9 years)	Energy and protein intakes recorded by dietitian after each meal for 5 days at each time point (0, 1 and 2 months) in rehabilitation unit	Group 1 (time 0 only *n* 7) 1860 (SE 50) Group 2 (0 and 1 month, *n* 13) 0: 1670 (SE 95) 1: 1810 (SE 140) Group 3 (0, 1 and 2 months) 0: 1405 (SE 95) 1: 1620 (SE 95) 2: 1715 (SE 70)	–	–

CI, confidence interval; FF, fracture of femur; FNF, fractured neck of femur; med., median; NSP, non-starch polysaccharide; THR, total hip replacement. For other abbreviations, see Table A2.1.

Table A2.12. Food intake in patients with renal disease.

Investigator	Type of patients/n	Assessment method	Energy intake (kcal day^{-1})	Protein intake (g day^{-1})	Other nutrient intake
Community					
Chazot et al., 2001, France	HD > 20 years (6 M, 4 F, mean 59.5 years, 53.3 kg) HD mean 51 months (6 M, 4 F, mean 58.6 years, 59.5 kg)	3-day food questionnaire	1865 (SD 520) (HD > 20 years) 35.1 (SD 8.3) kcal kg^{-1} ABW 27.7 (SD 5.2) kcal kg^{-1} IBW 1820 (SD 555) (HD < 20 years) 31 (SD 9.5) kcal kg^{-1} ABW 27.4 (SD 6.8) kcal kg^{-1} IBW	80.2 (SD 24.3) 1.53 (SD 0.48) g kg^{-1} ABW 1.20 (SD 0.3) g kg^{-1} IBW 70.4 (SD 20.6) 1.19 (SD 0.33) g kg^{-1} ABW 1.07 (SD 0.3) g kg^{-1} IBW	–
Cooper and Beaven, 1993, UK	HD (17 M, 10 F, mean 64, range 38–80 years, BMI N/R)	4-day dietary record	26.2 kcal kg^{-1} IBW	0.9 kg^{-1} IBW	–
Fraser et al., 1999, UK	HD (n 10, sex N/R, med. 60.5, range 30–75 years, med. BMI 23.5, range 19–35) Matched healthy controls (n 10, med. 50, range 22–71 years, med. BMI 22, range 19–30)	3-day dietary record	1640 (SD 285) (patients) 2400 (SD 535) (controls)	–	–
Lorenzo et al., 1995, Spain	HD, mean 68.2 range 6–200 months (28 M, 11 F, mean 48.9, range 10–74 years)	3-day dietary record (including 1 HD day)	26.8 (SD 11) kcal kg^{-1} ABW	1.02 (SD 0.4) g kg^{-1} ABW	Ca intake low
Hospital					
Sanders et al., 1991, USA	Chronic dialysis, hospitalized (HD, n 20; CAPD, n 2, 20 M, 2 F, mean approx. 56 years, mean approx. 70 kg)	2-week dietary record in hospital. Randomized to receive regular or renal (restricted) diet	1300 (SD 130) (reg.) 650 (SD 95) (renal)	58 (SD 4) (reg.) 31 (SD 4) (renal)	Reg: low intakes of vitamins D, B$_1$, C, folate, niacin and Ca Renal: low intakes of above plus vitamin B$_2$ and Fe

ABW, actual body weight; CAPD, continuous ambulatory peritoneal dialysis; HD, haemodialysis; IBW, ideal body weight; reg., regular diet. For other abbreviations, see Table A2.1.

Table A2.13. Food intake in surgical patients.

Investigator	Type of patients/n	Assessment method	Energy intake (kcal day^{-1})	Protein intake (g day^{-1})	Other nutrient intake
Hospital					
Barton et al., 2000a, UK	General surgical/n = 23 Ward study: daily mean 23 patients Subgroup: 6 M, 7 F, mean 66, range 35–76 years	Calculated by difference from whole ward food provision and wastage. Checked against 3-day weighed records in a subgroup	1350 (ward) 1415 (SD 415) (subgroup)	41	–
Jensen and Hessov, 1997, Denmark	Lower GI surgery, benign and malignant (n 87, age/sex N/R)	3-day dietary record plus interview just before discharge	25.7 kcal kg^{-1} (10.5–42.4)	0.9 g kg^{-1} (0.4–1.8) (14 en%)	–
Keele et al., 1997, UK	Moderate to major GI surgery, benign and malignant (23 M, 20 F, mean 60, range 19–86 years, mean wt 69.6, CI 4.3 kg)	7-day dietary record from day of resumption of oral intake	480 (day 5, n 43) 985 (day 6, n 42) 1240 (day 7, n 40) 1360 (day 8, n 31) 1420 (day 9, n 25) 1400 (day 10, n 17) 1425 (day 11, n 11)	13.4 31.1 41.9 46.3 48.9 47.7 45.5	–
Mancey-Jones et al., 1994, UK Abstract	Retrospective audit of GI surgical patients (n 490, age/sex N/R)	Nursing records	–	–	79% had restricted intake. 17% had restricted intake for > 7 days
Meguid et al., 1988, USA	Abdominal surgery, benign and malignant (n 464, range 16–90 years, sex N/R)	IONIP: number of days until patients began eating at least 60% of estimated energy requirements on 2 consecutive days	IONIP < 7 days: 28% IONIP 7–10 days: 17% IONIP > 10 days: 55%	–	–
Murphy, P.M. et al., 2001, UK Abstract	Post-oesophagogastrectomy for oesophageal cancer (9 M, 7 F, mean 61, SD 9 years, mean BMI 25.3)	Daily audit for 22 days postoperatively	Mean energy requirements were fully met on day 8 only, then dropped off to < 60% of requirements	–	–

Continued

Table A2.13. *Continued*

Investigator	Type of patients/n	Assessment method	Energy intake (kcal day⁻¹)	Protein intake (g day⁻¹)	Other nutrient intake
Rana *et al.*, 1992, UK	Moderate to major GI surgery, benign and malignant (13 M, 7 F, mean 64.5, SE 2.4 years, mean wt 66.1, SE 3 kg)	7-day dietary record from day of resumption of oral intake	885 (day 5, *n* 20) 905 (day 6, *n* 20) 1055 (day 7, *n* 20) 1190 (day 8, *n* 19) 1275 (day 9, *n* 17) 1220 (day 10, *n* 11) 1290 (day 11, *n* 9)	29.8 44.5 47.3 59.2 55.9 58.1 63.7	–
Trick, 2000, UK Abstract	Surgical patients (*n* 50, age/sex N/R)	24 h dietary recall 1 day preop. and twice postop. (3–5 days and 7–12 days)	–	–	Preop.: 76% failed to meet requirements Postop. d 3–5: 94% failed to meet requirements Postop. d 7–12: 82% failed to meet requirements
Community Maskell *et al.*, 1999, UK	Post-pancreatectomy, median 4 (1–30 months) (*n* 15, median 61, range 40–75 years, sex N/R)	7-day weighed food intake	Median 1914 (1154–2804) (median 88% of EAR)	Median 74 (48–117) (median 139% of EAR)	Low vitamin D and Se intake in some patients

CI, confidence interval; d, days; EAR, estimated average requirement; GI, gastrointestinal; IONIP, inadequate oral nutritional intake period. For other abbreviations, see Table A2.1.

Table A2.14. Food intake in paediatric patients.

Investigator	Type of patients/n	Assessment method	Energy intake (kcal day^{-1})	Protein intake (g day^{-1})	Other nutrient intake
Mixed diagnoses, hospital					
Hankard *et al.*, 2001, France (French)	Mixed: GM, GS and PS (*n* 58, > 6 months, age/sex N/R)	Part weighed/part questionnaire food record	Approx. 50 kcal kg^{-1} 66% had intakes below 75% of RDA	Approx. 2.0 g kg^{-1}	–
Cerebral palsy, community					
Dahl and Gebre-Medhin, 1993, Sweden	Cerebral palsy[a] (*n* 19) and MMC (*n* 12), mean approx. 8 years	3-day dietary record in rehabilitation centre	Only 2 (MMC) reached 100% of RDA, 20 had EI < 10th percentile of RDA	–	–
Thommessen *et al.*, 1991, Norway	Cerebral palsy (*n* 32, mean approx. 5.5, range 1–13 years)	4-day dietary record at home	6 had relative intakes of energy < 70% of RDA for age	–	–
Cystic fibrosis, community					
Anthony *et al.*, 1998, Australia	Cystic fibrosis (mild lung disease) (14 M, 11 F, mean 9.1, SD 1.2 years) Healthy siblings (12 M, 13 F, mean 9.8, SD 1.7 years)	7-day weighed food intake (combination of precise weighing and weighed inventory method) at home	2120 (SD 335) 74 (SD 14) kcal kg^{-1} 1950 (SD 260) 56 (SD 13) kcal kg^{-1}	–	–
Liver disease, community					
Chin *et al.*, 1992, Australia	ESLD awaiting liver transplant (9 M,18 F, med. 1.72, range 0.5–6.75 years)	3-day weighed food intake at home	Mean energy intake was 70% (SD 16) of RDI	–	Nutrient intake overall 70% of RDA for age
Malignancy, community					
Smith *et al.*, 1991, UK	Cancer (solid and haematological tumours) (52 M, 48 F, med. 5, range 0.3–16.5 years) Controls without sign. disease (31 M, 24 F, med. 4.2, range 0.3–16 years)	24 h parental diet recall for time preceding admission (62 patients and 23 controls)	Median intake as % RDA: 90 (18–140) % < 80% RDA: 44% Controls: 99 (70–123) % < 80% RDA: 4%	Median intake as % RDA: 107 (16–200) Controls: 146 (81–240)	–

Continued

Table A2.14. *Continued*

Investigator	Type of patients/n	Assessment method	Energy intake (kcal day⁻¹)	Protein intake (g day⁻¹)	Other nutrient intake
Malignancy, hospital					
Kurugöl et al., 1997, Turkey	Leukaemia, bone tumours and other tumours, remission (25) and active disease (20) (27 M, 18 F, mean 10.5, SD 5.4 years)	3-day dietary history in hospital	765 (SD 165) (R, 1–3 years) 540 (SD 25) (A, 1–3 years) 1220 (SD 470) (R, 4–6 years) 1110 (SD 465) (A, 4–6 years) 1475 (SD 300) (R, 7–10 years) 1095 (SD 710) (A, 7–10 years) 1535 (SD 365) (R, 11–14 years, M) 1440 (SD 150) (A, 11–14 years, M) 1820 (SD 130) (R, 11–14, F) 1780 (SD 100) (A, 11–14, F) 1570 (SD 170) (R, 15–18, M) 1330 (SD 625) (A 15–18, M) 1235 (SD 125) (R, 15–18 F) 1110 (SD 220) (A, 15–18, F) 95% consumed less energy than RDA	26.2 (SD 4.8) (R, 1–3 years) 15.3 (SD 3.4) (A, 1–3 years) 42.2 (SD 16.1) (R, 4–6 years) 36.3 (SD 8.0) (A, 4–6 years) 54.9 (SD 9.9) (R, 7–10 years) 36.3 (SD 28.2) (A, 7–10 years) 51.6 (SD 12.3) (R, 11–14 years, M) 48.9 (SD 5.2) (A, 11–14y, M) 55.0 (SD 1.0) (R, 11–14, F) 30.3 (SD 3.1) (A, 11–14, F) 48.4 (SD 20.8) (R, 15–18, M) 45.6 (SD 25.3) (A 15–18, M) 47.8 (SD 3.6) (R, 15–18 F) 39.9 (SD 4.3) (A, 15–18, F) 36% consumed less protein than RDA	High proportion of patients consumed low intakes of the micronutrients measured (vitamins A, C, B₁, B₂, niacin and Ca, Fe, Zn and Cu)
Renal disease, community					
Norman et al., 2000, UK	Chronic renal insufficiency (predialysis) (59 M, 36 F, age > 2 years)	3-day partially weighed dietary record at home	Energy intake in patients with normal GFR was 103% of EAR compared with 85% in children with severe CRI	2.3 g kg⁻¹ (normal GFR) 2.3 g kg⁻¹ (mild CRI) 2.2 g kg⁻¹ (moderate CRI) 2.0 g kg⁻¹ (severe CRI)	Ca and P intakes lowest in severe CRI. Mean Ca intake met RNI, but in some cases only reached 67% of RNI
Pereira et al., 2000, Brazil	ESRD (12 M, 18 F) (23 PD, 4 IPD, 19 CAPD, 7 HD, mean 9.3, SD 7.4 years)	3-day dietary record at home	90% had energy intakes < 100% of RDA	–	Dietary intake of water-soluble vitamins < 100% RDA in majority of children. All received one tablet day⁻¹ water-soluble vitamins, which resulted in intakes > RDA

ᵃOne subject received tube feeding.
A, active disease; CAPD, continuous ambulatory peritoneal dialysis; CRI, chronic renal insufficiency; EAR, estimated average requirement; EI, energy intake; ESLD, end-stage liver disease; ESRD, end-stage renal disease; GFR, glomerular filtration rate; GM, general medical; GS, general surgical; HD, haemodialysis; IPD, intermittent peritoneal dialysis; MMC, myelomeningocoele; N/R, not recorded; PD, peritoneal dialysis; PS, psychiatric; R, remission; RDA, recommended daily allowance; RDI, recommended dietary intake; RNI, reference nutrient intake; sign., significant; SD, standard deviation.

Appendix 3

A Detailed Analysis of the Effects of Oral Nutritional Supplements in the Hospital Setting

Chapter 6 provided an overall summary of the effects of oral nutritional supplements (ONS) obtained from a combined analysis of different groups of patients in the hospital setting. Here, a more detailed review is provided, according to individual patient groups.

Chronic Obstructive Pulmonary Disease (COPD)

COPD is a major cause of hospitalization, which is associated with high morbidity and mortality. The disorder is characterized by the presence of chronic and irreversible air-flow obstruction, typically associated with excess sputum production, breathlessness, fatigue, muscle wasting, recurring infections of the airways and anorexia. Nutritional intake is frequently compromised by the symptoms of COPD, which may limit the quantity of food ingested and may impair a patient's ability to prepare or to eat food. As a consequence, weight loss and deterioration in functional performance frequently occur in patients with COPD. More information on the prevalence of disease-related malnutrition (DRM) is given in Chapter 2. This section reviews the evidence of the effectiveness of ONS in the treatment of patients with COPD in hospital and does

not consider the studies of COPD patients in the community, which are addressed in Appendix 4.

COPD: present analysis

Of the two hospital-based randomized controlled trials (RCT) of ONS, one involved patients suffering from an acute exacerbation of COPD (Saudny-Unterberger et al., 1997) and the other patients during rehabilitation or recovery from an acute exacerbation (Schols et al., 1995) (total patient n 127). In both patient groups, ONS were well tolerated. Information on the ONS used is documented in Table A3.1[1], the study characteristics have been summarized in Table A3.2 and the main outcomes of ONS in Table A3.3. Each of the four review questions is addressed in turn, with a summary in Box A3.1.

(I) What effect do ONS have on the voluntary food intake and total energy intake of patients with COPD in hospital?

The studies reviewed suggest that ONS can significantly improve total energy and protein intakes in hospitalized COPD patients (Schols et al., 1995; Saudny-Unterberger et al., 1997). Specifically, in patients suffering from an acute exacerba-

> **Box A3.1.** Key findings: effect of ONS in hospital patients with COPD.
>
> Nutritional intake: ONS can improve total energy and protein intakes and may improve appetite and food intake.
>
> Body weight: use of ONS can lead to weight gain in COPD patients. Non-response to supplementation may be due to the presence of an elevated inflammatory response.
>
> Body function: functional benefits include ventilatory function, respiratory muscle strength and walking distances and can occur in patient groups with a body mass index (BMI) < 20 kg m^{-2} or > 20 kg m^{-2}. There are no apparent detriments of using ONS in hospitalized COPD patients.
>
> Clinical and financial outcome: the effects of ONS on clinical outcome and cost efficacy have yet to be assessed in this patient group.

tion of COPD (BMI > 20 kg m^{-2}), a combination of commercial liquid sip feeds and puddings, plus food snacks, significantly improved energy and protein intakes when expressed as a function of body weight (+ 10 kcal kg^{-1} and + 0.35 g kg^{-1} protein daily) compared with an unsupplemented group (Saudny-Unterberger *et al.*, 1997; see Table A3.3). Although the quantity of ONS prescribed and consumed was undocumented, the total energy and protein intake in supplemented patients exceeded that of unsupplemented patients by 355 kcal and 10 g, respectively. In a separate 8-week in-patient rehabilitation programme, stable patients with COPD were presented with an energy-dense ONS (420 kcal and 15 g protein day^{-1}, 2.1 kcal ml^{-1}) and encouraged to eat normal food. Total energy intake was significantly increased in both depleted and non-depleted patients, who were ~84% and ~102% of their ideal body weight (IBW), respectively (see Table A3.3; Schols *et al.*, 1995; see Fig. 6.5 in Chapter 6). On average, ONS increased total energy intake by 428 kcal (114% of ONS energy, method (ii) Chapter 5) in the depleted patient group and by 620 kcal (161% of ONS energy, method (ii) Chapter 5) in the non-depleted group. Hence, the voluntary food intake in both depleted and non-depleted supplemented COPD patients was greater than in unsupplemented patients, raising the possibility that supplementation may have stimulated appetite and food intake. A similar increase in food intake and total energy intake was observed in a further group of patients receiving an ONS in combination with 25–50 mg of nandrolone decanoate given on four occasions during the study. Checks of compliance with ONS were made in both trials using daily food records.

Although the intake of other nutrients (vitamins, minerals, etc.) was not reported in either of the trials reviewed, the ONS used in these trials were nutritionally complete (e.g. Nutridrink, Ensure Plus), and so it is likely that intakes of micronutrients were also improved.

(II) What effect do ONS have on the body weight and composition of patients with COPD in hospital?

The existing information indicates that ONS of hospitalized COPD patients can aid body-weight gain. Combined analysis of data from the two hospital trials reviewed (total *n* 159) (Schols *et al.*, 1995; Saudny-Unterberger *et al.*, 1997) indicated a mean % weight change (weighted for sample size) in supplemented patients of + 2.9% compared with 0% in unsupplemented groups of patients. Meta-analysis was not undertaken due to limited data. Specifically, patients with stable or an acute exacerbation of COPD who were taking an ONS gained small amounts of weight, whereas unsup-

Table A3.1.[1] Oral nutritional supplements used in randomized controlled trials of patients with COPD in hospital.

Trial	ONS	ONS energy density (kcal ml^{-1})	ONS prescribed	ONS energy (kcal) intake	ONS protein (g) intake	Toleration
Saudny-Unterberger et al. (1997)	Ensure Ensure Plus (Abbott) Puddings and snacks	1 1.5 –	To meet requirements of 1.5 × REE or 1.7 × REE (BMI < 20)	–	–	No side-effects (breathlessness or GI discomfort)
Schols et al. (1995)	Mixture of Nutridrink, Protifar, Fantomalt, oil (seven mixtures of different flavours); 14% P, 35% CHO, 51% F	2.1	420 kcal, ~15 g P	Depleted S^1 375 S^2 378 Non-depleted S^1 389 S^2 399	Depleted S^1 ~13 S^2 ~13.5 Non-depleted S^1 ~13.9 S^2 ~14.3	Well tolerated

S^2 received the same ONS as S^1, with the addition of steroid injections.

BMI, body mass index; CHO, carbohydrate; F, fat; GI, gastrointestinal; P, protein; REE, resting energy expenditure; S, supplemented.

Table A3.2. Trial characteristics: hospital-based randomized controlled trials of oral nutritional supplementation in COPD patients.

Trial and patient group	Design	No. S	No. US	Initial BMI S group	Initial BMI US group	Duration of ONS	Dietary counselling	Control group
Saudny-Unterberger et al. (1997) Acutely ill COPD	10001	14	10	23.4	25.7	2 weeks (cont. at home if discharged)	Received food snacks or ONS	Hospital diet
Schols et al. (1995) In-patient pulmonary rehab. programme (not in hospital)	10001	S^1 33 S^2 32 ONS + steroids[a]	38[b]	No data. Trial included depleted (av. 84% IBW) and non-depleted patients (av. 102% IBW)		8 weeks minimum	All encouraged to eat regular meals	Normal meals Pulmonary rehabilitation programme

[a] S^2 received 25–50 mg nandrolone decanoate injected intramuscularly on days 1, 15, 29, 43.

[b] US group received placebo injection intramuscularly on days 1, 15, 29, 43 (control for steroid).

av., average; BMI, body mass index; cont., continued; IBW, ideal body weight; rehab., rehabilitation; S, supplemented; US, unsupplemented.

Table A3.3. Main findings of randomized controlled trials of oral nutritional supplementation in hospitalized COPD patients.

Trial	Energy/protein intake	Wt change S	Wt change US	Function	Outcome	Finance
Saudny-Unterberger et al. (1997)	TEI (kcal kg^{-1} day^{-1}): S 39 (2) kcal kg^{-1} day^{-1}, US 29 (3) kcal kg^{-1} day^{-1} (S vs. US $P < 0.004$) TEI (kcal, US weighed more than S) S 2370 (125) kcal US 2015 (105) kcal (S vs. US $P < 0.052$) TPI (g kg^{-1} day^{-1}) S 1.54 (0.1) g, US 1.19 (0.11) g ($P < 0.025$) TPI (g) S 94 (6) g, US 84 (6) g (NS)	+0.21 (0.68) kg or +0.29 (0.93) % (S vs. US NS)	−0.08 (0.2) kg or −0.13 (0.32)%	FEV$_1$ (% predicted, pulmonary function): NS change in S (+4.6) or US (−1.5) (S vs. US NS) FVC (% pred.): sig. improvement in S (+8.7) vs. US (−3.5) (S vs. US sig.) $P_I$max, $P_E$max (respiratory muscle strength): NS change in S (S vs. US NS, n too small) Hand-grip strength: no sig. changes Breathlessness: improved sig. in S (+13.7 mm) and NS in US (+7.7), (S vs. US NS) Well-being: improved sig. in S (+12) vs. US (−10), (S vs. US $P < 0.066$) Walking distance: NS increase in S (252 m) or US (200 m), (S vs. US NS)	–	–
Schols et al. (1995)	**Depleted group:** S^1 1990 (450) kcal (TEI 2365, 174% REE) S^2 2000 (370) kcal (TEI 2378, 168% REE) (S vs. US sig.) US 1937 (420) kcal (144% REE) S^1 % ONS energy 114% additive S^2 % ONS energy 117% additive **Non-depleted group:** S^1 2083 (410) kcal (TEI 2472, 156% REE) S^2 2076 (389) kcal (TEI 2475, 158% REE) (S vs. US sig.) US 1846 (380) kcal (119% REE) S^1 % ONS energy 161% additive S^2 % ONS energy 158% additive TEI for S$^{(1 + 2)}$ 170% REE, US 57% (sig.)	**Non-depleted** S^1 +1.1 (2.4) kg (sig.) (1.56 (3.40)%) S^2 +1.2 (2.7) kg (sig.) (1.77 (3.98)%) (S$^{(1 + 2)}$ vs. US sig.) FFM S^1 +0.5 (3.1) kg (NS) S^2 +1.4 (2.6) kg (sig.) (S vs. US sig.) MAMC sig. increase in S^2 **Depleted** (figures read from graph) S^1 +2.8 (0.6) kg (sig.), (5 (1.11)%) S^2 +2.3 (0.5) kg (sig.), (4.15 (0.92)%) (S vs. US sig.) FFM S^1 +1.9 (2.5) kg (sig.) S^2 +1.9 (1.9) (sig.) S$^{(1 + 2)}$ vs. US (sig.) S^1 sig. greater gain in fat mass than S^2 Inc. in CHI and MAMC in both S groups (S^2 vs. US sig.)	−0.4 (2.4) kg or −0.54 (3.26)% −0.2 (2.1) kg +0.5 (0.4) kg or +0.92 (0.74)% −0.6 (1.5) kg	No change in FEV$_1$ in either S group S$^{(1 + 2)}$ sig. improvements in $P_I$max at 4 weeks and S^2 at 8 weeks (S^1 vs. S^2 NS) (similar changes in depleted and non-depleted patients) Sig. improvements in walking distance in depleted (173 m, 29%) and non-depleted (147 m, 24%), S^1 vs. S^2 NS) No differences in corticosteroid users	–	–

TEI, total energy intake; S, supplemented; US, unsupplemented; TPI, total protein intake; REE, resting energy expenditure; NS, not significant; sig., significant; FFM, fat free mass; MAMC, mid-arm muscle circumference; CHI, creatinine–height index; FEV$_1$, forced expiratory volume in 1 s; $P_I$max., maximal inspiratory pressure; $P_E$max., maximal expiratory pressure; Inc., increase.

plemented patients typically lost weight in the studies reviewed (Schols *et al.*, 1995; Saudny-Unterberger *et al.*, 1997; see Table A3.3). However, the weight changes in the supplemented patients were only significantly greater than those in unsupplemented patients in the longer 8-week trial (e.g. + 1.5 kg (non-depleted); + 2.5 kg (depleted); see Table A3.2 for definition) (Schols *et al.*, 1995). In this trial, although quantitative changes in body weight were similar to those of patients who received additional steroid treatment, patients receiving only an ONS gained less fat-free mass (FFM) and more fat mass. These compositional differences were especially evident in patients who were nutritionally depleted at the start of the trial (< 90% IBW; see Table A3.3). A further analysis of this trial has indicated that patients who did not gain weight with ONS (non-response: weight change < 2%, *n* 5) were older, had lower baseline energy intakes and were greater users of continuous supplemental oxygen than those who did respond (weight gain > 5%, *n* 10). These patients had higher fasting plasma glucose, lipopolysaccharide-binding protein and soluble TNF receptor 55 and 75 concentrations (indicative of a systemic inflammatory response) (Creutzberg *et al.*, 2000).

(III) What effect do ONS have on the body function of patients with COPD in hospital?

Trials of ONS in hospitalized COPD patients indicate that significant functional benefits can occur, in addition to improvements in energy intake and body weight. For example, one study reported that, after just 2 weeks of ONS (plus food snacks), there were significant improvements in % of predicted forced ventilatory capacity (FVC) (compared with unsupplemented patients) and in breathlessness and well-being scores (longitudinal improvements) (Saudny-Unterberger *et al.*, 1997). Although changes in respiratory muscle strength (maximal inspiratory pressure ($P_I$max)) and walking distance were not significant after 2 weeks of ONS (Saudny-Unterberger *et al.*, 1997), in another trial they both

significantly improved after 8 weeks of ONS in 'depleted' and 'non-depleted' patients, as well as in steroid and non-steroid users (Schols *et al.*, 1995).

An in-patient, placebo-controlled, metabolic study has also assessed the short-term effects of ONS consumption (2.09 MJ) on measurements of respiratory function in stable COPD patients (Vermeeren *et al.*, 2001). In this trial, no adverse effects of consuming ONS (either 60% energy from fat or 60% carbohydrate taken over a 5 min period) on pulmonary function and no differences in the pulmonary responses following the two supplement types were reported. Subjective assessments suggested that fatigue and pain did not change significantly after either ONS, although there was a significantly greater increase in breathlessness after the high-fat than after the high-carbohydrate ONS (Vermeeren *et al.*, 2001).

(IV) What effect do ONS have on the clinical and financial outcome of patients with COPD in hospital?

In the two trials reviewed (Schols *et al.*, 1995; Saudny-Unterberger *et al.*, 1997), no data were presented on the impact of ONS on clinical and economic outcomes in hospitalized COPD patients. As ONS are able to improve the functional capacity of COPD patients, it is possible that recovery times and length of hospital stay will be shortened, with consequent financial savings (estimated cost of 1 day in hospital in the UK £250). Further research into the clinical and cost-effectiveness of ONS in COPD patients is needed.

COPD: other reviews/meta-analyses

A meta-analysis (Ferreira *et al.*, 2000) of nutritional support trials in COPD patients suggested small but positive effects on weight (effect size + 1.65 kg), muscle circumference (+ 0.3 cm) and 6 min walking distance (+ 3.4 m), although these differences were not significant. However, of the nine trials that were included, only one trial of ONS was undertaken in hospitalized patients (Schols *et al.*, 1995). This analysis also alluded to the need for large trials that investigate functional outcome measures (particularly quality of life) following nutritional support in this patient group (Ferreira *et al.*, 2000).

Elderly

The elderly represent the fastest-growing segment of the population. Furthermore, approximately half of the hospitalized patients in the UK are over 65 years. Even older subjects in the general population suffer from frequent nutrient deficiencies (Finch *et al.*, 1998), the causes of which are multiple (social, psychological, physiological, disease-related (Morley, 1998)). More specifically, changes in taste perception and appetite control may adversely affect the nutritional status of the elderly (Hetherington, 1998). Hospitalized elderly patients are at even greater nutritional risk because of acute illness or injury (for prevalence and consequences of malnutrition, see Chapter 2). Deterioration in nutritional state also frequently occurs in elderly patients during their hospital stay (Larsson *et al.*, 1990). Therefore, the use of nutrition to improve or maintain nutritional and functional status should be recognized as an important component of the care of elderly patients in hospital. Although there are many ways of providing nutritional support, ONS are frequently used because they are readily available and easy to administer at virtually any time of day. The efficacy of ONS in elderly patients in hospital is discussed below, following a systematic review of the evidence. The effectiveness of ONS in elderly patients in the community is considered separately in Appendix 4.

Elderly: present analysis

This review involved 12 RCT (total patient *n* 1146) (Banerjee *et al.*, 1978, 1981; McEvoy and James, 1982; Larsson *et al.*, 1990; Ek *et al.*, 1991; Unosson *et al.*, 1992;

Hankey *et al.*, 1993; Hubsch *et al.*, 1994; Carver and Dobson, 1995; Reilly, J.J. *et al.*, 1995; Volkert *et al.*, 1996; Potter *et al.*, 2001) and five non-randomized trials (NRT) (*n* 749). The RCT are summarized in Tables A3.4–A3.6, Box A3.2 and discussed in greater detail below, in relation to the four review questions, and the five NRT (Katakity *et al.*, 1983; Elmstahl and Steen, 1987; Ovesen, 1992; Bos *et al.*, 2000; Bourdel-Marchasson *et al.*, 2000) are summarized briefly in Tables A3.7, A3.8 and A3.9.

In the RCT of ONS in elderly hospitalized patients, the duration of ONS ranged from 3 weeks (Hubsch *et al.*, 1994) to 26 weeks (Larsson *et al.*, 1990; Ek *et al.*, 1991; Unosson *et al.*, 1992) (potentially three reports of the same trial). Although there appeared to be no side-effects with ONS, regular ingestion of the prescribed amount was a problem in a number of trials (McEvoy and James, 1982; Larsson *et al.*, 1990; Unosson *et al.*, 1992; Carver and Dobson, 1995; Volkert *et al.*, 1996). In at least one trial, this was due to the failure of nurses to add powdered ONS to food (Hankey *et al.*, 1993). In one trial, problems with compliance were overcome by prescribing the ONS on drug charts so that nurses could administer and record consumption of the feed as with any other prescribed product (Potter *et al.*, 2001).

No information on nutritional status was provided in half of the RCT. In the other trials, nutritional status was considered to be poor since the average BMI was < 20 kg m^{-2} or IBW was $< 90\%$ (McEvoy and James, 1982; Larsson *et al.*, 1990; Unosson *et al.*, 1992; Carver and Dobson, 1995; Reilly, J.J. *et al.*, 1995; Volkert *et al.*, 1996; see Tables A3.5 and A3.8). For more information on the prevalence of malnutrition in the elderly, see Chapter 2.

(I) What effect do ONS used in elderly patients in hospital have on voluntary food intake and total energy intake?

The evidence suggests that ONS, varying in type and composition, can improve total nutrient intake in hospitalized elderly. In

---

> **Box A3.2.** Key findings: effect of ONS in elderly hospital patients.
>
> Nutritional intake: ONS can improve intakes of energy, protein and micronutrients without substantially reducing food intake.
>
> Body weight: ONS can lead to weight gain or attenuate weight loss in patients who are (BMI < 20 kg m^{-2}) or are not (BMI > 20 kg m^{-2}) underweight. Muscle mass may be improved.
>
> Body function: functional benefits with ONS include increased activities of daily living and Norton scores of activity and benefits are seen in patient groups who are or are not underweight (BMI < or > 20 kg m^{-2}). ONS may reduce the likelihood of pressure ulcer formation but RCT are required.
>
> Clinical outcome: there are no apparent detriments of using ONS in the elderly. Mortality is significantly reduced with ONS (odds ratio 0.58; 95% CI 0.4–0.83) and hospital stays may be reduced.
>
> Financial outcome: retrospective calculations suggest that financial savings may occur.

the studies reviewed, a range of sweet and savoury ONS, in the form of sip feeds or powders reconstituted to form drinks, were used. The energy density of these ONS ranged from 1.0 to 1.5 kcal ml^{-1} (see Tables A3.4 and A3.7) and the amounts prescribed ranged from 265 kcal (Banerjee *et al.*, 1978) to 652 kcal (Hankey *et al.*, 1993). However, only four studies reported average daily ONS intake (231–596 kcal) (Hubsch *et al.*, 1994; Carver and Dobson, 1995; Reilly, J.J. *et al.*, 1995; Volkert *et al.*, 1996). Refer to Table A3.4 for more details.

Notably, significant improvements in energy, protein and/or micronutrient (range of vitamins and minerals) intakes were observed in five trials, either compared with a control group (Banerjee *et al.*, 1978; Volkert *et al.*, 1996; Potter *et al.*, 2001) or with baseline intakes before supplementation (Unosson *et al.*, 1992; Hankey *et al.*, 1993). In these studies, nutritional status was reported as follows: < 90% of IBW or BMI < 20 kg m^{-2} (Unosson *et al.*, 1992; Volkert *et al.*, 1996); 'severely undernourished' to 'adequately nourished' (Potter *et al.*, 2001); or unknown (Banerjee *et al.*, 1978; Hankey *et al.*, 1993) (see Table A3.6). Other studies also showed that patients given ONS had greater energy and nutrient intakes (e.g. protein, calcium, iron, vitamins) than those who were unsupplemented (Hubsch *et al.*, 1994; Reilly, J.J. *et al.*,

1995). It was not possible from the data provided to quantitatively assess the impact of ONS on voluntary food intake in any of these trials. However, information from a couple of trials (Reilly, J.J. *et al.*, 1995; Potter *et al.*, 2001) implied that ONS did not reduce food intake in supplemented compared with unsupplemented patients (e.g. voluntary food intake 25 and 24 kcal kg^{-1} day^{-1}, respectively in one trial (Reilly, J.J. *et al.*, 1995)). Daily checks on compliance and/or records of ONS intake were reported only in some trials (Hubsch *et al.*, 1994; Carver and Dobson, 1995; Reilly, J.J. *et al.*, 1995; Volkert *et al.*, 1996; Potter *et al.*, 2001) (glucose polymer only (Hankey *et al.*, 1993)).

It has been suggested that glucose and other predominantly carbohydrate-based ONS may be effective at improving the total energy intake of elderly people (MacIntosh *et al.*, 2000). This suggestion has been made on the basis that older individuals tend to reduce their habitual energy intake following supplements to a lesser extent than younger adults (MacIntosh *et al.*, 2000). However, in a trial involving a carbohydrate-only supplement (glucose drink) in the elderly, compliance was poor (Hogarth *et al.*, 1996) and outcome was not improved. In terms of the timing of supplementation, a short-term controlled study in healthy elderly subjects suggests that total

Table A3.4. Oral nutritional supplements used in randomized controlled trials of elderly patients in hospital.

Trial	ONS	ONS energy density	ONS prescribed	ONS energy (kcal) intake	ONS protein (g) intake	Toleration
Banerjee et al. (1978)	Complan	4.4 kcal g^{-1}	265 kcal, 18.6 g P	–	–	–
Banerjee et al. (1981) (same as 1978)	Complan	4.4 kcal g^{-1}	265 kcal, 18.6 g P	–	–	–
Carver and Dobson (1995)	Fortisip 13% P, 48% CHO, 39% F	1.5 kcal ml^{-1}	600 kcal, 20 g P	596 kcal 600 kcal (n 19) ~510 kcal (n 1)	19.9 g 20 g (n 19) ~17 g (n 1)	n 2 withdrawn as reluctant to take ONS
Ek et al. (1991)	Biosorb drink 4 g P, 11.8 g CHO, 4g F per 100 ml	1 kcal ml^{-1}	400 kcal, 16 g P	–	–	–
Hankey et al. (1993)	Build Up Maxijul glucose polymer	–	Build Up 652 kcal Maxijul up to 357 kcal	Build Up not measured Maxijul 222 (27) kcal	0 g	Build Up enjoyed by all Maxijul powder – poor compliance of nursing staff to incorporate into drinks (36–93% prescribed used)
Hubsch et al. (1994)	7.5 g P, 15 g CHO, 3.5 g F per 100 ml	~1.2 kcal ml^{-1}	476 kcal, 30 g P	231 (87–476) kcal	14.5 (5.4–30) g	–
Larsson et al. (1990)	Biosorb drink 4 g P, 11.8 g CHO, 4 g F per 100 ml	1 kcal ml^{-1}	400 kcal, 16 g P	–	–	n 39 withdrawn as refused ONS
McEvoy and James (1982)	Build Up	–	644 kcal, 36.4 g P	–	–	–
Potter et al. (2001)	Entera 6.25 g P per 100 ml	1.5 kcal ml^{-1}	540 kcal, 22.5 g P	50% consumed 430–540 kcal 25% consumed at least 270 kcal	50% took 17.9 g–22.5 g 25% took at least 11.3 g	Given three times daily (8 a.m., 2 p.m., 6 p.m.) and well tolerated. Compliance similar between groups, with low intake mostly due to medical reasons and not unpalatability of ONS
Reilly, J.J. et al. (1995)	– Commercial sip feed	1.5 kcal ml^{-1}	450 kcal, ?P	~432 kcal[a]	–	n 4 refused ONS
Unosson et al. (1992)	Biosorb drink 4 g P, 11.8 g CHO, 4 g F per 100 ml	1 kcal ml^{-1}	400 kcal, 16 g P	–	–	n 35 withdrawn as refused ONS
Volkert et al. (1996)	Variety used Soups (7 g P) and sweet drinks (8 g P) (per 100 ml)	Soup: 1.22 kcal ml^{-1} Sweet drinks: 1.2–1.28 kcal ml^{-1}	500 kcal, 30 g P	251 (89–500) kcal Compliers (n 11) 285 (123–500) kcal and non-compliers (n 9) 209 (89–314) kcal	15.3 g (5.4–30) Compliers 17.4 g (7.5–30) Non-compliers: 12.8 g (5.4–19.1)	If taken, well tolerated. Compliers (n 11) good acceptance, non-compliers (n 9) had poor acceptance

[a] Average ONS intake 12 kcal kg^{-1} body weight (average weight 36 kg).
CHO, carbohydrate; F, fat; P, protein.

Table A3.5. Trial characteristics: hospital-based randomized controlled trials of oral nutritional supplementation in elderly patients

Trial and patient group	Design	No. S	No. US	Initial BMI S group	Initial BMI US group	Duration of ONS	Dietary counselling	Control group
Banerjee et al. (1978) Long-stay elderly	10001	24	26	–	–	14 weeks	–	Hospital diet
Banerjee et al. (1981) Long-stay elderly (same patients as 1978)	10000	24	26	–	–	14 weeks	–	Hospital diet
Carver and Dobson (1985) Elderly with senile dementia	10101	23	23	17.9	17.9	12 weeks	–	200 ml vitamin solution twice daily (same vitamins as in ONS)
Ek et al. (1991)[a] Long-term medical	10000	?403 in total		28.5% defined as malnourished on entry to trial		Duration of H stay (max. 26 weeks)	–	Both S and US groups received standard hospital diet (2200 kcal day^{-1})
Hankey et al. (1993) Continuing care	10001	10	10	~47 kg (no BMI)	~40 kg	8 weeks	–	Standard hospital food
Hubsch et al. (1994) Malnourished elderly	10000	35	37	–	–	3 weeks	–	Hospital diet
Non-English **Larsson et al. (1990)**[a] Long-term medical	10001	202	241	IBW 86 (1.1)% MN: 72.9%[b] noMN: 91.9% IBW < 85%	IBW 90 (1.1)% MN: 77.5%[b] noMN: 93.8% IBW < 85%	Max. 26 weeks	–	Standard hospital diet (2200 kcal day^{-1})
McEvoy and James (1982) Acutely ill elderly	10001	26	25	BMI < 85%	BMI < 85%	4 weeks	–	Standard hospital diet
Potter et al. (2001) Elderly emergency admissions (median age 83 (61–99 years))	11001	(i) 34 (ii) 90 (iii) 62	(i) 40 (ii) 87 (iii) 68	(i) BMI < 5th percentile[b] (ii) BMI > 5th percentile < 25th percentile (iii) BMI > 25th percentile < 75th percentile		~16 days (length of hospital stay)	–	–
Reilly J.J. et al. (1995) Abstract Acutely sick elderly	10000	20	17	All defined as MN, BMI < 25th percentile and/or AMA < 17 cm^2		Max. 14 days or until discharge	–	Standard care
Unosson et al. (1992)[a] Long-term medical	11001	197	233	% IBW < 90% (30% defined as MN)	% IBW < 91% (23% defined as MN)	Max. 26 weeks	–	Standard hospital diet (2200 kcal day^{-1})
Volkert et al. (1996) Acute care	11001	20	26	Compliers 19.8 (1.5)[c] Non-compliers 19.1 (2.3)[c]	19.3 (2.6)	28 (13) days	–	Standard hospital diet (1850 kcal, 65 g P day^{-1})

[a] It is likely that these are separate accounts of one trial.
[b] Group (i) significantly younger than groups (ii) and (iii).
[c] Measurements in only n 19 due to oedema, inability to weigh.
For purposes of analysis, BMI assumed to be < 20 kg m^{-2} for (i) (Potter *et al.*, 2001) or MN (Larsson *et al.*, 1990) and > 20 kg m^{-2} for (iii) or noMN. AMA, arm muscle area; H, hospital; MN, malnourished; noMN, not malnourished; P, protein; S, supplemented; US, unsupplemented.

Table A3.6. Main findings of randomized controlled trials of oral nutritional supplementation in hospitalized elderly patients.

Trial	Energy intake	Body weight S	Body weight US	Body function	Clinical outcome	Finance
Banerjee *et al.* (1978)	'Dietary observations showed that many pt ate less during the supplementary period' S greater increase in protein, Ca, Fe, vit. D, C, B_1, B_2, nicotinic acid (sig. vs. US). Energy, fat and CHO intakes NS. Energy intakes high pre-ONS (>1700 kcal, 52 g P)	– TSF increased (sig. vs. US)	–	Changes in albumin, transferrin NS different between S and US	–	–
Banerjee *et al.* (1981)	As above	As above	As above	No changes in albumin, prealbumin, transferrin or complement in S or US (NS) No difference in % T- and B-cell lymphocytes between S and US (unreliable methodology as total cell counts not done, small *n*)	–	–
Carver and Dobson (1985)	– 'no suggestion that their intakes differed'	+3.5 (1.8) kg (*n* 20) or +7.5 (3.9)% MAMC +0.5 (0.9) cm, TSF +1.5 (1.5) mm (sig.) (Wt and MAMC, S vs. US ?)	+0.6 (1.7) kg (*n* 20) or 1.3 (3.8)% No changes in MAMC/TSF	–	–	–
Ek *et al.* (1991)[a]	–	–	–	9.9% of S (vs. 12% of US) developed pressure ulcers. Total no. of sores: S 67; US 83; % of ulcers improved: S 51.3%; US 43.9%; % healed: S 41.8%; US 30.3% (all NS) (small numbers as only 1/3 followed for 26 weeks)	–	–
Hankey *et al.* (1993)	TEI and TPI increase from 1069 kcal/39.2 g (pre-ONS) to 1740 kcal/64 g (post-ONS) in S (sig.) (S vs. US ?) S: sig. increase in vit. B_2, nicotinic acid, biotin, B_6, B_{12}, D, A, E and Ca and Fe (*n* 7) US NS increases in any nutrients (*n* 7)	NS change in wt (~+1 kg or 2.1%) or MAC AMC increased sig. in S at 4 and 8 weeks (~+3 cm) (no S vs. US comparisons)	NS change in weight (0 kg or 0%) or MAC Sig. reduction in TSF, no change in AMC (*n* 7)	NS changes in albumin in S or US (*n* 7)	–	–
Hubsch *et al.* (1994)	S group higher intakes of kcal, P, Ca, Fe, vit. A, B_1, B_2, B_6, C (? sig.)	–0.1 kg or –0.22% (inconsistent with data below) LBM +0.7 kg FM +0.3 kg (sig. vs. US)	–0.8 kg or –1.84% LBM –0.5 kg FM –0.3 kg	S: greater increase in ADL scores (45 to 70) than US (40 to 50) (NS)	–	–

Study						
Larsson *et al.* (1990)[a]	–	MN: NS change in wt index, TSF or MAMC noMN: less wt loss at 8 and 26 weeks, less decrease in MAMC than US (sig.) MN: at 8 weeks: 41% of S no longer MN vs. 18% of US (sig.) NoMN: at 26 weeks: 8.3% MN in S vs. 26.1% in US (sig.)	MN: no sig. change in wt index, TSF and MAMC	S (MN and no MN): sig. increase in no. pts with reactivity to delayed hypersensitivity skin test S: greater increase in prealb. in MN group than US (sig.) Acute-phase proteins decreased in all groups (no effect of ONS)	noMN: lower mortality rate in S (8.6%) vs. US (18.6%) (sig.) MN: lower mortality rate in S (29%) vs. US (37%) (NS) Higher mortality rate in MN vs. noMN group (sig.)	–
McEvoy and James (1982)	–	+2.6 (2.4) kg (sig. vs. US) or +5.2 (4.8)%[b] Sig. greater increase in TSF and MAC vs. US. Increase in MAMC S vs. US NS	−0.2 (1.5) kg or −0.4 (3.0)%[b]		–
Potter *et al.* (2001)	TEI was sig. increased in S vs. US (+331 kcal (+133, +506 kcal 95% CI); NS difference between groups) VFI was similar in S (1078 kcal) and US (1090 kcal) Measurements in *n* 94	+1 (5.6)% (S vs. US sig.) (i) +3.4 (6.0)% (ii) +0.3 (5.9)% (iii) +1.0 (4.6)% Less deterioration in AMC in S vs. US (NS) AMC −0.4 (6.6) cm	−1 (6.1)% (i) −1.3 (7.6)% (ii) −0.8 (5.9)% (iii) −1.2 (5.2)% AMC −1.6 (6.1) cm	NS difference in proportion with improving functional status (Barthel scores) between S (68%) and US (64%) overall but a sig. difference in group (i) (S 68% vs. US 39%) NS change in micronutrient concentrations in any group	NS trend towards lower mortality in S (21 (11)%) vs. US (33 (17)%) but a sig. reduction in mortality in group (i) (S 5% vs. US 14%) No differences in place of discharge between S and US NS reduction in length of H stay (S 16 days, US 18 days) overall, but a sig. reduction in group (iii) (S 13.5 days US 21 days)	–
Reilly, J.J. *et al.* (1995)	S TEI 37 (2.9–56) kcal kg^{-1} day^{-1}[c] S VFI 25 kcal kg^{-1} day^{-1} US VFI 24 kcal kg^{-1} day^{-1} (10–66)	Trend towards less deterioration of wt and AMA in S vs. US (NS)	–	–	–

Continued

Table A3.6. *continued*

Trial	Energy intake	Body weight S	Body weight US	Body function	Clinical outcome	Finance
Unosson *et al.* (1992)	Food and fluid intakes increased at 4 weeks vs. baseline in S group (sig.)	–	–	Only one sig. difference between groups – Norton scores of activity at 8 weeks in well-nourished pt group: S had greater improvement in activity, maintained at 8 weeks with greater % ambulant or walking with help and fewer chair-bound and bedridden than US. Both S and US: general physical condition improved at 4 and 8 weeks, sig. vs. baseline). S: activity score improved at 4 and 8 weeks (sig.); US: mobility at 8 weeks (sig.)	S: lower mortality (14%) than US (22%, sig.) S patients, with Norton score ≤ 22 on admission, lower mortality rate (17.8%) than US (35.7%) S patients with reduced food/fluid intake on admission (≤ 3) had a lower mortality rate (21.6%) than US (53.4%)	–
Volkert *et al.* (1996)	TEI: compliers (C): 1170 (318) kcal, 50 g (14.9) P; non-compliers (NC): 1240 (314) kcal, 45 g (11.9) P (C vs. NC NS) US: 995 (409) kcal, 32.8 (14.1) g P Both S groups sig. higher intakes of Ca, Mg, Fe and vits D, E, C, B$_1$, B$_2$, B$_6$, B$_{12}$, folate vs. US. Compliers sig. higher protein and K than US	C: +0.4 kg or +0.85% NC: −1.6 kg (sig. loss compared with baseline) (6 months after discharge, sig. wt gain for C (+3.4 kg) and NC (+3 kg), NS vs. US)	−0.1 kg or −0.23% (6 months after discharge, +2.9 kg)	ADL (C *n* 9) Sig. greater % (64%) of S improved ADL than US (23%) C: ADL scores increased from 45 (15–95) to 70 (25–95); NC ADL scores from 60 (5–95) to 70 (20–95) vs. US from 45 (0–90) to 50 (5–95) (S vs. US NS) Greater proportion of independent pts (> 65) in C and NC vs. US (sig.) at end of trial. In C, decrease in % of dependent pts (36% to 18%) and increase in independent pts (36% to 63%). Smaller but similar changes in US. No such changes in NC	–	–

[a] Three reports of one patient group.
[b] Assumes an original body weight of 50 kg.
[c] S group. If assume weight of 36 kg (calculated from ONS data): S TEI 1332 kcal, VFI 900 kcal; (US VFI 864 kcal if similar weight to S group).
ADL, activities of daily living; AMA, arm muscle area; AMC, arm muscle circumference; CHO, carbohydrate; CI, confidence interval; FM, fat mass; H, hospital; LBM, lean body mass; MAMC, mid-arm muscle circumference; MAC, mid-arm circumference; MN, malnourished; MUAMC, mid-upper-arm muscle circumference; noMN, not malnourished; NS, not significant; P, protein; prealb., prealbumin; pt, patients; S, supplemented; sig., significant; TEI, total energy intake; TPI, total protein intake; TSF, triceps skin-fold thickness; US, unsupplemented; VFI, voluntary food intake

Table A3.7. Oral nutritional supplements used in trials of elderly patients in hospital (non-randomized data).

Trial	ONS	ONS energy density	ONS prescribed	ONS energy (kcal) intake	ONS protein (g) intake	Toleration
Bos *et al.* (2000)	Nutrigil HP (Jacquemaire-Sante, BSA) Per 100 ml: 7.5 g P, 12.5 g CHO, 2.3 g F, vitamins and minerals	~1 kcal ml⁻¹	397 kcal, 30 g P 400 ml	374 kcal	28.3 g P	–
Bourdel-Marchasson *et al.* (2000)	Variety of ONS from Nutricia, Clintec-Sopharga, Jacquemaire-Sante	1 kcal ml⁻¹	400 kcal, ~23 g	day 2 179; day 5 182; day 8 191; day 11 217; day 15 193 kcal 60% took ONS 1 week, 99% in 2 weeks	day 2 10.5 day 5 10.4 day 8 11.2 day 11 13.0 day 15 11.6	–
Elmstahl and Steen (1987)	S¹ Semper (17% P, 53% CHO, 30% F; per 100 kcal: 4 g P, 13 g CHO, 3 g F)	1.19 kcal ml⁻¹	500 kcal, 20 g P	407 kcal (342 ml)	16.3 g	–
	S² Clinifeed ISO (Roussel) 2 flavours (11% P, 52% CHO, 37% F; per 100 kcal 3 g P, 13 g CHO, 4 g F)	1 kcal ml⁻¹	500 kcal, 15 g P	405 kcal (405 ml)	12.2 g	
	S³ Caloreen + Hospital dietary supplement (4% P, 69% CHO, 27% F; per 100 kcal 1 g P, 17 g CHO, 3 g F)	2 kcal ml⁻¹	500 kcal, 5 g P	440 kcal (220 ml)	4.4 g	
Katakity *et al.* (1983)	Cow & Gate powder reconstituted with water to form malted drink (usually made up with milk)	? 0.45 kcal ml⁻¹	204 kcal, 9 g P (? 750 ml)	–	–	–
Ovesen (1992)	S¹ Nutrison Standard (Nutricia)	1 kcal ml⁻¹	800 kcal, 32 g P	300 (200–400) kcal (calculated 286 kcal) (300 (200–400) ml)	12 (8–16) g	*n* 10 GI intolerant to S. Both
	S² Nutrison Energirig (Nutricia) 1 flavour only	1.5 kcal ml⁻¹	1200 kcal, 32 g P	600 (375–750) kcal (calculated 583 kcal) (400 (250–500) ml)	16 (10–20) g	S high taste ratings and no change over trial period

CHO, carbohydrate; F, fat; GI, gastrointestinal; P, protein; S, supplemented.

Table A3.8. Trial characteristics: hospital-based trials of oral nutritional supplementation in elderly patients (non-randomized data).

Trial and patient group	Design	No. S	No. US	Initial BMI S group	Initial BMI US group	Duration of ONS	Dietary counselling	Control group
Bos et al. (2000)	B	17	6	20.7 (3.9) 13 (9)% wt loss	20.2 (2.5) 12 (6)% wt loss	10 days	–	Standard diet
Bourdel-Marchasson et al. (2000) Acutely ill	B	295	377	– 60.2 kg	– 55.2 kg	15 days or discharge	No, but assisted during meals	Standard diet (1800 kcal), usual nutritional care
Elmstahl and Steen (1987) Long-term care	C[a]	S^1 8 S^2 9 S^3 11	–	– 48.2 (7.6) kg	–	8 weeks	–	–
Katakity et al. (1983) Stable, long-term	B	12	–	–	–	12 weeks	–	–
Ovesen (1992) Elderly with poor appetite	C[a]	24	–	S^1 50 (38–74) kg S^2 55 (42–68) kg	–	10 days	–	–

[a] Trials comparing different supplements (S^1, S^2, S^3), within-group data used only.
S, supplemented; US, unsupplemented.

Table A3.9. Main findings of oral nutritional supplementation trials in hospitalized elderly patients (non-randomized data).

Trial	Energy intake	Wt change S	Wt change US	Function	Outcome	Finance
Bos *et al.* (2000)	S TEI: 1768 kcal 71 g P; VFI: 1395 kcal, sig. increase from baseline (28 to 35 kcal kg⁻¹ wt) US VFI 1476 kcal 54 g P, little change vs. baseline (28–29 kcal kg⁻¹ wt), (S vs. US sig.)	+0.8 kg (S vs. US NS) +1.2 kg FFM (S vs. US sig.) −0.4 kg FM	+0.2 kg 0 kg FFM +0.2 kg FM	*ONS led to increases in protein synthesis kg⁻¹ wt in fasted state; increase in net protein balance in fed state – sig. increase in net diurnal protein balance after ONS. In fed state net protein balance positively correlated with protein intake (r^2 0.46)*	–	–
Bourdel-Marchasson *et al.* (2000)	S sig. higher TEI and TPI on days 2, 5, 8, 11 than US. By day 15, only TPI sig. higher vs. US Day 2 S 1081 US 957 kcal; 46, 38 g P Day 5 S 1181 US 1022 kcal; 50, 42 g P Day 8 S 1193 US 1044 kcal; 50, 42 g P Day 11 S 1266 US 1110 kcal; 54, 46 g P Day 15 S 1188 US 1102 kcal; 51, 44 g P (suggests 79, 100, 88, 79, 52% ONS energy additive vs. US)	–	–	Pressure ulcer cumulative incidence: Day 5 S 16% US 25% (? sig.) Day 10 S 27% US 37% (? sig.) Day 15 S 40% US 48% (? sig.) S vs. US no difference in erythema formation S a 'protective factor' for pressure ulcer development vs. US from multivariate analysis	Similar incidence of death (S *n* 25 vs. US 22, NS)	–
Elmstahl and Steen (1987)	S¹ 1214 (pre)–1453 (post) kcal (+239, 59% ONS); S² 1316 (pre)–1568 (post) kcal (+252, 62% ONS); S³ 1215 (pre)–1623 (post) kcal (+408, 93% ONS). NS changes in % energy from CHO, P or F between groups or vs. pre-ONS S¹ sig. inc. in protein (+10 g), vits A, D, B₂, B₁ and Ca and Fe S² sig. inc. in protein (+4 g), vits C, B₂ and Ca and Fe S³ sig. inc. in vits A, D, B₂, B₁ and Ca and Fe Mean pre-ONS 1247 (186) kcal; post-ONS 1557 (?) (*n* 28) Intake of energy from snacks decreased 20%–11%	S¹ 1.1 kg S² 1.4 kg S³ 0.7 kg (all sig. vs. pre-ONS) NS. changes in MAC, TSF	–	Sig. increase in haptoglobulin and ceruloplasmin in post-ONS vs. pre-ONS (signs of inflammation)	–	–

Continued

Table A3.9. *Continued*

Trial	Energy intake	Wt change S	Wt change US	Function	Outcome	Finance
Katakity *et al.* (1983)	–	–	–	Sig. increase in HGS during period of ONS and subsequent fall when ONS stopped (4-week assessment period): pre 16 kg, during 22 kg, after 17 kg. No change in dark adaptation or cognitive function (digit coding, reaction times). Increase in vit. C blood and plasma conc. during ONS, sig. drop post-ONS. Sig. improvement in vit. B$_1$, folate (serum) and vit. D status during ONS, lost post-ONS	–	–
Ovesen (1992)	pre-ONS day 3 ONS day 10 ONS (calculations from graph) S^1 1142 – 1214 – 1380 VFI (+238 kcal) S^1 1142 – 1618 – 1666 TEI (+524 kcal) (%ONS 183%) S^2 1000 – 976 – 988 VFI (−12 kcal) S^2 1000 – 1595 – 1595 TEI (+595 kcal) (% ONS 98%) All TEI (day 3, day 10) sig. vs. pre-ONS S^1 increased VFI to outweigh the kcal density of S^2	–	–	–	–	–

CHO, carbohydrate; conc, concentration; F, fat; FFM, fat-free mass; FM, fat mass; HGS, hand-grip strength; inc., increase; MAC, mid-arm circumference; NS, not significant; % ONS, per cent ONS energy additive to food intake; P, protein; S, supplemented; sig., significant; TEI, total energy intake; TPI, total protein intake; TSF, triceps skin-fold thickness; US, unsupplemented; VFI, voluntary food intake; vit., vitamin.

energy intake is greater if a supplement is given > 60 min before a test meal than if given together with the meal (Wilson *et al.*, 2002). Longer-term trials in elderly individuals with disease are lacking.

(II) What effect do ONS used in elderly patients in hospital have on body weight and composition?

This analysis showed that ONS in elderly hospital patients can lead to improvements in body weight and composition. The changes in body weight following ONS in elderly patients in hospital (reported in seven trials; McEvoy and James, 1982; Larsson *et al.*, 1990; Hankey *et al.*, 1993; Hubsch *et al.*, 1994; Carver and Dobson, 1995; Volkert *et al.*, 1996; Potter *et al.*, 2001) were variable, potentially due to differences in diagnoses and treatments, initial nutritional status or the quantity or duration of ONS prescribed in the various trials (see Table A3.4–A3.6).

An analysis of average % weight change data (weighted for sample size) from five studies (*n* 860) (Larsson *et al.*, 1990; Hankey *et al.*, 1993; Hubsch *et al.*, 1994; Carver and Dobson, 1995; Potter *et al.*, 2001) indicated an attenuation of weight loss with ONS (supplemented patients + 0.14% versus unsupplemented patients − 3.2%, $P < 0.04$ independent *t* test). Meta-analysis of three RCT (six data sets) (Larsson *et al.*, 1990; Carver and Dobson, 1995; Potter *et al.*, 2001) comparing ONS with routine care, using a fixed-effects model, indicated an effect size with supplementation of 0.52 (95% confidence interval (CI) 0.16–0.88), with no significant heterogeneity between studies.

Individually, in three trials in which a significant increase in weight was observed, either over the period of supplementation (senile dementia patients (Carver and Dobson, 1995)) or compared with a control group (acutely ill elderly (McEvoy and James, 1982; Potter *et al.*, 2001)), the patient groups were more 'undernourished' than in other trials (BMI < 17.9 kg m^{-2} (Carver and Dobson, 1995); < 85% IBW (McEvoy and James, 1982); BMI < 5th percentile (group

(i), Potter *et al.*, 2001)). Indeed, in a large supplementation trial, in which patients were stratified according to BMI percentiles, the 'severely undernourished' patients (BMI < 5th percentile) showed a greater response to supplementation (difference of + 4.7% versus unsupplemented patients in group (ii)) than the better-nourished patients (+ 1.1% in group (ii) BMI > 5th − < 25th percentile; + 2.2% in group (iii) BMI > 25th − < 75th percentile). This was one of the few trials for which the sample size was determined in advance, on the basis of weight change, by power calculations. In contrast, a large investigation in long-term elderly medical patients (Larsson *et al.*, 1990) found that those who were defined as 'well nourished' appeared to respond to ONS more favourably than the 'malnourished'. Unlike the 'malnourished' group, the 'well-nourished' patients had significantly smaller weight loss and less loss of muscle mass (mid-arm muscle circumference (MAMC)) compared with unsupplemented patients. Furthermore, these patients also exhibited improvements in outcome compared with the unsupplemented control group (see question IV). Such changes were not observed in the 'malnourished' group (see Table A3.6), although, over the supplementation period, the proportion of supplemented patients who were malnourished became significantly less than the unsupplemented patients in both the 'malnourished' and 'well-nourished' groups (criteria for 'malnourished': < 85% IBW and other anthropometric and biochemical criteria). It is difficult to interpret the relationship between the efficacy of ONS and the nutritional status of elderly patients in hospital for a number of reasons. In addition to many confounding factors (including disease type and severity, oedema), the lack of universally agreed criteria for the definition of risk of malnutrition in hospital patients hinders comparisons between different study groups (see Chapter 1). Also, different numbers of patients in 'malnourished' and 'well-nourished' groups may explain the lack of significant changes to outcome in some groups (e.g. Larsson *et al.*'s (1990) trial).

The long-term impact of ONS on body weight, after discharge from hospital, has also been considered in some studies. For example, in one supplementation trial, weight increased by only a small, non-significant degree during the period of hospitalization (Volkert *et al.*, 1996) but this was followed by a greater and significant longitudinal weight gain during the subsequent period after discharge (see Table A3.6). Some studies also reported that ONS produced significant improvements in muscle mass (Hankey *et al.*, 1993; Hubsch *et al.*, 1994; Carver and Dobson, 1995), mostly by using upper-arm anthropometry. Very few trials considered the potentially confounding effects of oedema on body weight and composition measurements. One trial, in acutely ill elderly patients, performed an analysis of weight changes, after excluding those with potentially confounding conditions (i.e. those that may lead to changes in body weight), to take into account the possible involvement of fluid shifts. This subgroup analysis indicated significantly greater weight changes in supplemented (+ 2%) versus control (− 0.8%) patients and mirrored the analysis of the study group as a whole (+ 1%, − 1%, respectively) (Potter *et al.*, 2001).

(III) What effect do ONS used in elderly patients in hospital have on body function?

Improvements in a number of functional parameters following ONS were observed in most of the trials that made such assessments (Larsson *et al.*, 1990; Ek *et al.*, 1991; Unosson *et al.*, 1992; Hubsch *et al.*, 1994; Volkert *et al.*, 1996; Potter *et al.*, 2001). These included improvements in activities of daily living (ADL) (patients' BMI < 20 kg m^{-2} (Volkert *et al.*, 1996) or unknown (Hubsch *et al.*, 1994)), with a greater proportion of patients becoming independent in the supplemented than in the unsupplemented groups. Similarly, improvements in Norton scores of activity were observed in another trial (patients < 90% IBW) (Unosson *et al.*, 1992). ONS patients had greater improvements in activity, with a greater proportion becoming ambulant, with

or without help, and a smaller proportion remaining chair-bound/bedridden than in the control group (Unosson *et al.*, 1992). However, these improvements were evident in the 'well-nourished' group and not in those defined as 'malnourished' (criteria for 'malnourished': < 85% IBW and other anthropometric and biochemical criteria). These statistical differences may have been due to the two- to threefold greater numbers of patients in the 'well-nourished' than in the 'malnourished' groups.

In contrast, another trial (Potter *et al.*, 2001) reported that only in the severely 'undernourished' supplemented group (group (i)) were functional recovery rates (Barthel scores) significantly greater than in unsupplemented patients. Such differences were not seen in the better nourished groups ((ii) and (iii)). In a further report (BMI of patients unknown) (Ek *et al.*, 1991), those patients receiving ONS were less likely to develop pressure ulcers than were unsupplemented patients (9.9% vs. 12%) and were more likely to have fewer pressure ulcers (67 vs. 83) and a greater proportion of ulcers healed (51% vs. 44%). The improvements in patients' activity levels (as reported by Unosson *et al.*, 1992) may have been a contributory factor. However, none of these differences were statistically significant, possibly due to the small numbers of patients. Significant improvements in some biochemical and immunological parameters were also observed following ONS (report by Larsson *et al.*, 1990; see Table A3.6).

Further trials of ONS in elderly patients, with sufficient power to detect changes in functional measurements, are needed. Analysis of changes in body functions in patient groups according to their nutritional status and clinical status would also be useful.

(IV) What effect do ONS used in elderly patients in hospital have on clinical and financial outcome?

ONS may have a favourable impact on the clinical outcome of hospitalized elderly by reducing mortality (see Fig. 6.12 in Chapter 6) and hospital stays.

MORTALITY

A meta-analysis of mortality data from studies of ONS in the hospital setting (Larsson *et al.*, 1990; Unosson *et al.*, 1992; Volkert *et al.*, 1996; Potter *et al.*, 2001) suggests a significant reduction in mortality in supplemented (13% (82/615)) versus unsupplemented (26% (147/703)) patients (odds ratio 0.58 (95% CI 0.40–0.83)[2]. Two reports (Larsson *et al.*, 1990; Unosson *et al.*, 1992) assessed the effect of a maximum of 26 weeks of ONS in hospitalized elderly (patients < 90% IBW) on clinical outcome. Unosson *et al.* (Unosson *et al.*, 1992) found that long-term elderly medical patients had a significantly lower mortality if taking ONS (14%) than if not (22%). More detailed analysis of mortality according to patients' nutritional status (presented by Larsson *et al.*, 1990) indicated that the 'well-nourished' group taking ONS had a significantly lower mortality rate (8.6%) than those not supplemented (18.6%). In the same study, a similar, but non-significant trend towards lower mortality was also observed in the 'malnourished' group receiving ONS (29% vs. 37% unsupplemented; see Table A3.6) (although the differences in significance may have been due to the two- to threefold greater number of patients in the 'well-nourished' than in the 'malnourished' group). In contrast, in acutely ill patients, only the most undernourished (BMI < 5th percentile) supplemented patients had significantly lower mortality rates (5% versus 14% for unsupplemented) (Potter *et al.*, 2001). These may represent genuine differences or simply be an artefact of the many different ways investigators have defined malnutrition. (For a discussion of the issues, refer to Chapter 1.)

LENGTH OF HOSPITAL STAY

This review suggests that length of stay can be shortened by the use of ONS in elderly patients. Early nutritional intervention in elderly patients at nutritional risk (primarily using ONS and snacks, enteral tube feeding (ETF) and parenteral nutrition (PN) in some) led to a significant shortening of hospital length of stay versus those given delayed or no nutrition (Treber and Harris, 1996). More specifically, a significant reduction in hospital stay with ONS (by 7.5 days compared with a control group (13.5 days vs. 21 days)), in acutely ill elderly patients, was found in 'well-nourished' patients (group (iii)) but not in the 'moderately' or 'severely' undernourished patients (Potter *et al.*, 2001). This difference could not be explained by diagnoses or destination after discharge (although there were more unsupplemented patients discharged to institutions (12% versus 7%, not significant), which could have delayed discharge). Changes in body weight following ONS in this group were only small (+ 1%), and therefore the mechanisms by which ONS may have hastened recovery require investigation (however, the significance value of $P < 0.05$ may be invalid if multiple statistical testing has not been taken into account). It may be that the provision of an essential nutrient (e.g. protein or a micronutrient) or a critical intake of energy at a specific time in recovery can improve a patient's outcome, independent of changes in gross body weight and composition. Further research is required.

FINANCIAL OUTCOME

No financial data was presented in any study, although it is reasonable to suggest that effective use of ONS might result in cost savings by reducing patient's utilization of health-care resources (both in hospital and post-discharge). For example, in a number of studies, supplemented patients were shown to have greater levels of independence and activity (i.e. fewer chair-bound/bedridden) than unsupplemented patients (Unosson *et al.*, 1992; Volkert *et al.*, 1996). Consequently, the supplemented patients might have required less nursing or therapy time, both during hospitalization and after discharge, although further research is needed to verify this. Cost savings are also likely if early nutritional intervention can reduce length of hospital stay (Treber and Harris, 1996). The retrospective cost analysis undertaken as part of this review (see Chapter 6), using data provided in one trial (Potter *et al.*, 2001), suggested a cost saving per patient of £452 (assuming that the cost of hospital stay is £250 per day and that the cost of ONS is £3 per day (see Chapter 6)).

The effects of ONS on the incidence and healing of pressure ulcers may be another potential area for cost savings (Ek *et al.*, 1991). Pressure ulcers are a huge financial burden on health-care systems (Preston, 1991) and so it is likely that sizeable savings can be made if ONS can reduce their incidence and improve their healing. However, such financial analyses often represent the direct cost to the health service alone and do not take into account the economic consequences associated with well-being and overall quality of life (e.g. quality-adjusted life years (QALY)). Further research is therefore needed.

Elderly: other analyses

Enteral nutritional support has been shown to be effective at increasing body weight in elderly patient groups according to a recent meta-analysis (Potter, 2001). The pooled, weighted, mean difference for weight change in supplemented compared with unsupplemented patients was + 2.06% (95% CI 1.63–2.49%). However, it is difficult to assess the specific effects of ONS from this analysis, as many of the trials involved patients given ETF or food snacks. Furthermore, many of these trials were undertaken in the community setting and the patient group was highly diverse (included patients with COPD, liver disease, cancer and orthopaedic patients). In an attempt to overcome the confounding effects of trials using different types of nutritional support in different health-care settings, Chapter 6 has presented results of trials of ONS only, according to the diagnostic group of patients and the health-care setting. These diagnostic groups have been considered individually, as well as cumulatively (see Chapter 6). Meta-analysis of trials in sick elderly patients with non-malignant and non-surgical conditions suggested that there was a significantly lower risk of mortality in patients receiving oral nutrition (ONS or food snacks) compared with 'unsupplemented' patients, with an odds ratio of 0.61 (95% CI 0.45–0.82) (Potter, 2001). Following this meta-analysis (Potter, 2001), it was concluded:

Given that oral supplementation is a non-toxic intervention and that it has reproducible benefits, there is sufficient evidence to recommend that sick elderly patients who are able to swallow but are under-nourished on admission to hospital are considered for prescription of oral supplementation.

Liver Disease

Malnutrition frequently occurs in patients with liver disease and the severity of malnutrition typically depends on the degree of liver failure (Mendenhall *et al.*, 1984b; Cabre and Gassull, 1993). Anorexia, chemosensory disturbances and food intakes that are inadequate to meet increased nutritional requirements are problems in patients with liver disease (Deems *et al.*, 1993; Verboeket-Van de Venne *et al.*, 1993) and dietary restrictions are frequently prescribed in the management of ascites and encephalopathy, which may further limit nutritional intake (Thomas, 1994). In addition to the effects of disease on nutritional status, in patients with alcoholic liver disease, excessive alcohol intake may also contribute to the development of specific nutrient deficiencies and weight loss. The evidence that suggests that malnutrition in patients with liver disease adversely affects clinical outcome (see Chapters 2 and 4) supports the need for effective nutritional intervention to prevent or treat patients who are malnourished or at risk of malnutrition. This section aims to address the evidence of efficacy of ONS use in patients with liver disease who are treated in hospital (Box A3.33). The use of ONS in patients with liver disease who are treated as hospital outpatients is addressed in Appendix 4.

Liver disease: present analysis

In 1941, Patek and Post reported that both survival and bodily functions (at 6 months and 1 and 2 years) were better when patients with liver disease (cirrhosis) were given a high-energy and protein diet supplemented with a milk-based liquid ONS enriched with yeast and sugar than with the conventional management (a low-protein, low-fat diet). More recent investigations, which are included in the current systematic review, include three RCT (total *n* 391) and four NRT in patients with alcoholic liver disease (two RCT: Bunout *et al.*, 1989; Mendenhall *et al.*, 1993; 2 NRT: Mendenhall *et al.*, 1985; Roselle *et al.*, 1988) and cirrhosis (two NRT: Christie *et al.*, 1985; Okita *et al.*, 1985) and in patients undergoing liver transplantation (one RCT: Le Cornu *et al.*, 2000). Details of the studies are summarized in Tables A3.10–A3.15. The RCT are discussed in more detail below, addressing the four review questions. The specific use of supplements containing only branched-chain amino acids is not considered here.

Of the three RCT in patients with liver disease, only one trial restricted ONS to the period of hospitalization (Bunout *et al.*, 1989). Those patients undergoing liver transplantation received ONS as out-patients (duration unspecified) prior to hospital admission (Le Cornu *et al.*, 2000) and, in Mendenhall's study of alcoholic liver disease, ONS continued in patients after their discharge from hospital (Mendenhall *et al.*, 1993).

(I) What effect do ONS have on the voluntary food intake and total energy intake of patients with liver disease in hospital?

This review suggests that ONS are an effective means of improving the nutritional intake of patients with liver disease (see Tables A3.12 and A3.15). In all RCT, ONS increased total energy and protein intakes (significantly in two trials (Bunout *et al.*, 1989; Mendenhall *et al.*, 1993)) compared with an unsupplemented group. Indeed, in all trials, reported ONS intake was large ($\geq$ 600 kcal: Bunout *et al.*, 1989; Le Cornu *et al.*, 2000; > 1000 kcal: Mendenhall *et al.*, 1993). Furthermore, Mendenhall *et al.* (1993) were able to show that improvements in energy and protein intakes in the hospitalization period occurred regardless of the nutritional status of patients (mild, moderate and severe protein-energy malnutrition, defined by a number of anthropometric and biochemical parameters). However, in this trial (Mendenhall *et al.*, 1993) patients received a simultaneous course of oxandrolone, an anabolic steroid, in addition to ONS, and in another trial (Le Cornu *et al.*, 2000) patients were also given dietary advice to improve energy intakes.

It was possible to estimate the effect of ONS on voluntary food intake in two

---

Box A3.3. Key findings: effect of ONS in hospital patients with liver disease.

Nutritional intake: ONS can improve patients' total intakes of energy and protein, particularly when accompanied by steroid use or dietary advice. ONS provide largely additional energy (> 50% additive) to voluntary food intake in patients with chronic liver disease but may be less effective when used pre-liver transplant.

Body weight: ONS may improve nutritional status (including muscle mass). Changes in body weight can be an unreliable outcome measure in this patient group.

Body function: improvements in hand-grip strength and in liver function may occur. There are no reported detriments of using ONS in this patient group.

Clinical outcome: mortality rates may be reduced in patients with alcoholic liver disease who are given ONS (combined analysis suggests a 5% reduction from 37% to 32%). There is no evidence of benefit to clinical outcome of using ONS pretransplant.

Financial outcome: there is no information about cost efficacy in this group.

Table A3.10. Oral nutritional supplements used in trials of patients with liver disease in hospital.

Trial	ONS	ONS energy density	ONS prescribed	ONS energy (kcal) intake	ONS protein (g) intake	Toleration
Bunout *et al.* (1989)	ADN (casein, maltodextrins, MCT, sunflower oil) 97 kcal, 3.4 g P, 46 mg Na per 100 ml	0.97 kcal ml⁻¹	To enable total intakes of 50 kcal kg⁻¹ and 1.5 g protein kg⁻¹	–	–	–
Le Cornu *et al.* (2000)	Specially formulated Nutricia feed 4 g P, 6.7 g F, 1.95 mmol Na, 5 mmol K per 100 ml	1.5 kcal ml⁻¹	750 kcal, 20 g P (500 ml)	Reported intake 600 kcal Reported vol. 339 ml = 509 kcal, (0–500 ml range)	16 g (Mean vol. 339 ml = 13.6 g)	–
Mendenhall *et al.* (1993)	Hepatic Aid (BCAA-rich ONS)	–	1600 kcal, 60 g P + 80 mg day⁻¹ of oxandrolone (As out-patients, 1200 kcal, 45 g P + 40 mg day⁻¹)	Mild PEM: S 1114 kcal US 190 kcal Moderate PEM: S 1207 kcal US 187 kcal Severe PEM: S 1063 kcal US 178 kcal	Mild PEM: 42 g Moderate PEM: 45 g Severe PEM 40 g	Occasional GI complaints (nausea, diarrhoea, bloating)

BCAA, branched-chain amino acid; F, fat; GI, gastrointestinal; MCT, medium-chain triglycerides; P, protein; PEM, protein-energy malnutrition; S, supplemented; US, unsupplemented.

Table A3.11. Trial characteristics: hospital-based trials of oral nutritional supplementation in patients with liver disease.

Trial and patient group	Design	No. S	No. US	Initial BMI S group	Initial BMI US group	Duration of ONS	Dietary counselling	Control group
Bunout et al. (1989) Alcoholic liver disease	10001	17	19	26.9 (ascitic)	28.1 (ascitic)	20 (3) days (until discharge or death)	No – unless encephalopathy developed and protein intake was reduced (S and US)	Standard diet (not to exceed 35 kcal kg^{-1} and 0.8 g protein kg^{-1})
Le Cornu et al. (2000) Pre-transplantation ONS (home–hospital–home). ONS in the OP setting prior to transplant	11001	42	40	All patients recruited < 25th percentile for MAMC		? (months) From OP appointment until transplant S 77 days (1–395) US 45 days (1–424)	Yes – 'usual dietary advice'	Dietary advice to increase energy and protein as appropriate
Mendenhall et al. (1993) Alcoholic hepatitis ONS plus anabolic steroid (oxandrolone)	10111	137	136	All patients described as having abnormal nutritional status (34% to 92% of PEM score) 3.7% mild 48.3% moderate 48% severe		30 days in hospital 60 days as out-patient	–	Low-calorie, low-protein food ONS (264 kcal, 6.8 g P) and placebo tablet in hospital. Both groups had standard hospital diet and multi-vit. and min. supplement

min., mineral; multi-vit., multi-vitamin; OP, out-patients; P, protein; PEM, protein–energy malnutrition; S, supplemented; US, unsupplemented.

Table A3.12. Main findings of oral nutritional supplementation trials in hospitalized patients with liver disease.

Trial	Energy intake	Wt change S	Wt change US	Function	Outcome	Finance
Bunout et al. (1989)	Greater TEI and TPI in S (S vs. US sig.) S 2707 (71) kcal; US 1813 (121) kcal S 80 (3) g; US 47 (3.8) g protein (protein intake lowered in n 3 due to encephalopathy)	−6.29 (1.5) kg or −8.82 (2.1)% S vs. US (NS) (Significant reduction in ascites in both S and US.) TSF and MAMC NS changes	−4.65 (1.8) kg or −6.23 (2.41)%	NS changes in biochemical parameters (albumin, AAT, ALP) except a sig. increase in haematocrit in S (? related to fluid shifts/ascites)	Lower mortality in S (n 2) than US (n 5) P < 0.07	—
Le Cornu et al. (2000)	S (all) 2419 (1093–4944) kcal: 79.8 (35.2–183.1) g P (ONS ~20% of TEI). If 509 kcal as ONS, 36% of energy is additive (+ 185 kcal). If 600 kcal as ONS, 31%. additive US (all) 2234 (863–4669) kcal: 86.5 (11.6–132.4) g P (all S vs. US NS) TEI from B/line to transplant (n 5) S 1840 kcal to 2495 kcal (+ 555 kcal) US 2473 kcal to 2718 kcal (+ 245 kcal)	— Sig. increase in MAC and MAMC (S vs. US ?) Pre-transplant (after ONS): sig. more S than US with MAMC < 5th percentile	— Sig. increase in MAC and MAMC	S sig. increase in HGS (no change in US) (S vs. US ?) (evidence of deteriorating renal function during ONS period in S group with increasing urea)	Fewer deaths in S (n 5) than US (n 9) from start of trial to 6 months post-transplant Pre-transplant, 9 deaths (2 S, 7 US, P < 0.067) Post-transplant, 5 deaths (3 S, 2 US, NS) No difference between S and US in outcome after transplant: time on ventilator, time in ICU, time in hospital, episodes of post-transplant rejection	—
Mendenhall et al. (1993)	S mild PEM: TEI 2297 kcal, 91 g P, VFI 1183 kcal S moderate PEM: TEI 2575 kcal, 100 g P, VFI 1368 kcal S severe PEM: TEI 2077 kcal, 80 g P, VFI 1014 kcal US mild PEM: TEI 1912 kcal, 73 g P, VFI 1722 kcal US moderate PEM: TEI 1425 kcal, 54 g P, VFI 1238 kcal severe PEM: TEI 1535 kcal, 59 g P, VFI 1357 kcal Sig. increase in TEI and TPI (S vs. US), especially in the hospitalization period, regardless of nutritional status (53% S vs. 15% US > 2500 kcal)	— Moderate PEM: 72% (S vs. US sig.)	53% stabilized or improved PCM scores	S most successful in moderate PEM group: at 6 months, 72% stabilized or improved liver disease (bilirubin level, prothrombin time) (52% S vs. US, sig.). Not seen in severe PEM group (mild PEM, no data, small sample size)	Mortality rate at 6 months S 35%; US 39% (NS) (mortality related to level of MN and caloric intake during hospitalization) Mild PEM: (S n 5) sample size too small for survival analysis Moderate PEM: after 1 month ONS in hospital, 9% mortality in S vs. 20.9% US (S vs. US sig.). At 6 months, 20% S, 37% US (sig.), median survival 49 months vs. 26 months (sig.). Severe PEM: no differences in survival noted. (Results similar to previous trial when only steroids given for 1 month (Mendenhall et al., 1984a). When the results from the 2 trials were combined according to energy intake, in the moderate PEM group, the combination of steroid and energy intakes > 2500 kcal resulted in a sig. improvement in mortality (4% vs. 28% sig.) but steroid use plus an inadequate intake had no effects vs. the placebo group. Severe PEM with an adequate kcal intake had a 19% mortality at 6 months vs. 51% in those with an energy intake < 2500 kcal)	—

AAT, alanine aminotransferase; ALP, alkaline phosphatase; HGS, hand-grip strength; ICU, intensive-care unit; MAC, mid-arm circumference; MAMC, mid-arm muscle circumference; MN, malnourishment; NS, not significant; P, protein; PCM, protein calorie malnutrition; PEM, protein-energy malnutrition; S, supplemented; sig., significant; TEI, total energy intake; TPI, total protein intake; US, unsupplemented; VFI, voluntary food intake.

Table A3.13. Oral nutritional supplements used in trials of patients with liver disease in hospital (non-randomized data).

Trial	ONS	ONS energy density	ONS prescribed	ONS energy (kcal) intake	ONS protein (g) intake	Toleration
Christie *et al.* (1985)	S[1] Travasorb-Hepatic (50% of protein from BCAA) S[2] Ensure + 60 g l^{-1} Polycose (18% protein from BCAA, Abbott)	–	Up to 60 g P	S[1] 2514 kcal S[2] 2421 kcal	S[1] 43.1 g S[2] 47.9 g	Problems consuming the large volumes Preference for energy-dense ONS expressed. Isolated cases of bloating (*n* 1), diarrhoea (*n* 1), unpalatability (*n* 2)
Mendenhall *et al.* (1985)	Hepatic-Aid 220 kcal from P (in form of amino acids, enriched in BCAA) 2000 kcal from CHO and F	–	2240 kcal	2197 kcal	55 g	Bloating, diarrhoea (*n* 2)
Okita *et al.* (1985)	SF-1008C (Otsuka Pharmaceutical, Tokyo) per 100 g 27 g P, 62 g CHO, 7 g F, 419 kcal	4.19 kcal g^{-1}	630 kcal 40 g P (150 g, 50 g in 175 ml water)	–	–	Well tolerated and easily ingested
Roselle *et al.* (1988)	Hepatic-Aid	–	2200 kcal	–	–	–

BCAA, branched-chain amino acids; CHO, carbohydrate; F, fat; P, protein; S, supplemented.

Table A3.14. Trial characteristics: hospital-based trials of oral nutritional supplementation in patients with liver disease (non-randomized data).

Trial and patient group	Design	No. S	No. US	Initial BMI S group	Initial BMI US group	Duration of ONS	Dietary counselling	Control group
Christie *et al.* (1985) Double-blind crossover, stable cirrhosis[a]	B	8 (only 6 crossover)	–	125% IBW[d]	–	S[1] 7.3 days S[2] 6.1 days 3 days no ONS in between	40 g P diet, ONS introduced gradually to maximum tolerated P intake	–
Mendenhall *et al.* (1985) Moderate or severe alcoholic hepatitis[a]	B	18[b]	34	95.2% IBW (ascites present in 89%)	104% IBW (ascites present in 85%)	30 days	No – S group given minimum 1000 kcal hospital diet	2500 kcal hospital diet
Okita *et al.* (1985) Liver cirrhosis	B	10	–	–	–	2 weeks	No – given low-protein diet (1500 kcal, 40 g P)	–
Roselle *et al.* (1988) Alcoholic hepatitis[a,c]	C	12	–	–	–	30 days	No – given regular hospital diet (1000 kcal)	–

[a] Trials include period of hospitalization for alcohol withdrawal and simultaneous ONS.

[b] 5 withdrew during the first 10 days (non-compliance, poor toleration of ONS; original *n* 23). A further 4 did not take the ONS for 30 days and dietary intake data presented for *n* 14 only.

[c] Data compared with pre-ONS period (larger *n* of 23).

[d] Most patients (7/8) ascitic.

P, protein; S, supplemented; US, unsupplemented.

Table A3.15. Main findings of oral nutritional supplementation trials in hospitalized patients with liver disease (non-randomized data).

Trial	Energy intake	Wt change S	Wt change US	Function	Outcome	Finance
Christie et al. (1985)	S¹ provided 64% of TEI and 56% TPI S² provided 69% of TEI and 65% TPI (S¹ vs. S² NS). Sig. increase in N balance in S¹ and S²	—	—	NS improvement in liver function. No deterioration or improvement in neurological status with S¹ but sig. reduction in PSEI with S²	—	—
Mendenhall et al. (1985)	TEI: S 3236 kcal (VFI 1039 kcal), 116% of est. requirements, 98 g P (n 14 who completed 30 days of ONS) US 2313 kcal, 82% of est. requirements, 81 g P (kcal and g P, S vs. US sig.)	Improvement in IBW +3% (sig. vs. US) Improvement in MAMC (+4%, S vs. US sig.)	Loss of % IBW (−4%) Loss of MAMC (−5%)	S: sig. increase in transferrin, RBP, total lymphocyte count and skin tests (S vs. US NS) S and US ascites, encephalopathy, bilirubin improved	NS diff. in mortality (S 16.7% n 3/18; US 20.6% n 7/34). 1st week of ONS no deaths vs. 7 in US group (numbers too small for analysis)	—
Okita et al. (1985)	Pre-ONS: 1621 (243) kcal, 74 (7.4) g P During ONS: 1932 (269) kcal, 85 (6.6) g P Post-ONS: 1604 (280) kcal, 73 (9.2) g P Sig. increase in kcal and P during ONS	—	—	Sig. improvement in number connection test vs. pre-ONS (sig.). Sig. decrease in AAA and methionine levels but no increase in BCAA levels. NS changes in N excretion, serum total protein, albumin or LFT. Sig. increase in pre-albumin	—	—
Roselle et al. (1988)†	No change in 'total calorie depletion scores' Sig. change in 'total protein depletion scores' (77.1 to 112.6) If combined, sig. improvement in nutritional score (83.6 to 105.3)	—	—	24% increase in CD4 cells (sig.), but decrease in CD3 and CD8 cells. No change in lymphocyte no./% or B cells. Improvement in disease severity (sig.)	—	—

† Data compared with pre-ONS period (larger n of 23).
AAA, aromatic amino acids; BCAA, branched-chain amino acid; est., estimated; LFT, liver function tests; N, nitrogen; P, protein; PSEI, anti-portal systemic encephalopathy index; RBP, retinol-binding protein; S, supplemented; TEI, total energy intake; TPI, total protein intake; US, unsupplemented; VFI, voluntary food intake.

RCT (Table A3.12). These suggested that the increase in total energy intake was equivalent to 31% of the ONS energy in pretransplant patients (Le Cornu et al., 2000), > 50% in 'mildly' and 'severely malnourished' patients with alcoholic hepatitis (52% in 'mildly malnourished' and 68% in 'severely malnourished' (Mendenhall et al., 1993)[3]) and 111% in 'moderately malnourished' patients (i.e. in addition to the ONS, supplemented patients had greater food intakes than unsupplemented patients (Mendenhall et al., 1993)[3]). However, checks of compliance with supplementation were not recorded in any of the randomized trials. There were also few data on patients' ability to tolerate supplements (see Tables A3.10 and A3.13), with the exception of occasional reports of gastrointestinal complaints in patients taking a branched-chain amino acid-enriched supplement (Mendenhall et al., 1993). Furthermore, in one NRT the efficacy of using higher-energy-density sip feeds with small, more tolerable volumes was suggested (Christie et al., 1985).

(II) What effect do ONS have on the body weight and composition of patients with liver disease in hospital?

The use of ONS in patients with liver disease may lead to improvements in nutritional status. However, the measurement of body weight as an outcome parameter following ONS is largely unreliable in patients with liver disease due to the confounding effects of ascites. Indeed, the changes in weight following a period of ONS, reported in only one trial, were attributed to a reduction in ascites (Bunout et al., 1989), which occurred to a greater extent in supplemented patients. However, significant improvements in upper-arm anthropometry (Le Cornu et al., 2000) and in protein-calorie malnutrition scores (using a number of other anthropometric and biochemical parameters) (Mendenhall et al., 1993) were noted in supplemented patients and not in unsupplemented patients.

(III) What effect do ONS have on the body function of patients with liver disease in hospital?

Few functional parameters have been assessed in the trials reviewed. Significant longitudinal improvements in hand-grip strength were observed in pretransplant patients (Le Cornu et al., 2000) and in liver function in a 'moderately malnourished' group of supplemented patients (Mendenhall et al., 1993). Similar changes were not seen in those who were 'severely malnourished'. Further research is needed.

(IV) What effect do ONS have on the clinical and financial outcome of patients with liver disease in hospital?

ONS may improve the clinical outcome of patients hospitalized with liver disease. A combined analysis of data from two trials shows a lower mortality rate in supplemented (32%) than in unsupplemented (37%) patients with alcoholic liver disease (Bunout et al., 1989; Mendenhall et al., 1993). However, significant reductions in mortality were only achieved in the larger trial (Mendenhall et al., 1993) (see Fig. 6.13 in Chapter 6). Notably, a group of 'moderately malnourished' patients had significantly lower mortality (9%) than unsupplemented patients (21%) after 1 month of ONS in hospital (combined with oxandrolone) and at 6 months after discharge from hospital (20% vs. 37%), with significantly longer median survival times (49 months vs. 26 months) (Mendenhall et al., 1993). No such improvements were evident in the 'severely malnourished' group (Mendenhall et al., 1993). Further analysis of these data and those of a previous trial by the same authors (Mendenhall et al., 1984a), when an anabolic steroid was given for 1 month without ONS, suggested that only with the combination of steroid and adequate calorie intake (> 2500 kcal) was mortality significantly improved (Mendenhall et al., 1993). Steroid treatment alone had no effect on mortality when energy intake was inadequate. In supplemented patients undergoing liver transplantation (Le Cornu et al., 2000), no differences in clinical outcome after transplantation were observed between supplemented and unsupplemented patients (e.g. no difference in time on ventilator, time in the intensive care unit (ICU), time in hospital) although mortality was lower (12% versus 23%, not significant). Overall, small numbers of patients at follow-up in some of the trials reduced the statistical power of the studies to detect significant changes in clinical outcome. Therefore, the mortality results from these three studies were combined in a meta-analysis. This suggested that the odds ratio for mortality with ONS in patients with liver disease was 0.74 (95% CI 0.29–1.92; n 391) (no significant heterogeneity, fixed-effects model). Therefore, larger trials in patients with liver disease are needed to assess whether ONS can reduce mortality significantly, ideally undertaken in those with specific types of liver disease. Research into the cost efficacy of ONS in this patient group is also required.

Neurology/General Medical

Despite the impact of neurological disease on a patient's ability to eat (e.g. poor appetite, dysphagia, limited communicative ability and difficulties in physically preparing or eating meals), there is a remarkable lack of information about the importance of nutritional support in this patient group, who are at risk of malnutrition (see Chapter 2 for prevalence). Stroke (cerebrovascular accident (CVA)) patients are especially at risk of malnutrition, partly because they are usually elderly and may have pre-existing nutrient deficiencies and partly because of the neurological deficits produced by the CVA. These deficits impair food intake by causing weakness and inability to bring food to the mouth, by causing swallowing difficulties and impairing consciousness and communication. The use of puréed diets, which are often given to such patients, is known to further compromise intakes (Brynes *et al.*, 1998).

Malnutrition has also been documented in mixed groups of general medical patients (see Chapter 2), and the nutritional status of

such patients frequently deteriorates while they are in hospital. Amongst the reasons are the effects of disease, drugs, hospitalization (unfamiliar surroundings, hospital food and rigid mealtimes) and emotional problems (anxiety, stress and loneliness), all of which may limit food intake (Association of Community Health Councils for England and Wales, 1997). Nutritional support, including the use of ONS, is often required in a variety of general medical patients to prevent or treat malnutrition.

Neurology/general medical: present analysis

Only one RCT (total patient n 61) in mixed general medical patients and one in CVA patients (total patient n 42) (McWhirter and Pennington, 1996; Gariballa *et al.*, 1998a) were reviewed and summarized in Tables A3.16–A3.18 and Box A3.4. The four main review questions are addressed sequentially below.

(I) What effect do ONS have on the voluntary food intake and total energy intake of neurology/general medical patients in hospital?

ONS may improve total energy intakes in neurology/medical patients. Supplementation of patients with CVA (no swallowing difficulties) (Gariballa *et al.*, 1998a) and a mixed group of malnourished (criteria BMI < 20 kg m^{-2}, triceps skin-fold thickness (TSF)/MAMC < 15th percentile) general medical patients (McWhirter and Pennington, 1996) effectively increased total energy and protein intakes, with little effect on voluntary food intake. Both studies indicated that voluntary food intake in patients receiving an ONS (723 kcal: Gariballa *et al.*, 1998a; < 588 kcal: McWhirter and Pennington, 1996; see Tables A3.16 and A3.18) was not significantly different from that of control patients. Furthermore, ONS (both trials used commercial liquid sip feeds), given for 10 days (McWhirter and Pennington, 1996) or 4 weeks (Gariballa *et al.*, 1998a), were well tolerated in both patient groups (Table A3.16), except that only 50% of CVA patients took

---

Box A3.4. Key findings: effect of ONS in neurology/general medical hospital patients.

Nutritional intake: supplementation of medical (including CVA) patients who are able to eat and drink is an effective way of increasing total energy and protein intakes, with little suppression of voluntary food intake. The effects of different types of ONS in neurological patients with dysphagia have not been assessed.

Body weight: ONS can significantly increase weight and muscle mass in general medical patients and attenuate weight loss in CVA patients.

Body function/clinical outcome: supplementation of CVA patients may improve functional status, shorten hospital stays, lower rates of complications and reduce mortality rates. Further research in larger trials is needed to confirm these findings. There are no apparent detriments of using ONS in this patient group.

Further research: large RCT are needed in those with other neurological diseases (multiple sclerosis, Parkinson's disease), for which little is known about the efficacy of ONS.

ONS for the full duration of the trial (4 weeks) (Gariballa *et al.*, 1998a). The % of ONS energy additive to food intake (calculated from data in one trial only) was 73% (McWhirter and Pennington, 1996).

(II) What effect do ONS have on the body weight and composition of neurology/general medical patients in hospital?

ONS can prevent the weight loss that is often seen in general medical (including CVA) patients. The two trials reviewed (McWhirter and Pennington, 1996; Gariballa *et al.*, 1998a) reported that patients receiving ONS gained weight, whereas unsupplemented patients lost weight, although the difference was only significant in one of the trials involving general medical patients (McWhirter and Pennington, 1996) (supplemented + 2.9%, unsupplemented −2.5%; see Table A3.18). The same trial reported that the MAMC improved in supplemented patients but declined in those who were unsupplemented (McWhirter and Pennington, 1996).

(III) What effect do ONS have on the body function of neurology/general medical patients in hospital?

Only the one trial (Gariballa *et al.*, 1998a) in CVA patients made assessments of function post-supplementation. Patients receiving an ONS were found to have similar improvements in Barthel scores to unsupplemented patients. However, the supplemented group was reported to maintain significantly better iron and albumin status.

(IV) What effect do ONS have on the clinical and financial outcome of neurology/general medical patients in hospital?

Hospital stays, mortality rates and complication rates may be reduced in patients with a CVA (Gariballa *et al.*, 1998a; see Table A3.18). In an RCT of CVA patients, supplemented patients were reported to have a shorter length of hospital stay (by an average of 18 days), a lower mortality rate (10% versus 30%) and a slightly lower rate of infectious complications (45% versus 55%) during the period of hospitalization than unsupplemented patients, but none of these differences were significant. In addition, a greater number of supplemented patients were discharged to their own home (60% versus 40% of unsupplemented) (Gariballa *et al.*, 1998a). None of these differences reached statistical significance, probably because of the small numbers of patients in the study. If similar results were obtained with larger numbers of patients, the economic implications associated with shorter hospital stays and reduced utilization of health-care resources in the community would be considerable. Larger, adequately powered trials are needed.

Table A3.16. Oral nutritional supplements used in randomized controlled trials of neurology and general medical patients in hospital.

Trial	ONS	ONS energy density	ONS prescribed	ONS energy (kcal) intake	ONS protein (g) intake	Toleration
Gariballa *et al.* (1998a)	Fortisip	1.5 kcal ml⁻¹	≤ 600 kcal, 20 g P (? administered twice a day)	Est. 723 kcal (95% CI 498–947)	Est. 21 g (95% CI 11.7–30.3)	Good, no failures or withdrawals
McWhirter and Pennington (1996)	Tonexis (Clintec) 3.75 g P, 13.8 g CHO, 3.33 g F per 100 ml	1 kcal ml⁻¹	To meet est. energy requirements	588 kcal Av. 74% of prescription	23.9 g	Well tolerated, 2 failures to comply

CHO, carbohydrate; Est., estimated; F, fat; P, protein.

Table A3.17. Trial characteristics: hospital-based randomized controlled trials of oral nutritional supplementation in neurology and general medical patients.

Trial and patient group	Design	No. S	No. US	Initial BMI S group	Initial BMI US group	Duration of ONS	Dietary counselling	Control group
Gariballa *et al.* (1998a) Acute stroke patients	11001	21	21	– Wt 57.3 (9.1) kg	– Wt 57 (8.85) kg	4 weeks (only *n* 10 took ONS for 4 weeks)	–	Hospital diet
McWhirter and Pennington (1996) Malnourished medical (data from ETF intervention group not included, see Appendix 5)	10001	35	26	All described as malnourished		9.7 days	–	Hospital diet

ETF, enteral tube feeding; S, supplemented; US, unsupplemented.

Table A3.18. Main findings of randomized controlled trials of oral nutritional supplementation in hospitalized general medical and neurology patients.

Trial	Energy intake	Wt change S	Wt change US	Function	Outcome	Finance
Gariballa *et al.* (1998a)	S greater energy intake (1807 (318) kcal) than US (1084 (343) kcal) ONS 67% increase in kcal and 47% increase in P 'Supplements were not associated with significant reduction in voluntary oral intake during the trial period'	+0.2 kg (−1.1, 1.4) kg or +0.35% (average 2, 4 and 12 weeks after start of ONS, S vs. US NS) TSF and MAMC NS change (S vs. US NS)	−0.7 kg (−2.7, 1.4) kg or −1.23% TSF and MAMC NS change	Higher Barthel scores (functional state) in S group before and after ONS (NS) S maintained better Fe and albumin status (sig. vs. US)	S shorter hospital stay than US (NS) S lower number of infective complications than US (NS) during hospital stay S greater number discharged to own home (60% vs. 40% US, NS) S lower mortality at 12 weeks (10% *n* 2) than US (35% *n* 7) (small *n* for these outcomes)	–
McWhirter and Pennington (1996)	S: TEI 1680 kcal, 77.9 g P S: VFI 1090 kcal, 54 g P US: VFI 1250 kcal, 39.5 g P (VFI: S vs. US NS) % pt taking > 80% est. requirements: TEI: S 71% US 4%; TPI S 91% US 15% (Third arm of trial received ETF)	+ 2.9% (S vs. US sig.) MAMC + 1.66% (S vs. US sig.)	− 2.5% MAMC − 22.8%	–	–	–

est., estimated; MAMC, mid-arm muscle circumference; P, protein; S, supplemented; TSF, triceps skin-fold thickness; TEI, total energy intake; TPI, total protein intake; US, unsupplemented; VFI, voluntary food intake.

Oral and Maxillofacial Surgery

Orthognathic surgery and mandibular fractures typically require intermaxillary fixation to prevent the movement of the mandible. Consequently ingestion and mastication of food are severely impaired, often for more than 1 month (Kendell *et al.*, 1982). As dietary intake can be severely compromised in such patients, provision of nutrition in a form that can be easily taken by the patient and that enables them to meet their nutritional requirements becomes essential. The use of liquid ONS that are energy- and nutrient-rich is one such strategy for orthognathic patients. The efficacy of such intervention has been investigated in only a few trials and these are reviewed below.

Oral and maxillofacial surgery: present analysis

Three RCT (two undertaken by the same research group (Kendell *et al.*, 1982; Olejko and Fonseca, 1984)) investigated the effects of postoperative ONS in the orthognathic surgical patient (Kendell *et al.*, 1982; Olejko and Fonseca, 1984; Antila *et al.*, 1993). The findings and details of these studies, which traversed both hospital and home settings, are summarized in Box A3.5 and Tables A3.19–A3.21. In these studies, a commercial liquid sip feed (1.5 kcal ml^{-1}; see Table A3.19), prescribed to meet 50% of estimated energy requirements postoperatively, was given in combination with

verbal and written dietary advice. The same advice was also given to the control groups. In addition, supplementation was also given for 4 weeks preoperatively in one trial (Olejko and Fonseca, 1984).

(I) What effect do ONS have on the voluntary food intake and total energy intake of orthognathic patients in hospital?

ONS, in the form of sip feeds, improve the intakes of energy and a variety of nutrients (including vitamins and minerals) in orthognathic patients. Postoperative ONS in mandibular fracture and orthognathic surgical patients was shown in all the reviewed trials (Kendell *et al.*, 1982; Olejko and Fonseca, 1984; Antila *et al.*, 1993) to substantially improve intakes of energy (see Table A3.21). Intakes of a number of micronutrients were also significantly greater in supplemented compared with unsupplemented patients (e.g. vitamins B_1 and B_2, niacin, folate, zinc, copper, selenium and iron) in these trials. There was also a trend towards increased protein intakes in patients supplemented postoperatively. Preoperative supplementation in patients prior to orthognathic surgery, who as a group were not malnourished (BMI 21.6 kg m^{-2}), appeared to have little effect on energy/nutrient intakes (see Table A3.21), compared with those who were unsupplemented (Olejko and Fonseca, 1984). Despite this, the authors reported that patients supplemented preoperatively had significantly greater weight gain than those not given an ONS at that time (see Question II, p. 490).

Box A3.5. Key findings: effect of ONS in oral/maxillofacial hospital patients.

Nutritional intake: ONS can be used to increase energy, protein and micronutrient intakes postoperatively, but have little apparent effect on intake or clinical benefit when used prior to surgery.

Body weight: ONS can attenuate the weight loss (by 4%) typically seen postoperatively.

Body function and clinical outcome: the effects of ONS on body function or clinical outcome have not been investigated and so further RCT are needed to evaluate both the clinical and cost-effectiveness of this mode of treatment.

Table A3.19. Oral nutritional supplements used in randomized controlled trials of orthognathic patients in hospital.

Trial	ONS	ONS energy density	ONS prescribed	ONS energy (kcal) intake	ONS protein (g) intake	Toleration
Antila et al. (1993)	Enteropolar TEHO, Medipolar, Finland (6.8 g P, 5.3 g F, 18.8 g CHO per 100 ml)	1.5 kcal ml^{-1}	To meet 75% of patients' REE	–	–	–
Kendell et al. (1982)	Ensure plus (Abbott) 14.7% P; 32% F; 53.3% CHO	1.5 kcal ml^{-1}	50% of estimated energy requirement	–	–	–
Olejko and Fonseca (1984)	Nutritionally complete liquid (commercial) 14.7% P; 32% F; 53% CHO	1.5 kcal ml^{-1}	50% of estimated energy requirement (postop.) 354 kcal (preop.)	–	–	–

CHO, carbohydrate; F, fat; P, protein; postop., postoperative; preop., preoperative; REE, resting energy expenditure.

Table A3.20. Trial characteristics: hospital-based randomized controlled trials of oral nutritional supplementation in orthognathic patients.

Trial	Design	No. S	No. US	Initial BMI S group	Initial BMI US group	Duration of ONS	Dietary counselling	Control group
Antila et al. (1993)	10000	8	9		23.0	28 (9) days (intermaxillary fixation) 39 (7) days (orthognathic)	Nutritional counselling for S and US (usual oral instructions and recommendations on blenderizing foods)	Nutritional counselling as for S
Kendell et al. (1982)	10001	12	12	22.2 (average BMI for whole group)		42 days (mean 4.34 days in hospital)	Verbal and written advice to both groups	Standard diet
Olejko and Fonseca (1984)	10001	8 postop. 8 pre- and postop.	8	21.6 postop. 20.6 pre/postop.	24.7	4 weeks pre- and/or 6 weeks postop.	Verbal and written advice to both groups	Standard diet

preop., preoperative; postop., postoperative; S, supplemented; US, unsupplemented.

Table A3.21. Main findings of randomized controlled trials of oral nutritional supplementation in hospitalized orthognathic patients

Trial	Energy intake	Wt change S	Wt change US	Function	Outcome	Finance
Antila *et al.* (1993)	S sig. higher intake of E (2951 vs. 1867 kcal), zinc, copper, selenium and iron than US and NS higher P intake (122 g vs. 71 g)	−3.8 (2.7)%[a] (S vs. US ?) Sig. increase in subscapular skin-fold (S vs. US sig. at 6 weeks) NS differences in other anthropometric parameters	−6 (3.8)%[a]	NS difference between S and US for serum trace elements and leucocyte zinc	−	−
Kendell *et al.* (1982)	S: higher E (90.4% vs. 53.8% RDA, sig.) and P (NS) intake than US group. Sig. higher B_1, B_2, niacin, zinc and folate	−2.50% (NS less than US)	−7.90%	−	−	−
Olejko and Fonseca (1984)	Preop. (includes ONS): S prepost 2315 kcal, 84 g P; S post 2410 kcal, 81 g P; US 2878 kcal, 97 g P Postop.: S prepost 3067 kcal, 112 g P; S post 2973 kcal, 116 g P; US 1847 kcal, 55 g P. Change: S prepost. +752 kcal, 28 g P; S post.: +563 kcal, 35 g P; US −1031 kcal, 42 g P. Decreased fat intakes (sig. in US), increased CHO intake S (?NS). Better Fe, B_1 and niacin intakes in S group	− Over 10-week period, sig. less wt loss than US (no data) Preop.: +3.1% (S vs. US sig.)	−9.70% Sig. greater wt loss vs. both S groups over 10 weeks Preop.: sig. less wt gain than S (no data)	−	−	−

[a] Maximum weight loss figures for supplemented and unsupplemented groups.

CHO, carbohydrate; E, energy; NS, not significant; P, protein; postop, postoperative; preop., preoperative; prepost, took ONS before and after orthognathic surgery; RDA, recommended daily allowance; S, supplemented; sig., significant; US, unsupplemented.

(II) What effect do ONS have on the body weight and composition of orthognathic patients in hospital?

This review suggests that ONS given post-operatively appear to curtail the weight loss associated with oral and maxillofacial surgery. Patients receiving ONS lost less weight than those who were unsupplemented in all trials (Kendell *et al.*, 1982; Olejko and Fonseca, 1984; Antila *et al.*, 1993) (see Table A3.21; significant in one trial only (Olejko and Fonseca, 1984)). However, there was no difference in overall weight loss between those receiving a pre- and postoperative supplement and those receiving ONS postoperatively only.

Combined analysis of % weight change (data from two trials (Kendell *et al.*, 1982; Antila *et al.*, 1993), *n* 41; weighted for sample size) indicated an attenuation of weight loss when ONS were used (supplemented patients −3% versus unsupplemented patients −7%).

(IV) What effect do ONS have on the functional, clinical and financial outcome of orthognathic patients in hospital?

The use of ONS postoperatively did not significantly change some measures of metabolic function (serum trace element or leucocyte zinc concentrations) compared with the control patients (Antila *et al.*, 1993). No other functional measures or clinical or financial outcome measures were assessed in these trials and so further research is required in this patient group.

Orthopaedics

Epidemiological studies from a number of European countries highlight the considerable (and increasing) number of admissions of elderly patients with fractured neck of femur (Boyce and Vessey, 1985; De Deuxchaisnes and Devogelaer, 1988). In addition to demographic changes, malnutrition may be an important determinant of both the incidence and the complications associated with hip fracture in the elderly

(Delmi *et al.*, 1990). Indeed, elderly patients with hip fracture are often malnourished on admission to hospital (see Chapter 2). Loss of muscle and fat mass and the weakness and lack of coordination often associated with malnutrition may contribute to falls. Furthermore, in elderly patients, those given ONS have been reported to have fewer falls (see section on the elderly in Appendix 4). Once patients are admitted to hospital, nutritional intakes can also be poor (Hessov, 1977; see Chapter 3). Furthermore, nutritional support by ETF (Bastow *et al.*, 1983) in hospitalized fractured neck of femur patients has been shown to significantly improve clinical outcome and this is discussed in more detail in Chapter 7. However, how effective is the use of ONS in this patient group? An investigation highlighting the negative energy and protein balance of elderly patients hospitalized with fractured neck of femur suggested that (Jallut *et al.*, 1990):

> such patients would benefit from an oral supplementation above their spontaneous food intake providing an extra 200–300 kcal/day containing 20 g of protein/day.

Orthopaedics: present analysis

Studies of ONS use versus no nutritional support or versus a 'placebo' supplement (Tkatch *et al.*, 1992; Schurch *et al.*, 1998) in elderly fractured neck of femur patients were systematically reviewed and are described below. Six RCT (total *n* 296 patients) (Stableforth, 1986; Moller-Madsen *et al.*, 1988; Delmi *et al.*, 1990; Brown and Seabrook, 1992; Tkatch *et al.*, 1992; Schurch *et al.*, 1998) and three NRT (total *n* 230 patients (Williams *et al.*, 1989; Doshi *et al.*, 1998; Lawson *et al.*, 2000); repeat reports of the same patient group not counted (Doshi *et al.*, 1998; Lawson *et al.*, 2000)) were reviewed and are summarized in Box A3.6 and Tables A3.22–A3.27. A summary of the findings of the NRT has been documented in Tables A3.25–A3.27 and the main findings from the RCT are discussed below, addressing each of the four review questions.

Table A3.22. Oral nutritional supplements used in randomized controlled trials of orthopaedic patients in hospital.

Trial	ONS	ONS energy density	ONS prescribed	ONS energy (kcal) intake	ONS protein (g) intake	Toleration
Brown and Seabrook (1992)	Fresubin (Fresenius)	–	–	–	–	–
Delmi et al. (1990)	250 ml ONS: 20.4 g P from milk; 5.8 g F; 29.5 g CHO; Ca 0.525 g, Mg 70 mg	1 kcal ml^{-1}	254 kcal	254 kcal	20.4 g	Well tolerated. No side-effects
Moller-Madsen et al. (1988)	Newly developed 5 g P/100 kcal per 100 ml	1 kcal ml^{-1}	3 times per day ?amount	–	–	Well tolerated
Schurch et al. (1998)	Meritene (Sandoz) powder[a]	3.85 kcal g^{-1}	250 kcal, 20 g P	–	–	Well tolerated and no major side-effects (compliance checks made)
Stableforth (1986)	Carnation Instant Breakfast (Nestlé) Per 100 ml: 6.2 g P, 13.3 g CHO, 3.7 g F	1.2 kcal ml^{-1}	320 kcal (300 ml) or ? prescribed *ad libitum*	–	–	Large amounts of ONS impractical as 'lighter patients lost their appetite for ward food and some of the iller patients became nauseated'
Tkatch et al. (1992)	250 ml ONS: 20.4 g P from milk 5.8 g F, 29.5 g CHO, 0.525 g Ca, 70 mg Mg	1 kcal ml^{-1} (assumed same as ONS used by Delmi et al., 1990)	S: 254 kcal, 20.4 g P US: 116 kcal, 0 g P (placebo)	–	–	–

[a] Patients all received a single oral dose of vitamin D (200,000 IU) at the start of the trial.
CHO, carbohydrate; F, fat; IU, international units; P, protein; S, supplemented; US, unsupplemented.

Table A3.23. Trial characteristics: hospital-based randomized controlled trials of oral nutritional supplementation in orthopaedic patients.

Trial	Design	No. S	No. US	Initial BMI S group	Initial BMI US group	Duration of ONS	Dietary counselling	Control group
Brown and Seabrook (1992) Abstract Femoral neck fracture	10000	5	5	17	17	No data	–	Hospital diet
Delmi et al. (1990)[a] Femoral neck fracture	10000	27	32	–	–	32 days	–	Hospital diet
Moller-Madsen et al. (1988) Letter Femoral neck fracture	10000	25 in total for both S and US	–	–	–	–	–	Hospital diet
Schurch et al. (1998) Recent hip fracture	11101	41	41	24.2 (4.4)	24.4 (3.5)	5 days per week for 6 months	–	Placebo ONS with no protein but isocaloric (? micronutrient content)
Stableforth (1986) Femoral neck fracture	10000	24	34	– 65 kg	– 53 kg	10 days	–	Ward diet
Tkatch et al. (1992) Osteoporobic fracture of proximal femur	10001	33	29	–	–	38.2 days	–	US group a placebo, 116 kcal, no protein, and the same micronutrients as ONS

[a] A preliminary report supporting the efficacy of an ONS in a subset of patients (n 7, French language, Gegerie et al., 1986) has not been reviewed.
S, supplemented; US, unsupplemented.

Table A3.24. Main findings of randomized controlled trials of oral nutritional supplementation in hospitalized orthopaedic patients.

Trial	Energy intake	Wt change S	Wt change US	Function	Outcome	Finance
Brown and Seabrook (1992)	S had greater TEI and TPI than controls. Both groups did not meet their nutritional requirements (no data)	Wt loss less than US (no data)	Wt loss (no data)	–	Quicker recovery and shorter hospital stay than controls (by 26 days) (NB. Data from several groups assessed as one)	–
Delmi et al. (1990)	TEI, TPI and calcium intakes increased vs. baseline by 23%, 62% and 130% in S group. Food intake was not reduced in S group (S and US 1100 kcal). No statistical comparisons with US	–	–	–	Shorter hospital stay – 24 days vs. 40 days (sig. vs. US group) Better clinical course in 2nd hospital (sig.) and after 6 months (sig.) (complications/death % favourable course) Diff. NS. in orthopaedic ward	–
Moller-Madsen et al. (1988)	Sig higher TEI (1309 vs. 1094 kcal) and sig. higher TPI (52 vs. 37 g day^{-1}) than US	No difference between S and US				–
Schurch et al. (1998)	– NS difference in intakes from diet of calcium and phosphorus between groups (excluding ONS intake)	–	–	Sig. greater increase in IGF-1 and prealb. and an attenuation of the loss in proximal femur bone mineral density (-2.29% (S) vs. -4.71% (US[a]), sig.) NS difference in osteocalcin, calcium, phosphate, PTH or vitamin D concentrations or in DCH (S vs. US[a] NS)	Sig. shorter stay in rehabilitation wards (S 33 days vs. US[a] 54 days, sig.)	–
Stableforth (1986)	TEI: S 1075 kcal, US 887 kcal (NS) kcal kg^{-1} wt: S 19.1 US 17.7 kcal kg^{-1} (NS) TPI: S 40 g, US 27 g (sig.) S 121 mg N kg^{-1} vs. US 90 mg N kg^{-1} (sig.) 5/6 pts with positive N balance were taking ONS. In trochanteric fractures, N balance: US (n 15) -636 mg N kg^{-1} S (n 8) -165 mg N kg^{-1} (sig.) (data not provided for all)	Small changes in body weight ~ -5% loss (no other data)	–	–	–	–
Tkatch et al. (1992)	–	–	–	Sig. greater increase in osteocalcin in S. NS difference in BMD levels but no S pt had sig. loss in the femoral shaft at 7 months (sig. vs. US). These differences not seen at other bone sites	More pts with favourable course in S (79%, 48%) at recovery H and at 7 months than US (36%, 20%) (sig.). Lower death rate in S (NS), and all deaths in S in the immediate postop. period. Length of hospital stay shorter in S (69 days vs. 101 days, sig.) than in US. More S pts returned home (67% vs. 45%, NS). No diff. in no. of fractures (favourable course = none or 1 minor complication) (unfavourable course = 1 or more major complications)	–

[a] US given a placebo supplement that was isocaloric with the ONS (S) but protein-free.

S, supplemented; US, unsupplemented; TEI, total energy intake; TPI, total protein intake; IGF-1, insulin-like growth factor-1; sig., significant; NS, not significant; prealb., prealbumin; BMD, bone mineral density; DCH, delayed cutaneous hypersensitivity; H, hospital; N, nitrogen; pts, patients; PTH, parathyroid hormone.

Table A3.25. Oral nutritional supplements used in trials of orthopaedic patients in hospital (non-randomized data).

Trial	ONS	ONS energy density	ONS prescribed	ONS energy (kcal) intake	ONS protein (g) intake	Toleration
Doshi et al. (1998)[a]	Assume Fortisip and Enlive	–	– (assume as below)	–	–	Median compliance 14.9%
Lawson et al. (2000)	Fortisip (Nutricia)	1.5 kcal ml^{-1}	600 kcal, 20 g P (400 ml)	234 kcal	~7.8 g	Compliance poor (100% = 2 ONS, average compliance 21%). Only n 4 had 61–80% compliance; 39% of pts discontinued ONS at some point. Compliance varied with BMI and ONS type (BMI < 25: 19% compliance; BMI > 25: 32%); n 37 chose Fortisip, 76% changed to Enlive and 16% stopped ONS; n 18 chose Enlive, 11% changed to Fortisip and 44% stopped ONS
	Enlive (Abbott) (range of flavours)	1.25 kcal ml^{-1}	600 kcal, 19 g P (480 ml)			
Williams et al. (1989)	Ensure (Abbott)	1 kcal ml^{-1}	500–750 kcal, 17.6–26.4 g P (2–3 cans, 500–750 ml)	400 kcal (1.6 cans)	14.1 g	n 11 refused ONS or took only 20–100 ml and were excluded (data analysed as 'non-compliant' group)

[a] Doshi et al. (1998) an abstract report of Lawson et al. (2000).
P, protein; pts, patients.

Table A3.26. Trial characteristics: hospital-based trials of oral nutritional supplementation in orthopaedic patients (non-randomized data).

Trial and patient group	Design	No. S	No. US	Initial BMI S group	Initial BMI US group	Duration of ONS	Dietary counselling	Control group
Doshi *et al.* (1998)[a] Abstract	B	84	97	–	–	–	–	–
Lawson *et al.* (2000) Non-targeted ONS in postop. orthopaedic patients	B	84	97	26.2 (16.2–31.8) *n* 50	–	6.7 days (median 4)	–	Standard hospital diet
Williams *et al.* (1989) Elderly admitted for surgery for fractured neck of femur or for elective total hip replacement	B	19	19 + 11 non-compliant	'High-risk' patients (assessed using a nutritional risk questionnaire)	–	~20 days (ONS from admission to discharge)	–	Normal foods

[a] Doshi *et al.* (1998) an abstract report of Lawson *et al.* (2000).
postop., postoperative; S, supplemented; US, unsupplemented.

Table A3.27. Main findings of oral nutritional supplementation trials in hospitalized orthopaedic patients (non-randomized data).

Trial	Energy intake	Wt change S	Wt change US	Function	Outcome	Finance
Doshi *et al.* (1998)	S sig. greater kcal (1523 kcal) than US (1289 kcal) (*n* 48)	–	–	–	Sig. fewer major complications in S vs. US Fewer wound/joint infections (7.6 vs. 21.5%) Less severe anaemia (0 vs. 6.3%) Fewer pressure sores (0 vs. 5.1%) Less bone-fusion problems (0 vs. 5.1%) (no difference in pneumonia) Sig. fewer minor complications in S vs. US – wound inflammation and urinary tract infection (S 10.1% vs. US 21.5%)	–
Lawson *et al.* (2000)	S sig. greater kcal (1523 kcal) than US (1289 kcal) Protein: S 62 g US 52 g (NS) (*n* 48) Report average increase 234 kcal day^{-1} (78% of ONS energy)	–	–	–	–	–
Williams *et al.* (1989)	–	No change in TSF or MAMC	Sig. decrease in TSF and MAMC (sig. decrease in MAMC in non-compliant)	NS changes in HGS in S or US or non-compliant groups	S: shorter hospital stay (18.4 days vs. 20.2 days, S vs. US NS) S – quicker time to mobilization (by 1.5 days) and greater % discharged on sticks (by 11%) or as independent (by 10%) (S vs. US NS)	–

HGS, hand-grip strength; MAMC, mid-arm muscle circumference; NS, not significant; S, supplemented; sig., significant; TSF, triceps skin-fold thickness; US, unsupplemented.

Four out of six RCT involved the use of sip feeds (see Table A3.22) (Moller-Madsen *et al.*, 1988; Delmi *et al.*, 1990; Brown and Seabrook, 1992; Tkatch *et al.*, 1992) and two trials used powder reconstituted to form a drink (Carnation Instant Breakfast (Stableforth, 1986) and Meritene (Sandoz) (Schurch *et al.*, 1998)). The energy density of these ONS ranged from 1.0 to 1.2 kcal ml^{-1}, although the patients' actual intake of supplement was documented in only one RCT (Delmi *et al.*, 1990). Supplementation periods ranged from 10 days (Stableforth, 1986) to 6 months (Schurch *et al.*, 1998) (where documented) and toleration of ONS was mostly good (with the exception of large volumes of reconstituted-milk drink suppressing appetite (Stableforth, 1986), see Table A3.22).

(I) What effect do ONS have on the voluntary food intake and total energy intake of orthopaedic patients in hospital?

This review indicates that ONS can effectively increase the nutritional intake of patients hospitalized with fractured neck of femur. Oral nutritional supplementation of fractured neck of femur patients in hospital improved energy, protein (Stableforth, 1986; Moller-Madsen *et al.*, 1988; Delmi *et al.*, 1990; Brown and Seabrook, 1992) and calcium intakes (Delmi *et al.*, 1990) in the four trials that

made such assessments, although in only two trials were total energy (Moller-Madsen *et al.*, 1988) and protein intakes (Stableforth, 1986; Moller-Madsen *et al.*, 1988) described as significantly greater for all supplemented patients, compared with the unsupplemented group (see Table A3.24). Similarly, a dietary survey found that the addition of one ONS (254 kcal, 20 g protein) to the diets of elderly orthopaedic patients (*n* 7) increased their energy intakes by 23%, protein by 62% and calcium by 131% (Gegerie *et al.*, 1986). However, Stableforth (1986) indicated that ONS might have been more effective in a subgroup of patients with trochanteric fracture, in whom significant improvements in total energy and protein intakes were observed. Despite the use of ONS, total energy and protein intakes remained insufficient to meet nutritional requirements in a number of trials (e.g. Stableforth, 1986; Brown and Seabrook, 1992).

The impact of ONS on food intake could only be estimated quantitatively in one of the trials reviewed. Delmi *et al.* (1990) stated that the voluntary food intake was the same in supplemented and unsupplemented patients, implying that 100% of the ONS energy was additive (i.e. no suppression of oral intake). It was not possible to relate changes in total energy intake to patients' nutritional status due to a lack of anthropometric information in most of the

---

Box A3.6. Key findings: effect of ONS in hospital orthopaedic patients.

Nutritional intake: ONS can significantly improve intakes of energy, protein and calcium, although total nutritional requirements may remain unmet. Voluntary food intake is not suppressed by ONS.

Body weight: a lack of assessment of changes in body weight and nutritional status with ONS in these orthopaedic trials prevents any conclusions being drawn. Further research is needed.

Body function: protein-containing ONS (compared with isocaloric protein-free placebos) may attenuate the loss of bone mineral density in the femur, although the mechanisms involved are under investigation.

Clinical outcome: significantly quicker recovery times, shorter stays in hospital and better clinical outcomes (fewer complications) are observed when mixed macronutrient (including protein) ONS are used. There is a consistent trend towards reduced mortality.

trials reviewed (Stableforth, 1986; Moller-Madsen *et al.*, 1988; Delmi *et al.*, 1990; Tkatch *et al.*, 1992).

(II) What effect do ONS have on the body weight and composition of orthopaedic patients in hospital?

Insufficient information in the trials reviewed prevented any quantitative assessment of the impact of ONS on body weight or body composition. It appears that weight loss typically occurred in these patients, despite ONS. However, Brown and Seabrook (1992) indicated that those patients receiving ONS lost less weight than the unsupplemented patients, but they provided no data (see Table A3.24). More research is needed.

(III) What effect do ONS have on the body function of orthopaedic patients in hospital?

Only two trials (Tkatch *et al.*, 1992; Schurch *et al.*, 1998) made any functional assessment in hospitalized patients with fractured neck of femur following ONS (254 kcal, 20 g protein) or a protein-free 'placebo' supplement (116 kcal with the same micronutrient content as the ONS) (Table A3.24). Supplementation for 6 months led to a significant attenuation of bone mineral density loss in the proximal femur (-2.29%) compared with the control group given the 'placebo' (-4.71%) (Schurch *et al.*, 1998). Shorter-term ONS (< 40 days) also led to significantly fewer supplemented patients losing bone mass in the femoral shaft compared with those who received a 'placebo' (Tkatch *et al.*, 1992), although no such changes were seen at other bone sites. The supplemented patients also had greater increases in osteocalcin (Tkatch *et al.*, 1992) and insulin-like growth factor 1 (IGF-1) (Schurch *et al.*, 1998) concentrations in some trials, although these were not consistently observed (Schurch *et al.*, 1998). Therefore, further trials are needed to investigate the impact of ONS on bone density and their potential mechanism of action and on other functional outcomes in this group of patients.

(IV) What effect do ONS have on the clinical and financial outcome of orthopaedic patients in hospital?

Improvements in clinical outcome have been consistently demonstrated in fractured neck of femur patients receiving nutritional support. Findings from the studies of ONS in hospitalized orthopaedic patients are no exception. The four trials that made assessments of clinical outcome (Delmi *et al.*, 1990; Brown and Seabrook, 1992; Tkatch *et al.*, 1992; Schurch *et al.*, 1998) were able to show that ONS (compared with no nutrition or a protein-free placebo supplement) led to significantly quicker recovery times with shorter stays in hospitals/rehabilitation (by 16 days (Delmi *et al.*, 1990), 21 days (Schurch *et al.*, 1998), 26 days (Brown and Seabrook, 1992) and 30 days (Tkatch *et al.*, 1992)). Furthermore, following discharge, patients who had received an ONS during their hospital stay had a better clinical outcome than those who were unsupplemented (Delmi *et al.*, 1990; Tkatch *et al.*, 1992). The proportion of patients with a 'favourable course' (no complications or only one minor complication, such as lower urinary tract infection or superficial phlebitis) was greater in supplemented than in unsupplemented patients during acute care (orthopaedic hospital, ~70% vs. 48%), and significantly greater in the recovery hospital (~53% vs. 12%) and at 6 months (~60% vs. 25%) (Delmi *et al.*, 1990). Similar improvements in clinical outcome were reported by Tkatch *et al.* (1992), from the same research group (see Table A3.24). They also indicated a trend towards lower mortality rates in supplemented patients. The authors of this study attributed these improvements in clinical outcome to the protein content of the supplement, as the unsupplemented group were given a placebo that was free from protein but with the same micronutrient composition. However, the placebo was also lower in energy than the ONS used in this trial (by 138 kcal daily, equivalent to a difference of 5244 kcal over the study period) and so it is difficult to attribute the benefits to the effect of protein alone. Further interpretation of these findings is limited as no data on total energy intake or weight changes were provided in this study (Tkatch *et al.*, 1992).

Although no financial data were presented in any of these trials, retrospective cost analysis was undertaken (see Chapter 6). This suggested that savings of between £3842 (Delmi *et al.*, 1990) and £8179 (Tkatch *et al.*, 1992) per patient could be made when ONS reduced complications and length of stay. These calculations assumed a daily hospital cost of £250, an additional cost of £80 for treating one complication and £3 for the supplement.

Overall, larger RCT in fractured neck of femur patients and other types of orthopaedic patients are required to address the clinical and cost-effectiveness of ONS across hospital and rehabilitation settings so that definitive recommendations for the nutritional treatment of this group can be formed.

Orthopaedics: other reviews

One of the findings of a Cochrane review of five RCT of ONS in fractured neck of femur patients was that:

> Oral multinutrient feeds (providing non-protein energy, protein, some vitamins and minerals) . . . may reduce unfavourable outcome (death or complications) (14/66 versus 27/73; relative risk 0.52, 95% confidence interval 0.32 to 0.84).
>
> (Avenell and Handoll, 2001)

However, it was suggested that larger, well-designed trials were needed to confirm the benefits of ONS in this patient group (Avenell and Handoll, 2001). Indeed, in our review, attention to the methodological quality of the studies reviewed (see Chapter 6) has highlighted the prevalence of poorly designed randomized trials (low Jadad scores, with four randomized trials with a score of 1) and non-randomized trials.

Surgery (Gastrointestinal and Vascular)

Patients undergoing major surgical procedures are at increased nutritional risk, mostly because dietary intake is reduced postoperatively (Hackett *et al.*, 1979). This is due to a variety of causes (see Chapter 3), including frequent 'nil by mouth' routines and the physical and psychological effects of medication, as well as surgery and hospitalization. Furthermore, patients who are malnourished before surgery are at increased risk of morbidity and mortality (see Chapter 4). As there is a high risk of malnutrition in surgical patients, particularly postoperatively (see Chapter 2), nutrition has an important role to play in the treatment of at-risk patients both pre- and postoperatively. Although ONS are widely used in the nutritional support of surgical patients, a review of the evidence of their efficacy in this group is required. Although ETF (see Chapter 7) and PN (Chapter 9) can also be used (and are often required), it has been stated that:

> Oral dietary supplements taken together with a normal diet has the attraction of simplicity with the added advantage that this mode of nutritional support is relatively free of complications.
>
> (MacFie *et al.*, 2000)

Surgery: present analysis

Six RCT (total patients *n* 347) of ONS in patients undergoing elective minor or major gastrointestinal surgery (Rana *et al.*, 1992; Murchan *et al.*, 1995; Elbers *et al.*, 1997; Keele *et al.*, 1997; Beattie *et al.*, 2000; MacFie *et al.*, 2000) or vascular surgery (Beattie *et al.*, 2000) were reviewed. The details of the studies and their findings are shown in Tables A3.28–A3.30 and Box A3.7, and the findings are discussed below. Studies of patients undergoing orthopaedic and orthognathic surgery are reviewed earlier in this appendix. In addition, three NRT in gastrointestinal or vascular surgical patients were reviewed (total *n* 117) (Wara and Hessov, 1985; Moiniche *et al.*, 1995; Eneroth *et al.*, 1997) and the key points are summarized in Tables A3.31–A3.33.

Table A3.28. Oral nutritional supplements used in hospital-based randomized controlled trials in surgical patients.

Trial	ONS	ONS energy density	ONS prescribed	ONS energy (kcal) intake	ONS protein (g) intake	Toleration
Beattie et al. (2000)	Ensure plus (Abbott)	1.5 kcal ml^{-1}	600 kcal, 25 g P	300–600 (by most pts)	12.5–25 (by most pts)	–
Elbers et al. (1997)	Protenplus (Fresenius)	1 kcal ml^{-1}	600 kcal, 54 g P	565	~51	–
Keele et al. (1997)	Fortisip (Nutricia) 13% P; 48% CHO; 39% F	1.5 kcal ml^{-1}	ad libitum	Days 1–7 246–349	Days 1–7 9–11.6	–
MacFie et al. (2000)	Fortisip (Nutricia)	1.5 kcal ml^{-1}	2 cartons of either ONS: 600 kcal 20 g P (max.)	Preop.: 507 (140) Postop.: 252 (195)	Preop.: 16.9 g Postop.: 8.4 g	Nausea postop. in small no. of pt Good compliance especially preop.
	Fortijuce (Nutricia)	1.25 kcal ml^{-1}	500 kcal 10 g P (min.)			
Murchan et al. (1995)[a]	Commercial sip feeds	1.5 kcal ml^{-1}	600 kcal 20 g P	–	–	–
Rana et al. (1992)	Fortisip (Nutricia) 13% P; 48% CHO; 39% F	1.5 kcal ml^{-1}	ad libitum	Days 1–3 470 (30) Days 1–7 471 (31)	18.7 (3.2) 15.7 (1)	–

[a] Preliminary report (abstract) of MacFie et al. (2000).
CHO, carbohydrate; F, fat; P, protein; preop., preoperative; postop., postoperative.

Table A3.29. Trial characteristics: hospital-based randomized controlled trials of oral nutritional supplementation in surgical patients.

Trial	Design	No. S	No. US	Initial BMI S group	Initial BMI US group	Duration of ONS	Dietary counselling	Control (US) group
Beattie et al. (2000) Elective GI or vascular surgery	11001	52	49	BMI < 20 + TSF/MAMC < 15th percentile and/or 5% wt loss in H	–	10 weeks post-discharge	–	Hospital diet
Elbers et al. (1997) Non-English, abstract reviewed	10000	10	10	26.3	24.7	3 weeks from day 5 post-surgery	–	Standard hospital diet
Keele et al. (1997) Moderate to major GI surgery	10001	43	43	23.5	25.1	Postop. until discharge, S: 10.8 days	–	Hospital diet
MacFie et al. (2000) Elective major GI surgery	10001	24 pre- and postop.; 24 preop.; 27 postop.	25	23 (17–30) 23 (15–31) 25 (17–34)	25 (21–35)	Preop.: 15 (5–59 days) Postop: 8 (0–20 days)	–	Usual hospital or home diet
Murchan et al. (1995) Abstract[a] Major GI surgery	10000	10 pre- and postop. 8 preop. 7 postop.	9	–	–	Preop. up to 14 days Postop. ?	–	Usual hospital or home diet
Rana et al. (1992) Moderate to major GI surgery	10001	20	20	22.3	23.7	7 days	–	Hospital diet

[a] Preliminary report (abstract) of MacFie et al. (2000).
H, hospital; MAMC, mid-arm muscle circumference; preop., preoperative; postop., postoperative; S, supplemented; TSF, triceps skin-fold thickness; US, unsupplemented.

Table A3.30. Main findings of randomized controlled trials of oral nutritional supplementation in hospitalized surgical patients.

Trial	Energy intake	Wt change S	Wt change US	Functional outcome	Clinical outcome	Finance
Beattie et al. (2000)	–	Sig. less wt loss (5.6% (3.4 kg) max.). Sig. less reduction in MAMC and TSF (S vs. US sig.)	Greater wt loss (9.8% (5.96 kg) max.)	Sig. less reduction in HGS in S vs. US. Sig. improvement in physical and mental health (SF-36) in S group	Less risk of chest and wound infections (NS) for S vs. US (6 vs. 13); fewer antibiotic prescriptions for S vs. US (7/52 vs. 15/49, NS). NS difference in length of stay	–
Elbers et al. (1997)	–	−7.1 (0.9) kg or −8.41 (0.9)% S lost greater wt preop. than US (11 vs. 9%) Body cell mass −1.77 kg (S vs. US sig.) Lean body mass −4.96 kg (S. vs. US NS)	−6.2 (0.7) kg or −8.2 (0.7)% Body cell mass −5.04 kg (S vs. US sig.) Lean body mass −6.13 kg	S greater increase in Spitzer index and Karnofsky index (measures of quality of life) than US at 3 weeks (S vs. US sig.) S greater increase in HGS (S vs.US NS)	NS difference in length of hospital stay (S vs. US NS)	–
Keele et al. (1997)	S and US food intake similar (S 1203 (301) kcal; US 1187 (349) kcal). S sig. higher TEI and TPI days 1–4 (e.g. day 4: S 1627, 55.5 g P; US 1359, 46.3 g P). S sig. higher P intake at day 7 than US (62.9 vs. 45.5 g)	Day 3 −1.5 kg Discharge −2.2 kg S lost sig. less wt than US (S vs. US sig.) Small sig. decrease in TSF and MAMC vs. preop. (S vs. US NS)	Day 3 −3 kg Discharge −4.2 kg Small sig. decrease in TSF and MAMC vs. preop.	S: maintained HGS, US had sig. reduction (vs. baseline) S: no increase in postop. fatigue (4.4; 4.5; 5.1), unlike US, who had sig. increases (3.9 (pre) 6.5 (day 3) 6.1 (day 7))	Sig. lower rate of postop. complications for S group (S 4; US 12)	–
MacFie et al. (2000)	TEI postop.: S 1640 (162) kcal, ?P; US 1268 (178) kcal, 46.2 g P. No difference in VFI (NS, n 5): S 1090 (143) kcal, 49.1 g P ONS: 1640–1090 = 550 (inconsistency in reported ONS intake, see Table A3.28)	−3.3 kg (S vs. US NS) Postop. to 4 weeks post-discharge −3.4 kg (S vs. US NS)	−4.1 kg Postop. to 4 weeks post-discharge −3.9 kg	S vs. US: no difference in HGS, psychological status or 6 month activity levels	No difference in postop. complications, mortality or duration of H stay between S vs. US	–
Murchan et al. (1995)	–	Preop.: +0.1 kg Postop.: sig. less wt loss than US (no data)	Preop.: −1.2 kg	S vs. US: no difference in HGS (NS)	Sig. shorter length of stay for S (12 (2) days) than US (18 (3) days) but no difference in complications	–
Rana et al. (1992)	S sig. higher oral E intake and TEI and TPI at days 1–3 and 1–7 Days 1–3 S 1132/43 g oral; 1607/59 g total; US 864/41 g total Days 1–7 S 1353/50 g oral; 1833/66 g total; US 1108/53 g total	Day 3 −1.1 (?) kg Day 7 −1.3 (?) kg	Day 3 −4.5 (1.2) kg Day 7 −4.7 (1.2) kg	Less decrease in HGS in S group (S vs. US sig.)	Lower incidence of infectious complications of chest/wound for S vs. US (sig. 3 vs. 10). No difference in H stay for S vs. US	–

E, energy; HGS, hand-grip strength; H, hospital; MAMC, mid-arm muscle circumference; NS, not significant; P, protein; preop., preoperative; postop., postoperative; S, supplemented; sig., significant; TEI, total energy intake; TPI, total protein intake; TST, triceps skin-fold thickness; US, unsupplemented; VFI, voluntary food intake.

Table A3.31. Oral nutritional supplements used in trials of surgical patients in hospital (non-randomized data).

Trial	ONS	ONS energy density	ONS prescribed	ONS energy (kcal) intake	ONS protein (g) intake	Toleration
Eneroth *et al.* (1997)[a]	Fortimel (Nutricia)	1 kcal ml⁻¹	To meet 2000 kcal	151 kcal (7% of total)	~15 g	–
Moiniche *et al.* (1995)	Fortimel (Nutricia)	1 kcal ml⁻¹	1000 kcal, 80 g P	~1000 kcal	80 g	–
Wara and Hessov (1985)	Rynkeby (protein-enriched fruit drink) Milk products (Cocoaquargdrink, Quargdrink)	0.64 kcal ml⁻¹ 0.64–0.86 kcal ml⁻¹	–	–	–	–

[a] Supplemented group received ONS and/or ETF (Nutrodrip Intensiv) and/or PN (Vitrimix, Tracel, Soluvit, Vitalipid Novum).
P, protein.

Table A3.32. Trial characteristics: hospital-based trials of oral nutritional supplementation in surgical patients (non-randomized data).

Trial and patient group	Design	No. S	No. US	Initial BMI S group	Initial BMI US group	Duration of ONS	Dietary counselling	Control group
Eneroth *et al.* (1997) Transtibial amputation for occlusive arterial disease	B	32	32 retro. matched controls	~10% wt loss in 3/12 *n* 27 low food intake *n* 18 'malnourished'	–	11 days (pre- and postop., aimed for 5 days preop.)	–	No supplementary nutrition (retrospective)
Moiniche *et al.* (1995) Colonic resection	C	17	–	–	–	4–6 days postop.	–	–
Wara and Hessov (1985) Colorectal surgery	B	18	18	–	–	12 days postop.	–	Liquid, bland diet before receiving normal food

preop., preoperative; postop., postoperative; retro., retrospective; S, supplemented; US, unsupplemented.

Table A3.33. Main findings of oral nutritional supplementation trials in hospitalized surgical patients (non-randomized data).

Trial	Energy intake	Wt change S	Wt change US	Function	Clinical outcome	Finance
Eneroth et al. (1997)	TEI: 2098 (176) kcal VFI: 1142 (563) kcal (55% of TEI) (n 28) (Some pts had ETF (403 (562) kcal, 19% of TEI) or PN (401 (456) kcal, 19% of TEI)	–	–	n 26 had healed stumps at 6 months (US n 13, S vs. US sig.) Excluding deaths, 2/23 S were not healed vs. 8/18 in US (sig.)	No differences in mortality (S n 9; US n 14 at 6 months) or length of hospital stay (S 36 (12–356 days); US 30 (4–269 days) (S vs. US NS)	–
Moiniche et al. (1995)	'All patients ate normally from the first postoperative day'	No change	–	–	–	–
Wara and Hessov (1985)	S 997 kcal, US 919 kcal (S vs. US NS) S 78% of BMR, US 71% of BMR (S vs. US sig.) S 43 g (0.67 g kg⁻¹), US 26 g (0.45 g kg⁻¹) P (S vs. US sig.)	–1.8 kg (S vs. US sig.)	–3.9 kg	–	–	–

BMR, basal metabolic rate; NS, not significant; P, protein; S, supplemented; sig., significant; TEI, total energy intake; US, unsupplemented; VFI, voluntary food intake.

Four RCT (Rana *et al.*, 1992; Elbers *et al.*, 1997; Keele *et al.*, 1997; Beattie *et al.*, 2000) investigated the effects of ONS given post-surgery to patients for 7 days to 10 weeks postoperatively. Two further reports (from the same research group) involved giving patients an ONS both pre- and post-operatively (Murchan *et al.*, 1995; MacFie *et al.*, 2000). In only one of the trials reviewed were patients who were at risk of malnutrition targeted (BMI < 20 kg m^{-2}, TSF/MAMC < 15th percentile and/or 5% weight loss during hospital admission) (Beattie *et al.*, 2000). All of the trials used ONS that were commercial liquid sip feeds, either milk- (1.5 kcal ml^{-1}) or juice-tasting (1.25 kcal ml^{-1}) varieties (see Table A3.28).

(l) What effect do ONS have on the voluntary food intake and total energy intake of surgical patients in hospital?

Postoperative supplementation of surgical patients can substantially improve nutritional intake. ONS used postoperatively significantly improved total energy and protein intakes in two trials (during days 1–7 (Rana *et al.*, 1992) and days 1–4 (Keele *et al.*, 1997)) and tended to do so in another trial (MacFie *et al.*, 2000). Three other reports (Murchan *et al.*, 1995; Elbers

et al., 1997; Beattie *et al.*, 2000) made no assessment of dietary intake. For more information see Table A3.30.

The impact of ONS on voluntary food intake was assessed in three trials (Rana *et al.*, 1992; Keele *et al.*, 1997; MacFie *et al.*, 2000), although only the data from two trials were clear enough to be used for quantitative calculation (Rana *et al.*, 1992; Keele *et al.*, 1997). In both of these trials, from the same research group, the supplements appeared to stimulate food intake over 7 days (calculated using method (ii), Chapter 5). Within these trials, ONS intake remained relatively constant (Keele *et al.*, 1997), while voluntary food intake and hence total energy and protein intakes improved gradually during the recovery period (e.g. from 878 kcal on day 1 to 1762 kcal on day 7) (Keele *et al.*, 1997). The improvements in intake occurred to a greater extent in supplemented than in unsupplemented patients. As one of the authors described it:

> the increase in energy intake occurred not just on account of that ingested from the supplements, but also as a consequence of increased intake from the standard hospital diet perhaps through improved appetite and well being.
>
> (Rana *et al.*, 1992)

Box A3.7. Key findings: effect of ONS in hospital surgical (gastrointestinal and vascular) patients.

Nutritional intake: postoperative use of ONS can substantially improve energy and protein intakes, although nutritional requirements may still remain unmet. Use of ONS postoperatively is reported to increase voluntary food intake relative to unsupplemented patients.

Body weight: ONS can attenuate the loss of body weight (average difference of +3%) associated with surgery and may reduce losses of muscle mass.

Body function: functional benefits associated with ONS include increases in hand-grip strength, improvements in physical and mental health and quality-of-life indices.

Clinical outcome: clinical outcomes are improved when ONS are used, with a consistent trend towards shorter stays in hospital, significantly fewer complications and reduced mortality. Benefits are documented in trials in which patients' average BMI is < 20 kg m^{-2} or > 20 kg m^{-2} and typically occur in trials in which patients lose less weight than controls. A lack of improvement in outcome may be due to the failure of ONS to increase energy intakes and improve body weight.

However, even with ONS, during the in-patient phase of the trials, total intakes of energy and protein typically remained 'inadequate' to meet the nutritional requirements of patients post-surgery (Keele *et al.*, 1997).

(II) What effect do ONS have on the body weight and composition of surgical patients in hospital?

The use of ONS in surgical patients, particularly postoperatively, appears to limit the losses of body weight and lean body mass that typically accompany surgery. Post-surgical intervention with ONS mostly resulted in supplemented patients losing less weight than unsupplemented patients (Rana *et al.*, 1992; Murchan *et al.*, 1995; Keele *et al.*, 1997; Beattie *et al.*, 2000; MacFie *et al.*, 2000) (documented as statistically significant in three trials (Murchan *et al.*, 1995; Keele *et al.*, 1997; Beattie *et al.*, 2000)).

Indeed, a combined analysis of % weight change in supplemented relative to unsupplemented patients (weighted for sample size, data from five trials (Rana *et al.*, 1992; Elbers *et al.*, 1997; Keele *et al.*, 1997; Beattie *et al.*, 2000; MacFie *et al.*, 2000), *n* 447) indicated an attenuation of weight loss in those given ONS (-4.6%) compared with those who were not (-7.0%; $P < 0.07$; independent *t* test). In the study of MacFie *et al.* (2000), weight loss was reduced in those patients who received an ONS preoperatively for 2 weeks but the changes did not reach statistical significance.

Losses in fat and/or lean mass (as measured by upper-arm anthropometry or bioelectrical impedance) were assessed in three trials and were typically found to be less in supplemented patients (significantly so in two trials (Elbers *et al.*, 1997; Beattie *et al.*, 2000)) than in unsupplemented patients.

(III) What effect do ONS have on the body function of surgical patients in hospital?

The functional outcome of surgical patients can be improved by giving ONS postoperatively. Reported benefits of using ONS postoperatively included increases in muscle strength and improved physical and mental health and quality of life. Functional benefits tended to occur in trials in which energy intakes were increased and body weight gain was greater (or weight loss less) relative to a control group.

Supplemented patients had greater increments (or smaller reductions) in hand-grip strength than unsupplemented patients in four out of six trials (Rana *et al.*, 1992; Elbers *et al.*, 1997; Keele *et al.*, 1997; Beattie *et al.*, 2000) significant versus a control group in one trial (Beattie *et al.*, 2000). The supplemented patients also showed significant longitudinal improvements in physical and mental health, using SF-36 (Beattie *et al.*, 2000), and less postoperative fatigue (Keele *et al.*, 1997) (see Table A3.30), which were not observed in the unsupplemented patients. Finally, compared with a control group, supplemented patients had significantly greater increases in a number of quality-of-life indices (Spitzer index and Karnofsky index) (Elbers *et al.*, 1997). In contrast, no improvements in patients' subsequent psychological status (hospital anxiety and depression (HAD) questionnaire) or activity levels were found in another trial, in which patients were given ONS pre- and/or postoperatively for a total of 2 weeks (MacFie *et al.*, 2000). However, this is not surprising as the assessments of functional outcome were not undertaken until 1 and 6 months after supplementation had been stopped (1 and 6 months, respectively, after discharge from hospital). Furthermore, ONS failed to significantly improve energy and protein intakes in this trial (MacFie *et al.*, 2000), unlike trials in which functional benefits were seen, when total energy intakes were significantly increased (Rana *et al.*, 1992; Keele *et al.*, 1997).

(IV) What effect do ONS have on the clinical and financial outcome of surgical patients in hospital?

Clinical outcome, including mortality, complication rates and length of hospital stay, can be improved with the use of ONS in surgical patients.

MORTALITY

Only two trials assessed mortality following ONS, but in one of these there were no deaths (Beattie *et al.*, 2000). In the other trial, involving a total of 100 patients, mortality was lower in supplemented (44%) than in unsupplemented (52%) patients but the difference was not significant (MacFie *et al.*, 2000). Large numbers of patients are necessary to demonstrate a significant difference in mortality, as discussed in Chapter 6. A meta-analysis of mortality data across surgical and other patient groups in the hospital setting (presented in Chapter 6) suggested that ONS could significantly reduce mortality, although the benefits were predominantly in those who were at risk of malnutrition (BMI < 20 kg m^{-2}). In MacFie *et al.*'s (2000) trial, the average BMI was > 20 kg m^{-2}.

COMPLICATION RATES

This review suggests that complication rates are typically reduced in patients given an ONS postoperatively (see Table A3.34). Our meta-analysis of complication rates in surgical studies (*n* 4: Rana *et al.*, 1992; Keele *et al.*, 1997; Beattie *et al.*, 2000; MacFie *et al.*, 2000) suggested an odds ratio of 0.38 (95% CI 0.15–1.01), with no significant heterogeneity between studies. More specifically, following short-term ONS, three trials of post-surgical patients found that the incidence of postoperative complications (infectious complications of chest and wound) was lower in those receiving an ONS compared with those who were unsupplemented (Rana *et al.*, 1992; Keele *et al.*, 1997; Beattie *et al.*, 2000) (documented as significant in one trial (Keele *et al.*, 1997)). Consequently, there was a non-significant trend towards supplemented patients receiving fewer antibiotic prescriptions postoperatively (13% versus 31% in unsupplemented) (Beattie *et al.*, 2000). The study of MacFie *et al.* (2000) found no significant differences in postoperative complications between supplemented and unsupplemented patients. The differences in clinical outcome between this study (MacFie *et al.*, 2000) and the other ONS trials do not

appear to be due to differences in the types of surgery performed, the types of ONS used or the duration of ONS. However, the lack of improvement in outcome in the trial of MacFie *et al.* (2000) may be due to the failure of ONS to significantly improve total energy intake in patients (Hessov, 2000), possibly because only small amounts of ONS were ingested by individuals who were generally better nourished than in the other trials. However, a lack of data indicating the nutritional status of individual patients in the different trials means it is difficult to assess this.

LENGTH OF STAY

Length of stay was consistently shorter in supplemented than in unsupplemented patients (see Table A3.35) in all trials that assessed it. However, the reductions were not significant in individual studies, partly because of the small number of subjects involved in each study (Rana *et al.*, 1992; Elbers *et al.*, 1997; Beattie *et al.*, 2000; MacFie *et al.*, 2000) and partly because the usefulness of length of hospital stay as an indicator of patient outcome may be limited, as it is affected by many external factors, such as delays in arrangements for subsequent care after discharge (e.g. social/community services).

FINANCIAL OUTCOME

Although no data on financial outcome were provided in any of these trials, cost savings in hospital surgical patients are likely if ONS reduce complication rates, prescription costs and length of hospital stay. Indeed, a retrospective cost analysis suggested reductions per patient of between £352 (Beattie *et al.*, 2000) and £532 per patient (Rana *et al.*, 1992) (see Chapter 6). Furthermore, it is possible that subsequent utilization of community health-care resources after discharge from hospital would be lower in supplemented patients, if, as the evidence suggests, deterioration in muscle strength and fatigue are less and physical and mental health/quality of life are improved to a greater extent post-surgery, relative to those who are unsupplemented. Prospective evaluation of

Table A3.34. Reduction in complication rates with oral nutritional supplementation in surgical patients.

Trial	Complication rates (%)		Type of complications
	Supplemented	Unsupplemented	
Beattie et al. (2000)	11[a]	26	Infective
Keele et al. (1997)	15[a]	50	Infective
MacFie et al. (2000)	15	8	Septic
Rana et al. (1992)	9[a]	28	Infective, GI perforation and multiple complications

[a] Significant reduction in complication rates in the supplemented group compared with the unsupplemented group.
GI, gastrointestinal.

Table A3.35. Reduction in length of stay with oral nutritional supplementation in surgical patients.

Trial	Reduction in length of stay with supplementation (expressed as per cent of unsupplemented patients' length of stay) (%)	Length of stay in unsupplemented patients
Beattie et al. (2000)	11	21 days
Keele et al. (1997)	18	13 days
MacFie et al. (2000)	23	13 days
Rana et al. (1992)	21	16 days

functional, clinical and financial outcomes following ONS in surgical patients is required across health-care settings (hospital to home) before conclusions can be made about the effects of ONS on these parameters.

Trials of other types of ONS used in surgical patients

ONS enriched with nutrients with immunomodulatory properties

A series of recent studies have reported the value of particular ONS enriched with potentially immune-enhancing nutrients preoperatively (arginine, omega-3 fatty acids, RNA), combined with postoperative ETF (Braga *et al.*, 1996, 1999; Gianotti *et al.*, 1999; Senkal *et al.*, 1999; Snyderman *et al.*, 1999; Tepaske *et al.*, 2001). These trials, undertaken in patients undergoing a variety of types of surgery (cardiac surgery, gastrointestinal and head and neck surgery for cancer), suggest that there may be benefits associated with using such formulations perioperatively (e.g. immunological changes (Braga *et al.*, 1999; Gianotti *et al.*, 1999; Tepaske *et al.*, 2001), changes in gut function (Braga *et al.*, 1996), reduced postoperative infections (Braga *et al.*, 1999; Senkal *et al.*, 1999; Snyderman *et al.*, 1999) and shorter lengths of hospital stay (Braga *et al.*, 1999)). However, due to the design of these investigations, it is not possible to ascertain whether the reported benefits are due to the use of ONS preoperatively or the use of similar formulations delivered by ETF postoperatively, or a combination of both. Further study is required to investigate the benefit, if any, of preoperative ONS enriched with nutrients with immunomodulatory properties. It would also be advantageous, both scientifically and clinically, to elucidate the role of the different nutrients individually, as opposed to the commonly used combinations of nutrients, and the mechanisms by which these nutrients might act to produce the changes in clinical outcome that have been observed (Reid, 2000).

Carbohydrate ONS used preoperatively

The use of a carbohydrate ONS (12.5% carbohydrate, primarily in the form of maltodextrins) preoperatively (2–3 h before elective surgery) may reduce postoperative insulin resistance. Preoperatively, discomfort may be reduced (hunger, thirst, anxiety) (Hausel *et al.*, 2001) and postoperatively well-being and muscle strength may be improved, although large RCT are needed to confirm these initial findings (Ljungqvist *et al.*, 2001). The intake of 400 ml of this type of ONS pre-elective surgery has been associated with no adverse effects, with gastric emptying being complete within 90 min and with no differences between patients' and controls' residual gastric volumes or gastric pH at the time of anaesthesia. A combined analysis of several studies, undertaken by the same group of workers, suggests that preoperative glucose drinks are associated with significantly shorter hospital stays (for a review, see Ljungqvist *et al.*, 2001; Nygren *et al.*, 2001). The same drinks also produce an improvement in postoperative glucose tolerance and insulin sensitivity, but the extent to which these are related to the duration of hospital stay is uncertain (see Chapter 1 for general discussion on glucose metabolism in experimental injury, critical care and elective surgery injury).

Patient Groups with No Randomized Controlled Data

Burns

No RCT of ONS versus no nutritional support in patients with burns were reviewed. The two trials with non-randomized data that were reviewed (Solem *et al.*, 1979; Demling and DeSanti, 1998) are summarized in Tables A3.36–A3.38. One of these trials suggested that the use of ONS in burns patients could protect against the development of Curling's ulcer (upper GI bleeding from ulcerative gastritis) (Solem *et al.*, 1979). The other trial (a comparison of two formulations) suggested that ONS

Table A3.36. Oral nutritional supplements used in trials of burns patients in hospital (non-randomized data).

Trial	ONS	ONS energy density	ONS prescribed	ONS energy (kcal) intake	ONS protein (g) intake	Toleration
Demling and DeSanti (1998)	S¹ Protein hydrolysate (Ensure HN or Sustacal, Abbott or Mead Johnson) (P 40 g, CHO 150 g, F 30 g l⁻¹) S² MET-Rx (low-carbohydrate, low-fat ONS; P 74 g, CHO 48 g, F 8 g l⁻¹) powder reconstituted to liquid	1 kcal ml⁻¹ Flexible	S¹ To meet 30–35 kcal kg⁻¹ and 1.3–1.5 g kg⁻¹ P S² To provide 70 g P daily (1.7–2 g kg⁻¹ P)	–	–	Better compliance with S² due to flexibility in adjusting flavour to suit patient preference. Compliance with S¹ much poorer (< 50%)
Solem et al. (1979)	Vivonex (Eaton Lab)	–	900 kcal, increased to 3000 kcal	–	–	–

CHO, carbohydrate; F, fat; P, protein; S, supplemented.

Table A3.37. Trial characteristics: hospital-based trials of oral nutritional supplementation in burns patients (non-randomized data).

Trial and patient group	Design	No. S	No. US	Initial BMI S group	Initial BMI US group	Duration of ONS	Dietary counselling	Control group
Demling and DeSanti (1998) Previous 30–50% burns in rehab.	B	15 S¹ 8 S² 7	–	–	–	3 weeks during rehab.	All given a high energy and protein diet	–
Solem et al. (1979) Severely burned, risk of Curling's ulcer	C	75?	–	–	–	After early postburn period until autografting	No – also received antacid treatment in early postburn period	–

rehab., rehabilitation; S, supplemented; US, unsupplemented.

Table A3.38. Main findings of oral nutritional supplementation trials in hospitalized burns patients (non-randomized data).

Trial	Energy intake	Wt change S	Wt change US	Function	Outcome	Finance
Demling and DeSanti (1998)	S[1] 30 (2) kcal kg^{-1} S[2] 31 (3) kcal kg^{-1}	S[2] sig. greater wt gain (1.9–2.9 lb week^{-1}) than S[1] (1.2–1.4 lb week^{-1}) over 3 week period	–	S[2] sig. greater increase in therapy index (measure of muscular strength and endurance) than S[1] (after 3 weeks, S[2] 8 (12) and S[1] 5 (1); index from 0 (greatest fatigue) to 10 (least fatigue))	S[2] shorter length of stay than S[1] (by 6 days, NS)	–
Solem *et al.* (1979)	–	–	–	Only 3/75 developed Curling's ulcer and none had classic Curling's ulcer (upper GI bleeding from ulcerative gastritis) S 'protects against clinically evident Curling's ulcer'	–	–

GI, gastrointestinal; NS, not significant; S, supplemented; sig., significantly; US, unsupplemented.

could easily be modified to suit patients' taste preferences, ensuring greater compliance. Such modifications led to significantly greater anthropometric and functional gains and shorter stays in rehabilitation than did the fixed high energy formulation (Demling and DeSanti, 1998). The use of ONS in burn patients requires further investigation using RCT.

Human immunodeficiency virus/acquired immune deficiency syndrome (HIV/AIDS)

No RCT of ONS in patients with HIV/AIDS in hospital were reviewed. Only two studies assessed the effects of ONS on a group of hospitalized patients with HIV/AIDS, comparing their nutritional and functional status before and after supplementation (non-randomized data reviewed and summarized in Tables A3.39–A3.41). One trial, in weight-losing HIV patients with chronic diarrhoea, indicated that improvements in weight and bowel function (improved stool frequency, reduced fat malabsorption) occurred if either a standard or a medium-chain triglyceride (MCT)-enriched ONS was used in isolation (no food intake) (Wanke et al., 1996). In contrast, a small abstract report of a similar study in patients with AIDS (Craig et al., 1994) indicated significant reductions in stool weight and stool fat and improvements in fat absorption only with the MCT-enriched ONS. A number of trials of ONS have been undertaken in patients with HIV/AIDS in the community setting and these are discussed in Appendix 4.

Malignancy

It has been suggested that provision of adequate nutrition makes a major contribution towards the clinical, biochemical and psychological status of the cancer patient in the face of the disease process (Shils, 1979). Patients with cancer may have numerous nutritional problems as a result of the effects of the disease and its treatment (radiotherapy, chemotherapy, surgery)

(Thomas, 1994). Anorexia and early satiety, fatigue, taste changes, mucositis, difficulties in ingesting and swallowing food, nausea and vomiting are among the factors that limit food intake in the cancer patient. Hence the nutritional status of patients with cancer is frequently compromised, with weight loss and malnutrition being common accompaniments of malignancy (see Chapter 2). Despite the problems of malnutrition in patients with most types of cancer and the widespread use of nutritional support as part of the treatment of this patient group, there is remarkably little information concerning the efficacy of using ONS to treat patients in hospital. No RCT comparing ONS with no nutritional support in hospital patients with cancer were reviewed. However, five NRT of ONS in patients with cancer in hospital were assessed (Bounous et al., 1971; Haffejee and Angorn, 1977; Cohn et al., 1982; Rickard et al., 1983; Barber et al., 1999b). These are summarized in Tables A3.42–A3.44. Four trials were in adults (Bounous et al., 1971; Haffejee and Angorn, 1977; Cohn et al., 1982; Barber et al., 1999b) and one trial in children (Rickard et al., 1979). In particular, the use of an elemental ONS in patients undergoing chemotherapy, with or without radiation, was associated with significantly less damage to the lower gastrointestinal tract compared with those who were unsupplemented (Bounous et al., 1971). In weight-losing pancreatic cancer patients, a fish oil-enriched ONS, given for 7 weeks, significantly improved energy intake, body weight, appetite and Karnofsky performance status compared with the pre-supplementation baseline (Barber et al., 1999b). None of the other trials reviewed made assessments of functional outcome measures. There is a lack of large, well-designed trials investigating the impact of ONS in specific groups of patients (i.e. specific sites and stages of cancer). Prospective evaluation is needed of the ability of ONS to influence functional and clinical outcomes in different groups of cancer patients in both hospital and community settings, while assessing the financial implications. Although the use of

Table A3.39. Oral nutritional supplements used in trials of patients with HIV/AIDS in hospital (non-randomized data).

Trial	ONS	ONS energy density	ONS prescribed	ONS energy (kcal) intake	ONS protein (g) intake	Toleration
Craig *et al.* (1994)	S¹ Lipisorb (Mead Johnson) S² Standard (unnamed) S¹ and S² 35% F (S¹ 85% of F MCT) (S¹ and S² differ only in fat composition)	1.3 kcal ml⁻¹	–	S¹ 2392 kcal S² 2398 kcal	–	–
Wanke *et al.* (1996)ᵃ	S¹ Lipisorb (Mead Johnson) S² Standard (unnamed) S¹ and S² 35% F (S¹ 85% of F MCT) (S¹ and S² differ only in fat composition)	–	To meet requirements of 1.2–1.5 × calculated BMR (no food intake)	– Only volume data. S¹: 1.7 (0.1) l (days 1–3) 1.8 (0.1) l (days 10–12) S²: 1.8 (0.8) l (days 1–3) 1.8 (0.1) l (days 10–12)	–	–

ᵃ Trial compares different ONS, within-group data used only.
BMR, basal metabolic rate; F, fat; MCT, medium-chain triglyceride.

Table A3.40. Trial characteristics: hospital-based trials of oral nutritional supplementation in patients with HIV/AIDS (non-randomized data).

Trial and patient group	Design	No. S	No. US	Initial BMI S group	Initial BMI US group	Duration of ONS	Dietary counselling	Control group
Craig *et al.* (1994) AIDS patients	C	S¹ 12 S² 12	–	– 62.2 kg	–	12 days	–	–
Wanke *et al.* (1996)ᵃ HIV with chronic diarrhoea	C	S¹ 12 S² 12	–	19.5 (2) 12.4% loss IBW	–	12 days	No – no food intake, non-caloric fluids only	–

ᵃ Trial compares different ONS, within-group data used only.
S, supplemented; US, unsupplemented.

Table A3.41. Main findings of oral nutritional supplementation trials in hospitalized patients with HIV/AIDS (non-randomized data).

Trial	Energy intake	Wt change S	Wt change US	Function	Clinical outcome	Finance
Craig et al. (1994)	S[1] 2392 kcal S[2] 2398 kcal (no food intake permitted)	S[1] −0.2 kg (NS) S[2] −0.5 kg (NS)	–	S[1] sig. reduction in stool weight, stool N, stool fat and sig. increases in fat absorption. No such changes with S[2]	–	–
Wanke et al. (1996)[a]	–	+0.2 kg m^{-2} for both S	–	Both S: 45% fewer stools, decreased stool fat and wt S[1] (MCT): decrease in stool no. (4 to 2.5), stool fat (14 to 5.4 g), stool wt (428 to 262 g) (sig. vs. baseline)	–	–

[a] Trial compares different ONS, within-group data used only.
N, nitrogen; NS, not significant; S, supplemented; sig., significant; US, unsupplemented.

Table A3.42. Oral nutritional supplements used in trials of patients with malignancy in hospital (non-randomized data).

Trial	ONS	ONS energy density	ONS prescribed	ONS energy (kcal) intake	ONS protein (g) intake	Toleration
Barber *et al.* (1999b)	Fish oil enriched ONS (Abbott) per 100 ml 131 kcal, 21% P, 61% CHO, 18% F	1.3 kcal ml⁻¹	610 kcal, 32.2 g P, 2.2 g EPA, 0.96 g DHA (2 cans 474 ml)	585 (370–610) kcal	30.6 (19.3–32.2) g	Some patients developed steatorrhoea and were treated with pancreatic enzymes. No other adverse events. ONS stopped due to dislike of taste (*n* 2), excessive weight gain (*n* 1), disease progression
Bounous *et al.* (1971)	3200-AS elemental diet (Mead Johnson) 233 g per 1000 kcal, 24 g P, 34.3 g F, 150 g CHO	1 kcal ml⁻¹	1600 kcal (370 g of ONS) sole source of nutrition but determined by patient[a]	1725 (1000–2360) kcal	–	Some patients were unable to take sufficient amounts orally and were tube fed. Some disliked the taste of the ONS and were not included in the trial
Cohn *et al.* (1982)	Variety	–	–	–	–	–
Haffejee and Angorn (1977)	Vivonex Standard (Eaton Labs) plus mineral/vitamin syrup	–	1200 kcal, 4 g N (4 packets)	–	–	Well tolerated, no GI distress
Rickard *et al.* (1983)	ONS (*?* unclear if given ETF in addition to ONS)	–	–	–	–	–

[a] *n* 2 took diet by gastrostomy.
CHO, carbohydrate; DHA, decosahexanoic acid; EPA, eicosapentanoic acid; F, fat; GI, gastrointestinal; N, nitrogen; P, protein.

$$ $$

Table A3.43. Trial characteristics: hospital-based trials of oral nutritional supplementation in patients with malignancy (non-randomized data).

Trial and patient group	Design	No. S	No. US	Initial BMI S group	Initial BMI US group	Duration of ONS	Dietary counselling	Control group
Barber *et al.* (1999b) Weight losing unresectable pancreatic cancer	C	20	–	19.8 (17.8–21.8)	–	7 weeks	–	–
Bounous *et al.* (1971) Management of intestinal lesions produced by 5-FU (< 5.25 g) in patients with cancer	B	9	12	–	–	4 days pre and during 5-FU[a]	–	Normal hospital food
Cohn *et al.* (1982) Head/neck, lung or GI cancer	C	12	8 (healthy age-matched controls)	19.1 (15.0–23.4)	–	–	High-calorie snacks and encouragement given to some patients with/without ONS	–
Haffejee and Angorn (1977) Intubation for cancer of the oesophagus	C	15	–	All defined as 'malnourished' (wt loss > 9 kg, decreased food intake for 2 weeks)	–	3 weeks post-intubation	Advice about chopping food (related to intubation). Given hospital diet (2500 kcal, 105 g P)	–
Rickard *et al.* (1983) Children with stage IV neuroblastoma, chemotherapy and radiotherapy	C	6	–	Described as 'nourished'	–	10 weeks	Yes (no details)	–

[a] *n* 2 took diet by gastrostomy.
5-FU, 5-fluorouracil; GI, gastrointestinal; P, protein; S, supplemented; US, unsupplemented.

Table A3.44. Main findings of oral nutritional supplementation trials in hospitalized patients with malignancy (non-randomized data).

Trial	Energy intake	Wt change S	Wt change US	Function	Clinical outcome	Finance
Barber *et al.* (1999b)[a]	TEI increased at 3 weeks (*n* 18) (S vs. baseline sig.). Median increase per patient 372 kcal (64% ONS energy) Pre-ONS: 1450 kcal (1048–2043) ONS: 1798 kcal (1355–2474)	At 3 weeks +1 kg (*n* 18) (−0.1 to 2.0) At 7 weeks +2 kg (*n* 13) (−0.4 to 4.6) (no ascites/oedema) LBM: At 3 weeks +1 kg (+0.6 to 1.4) At 7 weeks +1.9 kg (+1.0 to 3.0) NS changes in MAMC, TSF, fat mass	–	Sig. improvement in Karnofsky performance status vs. baseline Sig. improvement in appetite at 3 weeks Sig. improvement in plasma phospholipid EPA/DHA (indicator of compliance)	–	–
Bounous *et al.* (1971)	S 27.1 kcal kg^{-1} vs. US 20.4 kcal kg^{-1} (? sig.) S TEI 1725 kcal (1000–2360, all ONS) US TEI 1639 kcal (1000–2822, food) (S vs. US NS)	Weight maintained (0 kg)	−2.77 kg (sig. vs. baseline)	Less destruction of crypt epithelium in S Photographs of surface epithelium show epithelial cells better preserved in S (more mucin, dense cytoplasm, taller cells, fewer vacuoles), e.g. mean height of surface rectal epithelium better S 58.1 μm vs. US 42.1 μm (S vs. US sig.)	–	–
Cohn *et al.* (1982)	(A) > 1 kg wt gain: 2234 kcal 78.5 g P (*n* 5) (S vs. controls NS) (B) Within 1 kg wt change: 2407 kcal 89.2 g P (*n* 5) (S vs. controls NS) (C) > 1 kg wt loss: 1460 kcal 57.5 g P (*n* 2) (S vs. controls sig. lower)	Mean BMI 19.5 (15.5–23.6) Wt +0.9 kg (all) LBM −0.44 kg (all) (A) +3.5 kg, MAMC +4.4% TSF +7.3% (B) +0.10 kg, MAMC −2.3% TSF +10.2% (C) −3.4 kg, MAMC +4.7% TSF −13% (? sig. vs. baseline)	–	–	–	–
Haffejee and Angorn (1977)	– Positive N balance (pre −5 g vs. post +7 g ? sig.)	+3 kg (? sig.)	–	–	–	–
Rickard *et al.* (1983)	No specific data for patients receiving ONS	−0.17 (0.59) kg +0.33 (4.18)% Subscapular skin-fold −0.36 (0.46) mm	–	–	–	–

[a] Figures are median (interquartile range).
DHA, docosahexanoic acid; EPA, eicosapentanoic acid; LBM, lean body mass; MAMC, mid-arm muscle circumference; N, nitrogen; NS, not significant; P, protein; S, supplemented; sig., significant; TEI, total energy intake; TSF, triceps skin-fold; US, unsupplemented.

ONS in cancer patients in the community is discussed in Appendix 4, there is a lack of large, well-designed trials in specific subgroups of patients with cancer (i.e. specific sites and stages of cancer) that assess functional, clinical and financial outcomes.

Notes

[1] A dash has been used in tables throughout this appendix where information was not provided in the reviewed trial (and could not be calculated).

[2] When potential repeat reports were excluded (e.g. Larsson *et al.*, 1990 included and Unosson *et al.*, 1992 excluded), the odds ratio was 0.56 (95% CI 0.35–0.90), with no significant heterogeneity.

[3] Calculations disregard the small quantities of 'placebo' ONS consumed by unsupplemented patients in this trial (calculated using method (ii), Chapter 5).

See Chapter 5 for an explanation of the methodological coding of all trials.

Appendix 4

A Detailed Analysis of the Effects of Oral Nutritional Supplements in the Community Setting

Chapter 6 provided an overall summary of the effects of oral nutritional supplements (ONS) obtained from a combined analysis of different groups of patients in the community setting. Here, a more detailed analysis, addressing each review question, is provided, according to individual patient groups. The patient groups are presented alphabetically.

Chronic Obstructive Pulmonary Disease (COPD)

COPD is a common condition in developed countries (see Chapter 2). The acute exacerbations of this disease often lead to hospitalization and the effects of ONS in this setting have been addressed in Chapter 6 and Appendix 3. However, the chronic and debilitating nature of this disease means that large numbers of patients with COPD in the community are also troubled over prolonged periods of time by a poor appetite and a limited food intake, partly due to breathlessness and fatigue. Therefore, ONS are frequently recommended for use in COPD patients in the community setting.

COPD: present analysis

This section addresses the efficacy of ONS within the confines of the community (see

Box A4.1), based on the systematic review of 15 studies, nine of which incorporated a randomized, controlled design (Lewis et al., 1987; Norregaard et al., 1987; Efthimiou et al., 1988; Knowles et al., 1988; Donahoe et al., 1989; Otte et al., 1989; Fuenzalida et al., 1990; Rogers et al., 1992; Ganzoni et al., 1994; see Tables A4.1–A4.3[1] (randomized controlled trials (RCT)) and A4.4–A4.6 (non-randomized trials (NRT))).

(I) What effect do ONS have on the voluntary food intake and total energy intake of patients with COPD in the community?

ONS effectively increase total energy intakes in COPD patients, with > 50% of ONS energy additive to food intake (see Table A4.3). Supplementation increased total energy intake in all of the RCT reviewed (Lewis et al., 1987; Norregaard et al., 1987; Efthimiou et al., 1988; Knowles et al., 1988; Donahoe et al., 1989; Otte et al., 1989; Fuenzalida et al., 1990; Rogers et al., 1992; Ganzoni et al., 1994). The increase was significant in 56% of studies (Lewis et al., 1987; Efthimiou et al., 1988; Knowles et al., 1988; Fuenzalida et al., 1990; Rogers et al., 1992). The effects of ONS on habitual food intake could be calculated in only three studies (using methods (i), (ii) and (iii), see Chapter 5) (Lewis

---

Box A4.1. Key findings: effect of ONS in community patients with COPD.

Nutritional intake: ONS effectively increase total energy intake in COPD patients. The increase in total energy intake is equivalent to more than 50% of the supplement energy consumed.

Body weight: weight gain follows ONS in COPD patients and increases in muscle and fat mass may also occur.

Body function: improvements in function are most likely in trials in which significant weight gain is observed (no significant functional benefits unless weight gain is > 2 kg in underweight patients). Benefits include improved respiratory and skeletal muscle strength, walking distances and well-being. The efficacy of ONS in this patient group is partly due to the degree of undernutrition that is commonly present in COPD patients.

Stopping ONS: some of the benefits of ONS are lost once ONS are stopped and so continued monitoring is required.

Methodology: small sample sizes and lack of placebos limit the interpretation of data and there is a need for larger RCT.

Other treatments: in those who do not respond to ONS, adjunctive use of other treatments (e.g. exercise) may be beneficial.

---

et al., 1987; Norregaard *et al.*, 1987; Efthimiou *et al.*, 1988). These showed that > 50% of the energy supplied by an ONS was additional to the energy intake from food (Efthimiou *et al.* ~53%, Lewis *et al.* 57%, Norregaard *et al.* 83%). This is consistent with more anecdotal information which suggests that only a partial reduction in habitual food intake occurs during supplementation (Lewis *et al.*, 1987; Knowles *et al.*, 1988; Fuenzalida *et al.*, 1990).

Some idea of the change in energy intake with time could be obtained from two studies, both involving 8 weeks of supplementation (Lewis *et al.*, 1987; Knowles *et al.*, 1988). Lewis *et al.* (1987) showed a reduction in food intake during supplementation, while total energy intake was maintained. Data from Knowles *et al.* (1988) suggested that any change in food or ONS intake over time might depend on the pre-existing nutritional status or energy intake of the patients. It appears that greater total energy intakes can be achieved when ONS are given under closer supervision within the confines of a research setting as opposed to patient homes (Donahoe *et al.*, 1989; Fuenzalida *et al.*, 1990; Rogers *et al.*, 1992).

Assessments of dietary (food) intake during the supplementation period ranged from daily records (Lewis *et al.*, 1987; Fuenzalida *et al.*, 1990) to a 7-day food diary (Efthimiou *et al.*, 1988; Otte *et al.*, 1989), a 3-day record (Rogers *et al.*, 1992) or 24 h recalls (Knowles *et al.*, 1988). In the two abstracts the methodology was not detailed (Norregaard *et al.*, 1987; Donahoe *et al.*, 1989). There was also some uncertainty about compliance associated with ONS intake because this was mostly judged from patients' own records, often made over short periods of time only.

None of the studies undertook formal assessments of the effect of ONS on appetite. In the study of Lewis *et al.* (1987), patients complained of fullness associated with bloating if more than 280 kcal (2 kcal ml^{-1} feed) of supplement were consumed over a day. In Fuenzalida *et al.*'s (1990) study, complaints of bloating and flatus were also made by supplemented patients (1.5 kcal ml^{-1}).

(IA) IS THE TIMING OF SUPPLEMENTATION IMPORTANT? The studies (Stauffer *et al.*, 1986; Lewis *et al.*, 1987) that made suggestions about the timing of ONS consumption provided a variety of recommendations, including between

Table A4.1. Oral nutritional supplements used in randomized, controlled trials of patients with COPD in the community.

Trial	ONS	ONS energy density	ONS prescribed	ONS energy (kcal) intake	ONS protein (g) intake	Toleration
Donahoe *et al.* (1989)	–	–	–	–	–	–
Efthimiou *et al.* (1988)	Build Up (Nestlé)	1.13 kcal ml^{-1}	960 (640–1280) kcal	~681	~38	No problems
Fuenzalida *et al.* (1990)	Sustacal HC (Mead Johnson)	1 kcal ml^{-1}	Up to 1080 kcal	720–1080	–	Bloating and flatus the only complaints after 3 weeks of home ONS
Ganzoni *et al.* (1994)	Fresubin (Fresenius)	1 kcal ml^{-1}	–	–	–	–
Knowles *et al.* (1988)	Sustacal (Mead Johnson)	1 kcal ml^{-1}	To increase TEI by 50%	540 to 347[a]	–	–
Lewis *et al.* (1987)	Isocal HCN (Mead Johnson)	2 kcal ml^{-1}	960 kcal	497	–	Bloating and fullness
Norregaard *et al.* (1987)	Novo (enzymatically treated; Denmark)	1 kcal ml^{-1}	–	600	30	Described as palatable
Otte *et al.* (1989)	Novo (Denmark)	1 kcal ml^{-1}	400 kcal	–	–	–
Rogers *et al.* (1992)	Various (self-selected)	Various	–	–	–	–

[a]Last 4 weeks of supplementation, mean intake reduced from 540 to 347 kcal.
TEI, total energy intake.

Table A4.2. Trial characteristics: community-based randomized controlled trials of oral nutritional supplementation in COPD patients.

Trial	Design	No. S	No. US	Initial BMI S group	Initial BMI US group	Duration of ONS	Dietary counselling	Control group
Donahoe et al. (1989)[a] A COPD	10000	10	7	< 90% IBW	< 90% IBW	1 month (trial 4 months)	–	–
Efthimiou et al. (1988) Moderate to severe COPD, current or ex-smokers (mean FEV/FVC% 38%)	10001	7	7	80% IBW	81% IBW	3 months (trial 9 months)	ONS taken 'in addition to normal diet'	Continued with their normal diet
Fuenzalida et al. (1990)[a] Advanced COPD with FEV_1 30–50% of predicted	10001	5	4	79% IBW	79% IBW	6 weeks	–	Hospital diet alone on research ward
Ganzoni et al. (1994) A Non-English article, abstract reviewed COPD (av. FEV_1 0.8 l)	10000	14	16	–	–	12 months	Instructed to take a high-energy diet and to increase vitamin and calcium intakes	–
Knowles et al. (1988)[b] Severe COPD (FEV_1 < 50% of predicted)	11001	12	13	19.6–21.5 kg m^{-2} (61–108% IBW)	–	2 months (trial 4 months)	–	Crossover trial, no other intervention during unsupplemented period
Lewis et al. (1987) Severe COPD (FEV_1 < 1.2 l)	10001	10	11	86% IBW	85% IBW	8 weeks	No – ONS taken in addition to normal diet	Instructed to consume their normal diet and not encouraged to increase their food intake
Norregaard et al. (1987) A COPD (FEV_1 < 60% of predicted)	10000	9	7	< 90% IBW	< 90% IBW	5 weeks	–	Both groups received identical dietary instructions
Otte et al. (1989) Ambulant COPD (with FEV_1 < 70% of predicted)	10111	13	15	77% IBW	73% IBW	13 weeks	Encouraged not to change habitual diet	Placebo, same consistency and taste, 0.1 kcal ml^{-1} (400 ml dose). Encouraged not to change habitual diet

Rogers *et al.* (1992)[a] COPD with FEV$_1$/FVC < 0.60	10000	15	12	78% IBW	79% IBW	16 weeks	A nutritionally balanced meal plan providing an energy intake of 1.7 × REE in the research ward for first 4 weeks. At home, given regular nutritional counselling (intense diet education by a dietitian and nurse: appropriate meal plan to meet energy and protein requirements, portion sizes, symptom management, pulmonary education in relation to food intake)	Offered no meal plan or advice (self-selected their food) and living at home

[a]Part or all of the supplementation was carried out in a research ward/unit, often in a hospital.
[b]Crossover trial – 13 subjects received 8 weeks of supplementation followed by 8 weeks with no supplement, and 12 subjects were unsupplemented for 8 weeks and then supplemented for 8 weeks.
S, supplemented; US, unsupplemented; BMI, body mass index; A, abstract; IBW, ideal body weight; FEV, forced expiratory volume; FVC, forced ventilatory capacity; FEV$_1$, FEV in 1 s; REE, resting energy expenditure.

Table A4.3. Main findings of randomized controlled trials of oral nutritional supplementation in community COPD patients.

Trial	Energy intake	Body weight S	Body weight US	Body function	Clinical outcome	Finance
Donahoe et al. (1989)[a] A	'Adequate energy intake with ONS of 192% REE'	5.66% (sig.) (S vs. US ?) NS change in MAMC	−3.9% (NS)	Sig. improvement in respiratory muscle strength, hand-grip strength, 12 min walking distance in S. NS changes in US (S vs. US ?)	–	–
Efthimiou et al. (1988)	Sig. increase in TEI during ONS period compared with pre- and post-ONS periods (1429 kcal – 2118 kcal – 1474 kcal) in S (NS change in US group, S vs. US ?)	9.4% (sig.) Sig. increase in TSF and MAMC during ONS (NS changes in US, S vs. US ?)	0.2% (NS)	Sig. less breathlessness, lower oxygen cost of breathing and improved well-being (subjective) in S (NS changes in US, S vs. US ?) Sig. improvements in 6 min walking distance, respiratory muscle strength (inspiratory, expiratory and sternomastoid) and hand-grip strength in S (S vs. US ?) NS changes in FEV_1, FVC, TLC or KCO during or after ONS or in US	–	–
Fuenzalida et al. (1990)[a]	Sig. higher TEI for S and US during period in research unit compared with baseline intakes at home During stay in unit, S higher intake (52.6 kcal kg^{-1}) vs. US (43.7 kcal kg^{-1}) (S vs. US NS)	7.54 (2.3)% (sig.) Sig. increases in TSF and MAC	4.6 (2.7)%	Sig. improvements in respiratory muscle function during exercise, exercise duration, TLC and skin-test reactivity (sig. for both groups combined, analysis for S and US separately not reported due to small no.)	–	–
Ganzoni et al. (1994) A	Increase in TEI in S (NS) from 2136 kcal to 2505 kcal (+369 kcal) vs. a reduction in TEI in US (−310 kcal) (S vs. US ?)	13.8% (sig.) S vs. US NS Sig. increase in skin-fold thickness (S vs. US NS)	4.23% (NS)	NS difference between S and US for 6 min walking distance or ventilatory parameters (FVC, FEV_1)	–	–
Knowles et al. (1988)	Sig. increase in TEI in both ONS periods (by average +540 kcal, 28%) after 4 weeks of ONS, remaining sig. higher at 8 weeks only in those receiving ONS first in the crossover (average +347 kcal, 18%)	~ 2% (sig.) (S vs. US ?) NS change in TSF or MAMC during S or US	−1.4% (NS)	Sig. increase in respiratory muscle strength only in those with an increase in TEI > 30% during ONS NS changes in pulmonary function (FEV, FVC, residual volume, TLC) or respiratory muscle performance in those with changes in TEI < 30%	–	–

Study				
Lewis et al. (1987)	TEI and TPI sig. greater in S (2065 kcal, 80 g P) than US (1781 kcal, 58 g P) Reduction in VFI (~213 kcal, with ~57% of ONS energy additive)	2.86% (NS) (S vs. US ?) NS changes in MAMC or TSF	1% (NS)	NS change in maximal inspiratory or expiratory mouth pressures (measure of respiratory muscle function) or maximal sustained ventilatory capacity	–
Norregaard et al. (1987) A	Sig. increase in TPI (+27.3 g) and TEI (+500 kcal) to 2547 kcal and 90.5 g P in S group (NS change in US; S vs. US ?)	3.47% (sig.) (S vs. US ?) Sig. increase in FFM (+0.9 kg)	0% (NS)	Maximal voluntary ventilation improved in S (? sig.)	–
Otte et al. (1989)	VFI not reduced in S or US (similar to baseline at 2319 kcal (~205% BEE)) Assume TEI increased in S (no data)	3.29% (sig.) (S vs. US sig.) Sig. increase in skin-fold thickness at four sites (S vs. US sig.)	0.4%	None	–
Rogers et al. (1992)	Sig. increase in TEI (S 1.73 × REE vs. US 1.43 × REE; S vs. US sig.)	4.61% (sig.) (S vs. US sig.) Occasional periods of wt loss corresponding to disease exacerbation	–0.9%	Sig. improvements in respiratory muscle function (expiratory), hand-grip strength, 12 min walking distance (S vs. US sig.) Trend towards improvement in subjective scores of oxygen cost of breathing, dyspnoea compared with US. No difference in quality of life between groups	–

aImprovements in supplemented and unsupplemented patients given dietary encouragement.
S, supplemented; US, unsupplemented; A, abstract; REE, resting energy expenditure; sig., significant; NS, not significant; MAMC, mid-arm muscle circumference; TEI, total energy intake; TSF, triceps skin-fold thickness; FEV_1, forced expiratory volume in 1 s; FVC, forced ventilatory capacity; MAC, mid-arm circumference; TLC, total lung capacity; TPI, total protein intake; VFI, voluntary food intake; FFM, fat free mass; BEE, basal energy expenditure.

Table A4.4. Oral nutritional supplements used in non-randomized trials of patients with COPD in the community.

Trial	ONS	ONS energy density	ONS prescribed	ONS energy (kcal) intake	ONS protein (g) intake	Toleration
Openbrier et al. (1984)	Sustacal (Mead Johnson) Ensure (Abbott)	1 kcal ml^{-1}	750–1000 kcal	–	–	Only took prescribed amount early on in trial Decline in usage due to bland, sweet taste
Pardy et al. (1986)	Sustacal (Mead Johnson)	1 kcal ml^{-1}	–	–	–	–
Sridhar et al. (1994)	Build Up (Nestlé) Fortisip (Nutricia) Maxijul (SHS)	1.13 kcal ml^{-1} 1.5 kcal ml^{-1} 2 kcal ml^{-1}	–	–	–	2/9 (22%) withdrew due to intolerance to ONS (bloating and unacceptable taste)
Stauffer et al. (1986)	–	1.5 kcal ml^{-1}	1080 kcal	1045	–	–
Wilson et al. (1964)	3105F (Mead Johnson)	3.85 kcal g^{-1}	750 kcal, 45.4 g P	510	~30.9	Poorly tolerated in those with GI symptoms
Wilson et al. (1986)	Ready-prepared liquid supplement	–	To meet deficit between oral intake and 150% of predicted requirements	–	–	–

GI, gastrointestinal; P, protein.

Table A4.5. Trial characteristics: community-based non-randomized trials of oral nutritional supplementation in COPD patients.

Trial	Design	No. S	No. US	Initial BMI S group	Initial BMI US group	Duration of ONS	Dietary counselling	Control group
Openbrier *et al.* (1984) COPD FEV$_1$/FVC < 70% predicted	C	9	–	–	–	12–22 months	Yes – one teaching session with a dietitian about how to increase energy intake	–
Pardy *et al.* (1986) A Moderate to severe COPD (mean FEV$_1$ 38%)	C	25	–	81% IBW	–	2 months	Yes – encouraged to increase their baseline energy intake by 25% for 1 month and by 50% for a second month	–
Sridhar *et al.* (1994) COPD with FEV$_1$/FVC < 60% predicted	C	9	–	< 90% IBW[a]	–	4 months	Yes – pts advised on increasing their total energy intake to at least 50% > 1.3 × REE and protein intake to at least 1.5 g kg^{-1}	–
Stauffer *et al.* (1986) A Severe COPD FEV$_1$/FVC < 36% predicted	C	10	–	77% IBW	–	1 month	–	–
Wilson *et al.* (1964) COPD	C	43	–	–	–	1 month	–	–
Wilson *et al.* (1986) COPD with FEV$_1$/FVC < 70% predicted	C	3	–	75% IBW	–	2 weeks	–	–

[a]Or > 5% weight loss over 6 months.
BMI, body mass index; FEV$_1$, forced expiratory volume in 1 s; FVC, forced ventilatory capacity; IBW, ideal body weight; REE, resting energy expenditure; S, supplemented; US, unsupplemented.

Table A4.6. Main findings of non-randomized trials of oral nutritional supplementation in community COPD patients.

Trial	Energy intake	Body weight S	Body weight US	Body function	Clinical outcome	Finance
Openbrier et al. (1984)	–	−1.8 kg[a] (sig.)	–	–	–	–
Pardy et al. (1986)	n 13 increased TEI by > 50% (and n 12 by < 50%)	NS increase at 1 and 2 months (no data)	–	NS change in respiratory muscle strength or endurance, even in those increasing TEI by > 50%	–	–
Sridhar et al. (1994)	–	~+0.56 kg (NS)	–	NS change in FEV_1, respiratory muscle strength or VO_2 max	–	–
Stauffer et al. (1986)	Sig. increase in TEI from 1899 kcal to 2456 kcal. ~53% of ONS energy additive	0.4 kg (NS)	–	–	–	–
Wilson et al. (1964)	Sig. increase in TPI and TEI compared with baseline despite a sig. reduction in VFI. The severely dyspnoeic pt consumed lower TEI than the moderately dyspnoeic pt	–	–	–	–	–
Wilson et al. (1986)	All consumed energy in excess of their maintenance energy requirements	3.1 kg (sig.) Sig. increase in TSF and MAMC	–	Sig. improvements in hand-grip strength and maximal inspiratory mouth and transdiaphragmatic pressures Increased sense of well-being (?)	–	–

[a]Applies only to patients surviving (n 7).
S, supplemented; US, unsupplemented; sig., significant; NS, not significant; TEI, total energy intake; FEV_1, forced expiratory volume in 1 s; VO_2 max., maximum oxygen consumption; TPI, total protein intake; VFI, voluntary food intake; TSF, triceps skin-fold thickness; MAMC, mid-arm muscle circumference.

meals, sips through the day or all at once. It was not possible to conclude whether the timing of supplementation determined the extent to which ONS suppressed food intake, because of a lack of data.

(II) What effect do ONS have on the body weight and composition of patients with COPD in the community?

Nutritional supplementation with ONS leads to weight gain in patients with COPD, who are typically undernourished. Increases in muscle and fat mass may occur.

Nine RCT were conducted in COPD patients with body weights less than 90% of ideal (equivalent to a body mass index (BMI) less than ~20 kg m^{-2}). Eighty-nine per cent (*n* 8) (Norregaard *et al.*, 1987; Efthimiou *et al.*, 1988; Knowles *et al.*, 1988; Donahoe *et al.*, 1989; Otte *et al.*, 1989; Fuenzalida *et al.*, 1990; Rogers *et al.*, 1992; Ganzoni *et al.*, 1994) showed a significant gain in body weight over time and one showed a non-significant increase (1.5 kg) (Lewis *et al.*, 1987) (range of means 1.5 to 7 kg, see Table A4.3). In only two trials was weight gain significantly greater than in controls (Otte *et al.*, 1989; Rogers *et al.*, 1992). Oedema, which can be a common feature of COPD, confounds interpretation of body weight and changes in body weight. However, its presence or absence was not reported in these studies.

Per cent weight change for supplemented patients was 5.2% greater than for unsupplemented patients (data from nine RCT (*n* 187), weighted for sample size; *P* < 0.003; independent *t* test). Meta-analysis of % weight change (nine trials, a fixed standard deviation (SD) for % weight change of 3% for missing values) indicated a cumulative effect size of 1.53 (95% confidence interval of 1.13–1.92) (Lewis *et al.*, 1987; Norregaard *et al.*, 1987; Efthimiou *et al.*, 1988; Knowles *et al.*, 1988; Donahoe *et al.*, 1989; Otte *et al.*, 1989; Fuenzalida *et al.*, 1990; Rogers *et al.*, 1992; Ganzoni *et al.*, 1994). The pooling of these community studies high-

lighted much less heterogeneity than was observed from the hospital studies in COPD patients, for which the effect size was 1.25 (95% confidence interval 0.43–2.07).

In the eight studies (Lewis *et al.*, 1987; Norregaard *et al.*, 1987; Efthimiou *et al.*, 1988; Knowles *et al.*, 1988; Donahoe *et al.*, 1989; Fuenzalida *et al.*, 1990; Rogers *et al.*, 1992; Ganzoni *et al.*, 1994) that collected other anthropometric data on the upper arm (including triceps skin-fold thickness (TSF) and mid-upper arm muscle circumference), significant increments over time were documented in 50% (Norregaard *et al.*, 1987; Efthimiou *et al.*, 1988; Fuenzalida *et al.*, 1990; Ganzoni *et al.*, 1994).

(III)/(IV) What effect do ONS have on the body function and clinical outcome of patients with COPD in the community?

The use of ONS in COPD patients can improve functional outcome measures, including respiratory and skeletal muscle strength, walking distances and well-being.

Forty-four per cent (4/9) of the randomized controlled studies of COPD patients showed significant functional benefits associated with ONS use (Efthimiou *et al.*, 1988; Donahoe *et al.*, 1989; Fuenzalida *et al.*, 1990; Rogers *et al.*, 1992) (see Table A4.3). In three of these studies, supplementation was carried out in a research unit for part or all of the time (Donahoe *et al.*, 1989; Fuenzalida *et al.*, 1990; Rogers *et al.*, 1992). In all of these studies, the weight gain associated with supplementation exceeded 2 kg (2 to 4.4 kg). In studies where the weight gain was < 2 kg, no functional improvements occurred (see Fig. 6.20 in Chapter 6).

Only one study made some assessment of quality of life (QOL) (Rogers *et al.*, 1992) but no improvement was found despite the functional and structural benefits that accompanied supplementation. Two studies made assessments of general well-being, with conflicting results (Efthimiou *et al.*, 1988; Otte *et al.*, 1989).

No assessments of clinical outcome were made in this patient group.

(V) What are the effects of stopping ONS in patients with COPD in the community?

Only two studies made assessments of patients after supplementation was stopped (Efthimiou *et al.*, 1988; Knowles *et al.*, 1988), one for 3 months (Efthimiou *et al.*, 1988) and one for 2 months (Knowles *et al.*, 1988). They clearly showed total energy intake returning to baseline levels, accompanied by some weight loss. Efthimiou *et al.* (1988) also reported that some (but not all) of the functional benefits that occurred after 3 months of supplementation were lost after supplementation was stopped.

Summary of non-randomized community trials in patients with COPD

Six trials were non-randomized in design (Wilson *et al.*, 1964; Openbrier *et al.*, 1984; Pardy *et al.*, 1986; Stauffer *et al.*, 1986; Wilson *et al.*, 1986; Sridhar *et al.*, 1994). Most of these studies were carried out in malnourished patients (< 90% ideal body weight (IBW)) (Pardy *et al.*, 1986; Stauffer *et al.*, 1986; Wilson *et al.*, 1986; Sridhar *et al.*, 1994) or those who were losing weight (Sridhar *et al.*, 1994), although in two studies supplemented patients were not exclusively malnourished (Wilson *et al.*, 1964; Openbrier *et al.*, 1984) (see Tables A4.4–A4.6).

The duration of supplementation varied from 2 weeks (Wilson *et al.*, 1986) to 22 months (Openbrier *et al.*, 1984). The amount of ONS given daily varied between 750 kcal (3.15 MJ) (Wilson *et al.*, 1964; Openbrier *et al.*, 1984) and 1080 kcal (4.54 MJ) (Stauffer *et al.*, 1986), although in three studies (Pardy *et al.*, 1986; Wilson *et al.*, 1986; Sridhar *et al.*, 1994) no data on prescribed amounts were reported (Table A4.4). There was also little check on compliance with ONS intake. Three studies made some assessment of total energy intake during supplementation (Wilson *et al.*, 1964; Stauffer *et al.*, 1986; Wilson *et al.*, 1986). However, only Stauffer *et al.* (1986) were able to demonstrate a significant increase in total energy intake during supplementation compared with the baseline period (2456 kcal (10.3 MJ) vs. 1899 kcal (7.98 MJ)). These data suggested that, of the 1045 kcal (4.4 MJ) of ONS taken, approximately 53% (557 kcal) was additive to habitual intake of energy from food (compared with baseline). In this study, patients were advised to take the ONS between meals. Similarly, data from another study indicated that ~59% of the ONS energy was additional to that from food, again when compared to baseline (Wilson *et al.*, 1986). Of the studies that assessed functional outcomes (Openbrier *et al.*, 1984; Pardy *et al.*, 1986; Wilson *et al.*, 1986; Sridhar *et al.*, 1994), only one documented significant functional improvements (Wilson *et al.*, 1986). After 2 weeks of taking an *ad libitum* diet, with (*n* 3) or without supplementation (as needed to achieve total energy intakes 150% of basal energy expenditure), hand-grip strength and respiratory (inspiratory) muscle strength (maximal inspiratory pressure ($P_I$max)) had improved significantly and an increased sense of well-being occurred in 83% (*n* 5) of patients. Interestingly, this study, which was carried out in a research unit (total of 3 weeks), was also the only uncontrolled study to report a significant increase in weight (3.2 kg), TSF and mid-arm muscle circumference (MAMC). In contrast, deterioration in functional capacity (respiratory function) was observed in one study in which significant weight loss and poor compliance with supplementation occurred (Openbrier *et al.*, 1984).

In summary, from these six non-randomized, uncontrolled trials it was difficult to come to firm conclusions, as these trials frequently had only small numbers of patients participating. However, as in the controlled trials, where data were available it appeared that > 50% of ONS energy added to that taken from food and that a weight gain > 2 kg was associated with improvements in functional outcomes.

COPD: other meta-analyses/reviews

A meta-analysis of trials in COPD patients suggested that there were small but positive effects of nutritional support on weight

(+1.65 kg), muscle circumference (+0.3 cm) and 6 min walking distances (+3.4 m), although these differences were not statistically significant (Ferreira *et al.*, 2000). A narrative review of the effects of enteral nutrition (including ONS) in malnourished COPD patients suggested positive effects on body composition, muscular strength and respiratory function (Akner and Cederholm, 2001).

The findings of this review and other reviews (Ferreira *et al.*, 2000) suggest that larger, well-designed trials that investigate the effects of ONS on functional and clinical outcome parameters are essential to fully characterize the benefits of using ONS in COPD patients. For example, the studies reviewed tended to have low Jadad scores (score of 1 in four trials, score of 2 in three trials) and small sample sizes (*n* 9 to 30), with a notable absence of power statistics. For more information about study design and power calculation, refer to Chapter 10. Within larger studies, it may be possible to ascertain the efficacy of ONS in different subsets of patients with COPD. It may be that some patients will benefit more than others from ONS. For example, in one study of COPD patients in a hospital environment, those not responding to supplementation were those who were older and had a poor appetite and an elevated inflammatory systemic response (Creutzberg *et al.*, 2000). The reasons for non-response in community COPD patients have not been fully characterized as yet but deserve exploration.

Crohn's Disease (Adults and Paediatrics)

Crohn's disease is a chronic inflammatory disease of the gastrointestinal (GI) tract and the symptoms include diarrhoea, abdominal pain, fever and weight loss. The incidence of this disease is increasing (across Europe) but as yet there is no cure. Dietary treatment with ONS is used both therapeutically as a sole source of nutrition and as nutritional support to improve nutritional intake and prevent weight loss. This section addresses the impact of using ONS in adult and paediatric patients with Crohn's

disease living at home, typically after discharge from hospital.

Crohn's disease: present analysis

Three RCT (Harries *et al.*, 1983; O'Morain *et al.*, 1984; Lindor *et al.*, 1992) (see Tables A4.7–A4.9) and seven prospective NRT that lacked a control group receiving no nutritional support (Kirschner *et al.*, 1981; Logan *et al.*, 1981; Harries *et al.*, 1984; Raouf *et al.*, 1991; Akobeng *et al.*, 2000; Fell *et al.*, 2000; Geerling *et al.*, 2000b; see Tables A4.10–A4.12) have been systematically reviewed and the findings summarized according to the main review questions (see Box A4.2).

(I) What effect do ONS have on the voluntary food intake and total energy intake of patients with Crohn's disease in the community?

ONS may be used as a sole source of nutrition in the treatment of Crohn's disease or as an effective way of increasing total energy intake in those able to eat. ONS appear not to suppress food intake.

The one randomized trial (Harries *et al.*, 1983) that assessed total energy intake showed a significant increase during supplementation (see Table A4.9). Similarly, the non-controlled trials that assessed changes in total energy intake in adults (Harries *et al.*, 1984) and children (Kirschner *et al.*, 1981) documented increases, but these were not statistically evaluated (see Table A4.12). In the other trial that made observations of intake in children with Crohn's disease, when ONS were used as a sole source of nutrition, energy and protein intakes were 2500 kcal and 90 g, respectively (Fell *et al.*, 2000).

Although no assessments were made of the effect of supplements on appetite, it appeared that supplementation did not suppress food intake in the one trial that made such assessments (Harries *et al.*, 1983) (randomized, crossover design). On the contrary, calculations based on method (i) (see Chapter 5) suggested that the increase in food intake that occurred

---

Box A4.2. Key findings: effect of ONS in community patients with Crohn's disease.

Nutritional intake: ONS (nutritionally complete) can be used as a sole source of nutrition in both adult and paediatric patients with acute exacerbations of Crohn's disease. When used as a supplement to food intake, ONS may increase total energy intake without reducing food intake substantially.

Body weight and function: a rather limited evidence base suggests that ONS may increase body weight and muscle mass and growth in growth-retarded children and may improve functional outcome measures (quality of life).

Further research: well-controlled, adequately powered studies are needed in this patient group.

---

during supplementation was equivalent to ~35% of the supplement energy consumed.

Assessments of dietary intake were typically short (3 days) and checks on supplement compliance were mostly lacking, although one study made checks of returned ONS packets (Geerling *et al.*, 2000b).

(IA) IS THE TIMING OF SUPPLEMENTATION IMPORTANT?
No information was presented in any of these studies on the timing of supplement consumption, in relation to the time of day (morning, afternoon, evening) or the consumption of food, except in one study in which patients were recommended to take the supplement as several small feeds over 16 h of the day (Lindor *et al.*, 1992).

(II) What effect do ONS have on the body weight and composition of patients with Crohn's disease in the community?

ONS can increase body weight and may improve parameters of muscle mass in patients with Crohn's disease. In children, ONS can improve growth in those who are growth-retarded.

The two (out of three (Harries *et al.*, 1983; O'Morain *et al.*, 1984; Lindor *et al.*, 1992)) randomized studies that assessed the changes in weight with ONS versus no nutritional support documented significant weight gain over time (Harries *et al.*, 1983; O'Morain *et al.*, 1984) or compared with an unsupplemented group (Harries *et al.*, 1983) (see Table A4.9). The one trial that assessed other anthropometric parameters (MAMC) observed a significant increase (Harries *et al.*, 1983) (see Table A4.9). None of the ran-

domized studies presented information on nutritional status at the start of the study.

The two non-controlled trials in adult patients with Crohn's disease (Logan *et al.*, 1981; Harries *et al.*, 1984) reported weight gain (significant in only one (Harries *et al.*, 1984)) (see Table A4.12). The same study also observed a significant increase in MAMC (Harries *et al.*, 1984). Baseline nutritional status was also documented (~85% IBW).

The three NRT that observed changes in nutritional status with ONS in children documented improvements in weight (Akobeng *et al.*, 2000), weight and BMI SD scores (Fell *et al.*, 2000) and linear growth rates (Kirschner *et al.*, 1981), although none of these changes appeared to have been assessed for statistical significance (see Table A4.12).

(III)/(IV) What effect do ONS have on the body function and clinical outcome of patients with Crohn's disease in the community?

There is a need for better-designed RCT in patients with Crohn's disease to clarify the role of ONS in reducing Crohn's disease activity and other parameters, such as QOL. The main functional outcome measure in trials was the Crohn's disease activity index (CDAI). A reduction in this score was demonstrated in two RCT (Harries *et al.*, 1983; Lindor *et al.*, 1992) (see Table A4.9). In one of these studies, the response to ONS and steroid treatment was similar to the response following steroid treatment alone (Lindor *et al.*, 1992). Simpler, but

Table A4.7. Oral nutritional supplements used in randomized controlled trials of patients with Crohn's disease in the community.

Trial	ONS	ONS energy density	ONS prescribed	ONS energy (kcal) intake	ONS protein (g) intake	Toleration
Harries et al. (1983)[a]	Ensure Plus (Abbott)	1.5 kcal ml⁻¹	To increase energy intakes to 3000 kcal	550/560	22.9/23.3	17% unable to tolerate ONS (severe diarrhoea/unpalatability). Increase in stool frequency in first month (sig.)
Lindor et al. (1992)[a,b]	Vital HN	–	40 kcal kg⁻¹	–	–	44% (n 4) unable to tolerate ONS (a nasogastric tube used for those unable to take maintenance amount[b])
O'Morain et al. (1984)	Vivonex (Norwich Eaton Lab)	1 kcal ml⁻¹	~1980–2661 (40–60 kcal kg⁻¹ and 8–12 g N)	–	–	Two unable to tolerate, with one taking ONS via tube – withdrawn from analysis

aSteroid therapy continued in some patients during the trial.
bAn unspecified number of the supplemented group took the supplement via tube.
N, nitrogen.

Table A4.8. Trial characteristics: community-based randomized controlled trials of oral nutritional supplementation in patients with Crohn's disease.

Trial	Design	No. S	No. US	Initial BMI S group	Initial BMI US group	Duration of ONS	Dietary counselling	Control group
Harries et al. (1983)[a] Malnourished with Crohn's disease	10001	S 28[b]	–	85–88% IBW	–	2 months	–	Ordinary diet during control period
Lindor et al. (1992)[a] Active Crohn's disease	10001	S¹ 9 S² 8[a]	10[a]	–	–	1 month	No – ONS used as sole source of nutrition	S² given ONS as sole source of nutrition and prednisone (0.75 mg kg⁻¹) and US given prednisone alone and encouraged to eat as tolerated
O'Morain et al. (1984) Active Crohn's disease	10001	S 11	10[a]	–	–	1 month	No – ONS as sole source of nutrition	Given 0.75 mg kg⁻¹ prednisolone daily

aSteroid therapy given to some or all patients during the trial.
bCrossover trial.
IBW, ideal body weight; S, supplemented; US, unsupplemented.

Table A4.9. Main findings of randomized controlled trials of oral nutritional supplementation in patients with Crohn's disease in the community.

Trial	Energy intake	Body weight S	Body weight US	Body function	Clinical outcome	Finance
Harries *et al.* (1983)[a]	Sig. increase in TEI during ONS in both crossover groups (e.g. from 2610 kcal at baseline to 3360 kcal during ONS)	2.24 kg (sig.) (S vs. US sig.) Sig. increase in MAMC	1.74 kg	Improved well-being (NS) during the period of ONS	Decrease in CDAI (NS)	–
Lindor *et al.* (1992)[a]	–	–	–	–	NS difference in changes in CDAI between groups receiving steroid treatment and those receiving the ONS alone or with the steroid	–
O'Morain *et al.* (1984)[a]	–	1.5 kg (sig.)[b]	3.5 kg (sig.)	*Sig. increase in Hb and albumin, sustained in S but not US at 3 months*	Sig. reduction in average clinical scores at 1 week in S, continued at 3-month follow-up. Responses similar in S and US (steroid) groups	–

[a]Steroid therapy given to some or all patients during the trial.
[b]Values presented at end of 4 weeks of supplementation, follow-up 2 months later, weight maintained in S, wt gain continued in US (steroid).
CDAI, Crohn's disease activity index; Hb, haemoglobin; NS, not significant; ONS, supplemented; sig., significant; TEI, total energy intake; US, unsupplemented.

Table A4.10. Oral nutritional supplements used in non-randomized trials of patients with Crohn's disease (adults and paediatrics) in the community.

Trial	ONS	ONS energy density	ONS prescribed	ONS energy (kcal) intake	ONS protein (g) intake	Toleration
Akobeng *et al.* (2000)	S^1 standard (4% glutamine) S^2 glutamine-enriched (42% of amino acid) ($n = 4$ took by tube)	0.9 kcal ml^{-1} 0.9 kcal ml^{-1}	– –	S^1 1980 (216) S^2 2160 (306)	– –	n 2 were withdrawn due to persistent vomiting (n 1) and abdominal pain and refusal to take ONS (n 1)
Fell *et al.* (2000)	Polymeric casein ONS rich in TGF-β_2	1 kcal ml^{-1}	As a sole source of nutrition to match daily energy requirement	Median 2500 (1950–3000)	Median 90	n 2 nausea and n 3 constipation (n 1 also required intravenous glucose)
Geerling *et al.* (2000b)	S^1 standard S^2 enriched with antioxidants and other micronutrients S^3 Impact (antioxidants and omega-3 fatty acids)	– – –	S^1 612 kcal, 27.2 g P S^2 14 kcal, 27.4 g P S^3 648 kcal, 34.8 g P	– – –	– – –	Intolerance due to fullness in n 4
Harries *et al.* (1984)	Ensure Plus (Abbott)	1.5 kcal ml^{-1}	–	550	–	–
Kirschner *et al.* (1981)[a]	Ensure (Abbott) or Vivonex (Norwich Eaton Lab)	1 kcal ml^{-1}	600–1200	–	–	Patients chose the ONS they preferred the taste of. n 2 were given 4 weeks of PN
Logan *et al.* (1981)	Vivonex (Norwich Eaton Lab)	1 kcal ml^{-1}	1800	–	–	Described as unpalatable
Raouf *et al.* (1991)[a]	S^1 E028 (SHS) S^2 Triosorbon (whole protein; Merck), flavoured with Nesquick (Nestlé)	0.76 kcal ml^{-1} –	2000 kcal, 80 g P	–	–	–

[a]Steroid therapy continued in some patients during the trial.
P, protein; PN, parenteral nutrition; S, supplemented; TGF, transforming growth factor β_2.

Table A4.11. Trial characteristics: community-based non-randomized trials of oral nutritional supplementation in patients with Crohn's disease in the community.

Trial	Design	No. S	No. US	Initial BMI S group	Initial BMI US group	Duration of ONS	Dietary counselling	Control group
Akobeng et al. (2000) Children with active Crohn's disease (mean age of ONS group 10.8 (2.7) years). RCT comparing different ONS	C	S^1 9 S^2 9	–	– S^1 28.2 (9) kg S^2 39.6 (17.2) kg (no sd scores)	–	4 weeks	–	–
Fell et al. (2000) Children with active intestinal Crohn's disease	C	29 (aged 8.1–17.1 years)	–	Wt sd score –1.49 BMI sd score –1.48	–	8 weeks	No – used as sole source of nutrition	–
Geerling et al. (2000b) Crohn's disease (small bowel, < 5 years duration); RCT comparing different ONS	C	S^1 8 S^2 8 S^3 9	–	S^1 23.8 kg m^{-2} (20.3 to 30.8) S^2 21.2 kg m^{-2} (19.4 to 26.2) S^3 22.1 kg m^{-2} (19.2 to 25.4)	–	3 months	–	–
Harries et al. (1984) Adults with Crohn's disease	C	21 (33)	–	85% IBW	–	2–4 months	–	–
Kirschner et al. (1981)[a] Crohn's disease and growth retardation	C	7	–	–	–	< 12 months	–	–
Logan et al. (1981) Extensive jejunoileal Crohn's disease	C	7	–	86% IBW	–	28–56 days	No – used as sole source of nutrition	–
Raouf et al. (1991)[a] Active Crohn's disease; RCT comparing different ONS	C	24	–	–	–	3 weeks	No – used as sole source of nutrition	–

[a]Steroid therapy given to some or all patients during the trial.
IBW, ideal body weight; RCT, randomized controlled trial; S, supplemented; US, unsupplemented.

Table A4.12. Main findings of non-randomized trials of oral nutritional supplements in patients with Crohn's disease in the community.

Trial	Energy intake	Body weight S	Body weight US	Body function	Clinical outcome	Finance
Akobeng *et al.* (2000) Paediatrics	–	S[1] 1.05 kg S[2] 0.98 kg	–	NS difference in changes in orosomucoid conc. or platelet count	56% in S[1] and 44% in S[2] went into remission (S[1] vs. S[2] NS). PCDAI declined in all children in S[1] (av. –27.22) but increased in *n* 2 in S[2] (av. –7.86; S[1] vs. S[2] sig.)	–
Fell *et al.* (2000) Paediatrics	Sole source of nutrition with median TEI 2500 kcal and TPI 90 g	+0.42 wt SD score +0.73 BMI SD score	–	–	79% went into remission – macroscopic and histological healing associated with sig. decrease in ileal and colonic IL-1β mRNA, and sig. decrease in ileal interferon gamma mRNA, sig. increase in TGF-β₁ mRNA and sig. decrease in colonic IL-8 mRNA (i.e. downregulation of mucosal proinflammatory cytokine mRNA)	–
Geerling *et al.* (2000b)	–	–	–	Sig. increase in serum vit. E and C concentrations and whole-blood SOD activity in S[2] and S[3], not seen in S[1] Analysis of S[2] and S[3] combined: sig. increase in serum vit. C, E, Se, whole-blood SOD activity and total antioxidant status S3: sig. reduction in the proportion of AA and increased EPA and DHA in plasma phospholipids and adipose tissue	From two abstract reports (same trial)[a]: reduction in CDAI score in S (sig.). No change in quality of life in any groups. Improved muscle strength in S[2] and S[3] (sig.)	–
Harries *et al.* (1984)	Increase in TEI (?)	7% IBW (sig.)	–	Sig. reduction in serum orosomucoids, indicative of reduced disease activity	–	–
Kirschner *et al.* (1981)[b,c] Paediatrics	TEI improved from 1535 (148) kcal to 2493 (108) kcal (?)	–	–	Improved linear growth rate in all patients (?)	–	–
Logan *et al.* (1981)	–	Increase of 2% of IBW (NS)	–	47% mean reduction in gastrointestinal protein loss and increase in blood lymphocyte count (sig.) Increased energy and sense of well-being reported by pts	–	–

Continued

Table A4.12. *Continued*

Trial	Energy intake	Body weight S	Body weight US	Body function	Clinical outcome	Finance
Raouf *et al.* (1991)[b]	–	–	–	–	9/11 patients into remission (assessed by Bristol simple activity index) in S[2] and 9/13 patients into remission with S[1] (S[1] vs. S[2]?). On crossover, no relapses with S[2], 3/7 with S[1]	–

[a]Two abstract reports not specifically reviewed of the same trial (Geerling *et al.*, 1998b, c).
[b]Steroid therapy given to some or all patients during the trial.
[c]*n* 2 given a 4-week period of parenteral nutrition.
AA, arachidonic acid; CDAI, Crohn's disease activity index; DHA, docosahexanoic acid; EPA, eicosapentanoic acid; IL, interleukin; NS, not significant; PCDAI, paediatric Crohn's disease activity index; S, supplemented; sig., significant; SOD, singlet oxygen dismutase; TEI, total energy intake; TGF, transforming growth factor; TPI, total protein intake; US, unsupplemented;

less valid, scores also indicated reductions in Crohn's disease activities that were significant (O'Morain *et al.*, 1984). Similarly, in NRT in adults (Raouf *et al.*, 1991) and paediatrics (Akobeng *et al.*, 2000; Fell *et al.*, 2000), decreases in disease activity, determined by the paediatric CDAI, other scores or histologically, were also observed over time following ONS (see Table A4.12). However, these studies made comparisons with baseline disease activity without the use of suitable control groups, and so it was not possible to say whether the changes were due to supplementation *per se* or to a spontaneous reduction in disease activity. Also, patients often received concurrent steroid therapy.

In adults, other functional measures included non-significant increases in energy and sense of well-being (Harries *et al.*, 1983; Lindor *et al.*, 1992). Significant improvements in muscle strength following ingestion of antioxidant- and omega-3-enriched ONS have also been reported (abstract form only (Geerling *et al.*, 1998c)). The one trial in which QOL was formally assessed showed no benefit (abstract form only (Geerling *et al.*, 1998b)). In paediatric trials, a significant improvement in linear growth rates (growth velocity, height percentiles) was observed in growth-retarded children (Kirschner *et al.*, 1981; Fell *et al.*, 2000).

(V) What are the effects of stopping ONS in patients with Crohn's disease in the community?

Only one study continued to assess patients after the cessation of ONS (O'Morain *et al.*, 1984). The benefits observed (weight gain, improved clinical score) persisted for 2 months after the ONS were stopped, but the results were not compared with a control group.

Summary of non-randomized community trials in patients with Crohn's disease

We reviewed seven prospective NRT that lacked a control group receiving no nutritional support (Kirschner *et al.*, 1981; Logan *et al.*, 1981; Harries *et al.*, 1984; Raouf *et al.*,

1991; Akobeng *et al.*, 2000; Fell *et al.*, 2000; Geerling *et al.*, 2000b; see Tables A4.10–A4.12), three of which were predominantly in children (Kirschner *et al.*, 1981; Akobeng *et al.*, 2000; Fell *et al.*, 2000). An example is Kirschner *et al.*'s (1981) small study (*n* 7), conducted in children aged 11–15 years presenting with growth failure. Their diets were supplemented for up to 1 year with whole-protein or amino acid ONS (600–1200 kcal day^{-1}). In the 12 months preceding the study, growth rate was only 1.8 cm ($<$ 3rd percentile, should be $>$ 4 cm for this age group). With the increase in total energy intake (apparently +958 kcal from baseline, measured by an unspecified method) due to ONS, growth rate improved (to 6.2 cm year^{-1}, 20th percentile) in five children. Similar changes were also observed in the two other children, who, in addition to ONS, received peripheral parenteral nutrition for 4 weeks. None of the data were statistically evaluated. The other two trials in paediatrics also suggested that weight gain, improvements in growth and reductions in disease activity occurred over time, although the lack of unsupplemented groups limits the conclusions that could be formed. Both of these trials involved special formulas, enriched either with glutamine (42% protein as glutamine) (Akobeng *et al.*, 2000) (remission rates significantly less than those on the standard feed) or with transforming growth factor-β_2 (TGF-β_2) (associated with downregulation of mucosal proinflammatory cytokine mRNA, no comparison with a standard ONS) (Fell *et al.*, 2000).

The two trials (Logan *et al.*, 1981; Harries *et al.*, 1984) undertaken in malnourished adults demonstrated weight gain with ONS (see Table A4.12). However, this was significant in only one trial (Harries *et al.*, 1984), in which an increased total energy intake was documented in patients (*n* 21) reported to consume 550 kcal daily as an ONS for 2–4 months (see Tables A4.10 and A4.12). In this study, food intake was increased during the period of supplementation when compared with baseline, but the lack of a control group means changes in disease activity could not be excluded. In Logan *et al.*'s

(1981) trial, although patients were prescribed ~1800 kcal of an elemental diet for up to 2 months, the intake of ONS (described as unpalatable) and total energy intake (ONS + food) were not documented. Functional benefits (only anecdotal) included increased energy and well-being (Logan et al., 1981). A significant reduction in orosomucoid concentrations in one trial (Harries et al., 1984) was indicative of improved disease activity but no official scoring system for disease activity was used and there was no control group for comparison. In adults, two further trials were comparisons of different ONS types (Raouf et al., 1991; Geerling et al., 2000b) (two earlier abstract reports: Geerling et al., 1998b,c)). Geerling et al. reported significant increases in blood antioxidant status with an ONS enriched with antioxidants and changes in the fatty acid profile of plasma phospholipids and adipose tissue with an ONS enriched with omega-3 fatty acids. The functional relevance of these measures to clinical outcome was not explored in this patient group (mean BMI > 20 kg m^{-2}). The two abstract reports of this study (Geerling et al., 1998b,c) indicated that, compared with baseline data, CDAI scores were significantly reduced in those receiving the ONS enriched with omega-3 fatty acids and antioxidants. A significant improvement in muscle strength was also observed in patients who took either this ONS or the ONS enriched simply with antioxidants but no such changes occurred in those receiving the standard supplement. In addition, no change in rated QOL was found in any of the supplemented patients (see Table A4.12). Interpretation of these data was limited by the small number of patients (n 8–9), comparisons made only with baseline measurements and a lack of information on nutritional status, supplement and food intake.

Oral supplementation versus tube feeding

Other forms of nutritional support, such as enteral tube feeding (ETF), are also used in the treatment of patients with Crohn's disease, as a sole source of nutrition. A number of studies have looked at the use of ETF in patients with Crohn's disease, although most have been conducted in the hospital setting. The majority of these trials have assessed the impact of tube feeding on disease activity, comparing either different feed formulations (amino acid, peptide or whole protein feeds) (Rigaud et al., 1991; Royall et al., 1994; Mansfield et al., 1995) or different treatment types (e.g. steroid therapy) (Lochs et al., 1991). The results of these have been thoroughly reviewed elsewhere (Griffiths et al., 1995; Messori et al., 1996; King et al., 1997; Zachos et al., 2001). As with trials of ONS (Kirschner et al., 1981), ETF in children with Crohn's disease has resulted in improved growth (Morin et al., 1980; Belli et al., 1988). However, although studies using nasogastric tubes generally have better compliance and lower withdrawal rates (0–13%) than those using ONS (0–41%) (mostly due to the unpalatability of the commercial formulas used), there is a lack of suitably controlled studies comparing the two treatments. Interpretation of the effects of ONS or tube feeding on disease activity in patients with Crohn's disease has been hindered by inadequate study design. As outlined by King et al. (1997), the sample sizes in these studies are too small to provide sufficient power to discriminate differences between treatments (i.e. steroid versus dietary formulas) (see Chapter 7 for more details).

Cystic Fibrosis (Adults and Paediatrics)

Cystic fibrosis is a genetic condition caused by a mutation of the long arm of chromosome 7, which leads to abnormalities in the protein called cystic fibrosis transmembrane conductance regulator (CFTR). Transport across epithelial cell membranes and, more specifically, chloride transport are affected by this disease, which is characterized by pancreatic insufficiency and malabsorption, respiratory infections, poor appetite, growth retardation and wide-ranging nutritional deficiencies.

Consequently, nutritional support including ONS is often used in this patient group for long periods of time. Indeed, the Cystic Fibrosis Foundation Consensus Report (Ramsey *et al.*, 1992) recommends that:

> Emphasis should be placed on optimising feeding behaviours and adding oral supplements. If these measures are not successful within 3 months or if the patient's weight–height ratio declines to < 85% of ideal, more aggressive nutritional management should be considered.

Cystic fibrosis: present review

In an attempt to ascertain the efficacy of adding oral supplements to the diets of cystic fibrosis patients living at home, 13 studies were reviewed, of which only three involved randomization of patients (Sondel *et al.*, 1987; Kalnins *et al.*, 1996; Steinkamp *et al.*, 2000) (see Tables A4.13–A4.15). Three NRT included a control group of either healthy subjects (Shepherd *et al.*, 1983), age- and sex-matched patients (Berry *et al.*, 1975) or patients matched for disease severity in the absence of random selection (Yassa *et al.*, 1978). The majority conducted investigations without a control group in a supplemented group only (Allan *et al.*, 1973; Barclay and Shannon, 1975; Parsons *et al.*, 1983; Hayes *et al.*, 1995; Rettamel *et al.*, 1995; Kashirskaja *et al.*, 1996; Skypala

et al., 1998). One of the reasons for this concerns the ethical issues of withholding nutritional therapy in patients with varying degrees of growth failure. However, these studies are still important, as most have conducted valuable longitudinal assessments in the same patients, both before supplementation, when there was poor growth performance, and after supplementation. All the studies have been described and summarized below (see Box A4.3).

(I) What effect do ONS have on the voluntary food intake and total energy intake of patients with cystic fibrosis in the community?

ONS provide additional energy to that taken as food, leading to increases in total energy intakes in those with cystic fibrosis. Of the six studies that presented data on the effects of supplementation, in 83% (*n* 5) total energy intake increased (Parsons *et al.*, 1983; Shepherd *et al.*, 1983; Sondel *et al.*, 1987; Skypala *et al.*, 1998; Steinkamp *et al.*, 2000), significantly so in four of them (Parsons *et al.*, 1983; Sondel *et al.*, 1987; Skypala *et al.*, 1998; Steinkamp *et al.*, 2000) (see Table A4.15). In some cases however, the weight gain did not match the reported increase in total energy intake (e.g. Skypala *et al.*, 1998) (see Table A4.14).

There was limited information on the effects of ONS on appetite (Yassa *et al.*, 1978; Hayes *et al.*, 1995), although Yassa *et*

Box A4.3. Key findings: effect of ONS in community patients with cystic fibrosis.

The findings from predominantly non-randomized trials suggest the following.

Nutritional intake: in undernourished cystic fibrosis patients (adults and paediatrics), ONS can increase total energy intake without reducing food intake substantially. The increase in total intake may be equivalent to more than 80% of ONS energy, although large volumes of unpalatable formulations may reduce appetite.

Growth and body function: NRT consistently show that use of ONS is associated with increased growth in growth-retarded children and some functional changes (improved activity and pulmonary scores, anecdotal benefits to mood, sleep, hair, skin, energy and activity levels). In the trials reviewed, patients often chose to continue ONS after the studies had stopped.

Ethics: large, placebo-controlled trials comparing ONS with no nutrition intervention may not be ethically justifiable in children with severe growth failure.

Table A4.13. Oral nutritional supplements used in all trials of patients with cystic fibrosis in the community.

Trial	ONS	ONS energy density	ONS prescribed (kcal)	ONS energy (kcal) intake	ONS protein (g) intake	Toleration
Randomized controlled trials						
Kalnins et al. (1996)	Boost Plus (Mead Johnson)	–	To increase energy intake by 20% of predicted energy needs	At 1 month 462 At 3 months 756	–	57% continued to use ONS after the 3-month trial 63% had fullness and 25% appetite loss but not significantly more than with the dextrose placebo
Sondel et al. (1987)	Magnacal (Organon Pharmaceuticals)	2 kcal ml[-1]	30% RDI	635	–	
Steinkamp et al. (2000)	Fresubin (energy: 31% F, 16% P, 53% CHO, Fresenius)	1 kcal ml[-1]	To enable estimated energy requirements to be met (between 500 and 800 kcal)	628 (254)	–	–
Non-randomized trials						
Allan et al. (1973)	Beef serum hydrolysate and glucose polymer[a]	–	100% RDI and 50% RDI	–	–	No adverse effects but perseverance needed due to unpleasant taste of ONS. Needed flavouring
Barclay et al. (1975)	Albumaid and caloreen	–	100% RDI	–	–	8/12 (the oldest patients) found ONS monotonous and unpleasant
Berry et al. (1975)	As Allan et al., 1973[a]	–	50–70% RDI	–	–	Poor acceptance as ONS monotonous and unpleasant
Hayes et al. (1995)	–	–	600 kcal	–	–	ONS well tolerated – no increase in fullness and no reduction in appetite
Kashirskaja et al. (1996)	Home-made (food ingredients)	–	–	–	–	–
Parsons et al. (1983)	Milk-based beverages (no name)	1 kcal ml[-1]	–	31% of calculated energy requirement	–	Good acceptance due to ONS palatability

Reference	ONS				Comments
Rettammel et al. (1995)	–	2 kcal ml⁻¹	Maximum of 30% of est. daily energy requirement	471 to 1413	–	4 patients had mild symptoms of bloating and/or nausea, relieved by reducing volume and increasing frequency. 11 experienced fullness after ONS
Shepherd et al. (1983)	Vipep	1 kcal ml⁻¹	1000–1200 kcal	–	–	–
Skypala et al. (1998)	Scandishake (SHS) (powder reconstituted to drink)	2 kcal ml⁻¹	To increase TEI to 120% of baseline intake	659 (437–1167)	18 g (12–32 g)	Bloating and abdominal pain in 4 patients but resolved by enzymes
Yassa et al. (1978)	As Allan et al., 1973[a]	–	100% RDI	–	–	ONS was described as unpleasant

[a]The ONS used in these trials were 'home-made' and unpalatable. They are very unlike the nutritionally complete sip feeds available commercially nowadays.
CHO, carbohydrate; F, fat; P, protein; RDI, recommended daily intake; TEI, total energy intake.

Table A4.14. Trial characteristics: community-based trials of oral nutritional supplementation in patients with cystic fibrosis (including information on changes in body weight/growth with supplementation).

Trial	Design	No. S	No. US	Age	Duration of ONS	Initial z score (weight) or equivalent	Change in z score (weight) with S	Weight change after S (kg)	Initial z score (height)	Change in z score (height) with S
Randomized controlled trials										
Kalnins *et al.* (1996) A	10000	7	6	> 10 years	3 months	S 84% wt-for-ht US 84% wt-for-ht	NS change in S or US groups (+1% wt-for-ht)	–	–	–
Sondel *et al.* (1987)	10001	16	–	7 years–16 years	7 weeks	–	–	– (NS)	–	–
Steinkamp *et al.* (2000)	11000	16	20	> 4 years S 13.3 (3.8) years US 10.4 (4.3) years	3 months	S 83% wt-for-ht US 88% wt-for-ht	+2% wt-for-ht (S vs. US ?)	+1.2 kg (+3.7%) (sig.) US 0 kg (0%) Increase in body fat, NS change in LBM	–	–
Non-randomized trials										
Allan *et al.* (1973)	C	17 (100% RDA) 11 (50% RDA)	–	5 months–20 years 100% 6.6 years 50% 11.8 years	3 months–3 years	All –2.1 (0.89) 100% –2.2 (0.80) 50% –1.9 (1.1)	All +0.86 (sig.)[a] 100% +1.34 (sig.) 50% –0.02 (NS)	S (100%) 6.3 kg S (50%) 2.6 kg (both sig.)[a]	All –1.71 (0.99) 100% –1.74 (1.06) 50% –1.67 (0.94)	All +0.28 (NS)[a] 100% +0.5 (NS) 50% –0.11 (NS)
Barclay *et al.* (1975)	C	12	–	5 months–8 years	1 year	< 3rd–25th centile	< 3rd–> 90th centile	S < 2 years ~3.6 kg S > 3 years ~0.8 kg (?)	–	–
Berry *et al.* (1975)	B	15	15	7.67 years 10 months–18 years	1 year	S –2.0 (0.6) US –1.0 (1.1)	S +0.5 (sig.) (–0.2 to +2.3) US –0.2 (NS) (–0.9 to +0.3)	–	S –1.4 (1.0) US –1.0 (1.5)	S +0.3 (NS) (–0.3 to +3.0) US 0 (NS) (–0.7 to +0.6)

Study	Group	n		Age	Duration					
Hayes et al. (1995)	C	10	—	7 years–19 years	3 months	—	—	3.21 kg (?)	—	—
Kashirskaja et al. (1996)	C	42	—	4 months–15 years	1 year	S[1] <85% (wt-for-age) S[2] <76% (wt/ht-for-age)	S[1] +5% (to ~90%) (wt-for-age) S[2] +14% (to ~90%) (wt/ht-for-age)	—	—	—
Parsons et al. (1983)	C	8	—	5.51 years (1.4) (4.1–7.7)	1 year	−1.14 (0.65)	+1.44 (1.46) (sig.)	S 1.44 kg (sig.)	S −1.03 (1.52)	S +1.29 (2.01)(NS)
Rettammel (1995)	C	20 (15 <18 years 5 >18 years)	—	5 years–27 years	3 months	Children −1.00 (0.71) ($n7$); 92.4% of reference wt/ht ($n8$) Adults 72.1% reference wt/ht	NS change (children – no data)	<18 years (sig.) >18 years (NS) wt velocity (NS) (no data given) NS change in TSF or MAMC	S −0.83 (0.89)	NS change (no data)
Shepherd et al. (1983)[b]	B	7	—	5.2 years–13.2 years	6 months	S −1.23 (0.37)	+0.52 (0.67) (sig.)	+3.5 (2.5) kg Sig. increase in fat and muscle mass	S −0.91 (0.74)	S +0.23 (0.52) (sig.)
Skypala et al. (1998)	C	26 (11 <16 years)	—	18.5 years (9–34)	2 months	Children −0.75 (−1.41 to 0.31) <16 years 90.7% wt-for-ht Adults BMI 17.5 kg m^{-2}	Children +0.22 (sig.) <16 years +4.1% (sig.) Adults +0.4 kg m^{-2} (sig.)	+1.9 kg (sig.) Sig. increase in MAMC	Children 98% ht-for-age	Children – no change
Yassa et al. (1978)	B	28	15	8.0 years (3.2–16.0)	1 year	S −0.92 (0.15 SEM) US −0.82 (0.12)	S +0.32 (0.08 SEM) (sig.) US +0.01 (0.1) (NS)	—	S −1.01 (0.19) US −1.13 (0.27)	S +0.21 (0.06 SEM) (sig.) US −0.08 (0.08) (NS)

[a]Statistical calculations performed on raw data provided in the paper.

[b]Some patients took the supplement by tube (not separated from those taking the supplement orally); unsupplemented group: healthy controls not followed up over time. Figures in italics were calculated from the raw data and found to differ from those in the paper.

A, abstract; LBM, lean body mass; MAMC, mid-arm muscle circumference; NS, not significant; RDA, recommended daily allowance; S, supplemented; SEM, standard error (of estimate of mean value); sig., significant; TSF, triceps skin-fold; US, unsupplemented.

Table A4.15. Effect of oral nutritional supplements on total energy intake, functional and clinical outcome measures in cystic fibrosis patients.

Trial	Increase in total energy intake with ONS	Changes in functional and clinical outcomes
Randomized controlled trials		
Kalnins et al. (1996)	NS change in energy intake in S or US groups	No changes in respiratory function
Sondel et al. (1987)	Sig. increase in TEI from 2300 kcal to 2850 kcal (S vs. US sig.)	–
Steinkamp et al. (2000)	VFI did not change in S group and TEI was sig. increased (from 2105 kcal to 2733 kcal) (S vs. US ?) (~ 94% ONS energy additive (i))	No changes in respiratory function Improvement in essential fatty acid status
Non-randomized trials		
Allan et al. (1973)	–	Improved general activity, growth and nutrition, pulmonary and physical health (?)
Barclay et al. (1975)	–	Improved general well-being and activity (parental reports) (?)
Berry et al. (1975)	–	Improved clinical score (general activity, growth and nutrition) and bone age (sig.) Parents observe fewer abdominal cramps, improved sleeping pattern, greater energy and activity, improved school attendance, increased nail and hair growth
Hayes et al. (1995)	–	Lower occurrence of abdominal pain, rectal prolapse and stool frequency (sig.)
Kashirskaja et al. (1996)	–	Reduction in number of hospital admissions (sig.). Subjective parents' assessments of improved health and respiratory status, happier children, milder and less frequent exacerbations with more prompt response to treatment (also a concurrent increase in the use of antibiotics!)
Parsons et al. (1983)	Sig. increase in TEI with ONS. 'Supplements did not displace food intake significantly'	Reduced faecal energy loss
Rettammel et al. (1995)	TEI not significantly increased but sig. increases in intakes of vit. A, E, D, zinc and iron	–
Shepherd et al. (1983)[a]	Yes (?)	Improved clinical score (total, pulmonary, general scores) (sig.)
Skypala et al. (1998)	Sig. increase in TEI from 2665 kcal at baseline to 3208 kcal	–
Yassa et al. (1978)	–	Increased bone age (sig.)

[a]Some patients took the supplement by tube (not separated from those taking the supplement orally).

?, uncertain if statistically significant; NS, not significant; S, supplemented; sig., significant; TEI, total energy intake; US, unsupplemented; VFI, voluntary food intake.

al.'s (1978) study suggested that large amounts of an unpalatable dietary supplement (100% recommended daily intake (RDI) for energy) suppressed appetite (see Table A4.13). However, in three studies, the extent to which the ONS energy added or replaced the energy from food could be estimated (methods (i) and (iii), see Chapter 5). All of these (Parsons *et al.*, 1983; Sondel *et al.*, 1987; Steinkamp *et al.*, 2000) suggested that ≥ 80% of supplement energy was additive to dietary energy intake when compared with baseline, but it was not possible to assess whether the effect changed with time.

Assessments of compliance with ONS intake and calculations of food intake were mostly made from patient's own records, typically over short periods of time (24 h to 3 days) at intervals during the studies. Therefore there is some uncertainty about the accuracy of these results. It was also not possible to assess changes in the intake of supplement or food over time in the reviewed studies.

(IA) IS THE TIMING OF SUPPLEMENTATION IMPORTANT?
There was insufficient information about the effect of the timing of ONS on energy intake, appetite and associated functional changes. Four studies 'recommended' the timing of supplement consumption as follows: small sips at frequent intervals during the day (Berry *et al.*, 1975; Yassa *et al.*, 1978); during the afternoon/evening (Sondel *et al.*, 1987); and during the night (Hayes *et al.*, 1995), but no comparisons were made between the different schedules.

(II) What effect do ONS have on the body weight and composition of patients with cystic fibrosis in the community?

Information predominantly from NRT suggests that ONS may improve body weight and increase growth in growth-retarded children (see Table A4.14). Although RCT in large groups of patients are desirable, they may be difficult to achieve, both practically and ethically, in paediatric populations.

Of the three RCT reviewed, two indicated that small, non-significant increases

in weight-for-height followed 3 months of ONS in growth-retarded children and adolescents/young adults (Kalnins *et al.*, 1996; Steinkamp *et al.*, 2000). The other study showed no significant change in body weight, height or skin-fold thickness in children with cystic fibrosis (Sondel *et al.*, 1987). Seven of eight NRT in growth-retarded children showed significant improvements in growth, with increases in *z* scores for weight (Allan *et al.*, 1973; Berry *et al.*, 1975; Yassa *et al.*, 1978; Parsons *et al.*, 1983; Shepherd *et al.*, 1983; Skypala *et al.*, 1998) or improved weight/height-for-age (Kashirskaja *et al.*, 1996) (see Table A4.14). The other study (Rettamel *et al.*, 1995) demonstrated significant weight gain in children, but no improvement in the *z* score. Of the studies that assessed height (*n* 7) (Allan *et al.*, 1973; Berry *et al.*, 1975; Yassa *et al.*, 1978; Parsons *et al.*, 1983; Shepherd *et al.*, 1983; Rettamel *et al.*, 1995; Skypala *et al.*, 1998), only two showed a significant improvement (Yassa *et al.*, 1978; Shepherd *et al.*, 1983).

Two trials that assessed body fat and/or muscle mass (Shepherd *et al.*, 1983; Steinkamp *et al.*, 2000) indicated significant improvements following supplementation. Another four trials measured arm anthropometry (MAMC (Skypala *et al.*, 1998; Retammel *et al.*, 1995; Yassa *et al.*, 1978) and skin-fold thickness (Sondel *et al.*, 1987; Retammel *et al.*, 1995; Yassa *et al.*, 1978)), but only one demonstrated a significant increase (Skypala *et al.*, 1998) (see Table A4.14).

Of the two studies primarily undertaken in adults (Rettamel *et al.*, 1995; Skypala *et al.*, 1998), one showed a significant gain in weight (Skypala *et al.*, 1998) and the other no change (Rettamel *et al.*, 1995), despite being undertaken in patients at risk of malnutrition (< 72% weight-for-height).

(III)/(IV) What effect do ONS have on the body function and clinical outcome of patients with cystic fibrosis in the community?

A variety of functional changes may occur following ONS, although the evidence for such benefits is mostly from

NRT and often anecdotal. Of the three randomized trials reviewed (Sondel *et al.*, 1987; Kalnins *et al.*, 1996; Steinkamp *et al.*, 2000), one made no assessments of functional measures (Sondel *et al.*, 1987) and the other two found no significant changes in respiratory function (Kalnins *et al.*, 1996; Steinkamp *et al.*, 2000) (see Table A4.15). Improvements in essential fatty acid status in supplemented children and adults with cystic fibrosis were observed (Steinkamp *et al.*, 2000). Many of the non-randomized studies reported a variety of significant improvements in body functions or in clinical outcome (Berry *et al.*, 1975; Yassa *et al.*, 1978; Shepherd *et al.*, 1983; Kashirskaja *et al.*, 1996; Skypala *et al.*, 1998). These included clinical score (general activity and pulmonary scores), a reduction in the number of hospital admissions and a lower occurrence of GI complications. Other functional improvements were not statistically evaluated (Allan *et al.*, 1973). A variety of anecdotal benefits (Barclay and Shannon, 1975; Berry *et al.*, 1975; Parsons *et al.*, 1983; Kashirskaja *et al.*, 1996) were also documented and included improved sleeping patterns and mood, increased energy and activity, milder and less frequent disease exacerbations, less need for antibiotics and improved condition of hair and skin (see Table A4.15).

(V) What are the effects of stopping ONS in patients with cystic fibrosis in the community?

This was assessed in only one study, which reported that stopping ONS produced either loss of weight or a slower increase in height and weight (Yassa *et al.*, 1978). The advancement in bone age, documented during the supplementation period, continued after the supplements were stopped (Yassa *et al.*, 1978). However, this study did not include a control group for comparison. Three studies reported that patients chose to continue with ONS after the end of the study due to the benefits they experienced (Shepherd *et al.*, 1983; Kalnins *et al.*, 1996; Skypala *et al.*, 1998).

ONS, behavioural therapy or ETF?

Other therapies, both nutritional (e.g. ETF) and behavioural, have been used in cystic fibrosis patients, although their relative efficacy remains uncertain.

- The effects of ONS, described above, are in general agreement with the effects of ETF in patients with cystic fibrosis. Studies of home ETF in malnourished patients with cystic fibrosis have shown improvements in body weight (Bertrand *et al.*, 1984; Levy *et al.*, 1985; Boland *et al.*, 1986; Moore *et al.*, 1986; O'Loughlin *et al.*, 1986; Shepherd *et al.*, 1988; Steinkamp *et al.*, 1990; Smith, D.L. *et al.*, 1994; Steinkamp and von der Hardt, 1994), growth performance (Levy *et al.*, 1985; Moore *et al.*, 1986; O'Loughlin *et al.*, 1986; Steinkamp *et al.*, 1990) and muscle mass (Levy *et al.*, 1985; Boland *et al.*, 1986; O'Loughlin *et al.*, 1986; Shepherd *et al.*, 1986, 1988; Steinkamp *et al.*, 1990). Functional benefits have been demonstrated in most long-term tube feeding studies, and have included pulmonary function (Levy *et al.*, 1985; Shepherd *et al.*, 1988; Steinkamp *et al.*, 1990; Steinkamp and von der Hardt, 1994) (not improved in all studies (Boland *et al.*, 1986; O'Loughlin *et al.*, 1986; Smith, D.L. *et al.*, 1994)), a reduction in the number of pulmonary exacerbations (O'Loughlin *et al.*, 1986; Shepherd *et al.*, 1986) and increased well-being (O'Loughlin *et al.*, 1986). No functional benefits were found with short-term ETF (1 month) (Bertrand *et al.*, 1984). Another study (Dalzell *et al.*, 1992) (ONS and/or ETF for 1.35 years) found that, at long-term follow-up (up to 4 years after supplementation had stopped), there was no difference in the rate of deterioration of disease in supplemented and unsupplemented patients, although body weight and height *z* scores remained significantly greater and there was a trend towards lower mortality in those who had received nutritional intervention. No formal comparisons between ONS and ETF have been made (see Chapter 7 for more details).

- Studies have been conducted in children to assess the effect of behavioural therapy in increasing total energy intake (Stark et al., 1990, 1993). The behavioural approach has had similar benefits to ONS (body weight gain, etc. (Jelalian et al., 1998)). However, formal controlled trials comparing behavioural therapy with supplements, either alone or in combination with other nutritional interventions, are lacking.

In conclusion, the findings of this review and others (Smyth and Walters, 2002) are that there is clearly a need for well-designed, randomized trials, where ethically feasible, in patients (both adults and children) with cystic fibrosis, to ascertain the impact of using ONS in this patient group.

Elderly

The number of elderly people is continuing to rise and people are now living for longer than ever before. In the UK, approximately 16% of the population are aged over 65 years and this proportion is growing. The elderly are the single biggest users of the health service, mainly because they are more likely to develop ill health or disability. The elderly are also a group at high risk of malnutrition (see Chapter 2), due to the effects of age and disease plus socio-economic factors. Therefore nutritional support is often warranted in elderly individuals with disease living in nursing homes and other care homes and in those living at home. Although ONS are frequently used in such settings, how effective are they?

Elderly: present analysis

Ten RCT of ONS (~200–600 kcal for 4–24 weeks) in the elderly were reviewed (Box A4.4). These were undertaken in patients in nursing homes, in those recently discharged from hospital, in the free-living and in individuals with and without active

disease (Chandra and Puri, 1985; Meredith et al., 1992; Fiatarone et al., 1994; Woo et al., 1994; Gray-Donald et al., 1995; Volkert et al., 1996; Krondl et al., 1999; Fiatarone Singh et al., 2000; Lauque et al., 2000; Persson et al., 2000b). These trials are summarized in Tables A4.16–A4.18. Seven NRT in elderly patients receiving ONS at home, including those receiving meals on wheels and in nursing homes, were also reviewed and have been summarized in Tables A4.19–A4.21.

(l) What effect do ONS have on voluntary food intake and total energy intake in elderly patients in the community?

ONS significantly increase total energy intakes in the elderly, including free-living healthy individuals and those with disease. A greater proportion of ONS energy is additive to food intake in patients who are underweight (BMI < 20 kg m^{-2}) but suppression of food intake may increase if ONS are continued over long periods of time.

All of the RCT that assessed total energy intake (n 7: Meredith et al., 1992; Fiatarone et al., 1994; Woo et al., 1994; Gray-Donald et al., 1995; Krondl et al., 1999; Fiatarone Singh et al., 2000; Lauque et al., 2000) showed an increase with ONS and in four this was significant over time or compared with a control group (Meredith et al., 1992; Fiatarone et al., 1994; Woo et al., 1994; Lauque et al., 2000) (see Table A4.18). One of these trials involved simultaneous resistance exercise (Fiatarone et al., 1994) and in three of the trials the individuals were free-living with no signs of disease (Meredith et al., 1992; Gray-Donald et al., 1995; Krondl et al., 1999).

Of the five non-randomized studies that assessed energy intake (Lipschitz et al., 1985; Welch et al., 1991; Breslow et al., 1993; Gray-Donald et al., 1994; Yamaguchi et al., 1998), all showed an increase in total energy intake – significant in 80% (all but one (Lipschitz et al., 1985)) (see Table A4.21).

The one study that made formalized assessments of appetite during supplementation (Woo et al., 1994) observed a similar,

---

Box A4.4. Key findings: effect of ONS in elderly community patients.

Nutritional intake: ONS can increase total energy and nutrient intakes in healthy free-living elderly and in those with disease that are living at home or in institutions. There may be a reduction in voluntary food intake and total energy and nutrient intakes if ONS are used for long periods of time, especially in patients in nursing homes.

Timing of ONS: it is not possible to advise on the best time to provide ONS in elderly patients from the evidence currently available and it is possible that the recommendations may vary according to patients' age and clinical condition.

Body weight: ONS may improve body weight and muscle mass.

Body function: a variety of functional benefits follow intervention with ONS (increases in activities of daily living, immunological benefits, increases in vitality, reduced number of falls), some of which may occur after supplementation has stopped. Significant improvements in weight are typically observed when significant functional benefits are found.

Benefits according to BMI: improvements in energy intake, weight and function with ONS are more likely in patients who are underweight (BMI < 20 kg m^{-2}) and in those given resistance exercise with supplementation. In healthy individuals who are not underweight, total energy intake and body weight can be increased by ONS, the significance of which has not been assessed.

Clinical outcome: although clinical outcome has not been assessed in community elderly patients, in hospitalized elderly, ONS have been associated with reductions in mortality, length of hospital stay and reduced complication rates. Research in the community is required.

Other treatments: there are many other strategies that have been used to increase food intake in the elderly, including changing the energy and protein density of the diet, enhancing the smell or taste of foods and changing the environment for eating, particularly in institutions. The effect of these strategies compared with ONS is unknown and further investigation is needed.

---

significant improvement over time in both supplemented and unsupplemented patients. This suggests that appetite was not suppressed by ingestion of the supplement, which typically resulted in an increase in total energy intake. It was possible to assess the effect of supplementation on food intake in three trials of elderly patients with an IBW $< 90\%$ (BMI < 20 kg m^{-2}). One study found that habitual food intake was initially increased in the first 8 weeks of supplementation, and thereafter $> 90\%$ of the supplement energy remained additional to that taken from food (Lipschitz *et al.*, 1985). One trial suggested only ~40% of supplement energy was additive (Gray-Donald *et al.*, 1995), whereas Lauque *et al.* (2000) suggested that ~70% was additive. Trials in patients with a mean BMI > 20 kg m^{-2} suggested that a smaller proportion of the supplement energy (30–44%) was additive to food intake (Breslow *et al.*, 1993; Fiatarone *et al.*, 1994; Fiatarone Singh *et*

al., 2000) (see Chapter 5). However, the effect of ONS on voluntary food intake may vary over time. Indeed, in elderly nursing home residents, supplemented patients had significantly greater reductions in voluntary food intake (including a reduction in the intake of protein, vitamins and minerals from food) over the time span of the study (10 weeks) than unsupplemented patients, with the result that total energy intake, although higher in the supplemented patients, was not significantly so (Fiatarone Singh *et al.*, 2000). In another study in elderly nursing home residents (Lauque *et al.*, 2000), ONS consumption was less at weekends and after 50 days' duration. In addition, giving elderly patients some form of exercise (e.g. resistance exercises) while receiving an ONS may be beneficial. For example, when elderly nursing home residents were given resistance exercise during ONS (Fiatarone *et al.*, 1994), ~80% of ONS energy was additive to food intake.

Table A4.16. Oral nutritional supplements used in randomized controlled trials of the elderly in the community.

Trial	ONS	ONS energy density	ONS prescribed	ONS energy (kcal) intake	ONS protein (g) intake	Toleration
Chandra and Puri (1985)	–	–	–	–	–	–
Fiatarone et al. (1994)	Exceed (Abbott)	1.5 kcal ml^{-1}	360 kcal	S 353 S + EX 358	–	Diarrhoea (n 2)
Fiatarone Singh et al. (2000)	Exceed (Abbott) (energy: 60% CHO, 23% F, 17% P) or soft nutritional bar (n 4)	1.5 kcal ml^{-1}	360 kcal	267	–	High compliance
Gray-Donald et al. (1995)	Ensure Enrich Ensure Plus (all Abbott)	1 kcal ml^{-1} 1 kcal ml^{-1} 1.5 kcal ml^{-1}	500–700 kcal (2 cans)	329–494 (1.4 cans)	~12.2–22.1	36% of eligible sample refused to take a supplement
Krondl et al. (1999)	Boost (Mead Johnson)	1 kcal ml^{-1}	~201 kcal and 10 g P	202 kcal	~10.1	Well accepted and generally consumed in accordance with instructions, with all except 1 pt consuming the prescribed 5.5–6.5 cans per day Consistency, colour, sweetness rated highly
Lauque et al. (2000)	Clinutren products (Nestlé) Soup (200 kcal, 10 g P) Fruit drink (120 kcal, 7.5 g P) Dessert (150 kcal, 12 g P) 'HP' (200 kcal, 15 g P)	1 kcal ml^{-1} 0.6 kcal ml^{-1} 1 kcal ml^{-1} 1 kcal ml^{-1}	300–500 kcal	S^1 393 (23) S^2 430 (20)	– –	Compliance with ONS was good – 'convenient and well accepted' (slight reduction in consumption after day 50 and during weekends)
Meredith et al. (1992)	Two Cal HN (Abbott)	2 kcal ml^{-1}	480 kcal, ~20g P	–	–	–
Persson et al. (2000b) A	Semper	1 kcal ml^{-1}	200–600 kcal	Median 240 kcal (200–600)	–	–
Volkert et al. (1996)	Sweet formula	1.2 kcal ml^{-1}	–	–	–	–
Woo et al. (1994)	Ensure (Abbott)	1 kcal ml^{-1}	500 kcal	–	–	–

CHO, carbohydrate; EX, exercise; F, fat; P, protein; pt, patient.

Table A4.17. Trial characteristics: community-based randomized controlled trials of oral nutritional supplementation in the elderly.

Trial	Design	No. S	No. US	Initial BMI S group	Initial BMI US group	Duration of ONS	Dietary counselling	Control group
Chandra and Puri (1985) Free-living elderly with no signs of acute or chronic systemic disease	10001	15	15	–	–	4 weeks	'Nutritional advice' given as appropriate for each case	–
Fiatarone et al. (1994) Elderly (> 70 years) in residential care. Trial of resistance training and nutrition, part of FICSIT trial	10111	24 S / 25 EX + S	25 EX + placebo / 26 placebo	S 25.4 / S + EX 24.5	US + EX 24.9 / US 25.8	10 weeks	–	US given a placebo, flavoured liquid drink (4 kcal) and US + EX also given resistance training
Fiatarone Singh et al. (2000) Nursing home residents > 70 years, 52% cognitively impaired	10110	24	26	25.4 (0.7)	25.6 (0.5)	10 weeks	–	Placebo – non-nutritive drink (same volume as ONS)
Gray-Donald et al. (1995) Free-living elderly at risk of undernutrition	10001	24	24	19	19	12 weeks	Visited weekly when ONS were given	Visited weekly, some dietary advice given
Krondl et al. (1999) Healthy, free-living elderly, mean age 70 years (not requiring medical or dietetic treatment)	10001	35	36	25 (3)	24 (3)	16 weeks	–	Encouraged to continue with a regular eating pattern
Lauque et al. (2000) Elderly in nursing homes > 65 years	10001	S^1 13[a] / S^2 24	US^1 22 / US^2 19[a]	S^1 22.3 (0.7) / S^2 18.5 (0.5)	US^1 21.8 (0.9) / US^2 25.3 (0.8)	60 days	Pts strongly encouraged to consume ONS in addition to meals	–
Meredith et al. (1992) Sedentary male elderly (aged 61–72 years)	10000	6 (EX)	5 (EX)	24.8	25.4	12 weeks	–	–
Persson et al. (2000b) A Elderly on discharge from a hospital geriatric ward	10000	55 in total		19.4 (1.8)	20.9 (2.6)	4 months	Individualized counselling, stressing increase in fat intake	–
Volkert et al. (1996) Undernourished elderly followed from 1 month in hospital and up to 6 months post-discharge in the community	11001	20	26	19.8	19.3	1 month (H) 6 month (C)	–	–
Woo et al. (1994) Elderly (> 65 years) on discharge from an acute medical ward	11001	40	41	M 19.3 / F 20[b]	M 19.4 / F 19.9	1 month	–	Same follow-up as S

[a]Divided using the MNA tool into those not at risk of malnutrition (US^2), those at risk (S^1, US^1) (main comparison) and those who are malnourished (S^2).
[b]Results for male (M) and female (F).
A, abstract; C, community; EX, exercise in form of resistance training; H, hospital; MNA, Mini Nutritional Assessment; S, supplemented; US, unsupplemented.

Table A4.18. Main findings of randomized controlled trials of oral nutritional supplementation in the elderly in the community.

Trial	Energy intake	Body weight S	Body weight US	Body function	Clinical outcome	Finance
Chandra and Puri (1985)	–	+5.2 kg (sig.)	– (NS)	Higher rate of seroconversion and a higher mean antibody titre (sig.) following influenza virus vaccination in S	–	–
Fiatarone *et al.* (1994)	TEI sig. increased in S + EX only (primary effect of exercise). NS increase in S (S vs. US ?)	S +0.8 kg (sig.) EX + S +1.0 kg (sig.)	EX + placebo +0.2 kg (NS) Placebo –0.5 kg (NS)	NS change in mobility with ONS. Exercise led to sig. improvements in gait velocity, stair-climbing ability and overall physical activity	–	–
Fiatarone Singh *et al.* (2000)	Sig. decrease in VFI in S and US over time, sig. greater in S (–219 kcal) than US (–70 kcal), with TEI only 49 kcal greater in S group (TEI S vs. US NS) (~44% of ONS additive (i))	+1.44 (0.86)% (S vs. US sig.)	–1.37 (0.82)%	Sig. increase in Katz index of ADL in S and US (greater levels of dependency in basic activities such as toileting, eating, transfers, dressing, hygiene, bathing, S vs. US NS) NS changes in habitual physical activity, depressive symptoms, cognitive function, muscle strength or gait velocity or protein status In a subset of n 13, ONS had no effect on muscle fibre area or presence of intramuscular growth factor and indices of regeneration (IGF-1 and development of myosin isoforms)	NS change in no. of medications per day	–
Gray-Donald *et al.* (1995)	Increase in TEI NS (S vs. US NS). S intakes reported to be +214 kcal greater than US	+2.1 kg (?) (S vs. US sig.)	+0.6 kg (?)	Fewer falls (0%) in S group than US group (21%) (S vs. US sig.)	–	–
Krondl *et al.* (1999)	Sig. increase in TPI, Ca, Mg, K, phosphorus, Cu, vit. B_1, B_6 and folate in S (S vs. US NS). TEI increased by only 54 kcal in S	–	–	NS changes in SF-36 (quality-of-life index), except for sig. increase in vitality and general health perception in S (S vs. US ?) NS changes in general well-being questionnaire categories except for a sig. increase in general well-being in S (S vs. US ?) Sig. increase in Hb in ONS (women) and NS changes in zinc status in S or US	–	–

Continued

Table A4.18. Continued.

Trial	Energy intake	Body weight S	Body weight US	Body function	Clinical outcome	Finance
Lauque et al. (2000)	S[1] VFI reduced by −136 kcal but greater TEI than US[1] (1815 kcal vs. 1562 kcal; +257 kcal) S[2] VFI decreased by 42 kcal but sig. greater TEI than US groups (1877 vs. 1562 kcal (US[1]) or 1632 kcal (US[2])) Both S groups sig. increased TEI and TPI vs. US group (~71% of ONS additive (i))	S[1] +1.41 (0.5) kg (2.6 (0.92)%) S[2] (malnourished) +1.5 (0.4) kg	US[1] −1.3kg (−2.48%) US[2] (not malnourished) −0.5 kg	NS changes in grip strength	−	−
Meredith et al. (1992)	Sig. increase in TEI with S	+2.2 kg (sig.) (S vs. US sig.)	−1.6 kg	−	−	−
Persson et al. (2000b) A –	A –	+1.3 (3.7) kg (NS) (S vs. US sig.)	−2.7 (4.1) kg	Sig. improvement in ADL in S but not US (S vs. US NS) NS changes in total cholesterol or triglyceride after dietary counselling and ONS	−	−
Volkert et al. (1996)	–[a]	~+3.2 kg (sig.)	+2.9 kg (sig.)	More independent patients (ADL) in S group with good compliance than US (sig.)	−	−
Woo et al. (1994)	After 1 month of ONS, S group sig. higher intakes of E (1809 vs. 1452 kcal), P (61 g vs. 48 g), Ca, Fe, K, vit. B_1, B_2, niacin, C and A than US	+0.7 kg m^{-2} (sig.)[b] (S vs. US ?)	+0.23 kg m^{-2} (NS)	Greater ADL score 2 months after supplementation in S vs. US (S vs. US sig.) Mental test score improved after 1 month and life satisfaction after 2 months in S and US groups (S vs. US NS)	−	−

[a]No data for community setting (hospital only).
[b]Refers to data after 1 month of supplementation.
A, abstract; ADL, activities of daily living; E, energy; EX, exercise in the form of resistance training; Hb, haemoglobin; IGF-1, insulin-like growth factor 1; NS, not significant; P, protein; S, supplemented; sig., significant; TEI, total energy intake; TPI, total protein intake; US, unsupplemented; VFI, voluntary food intake.

Table A4.19. Oral nutritional supplements used in non-randomized trials of elderly patients in the community.

Trial	ONS	ONS energy density	ONS prescribed	ONS energy (kcal) intake	ONS protein (g) intake	Toleration
Breslow *et al.* (1993)	Sustacal (Mead Johnson) or Ensure (Abbott)	1 kcal ml⁻¹ 1 kcal ml⁻¹	720 kcal 720 kcal	770 601	29 37	Taste of Sustacal preferred. No diarrhoea
Bunker *et al.* (1994)	Protein Forte (Fresenius) (plus calogen (SHS) for those with BMI < 20 kg m⁻²)	1 kcal ml⁻¹	200 (+ 100) kcal	–	–	–
Cederholm and Hellstrom (1995)	Fortimel (Nutricia)	1 kcal ml⁻¹	400 kcal	–	–	–
Gray-Donald *et al.* (1994)	Ensure or Enrich (Abbott)	1 kcal ml⁻¹ 1 kcal ml⁻¹	~500 kcal	–	–	–
Lipschitz *et al.* (1985)	Ensure Plus (Abbott)	1.5 kcal ml⁻¹	1080 kcal	658–815	~27–34	–
Welch *et al.* (1991)	Enriched cereal, punch, milkshake, soup or pudding (Forta supplements)	–	–	–	–	Increase in total no. of stools in all patients
Yamaguchi *et al.* (1998)	– (40 g CHO, 15 g P, 9 g F per 237 ml)	1.27 kcal ml⁻¹	600 kcal, 30 g P	At 6 and 12 months 605 kcal At 18 months 443 kcal	–	The authors thought that taste fatigue may have been responsible for the declining consumption of ONS

CHO, carbohydrate; F, fat; P, protein.

Table A4.20. Trial characteristics: community-based non-randomized trials of oral nutritional supplementation in elderly community patients.

Trial	Design	No. S	No. US	Initial BMI S group	Initial BMI US group	Duration of ONS	Dietary counselling	Control group
Breslow *et al.* (1993) Elderly nursing home residents with pressure ulcers	B	8	5	20	22	8 weeks	Given standard nursing home diet	–
Bunker *et al.* (1994) Housebound elderly subjects (aged 70–85 years) with no known disease	B	27	31	–	–	12 weeks	Subjects told to consume ONS in addition to, not instead of, normal food	Given a capsule containing starch
Cederholm and Hellström (1995) Malnourished elderly out-patients with non-malignant disease (~74 years)	B	15	8	16.5	17.9	3 months	–	–
Gray-Donald *et al.* (1994) Undernourished elderly receiving home-care service (> 60 years)	C	14	–	16.6 (*n* 8) 22.9 (*n* 6)	–	12 weeks	Pts recommended to consume sufficient energy to lead to wt gain of 0.5 kg week^{-1}	–
Lipschitz *et al.* (1985) Elderly receiving meals on wheels at risk of undernutrition	C	12	–	80.7% IBW	–	16 weeks	–	–
Welch *et al.* (1991) Elderly nursing home residents (mean age 81 years) on a puréed diet	C	15	–	~17.3	–	6 months	No – but pts on puréed diets	–
Yamaguchi *et al.* (1998) Elderly receiving meals on wheels and at risk of malnutrition	B	32	30	24 (5) (range 17–30)	24 (3) (range 16–40)	18 months	–	Placebo ONS (105 kcal, no protein, 15 mg calcium)

pts, patients; S, supplemented; US, unsupplemented.

Table A4.21. Main findings of non-randomized trials of oral nutritional supplementation in elderly community patients.

Trial	Energy intake	Body weight S	Body weight US	Body function	Clinical outcome	Finance
Breslow et al. (1993)	TEI increased (NS)	–	–	Decrease in truncal pressure ulcer surface area and in particular stage IV ulcers (sig.)	–	–
Bunker et al. (1994)	–	–	–	NS change in DCH or lymphocyte populations (within normal ranges before ONS)	–	–
Cederholm and Hellström (1995)	–	2.5 kg (sig.) (S vs. US sig.) Sig. increase in TSF (sig. vs. US) and MAMC (NS vs. US)	1.6 kg (NS)	Sig. increase in hand-grip strength and DCH in S only (S vs. US NS)	–	–
Gray-Donald et al. (1994)	TEI sig. increased by 390 (500) kcal and TPI sig. increased by 20 (20) g	+1.82 kg (sig.)	–	Sig. improvement in general well-being and total lymphocyte count NS change in hand-grip strength	–	–
Lipschitz et al. (1985)	Substantial increase in TEI with ONS from 1290 kcal at baseline to 2283 kcal at 4 weeks	2.6 kg (?)	–	No improvement in total lymphocyte or T-lymphocyte counts Improvement in vitamin status (serum folate, vit. B_{12} and leucocyte ascorbate)	–	–
Welch et al. (1991)	Sig. increase in TEI from 88% of RDA to 123% and 130% at 3 months and 6 months. Sig. increase in TPI and intakes of A, D, E, C, B vitamins, Ca, phosphorus, Fe, Mg, Zn	2.1 kg (sig.)	–	–	–	–
Yamaguchi et al. (1998)	Sig. increase in energy and all nutrients (except fat and vit. A) vs. baseline at 6 and 12 months. Similar changes not seen in US, except sig. increase in zinc intake. At 18 months in S, intake of energy, folate, Fe, Mg and Zn sig. higher than baseline (S vs. US ?)	2.88 kg (–6.3 to +12.9 kg)	–3.2 kg (–8.15 to +1.85 kg)	–	–	–

DCH, delayed cutaneous hypersensitivity; RDA, recommended daily allowance; S, supplemented; TEI, total energy intake; TPI, total protein intake; US, unsupplemented.

There is some uncertainty about the extent of dietary compliance (food and supplement), partly because the assessments were made from patients' own records or from memory (which could be unreliable in elderly patients) and partly because they were carried out over short periods of time. However, some studies made an extra effort to count all the supplement cartons that were supplied and used (Gray-Donald et al., 1995; Volkert et al., 1996) and weighed food intake methods to assess dietary intake (Breslow et al., 1993; Fiatarone et al., 1994) were undertaken. In contrast, the methods used to assess supplement and food intake were not reported in some studies (Lipschitz et al., 1985; Cederholm and Hellström, 1995).

(IA) IS THE TIMING OF SUPPLEMENTATION IMPORTANT?
As many conflicting recommendations are made about the best time to give ONS to the elderly and comparisons of these timings have not been made, it is not possible to conclude which time is the most effective.

The timing of supplement consumption was detailed in many of the studies (Lipschitz et al., 1985; Welch et al., 1991; Meredith et al., 1992; Breslow et al., 1993; Fiatarone et al., 1994; Woo et al., 1994; Cederholm and Hellström, 1995; Volkert et al., 1996; Krondl et al., 1999; Fiatarone Singh et al., 2000). Mostly patients were instructed to take them between meals or in the early or late part of the evening. However, in one study patients were asked to take the supplement with their main meals (Breslow et al., 1993). However, no firm conclusions were reached about the importance of the timing of ONS consumption because of the lack of controlled data, with inadequate evaluation of compliance with the times of supplement intake.

(II) What effect do ONS have on the body weight and composition of elderly patients in the community?

ONS can improve body weight in elderly patients living at home or in nursing or residential homes and in those who do or do not have active disease.

All nine RCT that assessed body weight showed weight gain following ONS, which was statistically significant when compared with either baseline (Chandra and Puri, 1985; Fiatarone et al., 1994; Woo et al., 1994; Volkert et al., 1996) or a control group (Meredith et al., 1992; Gray-Donald et al., 1995; Fiatarone Singh et al., 2000; Persson et al., 2000b) in all but one trial (Lauque et al., 2000) (see Table A4.18). On average, % weight gain in supplemented patients was 2.33% more than for unsupplemented patients (weighted analysis of eight RCT (n 366); $P < 0.05$; independent t test). In one of these trials it was not possible to differentiate between the effect of the supplement and the resistance training that was given simultaneously (Fiatarone et al., 1994). Average % weight change (weighted mean) for supplemented patients with a BMI < 20 kg m^{-2} was 5% (three trials: Woo et al., 1994; Gray-Donald et al., 1995; Volkert et al., 1996), compared with 1.8% for those with a BMI > 20 kg m^{-2} (four trials: Meredith et al., 1992; Fiatarone et al., 1994; Fiatarone Singh et al., 2000; Lauque et al., 2000). Incidentally, similar weight gain was recorded in men receiving supplementation whether they initially had a low BMI (< 20 kg m^{-2}) (Fiatarone et al., 1994) or were well nourished (mean BMI 25 kg m^{-2}) (Meredith et al., 1992). However, the greatest % weight change in the group who were not underweight consisted of healthy subjects (BMI 25 kg m^{-2}) (Meredith et al., 1992).

Of the seven NRT that were carried out in the elderly, all of those that assessed changes in weight showed an increase (n 5) (Yassa et al., 1978; Lipschitz et al., 1985; Welch et al., 1991; Gray-Donald et al., 1994; Cederholm and Hellström, 1995), with significant changes versus baseline (Welch et al., 1991; Gray-Donald et al., 1994) or compared with a control group (Cederholm and Hellström, 1995) in some trials. Patients in these studies tended to have an initial BMI < 20 kg m^{-2} (see Table A4.21).

The documented weight gain during the study was frequently far smaller than might be expected from the reported increase in total energy intake with supplementation (for example, Lipschitz *et al.*, 1985). It is unclear whether this represents problems with compliance with supplement intake and dietary records, changes in energy expenditure or the presence of oedema.

Of the six studies (randomized and non-randomized) that made assessments of body composition using arm anthropometry, three suggested significant increases in fat mass (Chandra and Puri, 1985; Woo *et al.*, 1994; Cederholm and Hellström, 1995) and one a significant increase in muscle mass (Cederholm and Hellström, 1995).

(III)/(IV) What effect do ONS have on the body function and clinical outcome of elderly patients in the community?

A variety of functional benefits follow the use of ONS in elderly community patients, including a reduction in falls, increases in activities of daily living and immunological benefits.

Of the nine randomized, controlled studies in the elderly that assessed changes in functional outcomes, 78% (*n* 7) indicated significant benefits to function, either with time or versus a control group (Chandra and Puri, 1985; Woo *et al.*, 1994; Gray-Donald *et al.*, 1995; Volkert *et al.*, 1996; Krondl *et al.*, 1999; Fiatarone Singh *et al.*, 2000; Persson *et al.*, 2000b) (see Table A4.18). These included fewer falls (Gray-Donald *et al.*, 1995), more independence with activities of daily living (Volkert *et al.*, 1996; Fiatarone Singh *et al.*, 2000; Persson *et al.*, 2000b), immunological benefits (Chandra and Puri, 1985) and improvements in vitality and general health perception (Krondl *et al.*, 1999). One study even showed benefits only after ONS had stopped (Woo *et al.*, 1994) (see below). A couple of RCT failed to demonstrate improvements in muscle strength (Lauque *et al.*, 2000) or mobility (Fiatarone *et al.*, 1994) with ONS alone.

In all RCT showing significant functional benefits, weight was also significantly improved (either versus control or over time). Significant functional benefits were only observed when weight gain was > 2 kg (see Fig. 6.20 in Chapter 6).

Three out of five of the less controlled trials that made assessments of functional outcome measures showed benefits (see Table A4.21). These were improvements in pressure ulcers (Breslow *et al.*, 1993), hand-grip strength (Cederholm and Hellstrom, 1995) and general well-being (Gray-Donald *et al.*, 1994), but the interpretation of these findings was limited by the lack of control groups.

Anecdotal findings suggested that patients who were non-compliant with ONS may have had a poorer outcome (Volkert *et al.*, 1996) than those who were unsupplemented.

None of the studies assessed clinical outcome.

(V) What are the effects of stopping ONS in elderly patients in the community?

There may be improvements in body function even after ONS have stopped although this was assessed in only one study (patients' BMI < 20 kg m^{-2}) (Woo *et al.*, 1994). This trial suggested better functional measurements (activities of daily living, sleeping) in the supplemented patients 2 months after ONS had stopped than in the unsupplemented patients. Overall, there was a lack of controlled studies assessing the effects of stopping supplements on the various parameters.

Summary of non-randomized community trials in the elderly

Seven NRT carried out in elderly people were reviewed (Lipschitz *et al.*, 1985; Welch *et al.*, 1991; Breslow *et al.*, 1993; Bunker *et al.*, 1994; Gray-Donald *et al.*, 1994; Cederholm and Hellström, 1995; Yamaguchi *et al.*, 1998), two of which were undertaken in nursing homes (Welch *et al.*, 1991; Breslow *et al.*, 1993) and two in those receiving meals on wheels (Lipschitz *et al.*, 1985; Yamaguchi *et al.*, 1998) (see Tables A4.19–A4.21). Welch *et al.* (1991) observed significant increases in total energy intake and body weight in 15 undernourished elderly nursing home residents given a variety of commercial fortified food products, in addition to a puréed diet over a 6-month period. Similarly, free-living, undernourished, chronically ill elderly patients gained significantly more weight during 3 months of supplementation with a liquid sip feed than non-randomly allocated control patients (Cederholm and Hellström, 1995). No functional assessments were made in these studies. In contrast, Breslow *et al.* (1993) documented decreases in truncal pressure ulcer surface area, particularly stage IV ulcers, in eight elderly patients in a long-term care facility following 8 weeks of supplementation, although some took the formula by tube and the attrition rate had been high. Unusually, those patients who consumed the supplement orally took it with meals. Total energy intake, assessed using a weighed-food inventory, was increased (not significantly). However, our calculations suggested that, compared with baseline, only 30% of the energy consumed as a supplement was additional to food intake. Bunker *et al.* (1994) was unable to find any improvement in immune function (delayed cutaneous hypersensitivity and lymphocyte counts) after 3 months of supplementation (200 kcal) in housebound subjects (no disease), in a non-randomized study. The mean initial BMI of these patients was within the ideal range (mean BMI 22.4–25.2 kg m^{-2}), and the authors concluded that the lack of a significant change could have been because immune function was not sufficiently impaired in these individuals before supplementation began. Other studies included a 16-week trial of ONS in 12 underweight elderly patients receiving meals on wheels (Lipschitz *et al.*, 1985). Subjects who were instructed to take the ONS mid-morning, mid-afternoon and late evening increased their total energy and protein consumption by approximately 50% (1290 kcal, 56 g protein at baseline, 2283 kcal, 86 g protein at 4 weeks), although whether this was significant was not clear. Recorded intake of the supplement at 4 and 8 weeks was 75% of the prescribed amount, but this reduced to 61% by the 16th week. Associated with ONS was a > 10% increase in food energy

intake for the first 8 weeks of the study (i.e. no replacement) and, even by the 16th week, 93% of the supplement energy was additive to food intake if compared with baseline levels of intake. Unfortunately, in this study, the method of dietary assessment and the frequency with which it was carried out were not clarified. Despite the reported extra energy intake over 16 weeks, the calculated average weight gain was only 2.6 kg. Our own statistical calculations from the raw data suggested that the increase in weight was significant from 4 weeks onwards. Significant improvements were seen in biochemical indices, including indices of vitamin status. No improvements in immunological status were observed, and no other functional outcome measures were assessed. A similar trial in elderly people receiving meals on wheels indicated that ONS for an 18-month period increased intakes of energy and some micronutrients (folate, iron, magnesium, zinc) over this time period, accompanied by weight gain (versus weight loss in those given a placebo). Another study (Gray-Donald *et al.*, 1994), in home-bound elderly (*n* 14) who were underweight or losing weight, found significant increases in total energy and protein intake and in body weight after 12 weeks of dietary supplementation (intake assessed with 24 h dietary recalls). Functionally there was a significant improvement in psychological well-being, assessed subjectively using a 'general well-being schedule'.

Few general conclusions could be drawn from these non-randomized studies, due to inadequacies in their experimental design (lack of randomization, lack of appropriate placebo and blinding, small sample sizes). The effects of ONS on pressure ulcers and other functional outcome measures (e.g. QOL) have not been adequately evaluated and therefore require further study.

Increasingly, ONS are being developed for use in patients (adults and elderly) with specific diseases (e.g. diabetes mellitus, respiratory disease). For example, low-carbohydrate, fibre-containing ONS for diabetic patients have been found to be well tolerated in elderly patients with type II diabetes and to produce less hyperglycaemia than standard ONS (Galkowski *et al.*, 1989). The benefits of using such disease-specific supplements in elderly individuals remain to be elucidated using RCT.

ONS dietary intervention or ETF?

A huge variety of strategies to increase food intake have been investigated in the elderly, including changes to the energy and protein density of foods, enhancement of the smell or taste of food and changes to the environment, particularly for those in institutions.

- Many strategies for increasing food intake orally in these patients have been investigated (for a review, see Marcus and Berry, 1998).
- Controlled studies of food-composition manipulation/dietary counselling in elderly patients are few and have typically been carried out in hospital or nursing home settings (e.g. Winograd and Brown, 1990; Barton *et al.*, 2000b), maybe because this approach is only feasible in such institutionalized settings. Very few studies have undertaken formal comparisons between this approach and the use of ONS, particularly in the community (see Chapter 6).
- There appear to be few studies of the efficacy of ETF in this patient group carried out in the community setting. In the hospital setting, preliminary data suggested that ETF improved the outcome for elderly women following surgery for fractured neck of femur (Bastow *et al.*, 1983) (for more information, see Chapter 7). A controlled comparison of ETF with ONS in the community is lacking.

Elderly: other reviews

Similar to our findings, a review of different nutritional interventions in elderly individuals concluded that nutritional treatment in this patient group could yield positive

effects on body composition and, in some cases, on muscle strength, well-being and immune function (Akner and Cederholm, 2001). In addition, a meta-analysis of the effects of ONS in elderly patients with a range of diseases and across settings has also indicated the benefits of using this form of treatment (Milne *et al.*, 2001). This meta-analysis suggested that there were significantly lower rates of mortality in those given ONS (odds ratio 0.61 (95% CI 0.45–0.83)). In particular, the benefits were reported to be greater in patients who were described as 'undernourished', over 75 years and offered > 400 kcal day^{-1} for periods > 35 days. This review also pointed out the inadequacies in study design of many of the trials undertaken of supplementation in the elderly (Milne *et al.*, 2001).

Human Immunodeficiency Virus/Acquired Immune Deficiency Syndrome (HIV/AIDS)

Infection with HIV leading to AIDS results in severe immunosuppression. Consequently, a number of AIDS-related infections and cancers can lead to many nutritional problems. These include anorexia, difficulties in eating and persistent unintentional weight loss, often associated with GI symptoms (diarrhoea, vomiting, nausea) and malabsorption. Therefore, the greatest need for nutritional intervention to improve intake is likely to be in individuals with symptomatic HIV disease/AIDS. However, the trials below assessing the effectiveness of intervening with ONS have been undertaken in both symptomatic and asymptomatic patients with HIV. A number of organizations have recommended the use of ONS, as the quotes below suggest, but how effective are they?

> When nutrient intake is suboptimal, or significant weight loss is recorded, a more aggressive approach is necessary. In this instance, provide calorically dense, enteral formulas to supplement or replace the regular oral diet.
>
> (Task Force on Nutrition Support in AIDS, 1989)

Supplemental nutrition therapy is recommended for those symptomatic people who have had an unintentional 10% decrease in reference weight. Regimens used involve high protein and high calorie diets incorporating nutritious fluid supplements.

> AIDS Interest Group of the British Dietetic Association (Peck and Johnson, 1990)

Intensive counselling and the selective use of oral nutritional supplements can be an effective intervention.

> Position of the American and the Canadian Dietetic Association (Anon., 1994)

HIV/AIDS: present analysis

Three trials incorporated a randomized controlled or crossover design comparing ONS with no nutritional support (see Tables A4.22–A4.24) and 16 did not (see Tables A4.25–A4.27). The majority of ONS trials reviewed in HIV/AIDS patients in the community involved use of modified/enriched formulas, containing any of the following: arginine, RNA, omega-3 fatty acids or fibre (Gaare *et al.*, 1991; Chlebowski *et al.*, 1992, 1993; Singer *et al.*, 1992; Süttmann *et al.*, 1996; Pichard *et al.*, 1998); medium-chain triglyceride (MCT)-enriched formulas (Wandall *et al.*, 1992; Chan *et al.*, 1994; Rabeneck *et al.*, 1998); or peptide formulas (Hellerstein *et al.*, 1994; Richards *et al.*, 1996). Key findings from these trials are summarized in Box A4.5.

(l) What effect do ONS have on voluntary food intake and total energy intake in patients with HIV/AIDS in the community?

Using a range of different ONS (different forms and flavours) is an effective way of increasing total energy intake in HIV and AIDS patients. The use of one type of ONS over a couple of months can lead to reductions in food intake and compensation for ONS intake in these patients, particularly in those who are not underweight. ONS use can increase micronutrient intakes.

Two-thirds of the studies that measured total energy intake documented increases (Gibert *et al.*, 1999; Berneis *et al.*, 2000) (see Table A4.24). In the smaller one of these trials (*n* 15), the increase was small and not significant (Berneis *et al.*, 2000) (see Table A4.24). In contrast, in the larger trial (*n* > 300), total energy intake was significantly increased and voluntary food intake was comparable between supplemented and unsupplemented groups (Gibert *et al.*, 1999). In this study a range of ONS were given (NuBasics range, Nestlé) and investigators found that most of the ONS energy came from ONS drinks (69%) and less from bars (20%), soups (9%) and coffee (2%).

Changes in total energy and nutrient intake were assessed over time in six of the trials containing non-randomized data (see Table A4.27). Increases in total energy intake were reported in five trials (Chlebowski *et al.*, 1993; Richards *et al.*, 1996; Süttmann *et*

Box A4.5. Key findings: use of ONS in community patients with HIV/AIDS.

Nutritional intake: a variety of different types of ONS may be more effective at increasing total energy intakes in HIV/AIDS patients than the use of one type for prolonged periods of time. ONS can also increase micronutrient intakes.

Body function: few functional benefits have been found with the use of ONS in this patient group. The lack of benefits may be due to initially adequate nutritional status in patients with asymptomatic disease (most groups of patients studied not underweight, BMI > 20 kg m^{-2}) and the failure of ONS to increase total nutrient intake for a long enough period of time. Methodological issues (small sample sizes) could also be a factor.

Further research: some trials suggest that the use of modified ONS (enriched with nutrients with 'immunomodulatory' properties) may be beneficial (improved GI function, reduced hospitalization rate). Large RCT are needed.

Table A4.22. Oral nutritional supplements used in randomized controlled trials of patients with HIV/AIDS in the community.

Trial	ONS	ONS energy density	ONS prescribed	ONS energy (kcal) intake	ONS protein (g) intake	Toleration
Berneis *et al.* (2000)	Meritene Y (Novartis) (600 kcal, 26 g P, 88 g CHO, 17 g F; liquid)	–	600 kcal	–	–	–
Gibert *et al.* (1999)	S[1] Peptamen (Nestlé) (peptide, MCT ONS; 16% P, 33% F, 51% CHO)	1 kcal ml^{-1}	500 kcal	S[1] 310 kcal S[2] 345 kcal[a] (on trial visit or 409 kcal on self-report)	– –	S[1] 22% discontinued before end of trial vs. 7% in S[2] (reasons diarrhoea or nausea in 1/3 of pts). No side-effects with S[2]. 5% discontinued multivitamin supplement
	S[2] NuBasics (Nestlé; bars, soups, drinks)	1 kcal ml^{-1} (drinks)				
Rabeneck *et al.* (1998)	Lipisorb (MCT) (Mead Johnson)	1.3 kcal ml^{-1}	–	–	–	1 stopped S due to dislike of taste and 1 due to nausea and epigastric pain

[a]69% of energy from ONS drinks other than coffee, 20% from bars, 9% from soups, 2% from coffee drink ONS.
CHO, carbohydrate; F, fat; MCT, medium-chain triglycerides; P, protein; pts, patients.

Table A4.23. Trial characteristics: community-based randomized controlled trials of oral nutritional supplementation in patients with HIV/AIDS.

Trial	Design	No. S	No. US	Initial BMI S group	Initial BMI US group	Duration of ONS	Dietary counselling	Control group
Berneis *et al.* (2000) Stable HIV with no infections	10001	8	7	< 21 or wt loss ≥ 5% (? time period)		12 weeks	Yes – by a dietitian (taught principles of balanced nutrition and discussion of individual problems related to nutrition (diarrhoea, nausea, vomiting) and aspects of hygiene)	No nutritional treatment, only monitoring (no advice)
Gibert *et al.* (1999) HIV infection	11001	S[1] 178 S[2] 179	179	S[1] 23.5 (2.6) S[2] 23.2 (2.6) (wt stable)	23.4 (2.6)	4 months	–	Multivitamin and mineral supplement (also given to S[1] and S[2])
Rabeneck *et al.* (1998) HIV-infected men with no GI symptoms or other infections with wt loss > 10% in 6 months	10001	49	50	20.6	21	6 weeks	Individualized nutrition counselling given to S and US by a dietitian – told how to consume a diet with an energy intake 960 kcal above their estimated total energy expenditure. At 2-week visits, pts receiving further counselling if intakes were not meeting the target	Individualized nutrition counselling by a dietitian (see previous column)

pts, patients; S, supplemented; US, unsupplemented.

Table A4.24. Main findings of randomized controlled trials of oral nutritional supplementation in HIV/AIDS patients in the community.

Trial	Energy intake	Body weight S	Body weight US	Body function	Clinical outcome	Finance
Berneis *et al.* (2000)	S had small, NS increase in TEI (+48 kcal), suggesting VFI reduced US VFI reduced by 309 kcal (S vs. US NS)	+2% (NS) (S vs. US ?) Sig. increase in LBM (+2.7% of wt) and sig. decrease in fat mass (−2.7%)	−0.68% (NS) NS change in LBM or fat mass	No changes in lymphocyte CD4 count, plasma TNF-R55, TNF-R75 and interleukin R2 concentrations (S vs. US NS) No change in quality of life (S vs. US NS) *Reduction in leucine oxidation (protein catabolism) in S group (S vs. US sig.)*	–	–
Gibert *et al.* (1999)	ONS group sig. higher TEI than US (S¹ +325 kcal and S² +239 kcal), with similar VFI: S¹ VFI 3145 kcal; TEI 3458 kcal S² VFI 3026 kcal, TEI 3371 kcal US VFI 3139 kcal (S¹ and S² vs. US sig.; S¹ vs. S² NS)	S¹ +0.8% S² +1.1% (S vs. US NS) NS changes in BCM S¹ +0.7% S² +1.2%	+0.7% +0.6%	–	–	–
Rabeneck *et al.* (1998)	–	−0.1 kg (NS) Increase in FFM (S vs. US NS)	−0.1 kg (NS)	NS difference in quality of life (S vs. US NS). S had larger increases in HGS (S +2.8 kg, US +0.7 kg, NS). Sig. improvements in cognitive function in S (short-term recall and long-term storage; NS improvement in long-term retrieval)	–	–

?, uncertain if statistically significant; BCM, body cell mass; FFM, fat-free mass; HGS, hand-grip strength; LBM, lean body mass; S, supplemented; TEI, total energy intake; TNF, tumour necrosis factor; US, unsupplemented; VFI, voluntary food intake.

Table A4.25. Oral nutritional supplements used in non-randomized trials of patients with HIV/AIDS in the community.

Trial	ONS	ONS energy density	ONS prescribed	ONS energy (kcal) intake	ONS protein (g) intake	Toleration
Burger et al. (1994)	Biosorb drink or Biosorb 1500	1 kcal ml⁻¹ 1.5 kcal ml⁻¹	1000–1500 kcal	496 (363)ᵃ	–	Poor toleration in 5 patients – too viscous, poor taste, early satiety
Chan et al. (1994)	S¹ Standard (no MCT) S² Lipisorb (MCT)	1.3 kcal ml⁻¹	90% RDA	–	–	Less nausea with MCT formula (sig.)
Chlebowski et al. (1992) Aᵇ	S¹ Ensure HN (Abbott) S² Enriched peptide (fibre, omega-3)	1 kcal ml⁻¹ 1.2 kcal ml⁻¹	480 kcal 576 kcal	465 566	– –	Diarrhoea (39%) and nausea (17%). 3 stopped S due to diarrhoea and 1 due to taste
Chlebowski et al. (1993)ᵇ	S¹ Ensure (Abbott) S² Advera (Abbott)	1 kcal ml⁻¹ 1.28 kcal ml⁻¹	502–754 607–910 (2–3 cans)ᵃ	327–377 394–455	13–15 18–21	Safety/tolerance of supplements excellent – no untoward GI symptoms
Dowling et al. (1990)	–	–	–	48–238ᶜ	1–9	–
Fogaca et al. (2000)	Advera (Abbott), peptide-based, with omega-3 fatty acids	1.28 kcal ml⁻¹	–	909	42.66	–
Gaare et al. (1991) A	Impact (Novartis)	1 kcal ml⁻¹	1000–1500 kcal	–	–	–
Hellerstein et al. (1994) A	S¹ Whole protein S² Novel peptide	1.3 kcal ml⁻¹ 1.1 kcal ml⁻¹	616–924 521–783	–	–	Novel peptide feed well tolerated, no adverse clinical effects
Hoh et al. (1998)	S¹ Ensure (Abbott) S² Advera (Abbott) (peptide)	1 kcal ml⁻¹ 1.28 kcal ml⁻¹	S¹ 500–750 kcal S² 606–909 kcal	550–600	19–28	Both formulas well tolerated with no changes in stool frequency
Pichard et al. (1998)	S¹ Standard formula S² Enriched formula (7.4 g arginine, 1.7 g omega-3 fatty acids per ONS) (Sandoz)	–	606 in two servings	475 (424–525)	–	Improved anorexia/GI tolerance in S. 9/55 stopped due to poor tolerance of S, more common with the enriched formula
Richards et al. (1996) A	S¹ Whole protein S² Peptide	–	–	400	–	–
Singer et al. (1992) A	S¹ Replete (Novartis) S² Impact (Novartis)	1 kcal ml⁻¹ 1 kcal ml⁻¹	4–6 cans 948–1422	–	–	–
Stack et al. (1996)	Resource Plus (Novartis)	1.5 kcal ml⁻¹	–	555 (254–913) 670 (482–710)ᵈ 474 (168–888)ᵉ	20 (9.3–33.6) 24 (17.7–26.1)ᵈ 17 (10.4–32.6)ᵉ	–

| Süttmann *et al.* (1996) | S¹ Standard formula S² Impact (Novartis) | 1 kcal ml⁻¹ 1 kcal ml⁻¹ | 500+ | S¹ 695 (118) S² 638 (117) | ~27.8 g ~38 g | – |
| Wandall *et al.* (1992) | MCT formula (no name) | – | – | – | – | – |

ᵃThe value indicates the mean amount taken by subjects completing the trial (*n* 10). Mean amount taken by all subjects during the trial was 688 (301) kcal day⁻¹, range 333–1352 kcal day⁻¹.

ᵇAbstract could be preliminary report of larger trial.

ᶜAsymptomatic patients (CDC II) 48 kcal day⁻¹, symptomatic (CDC IV) 238 kcal day⁻¹.

ᵈSupplement intake in patients with secondary infections.

ᵉSupplement intake in patients with no secondary infection.

A, abstract; CDC, Centre for Disease Control; MCT, medium-chain triglycerides; RDA, recommended daily allowance; S, supplemented.

Table A4.26. Trial characteristics: community-based non-randomized trials of oral nutritional supplementation in patients with HIV/AIDS.

Trial	Design	No. S	No. US	Initial BMI S group	Initial BMI US group	Duration of ONS	Dietary counselling	Control group
Burger *et al.* (1994) HIV patients with chronic wasting, no infections or GI symptoms	C	34	–	–	–	3 months	Nutritional counselling, offered to all pts before the trial as part of standard clinical practice – ONS a 2nd step in treatment	–
Chan *et al.* (1994) A AIDS and fat malabsorption (RCT comparing different ONS)	C	S^1 12 S^2 12	–	–	–	12 days	–	–
Chlebowski *et al.* (1992) A HIV infection, no GI symptoms (RCT comparing different ONS)	C	49 total	–	–	–	68 days	–	–
Chlebowski *et al.* (1993) HIV infection, with or without AIDS (RCT comparing different ONS)	C	S^1 25 S^2 31	–	S^1 ~21.7 S^2 ~23	–	6 months	ONS recommended in conjunction with a dietitian-directed dietary counselling programme based on standard nutrition principles	–
Dowling *et al.* (1990) Asymptomatic and symptomatic AIDS	C	Asymptomatic 17 Symptomatic 17	–	23.9 20.6	–	12 weeks	Pts encouraged to follow high-protein and energy diet with regular meals and snacks	–
Fogaca *et al.* (2000) AIDS, no diarrhoea or opportunistic infections	C	12	–	18.5 (2.77)	–	6 weeks	Received standardized dietary counselling to maintain normal intake (at ~1800 kcal day^{-1})	–
Gaare *et al.* (1991) A Weight loss secondary to AIDS	C	10	–	–	–	3 months	–	–
Hellerstein *et al.* (1994) A HIV and AIDS (RCT comparing different ONS)	C	39 total	–	–	–	1.5 months	–	–
Hoh *et al.* (1998) Blinded RCT comparing 2 ONS types in HIV and AIDS patients with weight loss and subjective GI symptoms	B (non-random US)	S^1 22 S^2 17	13	S^1 21.5 (0.4) S^2 21.6 (0.6)	20.6 (0.6)	6 weeks	–	Non-ONS group followed at similar time intervals
Pichard *et al.* (1998) HIV-infected (RCT comparing different ONS)	C	S^1 28 S^2 27	–	S^1 22.6 S^2 21.8	–	6 months	General information on optimal food intake provided at start of trial by a dietitian	–

Richards *et al.* (1996) A Malabsorption (RCT comparing different ONS)	C	S[1] 28 S[2] 27	—	—	—	18 months	—
Singer *et al.* (1992) A AIDS (RCT comparing different ONS)	C	S[1] 13 S[2] 15	—	—	—	3 months	—
Stack *et al.* (1996) HIV, with and without AIDS	C	17 7[a] 10[b]	—	21.2/98% IBW	—	6 weeks	Received dietary counselling regarding an optimal diet for HIV persons – high-protein diet and selection of foods to minimize GI complications
Süttmann *et al.* (1996) Symptomatic HIV infection (RCT comparing different ONS)	C	10[c]	—	22.3	—	8 months	—
Wandall *et al.* (1992) HIV/AIDS without GI infections	C	19	—	—	—	4 weeks	—

[a]Supplement intake in patients with secondary infections.
[b]Supplement intake in patients with no secondary infection.
[c]Crossover trial (4 months with each ONS).
A, abstract; pts, patients; S, supplemented; US, unsupplemented.

Table A4.27. Main findings of non-randomized trials of oral nutritional supplementation in patients with HIV/AIDS in the community.

Trial	Energy intake	Body weight S	Body weight US	Body function	Clinical outcome	Finance
Burger et al. (1994)	–	No increase	–	–	–	–
Chan et al. (1994) A	–	Increase (no data)	–	Sig. reduction in stool weight and stool fat in S^1 and S^2	–	–
Chlebowski et al. (1992) A	–	No (subjective data only)	–	Increase in subjectively rated well-being and energy level (? sig.)	–	–
Chlebowski et al. (1993)	Increase in TEI (?)	S^1 –0.68 kg S^2 +1.8 kg (S^1 vs. S^2 sig.)	–	–	Sig. lower hospitalization rate in S^2 in last 3–6 months of ONS than S^1	–
Dowling et al. (1990)	No increase in TEI in either group (asymptomatic or symptomatic)	2.6 kg (NS) 1.4 kg (NS)	–	–	–	–
Fogaca et al. (2000)	–	+0.92 kg (NS) Sig. increase in TSF (+2 mm)	–	No. of peripheral blood T cells, albumin, transferrin and no. CD3+, CD4+ and CD8+ cells in jejunal mucosa stable. Intestinal morphometry stable (no. lamina propria cells, intra-epithelial lymphocytes) but sig. decrease in villus : crypt ratio	–	–
Gaare et al. (1991) A	–	No	–	–	–	–
Hellerstein et al. (1994) A	–	–	–	Sig. higher % lymphocyte count and sig. reduction in stool frequency in S^2	Sig. fewer hospitalizations (sig. in S^2)	–
Hoh et al. (1998)	Sig. increase in TEI (by 10–15%) and TPI in both S^1 and S^2 and increased intakes of vitamins and trace elements. Sig. reduction in VFI but not equivalent to intake from ONS (S^1 ~67% additive; S^2 ~36% additive) Sig. increase in vit. C, B_{12}, B_6, Mg, Cu, Mn in S^2 only NS change in VFI in US	–0.3% NS change in % body fat or FFM	–	NS changes in Karnofsky scores or CD4+ T-cell counts	–	–

Reference					
Pichard et al. (1998)	Transient increase in TEI for 1–2 months only (? sig.) but reports of improved appetite	S^1 +1.9 kg (NS) S^2 +2.2 kg (NS)	–	Improvement in GI symptoms (? sig.)	–
Richards et al. (1996)	Increase in TEI (? sig.)	Wt maintenance (no data)	–	7.4 × greater risk of > 50% drop in CD4 count in S^1 vs. S^2 (sig.)	–
Singer et al. (1992) A	–	S^1 +1.45 kg (? sig.) S^2 +1.68 kg (? sig.) (S^1 vs. S^2 NS)	–	Improved immunoglobulin A (sig.) and β_2 microglobulin (NS) with S^2	–
Stack et al. (1996)	–	+1.1 kg (? sig.) −0.16 kg[a] +2.1 kg[b]	–	—	–
Süttmann et al. (1996)	Increase in TEI (NS)	S^1 −0.5 kg S^2 +2.9 kg (S^1 vs. S^2 sig.)	–	Sig. increase in serum concentrations of soluble TNF-R proteins in S^2	–
Wandall et al. (1992)	–	+1 kg (sig.)	–	—	–

[a]Patients with secondary infections.
[b]Patients with no secondary infection.
A, abstract; FFM, fat-free mass; NS, not significant; S, supplemented; sig., significant; TEI, total energy intake; TNF, tumour necrosis factor; TPI, total protein intake; US, unsupplemented; VFI, voluntary food intake.

al., 1996; Hoh *et al.*, 1998; Pichard *et al.*, 1998), but in only one trial was the increase evaluated as statistically significant (Hoh *et al.*, 1998). Furthermore, significant increases in some vitamins and minerals were observed with ONS, particularly with micronutrient-enriched ONS (Hoh *et al.*, 1998). However, significant reductions in voluntary food intake did occur, with between 36% and 67% of ONS energy being additive (depending on the ONS used; method iii). In other trials, the effect of ONS on food intake has been greater, particularly increasing over time. Pichard *et al.* (1998) showed almost complete replacement of the energy from food by the ONS after 2 months, whereas another trial found that ~20% of supplement energy was additional to that from food (Süttmann *et al.*, 1996). In these trials, the mean BMI of the patient group was > 20 kg m^{-2} (see Chapter 5 for method calculation).

There appeared to be insufficient monitoring of supplement usage in these studies (as in all) to ensure patients' compliance and accurate dietary records, except in one trial in HIV/AIDS weight-losing patients, in which can counts were carried out to assess ONS consumption (Hoh *et al.*, 1998).

The one trial that subjectively assessed appetite during the period of supplementation reported an improvement in anorexia (not statistically evaluated) (Pichard *et al.*, 1998), although this was associated with only a transient increase in total energy intake, and it was unclear whether an improvement in clinical condition also occurred.

(IA) IS THE TIMING OF SUPPLEMENTATION IMPORTANT?

No details about the time of supplement consumption were provided in any of these studies, so assessment of the effect of supplement timing on outcome variables was not possible. Research is needed.

(II) What effect do ONS have on the body weight and composition of patients with HIV/AIDS in the community?

From the studies reviewed, ONS appear to have little effect on body weight in patients with HIV and AIDS who are within the ideal weight range (BMI 20–25 kg m^{-2}). The effects of drug therapy (highly active anti-retroviral therapy (HAART)) have not been explored and may confound these results.

Of three RCT reviewed (Rabeneck *et al.*, 1998; Gibert *et al.*, 1999; Berneis *et al.*, 2000), two showed weight gain during supplementation, but the increases were not significant (Gibert *et al.*, 1999; Berneis *et al.*, 2000) (see Table A4.24). Analysis of % weight change data from three RCT showed similar results for both supplemented (+0.9%) and unsupplemented (+0.5%) patients (no significant difference). Pre-existing nutritional status was documented in most of these studies and tended to be in the ideal range, with the mean BMI of the patients often > 20 kg m^{-2} at the start of the trial.

Compartmental measurements of body composition suggested increases in lean body mass (LBM) (Rabeneck *et al.*, 1998; Berneis *et al.*, 2000) or body cell mass (Gibert *et al.*, 1999), although these were significant changes in only one 3-month trial of ONS, with the largest prescribed ONS intake (600 kcal day^{-1}) (see Table A4.24).

HAART, which dramatically reduces the incidence of tissue wasting and was being introduced at the time of these studies, may have had confounding effects (Keithley and Swanson, 2001).

(III)/(IV) What effect do ONS have on the body function and clinical outcome of patients with HIV/AIDS in the community?

Few functional benefits have been documented in this patient group following the use of ONS. This may be because increases in total energy intake and weight are not sustained and consequently, improvements in structure and/or function do not result.

Few studies assessed functional outcomes and none showed any significant detriments. Only two RCT made assessment of body functions following ONS. One trial documented greater improvements in hand-grip strength than in unsupplemented patients (not significant) and improvements in some aspects of cognitive function over time in supplemented patients (Rabeneck *et al.*, 1998). One trial was unable to find immunological benefits following ONS or differences in QOL between supplemented and unsupplemented groups (Berneis *et al.*, 2000). No assessments of clinical outcome were made. From the non-randomized data, improvements in GI function (Chan *et al.*, 1994; Hellerstein *et al.*, 1994; Pichard *et al.*, 1998) and in immunological status (Singer *et al.*, 1992; Hellerstein *et al.*, 1994) (not a consistent observation (Hoh *et al.*, 1998; Fogaca *et al.*, 2000)) and a reduction in the number of hospitalizations (Chlebowski *et al.*, 1993; Hellerstein *et al.*, 1994) were demonstrated, typically in studies comparing two formula types. Increased well-being (Chlebowski *et al.*, 1992) was also documented, but the reports were only anecdotal. Most studies which assessed aspects of QOL did not report a benefit (Singer *et al.*, 1992; Hoh *et al.*, 1998; Pichard *et al.*, 1998).

(V) What are the effects of stopping ONS in patients with HIV/AIDS in the community?

None of the studies reported following up patients after the ONS were stopped.

Summary of non-randomized community trials in patients with HIV/AIDS

Fifteen NRT of ONS were reviewed, including longitudinal data from nine RCT comparing different types of ONS (Dowling *et al.*, 1990; Gaare *et al.*, 1991; Chlebowski *et al.*, 1992, 1993; Singer *et al.*, 1992; Wandall *et al.*, 1992; Burger *et al.*, 1994; Chan *et al.*, 1994; Hellerstein *et al.*, 1994; Richards *et al.*, 1996; Stack *et al.*, 1996; Süttmann *et al.*, 1996; Hoh *et al.*, 1998; Pichard *et al.*, 1998; Fogaca *et al.*, 2000). Of the remainder of trials (*n* 6), patients with various stages of HIV infection were included in some (Burger *et al.*, 1994; Stack *et al.*, 1996), whereas in others they were categorized according to disease stage and studied separately (Dowling *et al.*, 1990). Typically, the numbers of patients in each study were small (see Table A4.26). Duration of supplementation varied from just 4 weeks (Wandall *et al.*, 1992) to 3

months (Dowling *et al.*, 1990; Gaare *et al.*, 1991; Burger *et al.*, 1994). The ONS intake (only reported in three studies (Dowling *et al.*, 1990; Burger *et al.*, 1994; Fogaca *et al.*, 2000)) varied from as little as 48 kcal (Dowling *et al.*, 1990) to 909 kcal (Fogaca *et al.*, 2000) (see Table A4.25). Not surprisingly, although four studies documented an increase in weight (Dowling *et al.*, 1990; Burger *et al.*, 1994; Wandall *et al.*, 1992; Stack *et al.*, 1996), in only one was it statistically significant, even though it was only 1 kg (Wandall *et al.*, 1992). In the only study that made any assessment of total energy intake, no significant increase was achieved during supplementation (Dowling *et al.*, 1990). This could have been due to the adequate nutritional status of patients at the start of the study (BMI 20.6–23.9 kg m^{-2}), with only small ONS volumes consumed. No functional improvements were reported in any of these studies.

The longitudinal data from RCT comparing different types of ONS in HIV patients suggested that energy (Chlebowski *et al.*, 1993; Hoh *et al.*, 1998), protein (Hoh *et al.*, 1998) and micronutrient intakes (Hoh *et al.*, 1998) could be improved in supplemented HIV patients. However, in one study (in which baseline energy intakes were high), ONS energy (~475 kcal) increasingly replaced food intake over the supplementation period, so that total energy was not increased after 6 months (Pichard *et al.*, 1998). Weight gain was observed in some studies (Chlebowski *et al.*, 1993; Süttmann *et al.*, 1996), although often in small amounts (e.g. Chlebowski *et al.*, 1993) relative to the duration of supplementation. In a couple of trials in patients with weight loss, weight was either maintained (Richards *et al.*, 1996; Hoh *et al.*, 1998) or lost with supplementation. Due to differences in patients' disease staging and their initial nutritional status within trials, it is difficult to clarify the impact of ONS on intake and weight. For example, ONS are unlikely to benefit patients who are weight-stable, not underweight (BMI > 20 kg m^{-2}) and do not have symptomatic disease. Similarly, a number of functional benefits have been observed, particularly in patients taking enriched ONS (see Tables A4.25 and A4.27), although the significance of some of these changes (i.e. subjective improvements in well-being (Chlebowski *et al.*, 1992) and immunological changes (e.g. Süttmann *et al.*, 1996)) is unclear. In one trial, a significant reduction in hospitalizations was observed in the last 3 months of supplementation (Chlebowski *et al.*, 1993). For more information, refer to Tables A4.25–A4.27.

Oral supplementation, dietary intervention or ETF?

There are alternative ways of increasing patients' total energy and nutrient intakes, including dietary counselling and ETF. The comparative effectiveness of these interventions has not been fully assessed yet.

- Studies of dietary counselling (without supplements) have indicated that this alone can increase or maintain adequate energy and protein intake from food and improve the nutritional status of patients with HIV/AIDS (Burger *et al.*, 1993; Schwenk *et al.*, 1994), although this is not a universal finding (Chlebowski *et al.*, 1995; Schwenk *et al.*, 1999b). Also, in many trials that have assessed the effects of ONS, patients have also received dietary counselling (see Chapter 6).
- A number of studies have shown increases in body weight, body cell mass and total body fat with ETF in malnourished AIDS patients, in hospital (Kotler *et al.*, 1991) and at home (Süttmann *et al.*, 1993). In children, increases in weight-for-age and weight-for-height have been documented (Henderson *et al.*, 1994). However, these findings were not universal. Most of these studies involved small numbers of patients, and few have adequately assessed functional outcome measures, such as QOL (Brantsma *et al.*, 1991) (see Chapter 7).
- There is a lack of controlled studies comparing the efficacy of dietary counselling or ETF with commercial ONS.

The main focus of most of the ONS studies in HIV/AIDS patients has been the benefits of use of feeds enriched with MCT, omega-3 fatty acids and/or micronutrients. Fundamental and yet important parameters, such as the effects of ONS *per se* on body composition, habitual food and total energy intake, have tended to be overlooked, as has the clinical course of these patients. As yet, few have demonstrated any significant functional benefits, possibly for a number of reasons: (i) patients were within the ideal BMI range at the start of the study; (ii) ONS may not have continued for a long enough period of time; (iii) ONS did not significantly increase nutrient intake, either because of reductions in habitual food intake or due to non-compliance; and (iv) small sample sizes are likely to have been insufficient in some studies to detect clinically significant changes. In future research, power statistics to calculate relevant sample sizes for specified end-points, homogeneous samples of patients (e.g. CD4 counts) and assessments of clinical and functional outcomes are needed. The need for controlled research in more representative samples of the symptomatic HIV-infected population has also been highlighted (Keithley and Swanson, 2001).

Liver Disease

Malnutrition is prevalent in patients with advanced chronic liver disease (CLD) and may be associated with a worse prognosis for patients (Mendenhall *et al.*, 1985, 1993) (see Chapter 2). In addition, treatment often incurs many dietary restrictions (including fluid, sodium, protein), which may further limit energy intake, in addition to the many other factors limiting food intake in CLD patients (e.g. anorexia, encephalopathy). Nutritional support is often required in this patient group to help maximize nutritional intake, and ONS are one mode of nutritional intervention used in clinical practice.

Liver disease: present analysis

Only two RCT were reviewed that addressed the efficacy of ONS in patients with CLD in the community setting (Simko, 1983; Hirsch *et al.*, 1993) (see Tables A4.28–A4.30). Supplementation for 3 months (Simko, 1983) to 1 year (Hirsch *et al.*, 1993) in relatively large quantities (> 800 kcal) was well tolerated. The efficacy of ONS has been considered below for each of the review questions and summarized in Box A4.6.

(I) What effect do ONS have on the voluntary food intake and total energy intake of patients with liver disease in the community?

ONS can increase total energy and protein intakes in patients with CLD, although the effects on voluntary food intake are unknown. Both trials demonstrated significant increases in total energy intake when compared with baseline and with the unsupplemented group (see Table A4.30). One study (Hirsch *et al.*, 1993) also observed large increases in protein intake, which were again significantly greater when compared with baseline and with the placebo group. The effects of ONS on habitual food intake and appetite were not recorded.

(IA) IS THE TIMING OF SUPPLEMENTATION IMPORTANT? No details were provided in the studies about the timing of supplementation during the day or the relation to food consumption.

(II) What effect do ONS have on the body weight and composition of patients with liver disease in the community?

Body weight is an unreliable indicator of nutritional status in patients with ascites. Alternative assessments, including muscle mass, are required. The trials reviewed (Simko, 1983; Hirsch *et al.*, 1993) showed increases in weight, mid-arm circumference

(MAC) and TSF in the supplemented patients (see Table A4.30). However, the increase in body weight over time was significant in only one study (Hirsch *et al.*, 1993) and the difference in weight gain between supplemented and unsupplemented groups was not significant. In fact, unsupplemented patients gained more weight (+8.24%) than the supplemented patients (+6.14%) in a weighted analysis of data from these two trials but the possible confounding effects of fluid retention have to be considered. In the one study (Simko, 1983) that assessed muscle mass (MAMC), an increase was observed but this was not significant.

(III)/(IV) What effect do ONS have on the body function and clinical outcome of patients with liver disease in the community?

ONS can reduce infection rates and hospitalization rates in patients with CLD (see Table A4.30). Only one trial assessed the impact of ONS on outcome measures (Hirsch *et al.*, 1993). A significant reduction in the incidence of severe infections and related hospitalization occurred in those taking the supplement compared with those taking the placebo. Functionally, this trial found that patients taking an ONS had earlier improvements in hand-grip strength than unsupplemented patients. No differences were found in mortality or total number of days in hospital in this same trial (Hirsch *et al.*, 1993).

(V) What are the effects of stopping ONS in patients with liver disease in the community?

Neither trial assessed any changes in these patients once ONS were stopped.

Box A4.6. Key findings: effect of ONS in community patients with chronic liver disease.

Nutritional intake, body weight, function and clinical outcome: ONS can increase total energy and protein intakes in patients with chronic liver disease. This can result in reductions in infection rates and hospital admission rates. Due to the limited number of studies in this diagnostic group, further investigation is warranted.

Table A4.28. Oral nutritional supplements used in randomized controlled trials of patients with liver disease in the community.

Trial	ONS	ONS energy density	ONS prescribed	ONS energy (kcal) intake	ONS protein (g) intake	Toleration
Hirsch et al. (1993) Simko (1983)	ADN Hepatic-Aid (powder ONS rich in BCAA, 10% energy from P, 70% CHO, 20% F)	1 kcal ml^{-1} –	1000 kcal Minimum of 60 g of ONS (~2400 kcal[a])	889 ~1480–1800[a]	– 37 (2) over 3 months 45 (5) in last 2 weeks	Diarrhoea in one patient No adverse effects found

[a]Calculated from ONS protein intake prescribed and taken.
BCAA, branched-chain amino acids; CHO, carbohydrate; F, fat; P, protein.

Table A4.29. Trial characteristics: community-based randomized controlled trials of oral nutritional supplementation in patients with liver disease.

Trial	Design	No. S	No. US	Initial BMI S group	Initial BMI US group	Duration of ONS	Dietary counselling	Control group
Hirsch et al. (1993) Out-patients with symptomatic alcoholic cirrhosis	10001	26	25	–	–	1 year	Instructed to consume ONS in addition to normal diet	Given a placebo capsule
Simko (1983) Advanced liver disease and history of hepatic encephalopathy	10001	7	3	–	–	3 months	–	Given a placebo powder Both S and US blinded to intervention

S, supplemented; US, unsupplemented.

Table A4.30. Main findings of randomized controlled trials of oral nutritional supplementation in patients with liver disease in the community.

Trial	Energy intake	Body weight S	Body weight US	Body function	Clinical outcome	Finance
Hirsch *et al.* (1993)	S sig. greater TEI (2469 kcal) and TPI (74 g) than US (1580 kcal, 45 g P)	+6.29% (+4.2 kg) (sig.)[a] (S vs. US NS) Sig. increase in TSF (S vs. US NS)	+9.0% (6.1 kg) (sig.)[a] Sig. increase in TSF	Sig. improvement in HGS in both groups, but improvement earlier in S	Sig. lower frequency of hospitalization in S patients (S 0.85 (23 occasions); US 1.6 (35 occasions)) with a sig. lower incidence of severe infections causing hospitalization in S (S 2; US 9) NS lower mortality (S 3, US 6) NS difference between S and US for medication requirements for encephalopathy	–
Simko (1983)	ONS did not affect protein intake from food (NS increase) and sig. increased TEI (S vs. US sig.)	+5.6 (5)% (NS) Sig. increase in TSF (S vs. US NS)	+1.8 (3.4)% (NS)	No deterioration in grade of encephalopathy in S. NS changes in Hb or TLC in either S or US but sig. greater increase in transferrin in S (vs. US)	–	–

[a]Ascites (causing hospital admission in US (*n* 11) and S (*n* 8) patients) may have affected measurements of weight.
Hb, haemoglobin; HGS, hand-grip strength; P, protein; TEI, total energy intake; TLC, total lymphocyte count; TPI, total protein intake; S, supplemented; US, unsupplemented.

Oral supplementation, dietary intervention or ETF?

ETF is another effective means of increasing nutritional intakes in patients with CLD.

- ETF has been advocated in malnourished patients with CLD. Several studies have reported putative benefits with ETF: significant improvements in Child's score (hepatic reserve) (Cabre et al., 1990); liver function (Smith et al., 1982) (including antipyrine half-life, serum bilirubin and encephalopathy scores in patients with alcoholic disease (Kearns et al., 1992)); and mortality (Cabre et al., 1990). These short-term studies have been conducted in hospital patients. There are a lack of similar data in the community and also a lack of studies formally comparing ETF with ONS. A hospital-based study (Calvey et al., 1984) reported that the energy delivered by tube (no oral intake) was significantly greater than the amount consumed orally as a supplement (large volumes (2 l) of a low-sodium feed), but no functional outcomes were assessed (see Chapter 7).

Malignancy

Cancer is one of the main causes of mortality in the Western world (see Chapter 2). In addition to the effects of the tumour, the treatments for cancer (e.g. surgery, radiotherapy, chemotherapy) can reduce appetite or impair the ability to eat and drink. Consequently, intakes below recommendations (Ovesen et al., 1991) can lead to progressive loss of weight and functional ability. Lack of appetite and weight loss is also a particular problem in patients in the terminal phase of their illness. Food and nutritional support for community patients with cancer may be valuable as an active treatment or when used palliatively (Seligman et al., 1998). This section looks at the use of ONS in patients with a variety of stages and types of cancers.

Malignancy: present analysis

A total of 17 studies in patients with cancer receiving ONS were reviewed (for a summary of key findings see Box A4.7). Nine were randomized, controlled trials (Bounous et al., 1975; Douglass et al., 1978; Brown et al., 1980; Foster et al., 1980; Elkort et al., 1981; Evans et al., 1987; Flynn and Leightty, 1987; Arnold and Richter, 1989; Nayel et al., 1992) and eight were not (Bounous et al., 1973; Baker et al., 1977; Crossland and Higgins, 1977; Wallner et al., 1990; Ovesen and Allingstrup, 1992; McCarter et al., 1998; Barber et al., 1999a, 2000) (see Tables A4.31–A4.33 (RCT) and A4.34–A4.36 (NRT)). The majority of studies included patients with more than one type of cancer and at various stages of the disease. Some studies gave no details about the cancer staging (Bounous et al., 1975; Foster et al., 1980; Nayel et al., 1992; McCarter et al., 1998) but most studies involved patients who were also receiving radiotherapy, chemotherapy or both.

(I) What effect do ONS have on the voluntary food intake and total energy intake of patients with malignancy in the community?

Improvements in total energy intake and in food intake may occur with the use of ONS in cancer patients, although increments may not be sustained over time.

Supplementation increased total energy intake in three RCT and significantly in two of these (Evans et al., 1987; Arnold and Richter, 1989). In one NRT (Ovesen and Allingstrup, 1992), total energy intake was significantly increased only in patients given one type of ONS (peptide feed) (see Table A4.36).

No formal assessments were made of the effect of supplements on appetite but Nayel et al. (1992) recorded anecdotally that the loss of appetite in supplemented and unsupplemented patients was similar. In addition, it was possible to calculate the effect of ONS on habitual food intake in a few studies (one RCT: Douglass et al., 1978; one NRT: Ovesen and Allingstrup, 1992). These indicated that more than 90% of supplement energy was

> **Box A4.7.** Key findings: effect of ONS in community patients with malignancy.
>
> Nutritional intake: improvements in total energy intake and food intake may occur in patients taking ONS, although over time the increments may not be sustained.
>
> Body weight: the effects of ONS on body weight are variable and likely to be confounded by the heterogeneity of patients, the types of cancer and the lack of information about oedema.
>
> Body function: trials have failed to show significant improvements in function (not widely assessed) and clinical outcome (trials typically too small, inadequate statistical power). Detriments may occur if ONS are used inappropriately in weight-stable, overweight cancer patients (e.g. cancer of the breast).
>
> Further research: large, well-designed RCT in homogeneous patient groups are needed to characterize the effects of ONS on structural and functional measures and clinical outcome.

additional to the energy intake from food when compared either with the control group or with baseline (methods (ii) and (iii), see Chapter 5). In these two trials (Douglass *et al.*, 1978; Ovesen and Allingstrup, 1992), food intake was greater during supplementation than at baseline. Although this could have resulted from an improvement in the clinical condition, no such changes were seen in the control groups.

The only studies that assessed change in supplement intake over time showed a reduction in the contribution of supplement intake to total energy intake (one RCT: Arnold and Richter, 1989; one NRT: Ovesen and Allingstrup, 1992; see Tables A4.33 and A4.36).

Supplement intake was typically calculated from patients' own records, often made for 24 h, but these could provide an unreliable estimate of actual consumption, as assessments of compliance were scanty. Some studies did not even report the amount of supplement taken (e.g. Brown *et al.*, 1980; Elkort *et al.*, 1981; Evans *et al.*, 1987; Wallner *et al.*, 1990; Nayel *et al.*, 1992; see Table A4.31).

(IA) IS THE TIMING OF SUPPLEMENTATION IMPORTANT?
Times at which patients were advised to consume supplements in these studies included between meals (Douglass *et al.*, 1978; Ovesen and Allingstrup, 1992) and frequently through the day (Bounous *et al.*, 1975). It was not clear whether the authors verified this with patients at the end of the study.

Insufficient data exist to reach conclusions about the timing of supplementation in patients with cancer. In particular, no information exists about the extent to which outcome measures are influenced by the timing of supplement consumption in patients with different types and stages of cancer, receiving different treatments.

(II) What effect do ONS have on the body weight and composition of patients with malignancy in the community?

The available information from heterogeneous groups of cancer patients suggests that changes in weight in supplemented patients are variable and may or may not be greater than in unsupplemented patients. More controlled investigations are needed in homogeneous groups of patients.

Of nine RCT, only one (Foster *et al.*, 1980) gave data on initial nutritional status, with patients being ~110% of IBW (see Table A4.32).

The effects of ONS on body weight were variable and generally confounded by the heterogeneity of patients and types of cancer and the lack of information about oedema. However, eight out of nine randomized studies investigated the changes in weight occurring during supplementation but only two trials showed a significantly greater gain in weight in supplemented than in control patients (Bounous *et al.*, 1975; Nayel *et al.*, 1992) (see Table A4.33). Four studies reported

Table A4.31. Oral nutritional supplements used in randomized controlled trials of patients with malignancy in the community.

Trial	ONS	ONS energy density	ONS prescribed	ONS energy (kcal) intake	ONS protein (g) intake	Toleration
Arnold and Richter (1989)	Sustacal (Mead Johnson)	1 kcal ml⁻¹	960–1080 kcal	At 3 weeks 626 At 6 months 167	At 3 weeks 36.7 At 6 months 8.35	Milky quality exacerbates mucus production
Bounous *et al.* (1975)	Flexical (Mead Johnson)	0.8 kcal ml⁻¹	1475–2400 kcal	909–2500	–	–
Brown *et al.* (1980)[a]	Vivonex HN (Eaton Lab)	1 kcal ml⁻¹	900 kcal	–	–	41% (*n* 21) unable to tolerate S – bloating, nausea, vomiting Comments of unpalatability and time-consuming to ingest
Douglass *et al.* (1978)	Vivonex HN (Eaton Lab)	1 kcal ml⁻¹	900 kcal	641	–	Nausea (*n* 3) and discontinued S
Elkort *et al.* (1981)	Isocal and Sustacal (Mead Johnson)	1 kcal ml⁻¹ 1 kcal ml⁻¹	500 kcal	–	–	Patients changed to Sustacal – improved compliance due to sweeter taste
Evans *et al.* (1987)	S^1 Isocal HCN (Mead Johnson) S^2 Isocal plus protein mix (Pro-Mix)[b]	1 kcal ml⁻¹	S^1 and S^2 Isocal to increase intakes to 1.7–1.9 × BEE S^2 Pro-mix to provide 25% of energy as protein	–	–	–
Flynn and Leightty (1987)	–	–	–	–	–	–
Foster *et al.* (1980)[a]	Vivonex HN (Eaton Lab)	1 kcal ml⁻¹	900 kcal	–	–	–
Nayel *et al.* (1992)	Ensure Powder (Abbott)	–	–	–	–	Supplement unpalatable

[a]Same research group.
[b]Also given zinc and magnesium supplements in addition to protein mix.
BEE, basal energy expenditure; S, supplement.

Table A4.32. Trial characteristics: community-based randomized controlled trials of oral nutritional supplementation in patients with malignancy.

Trial	Design	Cancer/treatments	No. S	No. US	Initial BMI S group	Initial BMI US group	Duration of ONS	Dietary counselling	Control group
Arnold and Richter (1989)	10001	Head and neck (all stages); radiotherapy	23	27	–	–	10 weeks	All pts encouraged to eat their normal diet *ad libitum* plus intensive counselling (including advice on full liquid, puréed or soft diets where appropriate)	Given dietary counselling (see previous column)
Bounous *et al.* (1975)	1–1001	Abdominal/pelvic (stages unknown); radiotherapy	9	9	–	–	22–40 days	No – ONS sole source of nutrition	Ate a normal diet
Brown *et al.* (1980)	10000	Intra-abdominal (all stages); radiotherapy	51	17	–	–	33–42 days	Advice to reduce fibre intake whilst maintaining energy intakes	Advice to reduce fibre intake whilst maintaining energy intakes
Douglass *et al.* (1978)	11001	Gastrointestinal (1 stage); radiotherapy	13	17	–	–	16 days	Both S and US advised on maintaining nutritional intake and taking between-meal snacks	Advised on maintaining nutritional intake and taking between-meal snacks
Elkort *et al.* (1981)	10000	Breast (all stages); chemotherapy	12	14	–	–	12 months	– Self-selected diet	Normal, self-selected diet
Evans *et al.* (1987)	11000	Non-small-cell lung (I) (all stages); chemotherapy, radiotherapy	S1 11(c) 21(I) S2 18(c) 18(I)	16 (c) 25 (I)	–	–	12 weeks	Dietary counselling to consume an energy intake of 1.7–1.95 × BEE in both S1 and S2, with use of ONS (Isocal drink) if required in S1 and with use of protein supplements (Pro-Mix as 25% of energy intake), Zn and Mg supplements in S2	Dietary counselling to consume an energy intake of 1.7–1.95 × BEE either provided with printed nutritional information or instructed by dietitians
Flynn and Leightty (1987)	10001	Head and neck (all stages); preoperative	19	17	–	–	10–21 days	Yes – given nutritional counselling including additional advice on how to meet their nutritional requirements	Nutritional counselling with suggestions on ways to cope with eating problems
Foster *et al.* (1980)	10000	Abdominal (stages unknown); radiotherapy	20	12	110%[a]	107%[a]	44 days	Given standard recommendations to reduce fibre intake	Standard recommendations to reduce fibre intake
Nayel *et al.* (1992)	10001	Head and neck (stages unknown); radiotherapy	11	12	–	–	10–31 days	–	–

[a] % usual body weight.
BEE, basal energy expenditure; S, supplemented; US, unsupplemented.

Table A4.33. Main findings of randomized controlled trials of oral nutritional supplementation in patients with malignancy in the community.

Trial	Energy intake	Body weight S	Body weight US	Body function	Clinical outcome	Finance
Arnold and Richter (1989)	Increase in TEI and TPI (S vs. US sig.) and similar VFI in S and US (which reduced over time)	−4.2 kg[a] (S vs. US NS)	−3.5 kg[a]	–	No difference in tumour response, side-effects, complications or mortality between S and US	–
Bounous et al. (1975)	NS difference in TEI between S and US, although S group closer (but below) ideal energy intake	+1.6 kg (S vs. US sig.)	−3.46 kg	Lower incidence of radiation induced diarrhoea in S vs. US (?) Sig. less reduction in TLC and Hb in S vs. US	–	–
Brown et al. (1980)	–	−0.5 kg (S vs. US NS) −1.7 kg in those unable to tolerate ONS	−1.6 kg	–	–	–
Douglass et al. (1978)	Increase in TEI from ~1500 kcal to ~2000 kcal in S, with ONS providing ~31% of energy intake (TEI 50% more than in US, ~1300 kcal)) (?)[b]	−6 (−2 to −12)% (?)	−5 (−10 to +9)% (?)	Trend towards improved DCH in S (NS)	No difference in survival between S and US	–
Elkort et al. (1981)	–	+1.18 kg (?)	1.54 kg (?)	NS difference in GI or haematological toxicity from chemotherapy (S vs. US NS)	NS difference in disease response to treatment	–
Evans et al. (1987)	S (S1 and S2) sig. increase in TEI in both l and c groups although 68% of pts were unable to consume 90% of their prescribed intake. VFI was similar in US (with counselling) and S1 and S2	S1 and S2 l −1.2%[c] S1 and S2 c +0.8%[c] (S vs. US NS)	l −3.1%[c] c +2.1%[c]	NS differences in tumour response rate or chemo-therapy toxicity	NS differences in survival times (interim analysis showed S1 had sig. worse survival than US or S2 and this arm of the trial was stopped early)	–
Flynn and Leightty (1987)	–	–	–	–	Fewer complications, shorter length of stay (by 3 days) in S (S vs. US ?)	–
Foster et al. (1980)	–	−1.0 kg (sig.) (S vs. US NS)	−1.4 kg (sig.)	–	–	–
Nayel et al. (1992)	–	+6.3%[a] (S vs. US sig.) Increase in TSF and MAC (S vs. US sig.)	−1.1%[a]	–	Less treatment delay, with a lower incidence of severe mucosal reactions in S (NS)	–

[a]Calculated mean.
[b]Analysis performed on 7 S and 7 US patients.
[c]Median presented.
?, uncertain if statistically significant; c, colorectal cancer; DCH, delayed cutaneous hypersensitivity; Hb, haemoglobin; l, non-small-cell lung cancer; NS, not significant; S, supplemented; sig., significant; TEI, total energy intake; TLC, total lymphocyte count; TPI, total protein intake; US, unsupplemented; VFI, voluntary food intake.

Table A4.34. Oral nutritional supplements used in non-randomized trials of patients with malignancy in the community.

Trial	ONS	ONS energy density	ONS prescribed	ONS energy (kcal) intake	ONS protein (g) intake	Toleration
Baker *et al.* (1977) A	Sustacal (Mead Johnson)	1 kcal ml^{-1}	–	–	–	–
Barber *et al.* (1999a)	Fish-oil-enriched (Abbott)	1.29 kcal ml^{-1}	619 kcal, 32.2 g P (+ 2 g EPA and 1 g DHA)	–	–	–
Barber *et al.* (2000)	Fish oil-enriched (21% P, 61% CHO, 18% F) (Abbott)	1.28 kcal ml^{-1}	607 kcal, 32.2 g P (2.2 g EPA, 0.96 g DHA per daily dose)	Median ~577	~31	Patients tolerated ONS well
Bounous *et al.* (1973) A	Elemental (no name)	–	–	26 kcal kg^{-1}	–	–
Crossland and Higgins (1977) A	Sustacal	1 kcal ml^{-1}	1080 kcal	–	–	–
McCarter *et al.* (1998)	S^1 Standard	1 kcal ml^{-1}	750 kcal	670	–	Cramping: (S^1) 55%, (S^2) 7%, (S^3) 38%
	S^2 Arginine-enriched	1 kcal ml^{-1}	750 kcal	653	–	Distension: (S^1) 55%, (S^2) 29%, (S^3) 62%
	S^3 Arginine/omega-3-enriched	1 kcal ml^{-1}	750 kcal	630	–	Abdominal cramps (*n* 3)
Ovesen and Allingstrup (1992)	S^1 Whole protein (Top Up)	1 kcal ml^{-1}	500+ kcal	419–222	20.8–11.2	
	S^2 Protein hydrolysate (Salvimulsin MCT)	1 kcal ml^{-1}		610–558 (1st and 2nd months)	32–28.8 (1st and 2nd months)	
Wallner *et al.* (1990)	Slim-Fast	1 kcal ml^{-1}	520–1040 kcal	–	–	Bloating (*n* 1)

A, abstract; CHO, carbohyrate; DHA, docosahexanoic acid; EPA, eicosapentanoic acid; F, fat; P, protein.

Table A4.35. Trial characteristics: community-based non-randomized trials of oral nutritional supplementation in patients with malignancy.

Trial	Design	Cancer/ treatments	No. S	No. US	Initial BMI S group	Initial BMI US group	Duration of ONS	Dietary counselling	Control group
Baker et al. (1977)	B	Breast (stages unknown); chemotherapy	6	6	–	–	3–9 months	No – self-selected diet	Self-selected diet only
Barber et al. (1999a)	B	Advanced pancreatic cancer; palliative care	18	18	–17.9% wt loss pre-trial (? time span) (S vs. US sig.)	–11.8% wt loss pre-trial (? time span)	3 weeks	–	Received 'full supportive care'
Barber et al. (2000)	C	Advanced pancreatic cancer; palliative care	16	–	17.7% wt loss pre-trial	–	3 weeks	–	–
Bounous et al. (1973) A	B	Abdominal (stages unknown); radiotherapy	4	6	–	–	6 weeks	–	–
Crossland and Higgins (1977) A	C	Head and neck (stages unknown); radiotherapy	30	–	–	–	6 weeks	–	–
McCarter et al. (1998) (RCT comparing three different ONS)	C	Oesophagus, stomach, pancreas (stages unknown); preoperative	S^1 11 S^2 14 S^3 13	–	S^1 94.5% IBW S^2 97.8% IBW S^3 94% IBW	–	1 week	Advised to consume in addition to meals	–
Ovesen and Allington (1992) (RCT comparing two different ONS)	C	Lung, ovary, breast (advanced stage); chemotherapy (n 12)	S^1 8 S^2 12	–	–	–	2 months	All seen by a dietitian and dietary counselling continued on an individual basis	–
Wallner et al. (1990)	B	Lung (l) and head/neck (h) (several stages); radiotherapy	l 20 h 20	l 20 h 20	l 26.3 h 23.5	–	7 weeks	Pts encouraged to consume other liquids/ solid food ad libitum	–

A, abstract; S, supplemented; US, unsupplemented.

Table A4.36. Main findings of non-randomized trials of oral nutritional supplementation in patients with malignancy in the community.

Trial	Energy intake	Body weight S	Body weight US	Body function	Clinical outcome	Finance
Baker et al. (1977)	–	–	–	–	–	–
Barber et al. (1999a)	'It is likely that the patients receiving the ONS consumed more calories and protein than those receiving supportive care' – no data	+1 kg (–0.1 kg to +2 kg) (+1.82%)	–2.8 kg (–3.7 kg to –1.7 kg) (–4.8%)	Sig. increase in transferrin in S but sig. decrease in albumin, transferrin and prealbumin and sig. increase in CRP in US	–	–
Barber et al. (2000)	–	+1 kg (median) (–0.25 to +1.75 kg, sig.) Increased LBM +0.75 kg (median) (0.1 kg to +1.6 kg)	–	*No change in overall REE. EE in response to feeding sig. increased and fat oxidation reduced to values similar to healthy control group Sig. increase in fasting insulin conc., NS change in fasting cortisol or glucose conc.*	–	–
Bounous et al. (1973) A	–	–	–	–	–	–
Crossland and Higgins (1977) A	–	–	–	Increased sense of well-being (?)	–	–
McCarter et al. (1998)	–	–	–	NS changes in mean lymphocyte mitogenesis, peripheral blood mononuclear cell production of cytokines (no differences between different ONS)	NS differences between groups in infectious or other complications or hospital stays	–
Ovesen and Allington (1992)	Increase in TEI in both groups, but sig. in S^2 only	S^1 –0.9 kg (NS) S^2 +1 kg (NS)	–	–	–	–
Wallner et al. (1990)	–	l –0.3 kg (S vs. US sig.) h –0.7 kg (S vs. US NS)	l –1.3 kg h –1.0 kg	–	–	–

conc., concentrations; CRP, C-reactive protein; EE, energy expenditure; h, head/neck cancer; l, lung cancer; NS, not significant; REE, resting energy expenditure; S, supplemented; sig., significant; TEI, total energy intake; US, unsupplemented.

that supplemented patients gained more weight or lost less weight than controls, but these changes were either not statistically significant (Brown et al., 1980; Foster et al., 1980; Evans et al., 1987) (lung) or not statistically evaluated (Bounous et al., 1975). The other trials showed a tendency for a greater gain/less loss in control patients (Douglass et al., 1978; Elkort et al., 1981; Evans et al., 1987; Arnold and Richter, 1989) (colorectal), although these were again not statistically significant. A weighted analysis of % weight change (from five RCT: Douglass et al., 1978; Foster et al., 1980; Elkort et al., 1981; Arnold and Richter, 1989; Nayel et al., 1992) suggested similar weight changes in supplemented and unsupplemented groups of patients (−2.0% versus −2.8%, no significant difference).

Four trials made some assessment of the changes in body composition with ONS (RCT: Elkort et al., 1981; Nayel et al., 1992; NRT: Ovesen and Allingstrup, 1992, Barber et al., 2000) (see Tables A4.33 and A4.36), but none reported significant improvements.

(III)/(IV) What effect do ONS have on the body function and clinical outcome of patients with malignancy in the community?

Trials have failed to show significant improvements in function or clinical outcome in cancer patients. This could be due to a lack of power from small studies, particularly in light of the heterogeneity of patient types.

There was remarkably little information about the effects of ONS on functional outcome measures and quality of life (see Table A4.33). Survival and tumour response rates appeared not to be influenced by supplementation, although power calculations would suggest that sample sizes were too small to detect changes in such parameters (Douglass et al., 1978; Elkort et al., 1981; Evans et al., 1987; Arnold and Richter, 1989). The reported functional benefits included fewer complications associated with radiotherapy treatment (Bounous et al., 1975;

Nayel et al., 1992) and surgical resection (Flynn and Leightty, 1987), and a slight reduction in the length of stay (Flynn and Leightty, 1987). None of these differences were statistically evaluated. It was suggested that some types of supplements (Elkort et al., 1981; Flynn and Leightty, 1987) might actually be detrimental in certain cancer patients. However, there was insufficient evidence to support this notion, as both studies involved an inadequate number of patients, some of whom were overweight. Indeed, the authors of these studies concluded that supplementation was inappropriate in such patients (Elkort et al., 1981; Flynn and Leightty, 1987). Therefore, it seems pragmatic not to recommend ONS to overweight cancer patients who are weight stable.

Supplementation of cancer patients generally did not produce functional benefits, but this may be partly because few studies systematically addressed these outcome measures, and those that did involved small groups of patients, or heterogeneous groups of patients in whom compliance with ONS was usually inadequately assessed.

(V) What are the effects of stopping ONS in patients with malignancy in the community?

Only two cancer trials made minor assessments of the effects of stopping supplements. One showed similar weight loss in supplemented and unsupplemented patients 14 weeks after supplementation had been stopped (Arnold and Richter, 1989). The other (Bounous et al., 1975) found that the change in weight and biochemical parameters persisted for 8 days after cessation of supplementation.

Summary of non-randomized community trials in patients with malignancy

Eight trials with non-randomized data were reviewed (summarized in Tables A4.34–A4.36). These involved patients with various types and stages of malignancy arising from the breast (Baker et al., 1977), GI tract (Bounous et al., 1973;

McCarter *et al.*, 1998), pancreas (Barber *et al.*, 1999a, 2000), head and neck (Crossland and Higgins, 1977; Wallner *et al.*, 1990) and lung (Wallner *et al.*, 1990). Three of these were reported as abstracts and so provided little information (Bounous *et al.*, 1973; Baker *et al.*, 1977; Crossland and Higgins, 1977). The studies were conducted during courses of chemotherapy (Baker *et al.*, 1977), radiotherapy (Bounous *et al.*, 1973; Crossland and Higgins, 1977; Wallner *et al.*, 1990), palliative care (Barber *et al.*, 1999a, 2000) or preoperatively (McCarter *et al.*, 1998) and the majority were of short duration (1–6 weeks). Details of supplements used can be seen in Table A4.34. Overall, these reports were lacking in crucial information relevant to this review, such as pre-existing nutritional status, changes in body structure and energy intake following supplementation and the amount of supplement taken. For example, very few studies documented pre-existing nutritional status (> 90% IBW: Wallner *et al.*, 1990; McCarter *et al.*, 1998) or recent weight loss (Barber *et al.*, 1999a, 2000) (see Table A4.35). In one of these trials (Wallner *et al.*, 1990), patients with lung cancer (initial BMI between 23 and 27 kg m^{-2}) receiving supplementation lost significantly less weight than those who were unsupplemented. Supplemented patients suffering from cancer of the head and neck had similar weight loss to the unsupplemented patients (Wallner *et al.*, 1990). In a couple of other trials, significant weight gain did occur with supplementation over time (Ovesen and Allingstrup, 1992; Barber *et al.*, 2000). Only one trial (Ovesen and Allingstrup, 1992) assessed changes in energy intake and indicated significant improvements in those patients consuming a peptide-based ONS during chemotherapy (see Table A4.36).

One of the few studies that made functional assessment reported an increased sense of well-being (and a decrease in weight loss) in patients receiving an ONS during 6 weeks of radiotherapy, although the changes were not statistically evaluated (Crossland and Higgins, 1977) (see Table A4.36). McCarter *et al.* (1998), in a small

trial of preoperative supplementation for 1 week, were unable to demonstrate any significant improvements in some immune parameters between three different ONS, although average ONS intake was reported to be > 600 kcal. Ultimately, as energy intake was typically not assessed (either dietary, supplement or total) in these studies, it was difficult to draw any conclusions about the effect of ONS on these parameters.

In conclusion, interpretation of these study findings was limited by involvement of a mixed group of patients with different cancer types and the limited amount of information provided. Therefore, conclusions about the effect of oral supplements on total energy intake, appetite and body function are difficult to form. Where information is provided about body structure, a positive effect of supplements has been noted. Ultimately further research in well designed trials is needed.

Oral supplementation, issues of palatability, dietary intervention and ETF

Dietary counselling and ETF are other strategies that may be used in cancer patients as ways to increase intake. The relative efficacy of these strategies, compared with ONS, requires investigation.

- A number of studies have assessed the palatability and acceptability of supplements in patients with various forms of cancer, who often suffered from anorexia, inadequate food intakes and the presence of taste changes induced either by the disease or by its treatment (Brown *et al.*, 1986; Parkinson *et al.*, 1987; Bolton *et al.*, 1990, 1992). These supplements have either been incorporated into food (Parkinson *et al.*, 1987) or taken singly (Brown *et al.*, 1986; Bolton *et al.*, 1990). Unfortunately, the assessments of palatability and preference have often been made over relatively short periods (< 1–3 days), often with small volumes of feed (e.g. 15 ml: Brown *et al.*, 1986) and so the long-term clinical relevance of the observations is unclear.

- Controlled studies comparing the effect of different types of ONS (composition, energy density) on food intake and appetite in patients are also lacking in the community. In the hospital setting, one trial comparing formulas of differing energy density in anorectic cancer patients observed no difference in total energy intakes (Ovesen, 1992).
- Although dietetic counselling has been reported to improve anthropometric parameters and total energy intake in cancer patients compared with control patients (Macia *et al.*, 1991), there remains a lack of controlled studies comparing the effects of oral commercial supplements with those involving foodstuffs in the community (see Chapter 6). Unfortunately, one study that involved both nutritional counselling and supplementation assessed very few outcome measures (body weight, energy intake, body function) (Flynn and Leightty, 1987).
- ETF is another therapeutic option for cancer patients with anorexia and inadequate energy intakes. One study showed benefits with ETF compared with oral feeding (including the use of oral supplements) in patients with head and neck cancer receiving radiation therapy (Hearne *et al.*, 1985) (see Chapter 7). There is a lack of controlled comparisons between cancer patients receiving ONS and those receiving ETF.

Renal Disease

Malnutrition is common in patients with end-stage renal disease, whether they are treated with haemodialysis or continuous ambulatory peritoneal dialysis (CAPD) (Mattern *et al.*, 1982; Bergstrom and Lindholm, 1993; see Chapter 2). Chronic anorexia and low nutritional intakes, combined with the effects of disease and dialysis, over prolonged periods of time, are contributing factors (Bergstrom and Lindholm, 1993). Therefore, effective forms of nutritional support to increase nutrient intake in these patients, who are typically out-patients living in their own homes, are warranted. How effective are ONS in this patient group?

Renal disease: present analysis

Two RCT and ten NRT were systematically reviewed to assess the efficacy of ONS in patients with renal disease (see Box A4.8). Most trials were undertaken in patients with chronic renal failure receiving dialysis (either haemodialysis or CAPD). ONS were typically well tolerated and the duration of supplementation ranged from 2 weeks to 6 months (see Tables A4.37–A4.39).

(I) What effect do ONS have on the voluntary food intake and total energy intake of patients with renal disease in the community?

ONS can increase energy and protein intakes in patients with chronic renal disease, including those on haemodialysis and CAPD. Data from RCT are needed.

Box A4.8. Key findings: effect of ONS in community patients with chronic renal disease.

Due to a lack of data from well-designed RCT in this patient group, it is difficult to form conclusions about the efficacy of ONS.

Nutritional intake and body weight: ONS may improve total energy and protein intakes and body weight in this patient group, but RCT are needed.

Body function and clinical outcome: the extent to which ONS use in patients with chronic renal failure can improve functional or clinical outcome is unknown and studies are required (one small RCT suggests that the duration of hospital admissions may be reduced).

Table A4.37. Oral nutritional supplements used in all trials of patients with renal disease in the community

Trial	ONS	ONS energy density	ONS prescribed	ONS energy (kcal) intake	ONS protein (g) intake	Toleration
Randomized controlled trials						
Kuhlmann et al. (1997) A	Renamil or Renapro (Rencare Bartz, Germany)	–	–	–	–	–
Wilson et al. (2001)	NuBasics (Nestlé) – drinks, soups or bars	1 kcal ml⁻¹ (drinks)	To increase P intake to 1.2 g kg⁻¹ and to meet energy requirements	–	–	–
Non-randomized trials						
Cockram et al. (1998)	S¹ Magnacal (Sherwood Medical) S² Nepro (Abbott) S³ FOS and beta-carotene ONS (3.7 g FOS, 750 iu vitamin A as beta-carotene per 237 ml)	– – –	To achieve intakes of 30 kcal kg⁻¹	S¹ 995/2375 (days 8–11/days12–21) S² 995/2280 S³ 995/2375	S¹ 69.7–83 S² 69.7–79.7 S³ 69.7–83	Intake averaged 99–93% of target volumes. Flatulence and diarrhoea occurred but NS changes in any GI symptoms vs. baseline in any group
Cuppari et al. (1994)	Liotécnica (Brazil; 10% P, 35% F, 55% CHO; powder reconstituted to drink)	1 kcal ml⁻¹	800 kcal, 19.6 g P	14 kcal kg⁻¹ day⁻¹ ~ 685 kcal	0.35 g kg⁻¹ day⁻¹ ~ 17 g	Well tolerated
Lynch et al. (1983)	Sumacal	2 kcal ml⁻¹	720 kcal	–	–	'Generally well tolerated without adverse effect'
Mareckova et al. (1995) A	Nutrilac Renal	–	To meet 20% of energy requirements	–	–	–
Ortiz et al. (1992)	Complete liquid ONS	–	236 ml	–	–	No side-effects
Patel and Raftery (1997)	Ensure Plus (Abbott) ProteinForte (Fresenius)	1.5 kcal ml⁻¹ 1 kcal ml⁻¹	200–300 kcal, 13–20 g P	–	–	–
Patel et al. (2000)	Ensure Plus (Abbott), Fortipudding (Nutricia), ProteinForte (Fresenius)	1.5 kcal ml⁻¹ 1.32 kcal g⁻¹ 1 kcal ml⁻¹	To meet intakes of 1.2 g kg⁻¹ P and 35 kcal kg⁻¹	~ 321 kcal	–	–
Smathers et al. (1992)	Sustacal (Mead Johnson), Instant Breakfast drink (Carnation), Ensure, Ensure Plus (Abbott)	–	Two to three 237 ml servings	–	–	Generally well accepted given between meals
Young et al. (1978)	Calnutrin (ONS with CHO, EAA and 0.3 g tyrosine) as powder drink	–	400 kcal	–	–	Several pts experienced nausea from the 2 ONS day⁻¹
Yulo et al. (1997) A	Benefit Bar	–	240 kcal	–	–	All tolerated ONS

CHO, carbohydrate; EAA, essential amino acids; F, fat; FOS, fructo-oligosaccharides; P, protein; iu, international units.

Table A4.38. Trial characteristics: community-based trials of oral nutritional supplementation in patients with renal disease (randomized controlled and non-randomized data).

Trial	Design	No. S	No. US	Initial BMI S group	Initial BMI US group	Duration of ONS	Dietary counselling	Control group
Randomized controlled trials								
Kuhlmann et al. (1997) A Malnourished haemodialysis patients	10000	4	4	–	–	3 months	–	–
Wilson et al. (2001) Malnourished haemodialysis patients with mild hypoalbuminaemia (duration of HD > 3 months)	10001	18	14	–	–	6 months	Yes – advice on liberalization of energy and P intakes	Dietary counselling (as given for intervention group)
Non-randomized trials								
Cockram et al. (1998) ESRD for at least 3 months and no recent hospitalizations (pts with evidence of malnutrition excluded)	C (RCT of different ONS)	S¹ 27 S² 26 S³ 26	–	Patients with evidence of malnutrition excluded	–	14 days	No – ONS given as sole source of nutrition	–
Cuppari et al. (1994) HD pts with signs of severe malnutrition	C	14 (n 10 finish)	–	86% IBW	–	4 months	All pts given advice to increase E and P intakes in HD unit (preceded ONS)	–
Lynch et al. (1983) Maintenance haemodialysis	C	9	–	–	–	3 months	–	–
Mareckova et al. (1995) A (non-English article, abstract reviewed) HD patients	C	–	–	–	–	3 weeks	–	–
Ortiz et al. (1992) A (non-English article, abstract reviewed) HD patients	C	6	–	–	–	2 months	–	–
Patel and Raftery (1997) CAPD pts (comparison of those already on ONS (for ~8 months) vs. those not on ONS due to lack of indication or refusal)	B	10[a]	12	22 (3)	26 (3)	8 weeks	–	–
Patel et al. (2000) Stable HD pts with low dietary protein intake	C	17	–	25.4 (3.4) (range 20.9–32)	–	2 months	–	–

Smathers et al. (1992) Peritoneal dialysis, socio-economically deprived, poor protein intake and/or peritonitis	C	13	–	–	–	3 months	ONS given after aggressive dietary counselling to increase HBV protein intake failed	–
Young et al. (1978) Chronic renal failure	C	7	–	–	–	2 months (1 month with added EAA)	–	–
Yulo et al. (1997) A Malnourished haemodialysis patients	C	25	–	–	–	6 months	–	–

[a]S sig. older than US group.

A, abstract; E, energy; EAA, essential amino acids; ESRD, end-stage renal disease; HD, haemodialysis; HBV, high biological value; P, protein; S, supplemented; US, unsupplemented.

Supplementation increased total energy intake in the one RCT (abstract) that made such an assessment, but this was not statistically evaluated (Kuhlmann *et al.*, 1997). All of the NRT trials that assessed changes in nutritional intake showed significant improvements in total energy intake with ONS (Lynch *et al.*, 1983; Cuppari *et al.*, 1994; Mareckova *et al.*, 1995; Patel and Raftery, 1997; Patel *et al.*, 2000), and most (80%, *n* 4) documented significant increases in total protein intakes too (Cuppari *et al.*, 1994; Mareckova *et al.*, 1995; Patel and Raftery, 1997; Patel *et al.*, 2000) (see Table A4.39). In one of these trials, dietary counselling to increase energy and protein intakes was also given (Cuppari *et al.*, 1994) (see Table A4.38).

No formal assessments were made of the effects of ONS on appetite. However, two NRT (Cuppari *et al.*, 1994; Patel *et al.*, 2000) suggested that voluntary food intake was unchanged (over a 2-month period) or improved (after 4 months) during the period of supplementation when compared with baseline (> 90% of ONS energy additive (iii) (see Chapter 5)), although the lack of a control group means that improvements in clinical condition could have contributed. Over a 2-month ONS period, voluntary food intake remained unchanged.

Although ONS were typically well tolerated, as Table A4.37 shows, very few studies reported ONS intakes (three NRT: Cuppari *et al.*, 1994; Cockram *et al.*, 1998; Patel *et al.*, 2000).

(IA) IS THE TIMING OF SUPPLEMENTATION IMPORTANT?
Conclusions about the best timing for consuming ONS in this patient group cannot be made. Although one trial (Smathers *et al.*, 1992) advised patients to take ONS between meals, no assessments of food and supplement intakes were reported.

(II) What effect do ONS have on the body weight and composition of patients with renal disease in the community?

There is insufficient evidence to say conclusively that ONS increase body weight/improve body structure in patients with renal disease, due to a lack of RCT. Greater weight gain in supplemented patients than in unsupplemented patients was evident in the one RCT that made such assessments, although the differences were small and not statistically analysed (Kuhlmann *et al.*, 1997). The initial nutritional status was also not described.

Weight gain was also documented in four other trials, but these lacked a control group (Lynch *et al.*, 1983; Ortiz *et al.*, 1992; Cuppari *et al.*, 1994; Patel *et al.*, 2000). Similarly, the trials that documented increases in body fat (using upper-arm anthropometry) (Ortiz *et al.*, 1992; Cuppari *et al.*, 1994) or a lack of change in muscle mass (Cuppari *et al.*, 1994) were also non-randomized.

(III)/(IV) What effect do ONS have on the body function and clinical outcome of patients with renal disease in the community?

It is not known whether ONS can improve functional or clinical outcome measures in patients with renal disease, including those on dialysis, due to a lack of assessments and an absence of well-designed RCT. Although a number of biochemical and metabolic changes were observed following a period of ONS in patients with renal disease (e.g. changes in albumin, transferrin, urea kinetics), there was no record of any functional outcome measures. Case-studies in the literature have indicated that improvements in cell-mediated immunity may follow 3 months of ONS (Hak *et al.*, 1982).

The only trial that made some assessment of clinical outcome showed a shorter length of hospital stay (by 36 days) in supplemented than in unsupplemented patients on haemodialysis (RCT; difference not significant, small sample size) (Wilson *et al.*, 2001). These patients were also given dietary counselling.

(V) What are the effects of stopping ONS in patients with renal disease in the community?

In patients with renal disease, some retention of weight gain may occur after ONS

Table A4.39. Main findings of trials (randomized controlled and non-randomized) of oral nutritional supplementation in patients with renal disease in the community.

Trial	Energy intake	Body weight S	Body weight US	Body function	Clinical outcome	Finance
Randomized controlled trials						
Kuhlmann *et al.* (1997) A	Increase in TEI in S (? sig.)	+1.17 kg (S vs. US ?)	+0.25 kg	–	–	–
Wilson *et al.* (2001)	–	–	–	Took S 3.2 (1.7) months to 'replete' (= albumin ≥ 3.8 g day^{-1} for 2 months) vs. 3.5 (1.2) months for US In 3-month follow-up, 61% of S achieved and maintained repletion even though ONS had been stopped (vs. 14% US, S vs. US ?)	S shorter hospital stay (71 days) than US (107 days) (S vs. US NS)	–
Non-randomized trials						
Cockram *et al.* (1998)	–	–	–	S[3] had less constipation than S[1] and S[2] Increase in serum calcium and calcium–protein product in S[2] and S[3]	–	–
Cuppari *et al.* (1994)	TEI sig. increased from 27 kcal kg^{-1} to 43 kcal kg^{-1} at day 120 (increase of 59%) TPI sig. increased from 1 g kg^{-1} to 1.57 g kg^{-1} (increase of 4.7%) (VFI increased (NS) during ONS from 27 kcal kg^{-1} to 30 kcal kg^{-1}) ONS > 100% energy additive	+3.1% (sig.) Sig. increase in MAC (+3.5%), TSF (+21.5%), % body fat (13.8%) and body fat (19.4%) No change in MAMA or LBM	–	*Sig. increase in PCR (1.06 to 1.22)* *No change in biochemical or haematological indices*	–	–
Lynch *et al.* (1983)	Sig. increase in TEI (from 1983 kcal to 2630 kcal in 1st week)	+1.51 kg (sig.)	–	–	–	–
Mareckova *et al.* (1995) A	Sig. increase in TEI (25.9 to 30 kcal kg^{-1}) and TPI (0.87 to 0.95 g kg^{-1})	–	–	*Sig. increase in serum albumin and Whitehead's quotient. Sig. increase in plasma EAA and BCAA*	–	–
Ortiz *et al.* (1992)	–	+2 kg (sig.) Sig. increase in TSF	–	*No change in urea kinetics*	–	–

Continued

Table A4.39. *Continued*

Trial	Energy intake	Body weight S	Body weight US	Body function	Clinical outcome	Finance
Patel and Raftery (1997)	Sig. increase in TEI from 27 kcal kg^{-1} to 33 kcal kg^{-1} (all patients increased energy intake, S vs. US sig.) Sig. increase in TPI (0.92 to 1.24 g kg^{-1}; S vs. US sig.) NS changes in phosphorus, potassium or sodium intakes	–	–	–	–	–
Patel *et al.* (2000)	Sig. increase in TEI from 1202 (230) kcal to 1500 (251) kcal and TPI (48 (11) g to 72 (9) g) VFI unchanged (–23 kcal, ~93% ONS energy additive) after 2 months of ONS and at 8 months (ONS stopped for 6 months)	+0.2 kg at 2 months +1.3 kg at 8 months (sig. increase after ONS stopped)	–	*Sig. increase in PCR (returned to baseline after ONS stopped)*		–
Smathers *et al.* (1992)	–	–	–	*54% had increase in serum albumin conc. (+4.7 g l^{-1})*	–	–
Young *et al.* (1978)	–	–	–	*Only when S continued with EAA was there a sig. increase in plasma transferrin, prealbumin and albumin (values maintained after ONS stopped for 1 month) NS changes in other acute-phase proteins*	–	–
Yulo *et al.* (1997) A	–	–	–		–	–

PCR, protein catabolic rate; S, supplemented; US, unsupplemented; TEI, total energy intake; sig., significant; NS, not significant; TPI, total protein intake; VFI, voluntary food intake; EAA, essential amino acids; BCAA, branched-chain amino acids; A, abstract; MAMA, mid-arm muscle area.

have stopped but more research is required to ascertain this. A couple of trials made assessments after ONS had stopped (Patel *et al.*, 2000; Wilson *et al.*, 2001). In one trial, weight gain (further 1.3 kg) had continued 6 months after ONS had stopped, although the improvement in protein catabolic rate was not sustained once ONS were stopped (Patel *et al.*, 2000). In the other, randomized, trial (Wilson *et al.*, 2001), at the 3-month follow-up after ONS had stopped, supplemented patients were more likely to have achieved or maintained 'repletion' (61%) than unsupplemented patients (14%) (maintaining serum albumin within ideal range). No assessments of nutritional intake or body function were made after ONS had stopped.

Summary of non-randomized community trials in patients with chronic renal disease

Ten NRT that compared ONS with no nutritional support in patients with chronic renal disease were also reviewed (these are summarized in Tables A4.37–A4.39). A small clinical trial (*n* 11) (Lynch *et al.*, 1983) evaluated the effect of offering to patients undergoing haemodialysis a maltodextrin caloric liquid supplement. Compared with a 2-week baseline period, patients gained statistically significant amounts of weight after 12 weeks of supplementation (see Table A4.39). The authors were able to verify an absence of oedema/lack of fluid accumulation as the cause. During the first week of supplementation, total energy intake, assessed by 3-day diet diaries, was also significantly increased (1983 to 2630 kcal) compared with baseline. Whether this significant increase persisted over the study duration was not clear, although from graphic representation it appeared that some decline in total energy intake occurred but accurate quantification was not possible. Although the authors commented that there was no apparent decrease in normal food intake, no data were given. Furthermore, no functional assessments were made in the study.

Indeed, none of the trials presented any data on changes in function or clinical outcome with ONS. However, four other trials did present information on the changes in energy intake with ONS (Cuppari *et al.*, 1994; Mareckova *et al.*, 1995; Patel and Raftery, 1997; Patel *et al.*, 2000), and all indicated significant increases in both energy and protein intakes. Two of these trials also documented little change or an increase in voluntary food intake during supplementation (Cuppari *et al.*, 1994; Patel *et al.*, 2000). Significant weight gain was also documented in a further three trials (Ortiz *et al.*, 1992; Cuppari *et al.*, 1994; Patel *et al.*, 2000) (in addition to Lynch *et al.*, 1983, described above), although in one trial this only occurred after ONS had been stopped (Patel *et al.*, 2000).

Although this review concentrates primarily on mixed, macronutrient ONS, the use of a single macronutrient ONS can also produce benefits. A couple of trials in patients on haemodialysis have documented increases in total energy intake and body weight (fat and lean mass) with the use of glucose polymers added to drinks and food (Allman *et al.*, 1990; Milano *et al.*, 1998). The weight gain was sustained after supplementation had stopped in both of these trials.

Renal disease: other reviews

A review of studies of enteral nutrition in patients with chronic renal failure indicated that positive effects on anthropometric and biochemical variables occurred (Akner and Cederholm, 2001), as this quote also reflects:

> Preliminary studies indicate that ONS has a positive effect on nutritional status of patients with end stage renal disease and could potentially decrease ... costs in this population   (Fedje *et al.*, 1996)

There is, however, a need for RCT to assess the impact of ONS on functional and clinical outcome parameters in patients with chronic renal disease, on different forms of dialysis.

Other Conditions

This section merely summarizes a number of other trials of supplementation programmes in a variety of different disease and treatment categories (see Tables A4.40–A4.42 for studies in GI surgical and congestive heart failure patients and Tables A4.43–A4.45 for studies in children failing to thrive).

Post-GI surgery

Box A4.9. Key findings: effect of ONS in community patients post-gastrointestinal surgery.

Nutritional intake: ONS use in surgical patients discharged from hospital can effectively increase total energy and protein intakes. Voluntary food intake appears not to be suppressed and may even be increased during ONS.

Body weight: ONS can significantly improve body weight and muscle mass.

Body function and clinical outcome: the benefits of ONS regarding functional or clinical outcomes, when used in surgical patients after discharge into the community, have not been fully investigated. No improvements in well-being have been found, although assessments close to the time of discharge have not been made (i.e. within 1 month).

Jensen and Hessov, 1997 (randomized controlled)

This well-designed study categorized a wide range of patients undergoing GI surgery according to age ($<$ and $>$ 75 years) and type of surgery (elective or acute emergency). It also randomized them at discharge to receive either ONS plus dietary counselling with the aim to increase total protein intake (to 1.5 g protein kg^{-1} body weight) or to a control group (given no supplement or dietary counselling) (see Table A4.41). The mean BMI

for each of the patient groups varied between 22 and 26 kg m^{-2} and the rates of weight loss before starting the study also varied between groups (1.7–6.9% over 3 months). Food intake was assessed using a 3-day food record and compliance checked by home visits if needed. Four months after discharge, ONS was found to be associated with a significant increase in absolute total energy intake in those under 75 years (+262 kcal (1.1 MJ)) and those over 75 years (+643 kcal (2.7 MJ)) compared with controls, although these increases were not significant when calculated in relation to LBM (see Table A4.42). This could be due to the heterogeneity of patients in respect of nutritional status and the type of surgery undertaken. Similarly, protein intakes were significantly increased by ~22% compared with the unsupplemented patients. Both supplemented and unsupplemented (control) patients increased their food intake during the period of study, and so calculation of the effect of the supplemental energy on food intake needed to encompass this. In the supplemented patients $<$ 75 years, comparison with the control group suggested that 53% of the supplement energy was additional to that from food (in those who were $>$ 75 years, the amounts of supplement taken were too small). Unlike most studies, this one undertook some assessment of appetite, although this was global and not specifically related to the intake of supplements. During the last week of hospital stay, 68% of patients scored their appetite as being below normal but, at follow-up, most reported a normal appetite. After 4 months, supplemented patients (all types) had a significantly greater increase in weight than unsupplemented patients (see Table A4.42), with significantly greater increases in LBM (1.4 kg more than controls) and fat mass as well. The authors also reported on the structural changes that occurred in the subgroups of patients. Supplemented elective patients ($<$ 75 years) had significantly greater gains in weight, LBM and fat mass at 4 months than controls. Supplemented patients ($<$ 75 years) who had undergone surgery for an acute condition had 3.2 kg

Table A4.40. Oral nutritional supplements used in randomized controlled trials of other conditions (GI surgery/congestive heart failure).

Trial	ONS	ONS energy density	ONS prescribed	ONS energy (kcal) intake	ONS protein (g) intake	Toleration
Jensen and Hessov (1997)	Top Up special or Plus One (Ferrosan, Søberg, Denmark)	1 kcal ml⁻¹ 0.6 kcal ml⁻¹	To help meet protein intake of 1.5 g kg⁻¹	25–34 kJ kg⁻¹ LBMᵃ	–	–
Keele *et al.* (1997)	Fortisip (Nutricia)	1.5 kcal ml⁻¹	*Ad libitum*	S-S 47–231 US-S 84–221	S-S 1.71–8.55 US-S 2.74–7.41	–
Broqvist *et al.* (1994)	Biosorb 1500 (Pharmacia)	1.5 kcal ml⁻¹	750 kcal, 30 g P	~570	~23	–

ᵃSubdivided by age (< and > 75 years).
P, protein; S-S, supplemented as in-patient and out-patient; US-S, supplemented as out-patient only.

Table A4.41. Trial characteristics: community-based randomized controlled trials of oral nutritional supplementation in patients with other conditions.

Trial	Design	No. S	No. US	Initial BMI S group	Initial BMI US group	Duration of ONS	Dietary counselling	Control group
Jensen and Hessov (1997) Post-GI surgery	10001	13 (a) 27 (e)	22(a) 25(e)	<75 years S 22.4 (a) S 25.5 (e) >75 years 22.7 (a) 23.7 (e)	<75 years 26.4(a) 22.8(e) >75 years 21.9(a) 24.4(e)	4 months	Yes – dietitian advised about choice of food and ONS to increase nutritional intake, especially protein	Discharged without dietetic advice
Keele *et al.* (1997) Post-GI surgery	10001	43	43	22.8–23.6ᵇ		4 monthsᵃ	– Pts selected their own food at mealtimes and drinks and snacks were readily available	Standard hospital diet prior to discharge
Broqvist *et al.* (1994) Congestive heart failure	10110	9	13	94% IBW	100% IBW	8 weeks	No – pts told not to change their dietary habits	500 ml diluted placebo

ᵃOut-patient phase of trial, randomly allocated to supplementation for ~7 days in hospital, randomized on discharge to supplementation or control group and followed up after 4 months.
ᵇMean data for groups at the end of the in-patient phase.
(a), acute patients; (e), elective patients; pts, patients; S, supplemented; US, unsupplemented.

Table A4.42. Main findings of randomized controlled trials of oral nutritional supplementation in patients with other conditions in the community.

Trial	Energy intake	Body weight S	Body weight US	Body function	Clinical outcome	Finance
Jensen and Hessov (1997)	Sig. increase in TEI in < 75 years (+262 kcal) and > 75 years (+643 kcal) (S vs. US sig.). Sig. increase in TPI. Increase in VFI in S and US In < 75 years, ~53% of ONS additive	+ 4.6 (2.6–6.6) kg (sig.) (S vs. US sig.) LBM +3.1 (2.1–4.1) kg (S vs. US sig.)	+ 1.9 (0.7–3.1) kg (sig.) LBM +1.7 (0.9–2.5) kg	–	–	–
Keele et al. (1997)	Sig. higher TEI in S-S 1 month post-discharge than in US-US and S-US. Sig. higher TEI in US-S 4 months post-discharge than S-US Increase in TPI NS at any month NS difference in VFI between S and US during hospital ONS period, with S having sig. greater TEI and TPI for 1st 4 days	S-S 4.5 kg[a] US-S 4.5 kg (S vs. US NS) S-US 3.0 kg (see ONS hospital review)	US-US 3.2 kg	NS improvements in well-being post-discharge with ONS (S-S; US-S) (see hospital ONS review for functional changes during hospital period)	–	–
Broqvist et al. (1994)	Sig. increase in TEI, TPI and fat intake (S vs. US sig. for TEI) (TEI 2420 kcal vs. US 1908 kcal) VFI did not change in either S or US	+1.17% Sig. increase in TSF	–0.26%	NS change in max. work capacity or in respiratory gas data (expiratory minute volume : oxygen uptake) No changes in concentrations of ATP, creatine or glycogen in muscle	–	–

[a]Calculated from graph, change from discharge weight.

S-S, supplemented as in-patient and out-patient; US-S, supplemented as out-patient only; S-US, supplemented as in-patient and not as out-patient; US-US, not supplemented; S, supplemented; US, unsupplemented; sig., significant; NS, not significant; TEI, total energy intake; TPI, total protein intake; VFI, voluntary food intake.

Table A4.43. Oral nutritional supplements used in non-randomized trials of other conditions (failure to thrive).

Trial	ONS	ONS energy density	ONS prescribed	ONS energy (kcal) intake	Toleration
Tolia (1995)	Pediasure or Ensure (Abbott)	1 kcal ml⁻¹ 1 kcal ml⁻¹	–	–	3/7 patients changed to tube feeding due to insufficient oral intake

Table A4.44. Trial characteristics: community based non-randomized trials of oral nutritional supplementation in patients with other conditions (failure to thrive).

Trial	Design	No. S	No. US	Initial BMI S group	Initial BMI US group	Duration of ONS	Dietary counselling	Control group
Tolia (1995)	C	4	–	–	–	21–60 months	Increases in energy intake using normal dietary constituents had been tried initially in all infants but were unsuccessful	–

Table A4.45. Main findings of non-randomized trials of oral nutritional supplementation in patients with other conditions in the community (failure to thrive).

Trial	Energy intake	Body weight S	Body weight US	Body function	Clinical outcome	Finance
Tolia (1995)	Sig. increase in TEI (no data)	–	–	75% improved growth percentiles (weight, height or head circumference)	–	–

S, supplemented; US, unsupplemented; sig., significant; TEI, total energy intake.

greater weight gain than controls, but this was not significant. In this group of patients, following supplementation, the increase in LBM was significant only at the 2-month follow-up and the increase in fat mass was significant at the 4-month follow-up. In patients over 75 years (following elective or acute surgery), supplementation after discharge did not significantly increase weight, LBM or fat mass compared with the unsupplemented group. One possible reason for this is the small sample size of the acute surgical patients. Unfortunately, no associated functional assessments were undertaken.

Keele et al., 1997 (randomized controlled)

This study involved randomization of patients following GI surgery into one of four study groups: 1 – supplemented as in- and out-patients (S-S); 2 – unsupplemented as in- and out-patients (US-US); 3 – unsupplemented as in-patients, supplemented as out-patients (US-S); 4 – supplemented as in-patients, unsupplemented as out-patients (S-US) (Tables A4.40 and A4.41). Although patients were encouraged to take ONS *ad libitum* (small, frequent servings between meals), the average supplement intake was relatively small (< 231 kcal, Table A4.40) and declined during the 4 months of the study. The authors specifically pinpointed statistically significant differences between the groups in total energy intake (assessed with 4-day food diaries) as follows: group 1 (S-S) > group 3 (US-S) and group 2 (US-US) at the first month after discharge; group 3 (US-S) > group 4 (S-US) at 2 months after discharge. Overall, total energy intake in the two groups receiving the supplement was relatively constant over the 4 months (2179 to 2068 kcal in S-S, 2084 to 2323 kcal in US-S), and the energy from food was typically higher compared with the unsupplemented groups (not statistically evaluated). Hence energy from supplementation during the first 2 months of study was apparently additional to that taken orally. Our calculations suggested that from ~76 to 335% of the supplement energy was additive

(method (ii), see Chapter 5), but this could be subject to error because of the small amounts of supplement ingestion (from 47 to 230 kcal). Similarly, after 4 months, all comparisons between supplemented and unsupplemented groups indicated that the relatively small supplement energy intake remained entirely additional to food intake, with the increase in total energy intake ~134–335% of the supplement energy consumed. No significant increases in protein intake occurred during the 4 months of supplementation. All groups gained weight following discharge (Table A4.42) but the differences between supplemented and unsupplemented patients were not statistically significant. MAC, TSF, MAMC and hand-grip strength were also unchanged. Furthermore, no significant improvements in fatigue or well-being were achieved after 4 months of supplementation. Structural and functional improvements may have occurred more rapidly in the supplemented patients but this difference may have disappeared by the time of the assessment, which was 4 months after discharge.

A weighted analysis of % weight change from these two studies in post-surgical patients suggested that greater weight gain was evident in supplemented patients (+5.5% versus +2.8%).

Congestive heart failure

Broqvist et al., 1994 (randomized controlled)

In this double-blind, placebo-controlled trial, the supplemented group had significantly higher TSF than the placebo group after 8 weeks of ONS (560 kcal taken between meals), but no other significant changes in anthropometry were noted. However, patients were on average 98% of IBW at the start of the trial. ONS did not increase the low levels of adenosine triphosphate (ATP), creatine and glycogen in the muscle of these patients with congestive heart failure. In addition, despite significant increases in the daily intakes of energy and protein, ONS did not change the maximal work capacity or respiratory gas data (expiratory minute volume, oxygen uptake) in these patients.

A recent narrative review of the use of ONS and ETF in patients with chronic heart failure (total of four trials; two ONS trials) concluded that the nutritional treatment of protein-energy malnutrition (PEM) in this patient group had been insufficiently studied (Akner and Cederholm, 2001).

Paediatric – failure to thrive

Tolia, 1995 (uncontrolled)

The main result from this small study of ONS was an improvement in growth percentiles in 75% (*n* 3) of infants with failure to thrive over a period of up to 36 months (Tables A4.43–A4.45). This was associated with a significant increase in total energy intake, although no data were given.

Of the original seven patients selected for study, three were unable to take sufficient amounts orally and were tube-fed. Of those that did take the supplement orally, the only one that did not show improvements in growth had poor compliance. All attempts to wean patients off supplements were accompanied by weight loss.

General Review

Jamieson et al., 1997

This review examined the change in QOL (Nottingham health profile) experienced by different groups of patients receiving various types of nutritional support. The subjects, who were followed up as out-patients for a variety of chronic diseases, had either a BMI < 20 kg m^{-2} or between 20 and 25 kg m^{-2}. Unfortunately, analysis was not performed according to the type of nutritional support, and so it was not possible to examine the change in QOL experienced by patients receiving ONS alone. However, nutritional support produced significant improvements in all categories of QOL (energy, pain, emotion, sleep, social isolation, mobility) but only in patients with an initial BMI < 20 kg m^{-2}. These improvements were accompanied by gain in weight and LBM. No such improvements were observed in patients within the BMI range 20–25 kg m^{-2}.

Note

[1]A dash has been used in the tables throughout this appendix where information was not provided in the reviewed trial (and could not be calculated).

Appendix 5

A Detailed Analysis of the Effects of Enteral Tube Feeding in the Hospital Setting

Chapter 7 provided an overall summary of the effects of enteral tube feeding (ETF) obtained from a combined analysis of different groups of patients in the hospital setting. Here, a more detailed review, addressing each review question, is provided, according to individual patient groups. The patient groups are presented alphabetically.

Burns (Randomized and Non-randomized Data)

The exaggerated catabolic response that is typically seen in patients hospitalized with burn injuries, coupled with exudation of nutrients through the damaged skin, means that requirements for energy, protein and other nutrients are high (Bartlett *et al.*, 1977; Heibert *et al.*, 1981). These requirements are unlikely to be met by an oral diet as patients are frequently anorectic, and in the early stages after burn injury, gastric stasis may lead to poor tolerance of an oral diet. As this quote states,

> Failure to recognise and effectively provide nutritional therapy for these patients will result in rapid depletion of fuels and nutrients essential for their convalescence
> (Bartlett *et al.*, 1977).

Burns: present analysis

The efficacy of ETF in this group of patients has been investigated in two randomized controlled trials (RCT) and one non-randomized trial (NRT) in patients hospitalized with burn injuries (Chiarelli *et al.*, 1990; Hansbrough and Hansbrough, 1993; Jenkins *et al.*, 1994) (see Box A5.1). One RCT compared patients receiving early ETF following burn injury (within 4.4 h (n 29) (Chiarelli *et al.*, 1990)) with those receiving no nutritional support (n 20). The other RCT (Jenkins *et al.*, 1994) studied the use of ETF before, during and after operative procedures in burns patients (n 40) compared with withholding this form of nutritional support at such times (n 40) (see Tables A5.1–A5.3[1]). These studies suggested that ETF, via a nasoenteric tube, was well tolerated in patients hospitalized with acute burns for periods of up to 4 weeks (see Table A5.1). Other case reports have also indicated the value of ETF as part of the treatment of burns patients (Bartlett *et al.*, 1977).

The trials reviewed and discussed here are those that have used a 'standard', commercial, nutritional formula (Hansbrough and Hansbrough, 1993; Jenkins *et al.*, 1994) or a hospital-made formula (Chiarelli *et al.*, 1990). However, a number of trials compar-

Table A5.1. Enteral tube feeds used in trials of patients with burns in hospital (randomized and non-randomized data).

Trial	ETF	ETF energy density	ETF prescribed	ETF energy (kcal) provision	ETF protein (g) provision	Toleration	Timing and pattern of ETF
Randomized controlled trials							
Chiarelli *et al.* (1990)	Mixtures (emulsion of eggs, carrots, apples, meat, oil, cheese, vitamins) (i) 44 g P, 32 g F, 125 g CHO l⁻¹; (ii) 79 g P, 81 g F, 230 g CHO l⁻¹	(i) 0.94 kcal ml⁻¹ (ii) 1.9 kcal ml⁻¹	To meet energy requirements for wt maintenance	3112 (2750–3450)	125 (116–132)	Well tolerated	Early ETF, immediately after burn injury (4.4 h after burn) on admission to H
Jenkins *et al.* (1994)	High-protein modular tube feed	–	1.3 × REE	–	–	No aspiration	Continuous (?24 h) given before, during and after operative procedures
Non-randomized trials							
Hansbrough and Hansbrough (1993)	Criticare HNᵃ (elemental diet, Mead Johnson), changed to Traumacal (Mead Johnson) as tolerated	–	1.5 × predicted BEE	–	–	.	ETF started within 6–10 h after burn injury, stopped for operative procedures and resumed a few h after surgery

ᵃFormula dilution in first few h after admission. As full-strength elemental diet tolerated, patients changed on to Traumacal.
BEE, basal energy expenditure; CHO, carbohydrate; F, fat; h, hours; H, hospital; P, protein; REE, resting energy expenditure; wt, weight.

Table A5.2. Trial characteristics: hospital-based trials of enteral tube feeding in patients with burns (randomized and non-randomized data).

Trial	Design	Diagnosis	No. ETF	No. CON	Initial BMI ETF group	Initial BMI CON group	Duration of ETF	Tube type	Control group
Randomized controlled trials									
Chiarelli *et al.* (1990) Italy	1–1001	Acute burns (25–60% of body surface area)	10	10	–	–	Up to 28 days?	NG tube	Did not receive ETF until > 48 h after hospitalization (58 h after burn injury)
Jenkins *et al.* (1994) USA Perioperative ETF	10001	Acute burns > 10% total body surface area	40[a]	40	–	–	Up to 4 weeks	Nasoduodenal tube (Frederick Miller)	ETF withheld before, during and immediately after surgical procedures
Non-randomized trials									
Hansbrough and Hansbrough (1993) (country?)	C	Acute burns > 20% (i) 20–30% (ii) 31–44% (iii) > 44%	46	–	–	–	Up to 10 days	NG tube	–

[a]ETF: significantly larger proportion of patients with third-degree burns, significantly more surgical procedures and antibiotic therapy.
CON, control; BMI, body mass index; NG, nasogastric.

Table A5.3. Main findings of enteral tube feeding trials in hospitalized patients with burns (randomized and non-randomized data).

Trial	Energy/nutrient intake	Wt change ETF	Wt change CON	Function	Clinical outcome	Finance
Randomized controlled trials						
Chiarelli *et al.* (1990)	ETF intakes 3112 kcal in both groups (CON tube feeding started later). No cumulative data. Positive N balance occurred sig. earlier in ETF (8.8 days) vs. CON (24 days)	ETF vs. CON NS	−5.4% (± 3.3%)	–	Shorter H stay by 20 days (ETF 69 days, CON 89 days, ETF vs. CON NS)	–
Jenkins *et al.* (1994)	ETF cumulative energy balance: +2673 kcal sig. greater than CON (−7899 kcal)	–	–	*ETF required sig. less supplemental albumin with weeks 1 and 2 than CON to maintain serum levels*	ETF sig. fewer wound infections than CON (2 vs. 9, sig.) NS differences in length of stay (34 vs. 33 days), incidence of clinical sepsis, pneumonia or mortality (5 vs. 4 deaths)	–
Non-randomized trials						
Hansbrough and Hansbrough (1993)	On day 2: (i) TEI 1855 kcal; (ii) TEI > 2000 kcal; (iii) TEI > 2500 kcal. TEI markedly reduced on surgical day (NBM and ETF stopped)	–	–	–	–	–

CON, control; H, hospital; N, nitrogen; NBM, nil by mouth; NS, not significant; sig., significant; TEI, total energy intake.

ing the efficacy of specialized feeds with other enteral formulas have been undertaken in patients with burn injury (Gottschlich *et al.*, 1990; Saffle *et al.*, 1997). These are feeds typically enriched with nutrients that may influence the immune and inflammatory systems (omega-3 fatty acids, arginine, RNA, some micronutrients). These are discussed briefly later in this appendix.

Whilst some trials in this patient group have used hospital-made feeds for ETF (Chiarelli *et al.*, 1990; Dhanraj *et al.*, 1997), it is generally recognized that commercial formulas have a higher, more consistent nutrient density (macro- and micronutrients), are easier to administer (no preparation or mixing) and are less susceptible to contamination with microorganisms (in production or administration). The efficacy of ETF in burns patients is discussed below by addressing the four main review questions.

Box A5.1. Key findings: effect of ETF in hospital patients with burns.

Nutritional intake: ETF can provide a valuable source of nutrients in the postburn injury treatment phase, when patients are often nil by mouth. Continuous ETF regimens may be most effective at ensuring that nutritional requirements are met.

Body weight: weight loss may be reduced with ETF.

Clinical outcome: there may be benefits to clinical outcome (reduced complications, shorter hospital stays) in this patient group but large RCT are needed to fully assess the impact of ETF on various outcomes (functional, clinical, financial).

(I) What effect does ETF have on the voluntary food intake and total energy intake of patients in hospital with burns?

ETF enables patients with acute burn injury, who are frequently nil by mouth due to injury, unconsciousness and operative procedures (and postoperative ileus),

to maintain a substantial energy, nitrogen and micronutrient intake. The results of two RCT suggested that, by starting ETF early after burn injury (Chiarelli *et al.*, 1990) and continuing ETF throughout the perioperative periods (Jenkins *et al.*, 1994), cumulative energy and nitrogen balances were significantly greater than in those in whom ETF was withheld (Table A5.3). Indeed, one NRT (Hansbrough and Hansbrough, 1993) simply highlighted the marked reductions in total energy intakes that occurred on surgical days if ETF was stopped, especially when patients were nil by mouth for prolonged periods of time. In addition, a retrospective review of the early use of ETF after burn injury (< 48 h) in 25 patients indicated significantly higher energy and protein intakes compared with when ETF was delayed (Garrel *et al.*, 1991). In order to ensure that the nutritional requirements of burns patients are met, it was also suggested that continuous 24 h ETF was more effective than intermittent modes of feed delivery (Heibert *et al.*, 1981).

(II) What effect does ETF have on the body weight and composition of patients in hospital with burns?

With substantial improvements in energy balance produced by ETF, it is likely that ETF can attenuate the weight loss typically observed in patients with burn injuries. However, only one RCT made assessments of changes in weight with ETF in burns patients (Table A5.3). The findings suggested that weight loss was indeed less in those receiving ETF, although not significantly so (Chiarelli *et al.*, 1990).

(III) What effect does ETF have on the body function of patients in hospital with burns?

No assessments of function were made in the trials reviewed. Therefore, further investigations are needed to ascertain any functional benefits that may result from early ETF with standard and specially formulated feeds in burns patients.

(IV) What effect does ETF have on the clinical and financial outcome of patients in hospital with burns?

The use of ETF in patients following burn injury may benefit a patient's outcome in a number of ways. Starting ETF early in burns patients led to shorter hospital stays (by 20 days, not significant) in one RCT (Chiarelli *et al.*, 1990) (see Table A5.3). Similarly, a retrospective review also indicated that patients given early ETF (< 48 h after burn injury) had significantly shorter lengths of hospital care (39 days) versus those in whom ETF was delayed (76 days) (Garrel *et al.*, 1991). In the other RCT reviewed (Jenkins *et al.*, 1994), maintaining ETF before, during and after operative procedures in burns patients was associated with significantly fewer wound infections compared with those in whom ETF was withheld (ETF group had significantly greater burn injury, more surgical procedures and more antibiotic use). No financial assessments were made in the trials reviewed. However, retrospective calculation would suggest that savings are likely if hospital stays are shortened by 20 days (approximate cost saving of £5000 per patient at minimum costs of £250 day^{-1}) and if infection rates are lower (less treatment time, less use of antibiotics, dressings, etc.).

Ultimately, further well-designed RCT in sufficiently large numbers of patients are required to assess the impact of ETF on clinical outcome. Financial information must also be collected in order to determine the cost-effectiveness of the early use of ETF in this patient group.

Use of immunonutrition

As burn injury is associated with marked immune and metabolic changes, immune-enhancing enteral feeds (containing a mix of nutrients that may include arginine, glutamine, omega-3 fatty acids, RNA, antioxidants) may be beneficial (Martindale and Cresci, 2001), although as yet there is insufficient evidence from human studies to assess the effects of this type of feed

(Gottschlich *et al.*, 1990; Saffle *et al.*, 1997). These studies have been considered in meta-analyses of 'immunonutrition' trials of critically ill patients (Heyland, 2001b) (see later in this appendix for details).

Chronic Obstructive Pulmonary Disease (COPD) (Randomized and Non-randomized Data)

Despite the prevalence of disease-related malnutrition (DRM) in patients with COPD (see Chapter 2) and the concurrent need for effective means of nutritional support (Donahoe and Rogers, 1990; Schols and Wouters, 1995), there is little information about the effectiveness of ETF as a supplement to food intake in this patient group. Indeed, only one randomized trial of ETF (Whittaker *et al.*, 1990) and one non-randomized trial (in which patients received either ETF or parenteral nutrition (PN)) (Goldstein *et al.*, 1988) in patients with COPD in the hospital setting have been reviewed (see Tables A5.4–A5.6). Although both of these trials were small, they suggested that there were a number of benefits from using ETF in patients with COPD. As Table A5.6 shows, these included significant improvements in nutritional intake and anthropometric parameters and improvements in respiratory function (respiratory muscle endurance). However, further research is required to clarify these benefits. Well-designed trials in larger groups of patients with COPD in the hospital setting are needed to assess the impact of ETF on functional and clinical outcome measures in particular, with some analysis of the cost-effectiveness of this method of nutritional support.

Critical Injury and Illness (Randomized and Non-randomized Data)

Traditionally, it was assumed that the administration and potential benefits of ETF in the critical care setting was limited by gastric ileus and intolerance of ETF. Indeed, clinical observations from trials

Table A5.4. Enteral tube feeds used in trials of patients with COPD in hospital (randomized and non-randomized data).

Trial	ETF	ETF energy density	ETF prescribed	ETF energy (kcal) provision	ETF protein (g) provision	Toleration	Timing of ETF
Randomized controlled trials							
Whittaker et al. (1990)	Isocal	—	1000 kcal above VFI or to equal 1.7 × REE (whichever greater)	1000	–	Transient pharyngeal discomfort (n 3), pharyngitis (n 1)	Overnight
Non-randomized trials							
Goldstein et al. (1988)	Ensure HN (high CHO) Pulmocare (high fat) (Ross Lab)[a]	1.5 kcal ml⁻¹ 1.5 kcal ml⁻¹	1.7 × REE	~46.8 kcal kg⁻¹ body wt	~300 mg N kg⁻¹ body wt	–	24 h

^{a}Some patients were randomized to receive high fat or high CHO PN.
CHO, carbohydrate; N, nitrogen; REE, resting energy expenditure; VFI, voluntary food intake.

Table A5.5. Trial characteristics: hospital-based trials of enteral tube feeding in patients with COPD (randomized and non-randomized data).

Trial	Design	No. ETF	No. CON	Initial BMI ETF group	Initial BMI CON group	Duration of ETF	Tube type	Control group
Randomized controlled trials								
Whittaker et al. (1990) Canada	10111	6	4	17.6	18.5	16 days	Nasoduodenal/jejunal (fluoroscopic placement)	Tube-fed an equivalent volume of a dilute solution of Isocal providing <100 kcal night⁻¹
Non-randomized trials								
Goldstein et al. (1988) USA	B	10	6 (no lung disease)	18.2	18.5	1 week high-CHO ETF and 1 week high-fat ETF	Nasoduodenal	Surgical/anorectic patients on PN

BMI, body mass index; CHO, carbohydrate; CON, control.

Table A5.6. Main findings of enteral tube feeding trials in hospitalized patients with COPD (randomized and non-randomized data).

Trial	Energy/nutrient intake	Wt change ETF	Wt change CON	Function	Clinical outcome	Finance
Randomized controlled trials						
Whittaker *et al.* (1990)	TEI substantially increased in ETF group by 1093 kcal (VFI at baseline ~1364 kcal, TEI with ETF ~2489 kcal). CON group VFI unchanged	+4.77% (+2.4 kg, sig.) (ETF vs. CON sig.)	−1.32% (−0.6 kg)	Sig. increase in maximal expiratory pressure and mean sustained inspiratory pressure (endurance) (ETF vs. CON, sig.) NS changes in max. inspiratory pressure or abductor pollicis function (normal at baseline)	−	−
Non-randomized trials						
Goldstein *et al.* (1988)	TEI and nitrogen intake sig. higher in ETF group than CON group (calc. ETF 2260 kcal; CON 2036 kcal)	+1.8 g kg⁻¹ (similar to CON) MAMC, AMA (ns)	+3 g kg⁻¹	Sig. increase (of ~10%) in maximal inspiratory and expiratory pressures in ETF group only Sig. increase in hamstring strength and endurance strength in ETF and CON groups Increase in HGS and quadriceps strength in ETF group (ns)	−	−

AMA, arm muscle area; CON, control; HGS, hand-grip strength; MAMC, mid-arm muscle circumference; NS, not significant; sig., significant; TEI, total energy intake; VFI, voluntary food intake.

suggested that intolerance to ETF or, more specifically, nasogastric (NG) feeding often occurred in patients who were critically ill, including those with head injury (Montecalvo *et al.*, 1992; Weekes and Elia, 1996; Montejo, 1999), principally due to technical problems. One particular problem was the increased risk of gastro-oesophageal reflux and aspiration of gastric contents into the lungs in patients receiving large volumes of nutrition into the stomach. However, the advent of techniques/equipment to allow feeding into the duodenum and jejunum, improvements in feed compositions and improved ETF protocols has led to a much wider use of ETF in the critical care setting. Indeed, a study comparing jejunal with gastric ETF in the critical care setting found that patients fed by jejunostomy tube received a significantly higher proportion of their energy requirements and had a lower rate of pneumonia than patients fed by gastric tube (Montecalvo *et al.*, 1992). In addition, some feeding protocols to improve gastrointestinal (GI) tolerance in critically ill patients have been shown to be highly effective (Frost and Bihari, 1997; Pinilla *et al.*, 2001) (mandatory use of prokinetics, increased gastric residual-volume thresholds, use of jejunal feeding tubes). Ultimately, as the quote suggests,

> There are few absolute contraindications to early enteral feeding and with motivated staff, the use of prokinetics and the availability of jejunal feeding tubes, the majority of intensive care patients can be fed enterally.
>
> (Frost and Bihari, 1997)

Indeed, of the studies reviewed in patients with critical illness or injury, there were only minor GI problems with ETF (Mowatt-Larssen *et al.*, 1992) and the use of prokinetics for some patients was recommended (Kompan *et al.*, 1999).

Many trials have also investigated the optimal composition of feeds for patients who are critically ill. Although studies have assessed the use of elemental diets (Borlase *et al.*, 1992), more recently interest has fallen on the use of specialized feeds in the critically ill (Lin *et al.*, 1998), devel-

oped with a mix of nutrients to meet the specific needs of failing vital organs and body systems (Chiolero and Kinney, 2001). For more information, see the discussion later in this appendix.

ETF is used in critically ill patients for other reasons. For example, failure to provide enteral nutrients can lead to substantial reductions in biliary lipid concentrations. This may lead to impairments in lipid metabolism in critically ill patients who continue to fast or are solely intravenously fed, which are only normalized once ETF is given (de Vree *et al.*, 1999). ETF is also considerably cheaper than alternative methods of nutritional support, such as PN (see Chapter 9).

Critical illness and injury: present analysis

Six RCT in critically ill patients with severe trauma, head injury or multiple injuries were reviewed. These compared ETF introduced early in the treatment of patients (9.2 to < 72 h after trauma or surgery) (Seri and Aquilio, 1984; Moore and Jones, 1986; Chuntrasakul *et al.*, 1996; Kompan *et al.*, 1999; Taylor *et al.*, 1999; Minard *et al.*, 2000) with no or delayed nutritional support (see Box A5.2 and Tables A5.7–A5.9). Four NRT in injury patients (Clifton *et al.*, 1985; Grahm *et al.*, 1989; Kirby *et al.*, 1991; Mowatt-Larssen *et al.*, 1992) were also reviewed and have been summarized in Tables A5.7–A5.9.

(I) What effect does ETF have on the voluntary food intake and total energy intake of patients in hospital with critical illness/injury?

ETF can be an effective way of providing nutrition in critically ill, injured patients who have high nutritional requirements and yet are typically nil by mouth. All RCT in critically ill, injured patients that made such assessments highlighted the efficacy of ETF, often provided early after trauma, at providing significantly greater amounts of energy and protein than if nutritional support was delayed or not given (Moore and Jones,

---

> **Box A5.2.** Key findings: effect of ETF in hospital patients with critical illness/injury.
>
> Nutritional intake and body weight: in critically ill or injured patients, ETF via a jejunostomy can provide a substantially greater intake of energy, protein and other nutrients than routine care. As a result, weight loss may be reduced.
>
> Body function and clinical outcome: body function (e.g. immune function) and clinical outcome (e.g. mortality) may improve.
>
> Further research: research is needed to assess the impact of ETF on functional and clinical outcomes in both the short and long term (including the use of feeds with 'immune-enhancing' properties).

1986; Chuntrasakul *et al.*, 1996; Kompan *et al.*, 1999; Taylor *et al.*, 1999; Minard *et al.*, 2000). Indeed, critically ill/injured patients are often unable to eat so ETF is the sole source of nutrition unless PN is given.

One NRT also indicated the effectiveness of early ETF (< 36 h after admission) at improving energy and nitrogen balance in head-injured patients compared with giving ETF 'later', once gastric function had returned (Grahm *et al.*, 1989). Furthermore, compared with the negligible intakes that would occur in this patient group if ETF was not given, three longitudinal trials recorded total energy intakes in head-injured patients in excess of 1800 kcal (Clifton *et al.*, 1985; Kirby *et al.*, 1991; Mowatt-Larssen *et al.*, 1992).

(II) What effect does ETF have on the body weight and composition of patients in hospital with critical illness/injury?

ETF is likely to attenuate some of the weight loss typically associated with patients who are critically ill. Two RCT suggested that weight loss was reduced in those given ETF (by 5.2% (Moore and Jones, 1986) and 6.8% (Chuntrasakul *et al.*, 1996) versus a control group) and significantly so in one trial (Chuntrasakul *et al.*, 1996) (Table A5.9). One other RCT found no changes in upper-arm anthropometry in abdominal trauma patients with ETF (Seri and Aquilio, 1984). Similarly, in one of the NRT, patients given 'early' ETF had weight gain (+2.9 kg) as opposed to weight loss in those in whom ETF was delayed (−1.1 kg)

(Grahm *et al.*, 1989). However, in this patient group it is likely that changes in body weight were confounded by fluctuations in fluid balance.

(III) What effect does ETF have on the body function of patients in hospital with critical illness/injury?

The provision of ETF for critically ill, injured patients may have a number of functional benefits (see Table A5.9). First, ETF may prevent increases in intestinal permeability that occur if an enteral source of nutrients is withheld (Kompan *et al.*, 1999). Secondly, ETF may improve some immunological or inflammatory markers (Moore and Jones, 1986; Taylor *et al.*, 1999), although this is not a consistent observation (Seri and Aquilio, 1984). Thirdly, ETF can reduce the need for PN in some patients (Moore and Jones, 1986). Larger prospective trials that assess the value of ETF in patients recovering from critical illness and trauma are required to assess the functional changes in this patient group.

(IV) What effect does ETF have on the clinical and financial outcome of patients in hospital with critical illness/injury?

This analysis suggests that the appropriate use of ETF in patients who are critically ill may improve clinical outcome. Many significant improvements in outcome were identified in the RCT that were reviewed (Table A5.9). These included:

Table A5.7. Enteral tube feeds used in trials of critically ill/injured patients in hospital (randomized and non-randomized data).

Trial	ETF	ETF energy density	ETF prescribed	ETF energy (kcal) provision	ETF protein (g) provision	Toleration	Timing of ETF
Randomized controlled trials							
Chuntrasakul *et al.* (1996)	Traumacal	Increased to reach 1.5 kcal ml⁻¹	ETF 1494 kcal CON 1475 kcal (To meet daily requirement)	Week 1 1886 (100) kcal Week 2 1850 (250) kcal	–	Low energy density and slow rate well tolerated earlier than usual	Continuous – received immediately after resuscitation or operation when haemodynamically stable (within 5 days of injury)
Kompan *et al.* (1999)	Jevity (Ross Lab), 17% P, 29% F, 54% CHO[a]	–	25–35 kcal kg⁻¹ body wt and 0.2–0.3 g N kg⁻¹ body wt	81% of ETF 'goal' given by end of 1 week	–	Cisapride required by all pts because of gastric residue	ETF started immediately (9.2 h after trauma)
Minard *et al.* (2000)	Impact with fibre (Novartis)	1 kcal ml⁻¹	21 kcal kg⁻¹ body wt and 0.3 g N kg⁻¹ body wt	1509 kcal	–	Minor feeding complications, including diarrhoea, distension and vomiting	< 72 h after trauma
Moore and Jones (1986)	Vivonex HN[a]	–	3000 kcal, 20 g N body wt	156% of BEE on day 4; 138% on day 7	–	*n* 12 intolerant to full jejunostomy feeding	Constant, started within 18 h
Seri and Aquilio (1984)	Liquid diet based on baby food (15% P, 34% F, 51% CHO)	1 kcal ml⁻¹	3000 kcal	–	–	–	Started 12 h postoperatively, with the aim of full feeding 72 h postop. (continuous 24 h infusion)
Taylor *et al.* (1999)	Fresubin 750 or Entera (pts < 12 years)	1.5 kcal ml⁻¹ 1.5 kcal ml⁻¹	To meet estimated energy and protein requirements	59% of requirement	0.24 g N kg⁻¹ body wt	Aspiration pneumonia in *n* 2 (*n* 1 ETF, *n* 1 CON)	Within 24 h of injury
Non-randomized trials							
Clifton *et al.* (1985)	Traumacal (22% P, 38% CHO, 41% F) or Magnacal (14% P, 50% CHO, 36% F) (Mead Johnson)	1.5 kcal ml⁻¹ 2 kcal ml⁻¹	To meet 150% of REE	3500 kcal	–	Occasional diarrhoea associated with antibiotic use	ETF started on 2nd day after injury

Reference	Feed		Aim	Energy delivered	Nitrogen/protein delivered	Comments	
Grahm *et al.* (1989)	Vital HN (Ross)	–	To meet estimated energy and protein requirements	–	–	Diarrhoea was not a problem and tubes were not displaced	Within 36 h of admission, continuous 24 h ETF
Kirby *et al.* (1991)	Vital (HN) (Ross) (10% F, 74% CHO, 16% P)	–	To meet estimated requirements	1867 kcal (1060–2600 kcal)	12.5 g N (7.1–18.5 g)	4.2 (2–8) days required to reach prescribed energy intake. Satisfactory feeding tolerance. Abdominal distension in n 1. Technical problems with tube	–
Mowatt-Larssen *et al.* (1992)	ETF^1 (peptide) Reabilan HN (O'Brien Pharmaceuticals) vs. ETF^2 (standard) Isocal HN (Bristol-Myers) + Promod (Ross)	–	Aim: 35 kcal kg^{-1} body wt	ETF^1 34.2 kcal kg^{-1} ETF^2 32.4 kcal kg^{-1b}	ETF^1 1.5 g kg^{-1} ETF^2 1.7 g kg^{-1b}	Diarrhoea on 6% of ETF days and elevated gastric residuals on 8–12% of days. Toleration of the two feeds similar	–

[a] Received additional PN to ensure nutritional requirements were met.
[b] Maximum nutrient intake obtained (? includes some oral intake).
BEE, basal energy expenditure; CHO, carbohydrate; CON, control; F, fat; N, nitrogen; P, protein; postop., postoperatively; REE, resting energy expenditure.

Table A5.8. Trial characteristics: hospital-based trials of enteral tube feeding in critically ill/injured patients (randomized and non-randomized data).

Trial	Design	Diagnosis	No. ETF	No. CON	Initial BMI ETF group	Initial BMI CON group	Duration of ETF	Tube type	Control group
Randomized controlled trials									
Chuntrasakul et al. (1996) Thailand	10001	Severe trauma (ISS 20–40)	21	17	–	–	2 weeks	NG tube (some received PN if ETF 'insufficient' but levels not defined)	Hypocaloric intravenous solution (5% dextrose, 1000 ml day^{-1})
Kompan et al. (1999) Slovenia	11001	Multiple injury (ISS >25; GCS ≥ 12), in shock	14	14	–	–	Up to 14 days or discharge	20F tubes changed to fine-bore NG tube when ETF established	Received 'late' ETF', 41 h after trauma. Within first 24 h, given PN
Minard et al. (2000) USA	10001	Severe closed head injury, GCS >3–11	12	15	–	–	ETF 13 days CON 8 days	Nasenteric tube (endoscopically placed)	Received 'late' ETF (given after gastric ileus resolved)
Moore and Jones (1986) USA	10001	Major abdominal trauma	32	31	75.8 (2.9) kg	71.4 (1.9) kg	63% on ETF for ≥ 5 days (range 5–20)	Needle-catheter jejunostomy	No ETF for first 5 days. 29% on PN for average of 22 days
Seri and Aquilio (1984) Italy	10001	Acute abdominal trauma (laparotomy)	10	8	Prognostic nutritional index 43–47% (AMC and TSF >100% of 'normal' for both groups)	–	7 days postop.	Needle-catheter jejunostomy (silicone catheter) placed during laparotomy	'Conventional nutritional treatment'
Taylor et al. (1999) UK	11001	Head injury requiring mechanical ventilation	42[a]	42[b]	–	–	9 days (CON 11 days)	ETF: Accusite pH sensor tube into intestine (34% of pts) or, if not feasible, gastric feeding tube (66%) CON: Orogastric or NG tube	Received ETF at a slow rate and increased as tolerated. ETF stopped if gastric residuals large
Non-randomized trials									
Clifton et al. (1985) USA	C	Acute severe head injury, GCS < 8	20 ETF[1] 10 ETF[2] 10	–	–	–	7 days	NG tube	–
Grahm et al. (1989) USA	B	Head injury, GCS < 10	17	15	–	–	Up to 7 days	Nasojejunal tubes (Keofeed II (IVAC), Flexiflo II (Ross)) or duodenography catheters (? NG tube in CON)	ETF initiated 'late', after day 3 when gastric function returned
Kirby et al. (1991) USA	C	Severe brain injury (GCS ≤ 8)	21	–	–	–	7.7 days (5–13 days)	Gastrojejunostomy	–
Mowatt-Larssen et al. (1992) USA	C	Acutely injured	28 ETF[1] 12 ETF[2] 16	–	ETF[1] 24.2 ETF[2] 26.2	–	5–10 days	Fine-bore NG (n 31), gastrostomy (n 4), jejunostomy (n 6)	–

[a] ETF group received tube feed at a rate to meet estimated energy and protein requirements in full from the start of feeding.

[b] CON group received ETF at slow rates (started at 15 ml h^{-1} and increased gradually as tolerated).

AMC, arm muscle circumference; BMI, body mass index; CON, control; GCS, Glasgow coma score; ISS, injury severity score; TSF, triceps skin-fold thickness.

Table A5.9. Main findings of enteral tube feeding trials in hospitalized critically ill/injured patients (randomized and non-randomized data).

Trial	Energy/nutrient intake	Wt change ETF	Wt change CON	Function	Outcome	Finance
Randomized controlled trials						
Chuntrasakul *et al.* (1996)	ETF sig. greater energy intake weeks 1 and 2 than CON (+1253 kcal week 1; 1133 kcal week 2)	Week 1 6.2 (1.12)% Week 2 −9.81 (1.5)% (ETF vs. CON sig. week 2)	Week 1 −10.3 (2.5)% Week 2 −16.6 (2.2)%	—	ETF: shorter ICU stay (by 0.21 days) and shorter period of ventilator use (< 1 day) vs. CON (NS) ETF fewer systemic complications than CON (no data) ETF fewer deaths (*n* 1) than CON (*n* 3) (NS)	—
Kompan *et al.* (1999)	ETF (early) received sig. more enteral feed daily than CON (late ETF) (e.g. day 4 1340 kcal vs. 703 kcal; day 7 81% vs. 61% of prescribed feeding goal)	—	—	CON sig. higher lactulose/mannitol ratio than healthy subjects on day 2 after trauma, an indication of increased intestinal permeability (not seen in ETF)	Sig. lower MOF scores in ETF (1.8) vs. CON (2.8) from day 4 onwards	—
Minard *et al.* (2000)	ETF (early) received sig. more enteral feed (1509 kcal day⁻¹) than CON (late ETF, 1174 kcal day⁻¹). 83% of ETF met > 50% 'goal' for ≥ 5 days (vs. 47% in CON)	—	—	—	Lower mortality in ETF than CON (8% vs. 27%, NS). NS difference in length of H or ICU stay, ventilator days, no. of infections per pt or pt with pneumonia between ETF and CON	—
Moore and Jones (1986)	ETF: 156% of BEE on day 4 and 138% on day 7 (vs. 36% and 35% in CON, ? sig.) N balance sig. improved in ETF (not in CON)	−2.64% (−2 kg) (ETF vs. CON ? sig.) Similar drop in MAMC in ETF and CON	−7.84% (−5.6 kg)	Sig. increase in TLC in ETF group (not seen in CON)	Sig. lower incidence of septic morbidity in ETF vs. CON (3 vs. 9) and sig. less sepsis (4% vs. 26%) Fewer of ETF group required PN than CON (12% vs. 29%, ? sig.) No difference in overall complication rates (ETF vs. CON NS) or length of stay (ETF 25 days vs. CON 29 days) or H costs (ETF US$16,280 vs. CON $19,636)	—
Seri and Aquilio (1984)	Sig. improvement in N balance (ETF vs. CON sig.)	NS changes in anthropometry (AMC, TSF) in ETF or CON	—	NS differences in TLC or delayed cutaneous hypersensitivity	Lower rate of septic complications in ETF (10%, *n* 1) than CON (25%, *n* 2; NS)	—

Continued

Table A5.9. *Continued*

Trial	Energy/nutrient intake	Wt change ETF	Wt change CON	Function	Outcome	Finance
Taylor *et al.* (1999)	ETF received sig. higher % of E and P requirements than CON (E 59% vs. 37%; P 69% vs. 38%)	–	–	ETF sig. reduction in CRP : albumin ratio after 6 days (not seen in CON)	ETF sig. lower no. of pts with an infective complication (61% vs. 85%) or more than one complication in total (37% vs. 61%) than CON. Tendency for more of ETF to have a good neurological outcome at 3 months than CON (61% vs. 39%, $P < 0.08$)	Calculated cost savings from reduced complication rates
Non-randomized trials						
Clifton *et al.* (1985)	Assume ETF intake 3500 kcal N intake for ETF[1] 17.6 g and ETF[2] 29 g, with greater N balance in ETF[2] (−5.3 g vs. −9.2 g)	15% fall in body wt (~ −11 kg)	–	–	–	–
Grahm *et al.* (1989)	Sig. greater TEI (2101 kcal) and lower E deficit for 7-day trial period of 3010 kcal for ETF vs. CON (TEI 1100 kcal, E deficit 10,194 kcal). Sig. higher N intake and sig. improvement in N balance in ETF vs. CON	+2.9 kg	−1.1 kg	–	ETF had lower incidence of bacterial infections (3 vs. 14) and fewer days on ICU (6 vs. 10) (ETF vs. CON sig.)	–
Kirby *et al.* (1991)	Average energy intake 1867 kcal (1060–2600 kcal) early after injury (? when)	–	–	–	–	–
Mowatt-Larssen *et al.* (1992)	Est. max. intakes with ETF: ETF[1] 2586 kcal, 113 g P ETF[2] 2573 kcal, 135 g P Sig. improvement in N balance in both groups	Sig. fall in PNI in both ETF groups	–	–	–	–

AMC, arm muscle circumference; BEE, basal energy expenditure; CON, control; E, energy; H, hospital; ICU, intensive care unit; MAMC, mid-arm muscle circumference; MOF, multiple organ failure; N, nitrogen; NS, not significant; P, protein; PNI, prognostic nutritional index; sig., significant; TEI, total energy intake; TLC, total lymphocyte count; TSF, triceps skin-fold thickness.

- A significantly lower mortality in head-injured patients when ETF was started within 72 h after trauma as opposed to delayed ETF after gastric ileus was resolved (Minard *et al.*, 2000).
- A significantly lower number of infective complications, significantly fewer patients with more than one complication and a trend towards better neurological outcome 3 months after head injury when ETF was given early in full within 24 h of head injury (at a rate to meet energy and protein requirements in full from the start) than with delayed ETF (Taylor *et al.*, 1999).
- A significantly lower incidence of sepsis and septic morbidity in abdominal-trauma patients given ETF in the first 5 days after admission compared with routine care (Moore and Jones, 1986).

Meta-analysis of three reviewed RCT (*n* 125: Chuntrasakul *et al.*, 1996; Minard *et al.*, 2000; Pupelis *et al.*, 2001) suggested that mortality may be reduced with ETF with an odds ratio (OR) of 0.23 (95% confidence interval (CI) 0.03–2.16) (not significant, small numbers). Similarly, meta-analysis of four of the RCT (*n* 192: Seri and Aquilio, 1984; Moore and Jones, 1986; Taylor *et al.*, 1999; Minard *et al.*, 2000) that provided data on complication rates indicated that there may be a reduced risk with an OR of 0.55 (95% CI 0.21–1.48) (not significant).

In one RCT in abdominal trauma patients, septic complication rates were lower in ETF patients, but not significantly so (Seri and Aquilio, 1984).

None of the trials reviewed that assessed the length of hospital or intensive care unit (ICU) stay (Moore and Jones, 1986; Minard *et al.*, 2000) found any significant changes as a result of ETF. However, it is likely that sample sizes of patients were insufficient to detect significant changes in this and other outcome parameters. (Only one trial reported power calculations to assess the sample size needed to assess changes in outcome (Taylor *et al.*, 1999).)

The one NRT reviewed that assessed outcome indicated that patients receiving 'early' ETF had a lower incidence of bacter-ial infections and fewer days on the ICU than those in whom ETF was delayed until gastric ileus resolved (Grahm *et al.*, 1989).

Ultimately, further trials are required to assess the impact of ETF on the clinical outcome of patients within the ICU and hospital settings and beyond into rehabilitation in the community. Larger trials are also needed that incorporate prospectively financial assessments of the cost-effectiveness of ETF in this patient group. One trial provided an estimation of the cost savings from using early ETF in head-injury patients:

- In the UK it is estimated that 3211 patients with head injuries per year require admission to the ICU and mechanical ventilation within 24 h of injury (Taylor *et al.*, 1999). If the improvements in outcome from Taylor *et al.*'s (1999) study (see Table A5.9) in head-injured patients were extrapolated to head-injury patients in the UK, an annual cost saving of > £4 million could accrue through 8734 fewer days in hospital. (This assumes that 34% of these patients meet the inclusion criteria, as in the study (34% of the 3211) and that 17% have a hospital stay between 20 and 100 days. Cost based on £500 day^{-1} (all-inclusive) for neurosurgical stay > 28 days.)

Critical illness/injury: other reviews

A meta-analysis of studies of a number of acutely ill patient groups (including head injury, trauma and medical ICU, five trials relevant to this section) suggests that early versus 'delayed' feeding may significantly reduce length of stay and complication rates (Marik and Zaloga, 2001), although significant heterogeneity exists between studies.

Role of feeds containing nutrients that may modulate immune function in critical illness

In addition to the use of standard formulas for feeding critically ill patients enterally, increasingly interest has focused on the use of 'immunonutrition' or 'immune-enhancing' feeds, as the quote below suggests:

> Arguably the most exciting developments in nutritional support of the critically ill have come from demonstrations that certain key nutrients can modulate immune, metabolic and inflammatory pathways if given in amounts in excess of what can be regarded as the 'norm'.
>
> (Heys and Wahle, 2001)

Meta-analyses have attempted to address the issue of efficacy of these feeds, which typically contain a mix of potentially immune-modulating nutrients (e.g. arginine, glutamine, omega-3 fatty acids, RNA, a variety of antioxidants), in critically ill patients (Beale *et al.*, 1999; Heys *et al.*, 1999; Heyland *et al.*, 2001b). In the most recent of these reviews, 'immunonutrition' in the critically ill (*n* 13 studies, including those on burns patients) was not associated with a reduction in complication rates compared with a standard feed (relative risk (RR) 0.96; 95% CI 0.77–1.20; nine trials), although there was a reduction in length of hospital stay (RR −0.47; 95% CI −0.93 to −0.01). There was also a trend towards higher mortality (RR 1.18; 95% CI −0.09 to 0.83; 13 trials) (Heyland *et al.*, 2001b), an association that was increased if only studies of higher methodological quality were examined. This finding raises the possibility, in severely ill patients with sepsis and inflammatory conditions, that it may not be beneficial to further stimulate the immune system, with the potential for detriment in such patients. Furthermore, the optimal mix and concentrations of different key nutrients (Reid, 2000) and the timing and use of these feeds in different patient groups remain to be elucidated with further RCT.

Elderly (Non-randomized Data)

Despite the frequency with which ETF is used in elderly hospitalized patients, there is a general lack of well-designed trials assessing the effectiveness of this mode of nutritional support in this patient group.

As no RCT have been reviewed, information from the NRT that have been reported are summarized in Tables A5.10–A5.12 and discussed briefly below. More information on ETF in elderly patients in the community can be found in Appendix 6.

ETF is a valuable therapy in elderly individuals in whom food intake is contraindicated, in that it allows one of the only means of nutritional supply, preventing starvation from developing. Indeed, ETF is frequently required in elderly patients with swallowing disorders to prevent tracheal aspiration and aspiration pneumonia (e.g. in patients with a cerebrovascular accident (CVA)). However, ETF can also be an effective means of increasing total nutrient intake in those in whom food intake is inadequate. The studies summarized in Tables A5.10–A5.12 highlight the use of ETF as a supplement to food intake in undernourished elderly patients in the clinical setting (Lipschitz and Mitchell, 1980; Treber and Harris, 1996) and later in this appendix the efficacy of ETF in CVA and orthopaedic patients is addressed.

ETF in undernourished, hospitalized elderly patients led to substantial increases in total energy (and nutrient) intake and food intake (Lipschitz and Mitchell, 1982), with patients reporting an increase in appetite. Subsequently, in this study, ETF led to improvements in nutritional parameters and measures of immune function, although the sample of patients was only small (*n* 7) (Lipschitz and Mitchell, 1982). In addition to functional benefits, it has been suggested that early (within 48 h of admission) nutritional intervention (including ETF) in elderly, undernourished patients may reduce the duration of hospital stay compared with giving nutrition late (> 72 h after admission) or not at all (Treber and Harris, 1996). Ultimately, large RCT are required in hospitalized elderly to assess the effects of using ETF as a supplement to food intake on functional, clinical and financial outcomes in this patient group. However, it has been suggested that the appropriate use of ETF will be cost-effective as the benefits to outcome are likely to exceed the small costs of feeding (Allison, 1995).

Table A5.10. Enteral tube feeds used in trials of elderly patients in hospital (non-randomized data).

Trial	ETF	ETF energy density	ETF prescribed	ETF energy (kcal) provision	ETF protein (g) provision	Toleration	Timing of ETF
Lipschitz and Mitchell (1982)	Ensure	1 kcal ml^{-1}	–	1800–2500 kcal	–	–	24 h
Treber and Harris (1996)	–	–	–	–	–	–	–

Table A5.11. Trial characteristics: hospital-based trials of enteral tube feeding in elderly patients (non-randomized data).

Trial	Design	Diagnosis	No. ETF	No. CON	Initial BMI ETF group	Initial BMI CON group	Duration of ETF	Tube type	Control group
Lipschitz and Mitchell (1982) USA Undernourished and hospitalized elderly	C	Malnutrition, weakness, confusion (some patients postoperative)	7	–	'Undernourished'	–	21 days ETF followed by 21 days of ONS	Small-bore polyethylene nasogastric tube	–
Treber and Harris (1996) Abstract USA Acute-care facilities	B	Pneumonia, heart failure, bowel procedures	98[a]	(i) 58 (delayed) (ii) 74 (no nutrition)	Of total group: 34% at potential risk and 21% at risk of undernutrition[b]	–	– Given early (within 48 h of admission)	–	(i) Nutrition delayed (> 72–96 h after admission) (ii) No nutrition given

[a]Total for patients receiving early nutritional intervention (includes patients given ETF, ONS, food snacks and PN).
[b]Used a mix of criteria to define risk of undernutrition including % IBW < 90% and low albumin.
BMI, body mass index; CON, control; IBW, ideal body weight; ONS, oral nutritional supplements.

Table A5.12. Main findings of enteral tube feeding trials in hospitalized elderly patients (non-randomized data).

Trial	Energy/nutrient intake	Wt change ETF	Wt change CON	Function	Clinical outcome	Finance
Lipschitz and Mitchell (1982)	VFI improved from 988 kcal before ETF to 1735 kcal after 21 days ETF (est. TEI 3535–4235 kcal). VFI maintained after ETF stopped (day 42 VFI 2414 kcal)	+16 kg (sig. increase over 42 days) (~2.6 kg day⁻¹!)	–	Improved immune function – sig. increase in TLC and improved cell-mediated immunity (intradermal skin tests) Correction of haematopoietic abnormalities, with improved stem-cell function (using bone marrow aspirates, marked increase in committed granulocyte/macrophage progenitor cell numbers after ETF vs. pre-ETF levels) (? sig.) Improved appetite and mobility and less confusion (subjective assessments)	–	–
Treber and Harris (1996)	–	–	–	–	Mean length of hospital stay was sig. shorter in the early nutrition intervention group (9.1 days, n 41) than those receiving delayed (12.3 days, n 28) or no nutrition (12.2 days, n 20) in those patients 'at risk of undernutrition'. These differences were not seen in patients classified as 'at potential risk of undernutrition'	–

CON, control; sig., significant; TEI, TLC, total lymphocyte count; total energy intake; VFI, voluntary food intake.

There is also little information about the tolerance of the elderly to ETF. Occasional reports of complaints include gastro-oesophageal reflux, aspiration pneumonia, clogged tubes and self-extubation (particularly with NG feeding) (Ciocon *et al.*, 1992; Guedon *et al.*, 1996). Elderly patients on ETF have also been reported to suffer from diarrhoea (Ciocon *et al.*, 1992), although consideration of all of the potential causes is typically not made (e.g. use of antibiotics, laxatives or other medications, hypoalbuminaemia, etc.) (Bowling, 1995).

There are also a number of ethical issues surrounding the use of long-term ETF and the insertion of percutaneous endoscopic gastrostomy (PEG) tubes in the elderly. In particular, there can be concerns about the use of long-term ETF in the severely disabled, the unconscious or the terminally ill patient. Issues relating to the ethics and the decision-making processes involved in ETF for elderly patients are beyond the scope of this report, but have been addressed in a number of reviews (Ouslander *et al.*, 1993, Krynski *et al.*, 1994; Bozzetti, 1996; Lennard-Jones, 1998).

Although the studies reviewed in this section were undertaken in elderly patients, studies of ETF in disease-specific groups (e.g. COPD, gastroenterology, neurology) also included the elderly and are addressed in separate sections within this appendix.

GI Disease (Randomized and Non-randomized Data)

ETF frequently provides nutritional support for patients with a wide range of GI conditions. In particular, ETF has been used in the treatment of patients with Crohn's disease to induce remission. Indeed, many trials have involved controlled comparisons of the efficacy of different enteral formulas (elemental, peptide, whole protein) versus steroid treatment in Crohn's disease, and meta-analyses of such trials in adults and children (Griffiths *et al.*, 1995; Messori *et al.*, 1996; Heuschkel *et al.*, 2000; Zachos *et al.*, 2001) are discussed briefly below.

GI disease: present analysis

ETF is also used as a supplement to food intake in patients in hospital with GI conditions. Trials that compared ETF with no nutritional support (routine clinical care) in such patients were reviewed (see Box A5.3 and Tables A5.13–A5.15) and included only one RCT, in patients with severe pancreatitis and peritonitis (Pupelis *et al.*, 2001). Both the RCT (Pupelis *et al.*, 2001) and the NRT (Yeung *et al.*, 1979a; Abad-Lacruz *et al.*, 1988; Afdhal *et al.*, 1989; Kudsk *et al.*, 1990; Rigaud *et al.*, 1991; Royall *et al.*, 1994) reviewed, in patients with Crohn's disease and other inflammatory bowel disease and in those post-surgery, suggested that ETF was well tolerated, with very few reports of GI symptoms in this patient group (see Table A5.13). In particular, two trials highlighted that ETF was safe and well tolerated in those with pancreatitis (Kudsk *et al.*, 1990; Pupelis *et al.*, 2001). In most of the trials reviewed, peptide or elemental feeds were used (see Table A5.13). Indeed, in patients with moderately impaired GI function, peptide-containing ETF may be better than whole-protein feeds (Rees *et al.*, 1992). Studies of ETF in GI surgical patients have also been reviewed and are summarized later in this Appendix.

(I) What effect does ETF have on the voluntary food intake and total energy intake of patients in hospital with GI disease?

ETF can be used in patients with GI disease to improve energy and nutrient intakes. In an RCT of postoperative patients with pancreatitis and peritonitis, those receiving ETF had significantly higher total energy intakes (average +822 kcal day^{-1}) than control patients given intravenous fluids (Pupelis *et al.*, 2001) (see Table A5.15). Two further trials (both non-randomized) indicated that ETF facilitated energy intakes in excess of 2000 kcal daily (Yeung *et al.*, 1979a; Rigaud *et al.*, 1991). In the majority of these trials, patients were nil by mouth and so the impact of ETF on food intake could not be

> **Box A5.3.** Key findings: effect of ETF in hospital patients with gastrointestinal disease.
>
> Nutritional intake: ETF can substantially increase energy intake in patients with pancreatitis and peritonitis and Crohn's disease. The impact on food intake has not been assessed.
>
> Body weight: body weight may be increased, but RCT are needed to assess the effects of ETF on both weight and body composition.
>
> Body function: ETF may reduce disease activity/inflammation in patients with Crohn's disease and hasten recovery of bowel function postoperatively in those with severe pancreatitis.
>
> Clinical outcome: in patients with pancreatitis/peritonitis, jejunal ETF significantly reduces rates of reoperation and mortality.
>
> Further research: RCT are needed to assess the impact of ETF in patients with different types of gastrointestinal disease.

investigated. Therefore, trials are needed that assess the efficacy of using ETF as a supplement to food intake where appropriate in patients with different GI conditions.

(II) What effect does ETF have on the body weight and composition of patients in hospital with GI disease?

The one RCT reviewed made no assessment of changes in weight or body composition with ETF (Pupelis *et al.*, 2001). Although longitudinal assessments showed that patients with GI disease receiving ETF gained significant amounts of weight (Afdhal *et al.*, 1989; Rigaud *et al.*, 1991; Royall *et al.*, 1994; Table A5.15), controlled trials are required. In particular, information about the changes in body composition (fat and muscle mass) with ETF should be gathered from RCT undertaken in GI-disease-specific groups so that changes in weight due to fluid fluctuations can be identified.

(III) What effect does ETF have on the body function of patients in hospital with GI disease?

The use of ETF postoperatively in patients with pancreatitis/peritonitis led to a quicker recovery of bowel function than in controls given routine clinical care (Pupelis *et al.*, 2001). No other functional outcomes were assessed. Although reductions in disease activity and significant reductions in inflammatory markers were observed in longitudinal trials of ETF in patients with Crohn's disease (Afdhal *et al.*, 1989; Rigaud *et al.*, 1991; Royall *et al.*, 1994; Table A5.15), controlled trials are needed to assess whether these occurred due to spontaneous changes in disease activity over time or due to ETF. Anecdotal reports have also suggested that nutritional support (including elemental ETF) may aid the healing of external GI fistulas compared with no nutritional support (Kaminsky and Deitel, 1975).

(IV) What effect does ETF have on the clinical and financial outcome of patients in hospital with GI disease?

Only one trial of a randomized, controlled design assessed changes in clinical outcome with ETF (Pupelis *et al.*, 2001). However, this trial highlighted a number of important improvements to outcome following ETF in postoperative pancreatitis patients (see Table A5.15). These included significantly lower rates of reoperation and significantly lower rates of mortality. Although there were no differences in length of hospital or ICU stay, such parameters are not always the best markers of outcome, being affected by many non-clinical factors (bed availability, discharge planning, etc.).

Table A5.13. Enteral tube feeds used in trials of patients with gastrointestinal disorders in hospital (randomized and non-randomized data).

Trial	ETF	ETF energy density	ETF prescribed	ETF energy (kcal) provision	ETF protein (g) provision	Toleration	Timing of ETF
Randomized controlled trials							
Pupelis *et al.* (2001)	Nutrison Standard or Nutrison Pepti	1 kcal ml⁻¹ 1 kcal ml⁻¹	> 300 kcal–1000 kcal	831 (±373)	–	–	Started in first 12 h postop.
Non-randomized trials							
Abad-Lucruz *et al.* (1988)	UNIASA (Spain) (74 g P, 91 g F, 221 g CHO per 2000 kcal)	–	–	58.3 kg⁻¹	0.37 g N kg⁻¹	Well tolerated. No ETF-related complications	–
Afdhal *et al.* (1989)	Trisorbon (16% P, 36% F, 48% CHO) MCT-enriched	1 kcal ml⁻¹	50 kcal kg⁻¹ wt	–	–	Well tolerated, mild bloating	Given nocturnally. Started on half-strength with full-strength ETF by day 3
Kudsk *et al.* (1990)	Vital HN	–	–	1.15 l (? energy density)	–	No dislodging or blocking of tubes, occasional diarrhoea, no increase in abdominal pain	–
Rigaud *et al.* (1991)	Comparison of Vivonex HN (elemental (E), 18% P, 0.8% F, 81.2% CHO) vs. Nutrison or Realmentyl (polymeric (P) feed, 18% P, 27% F, 55% CHO)	(E) 1 kcal ml⁻¹ (P) 1 kcal ml⁻¹	–	(E) 2286 kcal (P) 2311 kcal	16.2 g N 15.6 g N	All tolerated ETF well	–
Royall *et al.* (1994)	Vivonex (E) or Peptamen (SE)	–	–	35 kcal kg⁻¹	–	Intolerance to ETF on (E) (n 5) and (SE) (n 3) diets	–
Yeung *et al.* (1979a)	Flexical (Mead Johnson) (9% P, 61% CHO, 30% F)	1 kcal ml⁻¹	Up to 3500 kcal	–	–	Nausea and vomiting in a few pts on ETF	24 h

CHO, carbohydrate; (E), elemental feed; F, fat; MCT, medium-chain triglyceride; N, nitrogen; P, protein; (P), polymeric feed; postop., postoperative; (SE), semi-elemental feed.

Table A5.14. Trial characteristics: hospital-based trials of enteral tube feeding in patients with gastrointestinal disorders (randomized and non-randomized data).

Trial	Design	Diagnosis	No. ETF	No. CON	Initial BMI ETF group	Initial BMI CON group	Duration of ETF	Tube type	Control group
Randomized controlled trials									
Pupelis *et al.* (2001) Latvia	10001	Severe pancreatitis and peritonitis	30	30	–	–	–	Nasojejunal tube (Flocare, Nutricia)	Intravenous fluids until normal diet reintroduced
Non-randomized trials									
Abad-Lucruz *et al.* (1988) Spain	C	IBD[a]	8	–	'Malnourished'	–	21 days (12–28 days)	Fine-bore NG tube	–
Afdhal *et al.* (1989) Ireland	C	Severe Crohn's disease	11[b]	–	85% IBW	–	20 days	Fine-bore tube	–
Kudsk *et al.* (1990) USA	C	Postoperative for complications of pancreatitis (biliary surgery most common)	9	–	–	–	31 days	Jejunostomy	–
Rigaud *et al.* (1991) France	C	Active Crohn's disease[c]	30	–	~85% IBW	–	30 days (22–43 days)	NG tube	–
Royall *et al.* (1994) A Canada	C	Active Crohn's disease	40	–	–	–	21 days	Nasoduodenal tube	–
Yeung *et al.* (1979a) UK	B[c]	GI post-surgery	7	7[d]	–	–	15 days	Fine silicone rubber NG tube or jejunostomy (*n* 4)	PN (received more energy per kg wt than ETF (42.4 kcal kg[-1]))

[a] *n* 7 acute IBD (Crohn's disease, ulcerative colitis) and receiving steroid treatment; *n* 5 received antibiotics.
[b] Steroids withdrawn in *n* 9, low-dose prednisone given in *n* 2.
[c] Steroids given for days 1–14.
[d] Control group given PN.
A, abstract; BMI, body mass index; CON, control; IBD, inflammatory bowel disease; IBW, ideal body weight.

Table A5.15. Main findings of enteral tube feeding trials in hospitalized patients with gastrointestinal disorders (randomized and non-randomized data).

Trial	Energy/nutrient intake	Wt change ETF	Wt change CON	Function	Outcome	Finance
Randomized controlled trials						
Pupelis *et al.* (2001)	TEI sig. higher in ETF (1295 kcal vs. 473 kcal in CON). This includes PN (ETF 480 kcal; CON 473 kcal). No oral intake	–	–	Passage of first stool earlier in ETF (sig. vs. CON)	Sig. lower rate of reoperations in ETF (3.3% vs. 27% in CON due to unresolved peritonitis with relaparotomy) and a lower rate of other complications (NS vs. CON). Sig. lower mortality in ETF (3.3% vs. 23%). No difference in H (35 days vs. 36 days) or ICU (14 days vs. 16 days) stays	–
Non-randomized trials						
Abad-Lacruz *et al.* (1988)	–	NS change in TSF or MAMC	–	Sig. improvement in disease activity during course of trial. Sig. improvement in vitamin A, E, B_1 and B_2 status (no change in folate, biotin, vitamin C and β-carotene[a])	–	–
Afdhal *et al.* (1989)	TEI (ETF + low-residue diet) 5855 kcal, 182 g P	+3.1 kg (sig.) Sig. increase in TSF, NS increase in MAMC	–	Sig. reduction in disease activity score (uses subjective and objective scoring). Mean remission period 6 months (all who achieved remission relapsed within 9 months)	–	–
Kudsk *et al.* (1990)	–	–	–	Serum amylase levels reduced to normal within 5 days of ETF in all pts. ETF did not increase amylase at any time	–	–
Rigaud *et al.* (1991)	TEI and TPI from ETF: (E) 2286 kcal 16.2 g N (P) 2311 kcal 15.6 g N	1.8 kg (1.8 kg) (sig.) Sig. increase in TSF. No difference between (E) and (P)	–	Decrease in Crohn's disease activity with ETF (decreased CDAI, faecal output, steroid dose). Remission rates equivalent between 2 feeds ((E) and (P)). Reduction of inflammatory markers during ETF (sig., e.g. sedimentation rate)	–	–

Continued

Table A5.15. *Continued.*

Trial	Energy/nutrient intake	Wt change ETF	Wt change CON	Function	Outcome	Finance
Royall *et al.* (1994)	–	+1.7 kg (0.3 kg) (E) +2 kg (0.5 kg) (SE)	–	Sig. reduction in CDAI and inflammatory markers with ETF (both (E) and (SE) diets)	–	–
Yeung *et al.* (1979a)	TEI 2029 kcal (ETF) vs. 2421 kcal (CON on PN)	+0.2 kg (NS)	+3.2 kg (sig.) largely fluid change[b]	–	–	–

[a]Significantly lower levels of vitamin A, β-carotene and vitamin E in IBD patients than in healthy controls at start of trial. Plasma β-carotene was unchanged at the end of the trial.
[b]Control group given PN.

CON, control; CDAI, Crohn's disease activity index; (E), elemental feed; H, hospital; IBD, inflammatory bowel disease; MAMC, mid-arm muscle circumference; N, nitrogen; NS, not significant; (P), polymeric feed; sig., significant; TEI, total energy intake; TPI, total protein intake; TSF, triceps skin-fold thickness.

Although no prospective financial data were presented, considerable cost savings would have resulted from lower reoperation rates and lower complication rates in those receiving ETF in the RCT reviewed (Pupelis *et al.*, 2001).

Considering the wide range of GI diseases and the extensive use of ETF in this speciality, there is a lack of well-designed trials assessing the use of ETF versus routine clinical care in this patient group. In particular, assessments of changes in nutrient intake, body composition, function and outcome with ETF are needed, alongside financial evaluations of the effectiveness of this method of nutritional support.

GI disease: other analyses

Meta-analyses comparing ETF with steroid treatment in adults and paediatrics with Crohn's disease (hospital and community settings)

PATIENTS WITH CROHN'S DISEASE

A number of meta-analyses have compared the use of ETF with steroids as primary treatment in patients with active Crohn's disease (Griffiths *et al.*, 1995; Messori *et al.*, 1996). These suggest that corticosteroids may be more effective than ETF in the treatment of active Crohn's disease. However, compared with spontaneous or 'placebo-response' rates, exclusive ETF can be of therapeutic benefit, when tolerated, even though the efficacy may not equal that of steroid treatment (Griffiths *et al.*, 1995). One of the advantages of ETF is that it lacks the side-effects of corticosteroid treatment, which are particularly problematic in children and adolescents (see below). In addition, trials have failed to assess the quality of life of patients treated by the different modalities (Griffiths *et al.*, 1995). The interpretation of the effects of ETF on patients with Crohn's disease from individual trials has also been hindered by inadequate study designs. As outlined by King *et al.* (1997), the sample sizes in many studies that compared the efficacy of steroids with ETF were too small to provide sufficient power to discriminate differences between treatments.

Research is also required to ascertain the effects of modified nutritional formulas (including feeds enriched with antioxidants and omega-3 fatty acids) delivered enterally on the activity of Crohn's disease (trials with ONS of modified composition have been undertaken (Geerling *et al.*, 1998b,c, 2000b)).

CHILDREN WITH CROHN'S DISEASE

A recent meta-analysis has compared the efficacy of ETF (involving studies using elemental, semi-elemental and polymeric feeds) with steroids for periods of 3–15 weeks in the treatment of children with Crohn's disease (Heuschkel *et al.*, 2000). In five randomized trials (*n* 147), ETF was as effective as corticosteroids at inducing remission. Adding the findings of two NRT did not significantly alter these results. However, this meta-analysis suggested that ETF may have an advantage over steroid treatment as height velocities were greater in those children receiving ETF compared with those receiving steroids at short-term follow-up. Indeed, steroid use in children may adversely effect bone mineralization, growth and development (Heuschkel *et al.*, 2000). This review also highlighted the superior compliance of children to ETF compared with adults. For example, only 8% of children did not complete a course of ETF in the studies reviewed, whereas investigations in adults have suggested that up to 40% are withdrawn from ETF (Heuschkel *et al.*, 2000).

This section reviewed studies undertaken specifically in patients with GI disease. However, such patients may also have been studied within mixed groups of patients (e.g. general medical and surgical groups, see below).

General Medical/Mixed Diagnoses (Randomized and Non-randomized Data)

Estimates suggest that a substantial proportion of hospitalized patients across diagnoses are at risk of DRM (Stratton and Elia, 2000; see Chapter 2) and there are many reports of inadequate energy and nutrient intakes in this patient group (see Chapter 3). It is generally accepted that, in patients who are unable to eat, ETF is the most effective and safest means of providing a sole source of nutrition. However, the efficacy of supplementing intake with ETF in those able to eat has not been investigated in many well-designed RCT.

General medical/mixed diagnoses: present analysis

Only one RCT was reviewed (McWhirter and Pennington, 1996) and a further eight NRT (Bennegard *et al.*, 1983; Bastow *et al.*, 1985; Dresler *et al.*, 1987; Taylor, 1993; Hebuterne *et al.*, 1995; Schneider *et al.*, 1996; Gentile *et al.*, 2000; Winter *et al.*, 2000) were assessed and are summarized in Box A5.4 and Tables A5.16–A5.18. These trials incorporated patients with a wide range of diagnoses, including CVA, inflammatory bowel disease, anorexia nervosa and cancer.

Overall, the studies reviewed suggested that ETF was largely well tolerated (see Table A5.16; Dresler *et al.*, 1987; McWhirter and Pennington, 1996; Gentile *et al.*, 2000; Winter *et al.*, 2000). In a mixed group of medical patients (*n* 20), ETF was shown to be well tolerated whether given continuously over 24 h or in shorter 8 h cycles (Pinchcofsky-Devin and Kaminski,

1985b), although shorter schedules that allow periods of fasting and feeding are more physiological and may be beneficial metabolically (Pinchcofsky-Devin and Kaminski, 1985b).

However, ETF in the hospital setting is not without problems in this patient group. For example, temporary feeding interruptions, due to GI intolerance, feeding tube difficulties, cessation of feeding for medical procedures and inadvertent extubation may result in the prescribed energy goal of ETF not being met (Abernathy *et al.*, 1989), although this is more likely if patients are NG-fed (Abernathy *et al.*, 1989).

(I) What effect does ETF have on the voluntary food intake and total energy intake of general medical patients in hospital?

This analysis suggests that ETF is an effective way of increasing the energy and nutrient intakes of a variety of hospitalized patients. The trials reviewed in mixed groups of patients showed substantial increments in total energy intake with ETF compared with a randomized control group (McWhirter and Pennington, 1996) or compared with baseline intakes prior to ETF (Bennegard *et al.*, 1983; Bastow *et al.*, 1985; Hebuterne *et al.*, 1995; Schneider *et al.*, 1996; Table A5.18). A number of these trials also indicated that voluntary food intake was either not suppressed (versus a control group (McWhirter and Pennington, 1996) or uncontrolled data (Bennegard *et al.*, 1983)) or increased during the period

---

Box A.5.4. Key findings: effect of ETF in mixed groups of general medical hospital patients.

Nutritional intake: ETF can substantially increase total nutrient intake when used as a supplement to food and appears not to suppress appetite and food intake in patients with non-malignant disease.

Body weight: improvements in body weight and muscle mass may follow ETF.

Body function and clinical outcome: there may be functional benefits (immune function, intestinal absorption) with ETF and improvements to clinical outcome may be more likely if ETF is started earlier in the treatment of some patient groups.

Further research: studies in disease-specific groups may be more valuable than investigations of mixed patient groups.

Table A5.16. Enteral tube feeds used in trials of general medical patients in hospital (randomized and non-randomized data).

Trial	ETF	ETF energy density	ETF prescribed	ETF energy (kcal) provision	ETF protein (g) provision	Toleration	Timing of ETF
Randomized controlled trials							
McWhirter and Pennington (1996)	Clinifeed Favour (Clintec Nutrition)	1 kcal ml⁻¹	To meet est. energy requirements	843 (report 639 ml) 78% of prescribed	29.5	Diarrhoea (*n* 1), bloating (*n* 1), accidental removal of tube (*n* 1)	Overnight
Non-randomized trials							
Bastow *et al.* (1985)	Clinifeed Protein Rich (Roussel Lab) plus Neocal (oligosaccharide solution, Milner Scientific)	1.8 kcal ml⁻¹	1800, 60 g P	–	–	Occasional bloating	Overnight
Bennegard *et al.* (1983)	Clinifeed 400 (Roussel)	–	~1900 kcal, 70 g P (30–40 kcal kg⁻¹)	35 kcal kg⁻¹: ~1848 (cancer) ~2086 (non-cancer)	~68 (cancer) ~77 (non-cancer)	–	24 h
Dresler *et al.* (1987)	Isocal (Mead Johnson)	1 kcal ml⁻¹	120% of measured BEE	–	–	Tolerated with no diarrhoea or vomiting	18-hourly intervals
Gentile *et al.* (2000)	Polymeric, high-calorie formulas	1.5–2.0 kcal ml⁻¹	–	1395	–	No adverse consequences	–
Hebuterne *et al.* (1995)	Sondalis HP (Clintec Lab)	1.33 kcal ml⁻¹	To enable requirements to be met with combination of ETF and VFI	30.4 kcal kg⁻¹ IBW (<65 years) 29.4 kcal kg⁻¹ IBW (>65 years) 1935	1.51 g kg⁻¹ IBW (<65 years) 1.47 g kg⁻¹ IBW (>65 years)	Well tolerated in <65 years and >65 years. Diarrhoea in some pts and 2 cases of aspiration pneumonia	Overnight
Schneider *et al.* (1996)	Sondalis HP (Clintec Lab)	1.33 kcal ml⁻¹	–	–	–	Aspiration pneumonia (*n* 1)	Overnight
Taylor (1993)	Fresubin, Fresubin 750, OPD (Fresenius) or Pre-Nutrison (Nutricia)	Various	–	1500 (median)	–	–	–
Winter *et al.* (2000)	Vital or Alitraq (Ross Lab), followed by Ensure if tolerated	Various	30 kcal kg⁻¹ and 1.5 g P kg⁻¹ body wt	–	–	Intolerance to ETF in *n* 2 initially	–

BEE, basal energy expenditure; est., estimated; IBW, ideal body weight; P, protein; pts, patients; VFI, voluntary food intake.

Table A5.17. Trial characteristics: hospital-based trials of enteral tube feeding in general medical patients (randomized and non-randomized data).

Trial	Design	Diagnosis	No. ETF	No. CON	Initial BMI ETF group	Initial BMI CON group	Duration of ETF	Tube type	Control group
Randomized controlled trials									
McWhirter and Pennington (1996) UK	10001	Malnourished medical	25	26	All described as malnourished		11.8 days	NG tube	No nutrition intervention (one other group in trial given ONS)
Non-randomized trials									
Bastow *et al.* (1985) UK	C	Heterogeneous, undernourished – anorexia nervosa, cancer, TB	10	–	16.8	–	10–51 days	Fine-bore NG tube	–
Bennegard *et al.* (1983) Sweden *Metabolic investigation*	C	Cancer and general medical	13[a]	–	% IBW 67% (cancer) and 76% (non-cancer)	–	14 days	NG tube	–
Dresler *et al.* (1987) USA *Metabolic investigation*	C	Cancer and general medical	9[b]	–	> 10% wt loss (?over what time period)	–	14 days	Silastic intraduodenal tube	–
Gentile *et al.* (2000) Abstract Italy	C	Anorexia nervosa	39	–	12.9 (9.5–16.0)	–	59 (44) days	NG tube	–
Hebuterne *et al.* (1995) France[c]	C	Undernourished (anorexia, gastrectomy, IBD)	51 < 65 years 46 ≥ 65 years	–	All described as seriously undernourished (at least 10% wt loss in 3 months)	–	27 days	Fine-bore NG or NJ tube	–
Schneider *et al.* (1996) France	C	Gastrectomy, anorexia, cancer	20	–	14.7 (0.4)	–	14 days	Fine-bore polyurethane NG or NJ tube	–
Taylor (1993) UK	C	CVA, cancer, COPD	101	–	–	–	16 (34) days	NG tube – fine-bore or Ryles	–
Winter *et al.* (2000) South Africa	C	Crohn's, anorexia, TB	15[d]	–	13.41 (0.44)	–	2 weeks–3 months	NG tube	–

[a] *n* 8 cancer patients; *n* 5 non-cancer patients.
[b] *n* 5 cancer patients receiving radiotherapy; *n* 4 non-cancer patients (anorexia, depression, postoperative).
[c] Assumed BMI = 20 kg m^{-2} for categorization.
[d] *n* 2 required TPN for a period of time during treatment.
BMI, body mass index; CON, control; IBD, inflammatory bowel disease; IBW, ideal body weight; ONS, oral nutritional supplements; NJ, nasojejunal; TB, tuberculosis; TPN, total parenteral nutrition.

Table A5.18. Main findings of enteral tube feeding trials in hospitalized general medical patients (randomized and non-randomized data).

Trial	Energy/nutrient intake	Wt change ETF	Wt change CON	Function	Clinical outcome	Finance
Randomized controlled trials						
McWhirter and Pennington (1996)	TEI largely increased in ETF group (TEI 1863 kcal, 88.1 g P, ? sig.). Similar VFI in ETF and CON (1020 kcal ETF; 1250 kcal CON)	+3.3% (ETF vs. CON sig.) MAMC +2.1% (ETF vs. CON sig.)	−2.5% MAMC −2.79%	–	–	–
Non-randomized trials						
Bastow *et al.* (1985)	Increase in TEI due to ETF and an increase in VFI from 526–1240 kcal (pre-ETF) to 1472–2095 kcal (post-ETF)	+7.15 (3.5) kg (? sig.) Inc. in MAC and TSF (? sig.)	–	–	–	–
Bennegard *et al.* (1983)	ETF sig. improved TEI and energy balance: in cancer and non-cancer pts: cancer: pre −7.5; post +12.8 kcal kg⁻¹ (sig.), non-cancer: pre −4.6; post +14.8 kcal kg⁻¹ (sig.). ETF sig. increased N intake in both groups. VFI intake decreased sig. in cancer group only	+2.9 kg (cancer) (sig.) +3.3 kg (non-cancer) (sig.) Sig. increase in TSF and MAMC in non-cancer pts	–	–	–	–
Dresler *et al.* (1987)	–	Gain of ~4% of initial body wt (NS)	–	*(Metabolic investigation: ETF suppressed endogenous glucose production and whole-body protein catabolism in cancer and non-cancer patients)*	–	–
Gentile *et al.* (2000)	–	+5.6 (3.2) kg (sig.) BMI increased from 12.9 to 15.1 kg m⁻²	–	–	–	–
Hebuterne *et al.* (1995)[a]	ETF improved TEI in < 65 years and > 65 years to 288% of REE (< 65 years) and 282% (> 65 years) VFI sig. improved in both groups (+5 kcal kg⁻¹ in < 65 years and +2.3 kcal kg⁻¹ in > 65 years)	+4.2 kg (< 65 years) (sig.) +3.2 kg (> 65 years) (sig.) Sig. increases in TSF and MAC	–	–	–	–

Continued

Table A5.18. *Continued*

Trial	Energy/nutrient intake	Wt change ETF	Wt change CON	Function	Clinical outcome	Finance
Schneider *et al.* (1996)	TEI with ETF 3103 kcal (VFI 1168 kcal), with a sig. increase in energy intake over time	+1.6 kg (sig.) Sig. increases in TSF	–	Sig. improvements in humoral immunity (IgM, C3 and C4) and cell-mediated immunity (CD8, monocyte count, natural killer cell activity, skin tests)	–	–
Taylor (1993)	–	–	–	–	Pts (> 64 years) starved for > 5 days before ETF started had a sig. higher mortality than those starved for < 5 days during both the period of ETF and the H stay These pts also had longer H stays by 37 days than those starved 0–5 days. No account of disease severity made	Estimated savings of > £4519 per pt if NG feeding started earlier (starvation < 5 days)
Winter *et al.* (2000)	–	BMI increased to 16.1 (0.74) (? sig.)	–	Improved intestinal absorption (measured by xylose excretion), gastric acid output, pancreatic enzyme (lipase and amylase) output	–	–

aSimilar data reproduced in a later publication (Hebuterne, 1997): fat-free mass and body cell mass sig. improved following ETF (but to a sig. greater extent in < 65 years than in > 65 years). BMI, body mass index; CON, control; H, hospital; IgM, immunoglobulin M; inc., increase; MAC, mid-arm circumference; MAMC, mid-arm muscle circumference; N, nitrogen; NS, not significant; P, protein; REE, resting energy expenditure; sig., significant; ?sig., uncertain if statistically significant; TEI, total energy intake; TSF, triceps skin-fold thickness; VFI, voluntary food intake.

of ETF (uncontrolled data (Bastow *et al.*, 1985; Hebuterne *et al.*, 1995)). In cancer patients, although food intake was significantly reduced with ETF (Bennegard *et al.*, 1983), similar reductions were not seen in non-cancer patients (Bennegard *et al.*, 1983).

(II) What effect does ETF have on the body weight and composition of general medical patients in hospital?

The trials reviewed suggest that ETF of hospitalized patients leads to weight gain and may improve lean tissue mass. In the one RCT reviewed (McWhirter and Pennington, 1996), patients receiving ETF gained significantly more weight and muscle mass (mid-arm muscle circumference (MAMC)) than controls. All of the NRT that assessed body weight (Bennegard *et al.*, 1983; Bastow *et al.*, 1985; Dresler *et al.*, 1987; Hebuterne *et al.*, 1995; Schneider *et al.*, 1996; Gentile *et al.*, 2000; Winter *et al.*, 2000) found that patients receiving ETF gained weight, which was assessed as statistically significant in all but three trials (Bastow *et al.*, 1985; Dresler *et al.*, 1987; Winter *et al.*, 2000) (Table A5.18). Some trials also reported improvements in parameters of fat and muscle mass (Bastow *et al.*, 1985; Hebuterne *et al.*, 1995, Schneider *et al.*, 1996) (non-cancer patients only (Bennegard *et al.*, 1983)).

(III) What effect does ETF have on the body function of general medical patients in hospital?

There were no RCT that assessed functional changes with ETF and only two NRT that made such assessments (Schneider *et al.*, 1996; Winter *et al.*, 2000) (Table A5.18). These trials highlighted some functional benefits. Significant improvements in humoral and cell-mediated immunity (Schneider *et al.*, 1996) and in intestinal absorption (Winter *et al.*, 2000) were documented in severely undernourished patients receiving 2 weeks or more of ETF.

(IV) What effect does ETF have on the clinical and financial outcome of general medical patients in hospital?

Only one of the trials reviewed attempted to investigate the role of ETF in affecting patients' clinical outcome, with subsequent implications for cost (Taylor, 1993). An analysis by Taylor (1993) found that elderly patients (> 64 years) who were starved for more than 5 days before ETF was started had a significantly higher mortality and significantly longer hospital stays than those starved for shorter periods of time (< 5 days) (see Table A5.18). Consequently, they estimated that savings in excess of £4500 per patient could be made if ETF were started earlier.

Ultimately, well-designed RCT are needed to fully explore the clinical and cost efficacy of ETF in groups of patients in hospital. Ideally, studies in specific diagnostic groups, as opposed to mixed groups, should be undertaken in order to look at the changes in disease-specific functional and clinical outcome measures following ETF.

Liver Disease (Randomized and Non-randomized Data)

DRM is frequently a problem in patients with liver disease (see Chapter 2). Furthermore, the severity of malnutrition has been found to correlate with the severity of liver disease and 6-month mortality rates (Mendenhall *et al.*, 1985). Therefore, artificial nutritional support, and in particular ETF, is often required in these patients to prevent or treat malnutrition and the appearance of some of the major complications of liver disease (ascites, encephalopathy, severe infections) (Cabre *et al.*, 1990; Cabre and Gassull, 1993) as these quotes suggest:

> Appropriate and adequate nutritional support should play a role in the successful clinical management of alcoholic hepatitis.
>
> (Soberon *et al.*, 1987)

> Avoidance of even short periods of starvation ... and early nutritional support is mandatory in cirrhotic patients.
>
> (Müller, 1998)

However, how effective is ETF in patients with liver disease?

Liver disease: present analysis

Six RCT were reviewed that compared ETF with routine clinical care (no nutritional support) in patients with liver disease (Calvey *et al.*, 1984; Foschi *et al.*, 1986; Cabre *et al.*, 1990; Kearns *et al.*, 1992), including those post-liver transplant (Hasse *et al.*, 1995) and those treated for active oesophageal varices (de Ledinghen *et al.*, 1997) (see Box A5.5 and Tables A5.19–A5.21). In addition, three NRT (Smith *et al.*, 1982; Keohane *et al.*, 1983; Soberon *et al.*, 1987) were reviewed and are summarized in Tables A5.22–A5.24.

These trials indicated that ETF, using a variety of routes of feeding (into the stomach, duodenum or jejunum), was well tolerated in this patient group (Keohane *et al.*, 1983; Cabre *et al.*, 1990; Kearns *et al.*, 1992), including those with oesophageal varices (de Ledinghen *et al.*, 1997). For patients post-liver transplant, the routine use of jejunostomy feeding has been recommended (Pescovitz *et al.*, 1995). Very few GI complaints were reported in the studies reviewed (Smith *et al.*, 1982; Calvey *et al.*, 1984; de Ledinghen *et al.*, 1997) and there were no problems with oesophageal varices or the development of encephalopathy. Indeed, the presence of oesophageal varices is no longer a contraindication for ETF as fine-bore tubes are well tolerated (Cabre and Gassull, 1993; Thomas, 1994; de Ledinghen *et al.*, 1997). There were some practical issues in some of the trials, with patients failing to receive enough of their prescribed feed (Calvey *et al.*, 1984) and problems with tube placements (Kearns *et al.*, 1992; Hasse *et al.*, 1995). In the studies reviewed (see Tables A5.19 and A5.22), as in clinical practice (Thomas, 1994), modified enteral formulas (low-sodium, energy-dense or enriched with branched-chain amino acids (BCAA)) were sometimes used, depending on the disease state of the patients (e.g. low-sodium, energy-dense feed for an ascitic patient or a

feed enriched with BCAA for patients with hepatic encephalopathy (Thomas, 1994; Mizock, 1999)). The efficacy of ETF is addressed using the four main review questions.

> **Box A5.5.** Key findings: effect of ETF in hospital patients with liver disease.
>
> Nutritional intake: ETF can be used to significantly increase nutritional intake in patients treated for liver disease, including transplantation patients.
>
> Body weight: improvements in body weight have not been found in this patient group, probably due to the confounding effects of ascites.
>
> Clinical outcome: mortality and complication (infective and non-infective) rates may be reduced with ETF but larger trials are needed.

(I) What effect does ETF have on the voluntary food intake and total energy intake of patients in hospital with liver disease?

This analysis suggests that ETF in patients with liver disease and in those post-liver transplant can improve energy and nutrient intakes substantially. Of those trials that assessed changes in energy/nutrient intakes in various groups of patients with liver disease (cirrhosis (Cabre *et al.*, 1990; de Ledinghen *et al.*, 1997); alcoholic liver disease (Kearns *et al.*, 1992); post-liver transplant (Hasse *et al.*, 1995)), all showed improvements with ETF, which were assessed as significant in three of these trials when compared with the control group (Cabre *et al.*, 1990; Kearns *et al.*, 1992; Hasse *et al.*, 1995) (see Table A5.21). Similarly, two NRT indicated substantial increments in total energy intakes when ETF was given to patients with alcoholic liver disease (Smith *et al.*, 1982; Soberon *et al.*, 1987) (Table A5.24). In those RCT in which oral intake was encouraged, the contributions from food intake and ETF were not identified. However, one NRT did highlight an improvement in patients' food intake during 34 days of ETF (Smith *et al.*, 1982).

Table A5.19. Enteral tube feeds used in trials of patients with liver disease in hospital (randomized data).

Trial	ETF	ETF energy density	ETF prescribed	ETF energy (kcal) provision	ETF protein (g) provision	Toleration	Timing of ETF
Cabre *et al.* (1990)	Polymeric, BCAA-enriched feed developed for trial (UNIASA, Spain)	1.4 kcal ml^{-1}	2115 kcal, 71 g P	2115	71	ETF well tolerated by all. No encephalopathy	–
Calvey *et al.* (1984)	Maxipro HBV + Maxijoule LE (SHS) + Hepaticaid (Boots)	1 kcal ml^{-1}	2000 kcal, 10 g N	2000 kcal taken on 41% of days (ETF) and 28% of days (CON) (ETF vs. CON sig.)	–	~50% of pts were withdrawn (CON *n* 4; ETF *n* 7) due to failing to meet energy-intake goals. Similar rate of vomiting in ETF and CON. Diarrhoea in *n* 5 ETF	–
De Ledinghen *et al.* (1997)	Dripac Sondalis (Sopharga, France)	–	1665 kcal, 71 g P	2090 (903)	–	Well tolerated and no patients developed diarrhoea	Bolus over 3 h – NG feeding started day 1 after variceal treatment
Foschi *et al.* (1986)	Precision BR (semi-elemental feed, (Wander) 81.9% CHO, 10% peptides, 0.8% lipid)	–	–	–	–	–	–
Hasse *et al.* (1995)	Reabilan HN (Elan Pharma)	–	–	–	–	19 subjects withdrawn from trial (ETF 11; CON 8). Main reason in ETF group (*n* 7) was surgeons forgot to place NJ tube. *n* 4 had irritation from tube (ETF not stopped)	–
Kearns *et al.* (1992)	Isocal HCN (Mead Johnson)	2 kcal ml^{-1}	40 kcal and 1.5 g P kg^{-1} body wt	–	–	High energy and protein intakes from ETF tolerated well. ND tubes placed ~4 times	Constant ? 24 h

BCAA, branched-chain amino acid; CHO, carbohydrate; CON, control group; N, nitrogen; NJ, nasojejunal; ND, nasoduodenal; P, protein;.

Table A5.20. Trial characteristics: hospital-based trials of enteral tube feeding in patients with liver disease (randomized data).

Trial	Design	Diagnosis	No. ETF	No. CON	Initial BMI ETF group	Initial BMI CON group	Duration of ETF	Tube type	Control group
Cabre et al. (1990) Spain	10001	Cirrhosis	16	19	'Severely malnourished'	–	23.3 days	Fine-bore NG tube	2200 kcal, low-salt diet orally
Calvey et al. (1984) UK	10000	Cirrhosis	34	13[a]	–	–	4.5–9.5 days ETF 6 days CON	Compared 2 NG tubes: East Grinstead or Viomedex	Received same feed orally (2000 kcal, 10 g N – low-sodium feed)
De Ledinghen et al. (1997) France	10000	Alcoholic cirrhosis, bleeding oesophageal varices (underwent emergency sclerotherapy or banding ligation and octreotide)	12[b]	12[b]	26.9 (2.9)	25.5 (3.1)	8.6 (2.9) days	10F NG tube	Days 1–3 NBM after varices therapy day 4 standard low-sodium milk diet (800 kcal) day 5 mixed warm low-sodium diet (1400 kcal) day 6 standard low-sodium hospital diet (1800 kcal)
Foschi et al. (1986) Italy	10001	Obstructive jaundice, undergoing surgery, receiving PTBD	28[c]	32	–	–	20 days (prior to surgery)	K30 Pharmaseal nasoduodenal tube	Receiving PTBD
Hasse et al. (1995) USA/Israel	10001	Post-liver transplant	14	17	–	–	Started 12 h post-surgery and until oral intake met > 66% of nutritional requirements	Nasojejunal tube (10F)	Maintenance i.v. fluids until oral intake permitted
Kearns et al. (1992) USA	10001	Alcoholic liver disease	16	15	111% IBW[d]	125% IBW[d]	Up to 4 weeks	8F nasoduodenal tube	Regular diet

[a]Control group given ONS.

[b]clinically detected ascites in 42% (ETF) and 33% (CON) of pts. Assumed BMI < 20 for categorization and analysis.

[c]n 5 ETF + PN; n 4 PN (this group had sig. more diabetics and a longer duration of jaundice than CON).

[d]~75% of patients ascitic.

BMI, body mass index; CON, control; IBW, ideal body weight; i.v., intravenous; N, nitrogen; NBM, nil by mouth; ONS, oral nutritional supplements; PTBD, percutaneous transhepatic biliary drainage; sig., significantly.

Table A5.21. Main findings of enteral tube feeding trials in patients with liver disease in hospital (randomized data).

Trial	Energy/nutrient intake	Wt change ETF	Wt change CON	Function	Clinical outcome	Finance
Cabre et al. (1990)	ETF sig. higher TEI (2115 kcal) than CON (1320 kcal)	NS change in anthropometry	NS change in anthropometry	Hepatic reserve of ETF group improved sig. vs. CON (sig. reduction in Child's score)	Sig. lower mortality rate in ETF (2/16 (12%)) than CON (9/19 (47%)) but NS difference in rate of complications between ETF and CON (severe infection ETF 7/16 (44%); CON 7/19 (37%); GI bleed due to portal hypertension ETF 1/16 (6%); CON 4/19 (21%))	–
Calvey et al. (1984)	–	–	–	–	Incidence of variceal bleeding the same in ETF (1/44 pt-days) as in CON (1/45 pt-days)	–
De Ledinghen et al. (1997)	On day 7, ETF intake +422 kcal vs. CON (? sig.) (2090 kcal vs. 1669 kcal) On day 35 (OP follow-up), ETF consuming 364 kcal less than CON	+2.6%^{a} (+0.7 kg m^{-2}; ETF vs. CON NS) day 7 TSF +0.1 mm (ETF vs. CON ns) MAMC −0.6 cm (ETF vs. CON NS) (ETF NS differences at days 4, 7 and 35 vs. CON)	−4.7%^{a} (−1.2 kg m^{-2}) −0.3 mm −1.5 cm	NS differences in liver function between ETF and CON on day 4, 7 or 35 (Child–Pugh's score, LFT, number-correction test, ammonia concentrations)	Lower rate of rebleeding (n 1, 10%) in ETF than CON (n 4, 33%) (NS) Similar hospital stay (14.5 day ETF vs. 12.9 day CON, NS) Similar mortality rate (3 ETF vs. 2 CON, NS)	–
Foschi et al. (1986)	–	NS change in wt or TSF	–	–	Sig. lower rate of complications in ETF group (17.8% vs. 46.8% in CON) (infectious and non-infectious)	–
Hasse et al. (1995)	ETF sig. higher cumulative 12 day TEI and TPI (22,464 kcal, 927 g P) vs. CON (15,474 kcal, 637 g P) Calc. daily intakes (? sig.) ETF 1872 kcal, 77 g P CON 1289 kcal, 21 g P Daily TEI and TPI sig. higher in ETF vs. CON for first 6 days post-transplant	–	–	–	Sig. fewer viral infections in ETF (0%) than CON (18% of pts) Fewer bacterial (14% vs. 29%) and overall (21% vs. 47%) infections in ETF vs. CON (NS) Early ETF post-transplant did not affect hours on ventilator, length of stay in ICU or H (ETF 16 days vs. CON 18 days), rehospitalizations (0 in both groups) or rejection of transplant during 21 days postop.	Early ETF post-transplant did not affect H costs (prospective analysis)

Continued

Table A5.21. *Continued*

Trial	Energy/nutrient intake	Wt change ETF	Wt change CON	Function	Clinical outcome	Finance
Kearns *et al.* (1992)	ETF group consumed 200% of the energy and protein of the CON group (sig.) TPI ETF 103 g CON 50 g (sig.) TEI first 2 weeks: ETF 1.7 × REE; CON 0.8 × REE; TEI second 2 weeks: ETF 1.8 × REE (sig.); CON 1.2 × REE (sig.)	−2 kg (NS) (ETF vs. CON ? sig.)	−4 kg (sig.)	Improvement in grade of encephalopathy in ETF vs. deterioration in CON (sig. in first 2 weeks) No difference in LFT between groups Greater decrease in bilirubin in ETF (−49%) than CON (−12%) at 2 weeks (ETF vs. CON sig., trends continue at 4 weeks but NS) Sig. improvement in antipyrine elimination in ETF vs. CON	ETF lower mortality (13% week 1, 0% week 2) than CON (27%, 13%. NS) during 4 weeks of treatment. No difference in H length of stay (ETF 11 days, CON 12 days)	–

[a]Ascites present in > one-third of patients at start of trial.
CON, control; H, hospital; ICU, intensive care unit; LFT, liver function tests; NS, not significant; OP, out-patient; P, protein; postop., postoperative; REE, resting energy expenditure; sig., significant; ?sig., uncertain if statistically significant; TEI, total energy intake; TPI, total protein intake; TSF, triceps skin-fold thickness; TPI, total protein intake; .

Table A5.22. Enteral tube feeds used in trials of patients with liver disease in hospital (non-randomized data).

Trial	ETF	ETF energy density	ETF prescribed	ETF energy (kcal) provision	ETF protein (g) provision	Toleration	Timing of ETF
Keohane *et al.* (1983)	HepaticAid (BCAA-enriched formula)	–	~2688 kcal, 70 g P	–	–	No complications of ETF and use of tubes did not provoke oesophageal varices	Continuous 24 h
Smith *et al.* (1982)	Magnacal (Organon Nutritional Products, *n* 2) Type IIA (Modular, Ross, *n* 1) Type IIB (Modular, Mead Johnson, *n* 2)	2 kcal ml^{-1}	– – –	2170–2620 kcal (*n* 2) 3716 kcal (*n* 1) 2700–3400 kcal (*n* 2)	76–92 g (*n* 2) 143 g (*n* 1) 84–95 g (*n* 2)	Minor complications: constipation, diarrhoea, vomiting (*n* 5)	12 h period
Soberon *et al.* (1987)	Isocal HCN (45% fat, 15% P, 40% CHO; contains MCT and hydrolysed P)	2 kcal ml^{-1}	35 kcal kg^{-1} body wt	–	–	–	Continuous 24 h

BCCA, branched-chain amino acid; CHO, carbohydrate; P, protein.

Table A5.23. Trial characteristics: hospital-based trials of enteral tube feeding in patients with liver disease (non-randomized data).

Trial	Design	Diagnosis	No. ETF	No. CON	Initial BMI ETF group	Initial BMI CON group	Duration of ETF	Tube type	Control group
Keohane *et al.* (1983) UK	C	Cirrhosis in grade I to III hepatic coma	10	–	–	–	7.3 days (3–23 days)	Fine-bore NG tube (Clinifeed I, Roussel)	–
Smith *et al.* (1982) USA	C	Ascites due to alcoholic liver disease or cirrhosis	5	–	91.8% IBW (ascitic) Judged 'undernourished' by a number of criteria	–	34 days (14–62 days)	Dobbhoff nasoduodenal tube	–
Soberon *et al.* (1987) USA[a]	C	Anorectic alcoholic hepatitis	8	–	'Malnourished' TSF and MAMC < 25th/30th percentiles	–	3 days	Nasoduodenal tube	–

[a]Short-term metabolic trial in hospital patients.
BMI, body mass index; CON, control; IBW, ideal body weight; TSF, triceps skin-fold thickness.

Table A5.24. Main findings of enteral tube feeding trials in hospitalized patients with liver disease (non-randomized data).

Trial	Energy/nutrient intake	Wt change ETF	Wt change CON	Function	Outcome	Finance
Keohane *et al.* (1983)	–	NS improvement in any nutritional parameters	–	Sig. reduction in coma grading during period of ETF (also given lactulose and neomycin on admission)	–	–
Smith *et al.* (1982)	VFI increased from 1773 kcal (pre-ETF) to 2716 (post-ETF) (? whether VFI during ETF) ETF intakes 2170–3716 kcal	90.6% IBW Inc. in MAMA and MAFA (? sig.)	–	All showed clinical improvement with decreased ascites and normalized liver indices (bilirubin, prothrombin time, plasma ammonia, alkaline phosphatase)	–	–
Soberon *et al.* (1987)	ETF sig. increase in TEI and TPI and a fivefold increase in N balance Pre-ETF 830 kcal to ~1900 kcal with ETF	–	–	ETF did not worsen encephalopathy or affect fluid balance	–	–

CON, control; IBW, ideal body weight; inc., increase; MAMA, mid-arm muscle area; MAFA, mid-arm fat area; N, nitrogen; NS, not significant; sig., significant; TEI, total energy intake; TPI, total protein intake; VFI, voluntary food intake.

(II) What effect does ETF have on the body weight and composition of patients in hospital with liver disease?

Improvements in body weight following ETF were not found in the four RCT (Foschi *et al.*, 1986; Cabre *et al.*, 1990; Kearns *et al.*, 1992; de Ledinghen *et al.*, 1997) (Table A5.21) or the two NRT (Smith *et al.*, 1982; Keohane *et al.*, 1983) (Table A5.24) that made such assessments. Furthermore, although two trials indicated small improvements in parameters of muscle and fat mass relative to a control group (de Ledinghen *et al.*, 1997) or over time (NRT (Smith *et al.*, 1982)), these were not significant. However, small changes in body composition may be difficult to identify accurately with bedside assessment techniques, and the presence of ascites frequently complicates measurements of weight and other anthropometric parameters in liver disease patients. Therefore, in future studies, techniques that are capable of determining the proportions of different body compartments (fat, protein, water) should be included if more information is required about the changes in body composition that occur following ETF.

(III) What effect does ETF have on the body function of patients in hospital with liver disease?

The appropriate use of ETF in patients with liver disease may improve some functional parameters without producing any significant functional detriments. Following the use of ETF in patients with liver disease, two RCT demonstrated significantly greater improvements in liver function in those receiving ETF compared with controls (Cabre *et al.*, 1990; Kearns *et al.*, 1992), although this was not a consistent finding (de Ledinghen *et al.*, 1997) (Table A5.21). Improvements in clinical condition were also seen in two NRT, although there was no control group for comparison (Smith *et al.*, 1982; Keohane *et al.*, 1983) (see Table A5.24). Further RCT are required to assess the effect of ETF on functional parameters in patients with different types of liver disease and in those post-transplant. Ideally,

groups should be disease-specific and sufficiently large to have statistical power to detect functional changes.

(IV) What effect does ETF have on the clinical and financial outcome of patients in hospital with liver disease?

Improvements in clinical outcome may occur following the use of ETF in patients with liver disease and in patients post-liver transplant (see Table A5.21). From the RCT reviewed, no significant detriments were found and the improvements to clinical outcome observed included:

- Significantly lower rates of mortality in severely malnourished cirrhotics following ~20 days of ETF (Cabre *et al.*, 1990).
- Significantly lower rates of complications (infectious and non-infectious) in patients with obstructive jaundice receiving 20 days of ETF prior to surgery (Foschi *et al.*, 1986).
- Significantly fewer viral infections and fewer bacterial and overall complication rates in patients receiving ETF from 12 h post-liver transplant (Hasse *et al.*, 1995).

Meta-analysis of data from three RCT suggested that mortality rates (OR 0.42 (95% CI 0.05–3.44), *n* 90 (Cabre *et al.*, 1990; Kearns *et al.*, 1992; de Ledinghen *et al.*, 1997)) and complication rates (OR 0.36 (95% CI 0.07–1.81), *n* 126; (Foschi *et al.*, 1986; Cabre *et al.*, 1990; Hasse *et al.*, 1995)) may be reduced with ETF compared with routine clinical care. The reductions were not significant, possibly due to the small numbers involved in the analysis.

Those trials that assessed length of stay found no differences between intervention (ETF) and control groups (Kearns *et al.*, 1992; Hasse *et al.*, 1995; de Ledinghen *et al.*, 1997). Furthermore, Hasse *et al.*'s (1995) trial in post-transplant patients found that early ETF (within 12 h postoperatively) did not affect hospital costs (prospective analysis; average hospital charges ETF US\$93,857; control group US\$94,916). However, an American evidence-based review of the cost-effectiveness of enteral nutritional support in different disease states estimated that the cost of treating a patient who had liver surgery would be substantially lower if enteral nutrition (medical foods, ONS and ETF) were given (US$6500) than if not (US$17,000) (Nutrition Screening Initiative, 1996) (1994 US prices). Therefore, further financial evaluations would be beneficial in prospective RCT to assess the cost-effectiveness of ETF in patients with liver disease or in those undergoing liver transplantation.

Malignancy (Randomized and Non-randomized Data)

A large proportion of patients hospitalized with cancer suffer from malnutrition, as discussed in Chapter 2. The causes are multifactorial but commonly lead to weight loss and functional loss through impairing appetite and food intake. ETF can be a valuable way of supplementing the nutritional intake of cancer patients unable to maintain an oral intake to meet their requirements, either because of profound anorexia or physical eating difficulties. ETF can also be used as a sole source of nutrition in those unable to eat. Although there are a number of ethical issues related to the use of ETF in terminal cancer patients, these are beyond the scope of this review (for guidelines and information, refer to Bozzetti, 1996; Laviano and Meguid, 1996; Lennard-Jones, 1998).

Malignancy: present analysis

The efficacy of ETF as a supplement to nutritional intake in cancer patients in hospital has been investigated in this review. Although a number of trials in patients with various cancers (GI, head and neck, lung, leukaemia) were reviewed, only two were randomized trials (Tandon *et al.*, 1984; two reports: Van Bokhorst-de van der Schueren *et al.*, 2000b, 2001). One trial compared ETF (standard formula) with no nutritional support (Tandon *et al.*, 1984) (see Tables A5.25–A5.27) and the other

assessed the efficacy of preoperative ETF using standard and arginine-enriched formulas. A further four trials were non-randomized in design (Haffejee and Angorn, 1979; Lipschitz and Mitchell, 1980; de Vries *et al.*, 1982; Bruning *et al.*, 1988). A number of trials have also investigated the perioperative use of ETF in mixed groups of surgical patients, including those with cancer, and some studies have used specialized feeds containing nutrients thought to modulate inflammatory and immune parameters (see later in this appendix).

The trials reviewed suggested that ETF was mostly well tolerated (de Vries *et al.*, 1982; Bruning *et al.*, 1988) (Table A5.25). However, in one trial initial difficulties with feed delivery meant that patients were not meeting their energy requirements with ETF and consequently weight loss continued. This was overcome by increasing the prescribed dose of ETF to in excess of requirements (42 kcal kg^{-1} body weight) to ensure that patients met their nutritional requirements (Bruning *et al.*, 1988). The use of hospital-made formulas was associated with a case of infection and significantly more diarrhoea in patients with acute leukaemia than in controls (de Vries *et al.*, 1982). For these reasons, commercially produced, sterile feeds are usually recommended for ETF in cancer patients. The efficacy of ETF in hospital-based cancer patients is addressed using the four main review questions and summarized in Box A5.6.

(I) What effect does ETF have on the voluntary food intake and total energy intake of patients in hospital with malignancy?

This review suggests that ETF as a supplement to diet can improve appetite and food intake in cancer patients. Patients undergoing chemotherapy for GI cancer reported improvements in their appetite and food intake during 3 weeks of ETF, although no quantitative data were given in the paper (Tandon *et al.*, 1984) (Table A5.27). Similar changes were not seen in the control group receiving chemotherapy alone. In the other RCT reviewed (Van Bokhorst-de van der Schueren *et al.*, 2001), head and neck

---

Box A5.6. Key findings: effect of ETF in hospital patients with malignant disease.

Nutritional intake: ETF as a supplement to diet may improve appetite and food intake in patients with cancer, leading to significant improvements in total intake.

Body weight: ETF may aid weight gain or reduce weight loss in patients with malignancy, including those undergoing chemotherapy.

Body function and clinical outcome: functional benefits (immune function, well-being and better response to chemotherapy) and improvements in clinical outcome may follow ETF, but larger RCT are required in patients with different types of cancer and in those receiving different treatments (e.g. chemotherapy, radiotherapy).

---

cancer patients receiving an arginine-containing feed prior to surgery had greater appetite loss relative to the control group given no ETF (significant) and to those given a standard feed, in whom subjective increases in appetite were recorded (Van Bokhorst-de van der Schueren *et al.*, 2000b). However, in the main report of this study (Van Bokhorst-de van der Schueren *et al.*, 2001), total energy intakes were significantly greater in tube-fed (~110% of estimated basal energy expenditure (BEE)) patients than in controls (~79%), with voluntary food intakes accounting for ~10% of this. NRT in various groups of cancer patients (head and neck, leukaemia, oesophagus) indicated the effectiveness of ETF in maintaining energy and nutrient intakes in those with virtually no food intake (de Vries *et al.*, 1982; Bruning *et al.*, 1988) and in those given ETF as a supplement to an oral diet (Haffejee and Angorn, 1979) (Table A5.27). Indeed, patients with acute leukaemia expressed great relief at being tube-fed and not being forced to eat (de Vries *et al.*, 1982).

Since the prescribed amount of feed is sometimes not fully administered due to practical problems, in one study total ETF intake was increased by prescribing more feed (+~1100 kcal) (Bruning *et al.*, 1988).

(II) What effect does ETF have on the body weight and composition of patients in hospital with malignancy?

ETF may aid weight gain or reduce weight loss in patients with cancer, including those patients receiving chemotherapy (see Table A5.27). Weight-losing GI cancer patients receiving chemotherapy continued to lose significant amounts of weight if not given ETF (control group *n* 33), whereas those randomized to ETF gained small but significant amounts of weight (Tandon *et al.*, 1984; Table A5.27). Similarly, patients with acute leukaemia receiving ETF during chemotherapy had significantly less weight loss than a non-randomized control group (de Vries *et al.*, 1982). In contrast, when ETF was used preoperatively for 8 days in head and neck cancer patients, no significant changes in body weight, fat or muscle mass were found compared to the control group (Van Bokhorst-de van der Schueren *et al.*, 2001). Although other NRT assessed changes in weight and body composition with ETF (Haffejee and Angorn, 1979; Bruning *et al.*, 1988) (Table A5.27), the lack of randomized control groups prevented conclusions from being drawn. A retrospective review of cancer patients receiving radiotherapy suggested that ETF could help minimize weight loss due to the side-effects of this treatment in head and neck cancer patients, particularly if instituted before the onset of significant weight loss (Pezner *et al.*, 1987). Overall, there is a need for RCT to evaluate the changes in body weight and body composition (muscle and fat mass) that occur when ETF is used as a supplement to food intake. In this way the confounding effects of oedema, which often occurs in cancer patients (Kramer *et al.*, 1998), can be assessed.

Table A5.25. Enteral tube feeds used in trials of patients with malignancy in hospital (randomized and non-randomized data).

Trial	ETF	ETF energy density	ETF prescribed	ETF energy (kcal) provision	ETF protein (g) provision	Toleration	Timing of ETF
Randomized controlled trials							
Tandon et al. (1984)	Providal NG + Amidex-Pep solution (Dextromed, India) + fat and sugar	4 kcal ml⁻¹	3000–4000 kcal (plus allowed feed orally)	–	–	–	–
Van Bokhorst-de van der Schueren et al. (2000b, 2001)	ETF[1] standard feed (125 kcal and 6.25 g P per 100 ml) ETF[2] (as above, with 41% of P as arginine)	1.25 1.25	150% of calculated BEE	~100% of BEE	–	–	–
Non-randomized trials							
Bruning et al. (1988)	Nutrison High Energy	1.5 kcal ml⁻¹	(i) 32 kcal kg⁻¹ (ii) 43 kcal kg⁻¹	1.5 kcal kg⁻¹ body wt[a]	–	Failure of pts to receive planned dose due to pump-rate errors and blocked feeding tubes with drugs given (changed to larger tube size 10G and liquid drugs). Minority experienced GI complaints – fullness and nausea common early postop.	24h
de Vries et al. (1982)	Hospital-made pasteurized formula (89 g P, 62 g F, 280 g CHO per 2034 kcal) Nutrison RTS (Nutricia)	1.35 kcal ml⁻¹ 1 kcal ml⁻¹	–	2000–3000	–	Most pts accepted the tube very well and were relieved that they were not forced to eat One case of infection from hospital-made formula and 1 case of feeding into the lung. Sig. more diarrhoea in ETF vs. CON	24 h
Haffejee and Angorn (1979)	Vivonex + mineral/vitamin syrup	–	–	3700	20 g N	–	–
Lipschitz and Mitchell (1980)	–	–	–	3000	–	–	–

[a](i) Only 89% of planned dose of 32 kcal kg⁻¹ administered in n 8, so dose increased to 43 kcal kg⁻¹ (ii), of which 95% achieved.
BEE, basal energy expenditure; CHO, carbohydrate; F, fat; N, nitrogen P, protein; postop., postoperative; pts, patients; sig., significantly.

Table A5.26. Trial characteristics: hospital-based trials of enteral tube feeding in patients with malignancy (randomized and non-randomized data).

Trial	Design Diagnosis	No. ETF	No. CON	Initial BMI ETF group	Initial BMI CON group	Duration of ETF	Tube type	Control group
Randomized controlled trials								
Tandon et al. (1984) India	10001 Chemotherapy for advanced GI cancer	29	33	–	–	21 days	–	Chemotherapy alone
Van Bokhorst-de van der Schueren et al. (2000b, 2001)	10001 Surgery for head and neck cancer	ETF^1 15, ETF^2 17	17	42.6 (2.8) kg (20% wt loss, ? over what time period) — Pre-operative wt loss > 10% (? over what time period)	43.6 (4.3) kg 22% wt loss, ? over what time period)	Preop. 7–10 days Postop. 14 days	–	Given postop. ETF only with a standard feed (no preop. ETF)
Non-randomized trials								
Bruning et al. (1988) The Netherlands	C Head and neck cancer (postoperative)	20 (i) 8[a] (ii) 12	–	(i) 23.5 (ii) 24.4	–	21 days	Small-calibre (8G) NG tube (n 10), 10G NG tube (n 10)	–
de Vries et al. (1982) The Netherlands	B (retro?) Chemotherapy[b] for acute leukaemia	20	35	'Normal' n 5 'Mild depletion' n 13 (? only n 18) Nutritional state sig. poorer in ETF vs. CON group	'Normal' n 20 'Mild depletion' n 14 'Moderate depletion' n 1. Nutritional state sig. better in CON vs. ETF group	21 days	Nutricia NG tube (2 mm diameter)	Hospital diet. All patients (ETF and CON) were counselled by a dietitian
Haffejee and Angorn (1979) South Africa	C Cancer of the oesophagus	20	–	All 'undernourished' (defined by a variety of criteria)	–	21 days	–	–
Lipschitz and Mitchell (1980) A USA	B Chemotherapy for small cell lung cancer	7	7	'Moderately malnourished'		Over 2 chemo cycles (every 21 days)	–	Routine care

[a](i) First group of patients (group i) received only 89% of planned dose of 32 kcal kg^{-1} (n 8), so dose increased to 43 kcal kg^{-1} (of which 95% achieved) in subsequent pts (group ii).

[b]ETF started on the first day of induction chemotherapy in those patients with severe nausea or vomiting. Platelet and blood transfusions also given to some patients.

A, abstract; BMI, body mass index; chemo, chemotherapy; CON, control; postop, postoperative; preop, preoperative; retro, retrospective; sig., significantly.

Table A5.27. Main findings of enteral tube feeding trials in hospitalized patients with malignancy (randomized and non-randomized data).

Trial	Energy/nutrient intake	Wt change ETF	Wt change CON	Function	Clinical outcome	Finance
Randomized controlled trials						
Tandon *et al.* (1984)	Patients identified that appetite and oral intake improved during ETF (not seen to the same extent in CON)	+3.05% (+1.3 kg, sig.) (? ETF vs. CON)	−5.5% (−2.4 kg, sig.)	Absolute lymphocyte count and PHA skin response improved sig. (6.77 to 19.3 mm) in ETF and not in CON. No other differences between ETF and CON (TLC, immunoglobulins, T-cell count). Response to chemotherapy (objective and subjective rating) better in ETF vs. CON. Subjective feeling of well-being improved to a greater extent in ETF vs. CON (reduced analgesic requirement, improved performance status, increased appetite) (? sig.). Less GI toxicity from chemotherapy in ETF vs. CON (? sig)	Lower mortality in ETF vs. CON (21% vs. 39%) (? sig.)	–
Van Bokhorst-de van der Schueren *et al.* (2000b, 2001)	ETF sig. increased TEI (ETF[1] 110%, ETF[2] 113%) vs. CON (79% of BEE). Only ~10% of energy was provided as VFI in ETF groups. Symptoms of appetite loss less in ETF[1] and CON but increased in ETF[2] (arginine-containing) (ETF[2] vs. CON sig.)	Preop.: ETF[1] +0.5 kg ETF[2] +0.7 kg (ETF vs. CON NS) NS differences in changes in fat or muscle mass	−0.1 kg	NS differences in hand-grip strength or in immunological indices (lymphocyte count, T lymphocytes) Preop. to the day prior to surgery: Sig. increase in physical functioning, emotional functioning and dyspnoea symptoms in ETF[1] and ETF[2] (ETF[1] vs. CON sig.) (QLQ-C30; EORTC) NS differences in role, cognitive or social functioning or global health scores between groups NS changes or differences between groups in subjective assessments of physical fitness, mental health, daily and social activities and health At 6 months after surgery: Better cognitive function and less appetite loss in ETF[1] than ETF[2] (QLQ-C30) (? data for CON)	ETF[1] had lower complication rates (47%, 7/15) than CON (53%, 9/17) or ETF[2] (59%, 10/17) (fistula, wound complications, arterial bleeding, respiratory problems) NS differences in length of stay (ETF[1] 46 (30) days; ETF[2] 31 (23) days; CON 41 (32) days) NS differences in survival	–

Non-randomized trials

Study				
Bruning *et al.* (1988)	TEI (i) ~1905 kcal TEI (ii) ~3000 kcal (no VFI) (Both groups had lower TEI on days 1 and 2 postop.)	(i) −3.2 kg (sig.) − due to loss of BFM (ii) −0.4 kg (NS)	No change in malaise ratings or psychological complaint scale with ETF. 50% complained of thirst (No deficiencies of trace elements or vitamins. Reductions in urinary excretion of creatinine and 3-methylhistidine (sig. (i) only))	−
de Vries *et al.* (1982)	− Pts in ETF gp reported to have almost no VFI	−0.83% (ETF vs. CON sig.) Incidence of severe wt loss (> 5% in 21 days) sig. less in ETF vs. CON	−4.9% NS difference in no. of fever days between ETF and CON	−
Haffejee and Angorn (1979)	ETF increased TEI (reported intake from ETF ~3700 kcal, in addition to food intake not quantified)	+3.9 kg Inc. in TSF (? sig.)	Sig. increase in absolute and T-lymphocyte no., mitogenic response to PHA, serum C3, C4 and C3PA No change in B lymphocyte no. or total haemolytic complement No change in *in vivo* assessment of cellular immunity using skin tests	−
Lipschitz and Mitchell (1980)	−	−	Degree of neutropenia less after 1st and 2nd chemo cycles in ETF vs. CON (sig.). Greater rate of neutrophil recovery after 1st cycle of chemo in ETF vs. CON (sig.). Chemo had sig. less effect on bone marrow mitotic pool (myeloblasts, promyelocytes) and maturation pool in ETF vs. CON	−

BEE, basal energy expenditure; BFM, fat mass; chemo, chemotherapy; CON, control; NS, not significant; PHA, phytohaemagglutinin; preop., preoperative; sig., significant; TEI, total energy intake; TLC, total lymphocyte count; TSF, triceps skin-fold thickness; VFI, voluntary food intake.

(III) What effect does ETF have on the body function of patients in hospital with malignancy?

A number of functional benefits have been observed in cancer patients receiving ETF. The RCT reviewed suggested significant improvements in some markers of immune function, better objective and subjective responses to chemotherapy, greater improvements in well-being and less GI toxicity from chemotherapy than in those not given ETF (however, statistical comparisons between the two randomized groups were not presented) (Tandon *et al.*, 1984). The preoperative use of ETF (standard formula) in head and neck cancer patients led to significant improvements in some aspects of quality of life (physical and emotional functioning, EORTC) relative to a control group (Van Bokhorst-de van der Schueren *et al.*, 2000b). Although improvements were seen in those given an argi-nine-enriched feed, the differences compared with the control group were not significant (Van Bokhorst-de van der Schueren *et al.*, 2000b). No changes were seen in skeletal muscle strength either. Two NRT also suggested some improvement in immune markers with ETF (Haffejee and Angorn, 1979; Lipschitz and Mitchell, 1980) and better responses to chemotherapy than in control patients (Lipschitz and Mitchell, 1980) (see Table A5.27). Further research is required to assess the effect of ETF on body function in patients with different types of cancer and in those receiving different treatments (chemotherapy, radiotherapy, surgery).

(IV) What effect does ETF have on the clinical and financial outcome of patients in hospital with malignancy?

There may be some clinical benefits that result from the use of ETF in patients with cancer. Lower mortality rates were documented in patients receiving ETF (21%) during chemotherapy for advanced GI cancer compared with control patients (39%) (Tandon *et al.*, 1984) (Table A5.27). Whether this was statistically significant is

unclear. Indeed, the total numbers of patients in this trial were probably too small to assess significant changes in clinical outcome (probable type II error). Patients with head and neck cancer receiving ETF preoperatively had lower complication rates postoperatively (47%) than controls (53%) or those fed an arginine-enriched feed (59%), although it is not clear if these differences were significant (complications included fistula formation, wound and flap complications, bleeding and respiratory insufficiency) (Van Bokhorst-de van der Schueren *et al.*, 2001). In addition, no differences were observed in survival or hospital stays between groups. Therefore, larger RCT are required to confirm the benefits to clinical outcome observed in Tandon *et al.*'s (1984) trial, while assessing other clinical end-points (length of stay, complication rates, etc.). Ideally, studies should be undertaken in specific groups of patients (according to cancer site, stage-specific, treatment-specific).

No trials assessed the financial aspects of ETF. However, it can be hypothesized that improved responses to chemotherapy and improvements in immune function and well-being could translate into quicker recovery times and shorter hospital stays, producing some cost savings with ETF. Therefore, investigation of the cost-effectiveness of ETF in cancer patients is warranted.

Overall the trials reviewed were unable to properly assess changes in functional and clinical outcome measures with ETF because of limitations in study designs (small numbers, lack of randomization, lack of placebos). Further RCT are required in sufficiently large, homogeneous groups of cancer patients, including those receiving treatments (radiotherapy, chemotherapy) in hospital settings.

Use of immunonutrition

There is growing interest in the use of 'immune-enhancing' formulas for the nutritional support of cancer patients (e.g. GI and head and neck malignancies) (Daly *et al.*, 1995; Braga *et al.*, 1999; Snyderman *et al.*, 1999) undergoing surgery. A recent consensus has suggested that patients undergoing routine GI surgery for cancer should receive such feeds, particularly if they are malnourished (defined as an albumin < 3.5 g dl^{-1}) (Anon., 2001a). The consensus also suggests that malnourished patients undergoing major head and neck surgery may benefit. However, there is a need for further research in this area before definitive recommendations can be made.

Neurology – CVA (Non-randomized Data)

The importance of nutrition in the prevention and the treatment of stroke has recently been highlighted (Gariballa, 2000). In particular, ETF is a valuable means of providing nutrition for CVA patients, one-third of who may be dysphagic (Barer, 1989) and unable to eat or drink without risk of aspiration pneumonia. It could be that providing nutritional support via ETF in the early post-CVA period may, in improving nutritional intake, improve outcome (well-being/quality of life, recovery rate, etc.). However, controlled comparisons that assess the value of ETF in this patient group (compared with routine clinical care) are lacking. Similarly, the role of ETF in patients with other neurological conditions (Parkinson's disease, Huntingdon's chorea, multiple sclerosis (MS), motor neurone disease, etc.) has not been investigated in any depth.

No studies compared the efficacy of ETF at improving function and outcome with routine care in hospitalized CVA patients. Although it would be of benefit to examine the effects of ETF in CVA patients in RCT, it is difficult ethically to withhold nutritional support in this patient group or to insert a tube for placebo feeding.

The route of tube feeding may affect the efficacy of ETF in this patient group (Park *et al.*, 1992; Norton *et al.*, 1996). A number of case reports in stroke patients with prolonged swallowing difficulty have suggested that ETF using a PEG may improve

the outcome of late rehabilitation (Allison *et al.*, 1992). Some prospective, controlled studies (Park *et al.*, 1992; Norton *et al.*, 1996) have suggested that PEG feeding of stroke patients may be more effective than NG feeding. In these trials, stroke patients fed by PEG received a greater proportion of their nutritional requirements than those fed by NG tube (Park *et al.*, 1992; Norton *et al.*, 1996) (Tables A5.28–A5.30; see the individual papers for a discussion of the issues). One trial also indicated that patients' clinical outcome was better with PEG feeding (Norton *et al.*, 1996). Norton *et al.* (1996) suggested that stroke patients who were fed effectively (receiving 100% of their ETF requirement) by use of a PEG had lower mortality rates and higher discharge rates than those who were fed less effectively by NG feeding (receiving ~78% of their ETF requirement). Potentially, however, the inadequate assessments of swallow ability and the failure to instigate ETF until 14 days post-stroke in this trial may have affected patient outcome (Kerr *et al.*, 1996; Smithard, 1996). Indeed, one retrospective review has suggested that ETF of stroke patients within 72 h of admission is associated with a significantly shorter hospital stay (by ~10 days) (Nyswonger and Helmchen, 1992). However, prospective, controlled studies are required to investigate this.

Gastrostomy-fed patients with a stroke are mostly a severely disabled group and survival time after PEG placement is often short (Wanklyn *et al.*, 1995), although patients with a CVA are one of the largest groups receiving home ETF (UK data). National surveys of stroke patients receiving ETF have been undertaken in the community (Elia *et al.*, 2001a) and more details can be found in Appendix 6.

Further research is also required, where ethically possible, to ascertain the benefits of ETF in patients with all neurological conditions (e.g. MS, Parkinson's disease, Alzheimer's disease, etc.). Indeed, a recent case-report highlighted the benefits of ETF in patients with Alzheimer's disease. This same report also suggested that ETF was inadequately used in the clinical setting in

Table A5.28. Enteral tube feeds used in trials of neurology patients in hospital (non-randomized data).

Trial	ETF	ETF energy density	ETF prescribed	ETF energy (kcal) provision	ETF protein (g) provision	Toleration	Timing of ETF
Norton *et al.* (1996)	Nutrison (Nutricia)	1 kcal ml^{-1}	Assume 100% of est. energy requirements prescribed NG group received sig. smaller proportion of their prescribed feed (78%) than the PEG group (100%)	–	–	NG group required tube to be resited on average 6 times with 71% losing at least 1 day of feeding	–
Park *et al.* (1992)	Ensure (Ross) Peptamen for *n* 1 (Clintec)	1 kcal ml^{-1}	NG 1795 kcal PEG 1618 kcal	NG 981 (55% of prescribed) PEG 1511 (93% of prescribed)	–	NG – no complications; PEG – aspiration pneumonia (*n* 2), wound infection (*n* 1)	24 h

est., estimated; NG, nasogastric; PEG, percutaneous endoscopic gastrostomy; sig., significantly.

Table A5.29. Trial characteristics: hospital-based trials of enteral tube feeding in neurology patients (non-randomized data).

Trial	Design	Diagnosis	No. ETF	No. CON	Initial BMI ETF group	Initial BMI CON group	Duration of ETF	Tube type	Control group
Norton *et al.* (1996) UK	C	CVA and dysphagia[a]	16 PEG 16 NG	–	–	–	–	Nasogastric vs. PEG	–
Park *et al.* (1992) UK	C	CVA and dysphagia	19 PEG 19 NG	–	–	–	NG 5.2 days PEG 28 days	Nasogastric vs. PEG	–

aMethods for assessing swallowing function controversial. BMI, body mass index; CON, control.

Table A5.30. Main findings of enteral tube feeding trials in hospitalized neurology patients (non-randomized data).

Trial	Energy/nutrient intake	Wt change ETF	Wt change CON	Function	Clinical outcome	Finance
Norton *et al.* (1996)	–	PEG +2.2 kg NG − 2.6 kg (PEG vs. NG sig.)	–	–	PEG sig. lower mortality (*n* 2) than NG group (*n* 8) Discharge rates at 6 weeks sig. greater in PEG group (*n* 6) than NG group (*n* 0)	–
Park *et al.* (1992)	TEI PEG 1511 kcal and NG 981 kcal (without ETF patients would have nil intake due to dysphagia)	1st week: PEG +1.4 kg NG +0.6 kg Over trial: PEG +3.4 kg NG no data	–	–	–	–

CON, control; sig., significant; TEI, total energy intake.

patients with neurological conditions other than stroke who could otherwise benefit from this form of nutritional treatment (Barratt, 2000).

Other studies in mixed groups of patients (e.g. general medical, elderly) may have included those with neurological conditions (see the individual sections in this appendix (hospital studies) and in Appendix 6 (community studies)).

Orthopaedics (Randomized Data)

Improvements in outcome in fractured neck of femur patients have been shown following the use of oral nutritional supplements (ONS) (Delmi et al., 1990), as discussed in Chapter 6. Briefly, the findings presented in this section, although from a limited number of studies, also suggest that ETF in this patient group can influence outcome, reducing rehabilitation times and mortality (see Box A5.7).

Box A5.7. Key findings: effect of ETF in hospital orthopaedic patients.

Nutritional intake: ETF can significantly improve total intake in fractured neck of femur patients compared with routine clinical care. ETF appears not to suppress voluntary food intake.

Clinical outcome: rehabilitation times and hospital stays may be reduced and mortality rates may be lower with ETF, particularly in the underweight patient.

Further research: research is needed to assess the impact of ETF on nutritional status and outcome (functional, clinical and financial), both in the hospital setting and beyond.

Two RCT (Bastow et al., 1983; Sullivan et al., 1998) (see Tables A5.31–A5.33) investigating the impact of ETF on the outcome of patients with fractured neck of femur were reviewed. In both studies, ETF (~1000 kcal) was given overnight as a supplement to food intake and significantly improved total energy intake compared with a control group given routine clinical care.

In the earlier trial (Bastow et al., 1983), in which elderly women were underweight ('thin' or 'very thin'), rehabilitation times were reduced and hospital stays shortened (significantly so in 'very thin' patients, see Table A5.33). Also 'very thin' patients given ETF had a lower mortality rate, but this was not significant (which the authors felt could be due to the small sample size). In this group, significantly greater weight gain (+5 kg) was also observed with ETF compared with controls. This may have been because ETF did not suppress voluntary food intake in this trial, so that total energy intake was markedly increased. There may have been benefits of ETF to patients following discharge from hospital to community (as in ONS studies: see Chapter 6), but these were not assessed in this RCT.

In a more recent trial (Sullivan et al., 1998), in a group of patients (mostly male) who were, on average, not underweight (body mass index (BMI) ~24 kg m^{-2}), similar reductions in rehabilitation times were not seen. For example, there were no significant differences in hospital stays between ETF (38 days) and control (24 days) groups. Similarly, this study found no differences in rates of postoperative complications (88% vs. 80%) or life-threatening complications (25% vs. 30%). Rates of discharge to an institution, although lower in the ETF group, were not significantly so (50% vs. 57%). However, there was a lower mortality rate in patients given ETF in hospital (0% vs. 30%, not significant) and at 6 months (0% vs. 50%, significant). No information was provided about changes in nutritional status in this study.

Meta-analysis of mortality rates from three sets of data in two RCT (Bastow et al., 1983; Sullivan et al., 1998) suggested that there may be a reduction in mortality with ETF (OR 0.52 (95% CI 0.06–4.28)). The lack of significance could be due to small numbers in the analysis (n 140).

Ideally, larger, placebo-controlled studies are required to provide further information about the improvements in clinical outcome that may follow ETF and other forms of nutritional support (i.e. ONS) in fractured neck of femur patients, both within and beyond the environs of the hospital.

Table A5.31. Enteral tube feeds used in trials of orthopaedic patients in hospital (randomized data).

Trial	ETF	ETF energy density	ETF prescribed	ETF energy (kcal) provision	ETF protein (g) provision	Toleration	Timing of ETF
Bastow et al. (1983)	Clinifeed Iso (Roussel Lab)	1 kcal ml^{-1}	1000 kcal, 28 g P	1000	28	22% failed to tolerate NG tube. No aspiration and infrequent diarrhoea associated with antibiotics	Overnight
Sullivan et al. (1998)	Promote (Ross)	–	1031 kcal	896	–	No complications with the tube and no sig. diarrhoea.	11 h overnight, starting at 7 p.m.

P, protein; sig, significant.

Table A5.32. Trial characteristics: hospital-based trials of enteral tube feeding in orthopaedic patients (randomized data).

Trial	Design	Diagnosis	No. ETF	No. CON	Initial BMI ETF group	Initial BMI CON group	Duration of ETF	Tube type	Control group
Bastow et al. (1983) UK	10001	FNF (elderly women)	64	58	Described as 'thin' or 'very thin' 24.1 (4.8)	Described as 'thin' or 'very thin' 24.1 (7.8)	24 days 'thin' 28 days 'very thin'	Fine-bore NG tube	VFI only
Sullivan et al. (1998) USA	10001	FNF (elderly, mostly men)	8	10			15.8 (16.4) days	Fine-bore NG tube	Standard post-operative care

BMI, body mass index; CON, control; FNF, fractured neck of femur; VFI, voluntary food intake.

Table A5.33. Main findings of enteral tube feeding trials in hospitalized orthopaedic patients (randomized data).

Trial	Energy/nutrient intake	Wt change ETF	Wt change CON	Function	Clinical outcome	Finance
Bastow *et al.* (1983)	Large increase in TEI with ETF in 'thin' (2094 kcal) and 'very thin' (1928 kcal) groups vs. CON (1357 kcal and 1000 kcal). VFI slightly decreased in 'thin' group (sig.) but not 'very thin' group vs. CON	'Thin' +2.8 kg (ETF vs. CON NS) 'Very thin' +4.9 kg (ETF vs. CON sig). Sig. increases in TSF and MAC in 'very thin' groups	'Thin' +1.2 kg 'Very thin' +0.7 kg	–	Lower mortality in ETF ('very thin') vs. CON (NS) Shorter rehabilitation time (time taken to gain independent mobility) in ETF vs. CON (sig.). Shorter length of H stay in ETF ('very thin') vs. CON (29 days vs. 38 days, sig.)	–
Sullivan *et al.* (1998)	Sig. greater TEI (1845 kcal) with ETF than in CON (1028 kcal), VFI NS different in ETF (948 kcal) or CON (1019 kcal)	–	–	No difference in functional status between ETF and CON (mental test, ADL)	ETF reduced mortality in hospital (0% vs. 30%, NS) and at 6 months (0% vs. 50%, ETF vs. CON sig.) NS differences in rate of postop. complications (88% vs. 80%), life-threatening complications (25% vs. 30%), rate of discharge to an institution (50% vs. 57%), no. of medications (4.6 vs. 5.0) or length of stay (38 days vs. 24 days).	–

ADL, activities of daily living; CON, control; H, hospital; MAC, mid-arm circumference; NS, not significant; postop., postoperative; sig., significant; TEI, total energy intake; TSF, triceps skin-fold thickness; VFI, voluntary food intake.

Studies of ETF in mixed groups of surgical patients may have included orthopaedic patients (e.g. Moncure *et al.*, 1999) and these are discussed later in this appendix.

Paediatrics (Randomized and Non-randomized Data)

ETF plays a valuable part in the treatment of children at risk of DRM (Puntis, 2001). However, there is a lack of RCT in hospitalized paediatric patients that formally assess the efficacy of ETF as a supplement to food intake. Indeed, only one RCT in cystic fibrosis (CF) patients was reviewed (Shepherd *et al.*, 1988) and the remainder (*n* 7) were small NRT (*n* < 45) (Morin *et al.*, 1980; Yahav *et al.*, 1985; Smith *et al.*, 1986; Daniels *et al.*, 1989; Finch and Lawson, 1993; Chellis *et al.*, 1996; Leite and Fantozzi, 1998) (see Tables A5.34–A5.36). All of the studies reviewed showed ETF to be safe and efficacious when used in infants and children with a number of conditions (including critical illness, neurological deficits, intractable diarrhoea, CF, congenital heart disease, Crohn's disease (see Table A5.35)) and in a variety of hospital settings (Morin *et al.*, 1980; Smith *et al.*, 1986; Daniels *et al.*, 1989; Finch and Lawson, 1993; Chellis *et al.*, 1996; Leite and Fantozzi, 1998).

ETF from 3 days (Yahav *et al.*, 1985) to up to 3 months (Finch and Lawson, 1993) enabled children hospitalized with a variety of conditions (see Table A5.36) to improve energy and nutrient intakes (Morin *et al.*, 1980; Yahav *et al.*, 1985; Shepherd *et al.*, 1988; Daniels *et al.*, 1989; Finch and Lawson, 1993; Chellis *et al.*, 1996; Leite and Fantozzi, 1998), which in the majority of cases enabled estimated energy requirements to be met. Consequently, those trials that assessed changes in nutritional status with ETF (one RCT: Shepherd *et al.*, 1988; and four NRT: Morin *et al.*, 1980; Yahav *et al.*, 1985; Daniels *et al.*, 1989; Finch and Lawson, 1993) found weight gain, increases in height and improvements in other anthro-

pometric parameters. Although only one of these trials included a randomized control group (Shepherd *et al.*, 1988), an NRT (Daniels *et al.*, 1989) indicated that such changes did not occur when children with CF were not given ETF. Furthermore, this trial indicated that weight was subsequently lost when ETF was stopped on discharge from hospital (see below). In infants with congenital heart disease, prior to the start of ETF, a high-energy diet taken orally had been unable to stimulate weight gain (Yahav *et al.*, 1985).

All the trials of ETF in children in the hospital setting have been reviewed according to disease/diagnostic category and are summarized below. Trials of ETF in the community setting in children with a variety of diseases (including cerebral palsy, CF, liver disease, cancer, human immunodeficiency virus/acquired immune deficiency syndrome (HIV/AIDS)) have been summarized in Appendix 6.

Congenital heart disease

In growth-failing infants with congenital heart disease (aged 2–36 months old, *n* 11), ETF increased total energy intake from 88 to 169 kcal kg^{-1} body weight daily (using an energy-dense formula) over a 3–7-day period. This led to weight gain in all children (16–20 g kg^{-1} day^{-1}), with constant weight gain being observed when intake was > 170 kcal kg^{-1} day^{-1}. Previous attempts to increase weight using the high-energy formula taken orally had been unsuccessful. Heart rate and respiratory rate were transiently but significantly increased with ETF compared with the other diets, during which total intake was less (Yahav *et al.*, 1985).

Critical illness

In critically ill paediatric patients, ETF was well tolerated, with no documented complications (Chellis *et al.*, 1996; Leite and Fantozzi, 1998). In one trial, transpyloric feeding tubes placed at the bedside allowed

Table A5.34. Enteral tube feeds used in trials of paediatric patients in hospital (randomized and non-randomized data).

Trial	ETF	ETF energy density	ETF prescribed	ETF energy (kcal) provision	ETF protein (g) provision	Toleration	Timing of ETF
Randomized controlled trials							
Shepherd *et al.* (1988)	Criticare HM (Mead Johnson, semi-elemental)	1 kcal ml^{-1}	To achieve $\geq$ 140% of RDA for energy with oral intake	1000–1500	–	–	Nocturnal
Non-randomized trials							
Chellis *et al.* (1996)	Pediasure (Ross)	1 kcal ml^{-1}	To meet caloric requirements in 24 h	74% achieved prescribed energy goal in 24 h	–	Good – no complications (no aspiration), no nasal or GI mucosal injury	–
Daniels *et al.* (1989)	Vivonex elemental diet (Eaton Laboratories) plus glucose polymer	–	50% of est. energy requirement	374 kcal	–	Initial problems with tube or formula: vomiting, diarrhoea, nausea, bloating (*n* 8); behavioural difficulties (*n* 1);	Overnight
Finch and Lawson (1993)	Pediasure (Ross) (glucose polymer added in *n* 2)	1 kcal ml^{-1}	> 60% of est. energy requirements	–	–	*n* 5 had diarrhoea with ETF	–
Leite and Fantozzi (1998)	–	1 kcal ml^{-1}	100% of est. energy requirements	–	–	Diarrhoea in 15%, tube obstruction in 10%, bloating in 10%. No pneumonia, aspiration or GI bleeding	–
Morin *et al.* (1980)	Vivonex	–	80.5 (0.6) kcal kg^{-1} body wt	80.5 (0.6) kcal kg^{-1}	–	Well tolerated	22 h day^{-1} continuous
Smith *et al.* (1986)	Pregestimil (Mead Johnson) or Vivonex Standard (Norwich Eaton)	–	100% of est. energy requirements	–	–	–	–
Yahav *et al.* (1985)	Materna 15% (Trimalta, cow's milk-based formula) + Caloreen (Milner Scint Co) Total: 56% CHO, 38% F, 6% P	1.52 kcal ml^{-1}	–	–	–	Transient increase in heart rate and respiratory rate at the end of feeding	Intermittent (4 –6 times daily)

CHO, carbohydrate; est., estimated; F, fat; P, protein; RDA, recommended daily allowance.

Table A5.35. Trial characteristics: hospital-based trials of enteral tube feeding in paediatric patients (randomized and non-randomized data).

Trial	Design	No. ETF	No. CON	Initial BMI ETF group	Initial BMI CON group	Duration of ETF	Other treatments	Type of tube	Control group
Randomized controlled trials									
Shepherd *et al.* (1988) Australia	1–1000[a]	12	10	−0.94 z score for wt	−0.83 z score for wt	2–3 weeks	*Ad libitum* high-energy diet orally, antibiotics, physiotherapy	NG weighted silicone tube	Standard therapy and high-energy ward diet with enzymes
Non-randomized trials									
Chellis *et al.* (1996) USA	C	42	–	–	–	~6 days	–	Transpyloric feeding tube placed at bedside	–
Daniels *et al.* (1989) Austrailia	B	11	–	87.4% ideal wt-for-ht (75–100%)	–	13 (2.4) days	*Ad libitum* high-energy diet orally, antibiotics, physiotherapy	Fine-bore NG silastic feeding tube	Findings compared with pt's previous admission when no ETF given
Finch and Lawson (1993) UK	C	23 (only 18 ETF)	–	Failure to thrive in *n* 14 (< 3rd centile for ht and/or wt or > 1 wt centile less than ht)	–	1–3 months	–	–	–
Leite and Fantozzi (1998) Brazil	C	27	–	25% wasted and/or stunted	–	11 days (4–38 days)	–	Nasoduodenal polyurethane tube	–
Morin *et al.* (1980)	C	4	–	Growth retarded Ht < 3rd percentile, velocity of growth and wt gain < 3rd percentile	–	6 weeks	None (ETF sole source)	Silicone NG tube	–

Continued

Table A5.35. *Continued.*

Trial	Design	Diagnosis/ condition	No. ETF	No. CON	Initial BMI ETF group	Initial BMI CON group	Duration of ETF	Other treatments	Type of tube	Control group
Smith *et al.* (1986) USA	B[b]	Intractable diarrhoea > 2 weeks' duration (aged < 2 years)	16	29	–	–	–	Some received intravenous fluids	NG tube	Findings compared with admissions prior to a formal protocol for treatment being constructed
Yahav *et al.* (1985)	C	Congenital heart disease, growth failure (aged 2 months to 3 years)	11	–	60–90% wt-for-ht 60–100% ht-for-age	–	3–7 days	Those aged > 8 weeks given fruit, vegetables and meat	8F NG tube (polyvinyl chloride) – gravity feeding	Control period prior to NG feeding – given same formula orally

[a]Although patients were randomly assigned to treatment or control groups, those who declined ETF were entered into CON. Some patients were randomized on separate occasions to different groups.
[b]Retrospective control groups.
CON, control; CNS, central nervous system; NG, nasogastric.

Table A5.36. Main findings of enteral tube feeding trials in hospitalized paediatric patients (randomized and non-randomized data)

Trial	Energy/nutrient intake	Wt change ETF	Wt change CON	Function	Outcome	Finance
Randomized controlled trials						
Shepherd et al. (1988)	TEI increased with ETF from 86 kcal kg^{-1} (pre-ETF) to 112 kcal kg^{-1} (with ETF) No data on food intake	+4.76% (1.5 kg; sig. vs. pre-ETF) (ETF vs. CON NS) (sig. correlation between initial underweight and subsequent wt gain in ETF only)	+3.95% (1.2 kg)	Sig. increase in FEV$_1$ in both ETF and CON (ETF vs. CON NS) *Sig. increase in protein synthesis, catabolism and net deposition with ETF (sig. vs. pre-ETF and vs. CON)*	–	–
Non-randomized trials						
Chellis et al. (1996)	74% reached energy requirements within 24 h and the remainder in 48 h with ETF	–		–	–	Savings in charges of $425 daily per patient using ETF instead of PN. Total saving per patient of $2701 (prospective)
Daniels et al. (1989)	ETF sig. increased TEI from 116% of RDA (CON period) to 165% (expressed per kg body wt). TEI 795 kcal (±245 kcal). Small, sig. decrease in VFI with ETF	Sig. greater wt gain with ETF vs. pre-ETF period but wt lost after ETF stopped post-discharge		–	–	–
Finch and Lawson (1993)	Intake from ETF ~97% of EAR for energy (only 68% in overweight children). Some failure-to-thrive children also ate (7–25% of TEI)	Wt gain, growth (ht increase) and increases in TSF and MAC (? sig.)		–	–	–
Leite and Fantozzi (1998)	Est. energy requirements met by 7th day after admission with ETF (feeding started within 48 h of admission)	Nitrogen balance sig. improved		–	–	–
Morin et al. (1980)	ETF increased daily energy intake from 69.2 (9.3) to 80.5 (0.6) kcal kg^{-1}	+3.8 (0.5) kg (sig.) +1.8 (0.3) cm in ht (sig.) (greater than in 1 year period preceding ETF: +0.8 kg, +1.7 cm)		Improved growth (see earlier column) Complete remission of symptoms	–	–

Continued

Table A5.36. *Continued*

Trial	Energy/nutrient intake	Wt change ETF	Wt change CON	Function	Clinical outcome	Finance
Smith *et al.* (1986)	–	–	–	–	With ETF protocols: length of stay reduced by 26 days, 13 days fewer on TPN and 12 days fewer on PPN (NS)	Introduction of protocol to encourage use of ETF produced cost savings of US$14,750 per patient (prospective)
Yahav *et al.* (1985)	Increase in energy intake from 88.3 kcal kg^{-1} baseline to 169 (29) kcal kg^{-1} with ETF	13.3 (3.6) g kg^{-1} day^{-1} (all patients gained weight)	–	–	–	–

CON, control; EAR, estimated average requirement; est., estimated; FEV$_1$, forced expiratory volume in 1 s; ht, height; MAC, mid-arm circumference; NS, not significant; PPN, peripheral parenteral nutrition; RDA, recommended daily allowance; sig., significant; ?sig., uncertain if statistically significant; TEI, total energy intake; TPN, total parenteral nutrition; VFI, voluntary food intake.

paediatric patients to start ETF ~6.5 days earlier than if ETF had been withheld until the patients had stabilized sufficiently for transport to the radiology department for fluoroscopic placement (Chellis *et al.*, 1996). Bedside placement was also cheaper (by US$111 per patient). ETF enabled patients' energy requirements to be met and regular stool patterns to develop and reduced the use of PN. Consequently, the estimated savings in patients' charges were considerable (see Table A5.36), with a 37% reduction in patient-days on PN (Chellis *et al.*, 1996). In the other trial reviewed, ETF in critically ill children with acute neurological disease enabled their high nutritional requirements to be met safely and effectively (Leite and Fantozzi, 1998).

Crohn's disease

In a very small trial (*n* 4), children with growth retardation (aged 11–13 years) and Crohn's disease were given 6 weeks of ETF as a sole source of nutrition. ETF was well tolerated and enabled an increase in total energy intake, a significant increase in body weight, a significant improvement in height and complete remission of symptoms. The conclusions of this trial are limited due to the lack of a randomized control group. However, improvements in weight (+3.8 kg) and height (+1.8 cm) during the 6 weeks of ETF were significantly greater than recorded during the year preceding ETF (+0.8 kg, +1.7 cm).

Cystic fibrosis

ETF is recommended in the treatment of malnourished patients with CF (Pencharz and Durie, 2000). An RCT in growth-retarded CF patients highlighted the role of ETF as a supplement to food intake in those in hospital (Shepherd *et al.*, 1988). Total energy intake was markedly increased with ETF and significant longitudinal improvements in weight were observed (Table A5.36). However, similar increases were seen in the control group given a high-

energy diet orally (Shepherd *et al.*, 1988). Functionally, significant improvements in respiratory function forced expiratory volume in 1 s (FEV$_1$) occurred with ETF (also seen in control group) and increases in protein synthesis and deposition were also documented in the ETF group only (Shepherd *et al.*, 1988) (Table A5.36). In a non-randomized report, overnight ETF in a small group of children hospitalized with acute exacerbations of CF enabled total energy intakes and weight to be significantly improved compared to previous admissions when ETF was not given (Table A5.36) (Daniels *et al.*, 1989). However, long-term follow-up post-discharge in these patients suggested that weight gain was not sustained once ETF was stopped.

Other gastrointestinal conditions

The introduction of a protocol to improve the nutritional management of infants with intractable diarrhoea by using ETF (Smith *et al.*, 1986) led to reductions in length of hospital stay and resulted in fewer days of PN (centrally and peripherally administered). Consequently, calculated cost savings were US$14,750 per patient. However, this was not an RCT.

Ultimately, more trials in infants and children in disease-specific groups are needed to ascertain more fully the functional, clinical and financial benefits of using ETF in paediatrics. However, in cases of growth retardation, randomization of children to routine care (with no nutritional intervention) may not be ethically feasible.

Surgery (Randomized and Non-randomized Data)

Traditionally, the management of surgical patients included rest of the GI tract postoperatively. However, early case-studies, published in the 1940s, highlighted the efficacy of ETF in the surgical patient. ETF facilitated energy (3050–4700 kcal) and nitrogen (17.7–28 g) intakes that were substantially greater than those taken by control patients receiving standard management after surgery (nil by mouth and intravenous (i.v.) fluids) (Mulholland *et al.*, 1943). Consequently, the progressive loss of weight, fall in plasma protein concentrations and nitrogen deficits associated with standard management were prevented in those receiving ETF (Mulholland *et al.*, 1943). Furthermore, increased awareness of the continued functioning of the small intestine in the early postoperative period has led to the use of duodenal and jejunal ETF in surgical patients (refer to the consensus on 'Peri-operative artificial nutrition in elective adult surgery' by the French Society for Parenteral and Enteral Nutrition (FSPEN) and medical opinion leaders from across the world (FSPEN, 1996) and the ASPEN (2002) standards and guidelines). Indeed, it has been recommended that the traditional principles of preoperative cessation of feeding and waiting for gastric ileus to resolve postoperatively should be discarded and uninterrupted enteral nutrition given perioperatively (Bengmark, 1998).

Surgery: present analysis

Of the 11 RCT that were reviewed, all were undertaken in patients undergoing GI surgery and all received duodenal or jejunal ETF in the perioperative period (Sagar *et al.*, 1979; Hoover *et al.*, 1980; Ryan *et al.*, 1981; Smith *et al.*, 1985; Elmore *et al.*, 1989; Frankel and Horowitz, 1989; Schroeder *et al.*, 1991; Beier-Holgersen and Boesby, 1996; Carr *et al.*, 1996; Watters *et al.*, 1997; Singh *et al.*, 1998). These trials are summarized in Box A5.8 and Tables A5.37–A5.39 and are discussed below. The findings of a further three NRT (Yeung *et al.*, 1979b; Shukla *et al.*, 1984; Moncure *et al.*, 1999), undertaken in a variety of surgical patients (GI, orthopaedic, others), have been documented in Tables A5.40–A5.42.

The studies reviewed suggested that jejunal and duodenal ETF were largely well tolerated in the early postoperative period in patients undergoing GI surgery of various forms (Hoover *et al.*, 1980; Beier-Holgersen and Boesby, 1996; Carr *et al.*, 1996) or non-abdominal surgery (Moncure *et al.*, 1999), with only a minority of patients suffering some GI symptoms (Sagar *et al.*, 1979; Smith *et al.*, 1985) (see Table A5.37). However, in some trials there were practical/technical issues related to tubes, with problems of displacement in some patients (Hoover *et al.*, 1980; Smith *et al.*, 1985; Schroeder *et al.*, 1991). In particular, one trial had a number of tube-related problems and one death due to aspiration pneumonia (Smith *et al.*, 1985) and another reported significantly lower respiratory function (vital capacity) postoperatively in tube-fed patients (*n* 13) (Watters *et al.*, 1997). Incidentally, one NRT, conducted in India, in which GI symptoms were a particular problem, administered a hospital-made feed into the stomach (Shukla *et al.*, 1984), which patients found particularly repulsive in terms of both smell and taste. The efficacy of ETF in surgical patients is addressed by the four main review questions and in Box A5.8.

Box A5.8. Key findings: effect of ETF in hospital surgical patients.

Nutritional intake: ETF, primarily via the jejunal route, can substantially increase nutritional intake in the postoperative period, without suppressing food intake. Appetite and food intake may be improved by ETF.

Body weight: ETF can attenuate postoperative weight loss.

Body function: functional benefits include improved wound healing, benefits to immune function and earlier return of bowel function.

Clinical outcome: the results of meta-analysis suggest that there may be a significant reduction in complication rates with ETF compared with routine clinical care. Large RCT are required to confirm this. No significant detriments to clinical outcome have been noted.

Table A5.37. Enteral tube feeds used in trials of surgical patients in hospital (randomized data).

Trial	ETF	ETF energy density	ETF prescribed	ETF energy (kcal) provision	ETF protein (g) provision	Toleration	Timing of ETF
Beier-Holgersen and Boesby (1996)	Nutridrink (orange flavour) (Nutricia)	1.5 kcal ml^{-1}	Day 0 900 kcal, 30 g P Day 1 1500 kcal, 50 g P Day 2 2100 kcal, 70 g P Day 3 2700 kcal, 90 g P Day 4 2700 kcal, 90 g P	Day 0 900 Day 1 1500 Day 2 1800 Day 3 1500[a] Day 4 1500[a]	Day 0 30 Day 1 50 Day 2 60 Day 3 50[a] Day 4 50[a]	Well tolerated with incidence of nausea and vomiting similar in ETF and CON group	ETF started within 4 h postop.
Carr et al. (1996)	Fresubin (Fresenius)	1 kcal ml^{-1}	To meet est. energy and fluid requirements	1622 (375)	–	Full feeding achieved quickly and well tolerated with no excessive distension	Started on return from operating theatre, stopped on starting oral diet
Elmore et al. (1989)	Vivonex TEN (Norwich Eaton)	–	–	–	–	–	–
Frankel and Horowitz (1989)	Vivonex TEN (Norwich Eaton)	–	40 kcal kg^{-1} body wt (~2852 kcal)	–	–	–	Started in the recovery room and continued to 6 a.m. on 1st postop. day
Hoover et al. (1980)	Vivonex HN (Norwich Eaton)	1 kcal ml^{-1}	–	1350 (156)	9.05 g N	Tolerated by all, moderate diarrhoea (n 9), distension (n 1), broken catheter (n 1)	Started in the recovery room (full-strength feed used by days 7/8)
Ryan et al. (1981)	Vivonex HN (Norwich Eaton)	1 kcal ml^{-1}	–	1430	–	ETF discontinued in n 2 due to GI symptoms	Within 24 h of surgery?
Sagar et al. (1979)	Flexical (elemental, Mead Johnson)	1 kcal ml^{-1}	–	~1138	–	n 2 diarrhoea and nausea on 1st day of ETF, so feed diluted	ETF on 1st postop. day with half-strength feed
Schroeder et al. (1991)	Osmolite (Ross)	1 kcal ml^{-1}	–	–	–	Problems in n 4: placement problem/dislike of tube (n 2), drug-related nausea (n 2). No distension or diarrhoea	On arrival at ward postop.
Singh et al. (1998)	Low-residue milk-based diet[b]	1.148 kcal ml^{-1}	2296 kcal	–	–	Abdominal distension on day 1 of ETF in n 4. Jejunostomy leaks and suture line leaks in n 3 (re-exploration and jejunostomy removed)	Started from 12 to 24 h postop. with saline/dextrose solution, > 24 h low-strength feed gradually increased to full strength by 72 h (? time of day)

Continued

Table A5.37. *Continued*

Trial	ETF	ETF energy density	ETF prescribed	ETF energy (kcal) provision	ETF protein (g) provision	Toleration	Timing of ETF
Smith *et al.* (1985)	Isocal (Mead Johnson) 34 g P, 44 g F, 13 3g CHO l^{-1}	–	–	'Successful' ETF 1372 (336) 'Unsuccessful' ETF 354 (227)	–	n 5 problems with tube, n 6 GI symptoms ('unsuccessful' ETF), n 1 death[c]	Day 3 postop. (day 1–2 postop. given fluid)
Watters *et al.* (1997)	Jevity (Ross) 4.4 g P and 106 kcal 100 ml^{-1}	1.06 kcal ml^{-1}	The lesser of 2625 kcal or 125% of preoperative energy expenditure (calculated or measured)	Day 0 131 Day 1 504 Day 2 1008 Day 3 1470 Day 4 1260 Day 5 1155	–	n 8 (62%) abdominal distension or diarrhoea and feeding rate reduced	Full-strength ETF within 6 h after surgery at 20 ml h^{-1} and rate increased as tolerated to target rate on 2nd postoperative morning

[a]Nasoduodenal tube removed and feed taken orally.
[b]Skimmed-milk powder, sugar, vegetable oil (blenderized by hospital) plus proprietary vitamin supplements.
[c]High complication rate with jejunostomy ETF may be due to problems with placement procedure and subsequent care of catheter.
CHO, carbohydrate; CON, control; est., estimated; F, fat; N, nitrogen; P, protein; postop., postoperative.

Table A5.38. Trial characteristics: hospital-based trials of enteral tube feeding in surgical patients (randomized data).

Trial	Design	Procedure	No. ETF	No. CON	Initial BMI ETF group	Initial BMI CON group	Duration of ETF	Tube type	Control group
Beier-Holgersen and Boesby (1996) Denmark	10111	Major abdominal surgery for GI disease (gastric, oesophageal and colorectal)	30	30	24.8 (71.2 kg[a])	23.2 (86.5 kg[a])	5 days (3 days ETF, 2 days oral, follow-up for 30 days)	Nasoduodenal tube (Flocare, see Ch. 10)	Placebo feed via tube (orange-flavoured water, no nutrients)
Carr et al. (1996) UK	11001	Elective laparotomy for potential GI resection for chronic GI disease	14	14	24.1 (4.31)	22.1 (3.87)	6 days	Double-lumen nasojejunal tube	I.v. fluids and NBM until passage of flatus (i.v. fluids then stopped)
Elmore et al. (1989) USA	10000	Elective cholecystectomy	26[b]	(i) 36 (ii) 24 (iii) 28	–	–	Max. 3 days	Duodenal tube	(i) i.v. fluids; (ii) i.v. fluids and oesophagogastric decompression; (iii) placebo ETF and oesophagogastric decompression
Frankel and Horowitz (1989) USA	10001	Elective cholecystectomy for acute or chronic cholecystitis	25	25	–	–	<24 h	Nasoduodenal tube	No tube or decompression, sips of clear fluids evening of operation
Hoover et al. (1980) USA	10000	Extensive oesophageal, gastroduodenal, biliary or pancreatic procedures	27	22	–	–	Min. 10 days	Needle-catheter jejunostomy	I.v. isotonic glucose until oral diet adequate
Ryan et al. (1981)[c] USA	10001	Elective partial colectomy	7	7	166 lb ('well nourished')	144 lb	10 days	Needle-catheter jejunostomy	I.v. isotonic glucose for 6.6 days plus oral diet
Sagar et al. (1979) UK	11000	Major intestinal surgery	15	15	–	–	5 days	Nasoduodenal tube	Conventional management – i.v. fluids, NBM for 2 days, introduction of fluids, light diet on days 6/7 postop.
Schroeder et al. (1991) New Zealand	10001	Small or large bowel resection	16	16	– 70.5 (13.5) kg	68.4 (11.2) kg	56 h (tube removed 3rd postop. day)	Nasojejunal tube (placement added ~7 min to operation time)	Hypocaloric fluids and gradual introduction of oral diet
Singh et al. (1998)	10001	Non-traumatic intestinal perforation and peritonitis (sepsis scores 6–25, sig. higher in ETF)	21	22	20.6 (0.4) 8.3% wt loss (? time period)	21.2 (0.3) 5.5% wt loss	Until oral intake adequate (mean 6.5 days)	Jejunostomy 12F tube	Intravenous fluids and electrolyte supplements as needed

Continued

Table A5.38. *Continued*

Trial	Design	Procedure	No. ETF	No. CON	Initial BMI ETF group	Initial BMI CON group	Duration of ETF	Tube type	Control group
Smith *et al.* (1985) Australia	11001	Major abdominal surgery (major resection or bypass) for GI malignancy	25	25	– 61.6 (12.1) kg	– 62.1 (12.7) kg	Up to 10 days	Fine-bore needle catheter jejunostomy	Routine i.v. therapy
Watters *et al.* (1997) Canada	11001	Oesophagectomy or pancreatoduodenectomy	13	15	25.1 (3.1) Recent wt loss in *n* 3	24.3 (3.5) Recent wt loss in *n* 11	1st 6 postop. days	Jejunostomy	Received ETF at discretion of medical team, no sooner than 6th postop. day – standard hospital practice

[a]Median value.
[b]Received oesophagogastric decompression.
[c]Assumed BMI > 20 for categorization and analysis in the review.
CON, control; NBM, nil by mouth; postop., postoperative; sig., significantly.

Table A5.39. Main findings of enteral tube feeding trials in hospitalized surgical patients (randomized data).

Trial	Energy/nutrient intake	Wt change ETF	Wt change CON	Function	Clinical outcome	Finance
Beier-Holgersen and Boesby (1996)	ETF sole source of nutrition (NBM until 5th postoperative day) with TEI increasing from 900 to 1800 kcal from day 0 to day 2 postop.	–	–	ETF sig. earlier passage of stools than CON	ETF group had earlier discharge (by 2.5 days, ETF vs. CON, *P* < 0.08), a sig. lower rate of total postoperative complications and a sig. lower rate of infectious complications than CON. Slightly lower mortality and less PN use after ETF (NS vs. CON)	Lower median costs for ETF (~£1000) vs. CON (~£2000) per pt
Carr *et al.* (1996)	ETF sig. higher TEI (1622 kcal) than CON (377 kcal) and higher TPI (61 g vs. 0.8 g) with sig. higher N balance day 1 postop.	–0.5 kg Similar loss of MAC and TSF in ETF and CON	–1.8 kg	ETF sig. attenuation of gut permeability vs. CON Smaller drop in HGS in ETF (–6.7 kg) vs. CON (–9.6 kg) (NS)	NS difference in length of stay, days to oral intake or days to defecation Lower no. of complications in ETF group (NS)	'Postoperative enteral feeding may reduce the need for TPN and reduce expenditure'
Elmore *et al.* (1989)	–	–	–	–	NS difference in length of time of anaesthesia, length of time in postop. recovery, postop. requirement for analgesics/antiemetics or day of discharge in ETF vs. CON. NS difference in time to meet discharge criteria (oral diet, urination, defecation, afebrile, ambulant) in ETF vs. CON	–
Frankel and Horowitz (1989)	–	–	–	NS difference in time to return of GI function	NS difference in length of H stay, use of postop. analgesia or complications between ETF vs. CON	–
Hoover *et al.* (1980)	ETF sig. higher TEI and TNI vs. CON: ETF 1815 kcal 10.9 g N CON 810 kcal 1.7 g N VFI similar in both groups (ETF 350 kcal: CON 466 kcal)	–0.02 kg (ETF vs. CON sig.)	–3.8 kg	–	–	–
Ryan *et al.* (1981)	ETF sig. greater TEI 2283 kcal and TNI 14.1 g than CON (800 kcal, 3.4 g N) VFI ETF 757 kcal. CON 485 kcal (NS)	Wk 2: –3.7 (1.34)% Wk 4: –2.8 (1.16)% (ETF vs. CON sig.)	Wk 2: –5.6 (0.7)% Wk 4: –6.1 (1.35)%	–	NS higher rates of catheter-related sepsis in CON (i.v. therapy) than ETF. ETF sig. shorter need for i.v. catheter than CON (1.8 days vs. 6.6 days)	–

Continued

Table A5.39. Continued.

Trial	Energy/nutrient intake	Wt change ETF	Wt change CON	Function	Clinical outcome	Finance
Sagar et al. (1979)	ETF TEI much greater than CON (−1138 kcal vs. 462 kcal, ? sig.) in first 5 postop. days. After tube withdrawn and oral diet introduced, TEI greater in ETF (1560 kcal) vs. CON (900 kcal) (? sig.) (N balance less negative in ETF than CON postop.)	−0 kg[a] (−1 to +5.3 kg) (ETF vs. CON sig.)	−1.85 kg[a] (−5.8 kg to +0.5 kg)	NS difference in wound-infection rates	ETF sig. shorter length of H stay (median 14 days, 10–26 days) than CON (median 19 days, 10–46 days)	–
Schroeder et al. (1991)	ETF sig. higher TEI postop. (1179 kcal vs. 382 kcal, sig.)	−4.26 (4.1)% (3 kg (2.9); ETF vs. CON NS) Similar loss of total body protein, fat and water to CON	−6.14 (3.22)% (4.2 (2.2) kg)	Sig. higher wound healing rate in ETF vs. CON (hydroxyproline incorporation in Gortex tubes) NS difference in postop. fatigue scores, HGS, max. ventilatory volume, involuntary muscle function. NS shorter time to passage of flatus and first bowel motion (P < 0.07)	Shorter length of stay (ETF 10 days, CON 15 days, NS) and fewer complications (4 vs. 7, NS)	–
Singh et al. (1998)	ETF sig. greater energy intake than CON from day 1 onwards (day 1 +395 kcal; day 4 +1710 kcal; day 7 +2094 kcal greater)	–	–	–	NS difference in hospital stay between ETF (14 days) and CON (13 days) Sig. lower rate of septic complications in ETF vs. CON (overall complication rates NS different)	–
Smith et al. (1985)	–	~−2.92% (−1.8 kg) (successful, n 14) ~−5.52% (−3.4 kg) (unsuccessful, n 6) (ETF vs. CON NS)	~−3.54% (−2.2 kg)	–	NS difference in mortality (186 × 196) Similar rate of postop. surgical complications in ETF and CON Sig. longer stay in ETF (had to remain to finish 10 days ETF regimen) than CON (could be discharged before 10 days)!	–

| Watters *et al.* (1997) | No oral intake before 6th postop. day. No data on energy intake in ETF or CON | NS changes in wt in ETF or CON (no data) | – | Recovery of HGS and maximal inspiratory pressure similar in ETF and CON. Other respiratory variables (FEV_1, vital capacity) lower in ETF than CON (vital capacity sig. so) Higher postop. activity levels in CON than ETF (sig.), with tendency for quicker recovery times in CON (NS) NS differences in pain scores or narcotic administration, vigour scores or fatigue scores Sig. greater increase in Mg in ETF vs. CON | NS difference in no. anastomotic leaks (n 1 ETF, n 3 CON) Similar stay in ICU in ETF (2.9 days) and CON (2.3 days) and in hospital (17 (9) days vs. 16 (7) days) (ETF vs. CON NS) | – |

[a]Median weight loss.

CON, control; HGS, hand-grip strength; H, hospital; ICU, intensive care unit; MAC, mid-arm circumference; Mg, magnesium; N, nitrogen; NBM, nil by mouth; pt, patient; postop., postoperative; NS, not significant; sig., significantly; ?sig, uncertain if statistically significant; TEI, total energy intake; TNI, total nitrogen intake; TPN, total parenteral nutrition; TSF, triceps skin-fold thickness; VFI, voluntary food intake.

Table A5.40. Enteral tube feeds used in trials of surgical patients in hospital (non-randomized data).

Trial	ETF	ETF energy density	ETF prescribed	ETF energy (kcal) provision	ETF protein (g) provision	Toleration	Timing of ETF
Moncure *et al.* (1999)	Promote, Impact (ICU only), Replete, Peptamen, Deliver	–	–	day 0 1676 day 1 1581	day 0 89.6 day 1 92.6	No gastric reflux or aspiration. ETF safe if gastric reflux and constant suctioning of gastric contents carried out in perioperative period	ETF continued until transport to operating theatre (stopped 1.4 h before surgery and started 3 h after)
Shukla *et al.* (1984)	Providal NG (Dextromed, Bombay) 20% protein hydrolysate, 1% yeast, 75% CHO	–	–	3500–4000 (? Includes oral intake from food)	–	Nausea, vomiting and diarrhoea (due to high osmolarity of ETF, 3200–3500 mOsm) treated with drugs ETF stopped in *n* 7 due to uncontrollable diarrhoea, vomiting and severe aversion to smell and taste of ETF	Continuous, diurnal ETF for 10 days preoperatively
Yeung *et al.* (1979b)	Flexical (elemental diet, Mead Johnson) 22.5 g P hydrolysate, 153 g CHO, 34 g F l⁻¹	1 kcal ml⁻¹	2000–3500 kcal, to meet est. energy requirements	1692 (270)	–	Only 63% of those started (*n* 47) completed successful jejunostomy feeding (*n* 27) – reasons GI symptoms, death or unrelated to ETF	Usually within 48–72 h postop., half-strength

CHO, carbohydrate; est., estimated; F, fat; GI, gastrointestinal; P, protein; postop., postoperative.

Table A5.41. Trial characteristics: hospital-based trials of enteral tube feeding in surgical patients (non-randomized data).

Trial	Design	Procedure	No. ETF	No. CON	Initial BMI ETF group	Initial BMI CON group	Duration of ETF	Tube type	Control group
Moncure *et al.* (1999) USA	B	Non-abdominal surgery (tracheostomy, orthopaedics)	46[a]	36[a]	–	–	–	Jejunostomy tube	ETF stopped 11.6 h before and started 7 h after surgery
Shukla *et al.* (1984) India	B	Surgery for a variety of benign and malignant diseases	67	43	'Malnourished'	–	10 days	Nasogastric tube	Routine H diet
Yeung *et al.* (1979b) UK	B/C	Elective major colorectal or gastro-oesophageal surgery	27[b] 20[b]	20[b]	21.9	23	11 days	Fine-needle catheter jejunostomy	–

[a]Groups unbalanced for types of surgical procedure; [b]*n* 27 represents 63% of original sample of 43 who completed course of ETF. Subset of *n* 20 compared with a control group (*n* 20). CON, control; H, hospital.

Table A5.42. Main findings of enteral tube feeding trials in hospitalized surgical patients (non-randomized data).

Trial	Energy/nutrient intake	Wt change ETF	Wt change CON	Function	Clinical outcome	Finance
Moncure *et al.* (1999)	ETF received sig. more energy on day 0 (day of surgery, 1676 kcal vs. 791 kcal) and 1st postop. day (1581 kcal vs. 1152 kcal) than CON and sig. more protein on 1st postop. day (93 g vs. 64 g)	–	–	–	NS difference in mortality, length of stay in ICU or H or no. of ventilator days	–
Shukla *et al.* (1984)	ETF energy intakes 3500–4000 kcal day^{-1} (no data for VFI and energy from ETF, no data for CON group)	+0.50 kg (ETF vs. CON sig.) TSF and MAC increased (ETF vs. CON sig.)	−1.58 kg TSF and MAC decreased	ETF had sig. better cell-mediated immunity responses than CON (sig. greater TLC and response to skin tests) ETF sig. greater drop in IgG and IgA than CON	ETF lower wound-infection rate postop. (10.5% vs. 37% in CON ? sig.) Small differences in length of H stay (13 vs. 10 days) and mortality (11.7% vs. 6%) (ETF vs. CON ? sig.)	–
Yeung *et al.* (1979b)	TEI sig. greater (more than double) in ETF vs. CON as VFI in the 2 groups equal over 14 postop. days (data in a subgroup of 24 (12 ETF vs. 12 CON))	−0.8 kg (*n* 20) (ETF vs. CON ? sig.) Similar loss of body fat but sig. less change in MAMC (ETF vs. CON sig.)	−2.5 kg (*n* 20) Sig. loss of body fat (−0.8 kg)	–	Duration of H stay and complication rates similar in both groups	–

CON, control; H, hospital; ICU, intensive care unit; IgG, immunoglobulin G; MAC, mid-arm circumference; NS, not significant; postop., postoperative; sig., significant; ?sig., uncertain if statistically significant; TEI, total energy intake; TLC, total lymphocyte count; TSF, triceps skin-fold thickness; VFI, voluntary food intake.

(I) What effect does ETF have on the voluntary food intake and total energy intake of surgical patients in hospital?

ETF in the early postoperative period substantially improves nutrient intake, with the aim of providing a level of energy, protein and other nutrients to meet the high requirements of patients at this critical time of recovery. Those RCT that assessed total energy intake with ETF highlighted intakes significantly in excess of those taken by control patients given standard management (typically i.v. fluids) in the early postoperative period (up to 7 days postoperatively) (Sagar *et al.*, 1979; Hoover *et al.*, 1980; Ryan *et al.*, 1981; Schroeder *et al.*, 1991; Beier-Holgersen and Boesby, 1996; Carr *et al.*, 1996; Singh *et al.*, 1998) and beyond (Hoover *et al.*, 1980; Ryan *et al.*, 1981) (see Table A5.39). Similarly, the NRT, in a variety of surgical patients, also highlighted the greater energy and protein intakes of patients receiving ETF (by jejunostomy (Moncure *et al.*, 1999) or NG tube (Shukla *et al.*, 1984)) in the early postoperative period (Shukla *et al.*, 1984; Moncure *et al.*, 1999) (Table A5.42). Furthermore, those trials that assessed the introduction of an oral diet, either with ETF (Yeung *et al.*, 1979b; Hoover *et al.*, 1980; Ryan *et al.*, 1981) or after ETF was stopped (Sagar *et al.*, 1979), indicated that voluntary food intake was similar (even though ETF was given (Yeung *et al.*, 1979b; Hoover *et al.*, 1980)) or greater (both during (Ryan *et al.*, 1981) and after ETF was stopped (Sagar *et al.*, 1979)) than that of the control groups. These findings suggest that ETF does not substantially suppress food intake in postoperative surgical patients but, on the contrary, may stimulate appetite and resumption of an oral diet.

(II) What effect does ETF have on the body weight and composition of surgical patients in hospital?

Seven out of 11 RCT assessed changes in weight with ETF in postoperative surgical patients (Sagar *et al.*, 1979; Hoover *et al.*, 1980; Ryan *et al.*, 1981; Smith *et al.*, 1985;

Schroeder *et al.*, 1991; Carr *et al.*, 1996; Watters *et al.*, 1997). All except one (Watters *et al.*, 1997) of these investigations indicated that GI surgical patients fed via ETF (jejunal or duodenal feeding) lost less weight than control patients given routine i.v. treatment (Table A5.39). In three trials the differences between groups were statistically significant (Sagar *et al.*, 1979; Hoover *et al.*, 1980; Ryan *et al.*, 1981). Interestingly, in one of these trials, the attenuation of weight loss following 10 days of ETF (compared with controls) was still evident 2 and 4 weeks after the surgical procedure (Ryan *et al.*, 1981). Weight gain or less weight loss in patients receiving ETF versus controls was also found in two NRT, which indicated that losses of muscle (MAMC) (Yeung *et al.*, 1979b) and fat (triceps skin-fold thickness (TSF)) (Shukla *et al.*, 1984) were lower in ETF patients (Table A5.42). Despite the potentially confounding effects of fluctuations in fluid balance in post-surgical patients, only two RCT reported changes in muscle and fat mass (Schroeder *et al.*, 1991; Carr *et al.*, 1996) or water (Schroeder *et al.*, 1991). Over the relatively short postoperative period (3–6 days in these trials), similar changes were noted in ETF and control patients.

(III) What effect does ETF have on the body function of surgical patients in hospital?

Early ETF in the postoperative period may improve some, but not all body functions (see Table A5.39):

- In patients undergoing bowel resection, those receiving jejunal feeding had significantly higher wound healing rates than control patients (Schroeder *et al.*, 1991), although similar benefits were not observed in an earlier trial (Sagar *et al.*, 1979).
- In GI surgical patients, those given early jejunal feeding had a significantly smaller increase in gut permeability compared with the control group (Carr *et al.*, 1996). This trial also found smaller reductions in hand-grip strength (HGS) in the tube-fed patients (Carr *et*

al., 1996), although, as in one other trial (Watters *et al.*, 1997), changes were not significant.

- Return of bowel function was significantly earlier in enterally fed patients, as indicated by the passage of stools (Beier-Holgersen and Boesby, 1996), than in control patients, although this was not a universal observation (Frankel and Horowitz, 1989; Schroeder *et al.*, 1991).
- In malnourished surgical patients with benign and malignant conditions, cell-mediated immunity responses were significantly greater in those receiving ETF than in a non-randomized control group (Shukla *et al.*, 1984).
- Early ETF did not adversely or beneficially affect postoperative fatigue (Schroeder *et al.*, 1991; Watters *et al.*, 1997) or vigour (Watters *et al.*, 1997) scores compared with controls in GI surgical patients.

One small trial suggested that patients fed enterally by tube had lower postoperative vital capacity and lower activity levels than control patients (Watters *et al.*, 1997). None of the other trials showed any functional detriments with ETF.

The small size of most of these trials may result in functional changes not being detected (through insufficient statistical power). One trial that undertook power calculations (Watters *et al.*, 1997) was unable to meet the required number of patients calculated by their power statistics (20 per group) and the other (Elmore *et al.*, 1989) did not assess functional parameters. Consequently, larger RCT that include assessment of functional outcome measures following ETF in postoperative GI surgical patients are needed. Studies in patients undergoing other types of surgery are also required.

(IV) What effect does ETF have on the clinical and financial outcome of surgical patients in hospital?

There may be a number of benefits in clinical outcome if surgical patients are fed enterally in the early postoperative period. For example, patients fed duodenally following major abdominal surgery were discharged

from hospital ~2.5 days earlier, had a significantly lower rate of all complications and a significantly lower rate of infectious complications than the control group given a placebo feed (Beier-Holgersen and Boesby, 1996) (Table A5.39). Whilst some trials found length of stay was shorter in enterally fed patients (Sagar *et al.*, 1979; Schroeder *et al.*, 1991), in other trials no differences were observed (Smith *et al.*, 1985; Elmore *et al.*, 1989; Frankel and Horowitz, 1989; Carr *et al.*, 1996; Watters *et al.*, 1997; Singh *et al.*, 1998). Similarly, in some trials the rates of complication rates were lower (significantly: Singh *et al.*, 1998; or not significantly: Carr *et al.*, 1996) than or the same as (Smith *et al.*, 1985; Frankel and Horowitz, 1989; Watters *et al.*, 1997) in control patients. For example, Singh *et al.* (1998) documented significantly lower septic complication rates in enterally fed patients versus a control group, although overall complication rates did not differ (Singh *et al.*, 1998). In a small trial of elective colectomy patients, those receiving ETF had lower rates of catheter-related sepsis (not significant) than a control group given i.v. fluid (Ryan *et al.*, 1981). This raises the possibility that, in some studies, differences in outcome observed could be related to a detrimental effect of the treatment provided in the control arms (e.g. some forms of i.v. support (Lobo *et al.*, 2001)) as opposed to a benefit due to ETF. None of the trials suggested significant detriments to clinical outcome with ETF.

Meta-analysis of six RCT (*n* 241: Frankel and Horowitz, 1989; Schroeder *et al.*, 1991; Beier-Holgersen and Boesby, 1996; Carr *et al.*, 1996; Watters *et al.*, 1997; Singh *et al.*, 1998) that provided data on complication rates suggested a significant reduction, with an OR of 0.38 (95% CI 0.16–0.92). However, there was significant heterogeneity between studies using a fixed-effects model. Using the more conservative random-effects model, the reduction was not significant, with an OR of 0.25 (95% CI 0.05–1.31).

Whilst some of the NRT found no clinical advantages or disadvantages from early postoperative feeding (Yeung *et al.*, 1979b; Moncure *et al.*, 1999), one trial in malnourished surgical patients indicated a lower wound infection rate (see Table A5.42) and small, non-significant differences in hospital stay and mortality (Shukla *et al.*, 1984).

Overall, larger RCT are needed to assess changes in clinical outcome that follow the use of ETF in the early postoperative period in both GI and non-GI surgical patients. However, the consensus is that there appears to be little detriment from this practice, with the potential for benefit clinically and financially. Beier-Holgersen and Boesby (1996) were able to show prospectively that the costs for each patient receiving ETF were 50% (~£1000) of those of the control group (~£2000), including the relatively small costs of ETF. Indeed, it has been stated that: 'Post-operative enteral feeding may reduce the need for TPN and reduce expenditure' (Carr *et al.*, 1996).

In addition, retrospective calculations estimate that the health-care costs for patients undergoing liver or pancreatic surgery are substantially less for those given medical foods (including ETF or ONS) ($6500) than those not given them ($17,000), due to differences in complication rates (American data: Nutrition Screening Initiative, 1996). Therefore, further prospective investigations are required to highlight the cost-effectiveness of ETF in surgical patients.

The value of ETF in the perioperative period has been reviewed extensively and more details can be found in Campos and Meguid (1992), FSPEN (1996), Bengmark (1998), Torosian (1999), Bengmark *et al.* (2001) and ASPEN (2002).

The studies discussed above have primarily included standard commercial feeds, with a focus on adequate energy and protein provision (although in most cases nutritionally complete commercial formulas were used). In only one trial was a hospital-made diet used (Singh *et al.*, 1998). However, the future of nutritional support may involve a more comprehensive approach to nutrition, with a greater focus on the use of specific nutrients that can modify the metabolic and immune response to major surgery and injury (Torosian, 1999; Reid, 2000). Undoubtedly, further investigations are needed to elucidate more fully the benefits of perioperative nutritional support and the role of individual nutrients (including micronutrients) in different groups of surgical patients. Here are some observations made about perioperative nutritional support:

> First, the increasing availability of postoperative enteral nutrition, using naso-jejunal feeding tubes and other enteral access devices, may liberalise the indications for postoperative support by allowing relatively safe nutrition support during the post-operative period. Second, immune enhancing regimens seem to have value ... although their place has yet to be adequately defined.
>
> (Maxfield, 2001)

Surgery: other reviews

- A systematic review and meta-analysis of studies comparing any type of enteral (including oral) feeding started within 24 h of surgery, with nil by mouth, in elective GI surgical patients (Lewis *et al.*, 2001). This review of 11 studies (*n* 837) suggested that early oral (*n* 4) or tube (*n* 7) feeding (including use of immunonutrition feeds in one study) significantly reduced the risk of any type of infection (RR 0.72 (95% CI 0.54–0.98)) and mean length of stay (reduced by 0.84 days (0.36 to 1.33)). Risk reductions were observed for other complications (wound infection, anastomotic dehiscence and pneumonia) and mortality, but these were not significant. In addition, the risk of vomiting was increased with ETF (RR 1.27). The authors concluded that early feeding may be of benefit compared with nil by mouth. However, it is possible that the i.v. support given to control patients may have detrimental effects (Lobo *et al.*, 2001). Separate consideration of studies of oral and tube feeding in GI surgical patients may also be advantageous (see Appendix 3 for ONS).
- A meta-analysis of 15 studies (nine relevant to this section) undertaken in abdominal surgery patients (and others: burns, trauma, head injury) (Marik and Zaloga, 2001) suggested that early rather than 'delayed' use of ETF may reduce rates of infection and length of hospital

stay, although there was considerable heterogeneity between studies.

Immunonutrition in surgical patients

A recent consensus recommendation from a US summit on immune-enhancing enteral therapy stated that patients undergoing elective GI surgery (moderately or severely undernourished (albumin < 3.5 g dl^{-1}) undergoing major elective upper GI surgery; severely undernourished (albumin < 2.8 g dl^{-1}) undergoing lower-GI surgery) should receive early ETF with an 'immune-enhancing' diet (Anon., 2001a). In a recent meta-analysis of studies, immunonutrition was associated with significantly fewer infectious complications (RR 0.53 (95% CI 0.42–0.69)) in elective surgical patients with no effect on mortality (RR 0.99 (95% CI 0.42–2.34)), compared with critically ill patients, in which no effects on either outcome parameter were found (Heyland *et al.*, 2001b). Despite these benefits, the feed components that may be associated with such improvement in outcome and the mechanisms by which they act require further elucidation. In particular, the increased mortality risk found in well-designed studies in the critically ill and the recommendation that these feeds should not be used in septic patients invite caution until further research into the role of different feed components and their mechanisms of action has been undertaken.

Methods of ETF in surgical patients

The optimal route and pattern (e.g. nocturnal, bolus, intermittent, continuous) of ETF has been investigated in some groups of surgical patients. A small, controlled study suggested that intermittent, bolus ETF may be better metabolically (lower resting oxygen consumption, better cumulative nitrogen balance) than a continuous, 24 h regimen postoperatively in patients recovering from major head and neck surgery (Campbell *et al.*, 1983). There may also be advantages to the patient in terms of greater mobilization. Nevertheless, the optimal timing in other

groups of surgical patients and its impact on other outcome parameters (e.g. total nutrient intakes) remain to be elucidated.

The advent of gastrostomy and jejunal feeding has increased the flexibility of ETF in some groups of surgical patients. Furthermore, some patients have expressed a preference for the use of non-nasal routes of feeding. A survey of those (*n* 40) receiving ETF via a PEG after maxillofacial surgery (for cancer) found that patients preferred PEG feeding to NG feeding, particularly for aesthetic and psychological reasons (Koehler and Buhl, 1991), as the quote below expresses:

> Our experience with PEG has shown that this relatively simple technique offers the advantage of long-term adequate nutrition. The psychological and social advantages and the low cost in comparison with parenteral nutrition make PEG a very suitable method for adequate patient nourishment.
> (Koehler and Buhl, 1991)

This survey highlighted the fact that PEG feeding, which was started in hospital and easily continued at home (total ETF period 54–425 days), was associated with weight gain (3.1 kg at 4 weeks, 6.4 kg at 12 weeks). In addition, in those who were curatively operated (*n* 22), the length of hospitalization was shorter in the PEG-fed than in those non-PEG fed (Koehler and Buhl, 1991).

For information on studies undertaken specifically in patients undergoing orthopaedic surgery, refer to the section in this appendix.

ETF Using Disease-specific Feeds

Feeds designed to modulate immune and inflammatory parameters

Increasingly, feeds used for ETF are being formulated with specific nutrients for the treatment of disease-specific groups. In particular, feeds designed to modulate immune and inflammatory function have been developed for use in patients with critical illness and those post-surgery. These enteral-tube feeds are enriched with nutrients that may modulate inflammatory, metabolic and immune processes, including omega-3 fatty acids, amino acids (arginine and glutamine), antioxidants and RNA. Consequently, a large number of studies have investigated the efficacy of these feeds compared with feeds of standard composition in patients with critical illness (Brown *et al.*, 1994; Moore *et al.*, 1994; Bower *et al.*, 1995; Kudsk *et al.*, 1996; Atkinson *et al.*, 1998; Gadek *et al.*, 1999) and burns (Gottschlich *et al.*, 1990; Saffle *et al.*, 1997) and in cancer patients undergoing surgery (Daly *et al.*, 1988; Kemen *et al.*, 1995; Heslin *et al.*, 1997; Braga *et al.*, 1998; Gianotti *et al.*, 1999).

A discussion of the individual trials is beyond the scope of this report. However, a recent meta-analysis has investigated the efficacy of ETF with these specialized feeds compared with standard enteral feeds (Heyland *et al.*, 2001b). This review (2419 patients from 22 RCT) found that patients treated with feeds containing combinations of various nutrients (Impact (L-arginine, n-3 fatty acids, RNA), *n* 16 trials; Immun-Aid (L-arginine, L-glutamine, BCAA, *n*-3 fatty acids, RNA), *n* 2 trials; other (L-arginine and L-glutamine), *n* 4 trials) had an RR of mortality of 1.1 (95% CI 0.93–1.31) but significantly lower rates of infectious complications (RR 0.66 (95% CI 0.54–0.8)). Length of hospital stay was also shorter (effect size −0.63 (−0.94 to −0.32)). In light of the significant heterogeneity between studies, this review compared the effects of immunonutrition in two distinct patient groups: (i) critically ill; and (ii) surgical. In studies of both groups of patients, there were no effects on mortality. However, in well-designed trials in critically ill patients, there was a significantly higher RR of mortality with use of immunonutrition (RR 1.46 (95% CI 1.01–2.11)). There was also no effect of immunonutrition on infectious complication rates in the critically ill, but length of stay was reduced (effect size −0.47 (−0.93 to −0.01)). In contrast, significant reductions were seen in the elective surgical population.

Studies of ETF using similar disease-specific formulas have also been undertaken in other patient groups (e.g. head and neck cancer), with (Snyderman *et al.*, 1999) and without (Van Bokhorst-de van der Schueren *et al.*, 2001) benefit to outcome. Further work is needed in this area.

Even if there are genuine benefits from the use of these specialized feeds in some patient groups, it is difficult to attribute the benefits to any one specific nutrient (Reid, 2000). For example, in some of the studies reviewed, the feeds used differed from the standard formulas in a number of ways, in addition to the specific nutrients added (e.g. glutamine, omega-3 fatty acids). These included differences in energy and nitrogen contents and in the amounts of some micronutrients also thought to affect immune function (selenium, vitamin A and vitamin E). In addition, problems with study design exist, including inadequate randomization (e.g. not concealed), failure to analyse results on an intention-to-treat basis and lack of blinding.

Therefore, further well-designed trials are undoubtedly required to ascertain the benefits of using specific feeds for defined patient groups. In particular, enteral tube feeds with compositions that are clearly defined should be used in such trials with appropriately matched formulas for control patients. In addition to disease-specific targeting of ETF, the role of genotype in determining responsiveness to nutrients and ETF must now be considered. For further information about the use of feeds to modulate immune and inflammatory parameters, there are a number of reviews (McClave *et al.*, 1992; Keith and Jeejeebhoy, 1997; Zaloga, 1998; Standen and Bihari, 2000) and three meta-analyses (Beale *et al.*, 1999; Heys *et al.*, 1999; Heyland *et al.*, 2001b) that can be referred to. In addition, readers can consult a consensus on the use of 'immune-enhancing therapy' (Anon., 2001a).

Note

[1]A dash has been used in the tables throughout this appendix where information was not provided in the reviewed trial (and could not be calculated).

Appendix 6

A Detailed Analysis of the Effects of Enteral Tube Feeding in the Community Setting

Chapter 7 provided an overall summary of the effects of enteral tube feeding (ETF) obtained from a combined analysis of different groups of patients in the community setting. Here, a more detailed analysis, addressing each review question, is provided, according to individual patient groups. The patient groups are presented alphabetically. The majority of trials reviewed in the community setting were non-randomized in design. In some patient groups (e.g. obstructive chronic pulmonary disease (COPD), cancer), it may be reasonable to undertake randomized controlled trials (RCT) to establish the efficacy of ETF. In others, such as elderly patients with a cerebrovascular accident (CVA), RCT may be unethical, because oral feeding is likely to be harmful (e.g. leading to aspiration pneumonia and death). Therefore, lack of evidence from RCT does not mean that ETF should not be used in these groups of patients.

COPD (Randomized and Non-randomized Data)

Considering the incidence of disease-related malnutrition (DRM) in COPD patients, with difficulties with eating due to anorexia and breathlessness being commonplace, it is surprising that there are very few investigations of the efficacy of using ETF to improve nutritional intake in this patient group in the community setting.

Two small trials (one RCT (Donahoe et al., 1994) and one non-randomized trial (NRT) (Irwin and Openbrier, 1985)) were reviewed that assessed the efficacy of ETF in undernourished patients (< 90% ideal body weight (IBW)) with severe COPD (see Tables A6.1–A6.3[1]). Percutaneous endoscopic gastrostomy (PEG) feeding (Donahoe et al., 1994) appeared to be more acceptable and better tolerated than naso-enteric feeding (Irwin and Openbrier, 1985) in this patient group. In the RCT, patients given 4 months of nocturnal PEG feeding gained significant weight and fat mass over time, unlike the control patients maintained on standard hospital diets (Donahoe et al., 1994). However, this weight was subsequently lost after ETF was stopped (Table A6.3). No functional or clinical outcomes were assessed in this trial. In a very small sample of COPD patients fed naso-enterically for 4 weeks (n 4), a number of benefits were seen, including weight gain (n 4), increases in muscle mass (n 2), increases in inspiratory and expiratory pressures (n 4), reduced dyspnoea (n 1) and less disability (n 2) (Irwin and Openbrier, 1985). Furthermore, the frequency, duration and intensity of pulmonary-related hospital stays were found to be markedly reduced

678

Table A6.1. Enteral tube feeds used in trials of patients with COPD in the community (randomized and non-randomized data).

Trial	ETF	ETF energy density	ETF prescribed	ETF energy (kcal) provision	ETF protein (g) provision	Toleration	Timing of ETF
Randomized controlled trials							
Donahoe et al. (1994)	–	–	–	–	–	No adverse effects with placement of PEG or with home ETF	Nocturnal
Non-randomized trials							
Irwin and Openbrier (1985)	–	–	–	64 kcal kg⁻¹ wt (52–72 kcal kg⁻¹)	–	Sore throat (n 4), bloating (n 2 and ETF stopped in n 1), diarrhoea (n 1)	–

Table A6.2. Trial characteristics: trials of enteral tube feeding in patients with COPD in the community (randomized and non-randomized data).

Trial	Design	Diagnosis	No. ETF	No. CON	Initial BMI ETF group	Initial BMI CON group	Duration of ETF	Tube type	Control group
Randomized controlled trials									
Donahoe et al. (1994) A USA	10000	Severe COPD, FEV$_1$ 0.96 (± 0.4)	5[a]	6	75% IBW	75% IBW	Follow-up over 4 months of ETF and then 4 months of standard oral diet	PEG	Continued on standard oral diet
Non-randomized trials									
Irwin and Openbrier (1985) C A USA		Severe COPD, FEV$_1$ 0.5	4[b]	–	< 90% wt-for-ht	–	4 weeks	Naso-enteric	–

[a] 4 months ETF followed by 4 months of a standard oral diet.
[b] Only n 3 completed ETF for 4 weeks.
A, abstract; BMI, body mass index; FEV$_1$, CON, control; forced expiratory volume in 1 s.

Table A6.3. Main findings of enteral tube feeding trials in patients with COPD in the community (randomized and non-randomized data).

Trial	Energy/nutrient intake	Wt change ETF	Wt change CON	Function	Clinical outcome	Finance
Randomized controlled trials						
Donahoe *et al.* (1994)	–	+3.8 kg (sig. over time) (wt lost after ETF stopped for 4 months) Sig. increase in fat mass, not lean mass	NS change in wt, fat mass or lean muscle mass	–	–	–
Non-randomized trials						
Irwin and Openbrier (1985)	Used as a supplement to oral intake but no data given	Weight gain in *n* 4 (no data) – Increased muscle mass *n* 2 (no data)	–	Increased inspiratory and expiratory pressure in *n* 4; reduced dyspnoea *n* 1; decreased disability using Sickness Impact Profiles *n* 2	*n* 1 receiving longer-term ETF, intermittently over 18 months: frequency, duration and intensity of pulmonary-related H stays markedly reduced (pre-ETF 83 days, 6 months post-ETF 12 days)	–

CON, control; H, hospital; NS, not significant; sig., significant.

compared with the pre-ETF period (Irwin and Openbrier, 1985) (Table A6.3). Due to the currently limited evidence base, large RCT are needed to confirm these findings and to fully characterize the effectiveness of ETF compared with routine care in COPD patients in the community.

Cystic Fibrosis (CF) (Non-randomized Data)

Prospective evaluation in children (aged 5–10 years) with CF has suggested that their growth (in terms of height, fat-free mass and fat mass) is impaired longitudinally compared with healthy children (Stettler *et al.*, 2000) (particularly in boys). This particular publication did not discuss the use of nutritional support in these children and yet the studies reviewed (and discussed below) clearly indicate that oral nutritional supplements (ONS) and ETF can improve the growth of growth-retarded children and adolescents with CF, as the quote below suggests:

> We conclude that intensive nutritional support for 1 year has both short- and long-term effects on nutrition and growth, still evident some years after the cessation of this therapeutic modality. Supplementation for periods of longer than 1 year may produce greater gains and possibly prolong the improvement in pulmonary function observed.
>
> (Dalzell *et al.*, 1992)

One of the limitations of the current evidence base is the lack of RCT comparing ETF with routine clinical care (no RCT were reviewed). However, this is at least partly due to the ethical difficulties associated with randomizing children with growth failure to a placebo control arm of such a study. Instead, a number of NRT have been reported and these have been reviewed below.

Ten NRT (Shepherd *et al.*, 1983, 1986; Bertrand *et al.*, 1984; Levy *et al.*, 1985; Boland *et al.*, 1986; Moore *et al.*, 1986; O'Loughlin *et al.*, 1986; Dalzell *et al.*, 1992; Smith, D.L. *et al.*, 1994; Steinkamp and von der Hardt, 1994) of home ETF in patients with CF (adults, adolescents and children) were reviewed (Tables A6.4–A6.6). The existing information and the findings of the trials are summarized in Tables A6.4–A6.6 and Box A6.1. Nocturnal delivery of feed was consistently used in the studies reviewed and, in most reports, the nasogastric (NG) route was employed (seven studies: Shepherd *et al.*, 1983, 1986; Bertrand *et al.*, 1984; Moore *et al.*, 1986; O'Loughlin *et al.*, 1986; Dalzell *et al.*, 1992; Smith, D.L. *et al.*, 1994). The reviewed trials (in those with CF across age-groups) consistently showed ETF to be safe and typically well tolerated, with elemental, semi-elemental, whole-protein and medium-chain triglyceride (MCT)-enriched formulas being used. Furthermore, a retrospective audit of the use of overnight PEG ETF in adults and adolescents showed this method to be a safe, flexible and well-tolerated way of significantly improving the nutritional status of CF patients with severe pulmonary disease over a 12-month period (Ashworth *et al.*, 1996). The efficacy of ETF in this patient group was addressed using the four main review questions.

Box A6.1. Key findings: effect of ETF in community patients with cystic fibrosis.

Information from non-randomized trials suggests that ETF may:

- Improve nutritional intakes.
- Improve growth in growth-retarded children, body weight in adults and fat and muscle mass.
- Improve some objective (e.g. pulmonary function) and some subjective (e.g. well-being, activity) functional parameters.

RCT are needed where practically and ethically feasible.

Table A6.4. Enteral tube feeds used in trials of patients with cystic fibrosis in the community (non-randomized data).

Trial	ETF	ETF energy density	ETF prescribed	ETF energy (kcal) provision	ETF protein (g) provision	Toleration	Timing of ETF
Bertrand *et al.* (1984)	Vivonex (Eaton Lab) (Fat emulsion given once a week) (no enzymes added)	1 kcal ml⁻¹	–	106 kcal kg⁻¹ wt	–	All completed ETF with minimal discomfort or complaints	Continuous outside school hours (at least 16 h day⁻¹)
Boland *et al.* (1986)	Ensure (Ross) or Isocal (Mead Johnson) (powdered enzymes added to ETF)	1 kcal ml⁻¹	–	1000–2000	–	No serious complications (occasional local infection, granuloma formation, minor intermittent leakage) Nausea and vomiting in the morning after swallowing pulmonary secretions (*n* 2)	Nocturnal
Dalzell *et al.* (1992)	Calorie-dense	–	–	–	–	–	Nocturnal
Levy *et al.* (1985)	Vivonex (Eaton Lab) Flexical HN (Mead Johnson) (elemental) or Vital (Ross) (semi-elemental) (no enzymes)	1 kcal ml⁻¹ – –	~30% of estimated energy requirements	–	–	Generally well tolerated with minor complications (satiety, nausea, local tenderness) During second year of trial, all pts given Vital, which caused less gastric upset	ETF for 10–14 days in hospital, then discharged Nocturnal (10–12 h)
Moore *et al.* (1986)	Criticare HN (Mead Johnson)	1 kcal ml⁻¹ 0.67–1.5 kcal ml⁻¹ᵃ	To provide 2/3 of est. energy requirements (~100–150% of protein requirement)	–	–	'Safe and effective'	Nocturnal (8–12 h)
O'Loughlin *et al.* (1986)	Vital (Ross, 16.7% P, 9.3% F, 74% CHO, semi-elemental) (enzymes added to formula)	–	To meet 150% of est. requirements with food intake	–	–	–	ETF in H for 5–7 days before discharge Nocturnal (8–10 h)
Shepherd *et al.* (1983)	Vipep (Tuta Lab, Aus. elemental) 10% P, 22% F, 68% CHO	1 kcal ml⁻¹	To increase energy and protein intakes by 20–40%	1000–1200	–	Occasional complications with ETF, including vomiting with a coughing spasm and ejection of the NG tube	–

Shepherd *et al.* (1986)	Criticare (Mead Johnson), semi-elemental	1 kcal ml^{-1}	To meet 120–140% of RDA (including oral intake)	1000–1500	–	'Generally tolerated well.' Initial discomfort with tube. Early-morning fullness and some anorexia in first week	Nocturnal (10–12 h)
Smith, D.L. *et al.* (1994)	Nutrison Energy Plus (Nutricia) (enzyme dose taken at start of ETF)	1.5 kcal ml^{-1}	Prescribed 800–1200 ml	1564 (174)	–	9/14 developed hyperglycaemia, treated with small doses of short-acting insulin	Nocturnal (over 6 h) for 5 nights per week
Steinkamp and von der Hardt (1994)	Fresubin 750 MCT (Fresenius) 35% F, 20% P, 45% CHO (1–2 capsules of Creon per 100 ml at start of ETF)	1.5 kcal ml^{-1}	To meet measured REE	800–1500	–	No major side-effects/complications – occasional redness/tenderness at PEG site. Fullness, nausea and vomiting in the morning (n 4)	Nocturnal

[a]Energy density manipulated for children of different ages (diluted for youngest patients, fortified with maltodextrins for the three oldest children). est., estimated; P, protein; F, fat; CHO, carbohydrate; H, hospital; RDA, recommended daily allowance; REE, resting energy expenditure.

Table A6.5. Trial characteristics: trials of enteral tube feeding in patients with cystic fibrosis in the community (non-randomized data).

Trial	Design	Diagnosis	No. ETF	No. CON	Age range	Initial % wt-for-ht ETF group	Initial BMI CON group	Duration of ETF	Tube type	Control group
Bertrand et al. (1984) Canada	C	Cystic fibrosis, undernourished	10	–	3.5–12 years	84% wt-for-ht	–	4 weeks	Silicone nasogastric tube	–
Boland et al. (1986) Canada	C	Cystic fibrosis with moderate to severe lung disease, undernourished (resistant to ONS)	10	–	13.6 years (6.8–21.1 years)	80% wt-for-ht	–	10–36 months	Jejunostomy	–
Dalzell et al. (1992)[a] Australia	B	Cystic fibrosis, undernourished	10	14	9–20.2 years at follow-up	−1.6 z score for wt −1.0 z score for ht	−0.9 z score for wt −0.6 z score for ht	Median 1.35 years (follow-up period 5 years)	Nasogastric, converted to gastrostomy for long-term ETF	Better-nourished patients matched for sex, ht and FEV_1 at start of trial
Levy et al. (1985) Canada	B	Cystic fibrosis, moderate to severe lung disease, undernourished/ growth failing	14	10	12.9 years (4.9–21.5 years)	82% of std wt (wt velocity 28% and ht velocity 74% of standard[b])	–	Follow-up 1.1 years (0.8 year to 2.78 years)	Gastrostomy	Retrospective group (attempts were made to match by age, sex and clinical condition)
Moore et al. (1986) USA	C	Cystic fibrosis, growth failure, anorexia	8	–	8 months– 13 years	18% of std wt velocity and 47% of std ht velocity	–	3 months (follow-up 3 months after ETF stopped as well)	Nasogastric	–
O'Loughlin et al. (1986) Canada	C	Severe cystic fibrosis, malnourished	8[c]	–	7–27 years	77% IBW	–	Follow-up over 6.4 months	Nasogastric, passed every night by patient or parent	–
Shepherd et al. (1983) Australia	B	Growth retarded with cystic fibrosis	7[d]	8	5.2–13.4 years	−1.23 z score for wt	0 z score for wt	6 months	Nasogastric weighted silicone tube (n 3)	Healthy children
Shepherd et al. (1986)[a] Australia	B	Cystic fibrosis, undernourished, growth retarded	10[e]	14	8.9 years 3–13.2 years	~ −1.8 z score for wt (change of −0.41 during 1 year pre-ETF) ~ −1.2 z score for ht (change of −0.13 during 1 year pre-ETF)	~ −0.7 z score for wt ~ −0.5 z score for ht	1–2 years	Nasogastric weighted silicone tube (n 7), needle-catheter jejunostomy (n 2)	Height-, sex- and FEV_1-matched patients receiving conventional therapy

Smith, D.L. et al. (1994) UK	C	Advanced cystic fibrosis and undernourished	14	–	22.5 years 28–35 years	74% IBW	–	14.8 (± 4.5) months	Fine-bore nasogastric tube	–
Steinkamp and von der Hardt (1994)[f] Germany	C	Cystic fibrosis, extremely malnourished	14[f]	–	7–23 years	77.8% IBW	–	12 months	PEG	–

[a] Initial trial followed up patients for 1 year (Shepherd et al., 1986), with a subsequent 5-year follow-up in Dalzell et al. (1992).
[b] Using Tanner et al. (1966) standards.
[c] Previously unsuccessful use of ONS (n 7).
[d] n 3 received ETF and n 4 took the enteral formula orally.
[e] n 9 received ETF (in n 2 ETF started after ONS unsuccessful) and n 1 given ONS.
[f] n 9 of patients data at 6 month follow-up also reported in an earlier German publication not reviewed (Steinkamp et al., 1990).
BMI, body mass index; CON, control; FEV_1, forced expiratory volume in 1 s; std, standard.

Table A6.6. Main findings of enteral tube feeding trials in patients with cystic fibrosis in the community (non-randomized data).

Trial	Energy/nutrient intake	Wt change/growth ETF	Wt change CON	Function	Clinical outcome	Finance
Bertrand *et al.* (1984)	ETF as a sole source of nutrition sig. increased TEI from 67 kcal kg^{-1} (baseline) to 106 kcal kg^{-1} (with ETF)	Increased to 94% wt-for-ht with ETF (sig. increase) Decreased to 89% 2 months after ETF stopped Sig. increase in TSF/MAC but not MAMC	–	No improvement in exercise test (*n* 3 only), chest X-ray score (all), FEV_1 or FEF_{25-75} (*n* 5 only)	–	–
Boland *et al.* (1986)	–	+8.1% wt-for-ht (from start of trial to peak wt gain, sig.) vs. −6.3% during 6 months pre-ETF. Sig. increase in MAMC	–	Increased participation in daily activities and an improved sense of well-being (subjective, not rated). No decline in FVC but continued decrease in FEF (indicating continued progression of disease)	–	Use of standard, non-elemental feeds with enzymes, cheaper than elemental diets
Dalzell *et al.* (1992)	–	At 5 years: z score for wt −0.5 and for ht 0 (continued improvement in linear catch-up growth and weight gain) (ETF vs. CON sig.)	At 5 years: z score for wt −1.4 and for ht −1.7	Less deterioration of pulmonary function over 3 years in ETF than in CON (FEV_1), but NS. Difference over 3–5 years	ETF had lower mortality (NS) and lower H admissions (NS)	–
Levy *et al.* (1985)	Used as a supplement to food intake but no data given	+2% (sig. over 1 year) Sig. improvement in ht velocity (321%) and wt velocity (700%) Sig. increases in body fat and fat-free mass	−3% of standard[a] over 1 year	Pulmonary function (% of predicted FVC and FEV_1) did not change sig. in ETF over 1.1 years (*n* 10) but both declined sig. in CON (*n* 10) Marked increase in ability of ETF to participate in activities of daily living, even in those in whom lung function deteriorated	–	–
Moore *et al.* (1986)	Sig. increase in energy intake with ETF from 106 kcal kg^{-1} (pre-ETF) to 124 kcal kg^{-1}. Decreased to 115 kcal kg^{-1} 3 months after ETF stopped	+2.72 kg (sig. vs. −0.42 kg pre-ETF and −0.48 kg post-ETF) Ht and growth velocity increased by 60% (sig.) and wt velocity by 63% (NS) NS change in TSF, MAMC Gains not sustained once ETF stopped	–	Clinical scores increased sig. during ETF (composite score of case history, pulmonary physical findings, growth and nutrition). NS difference in the no. of 'sick' days during or after ETF	–	–

Reference	Energy intake	Weight/body composition		Functional/clinical outcomes	Comments
O'Loughlin *et al.* (1986)	TEI sig. increased with ETF (to 129% RDA vs. 101% pre-ETF) ETF constituted ~35% of energy intake and resulted in a small, NS decrease in oral intake from 95% to 84% of RDA	+5.6 kg (sig.)[b] Sig. increase in % IBW from 75 to 86% (n 10[b]), increase in total body fat and lean body mass (? sig.) In pts still growing (n 6), wt gain was associated with sig. increase in ht velocity	–	No change in pulmonary function tests (FEV_1, FEF_{25-75}, lung residual volume/total lung capacity, FVC) 88% (7/8 pts) had sig. improvements in well-being (1 unchanged) In pts gaining wt (n 7), episodes of pneumonia sig. decreased during ETF	–
Shepherd *et al.* (1983)	TEI increased with ETF: from 81 kcal kg⁻¹ (pre-ETF) to 103 kcal kg⁻¹ (with ETF). No data on food intake	+3.5 kg (± 2.5 kg) Sig. improvement in z score for wt (+0.52) and ht (+0.23) Sig. increase in MAC and TSF Sig. increase in body fat and muscle mass (using skin folds, urinary creatinine, total body potassium)	–	Sig. improvement in clinical scores (total, pulmonary, general) n 6 had a reduction in myofibrillar (muscle) protein degradation (NS)	(Because of the subjective benefits seen, 6/7 patients elected to continue with enteral nutrition after the trial)
Shepherd *et al.* (1986)	Used as a supplement to food intake but no data given	+0.88 change in z score for wt +0.2 change in z score for ht (ETF vs. CON sig. i.e. sig. greater change in z score for wt and ht with ETF vs. CON) Sig. catch-up in mean weight and height after 6 months ETF, continued for 1 year (no data given)	−0.07 −0.1	After ETF a sig. reversal of declining trend in pulmonary function (sig. vs. pre-ETF and vs. CON) Sig. reduction in no. of pulmonary exacerbations with ETF (vs. pre-ETF), not seen in CON Protein synthesis, in excess of breakdown, with net protein accretion after 1 month of ETF and a sig. reduction in the high rate of synthesis and breakdown with net anabolism after 6–12 months	–
Smith, D.L. *et al.* (1994)	–	+5.4 (± 4.4) kg (sig.) Good compliance (n 7) +6.85 kg Poor compliance (n 7) +3.85 kg (good vs. poor, sig.) % IBW increased to 81.6%	–	NS changes in FEV_1 or FVC (but those gaining the most wt showed improvements in FEV_1) (vs. pre-ETF, when lung function was declining)	–
Steinkamp and von der Hardt (1994)	–	+5.8 kg (sig.) at 6 months[c] +6 kg (sig.) at 12 months Sig. increase in MAMA, body fat and lean body mass	–	Considerable improvement in lung function: sig. increase in mean vital capacity, peak expiratory flow and FEV_1	–

[a] Using Tanner *et al.* (1966) standards.
[b] Includes 2 patients taking ONS and not receiving ETF.
[c] Data from earlier publication of n 9 patients followed up at 6 months.

CON, control; FEF, forced expiratory flow – an indication of small-airways disease progression; FEV_1, forced expiratory volume in 1 s; FVC, forced vital capacity; H, hospital; MAC, mid-arm circumference; MAMA, mid-arm muscle area; MAMC, mid-arm muscle circumference; NS, not significant; RDA, recommended daily allowance; sig., significant; TEI, total energy intake; TSF, triceps skin-fold thickness.

(I) What effect does ETF have on the voluntary food intake and total energy intake of patients in the community with CF?

ETF can be used effectively as a sole source of nutrition (Bertrand *et al.*, 1984) or as a supplement to food intake (Shepherd *et al.*, 1983; Moore *et al.*, 1986; O'Loughlin *et al.*, 1986) in those with CF. Using ETF in both of these ways, energy and nutrient intakes were improved, compared with pre-ETF intakes, as shown in all of the NRT reviewed that made such assessments (Shepherd *et al.*, 1983; Bertrand *et al.*, 1984; Moore *et al.*, 1986; O'Loughlin *et al.*, 1986) (Table A6.6). Indeed, in all four trials that reported longitudinal increases in energy intake, the improvements were statistically significant (Shepherd *et al.*, 1983; Bertrand *et al.*, 1984; Moore *et al.*, 1986; O'Loughlin *et al.*, 1986). However, in one trial, the increased total intake was not maintained once ETF was stopped (Moore *et al.*, 1986). Only one trial presented information about the changes in voluntary food intake with ETF (O'Loughlin *et al.*, 1986). This small (*n* 8) trial of patients, in whom the use of ONS had previously been unsuccessful, suggested that voluntary food intake was reduced by a small, non-significant degree with nocturnal NG tube feeding (Table A6.6).

(II) What effect does ETF have on the body weight and composition of patients in the community with CF?

ETF in growth-retarded children and adolescents with CF can lead to improvements in body weight and growth. All ten trials indicated increases in body weight following periods of ETF (duration 4 weeks to 3 years) (Shepherd *et al.*, 1983, 1986; Bertrand *et al.*, 1984; Levy *et al.*, 1985; Boland *et al.*, 1986; Moore *et al.*, 1986; O'Loughlin *et al.*, 1986; Dalzell *et al.*, 1992; Smith, D.L. *et al.*, 1994; Steinkamp and von der Hardt, 1994) (Table A6.6). Furthermore, all eight trials that assessed growth reported improvements (e.g. increases in weight and height velocity), which were statistically significant when compared with baseline (Shepherd *et al.*, 1983; Bertrand *et al.*, 1984; Levy *et al.*, 1985; Boland *et al.*, 1986; Moore *et al.*, 1986; O'Loughlin *et al.*, 1986) or with a non-random control group (Shepherd *et al.*, 1986; Dalzell *et al.*, 1992). A number of studies also indicated improvements in fat and muscle mass with ETF (fat mass: Shepherd *et al.*, 1983; Bertrand *et al.*, 1984; Levy *et al.*, 1985; O'Loughlin *et al.*, 1986; Steinkamp and von der Hardt, 1994; muscle mass: Shepherd *et al.*, 1983; Levy *et al.*, 1985; Boland *et al.*, 1986; O'Loughlin *et al.*, 1986; Steinkamp and von der Hardt, 1994), although improvements were not consistently observed in other studies (Moore *et al.*, 1986) (Table A6.6).

(III) What effect does ETF have on the body function of patients in the community with CF?

Functional improvements may occur in children, adolescents and adults with CF with the use of ETF. All trials reviewed made some assessment of functional outcomes following home ETF in patients with CF. Eighty per cent of trials showed improvements in some parameters (Shepherd *et al.*, 1983, 1986; Levy *et al.*, 1985; Boland *et al.*, 1986; Moore *et al.*, 1986; O'Loughlin *et al.*, 1986; Dalzell *et al.*, 1992; Steinkamp and von der Hardt, 1994) and 20% did not (Bertrand *et al.*, 1984; Smith, D.L. *et al.*, 1994) (see Table A6.6). Parameters that improved included subjective scores of well-being and estimates of activity levels (Levy *et al.*, 1985; Boland *et al.*, 1986; O'Loughlin *et al.*, 1986) and clinical scores (Shepherd *et al.*, 1983; Moore *et al.*, 1986). In some studies, indices of pulmonary function either improved more or declined less than control patients not given ETF or compared with pre-ETF periods (Levy *et al.*, 1985; Shepherd *et al.*, 1986; Dalzell *et al.*, 1992; Steinkamp and von der Hardt, 1994). Other studies found that ETF had no effect on pulmonary function (Bertrand *et al.*, 1984; Boland *et al.*, 1986; O'Loughlin *et al.*, 1986) and in one trial improvements were only evident in patients gaining the most weight (average +6.85 kg, Smith, D.L. *et al.,* 1994). Importantly, ETF did not have any significant adverse effects on body function. However, RCT are ultimately needed if the impact of ETF on functional outcomes in patients with CF in the community is to be addressed. Similar recommendations were made in a recent Cochrane review (Conway *et al.,* 2002).

(IV) What effect does ETF have on the clinical and financial outcome of patients in the community with CF?

Only one trial assessed the effect of ETF on clinical outcome (Dalzell *et al.,* 1992) (see Table A6.6). Compared with a non-randomized control group, tube-fed patients with CF had lower mortality rates and lower hospital admission rates, although these were not statistically significant differences. Lower hospital admission rates are likely to lead to cost savings, although none of the trials reviewed provided any financial data to assess the cost efficacy of ETF in patients with CF. Therefore, RCT are needed, as appropriate, if the impact of ETF on clinical and financial outcomes in patients with CF are to be identified.

Only studies undertaken in those with CF were reported in this section. For more information on studies in paediatrics with a variety of other conditions, see the paediatric section later in this appendix.

Diabetes Mellitus (Non-randomized Data)

Studies comparing ETF with no nutritional support have not typically been undertaken specifically in patients with diabetes mellitus. However, recently, changes in the formulations of feeds have been made to meet the specific needs of diabetic patients and those with impaired glucose tolerance. Subsequently, a number of studies comparing these new formulas (fibre-containing, MCT-rich, lower carbohydrate) with traditional standard formulas have been undertaken.

Tables A6.7–A6.9 summarize one such study.[2] However, as these investigations are beyond the scope of this review, similar trials of ETF in patients with type I or type II diabetes can be referred to individually (Harley *et al.,* 1989; Peters *et al.,* 1989; Sanz *et al.,* 1994). Furthermore, the issues surrounding the nutritional support of tube-fed patients with diabetes have been discussed and summarized in a *Clinical Nutrition* supplement (1998, Vol. 17, Suppl. 2).

Elderly (Non-randomized Data)

It is widely accepted that ETF can be a useful mode of treatment in appropriately selected elderly patients at risk of malnutrition, as this quote suggests:

> Artificial feeding by the enteral ... route is extremely effective, especially when carried out by an expert team and in appropriately selected patients in whom the outcome justifies the additional expenditure.
>
> (Allison, 1995)

Therefore, it is surprising that the efficacy of this mode of nutritional support has not been investigated in depth in elderly patients in community settings.

Only two NRT (one paper (Breslow *et al.,* 1993) and one abstract (Chernoff *et al.,* 1990)), which studied the use of ETF in institutionalized elderly with pressure ulcers, were reviewed (Tables A6.10–A6.12). Tube feeding was well tolerated in both reports, although in one trial the attrition rate over the 8-week study period was high (Breslow *et al.,* 1993) (see Table A6.10). ETF was found to increase energy and protein intakes versus baseline in the one trial that made assessments, using either standard (14% protein) or high-protein (24%) feeds (Breslow *et al.,* 1993) (see Table A6.12). In patients receiving the high-protein feed, the increase in protein intake with ETF was statistically significant. However, total energy intakes were similar in both ETF groups (who received ETF as a sole source of nutrition) to that of the patients taking the hospital diet plus ONS. The two groups of patients were not randomized with respect

Table A6.7. Enteral tube feeds used in trials of patients with diabetes in the community (non-randomized data).[2]

Trial	ETF	ETF energy density	ETF prescribed	ETF energy (kcal) provision	ETF protein (g) provision	Toleration	Timing of ETF
Craig *et al.* (1998)	Glucerna (fibre feed for patients with abnormal glucose tolerance, Ross 17% P, 33% CHO, 50% F, ETF[1]) vs. Jevity (standard fibre feed, Ross 17% P, 53% CHO, 30% F, ETF[2])	1 kcal ml⁻¹ \n 1 kcal ml⁻¹	To meet estimated energy requirements and adjusted to maintain body wt	–	–	No deleterious effects of using ETF[1] but lack of data on GI tolerance or on ability to manage tube	Continuous or intermittent ETF

CHO, carbohydrate; F, fat; GI, gastrointestinal; P, protein; wt, weight.

Table A6.8. Trial characteristics: trials of enteral tube feeding in patients with diabetes in the community (non-randomized data).

Trial	Design	Diagnosis	No. ETF	No. CON	Initial BMI ETF group	Initial BMI CON group	Duration of ETF	Tube type	Control group
Craig *et al.* (1998) USA	C[a]	Type 2 diabetics in long-term care (aged > 50 years)	30 \n ETF[1] 16 \n ETF[2] 14	–	–	–	Follow up for 3 months	'Enteral access device'	–

[a]Randomized trial comparing two enteral formulas (standard and diabetic). Longitudinal data reported for those completing the trial (*n* 30/34). BMI, body mass index; CON, control.

Table A6.9. Main findings of enteral tube feeding trials in patients with diabetes in the community (non-randomized data).

Trial	Energy/nutrient intake	Wt change ETF	Wt change CON	Function	Clinical outcome	Finance
Craig *et al.* (1998)	ETF used as a sole source of nutrition	ETF regimen prescribed to maintain weight. NS changes in wt reported	–	NS lower fasting serum glucose and HbA₁c with ETF[1]. Lower mean weekly capillary glucose measurements (from finger prick) with ETF[1] (sig. for 3 weeks of trial) Sig. higher HDL and trend towards lower TAG after 3 months in ETF[1]	Fewer fevers, pneumonia, urinary-tract infections, pressure ulcers and total infections with ETF[1] than with ETF[2] (NS) No difference in insulin use between formulas (numerically less with ETF[1] and tendency for reduced use over time)	–

CON, control; HbA₁c, haemoglobin A₁c; HDL, high-density lipoprotein; TAG, triacylglycerol.

Table A6.10. Enteral tube feeds used in trials of elderly patients in the community (non-randomized data).

Trial	ETF	ETF energy density	ETF prescribed	ETF energy (kcal) provision	ETF protein (g) provision	Toleration	Timing of ETF
Breslow *et al.* (1993)	Ensure (Abbott)(F^1 4% P) or Sustacal (Mead Johnson) (F^2 24% P)	1 kcal ml^{-1}	To meet estimated requirements as a sole source of nutrition	~1986 ± 646	~90 ± 35	Mild, occasional diarrhoea (*n* 2) (*n* 48 started in trial, but high attrition rate with only 28 completing (*n* 15 died))	–
Chernoff *et al.* (1990)	Replete (F^1 16% P; F^2 25% P)	–	–	–	F^1 57–90 F^2 92–150[a]	Both formulas well tolerated with no GI or metabolic side-effects	–

[a]Unclear if protein intake solely from ETF or if the contribution from an oral diet is included.
GI, gastrointestinal; P, protein.

Table A6.11. Trial characteristics: trials of enteral tube feeding in elderly patients in the community (non-randomized data).

Trial	Design	Diagnosis	No. ETF	No. CON	Initial BMI ETF group	Initial BMI CON group	Duration of ETF	Tube type	Control group
Breslow *et al.* (1993) USA	C	Elderly, malnourished with pressure ulcers (stage II to IV) in long-term care	28[a] F^1 13 F^2 15	–	F^1 22 F^2 20	–	8 weeks	–	Standard nursing home diet (~2000 kcal, 85 g P) plus ONS (720 kcal, 27–44 g P)[a]
Chernoff *et al.* (1990) A USA	C	Pressure ulcers in elderly long-term tube-fed institutionalized patients	12 ETF^1 6 ETF^2 6	–	–	–	8 weeks	–	–

[a]*n* 8 received F^1 (formula 1) by tube and *n* 7 F^2 by tube (the remainder were given the feeds orally as a supplement three times daily) – data presented for group as a whole only.
A, abstract; BMI, body mass index; CON, control; P, protein.

Table A6.12. Main findings of enteral tube feeding trials in elderly patients in the community (non-randomized data).

Trial	Energy/nutrient intake	Wt change ETF	Wt change CON	Function	Clinical outcome	Finance
Breslow *et al.* (1993)	Energy and protein intakes increased (NS) in both ETF and ONS vs. baseline (sig. increase in P intake in F^2 only). Total intakes similar in ETF and ONS groups (ETF: 1986 kcal, 90 g P; ONS: 1918 kcal, 87 g P)[a]	F^1 +1 kg m^{-1} F^2 +1 kg m^{-1} (NS change)	–	Sig. reduction in total truncal pressure ulcer surface area in F^2 but not in F^1, with the greatest reduction in those with the greatest energy and protein intakes. Sig. decrease in stage IV ulcer surface area in F^2 sig. greater than the small change seen in F^1	–	–
Chernoff *et al.* (1990)	–	'Weight was adequately maintained on both formulas'	–	On both formulas, ulcer size decreased (F^1 year ~42% and F^2 by ~73%), but the improvement was greater in F^2, with complete healing in *n* 4 (0 in F^1).	–	–

[a]ETF group given ETF as a sole source of nutrition and ONS group given ONS in addition to normal nursing-home diet.
CON, control; NS, not significant; P, protein; sig., significant.

to clinical condition and other confounding factors. In both of the reviewed trials, ETF led to weight stabilization or small gains in weight and a reduction in pressure ulcer size/area (see Table A6.12). However, the impact of ETF and other modes of nutritional support on the healing of pressure ulcers requires investigation in RCT in patients in nursing homes and other community settings and in hospitals. This appears to be a neglected area of investigation considering the widespread prevalence of pressure ulcers across Europe, the detrimental effects of pressure ulcers on patients' functional and clinical recovery (see Chapter 4) and the huge cost/resource implications for the care of such patients (Preston, 1991; O'Dea, 1995; Allman, 1997; Allman *et al.*, 1999). Trials are also needed in elderly patients to investigate the clinical and cost-effectiveness of ETF in different community settings.

It is also recognized that ETF may not always be ethically appropriate in some sick, elderly individuals (e.g. the terminally ill). For a review of some of the ethical issues surrounding withdrawing or withholding artificial nutrition, other articles should be referred to (Ouslander *et al.*, 1993; Krynski *et al.*, 1994; Bozzetti, 1996; Lennard-Jones, 1998).

Elderly patients may also have been included in studies of mixed groups of patients (e.g. general medical) and in other disease-specific groups (e.g. COPD or neurology) discussed elsewhere in this appendix.

Gastrointestinal (GI) Disease (Non-randomized Data)

Despite the importance of nutrition in the treatment of many GI diseases, there are few reports of the use of ETF in such patients resident in the community. In the one NRT that was reviewed (Mansfield *et al.*, 1995) (Tables A6.13–A6.15), 4 weeks of NG feeding in those with active Crohn's disease were associated with a number of patients entering remission, with each of the feeds used (elemental and peptide) being equally effective. Further well-designed research in patients with different GI disorders is war-

ranted if the efficacy of ETF in this patient group is to be explored, in the absence of confounding factors such as steroid use and spontaneous remission of disease activity.

In the clinical setting, ETF may be used in combination with steroids to enable patients with Crohn's disease to enter remission. Indeed, a number of meta-analyses have compared the efficacy of ETF with steroid treatment in patients with Crohn's disease in hospital and community settings (including Griffiths *et al.*, 1995; Heuschkel *et al.*, 2000) and these have been briefly summarized in Appendix 5.

Patients with GI disease may have also been included in studies undertaken in mixed groups of patients (e.g. general medical patients).

General Medical/Mixed Groups of Patients (Non-randomized Data)

Many investigations have reported the efficacy of ETF in mixed groups of patients with various diseases/conditions in the community (neurology, cancer, GI diseases, human immunodeficiency virus (HIV), post-surgery). A number of prospective studies (Tables A6.16–A6.18) and local and national surveys of patients receiving ETF in the community have been reviewed and are discussed briefly below.

The findings of the studies reviewed and of surveys of large groups of patients confirm that ETF can be safely and efficiently used in various community settings, including patients' own homes (as the following quote suggests) and nursing homes, and in diverse diagnostic groups (see Table A6.17): 'Naso-gastric tube feeding at home can be an acceptable, safe, economical and efficient treatment for nutritional depletion' (McIntyre *et al.*, 1983).

The GI tolerance of ETF is typically good (McIntyre *et al.*, 1983), patients are mostly able to cope with the procedure and are typically happy and confident caring for the tube (Bannerman *et al.*, 1999), which, in the majority of community-fed adults, is a PEG (Elia *et al.*, 2000a; British Artificial Nutrition Survey (BANS)).

Table A6.13. Enteral tube feeds used in trials of patients with gastrointestinal disorders in the community (non-randomized data).

Trial	ETF	ETF energy density	ETF prescribed	ETF energy (kcal) provision	ETF protein (g) provision	Toleration	Timing of ETF
Mansfield *et al.* (1995)	Elemental O28 (SHS) (ETF[1]) or Pepti-2000 LF (oligopeptide, ETF[2])	0.8 kcal ml[-1] 1 kcal ml[-1]	–	2250	–	*n* 6 could not tolerate NG tube (mostly men)	Started in hospital and discharged after ~6 days of ETF

Table A6.14. Trial characteristics: trials of enteral tube feeding in patients with gastrointestinal disorders in the community (non-randomized data).

Trial	Design	Diagnosis	No. ETF	No. CON	Initial BMI ETF group	Initial BMI CON group	Duration of ETF	Tube type	Control group
Mansfield *et al.* (1995) UK Hospital to home	C[a]	Active Crohn's disease	44[b] ETF[1] 22 ETF[2] 22	–	ETF[1] 83% IBW ETF[2] 92% IBW	–	4 weeks (ETF withdrawn if no improvement after 10 days)	Nasogastric	–

[a]Randomized trial comparing two enteral formulas.
[b]Steroids withdrawn at start of trial.
BMI, body mass index; CON, control.

Table A6.15. Main findings of enteral tube feeding trials in patients with gastrointestinal disorders in the community (non-randomized data).

Trial	Energy/nutrient intake	Wt change ETF	Wt change CON	Function	Outcome	Finance
Mansfield *et al.* (1995)	ETF given as a sole source of nutrition	ETF[1] No change ETF[2] increase to 95% IBW	–	*n* 16 entered remission with a reduction in intestinal inflammation (reduction in CDAI and bowel uptake of leucocytes,[a] reduced CRP). Marked response in first 10 days with slower improvement thereafter. *n* 22 did not respond (ETF[1] and ETF[2] were equally effective)	–	–

[a]Reduction in inflammatory activity on leucocyte scanning.
CDAI, Crohn's disease activity index; CON, control; CRP, C-reactive protein.

Table A6.16. Enteral tube feeds used in trials of mixed groups of patients with a variety of disorders in the community (non-randomized data).

Trial	ETF	ETF energy density	ETF prescribed	ETF energy (kcal) provision	ETF protein (g) provision	Toleration	Timing of ETF
Bannerman *et al.* (1999)	–	–	–	–	–	1 month: 73% felt they could cope with PEG and 83% were happy and confident caring for the PEG	–
Bastow *et al.* (1985)	Clinifeed Iso, Nutranel or a mix	Various	1.5 l (? 1500 kcal)	–	–	Well tolerated	Nocturnal
Edington *et al.* (1994)	Perative (Ross)	1.3 kcal ml⁻¹	1704 kcal	1472	–	31% (*n* 15) had 1 or more new GI symptoms during ETF (abdominal distension, diarrhoea, nausea, vomiting). Overall, 61% had 'good' response, 33% adequate, 6% poor	–
Jager-Wittenaar *et al.* (2000)	–	–	–	–	–	Well tolerated and alleviated symptoms of nausea. No aspiration or refeeding syndrome	Continuous, 24 h (started in hospital and then discharged home)
Pareira *et al.* (1954)	Mixture	1.46–2.34 kcal ml⁻¹	3500 kcal, 210 g P	–	–	Tolerance 'remarkably good'. Diarrhoea in 7% (total *n* 240 ETF, *n* 76 orally)	Continuous 24 h, changed to 4–6 aliquots after 1–3 weeks
Schneider *et al.* (2000a) A	–	–	–	–	–	–	–
Schneider *et al.* (2000c)	Polymeric feeds (*n* 36)	–	–	30 kcal kg⁻¹ wt	–	*n* 1 aspiration pneumonia. All complained of at least one episode of constipation (58%) or diarrhoea (42%). Other problems with tube migration, clogging, peristomal infection	Nocturnal (*n* 21), diurnal (*n* 17)
Von Herz *et al.* (2000)	–	–	–	–	–	–	–

A, abstract; GI, gastrointestinal; P, protein.

Table A6.17. Trial characteristics: trials of enteral tube feeding in mixed groups of patients with a variety of disorders in the community (non-randomized data).

Trial	Design	Diagnosis	No. ETF	No. CON	Initial BMI ETF group	Initial BMI CON group	Duration of ETF	Tube type	Control group
Bannerman et al. (1999) A UK	C	Mixed: neurology, head injury, cancer, cystic fibrosis	54	–	16 kg m^{-2} 'malnourished' (MAMC and/or TSF <10th centile)	–	Follow-up 1 and 6 months after PEG placement	PEG	–
Bastow et al. (1985) UK	C	Swallowing problems or anorexia associated with systemic disease	8	–	18. 8 kg m^{-2}	–	18–43 days	Fine-bore nasogastric tube	–
Edington et al. (1994) UK	C	IBD, malabsorption, HIV, cancer, post-operative, others	49[a]	–	–	–	3–28 days	Nasogastric tube	–
Jager-Wittenaar et al. (2000) A Netherlands	C	Pregnant women with hyperemesis gravidarum	12 9 went home	–	–	–	19 days 3–92 days	Nasogastric tube	–
Pareira et al. (1954) USA	C	Cancerous and non-cancerous cachexia	18 (with data, 240 studied[b])	–	% body wt loss 8–59% (? duration)	–	1–16 weeks	Nasogastric tube	–
Schneider et al. (2000a) A France	C	Mixed: head/neck cancer, amyotrophic lateral sclerosis, others	19	–	–	–	11 (3) weeks	PEG	–
Schneider et al. (2000c) France	C	Neurology, digestive disorders, head/neck cancer, others	38	–	17.5 kg m^{-2}	–	25 (5) months	PEG or surgical jejunostomy	–
Von Herz et al. (2000) A Germany	C	Mixed: neurology, head/neck disease, others	155	–	–	–	1 day, 2 months and 4 months after PEG insertion (n 56 only)	PEG	–

[a]Some patients were in hospital and some took the feed orally (? what proportion).
[b]Some patients fed in hospital and some took feed orally. Quantitative data for n 18 only.
A, abstract; CON, control; BMI, body mass index; IBD, inflammatory bowel disease; TSF, triceps skin-fold thickness.

Table A6.18. Main findings of enteral tube feeding trials in mixed groups of patients with a variety of disorders in the community (non-randomized data).

Trial	Energy/nutrient intake	Wt change ETF	Wt change CON	Function	Outcome	Finance
Bannerman *et al.* (1999)	–	1 month: Nutritional status of 47% improved and 50% deteriorated (using MAMA). All head/neck cancer pt deteriorated but all stroke patients improved	–	No change in SF-36[a] after 1 month ETF but for HAD[a] (*n* 15) scores: 44% more and 42% less anxious/ depressed, 14% no change 47% (*n* 9/19) at 1 month and 73% (*n* 8/11) at 6 months thought involvement in social activities had not improved since ETF Overall impact of PEG on quality of life: 1 month 53% (*n* 10) thought it was positive, *n* 2 negative; 6 months: *n* 8 thought it had a positive effect (none negative)	1 month: *n* 45 (83%) still alive and 76% of these were still receiving ETF via PEG, 4 resumed food intake 6 months: *n* 24 (44%) still alive	–
Bastow *et al.* (1985)	ETF used as a supplement to VFI. VFI increased from 931 to 1700 kcal during ETF	+6.45 (± 3.15) kg (? sig.) Increase in MAC and TSF (? sig.)	–	Rapid return to normal daytime activity was achieved and *n* 1 returned to work during ETF period (*Sig. increases in total protein and albumin*)	–	–
Edington *et al.* (1994)	*n* 30 (sole source of nutrition), *n* 17 as a supplement to usual diet, *n* 2 supplement to PN; TEI 2015 kcal, of which 73% from ETF and 551 kcal VFI	+0.1 (± 3.1) kg (NS) > 14 days ETF: +0.56 (± 3.8) kg (NS) 8–14 days ETF: +0.3 (± 2.5) kg (NS) <7 days ETF: −0.55 (± 3.1) kg (NS)	–	–	–	–
Jager-Wittenaar *et al.* (2000)	–	–	–	'The home treatment was very much appreciated by the patients'	Hospital stay was shortened compared with before the trial when ETF was not used	–
Pareira *et al.* (1954)	Appetite returned in 7 to 56 days. Most ate in addition to 3500 kcal of ETF (no data on VFI)	+2.54 kg (*n* 16) (? sig.) (*n* 64 with advanced cancer who lived > 1 week after starting ETF gained wt (no data))	–	(*Of those with advanced cancer, the majority became less of a nursing problem and quite a few who were bedridden became ambulatory*)	–	–

Continued

Table A6.18. Main findings of enteral tube feeding trials in mixed groups of patients with a variety of disorders in the community (non-randomized data).

Trial	Energy/nutrient intake	Wt change ETF	Wt change CON	Function	Clinical outcome	Finance
Schneider *et al.* (2000a) A	–	–	–	During ETF there was an improvement in all quality-of-life parameters: SF-36: mental component (sig.), physical component (sig.) EuroQol: visual analogue scale (sig.), EQ-5D (NS)	–	–
Schneider *et al.* (2000c)	ETF as the sole source of nutrition (*n* 15) or as a supplement (*n* 23). No data provided on intakes	BMI increased to 19.5 (± 0.6) kg m^{-2}	–	Quality-of-life scores (SF-36) for body pain, vitality and mental health the same as healthy population Sig. lower quality-of-life scores (SF-36) for ETF vs. normal population for physical functioning, general health, social functioning, emotional and physical roles. Sig. lower EuroQol scores than normal population (? valid comparison). Subjective assessment: home ETF was associated with improved or stable housework and social activities. Family relationships were stable in most patients. No improvement in work	Pt spent 1.9% of their time in hospital after starting ETF (in 46% of cases due to disease)	–
Von Herz *et al.* (2000)	–	Nutritional status stabilized for pts following PEG placement (no data)	–	Self-assessed quality of life (EORTC QLQ-C 30) increased sig. with regard to functional status and fatigue and constipation sig. decreased. Spitzer index (proxy rating) improved sig. for ETF for those assessing their own quality of life (*n* 67) and in those who were cognitively impaired (*n* 88), for whom the investigator assessed quality of life	–	–

[a]SF-36 (short form 36) and HAD (hospital anxiety and depression scale) used to assess health-related quality of life.
A, abstract; BMI, body mass index; CON, control; MAC, mid-arm circumference; MAMA, mid-arm muscle area; NS, not significant; PN, parenteral nutrition; pts, patients; ?sig., uncertain if statistically significant; sig., significant; TEI, total energy intake; TSF, triceps skin-fold thickness; VFI, voluntary food intake.

Prospective evaluations of the efficacy of ETF in patients with predominantly chronic conditions in the community are lacking. In most cases, this is likely to be due to the ethical difficulties of withholding ETF in patients in the control arm of such a trial. Eight NRT in mixed groups of patients receiving ETF were reviewed (Pareira *et al.*, 1954; Bastow *et al.*, 1985; Edington *et al.*, 1994; Bannerman *et al.*, 1999; Jager-Wittenaar *et al.*, 2000; Schneider *et al.*, 2000a,c; Von Herz *et al.*, 2000). As all of the trials reviewed were non-randomized, interpretation of the findings discussed below is limited. These trials have been summarized in Box A6.2 and Tables A6.16–A6.18.

Box A6.2. Key findings: effect of ETF in mixed groups of community patients.

National and local surveys suggest that ETF is increasingly being used to provide nutritional support for patients in the community, enabling discharge from the hospital setting to home or to care homes.

Information from non-randomized trials suggests the following:

- ETF can be used effectively as a sole source of nutrition (in patients in whom food intake is contraindicated) or as a supplement to food intake in the community environment.
- ETF may enable patients to maintain or gain weight.
- ETF may improve quality of life.

Without ETF, many of these patients would be expected to die or suffer from the effects of malnutrition. In such cases, RCT cannot be undertaken.

(I) What effect does ETF have on the voluntary food intake and total energy intake of patients in the community?

ETF, whether used as a sole source of nutrition or as a supplement, is a useful and effective way of maintaining or increasing nutritional intakes in community patients. The studies reviewed suggested that ETF was used effectively as a sole source of nutrition (Edington *et al.*, 1994; Schneider *et al.*, 2000a) or as a supplement to food intake (Pareira *et al.*, 1954; Bastow *et al.*, 1985; Edington *et al.*, 1994; Schneider *et al.*, 2000a) in patients with a variety of disorders in community settings (Table A6.18). In combination with ETF, the longitudinal surveys reviewed also suggested that appetite and voluntary food intake may improve over time (Pareira *et al.*, 1954; Bastow *et al.*, 1985). However, controlled trials in patients, in addition to healthy controls (Stratton and Elia, 1999b), are needed to fully assess the effects of ETF on total energy intake, appetite and voluntary food intake.

(II) What effect does ETF have on the body weight and composition of patients in the community?

ETF can be used to maintain or improve the nutritional status of a variety of patients. Of the studies reviewed that assessed body weight (*n* 6), in four, weight gain was quantitatively documented but not evaluated as statistically significant (Pareira *et al.*, 1954; Bastow *et al.*, 1985; Edington *et al.*, 1994; Schneider *et al.*, 2000a) and, in one, the nutritional status of patients stabilized with ETF (Von Herz *et al.*, 2000) (see Table A6.18). In a prospective survey, both improvement and deterioration in nutritional status (using arm anthropometry) were observed, possibly due to changes in the clinical condition of patients, many of whom died within 6 months of ETF (56%) (Bannerman *et al.*, 1999). However, another trial that measured arm anthropometry reported longitudinal increases in mid-arm circumference (MAC) and triceps skin-fold thickness (TSF) following ETF (Bastow *et al.*, 1985). Reports of case-studies have also highlighted the effectiveness of ETF as a supplement to diet in undernourished patients living at home (Main *et al.*, 1980; McIntyre *et al.*, 1983). For example, five patients were reported to have a mean rate of weight gain of 0.54 kg per week for 16 weeks with nocturnal NG feeding (McIntyre *et al.*, 1983). As these trials lacked a control group not given ETF for comparison, it is difficult to fully ascertain the impact of ETF on body weight and compositional changes in such patients.

(III) What effect does ETF have on the body function of patients in the community?

A number of trials studied the quality of life of patients after placement of PEG (Bannerman *et al.*, 1999; Jager-Wittenaar *et al.*, 2000; Schneider *et al.*, 2000a,c; Von Herz *et al.*, 2000). However, it is very difficult to draw conclusions about the impact of ETF via PEG on patients' quality of life, as data on the quality of life of such patients if ETF and PEG placement had not taken place are not available. Furthermore, these data may be difficult or impossible to obtain on ethical grounds. Not unexpectedly, one study suggested that the quality of life of tube-fed patients was lower than that of the normal healthy population (Schneider *et al.*, 2000a) (see Table A6.18). However this is an unrealistic comparison that does not take into account the effects of disease or other treatment modalities on quality of life. Other longitudinal studies suggested that quality of life might improve over the course of home ETF (Schneider *et al.*, 2000c; Von Herz *et al.*, 2000). Similarly, a study of the quality of life of out-patients receiving nutritional support (ETF, parenteral nutrition (PN) or ONS) indicated significant improvements in all quality-of-life scores (energy, pain, emotion, sleep, social isolation, mobility) in those who were underweight (body mass index ((BMI) < 20 kg m^{-2}) (Jamieson *et al.*, 1997). Other studies documented how much patients appreciated receiving ETF at home (Jager-Wittenaar *et al.*, 2000) or suggested that physical improvements ensued (Pareira *et al.*, 1954; Bastow *et al.*, 1985). In particular, ETF was associated with an improved ability to do housework and enjoy social activities (Schneider *et al.*, 2000a). No functional detriments were observed in the trials reviewed. For more details on functional changes during ETF, see Table A6.18.

(IV) What effect does ETF have on the clinical and financial outcome of patients in the community?

ETF has become an indispensable therapy for many patients, particularly for those in whom ETF is a sole source of nutrition, but also for those who have ETF in addition to an oral diet in order to meet their nutritional requirements and maintain nutritional status and body functions. The development of this technique for use in the home setting has enabled substantial numbers of patients to be discharged home or to a nursing home. This has benefits for patients (in terms of freedom from hospital, contact with family with the potential for improvement in quality of life) and for the health-care system (reduced hospital bed and resource use, cost savings). Indeed, Schneider *et al.* (2000a) documented that patients spent only 1.9% of their time in hospital after starting ETF (Table A6.18), a finding reflected by national surveys (Elia *et al.*, 2001b). In general, the outcome of patients on ETF is determined by their clinical condition. One small report (*n* 54) indicated that the majority of patients were still alive and continuing with ETF after 1 month at home and that some, although a small minority, resumed oral intake (Bannerman *et al.*, 1999). Outcome data from large numbers of patients receiving home ETF can also be obtained from national surveys and these are discussed below.

As highlighted above, cost savings may result from the use of ETF if patients previously cared for in hospital beds, using hospital resources while being fed, can now be discharged home. Furthermore, national surveys suggest that, once home, patients spend a very small amount of time in hospital (< 2% (Elia *et al.*, 1998, 2000a, 2001b)). Indeed, it has been estimated that savings of $> £90$ million can be made by the use of nutritional support in the home instead of the hospital setting in the UK each year (Elia, 1995).

Surveys of home ETF

Local and national surveys have reported growth in the use of ETF (in the community) as a means of nutritional support in patients with a wide variety of conditions. Examples have included local surveys from the UK (Weekes *et al.*, 1992; Hull *et al.*, 1993; McWhirter *et al.*, 1994a; Parker *et al.*, 1996a,b), France (de Ledinghen *et al.*, 1995; Schneider *et al.*, 2000b), Italy (Finocchiaro *et al.*, 1997) and Ireland (McNamara *et al.*, 2000). These local surveys have highlighted a number of issues:

- There is rapid growth in home ETF. An increasing number of patients are now being discharged home from hospital on ETF for domiciliary care because of technical and health-care advances.
- Early discharge of patients on ETF saves money/hospital resources, although the cost implications for community health care still need to be evaluated.
- Practical problems occur: there can be a lack of nutrition teams/poor organization of home nutrition support services, poor knowledge of ETF among community health-care professionals, doctors and nurses and a lack of follow-up.
- The diagnoses of patients receiving ETF across local and national boundaries vary, possibly due to the availability of resources, different treatment protocols and variations in disease incidence.
- Patients receiving ETF at home are typically a severely disabled, inactive, elderly group.
- Regular monitoring of nutritional status, including micronutrient status, is required in patients receiving long-term home ETF to ensure that deficiencies do not develop, that nutritional status is adequately maintained and that ETF is still required.

Widely reported national surveys, including those from Britain (Elia *et al.*, 2000a, 2001b) and the USA (Howard *et al.*, 1995), demonstrate the growth and safety of use of ETF in the community setting. They also provide some outcome data, such as mortality and quality of life.

British Artificial Nutrition Survey (BANS)

In Britain, home ETF is the dominant form of nutritional support, accounting for 65% of all the artificial nutrition (ETF and PN) used (in both hospitals and homes). The point prevalence of home ETF in the UK in the year 2000 was ~20,000, with an annual growth rate nearing 20%. The main diagnostic group was those with 'diseases of the central nervous system', with the conditions of CVA and cerebral palsy being the most common in adults and children, respectively. However, in the UK, ETF is increasingly being used in patients with cancer. In 2000, one in six adult patients on home ETF and one in four starting home ETF had cancer, typically oropharyngeal or oesophageal cancer. The most recent survey, published in 2001, indicated that patients spent < 1% of their time in hospital and that the majority were living in their own home (~60%). In addition, patients on home ETF in Britain are becoming increasingly elderly, with 60% aged over 60 years in 2000 and the commonest age band being 71–80 years. Therefore, it is not surprising that patients receiving home ETF are mostly disabled (51% of adults housebound or bedridden) and often dependent on others for their care (59% requiring total help with home ETF). In terms of outcome, 1-year mortality on home ETF varies depending on the diagnosis of patients, from 5% for cerebral palsy to 32% for CVA and 63% for motor neurone disease. Similarly, the rate of return to oral feeding depends on patients' condition (13% for CVA and 1% for motor neurone disease). For more information, the reader is referred to the most recent BANS report (Elia *et al.*, 2001b).

USA

In the USA there were ~152,000 patients receiving home ETF in 1992, with the use of home nutritional support doubling during 1989 and 1992 (home ETF and home PN) (Howard *et al.*, 1995). In particular, there has been an increased use of short-term home ETF. Retrospective calculations suggested that $357 million was spent on home enteral nutrition in 1992 in the USA (estimates were based on extrapolations from medical insurance data from Medicare). Overall, American data have highlighted the fact that this mode of treatment is relatively safe and that the best justification for using it at home is the predicted quality of survival of individuals, even for only a few months, as opposed to decisions based on the diagnosis of a patient. In America, the two main diagnostic groups receiving home ETF at the time of this survey were those with neurological disorders of swallowing, typically due to stroke or disorders of childhood. As in Britain, the majority of these patients (75%) were over 65 years of age. Estimated median survival for such patients (dysphagic, non-cancer patients) was 1.5 years. The other main group was those patients with cancer. Of these, estimates suggested that only ~20% experienced complete rehabilitation and 59% died. The information from this national survey, as with other local and national surveys, suggested that complications resulting in rehospitalization were few (0.9–2.7 per patient-year).

The information presented in this section relates to studies and surveys that were undertaken in patients with a variety of conditions. For studies undertaken in specific disease groups, refer to the individual sections in this appendix.

HIV/Acquired Immune Deficiency Syndrome (AIDS) (Non-randomized Data)

HIV infection and AIDS are a public health problem in European and other countries worldwide. Although weight loss is not universally observed in patients with HIV infection, in those who have developed AIDS, wasting, associated with anorexia, chronic diarrhoea, infections and fever, is a problem. Furthermore, time of death has been linked with the degree of wasting in patients with AIDS. Therefore, appropriate nutritional support, including ETF, to prevent or treat wasting in this patient group, may lead to improvements in clinical outcome (Green, 1995). However, no RCT comparing ETF with routine care in the community environment were reviewed.

Five NRT of PEG feeding for up to 10 months in patients with HIV (Ockenga *et al.*, 1994) or advanced AIDS (Brantsma *et al.*, 1991; Kotler *et al.*, 1991; Cappell and Godil, 1993; Süttmann *et al.*, 1993) were reviewed and the findings are discussed briefly below and summarized in Box A6.3 and Tables A6.19–A6.21. The confounding effects of drug therapy (e.g. highly active antiretroviral therapy (HAART)) or changes in disease conditions cannot be excluded, due to the poor design of the trials reviewed.

In most studies, patients were undernourished (Kotler *et al.*, 1991; Cappell and Godil, 1993; Süttmann *et al.*, 1993; Ockenga *et al.*, 1994) and receiving ETF in addition to an oral diet. ETF was typically well tolerated with a number of minor complications that were easily treated (see Table A6.19). Indeed, these small studies of patients with HIV and AIDS concluded that ETF via a PEG was relatively simple, safe and useful (Brantsma *et al.*, 1991; Cappell and Godil, 1993; Ockenga *et al.*, 1994), as this quote suggests: 'It is a safe, effective and comparatively cheap method of nutritional support, in or out of hospital' (Brantsma *et al.*, 1991).

The efficacy of ETF in this patient group was addressed by the four main review questions.

Box A6.3. Key findings: effect of ETF in community patients with HIV/AIDS.

Information from non-randomized trials suggests that ETF may do the following:

- Improve body weight and muscle and fat mass.
- Lead to functional benefits (immune, quality of life).

Although RCT in this patient group are ideally needed to assess the effectiveness of ETF, these may be difficult to undertake ethically in severely malnourished patients.

Table A6.19. Enteral tube feeds used in trials of patients with HIV/AIDS in the community (non-randomized data).

Trial	ETF	ETF energy density	ETF prescribed	ETF energy (kcal) provision	ETF protein (g) provision	Toleration	Timing of ETF
Brantsma et al. (1991)	Restore, Isocal, Top-up, Ensure Plus, elemental O28	–	2583 kcal (1250–3650 kcal)	–	–	No increase in diarrhoea with ETF. Wound infections (n 1, no antibiotics used)	–
Cappell and Godil (1993)	Vivonex (n 3), Ensure (3), Osmolite HN (2), Isocal (2) Osmolite (2) Tolerex (1) Pediasure (1)	–	–	Adults: 1882 (± 422) Paediatrics: 940 (± 202)	–	6 minor and 4 sig. complications related to PEG site. All rapidly resolved with treatment	–
Kotler et al. (1991)	Reabilan HN (peptide and MCT, Roussel)	1.32 kcal ml^{-1}	500 kcal day^{-1} above estimated requirements for 1 month, then increased by 150 kcal daily to tolerance	~2640	~116	'Well tolerated' but mild discomfort from tube in n 3 and mild–moderate diarrhoea in n 3 (easily controlled).	–
Ockenga et al. (1994)	–	–	–	–	–	Minor complications in 27% ETF and 14% of CON (non-HIV). 2 severe complications, no mortality	–
Süttmann et al. (1993)	Fresubin plus (15% P, 30% F, 55% CHO, MCT, Fresenius)	–	Increased in increments of 250–500 kcal to meet estimated requirements	~41.7 kcal kg^{-1} wt	–	Placement well tolerated. Initial inflammation at PEG site (n 7) quickly resolved, nausea and diarrhoea in n 5 controlled	Continuously over 12–16 h

CHO, carbohydrate; F, fat; MCT, medium-chain triglyceride; P, protein; sig., significant.

Table A6.20. Trial characteristics: trials of enteral tube feeding in patients with HIV/AIDS in the community (non-randomized data).

Trial	Design	Diagnosis	No. ETF	No. CON	Initial BMI ETF group	Initial BMI CON group	Duration of ETF	Tube type	Control group
Brantsma et al. (1991) Australia	C	Advanced HIV (AIDS and ARC, group IV)	14	–	–	–	8–299 days (mean 51.5 days)	PEG	–
Cappell and Godil (1993) USA Hospital to home	B	HIV, n 13 with AIDS (includes paediatrics, n 4) (prior to PEG, NG n 7, PN n 2, oral n 5)	14	21[a]	90% of adults and 100% of paediatrics 'undernourished' (< 5th wt-for-ht in adults and < 5th wt-for-age in paediatrics)	–	Follow up at 111 days (8–450 days)	PEG	Sex- and age-matched groups with PEG, no HIV, follow up for 65 days (3–222 days)
Kotler et al. (1991) USA Hospital to home	C	AIDS and profound anorexia	8	–	81% IBW	–	Up to 60 days	PEG	–
Ockenga et al. (1994) A Germany	B	HIV	37	27[a]	– (PEG placed for wt loss > 10% over 6 months in n 24)	–	Follow up for 194 days (6–781 days)	PEG	PEG (non-HIV–cancer/neurological)
Süttmann et al. (1993) Germany Hospital to home	C	Advanced HIV (AIDS and ARC, group IV)	14	–	17.3 (2.4)	–	75 days (6–228 days)	PEG	–

[a]Control group also receiving ETF via PEG (non-HIV patients).
A, abstract; ARC, AIDS-related complex; CON, control; PN, parenteral nutrition.

Table A6.21. Main findings of enteral tube feeding trials in patients with HIV/AIDS in the community (non-randomized data).

Trial	Energy/nutrient intake	Wt change ETF	Wt change CON	Function	Outcome	Finance
Brantsma et al. (1991)	–	+0.32 (−7.6 to +12.4 kg)[a]	–	'PEG appears to improve the quality and perhaps quantity of life for group IV HIV patients'	–	–
Cappell and Godil (1993)	–	+7.4% (NS)	–	–	30 days post-procedure mortality 0% in ETF and 14% in CON. 60 day mortality 14% in ETF and 19% in CON. No ETF deaths related to PEG	–
Kotler et al. (1991)	–	+3 kg (~6% above initial values) Sig. increase in TBK, index of body cell mass (+14%) and body fat	–	Total no. lymphocytes and CD8+ cells rose. No change in CD4+ cells or in immunoglobulin levels Improved clinical condition and mental function (observation)	All but one were discharged from hospital, with n 5 continuing ETF for 4–32 weeks and n 3 resuming normal intake. Survival probability at 6 months 0.5 and n 3 alive after 14 months	–
Ockenga et al. (1994)	–	–	–	–	No difference in mean survival time in ETF/HIV vs. CON (236 days vs. 278 days, NS) or in mortality (4 (11%) vs. 3 (11%))	–
Süttmann et al. (1993)	Patients consumed small or medium-sized amounts of regular food or restored eating in addition to ETF (no data)	+3.2 (2.7) kg (sig.). Sig. increase in body cell mass (BIA) and body fat Improvements independent of initial nutritional status	–	*(Sig. improvement in albumin and total iron-binding capacity)*	n 2 resumed oral diet alone, n 8 continued on total or supplementary ETF, n 4 died (not feeding-related)	–

[a]Extremes of weight change, often in short periods of time, likely to be due to fluid shifts.
BIA, bioelectrical impedance analysis; CON, control; NS, not significant; sig., significant; TBK, total body potassium.

(I) What effect does ETF have on the voluntary food intake and total energy intake of patients in the community with HIV/AIDS?

Only one trial briefly discussed the changes in energy intake with ETF (Süttmann et al., 1993), suggesting that patients continued to maintain an oral diet or increased their food intake during ETF (Table A6.21). None of the studies provided any quantitative information about total energy intake or voluntary food intake with ETF and so further controlled studies are needed if this issue is to be addressed.

(II) What effect does ETF have on the body weight and composition of patients in the community with HIV/AIDS?

ETF in undernourished patients with HIV and AIDS may lead to increases in body weight, including improvements in body cell mass and body fat content (see Table A6.21). All the trials that assessed body composition changes (n 4) showed weight gain with ETF (Brantsma et al., 1991; Kotler et al., 1991; Cappell and Godil, 1993; Süttmann et al., 1993). This was evaluated as statistically significant in one trial (Süttmann et al., 1993). In some patients, large changes in weight in relatively short periods of time were likely to be a reflection of fluid shifts (Brantsma et al., 1991) and measurements of body composition would have been a useful indicator of the compositional changes. In two trials, significant increases in body cell mass and body fat following home ETF were observed (Kotler et al., 1991; Süttmann et al., 1993) (see Table A6.21). However, as there were no RCT, it is difficult to distinguish the effect of ETF from the use of HAART or changes in disease condition that may also have led to changes in body weight and composition in these patients.

(III) What effect does ETF have on the body function of patients in the community with HIV/AIDS?

ETF in patients with HIV/AIDS may lead to functional benefits (see Table A6.21).

One small trial (n 14) claimed that ETF improved the quality of life of patients, although no subjective or objective assessments of this parameter were reported (Brantsma et al., 1991). Other small trials suggested that ETF led to immunological and biochemical benefits (Kotler et al., 1991; Süttmann et al., 1993) (see Table A6.21). Further well-designed (large samples, randomization, double-blinding) trials are needed in this patient group if the functional benefits that follow ETF are to be elucidated. For information on designing clinical trials, refer to Chapter 10.

(IV) What effect does ETF have on the clinical and financial outcome of patients in the community with HIV/AIDS?

There is a lack of controlled data comparing the effects of home ETF with no nutritional support on the clinical outcome of patients with HIV/AIDS. In addition, prospective evaluations of the cost-effectiveness of this mode of nutritional treatment in HIV/AIDS patients are lacking. Some of the studies reviewed made comparisons of clinical outcome with other disease groups. For example, Cappell and Godil (1993) indicated that mortality was lower in HIV patients fed by ETF than in non-HIV control patients also PEG-fed, whereas Ockenga et al. (1994) suggested that mean survival times and mortality rates were no different. Overall, however, RCT are needed that are large enough to have sufficient power to detect changes in outcome measures following ETF and that incorporate financial evaluation.

Malignancy (Randomized and Non-randomized Data)

Malnutrition is common in those with cancer (see Chapter 2) and, consequently, there is often a need for effective nutritional support. However, very few studies of ETF have been undertaken in this patient group in the community, with only one RCT (Hearne et al., 1985) and three NRT (Shike et al., 1989;

Fietkau *et al.*, 1991; Roberge *et al.*, 2000) being included in this review. All of these studies had been undertaken in patients with head and neck cancer, mostly during or after radiotherapy (Hearne *et al.*, 1985; Shike *et al.*, 1989; Fietkau *et al.*, 1991) (see Tables A6.22–A6.24). In this patient group, it appears that PEG feeding (Fietkau *et al.*, 1991) is better tolerated than NG feeding, particularly during irradiation of the head and neck region (Hearne *et al.*, 1985). Patients can also feel uncomfortable with an NG tube in the home environment and long to have it removed (Roberge *et al.*, 2000).

The findings of the reviewed studies are summarized in Box A6.4 and Tables A6.22–A6.24 and a number of issues concerning the efficacy of ETF are discussed below. Due to the small number of poorly designed trials and the lack of relevant assessments and statistical analysis, it is difficult to come to firm conclusions about the impact of ETF in cancer patients. The efficacy of this treatment has been assessed using the four main review questions.

(I) What effect does ETF have on the voluntary food intake and total energy intake of patients in the community with malignancy?

ETF may be an effective way of maintaining or improving the nutritional intake of patients with cancer, including those undergoing cancer treatments (e.g. radiotherapy). The one RCT reviewed showed that ETF maximized both energy and protein intakes to a greater extent than dietary counselling and the use of ONS (Hearne *et al.*, 1985) (Table A6.24). Further investigation is needed into the impact of ETF on voluntary food intake and total nutrient intake in patients with various types of cancer.

(II) What effect does ETF have on the body weight and composition of patients in the community with malignancy?

It appears that ETF can ameliorate the changes in nutritional status typically seen in patients undergoing radiotherapy,

either alone or in combination with other treatments. Indeed, a survey summarized in Table A6.25 highlighted that the body weight of PEG-fed patients with head and neck cancer stabilized or increased, in contrast with patients not given ETF in whom weight was lost (Fietkau *et al.*, 1991). Similarly, in the prospective studies reviewed, patients fed by ETF maintained or improved their nutritional status, either over time (Shike *et al.*, 1989) or compared with an orally fed control group (randomized (Hearne *et al.*, 1985); non-randomized (Fietkau *et al.*, 1991), Table A6.24). However, ETF may be less successful when used in patients with some types of cancers. For example, in patients with nasopharyngeal cancer, a similar degree of weight loss was seen in those enterally fed by NG tube to those orally fed, possibly due to the difficulties of having a tube in the head and neck region (Hearne *et al.*, 1985). PEG feeding may have been more effective. RCT are needed if conclusions about the impact of ETF on body weight or its effect on body composition are to be drawn.

(III) What effect does ETF have on the body function of patients in the community with malignancy?

Functional benefits may follow the use of ETF in patients with head and neck cancer in the community. Two NRT made some assessments of function following ETF (see Table A6.24). In one trial, although a group of PEG-fed patients had lower quality-of-life scores (Padilla's index) than orally fed patients at the start of treatment (radiotherapy), these scores remained stable during treatment (Fietkau *et al.*, 1991). In contrast, marked decline in the quality of life occurred in the orally fed group after radiotherapy (Fietkau *et al.*, 1991). In the other study, global health status and quality of life improved to a non-significant degree during home ETF (Roberge *et al.*, 2000). This trial also examined aspects of psychosocial function, which are often overlooked in patients receiving artificial feeding. Roberge *et al.*

Table A6.22. Enteral tube feeds used in trials of patients with malignancy in the community (randomized and non-randomized data).

Trial	ETF	ETF energy density	ETF prescribed	ETF energy (kcal) provision	ETF protein (g) provision	Toleration	Timing of ETF
Randomized controlled trials							
Hearne *et al.* (1985)	Commercial, isotonic formula	–	40 kcal and 1 g P kg⁻¹ wt in total	35–42 kcal kg⁻¹ wt (ETF only?)	1.2–1.6 g kg⁻¹ wt	Presence of tube in irradiated head and neck region might have increased radiation-induced toxic response	Most fed by intermittent gravity feeding (79%)
Non-randomized trials							
Fietkau *et al.* (1991)	–	–	–	–	–	No side-effects from ETF. Transient pain and local infection in small no. of patients undergoing PEG in the centre as a whole	PEG 2 weeks after radiotherapy started
Roberge *et al.* (2000)	Enterogil 500 Na 80	1 kcal ml⁻¹	–	2100	–	Digestive complaints were moderate: nausea (18%), reflux (33%), flatulence (43%). Psychological tolerance: 69% longed to have tube removed, 45% worried about accidental tube removal, 33% uncomfortable with body image	4 boluses during the day, each taking ~45 min (providing ~500 kcal)
Shike *et al.* (1989)	Commercial, nutritionally complete (predigested feeds for PEJ)	–	–	1748 ± 529	–	Unsuccessful placement (*n* 3), localized skin infection (*n* 3) initially. Aspiration pneumonia (*n* 1)	3–5 boluses (PEG), 8–10 h continuous infusion overnight (PEJ)

P, protein; PEG, percutaneous endoscopic gastrostomy; PEJ, percutaneous endoscopic jejunostomy.

Table A6.23. Trial characteristics: trials of enteral tube feeding in patients with malignancy in the community (randomized and non-randomized data).

Trial	Design	Diagnosis	No. ETF	No. CON	Initial BMI ETF group	Initial BMI CON group	Duration of ETF	Tube type	Control group
Randomized controlled trials									
Hearne *et al.* (1985)[a] USA	10001[b]	Advanced (stage III/IV) head and neck cancer undergoing Rtx	18	13[b]	80% usual wt	85% usual wt	During 8 weeks of Rtx	Nasoenteric, fine-bore silicone rubber or polyurethane	Oral diet (dietary counselling and oral nutritional supplements also given if needed)
Non-randomized data									
Fietkau *et al.* (1991)[c] Germany	C	Rtx for head and neck cancer	47[d]	134[e]	'Poor nutritional status'	Less undernourished than ETF	During 6 weeks of Rtx and for 18 weeks after	PEG	Oral diet (some may have received ETF as a supplement)
Roberge *et al.* (2000) France	C	Head and neck cancer	39	–	–	–	Monitored 1 and 4 weeks after discharge from H with ETF	Nasogastric (80%) and gastrostomy (20%)	–
Shike *et al.* (1989) USA	C	Head and neck cancer severe dysphagia caused by tumour, surgery, Rtx or Ctx	39	–	–	–	Follow up for 4.5 ± 6 months	PEG (*n* 36), PEJ (*n* 3)	–

[a]Similar publication by Daly *et al.* (1984) not reviewed.
[b]Comparison of ETF with oral nutritional support as CON group received dietary counselling and oral nutritional supplements.
[c]Findings from a smaller sample of the same patient group published earlier not reviewed (Fietkau, 1989).
[d]ETF group contained more stage IV patients (78% vs. 46%), more patients with dysphagia (56% vs. 23%) and received a greater radiation field size (sig.) than the CON group.
Final analysis on 14 ETF and 12 CON and not 'intention to treat' (*n* 4 crossing-over groups).
[e]Includes all patients taking food orally, with or without ETF.
Ctx, chemotherapy; CON, control; H, hospital; PEJ, percutaneous endoscopic jejunostomy; Rtx, radiotherapy.

Table A6.24. Main findings of enteral tube feeding trials in patients with malignancy in the community (randomized and non-randomized data).

Trial	Energy/nutrient intake	Wt change ETF	Wt change CON	Function	Outcome	Finance
Randomized controlled trials						
Hearne et al. (1985)[a]	ETF maintained higher TEI (35–42 kcal kg⁻¹) and TPI (1.2–1.6 g kg⁻¹) than CON (25–34 kcal kg⁻¹; 0.3–1.3 g P) consistently. No data on oral intake	Nasopharynx: –3.8%; All others: +0.2% (ETF vs. CON sig.)	–3.3%; –7.3%	–	No difference in duration of maximum radiation toxicity between ETF and CON, but earlier and higher incidence in ETF[b]	–
Non-randomized trials						
Fietkau et al. (1991)	–	+2 kg and increase in TSF (? sig.) No changes in MAMC in either ETF or CON	–3 kg during Rtx (wt remained constant after Rtx stopped)	Quality of life scores in ETF during Rtx steady but decreased sharply in CON. ETF improvement in biochemical parameters (prealbumin, RBP) not seen in CON	–	–
Roberge et al. (2000)	33% combined ETF with oral intake. No data on intakes	–	–	Global health status/quality-of-life scale score improved slightly with ETF. Scales that sig. improved were: constipation, coughing, social functioning, body image/sexuality. A number of patients experienced problems with psychosocial distress	–	–
Shike et al. (1989)	–	No residual tumour (n 7) and continue on ETF: +3.9 ± 1.3 kg. Receiving ETF during therapy for cancer and beyond (n 19): +4.0 ± 3.1 kg. No data for those with advanced disease (n 13)	–	–	–	–

[a]A very similar report by the same authors (Daly et al., 1984) indicated no difference in the survival curves for tube- vs. oral-fed patients (due to the similarity of these articles, Daly et al. (1984) has not been reviewed).

[b]Reason for earlier and higher incidence: ETF group contained more stage IV patients (78% vs. 46%), more patients with dysphagia (56% vs. 23%) and received a greater radiation field size (sig.) than the CON group. Final analysis on 14 ETF and 12 CON and not 'intention to treat' (n 4 crossing-over groups).

CON, control; MAMC, mid-arm muscle circumference; P, protein; Rtx, radiotherapy; RBP, retinol binding protein; sig., significant; TEI, total energy intake; TPI, total protein intake.

Table A6.25. Effect of ETF on body weight in patients with head and neck cancers after treatments, compared with controls (from Fietkau *et al.*, 1991).[a]

Cancer staging/therapy	Number of patients	PEG feeding: change in body weight	Without PEG feeding: change in body weight
Stage III	53	+1.5 kg	−2 kg
Stage IV	98	+0.5 kg	−3 kg
Sequential radiotherapy and chemotherapy	25	+0.5 kg	−3.5 kg
Additional interstitial radiotherapy	43	±0 kg	−3.5 kg
Surgery and radiotherapy	80	+1.5 kg	−1.5 kg

[a]Results not statistically analysed, non-random groups. RCT are needed if firm conclusions about the impact of ETF on body weight or its effect on bodily composition are to be made.

(2000) identified that tube-fed patients may have psychological difficulty with the presence of a feeding tube, particularly naso-enteric tubes (Roberge *et al.*, 2000). Socially, a small proportion of patients cited ETF as a reason for not visiting family or close relations and not going out in public (Roberge *et al.*, 2000), although overall there was still an increase in social functioning scores with ETF. Ultimately, randomized, controlled trials in head, neck and other cancer patients are needed that make assessments of functional measures, both physical and psychological, with ETF.

(IV) What effect does ETF have on the clinical and financial outcome of patients in the community with malignancy?

Only one trial assessed the clinical outcome of patients receiving ETF compared with oral feeding (Hearne *et al.*, 1985) (Table A6.24). No differences in the duration of maximum radiation toxicity were found between groups. In addition, none of the trials reviewed included any financial information relating to ETF. Therefore, RCT, where ethically feasible, are needed to assess the clinical and cost-effectiveness of ETF in patients with head and neck cancer and other types of cancer in the community setting.

Although this section has reviewed studies undertaken specifically in patients with cancer, other trials in mixed groups of patients may have included individuals with cancer (e.g. elderly and general medical; see sections in this appendix).

In some instances ETF may not always be appropriate in the terminally ill cancer patient and issues about withholding or withdrawing artificial nutritional support need to be considered (Lennard-Jones, 1998).

Box A6.4. Key findings: effect of ETF in community patients with malignant disease.

Nutritional intake: ETF may enable nutritional intake to be sustained or improved to a greater extent than dietary counselling or oral nutritional supplements in some groups of cancer patients.

Body weight: improvements in body weight or maintenance of nutritional status can be achieved with ETF. The route of feeding may be an important determinant of the effectiveness of the treatment (e.g. PEG feeding may be more effective than an NG tube in patients treated for head and neck cancer).

Body function: ETF may improve social functioning and quality of life compared with routine care.

Clinical outcome: the impact of ETF on patients' outcome has not been fully assessed and RCT are required where appropriate.

Ethics: ETF may not be appropriate in the end stages of cancer.

Neurology (Non-randomized Data)

No prospective trials in adult patients with neurological conditions such as CVA, Parkinson's and dementia were reviewed and yet ETF is widely used in such patient groups, as indicated by large national surveys from the USA (Howard *et al.*, 1995) and Britain (Elia *et al.*, 2000a, 2001b). Only one prospective trial was reviewed in patients in a persistent vegetative state (PVS) (see Tables A6.26–A6.28 and the discussion below). RCT are difficult to perform ethically in these patient groups, as ETF is often the only means of providing nutrition and fluid, especially when oral intake is contraindicated. Therefore, the use of home ETF in general in patients with some neurological diagnoses is discussed below

CVA

Although there are no prospective controlled studies in patients with CVA, surveys suggest that it is one of the commonest diagnoses in patients receiving home ETF, in both Britain and the USA. Indeed, in the UK, between 1996 and 1999, it was estimated that about 1.7% of all patients suffering from a CVA received home ETF (Elia *et al.*, 2001a). BANS found that, after 1 year of home ETF, 13% of CVA patients returned to oral feeding and ~30% died. The activity levels of these patients were limited (with > 70% being bedridden or housebound) and only ~20% were independent. However, overall, the time patients spent in hospital after discharge home with ETF was minimal (< 1%) which is likely to relieve pressure on the expensive hospital environment (Elia *et al.*, 2001a). Therefore, ETF of CVA patients in the community is likely to result in huge cost savings to the health-care system. The benefits to quality of life are currently being assessed by BANS.

Without ETF, many of these patients would be expected to die or suffer from the effects of malnutrition. In such cases, RCT cannot be undertaken. Also, in severely disabled patients with CVA who are unconscious or lead a very poor quality of life, the decision to withhold or withdraw ETF is an important ethical issue.

Dementia

There is a lack of consensus about the criteria for and the ethics of nutritional support for the patient with dementia. Some reviews suggest that ETF should not be used routinely in patients with advanced dementia (Finucane *et al.*, 1999; Anon., 2001b). However, a recent case report has highlighted the successful use of ETF in a dysphagic, demented patient with Alzheimer's disease (Barratt, 2000). This report also highlighted some of the ethical issues regarding the use of artificial feeding and challenged the traditional view of withholding such treatment in patients with dementia (Barratt, 2000). Overall, it is recommended that the appropriateness of ETF is considered for each individual patient, after careful consideration of the benefits and risk of this therapy in the short and long term (Anon., 2001b; McNamara and Kennedy, 2001). In particular, careful consideration must be given before ETF is started, as this method of treatment may be difficult to subsequently withdraw. Furthermore, there is a need for well-designed trials, where appropriate, to assess the efficacy of ETF in this patient group so that evidence-based guidelines can be developed.

PVS

One trial reviewed in patients with PVS demonstrated the safety and efficacy of home ETF as a sole source of nutrition at maintaining adequate energy intakes and nutritional status in this patient group (Wicks *et al.*, 1992) (Tables A6.26–A6.28). Without ETF or other non-oral forms of nutritional support, these patients would die from dehydration and starvation. However, in many patients with PVS, there are ethical issues about whether to withhold or withdraw ETF.

Table A6.26. Enteral tube feeds used in trials of neurology patients in the community (non-randomized data).

Trial	ETF	ETF energy density	ETF prescribed	ETF energy (kcal) provision	ETF protein (g) provision	Toleration	Timing of ETF
Wicks *et al.* (1992)	–	–	1880 kcal	1880	–	Peritonitis (*n* 1), tube site infection (*n* 2), tube displacement (*n* 2)	Overnight

Table A6.27. Trial characteristics: trials of enteral tube feeding in neurology patients in the community (non-randomized data).

Trial	Design	Diagnosis	No. ETF	No. CON	Initial BMI ETF group	Initial BMI CON group	Duration of ETF	Tube type	Control group
Wicks *et al.* (1992) UK	C	PVS	30	–	–	–	12 months	PEG	–

CON, control.

Table A6.28. Main findings of enteral tube feeding trials in neurology patients in the community (non-randomized data).

Trial	Energy/nutrient intake	Wt change ETF	Wt change CON	Function	Outcome	Finance
Wicks *et al.* (1992)	Assume 1880 kcal (without ETF patients with PVS would have nil intake)	Mean BMI increased from 19.05 to 21.23 in 1 year	–	–	–	–

CON, control.

Although this section has discussed the issues relating to ETF in patients with some neurological diseases, other trials in mixed groups of patients may have included individuals with such conditions (e.g. elderly and general medical sections in this appendix). However, there is still a need for specific consideration of the use of ETF in patients with different neurological diseases, including clinical and ethical issues, in both adults and children.

Paediatrics (Non-randomized Data)

National and local surveys have documented the widespread and increasing use of ETF in children with a variety of diseases in the community (Elia, 1996b, 1997b; McCarey *et al.*, 1996; Elia *et al.*, 1998, 2000a). In particular, small local surveys have suggested that ETF is safe and can be used effectively in children at home (Holden *et al.*, 1991). Specifically, parental and family views about home ETF have been very positive (Holden *et al.*, 1991; McCarey *et al.*, 1996) and children have been described as becoming 'more happy and active' after starting home nutritional support (Holden *et al.*, 1991). As this quote expresses, not only is ETF clinically effective, but it may also be cost-effective:

> Home enteral feeding represents an effective way of improving the nutritional status of children with chronic disease at home. It frees hospital beds and nursing resources, is well accepted by children and their families and is growing rapidly as an alternative to hospitalisation.
>
> (McCarey *et al.*, 1996)

The studies reviewed, in infants and children with a variety of different diagnoses, suggest that home ETF, using primarily NG or gastrostomy tubes, is easily and efficiently used. Due to the ethical difficulties associated with undertaking RCT in children, the evidence consists mostly of small, poorly designed NRT, and these are discussed briefly below according to diagnosis and summarized in Box A6.5 and Tables A6.29–A6.37.

Cerebral palsy

Children with cerebral palsy are increasingly being fed by tube at home, continuing with ETF into adolescence. It can be effective at increasing body weight and may influence outcome. A small RCT in ten children with cerebral palsy showed significantly greater weight gain (+6 kg) in those given ETF (1 kcal ml^{-1} formula, 82–150 kcal kg^{-1} day^{-1}) than those given a high-energy diet orally (−0.6 kg) (Patrick *et al.*, 1986; Tables A6.32–A6.34). When control patients were subsequently given ETF, weight gain significantly increased (+2.1 kg). It is unclear how long ETF was given for and no assessments of outcome were made in this study. On a more subjective note, a 6-year, retrospective review of cerebral palsy patients in America indicated that 94% of parents/carers believed that gastrostomy feeding was beneficial in the management of their child (McGrath *et al.*, 1992). Although the majority of children (70%) were totally dependent on carers, the authors commented that survival was unexpectedly high for this patient group (84% at 1 year, 68% at 4 years). Similarly, BANS showed that, at 1 year, 90% of cerebral palsy patients continued on home ETF, with a mortality of 6% (Elia *et al.*, 2001b).

Cystic fibrosis

ETF can be a very effective means of improving nutrient intakes and stimulating growth in growth-retarded children with CF (see earlier section on CF).

Gastrointestinal/liver disease

ETF may be an effective treatment for growth-retarded children with GI disease:

> We conclude that home nocturnal nasogastric feedings can achieve dramatic improvement in weight gain and linear growth in motivated adolescents with Crohn's disease and growth retardation.
>
> (Aiges *et al.*, 1989)

Five, small non-randomized trials of long-term home ETF (3 months to 2 years) in children with GI disorders (Crohn's disease (Belli *et al.*, 1988; Aiges *et al.*, 1989; Cosgrove and Jenkins, 1997); liver transplant (Chin *et al.*, 1990; Duche *et al.*, 1999)) and growth retardation were reviewed. ETF was well tolerated, with no serious complications, and, although three trials used NG feeding (Belli *et al.*, 1988; Aiges *et al.*, 1989; Chin *et al.*, 1990), PEG was the preferred method of feeding in one group of patients (Cosgrove and Jenkins, 1997).

The trials reviewed have been summarized in Tables A6.29–A6.31. The data provided suggested that ETF was an effective way of increasing total energy intakes when used as a supplement to food intake compared with baseline intakes (Belli *et al.*, 1988; Aiges *et al.*, 1989; Duche *et al.*, 1999). Furthermore, following 1–2 years of overnight ETF, increases in weight and height and growth were observed, either over time (Aiges *et al.*, 1989; Cosgrove and Jenkins, 1997; Duche *et al.*, 1999) or compared with a non-random control group managed conventionally without ETF (Belli *et al.*, 1988; Aiges *et al.*, 1989). In children undergoing liver transplant, 3 months of ETF (using a branched-chain amino acid (BCAA) formula) significantly increased z scores for weight – more so than a high-energy diet taken orally (Chin *et al.*, 1990).

Although few functional measures were assessed, significant improvements in clinical scores over time (Aiges *et al.*, 1989) or disease activity scores versus a control group (Belli *et al.*, 1988) (Crohn's disease activity index (CDAI)) were noted, although no differences in the number of relapses or in bone age were observed (Belli *et al.*, 1988). Reduced steroid use was also attributed to ETF in one trial in children with Crohn's disease (Cosgrove and Jenkins, 1997). However, steroid treatment in many of these trials (reported in three trials (Belli *et al.*, 1988; Aiges *et al.*, 1989; Cosgrove and Jenkins, 1997)) is also

likely to have affected appetite/food intake, weight and disease activity scores and so it is difficult to ascertain the true effects of ETF on these outcome measures. A retrospective analysis suggested that children with Crohn's disease who went into remission following bowel rest and ETF remained well for longer if they continued with nocturnal ETF after resuming a normal diet, compared with those who discontinued feeding (Wilschanski *et al.*, 1996).

The impact of ETF on clinical outcome in children with GI disease has not been assessed; although similar outcomes (mortality and hospital stay) were noted in an NRT in liver transplant patients, small sample sizes prevented meaningful statistical analysis (Chin *et al.*, 1990). Ideally, RCT comparing ETF with no nutritional support is required in paediatric patients with GI disorders. However, if patients suffer from or are at risk of growth retardation, failure to provide nutritional support would be unethical. In such cases, information provided by NRT has to be considered.

A number of studies have compared the efficacy of dietary treatment with steroid therapy of Crohn's disease in children, and a recent meta-analysis has summarized the findings (Heuschkel *et al.*, 2000) (see Appendix 5).

General/mixed diagnoses

The results of NRT suggest that ETF consistently improves growth in growth-retarded children and may have other benefits to the child. In a letter reporting the experience of home NG feeding in children aged between 2 months and 15 years with a variety of conditions (Navarro *et al.*, 1981), the authors stated that:

> The benefits of treatment [ETF] were improved nutritional status, functional digestive recovery, and rapid return to family life and even school attendances, with all the attendant psychological advantages. The economic advantage was also considerable in comparison to prolonged hospitalisation.
>
> (Navarro *et al.*, 1981)

Table A6.29. Enteral tube feeds used in trials of paediatric patients with GI and liver disorders in the community (non-randomized data).

Trial	ETF	ETF energy density	ETF prescribed	ETF energy (kcal) provision	ETF protein (g) provision	Toleration	Timing of ETF
Aiges et al. (1989)	Osmolite (Ross) or Isocal (Mead Johnson)	1 kcal ml^{-1}	85 kcal kg^{-1} body wt (ETF plus oral diet)	1000–1500 ml	–	n 2 mild dyspepsia, occasional nasal stuffiness with NG tube. No aspiration pneumonia	Nocturnal, stopped 30 min before waking to minimize effects on appetite
Belli et al. (1988)	Vivonex (Eaton)	–	70% of requirement by ETF and 30% orally	–	–	Very well tolerated, no renal, hepatic or metabolic complications. Compliance excellent	Nocturnal (for 15 h) given for 1 month periods three times in the year (during which no other diet permitted)
Chin et al. (1990)	ETF[1] Semi-elemental (Alfare (Nestlé)) ETF[2] BCAA-enriched (mix of Alfare (Nestlé), Heptamine (SHS), polyjoule and MCT oil)	1 kcal ml^{-1} 1 kcal ml^{-1}	To enable total intake to meet 120–150% of recommended daily intake	–	–	No adverse side-effects (diarrhoea or increased blood urea)	–
Cosgrove and Jenkins (1997)	Elemental O28 (SHS)	–	To meet 'clinical need' as a sole source of nutrition during relapse or as a supplement at other times	–	–	Happy with PEG vs. NG tube. Bloating (n 1), local sepsis and excess granulation tissue (n 4)	Nocturnal
Duche et al. (1999)	MCT-enriched formula: (16–18% Peptijunior (Mead Johnson), 18% Alfare (Nestlé) or 18% Pregestimil (Bristol-Myers), glucose polymer and MCT)	–	To meet 150–180 kcal kg^{-1} (including VFI) for children < 20 kg. Increase TEI by 30–40% on VFI for children > 20 kg	44–105 kcal kg^{-1} ETF	–	No serious complications. Mild wound infections in n 4 (easily treated)	Nocturnal (12 h)

BCAA, branched-chain amino acid; MCT, medium-chain triglyceride; TEI, total energy intake; VFI, voluntary food intake.

Table A6.30. Trial characteristics: trials of enteral tube feeding in paediatric patients with GI disorders in the community (non-randomized data).

Trial	Design	Diagnosis	No. ETF	No. CON	Age	Initial BMI ETF group	Initial BMI CON group	Duration of ETF	Tube type	Control group
Aiges *et al.* (1989) USA	B	Crohn's disease, growth-retarded[a]	8	6	14 years 5 months (13–17 years)	Growth-retarded: <3% ht-for-age Wt gain: +0.38 kg year^{-1}	Growth-retarded: <3% ht-for-age Wt gain: 1.2 kg year^{-1}	1 year (some stopped ETF temporarily during this time)	Nasogastric (8F silastic)	Matched for age and degree of growth retardation but refused ETF (includes 4 drop-outs from trial)
Belli *et al.* (1988) Canada	B	Crohn's disease, growth failure[a]	8[b]	4	9.8–14.2 years	<3rd percentile for ht, velocity of linear growth and of wt gain		1 year (followed a 1 year observation period)	Nasogastric silastic	Age- and disease-matched treated by conventional medical therapy
Chin *et al.* (1990)	B	Chronic liver disease, liver transplant	15	13	–	Underweight (z score < –1)	z score –0.55	90 days	Nasogastric	Given an MCT–milk formula orally ad lib plus high-energy diet
Cosgrove and Jenkins (1997) UK	C	Crohn's disease[a]	10[c]	–	14.4 years (median)(12.4–16.1 years)	Impaired growth (sd score for ht –1.4)	–	2 years (*n* 7) (*n* 3 continue on PEG feeding)	PEG	–
Duche *et al.* (1999) France	C	Severe cholestasis, pre-liver transplant	5	–	20 months–13 years	z score for wt –2.6 z score for ht –2.7	–	11–24 months prior to liver transplantation	PEG	–

[a]Some or all patients on steroid therapy.
[b]At the end of the month ETF period, a low residue diet was introduced for 15 days before a normal diet was allowed.
[c]Had previously been unsuccessful taking the formulas orally (*n* 10) or via an NG tube (*n* 2).
CON, control; MCT, medium-chain triglyceride; sd, standard deviation.

Table A6.31. Main findings of enteral tube feeding trials in paediatric patients with GI and liver disorders in the community (non-randomized data).

Trial	Energy/nutrient intake	Wt change/growth ETF	Wt change CON	Function	Clinical outcome	Finance
Aiges et al. (1989)	Pre-ETF oral intake 55–80% of their estimated energy requirement ETF provided an additional 1000–1500 kcal but no data were given of VFI	+11.75 kg (6.9–14.4 kg) (sig. vs. pre-ETF) Pre-ETF +0.38 kg (−2.8 kg to +3.2 kg) Height: +7 cm (sig.) All had increased ht velocity (n 6 achieved or exceeded the expected ht velocity)	+0.83 kg (−2.3 kg to +4.4 kg) Height: +1.5 cm (NS) (ETF vs. CON sig.)	Sig. improvement in clinical score due to a sig. increase in the nutritional component (other components remained unchanged)	–	–
Belli et al. (1988)	ETF sig. increased TEI by 25% from 106% (pre- and post-ETF) to 133% (with ETF)	+6.9 kg (± 1.5 kg) (210% of ideal predicted) (ETF vs. CON sig. and sig. vs. pre-ETF year, +2.7 kg) Height: +7 cm (± 0.8 cm) (126% of ideal predicted) (ETF vs. CON sig. and sig. vs. pre-ETF year, +2.7 cm) Sig. increase in TSF and MAMC (vs. pre-ETF)	−0.9 kg Height: −0.9 cm	Sig. lower CDAI scores for ETF vs. CON and compared with pre-ETF year (drop in CDAI immediately after first 1 month course of ETF) No difference in the no. of clinical relapses NS differences in bone age	(Similar intake of prednisone between ETF and CON)	–
Chin et al. (1990)	–	ETF[1] NS change in z score (−1.77 to −1.93) ETF[2] Sig. improvement in z score (−2.77 to 2.17) (ETF[2] vs. CON sig.)	Sig. improvement in z score (−0.55 to −1.1)	– (Use of NG tube did not alter rate of variceal bleeding and no change in encephalopathy with BCAA ETF)	Duration of post-transplant H stay no different between groups (no analysis as sample size too small)	–
Cosgrove and Jenkins (1997)	–	Assessments of weight not made (due to confounding effects of steroids) Median SD score for ht sig. improved from −1.4 (pre-ETF) to −1.1 (post-ETF)	–	–	Sig. reduction in prednisolone dose in all, with n 6 no longer requiring it	–
Duche et al. (1999)	TEI was increased with ETF to 100–180 kcal kg^{-1} (n 5, no statistics)	+350 g month^{-1} +0.53 cm month^{-1} (n 4, in n 1 ETF discontinued and liver transplant not carried out)	–	–	3 months after liver transplantation, n 4 alive and in good condition	–

CON, control; VFI, voluntary food intake; sig., significant; NS, not significant; TEI, total energy intake; MAMC, mid-arm muscle circumference; H, hospital; SD, standard deviation.

Other retrospective analyses have also highlighted the use of home ETF as a safe way of improving the growth of growth-retarded children with disease (Marin *et al.*, 1994; Kang *et al.*, 1998), although those with multisystem organ failure may benefit less (Marin *et al.*, 1994). In this analysis, two prospective NRT were reviewed (Greene *et al.*, 1981; Papadopoulou *et al.*, 1995) (report of a smaller subgroup not reviewed (Greene *et al.*, 1980)) and have been summarized in Tables A6.32–A6.34. These two trials of overnight long-term home ETF in groups of children with various disorders suggested that improvements in weight, weight-for-height, height-for-age, weight-for-age and arm anthropometry occurred over time (Greene *et al.*, 1981; Papadopoulou *et al.*, 1995). In particular, in stunted children (*n* 17), significant increases in weight-for-height *z* scores occurred following ETF and a significant correlation between the duration of ETF and the improvement in height-for-age *z* scores was noted (Papadopoulou *et al.*, 1995). In wasted children, significant increases in weight for age, MAC and TSF occurred with ETF (Papadopoulou *et al.*, 1995) and, in those who were adequately nourished but unlikely to maintain a satisfactory oral intake, weight-for-height, MAC and TSF were successfully maintained with home ETF (Papadopoulou *et al.*, 1995). Subjective improvements in function, noted by Greene *et al.* (1981), included a reduced requirement for haemodialysis in children with renal impairment and reductions in Crohn's disease activity. None of the trials reviewed assessed the changes in clinical outcome with ETF or its cost efficacy. The lack of control groups in the trials reviewed prevented firm conclusions from being made about the efficacy of ETF at improving growth, function and outcome in community-based children. Although larger, well-designed trials to assess these issues in children would be an advantage, these may not be possible ethically.

HIV/AIDS

ETF may be a useful adjunct to the treatment of children with HIV/AIDS, improving growth and potentially influencing outcome. Only one prospective NRT in children with HIV was reviewed (Henderson *et al.*, 1994), although children were included in the study by Cappell and Godil (1993) (see earlier section on HIV/AIDS). ETF via PEG or NG tube for an average of 8.5 months in growth-retarded children with HIV and AIDS led to significant improvements in weight-for-age, weight-for-height and arm fat area (see Tables A6.35–A6.37) (Henderson *et al.*, 1994). Improvements in height-for-age and mid-arm muscle area were also observed but were not statistically significant. In most of these children (11/18), ETF was used as a supplement to food intake (no data on energy intakes were provided) (Henderson *et al.*, 1994). Similarly, in a retrospective analysis, ETF in HIV-infected children was shown to improve weight and weight-for-height *z* scores, with progressive increases in energy intakes also being documented (Miller *et al.*, 1995). From this analysis, although gastrostomy feeding did not alter hospital stays, children who had the greatest increase in weight and fat mass had the greatest decrease in hospital stays after the gastrostomy was placed (Miller *et al.*, 1995). In addition, children with higher CD4 counts (age-adjusted) and lower weight-for-height *z* scores were more likely to respond positively to gastrostomy feeding and those responding favourably had a significant, 2.8-fold reduction in the risk of dying for every unit increase in weight *z* score (Miller *et al.*, 1995).

Malignancy

ETF may improve body weight and growth in growth-retarded children with cancer. Three NRT (two by the same author) indicated the benefits of using home ETF in children with cancer (Aquino *et al.*, 1995), including those receiving chemotherapy or radiotherapy (den Broeder *et al.*, 1998, 2000) (Tables A6.35–A6.37). In all studies, ETF for 10 weeks (den Broeder *et al.*, 2000) or up to 16 weeks (den Broeder *et al.*, 1998) or 10 months (Aquino *et al.*, 1995) led to significant improvements in body weight

Table A6.32. Enteral tube feeds used in trials of paediatric patients with various disorders in the community (non-randomized data).

Trial	ETF	ETF energy density	ETF prescribed	ETF energy (kcal) provision	ETF protein (g) provision	Toleration	Timing of ETF
Randomized controlled trials							
Patrick et al. (1986)	Isocal (Mead Johnson) or Ensure (Ross)	1 kcal ml⁻¹	–	82–150 kcal kg⁻¹	–	Use of NG tubes and high-energy intakes inhibited normal feeding, with some difficulties re-establishing normal feeding patterns	–
Non-randomized trials							
Balfe et al. (1990)	Similac PM 60/40 (Ross) + polycose, Promix and/or maize oil	–	–	–	–	Gastrostomy site infections (n 4), occasional vomiting and diarrhoea and problems with tubes falling out	–
Greene et al. (1981)[a]	Variety (Vivonex, Osmolite, Amin-Aid, Pregestimil)	–	–	–	–	No sig. metabolic disturbances, nausea, vomiting or diarrhoea. Poor appetite in first 2 weeks of ETF. Tube well tolerated by 2nd or 3rd day	Nocturnal
Papadopoulou et al. (1995)	–	–	–	–	–	Transient vomiting a relatively common problem (n 14). Distress at having tube (n 5), leakage with gastrostomy (2)	Nocturnal (n 28), continuously for 16–18 h (n 12), 24 h (n 4)

[a]Earlier report of a subgroup of these patients not reviewed (Greene et al., 1980).

sig., significant.

Table A6.33. Trial characteristics: trials of enteral tube feeding in paediatric patients with various disorders in the community (non-randomized data).

Trial	Design	Diagnosis	No. ETF	No. CON	Age	Initial BMI ETF group	Initial BMI CON group	Duration of ETF	Tube type	Control group
Randomized controlled trials										
Patrick *et al.* (1986)	10001	Cerebral palsy	5	5	2.8 to 15.8 years	32–79% of expected weight	–	–	Nasogastric	Standard treatment at start but given ETF after 5 weeks as benefits demonstrated in ETF groups
Non-randomized trials										
Balfe *et al.* (1990)	C	Chronic renal failure on peritoneal dialysis	20	–	3.9 (3.8) years	–	–	–	Gastrostomy (*n* 18) or NG (*n* 2)	–
Greene *et al.* (1981)	C	1: Chronic renal disease (3), short-bowel syndrome (2), cancer (6), IBD (2), congenital heart disease (1) 2: Inborn errors of metabolism (type I glycogen storage (9), homozygous type II hyperlipidaemia (2))	1: 14[a] 2: 11[a]	–	1: <1 year–18 years (*n* 3 >18 years) 2: 1 year–22 years	'Malnourished'	–	1: 1 to 8 months 2: 6 months to 5 years	Nasogastric	–
Papadopoulou *et al.* (1995)	C	Oncology (24), congenital heart disease (7), cystic fibrosis (4), gastroenterology (4), renal (2), neurology (2), other (1)	44 1: 17 2: 14 3: 13	–	48 months (median)	1: Stunted (−3.72 z score ht-for-age) 2: Wasted (−2.13 z score wt-for-age) 3: Adequately nourished but unlikely to maintain oral intake (0.34 z score wt-for-ht)	–	6 months (median, 1–44 months) 1: 15 months; 2: 4 months	Nasogastric (39), nasojejunal (1), gastrostomy (4)	–

[a]Predominantly paediatric patients (1: *n* 10; 2: unclear).
CON, control; IBD, inflammatory bowel disease.

Table A6.34. Main findings of enteral tube feeding trials in paediatric patients with various disorders in the community (non-randomized data).

Trial	Energy/nutrient intake	Wt change/growth ETF	Wt change CON	Function	Clinical outcome	Finance
Randomized controlled trials						
Patrick *et al.* (1986)	TEI 82 to 150 kcal kg^{-1}, with up to 10% of energy from VFI (no data for CON)	+6 kg (+33%, sig.) In CON pts given ETF after a delay, +2.1 kg (+13.4%, sig.) (ETF vs. CON, sig.)	−0.1 kg (−0.6%)	–	–	–
Non-randomized trials						
Balfe *et al.* (1990)	–	NS change in weight or height during ETF (z score for wt −2.38 (pre) vs. − 1.82 (post-ETF))	–	–	–	–
Greene *et al.* (1981)	Improvement in appetite after wt increase. No data on food intakes	1: 12/14 substantial wt gain; striking improvement in wt-for-ht index Of the paediatric pts (*n* 10), 8 increased wt (5–70%), 2 wt-stable 2: 'Growth stimulation' (no data)	–	*(1: Some pts had improved disease status (reduced requirement for haemodialysis, improved Crohn's disease)* *2: Reversal of metabolic anomalies)*	–	–
Papadopoulou *et al.* (1995)	–	1: NS increase in ht-for-age to −2.7 z score. In *n* 8 (stunted and wasted), sig. increase in wt-for-ht z scores. Sig. correlation between duration of ETF and improvement in ht-for-age 2: Sig. increase in wt-for-age z score to −0.93, MAC and TSF z score 3: NS increase in wt-for-ht, MAC or TSF	–	–	(In 35/44 children, the targets of the treating physician were achieved. In *n* 17 ETF continued)	–

CON, control; pt, patients; NS, not significant; sig., significant; TEI, total energy intake; VFI, voluntary food intake.

Table A6.35. Enteral tube feeds used in trials of paediatric patients with HIV or cancer in the community (non-randomized data).

Trial	ETF	ETF energy density	ETF prescribed	ETF energy (kcal) provision	ETF protein (g) provision	Toleration	Timing of ETF
HIV/AIDS							
Henderson et al. (1994)	Polymeric (n 6), lactose-free polymeric (n 2), protein hydrolysate (n 10)	–	50–100% of est. energy requirements (in addition to oral intake)	28–147 kcal kg^{-1} wt	1.6–4.1 g kg^{-1}	Stoma complications (n 3), gastrostomy leakage (n 2), intolerance (n 2), non-compliance (n 3)	Continuous (10–24 h, n 17) or bolus (n 1)
Cancer							
Aquino et al. (1995)	TwoCal HN, Pediasure, Ensure Plus (Ross)	1–2 kcal ml^{-1}	–	–	–	Well tolerated by all patients	8–16 h overnight
den Broeder et al. (1998)	–	–	–	106% of est. energy requirement	–	Diarrhoea in younger children (< 3 years) stopped after the first weeks of ETF. Vomiting associated with chemotherapy	Flexible and tailored to the pt routine
den Broeder et al. (2000)	Nutrison Pediatric Standard ETF[1] or Nutrison Pediatric Energy ETF[2] (Nutricia)	1 kcal ml^{-1} / 1.5 kcal ml^{-1}	To provide 100% or 150% of est. energy requirement (same volume of each feed given blinded)	ETF[1] 84% ETF[2] 112% of est. requirements	ETF[1] 1.27 g kg^{-1} ETF[2] 1.54 g kg^{-1}	Diarrhoea in younger children (< 3 years) stopped after the first weeks of ETF. Both formulas equally well tolerated	Nocturnal (10–12 h), started after dinner so appetite not reduced, plus a 2 h infusion during the day (after lunch)

est., estimated; pt, patients.

Table A6.36. Trial characteristics: trials of enteral tube feeding in paediatric patients with HIV or cancer in the community (non-randomized data).

Trial	Design	Diagnosis	No. ETF	No. CON	Age	Initial BMI ETF group	Initial BMI CON group	Duration of ETF	Tube type	Control group
HIV/AIDS										
Henderson et al. (1994) USA	C	HIV (AIDS n 11), growth failure, dysfunctional swallow (n 7), chronic diarrhoea (n 12)	18[a]	–	6 months (median) (3–159 months)	−2.13 z score for wt −1.07 z score wt-for-ht	–	8.5 months (median) (2 months– 2 years)	Nasogastric (n 4), gastrostomy (n 14, n 9 PEG)	–
Cancer										
Aquino et al. (1995) USA	C	Various cancers (newly diagnosed)	25	–	10.2 (2–21) years	Severely malnourished (>10% wt loss or <90% of 50th percentile for ht)	–	10.5 months (1–22 months)	Gastrostomy (18 surgical, 7 PEG)	–
den Broeder et al. (1998) Netherlands	B	Newly diagnosed with cancer (chemotherapy during the trial period)	7	14	6.6 years (2–12.3 years) CON 5.8 years (1.1–14.6 years)	91.7% of ideal wt	91.2% of ideal wt	Followed up over 16 weeks	Nasogastric	Retro – also received ETF (started by physician, no protocol followed)
den Broeder et al. (2000) Netherlands	C[b]	Cancer (chemotherapy or radiotherapy during the trial period)	27 12 ETF[1] 15 ETF[2]	–	5.7 ± 3.8 years ETF[1] 6.5 ± 4.5 years ETF[2]	ETF[1] −1.5 ETF[2] −1.5 z score wt-for-ht	–	10 weeks	Fine-bore silicone duodenal feeding tube into stomach	–

[a] n 11 received a trial of ONS prior to the start of ETF.
[b] Randomized trial comparing the efficacy of 2 ETF formulas.
CON, control; retro, retrospective.

Table A6.37. Main findings of enteral tube feeding trials in paediatric patients with HIV or cancer in the community (non-randomized data).

Trial	Energy/nutrient intake	Wt change/growth ETF	Wt change CON	Function	Clinical outcome	Finance
HIV/AIDS						
Henderson *et al.* (1994)	11/18 combined ETF with oral intake (no data on oral intake)	Sig. increase in wt-for-age from −2.13 to −1.46. Sig. increase in wt-for-ht from −1.07 to −0.13. Sig. increase in arm fat area. Increase in ht-for-age and MAMA NS	−	−	8 continued ETF, 3 died and 7 stopped (non-compliance, intolerance, leakage)	−
Cancer						
Aquino *et al.* (1995)	−	+12.9 (2.3)% of desirable body wt. No pt lost weight	−	−	−	ETF 9% of the cost of PN in an analysis of costs of ETF (n7) vs. PN (n7)
den Broeder *et al.* (1998)	−	+18.2 ± 8.4% (sig.) (ETF vs. CON sig.). % IBW 106% (ETF vs. CON sig.). All reached 'ideal' wt	+5.2 ± 7.3% (sig.). % IBW 75%	No difference in episodes of fever, although fewer episodes of fever without leucopenia in ETF (? sig.)	Same no. of Ctx courses in ETF and CON, but fewer delays in ETF. No dose reductions in ETF, 3 in CON	−
den Broeder *et al.* (2000)	Used as a supplement to food intake (data not reported)	Sig. increase in wt-for-ht z score from −1.5 to 0 (ETF[2]) and −1.5 to −0.6 (ETF[1]) (greater in ETF[2], sig. vs. ETF[1]). Wt-for-ht normalized in ETF[2]. Sig. increase in MAC, BSF and TSF in both groups (greater in ETF[2], sig. vs. ETF[1]). All parameters normalized in ETF[2]. Sig. increase in MAMA for 4 weeks in ETF[1] and for 10 weeks in ETF[2] (ETF[2] vs. ETF[1] sig.)	−	− (NS changes in serum proteins with ETF – albumin, prealbumin, transferrin, RBP)	−	−

BSF, biceps skin-fold; CON, control; Ctx, chemotherapy; MAMA, mid-arm muscle area; NS, not significant; PN, parenteral nutrition; RBP, retinol-binding protein; sig., significant.

(den Broeder *et al.*, 1998), compared with a retrospective control group not enterally fed (den Broeder *et al.*, 1998) or compared with baseline values pre-ETF (Aquino *et al.*, 1995; den Broeder *et al.*, 2000). In one of these trials, growth was also significantly improved longitudinally (den Broeder *et al.*, 2000). However, no functional or outcome benefits were reported. An analysis of costs for a subgroup of patients enterally fed (*n* 7) suggested that costs were 9% of those for a group of PN patients (*n* 7), although no information was provided about how well matched these groups were.

Renal disease

Improvements in weight and growth may follow the use of ETF in infants and children with renal failure. One small trial (see Tables A6.32–A6.34) in children with chronic renal failure, receiving peritoneal dialysis, showed no significant improvement in weight or height with ETF. However, the amount of feed taken and the duration of ETF were not documented (Balfe *et al.*, 1990). A number of short reports have indicated the efficacy of ETF in infants and children with chronic renal failure on peritoneal dialysis (O'Regan and Garel, 1990; Warady *et al.*, 1990, 1996). These suggested that ETF was typically used, in combination with oral intake, to increase nutrient intakes and allow normal or 'catch-up' weight gain appropriate for height and age in this patient group. Despite the efficacy of this treatment, infants fed by ETF early in life and/or for prolonged periods of time may develop eating difficulties. Therefore, strategies to overcome feeding dysfunction have been suggested and include encouragement of spontaneous oral intake during ETF, where possible (Strologo *et al.*, 1997).

Disability/mental retardation

No prospective trials were reviewed of ETF in paediatric patients with disability. However, retrospective analysis of the use of ETF in children with severe disabilities and mental retardation suggested that this mode of nutritional support might not always be clinically effective in some patient groups (Strauss *et al.*, 1997). Although difficult to undertake, prospective trials are needed to ascertain the best ways to maintain and improve the nutritional status of infants and children with mental retardation and growth failure.

Box A6.5. Key findings: effect of ETF in community paediatric patients.

Nutritional intake and growth: information, predominantly from NRT, suggests that ETF can be used safely to increase nutritional intake and to improve growth in infants and children with a variety of conditions (including cerebral palsy, cystic fibrosis, GI and liver diseases, HIV/AIDS, cancer, renal disease). Prolonged ETF in early life may lead to oral feeding dysfunction and strategies are needed to overcome this.

Body function and clinical outcome: the impact of ETF on functional and clinical outcomes requires examination, although it may be difficult to undertake RCT in children at high risk of malnutrition where nutritional intervention is withheld in the control arm.

Renal Disease (Non-randomized Data)

One small study of out-patients receiving haemodialysis (Sayce *et al.*, 2000) was reviewed (see Tables A6.38–A6.40). This, and a survey of patients on peritoneal dialysis (Ruddock, 2000), have suggested that PEG feeding can be safely and efficiently used in those with renal disease. Prospective follow-up of a group of haemodialysis patients in the UK showed that using ETF (presumably as a supplement to food intake) led to improvements in body weight and composition (see Table A6.40). Furthermore, hospital admissions for feeding-related complications were minimal (Sayce *et al.*, 2000).

A small, national UK survey of patients given continuous ambulatory peritoneal dialysis (CAPD) and PEG feeding indicated

Table A6.38. Enteral tube feeds used in trials of patients with renal disorders in the community (non-randomized data).

Trial	ETF	ETF energy density	ETF prescribed	ETF energy (kcal) provision	ETF protein (g) provision	Toleration	Timing of ETF
Sayce et al. (2000)	Nepro, TwoCal HN, Ensure Plus (Ross) Entera Fibre Plus (Fresenius)	Various	474–1722 kcal, 17–61 g P	–	–	Modification of types of feeds required to correct electrolyte imbalances in some patients, constipation, nausea and vomiting required use of higher-fibre feeds	Continuously overnight or bolus

HCDC, home care delivery company; P, protein.

Table A6.39. Trial characteristics: trials of enteral tube feeding in patients with renal disorders in the community (non-randomized data).

Trial	Design	Diagnosis	No. ETF	No. CON	Initial BMI ETF group	Initial BMI CON group	Duration of ETF	Tube type	Control group
Sayce et al. (2000) UK	C	Chronic renal disease, haemodialysis[a]	8	–	16.4[b]	–	Monitored for 3 months	PEG, Freka 9Fr (Fresenius)	–

[a]All haemodialysis patients treated with home gastrostomy feeding over a 4-year period.
[b]Median BMI 'using dry weight'.
CON, control.

Table A6.40. Main findings of enteral tube feeding trials in patients with renal disorders in the community (non-randomized data).

Trial	Energy/nutrient intake	Wt change ETF	Wt change CON	Function	Outcome	Finance
Sayce et al. (2000)	–	+5.3 kg (sig.) Sig. increase in TSF and MAMC	–	–	Mean no. of days in hospital 11.7 (average est. ~19–20 days for haemodialysis patients). Only 0.2% of hospital days due to feeding-related problems	–

CON, control; est., estimated; MAMC, mid-arm muscle circumference; TSF, triceps skin-fold thickness; sig., significant.

that ETF was more successful if patients were rested from CAPD after PEG placement and haemodialysed for 1–2 weeks (six sessions). Resting from CAPD or a short period of using smaller dialysis volumes and/or shorter dwell times with CAPD was recommended to allow healing of the gastrostomy. This survey also suggested that patients who had developed a poor nutritional status prior to starting ETF were less likely to be successfully fed by PEG. Therefore, it is recommended that gastrostomy feeding should be considered before patients become grossly malnourished (Ruddock, 2000).

Overall, there is a lack of information about the efficacy of ETF and other means of nutritional support (e.g. ONS) in patients with renal disease (either acute or chronic disease, in hospital and community settings). Therefore, RCT are required to ascertain the clinical and cost-effectiveness of ETF and other means of nutritional support in patients with renal disease across settings, including those undergoing haemodialysis or CAPD.

Notes

[1] A hyphen has been used in the tables throughout this Appendix where information was not provided in the reviewed trial (and could not be calculated).

[2] (Craig *et al.*, 1998; Tables A6.7–A6.9.) This is just one example of trials that have undertaken comparisons of standard enteral formulas with disease-specific feeds for use in diabetics. As such investigations are beyond the scope of this review, similar papers can be referred to individually (see diabetes section). The issues surrounding the nutritional support of tube-fed patients with diabetes have been discussed and summarized in a *Clinical Nutrition* supplement (1998, Vol. 17, Suppl. 2).

References

Abad-Lacruz, A., Fernandez-Banares, F., Cabre, E., Gil, A., Esteve, M., Gonzalez-Huix, F., Xioi, X. and Gassull, M.A. (1988) The effect of total enteral tube feeding on the vitamin status of malnourished patients with inflammatory bowel disease. *International Journal of Vitamin Research* 58, 428–435.

Abbasi, A.A. and Rudman, D. (1993) Observations on the prevalence of protein–calorie undernutrition in VA nursing homes. *Journal of the American Geriatric Society* 41, 117–121.

Abbott, D.F., Exton-Smith, A.N., Millard, P.H. and Temperley, J.M. (1968) Zinc sulphate and bedsores [letter]. *British Medical Journal* 2, 763.

Abelson, H.T. (1998) Oncology. In: Behrman, R.E. and Kliegman, R.M. (eds) *Nelson Essentials of Pediatrics.* W.B. Saunders, Philadelphia, pp. 583–608.

Abernathy, G.B., Heizer, W.D., Holcombe, B.J., Raasch, R.H., Schlegel, K.E. and Hak, L.J. (1989) Efficacy of tube feeding in supplying energy requirements of hospitalized patients. *Journal of Parenteral and Enteral Nutrition* 13, 387–391.

Abou-Assi, S., Craig, K. and O'Keefe, S.J. (2000) Prospective evaluation of nutritional management in patients with acute pancreatitis. *Clinical Nutrition* 19, 46.

Abrams, S.A. (2001) Chronic pulmonary insufficiency in children and its effects on growth and development. *Journal of Nutrition* 131, 938S–941S.

Acchiardo, S.R., Moore, L.W. and Latour, P.A. (1983) Malnutrition as the main factor in morbidity and mortality of hemodialysis patients. *Kidney International* 24, S199–S203.

Adams, S., Dellinger, E.P., Wertz, M.J., Oreskovich, M.R., Simonowitz, D. and Johansen, K. (1986) Enteral versus parenteral nutritional support following laparotomy for trauma: a randomised prospective trial. *Journal of Trauma* 26, 882–891.

Ader, R., Cohen, N. and Felten, D. (1995) Psychoneuroimmunology: interactions between the nervous system and the immune system. *Lancet* 345, 99–103.

Adler, M.W. (2001) Development of the epidemic: ABC of AIDS. *British Medical Journal* 322, 1226–1229.

Afdhal, N.H., Kelly, J., McCormick, P.A. and O'Donoghue, D.P. (1989) Remission induction in refractory Crohn's disease using a high calorie whole diet. *Journal of Parenteral and Enteral Nutrition* 13, 362–365.

Aggarwal, V. and Williams, M.D. (1998) Gastrointestinal problems in the immunosuppressed patient. *Archives of Disease in Childhood* 78, 5–8.

Agradi, E., Messina, V., Campanella, G., Venturini, M., Caruso, M., Moresco, A., Giacchero, A., Ferrari, N. and Ravera, E. (1984) Hospital malnutrition: incidence and prospective evaluation of general medical patients during hospitalisation. *Acta Vitaminology Enzymology* 6, 235–242.

Aiges, H., Markowitz, J., Rosa, J. and Daum, F. (1989) Home nocturnal supplemental nasogastric feedings in growth-retarded adolescents with Crohn's disease. *Gastroenterology* 97, 905–910.

Aker, S.N. (1979) Oral feedings in the cancer patient. *Cancer* 43, 2103–2107.

Akner, G. and Cederholm, T. (2001) Treatment of protein–energy malnutrition in chronic nonmalignant disorders. *American Journal of Clinical Nutrition* 74, 6–24.

Akobeng, A.K., Miller, V., Stanton, J., Elbadri, A.M. and Thomas, A.G. (2000) Double-blind randomised controlled trial of glutamine-enriched polymeric diet in the treatment of active Crohn's disease. *Journal of Pediatric Gastroenterology and Nutrition* 30, 78–84.

Alam, A.N., Sarker, S.A., Wahed, M.A., Khatun, M. and Rahaman, M.M. (1994) Enteric protein loss and intestinal permeability changes in children during acute shigellosis and after recovery: effect of zinc supplementation. *Gut* 35, 1707–1711.

Albanes, D. (1998) Height, early energy intake, and cancer. *British Medical Journal* 317, 1331–1332.

Alberino, F., Gatta, A., Amodio, P., Merkel, C., Di Pascoli, L., Boffo, G. and Caregaro, L. (2001) Nutrition and survival in patients with liver cirrhosis. *Nutrition* 17, 445–450.

Alexander, J.W., Gonce, S.J., Miskell, P.W., Peck, M.D. and Sax, H. (1989) A new model for studying nutrition in peritonitis: the adverse effect of overfeeding. *Annals of Surgery* 209, 334–340.

Al-Hudiathy, A.M. and Lewis, N.M. (1996) Serum albumin and age are predictors of length of hospital stay in surgical patients. *Nutrition Research* 16, 1891–1900.

Al-Jaouni, R., Hebuterne, X., Pouget, I. and Rampal, P. (2000) Energy metabolism and substrate oxidation in patients with Crohn's disease. *Nutrition* 16, 173–178.

Allan, J.D., Mason, A. and Moss, A.D. (1973) Nutritional supplementation in treatment of cystic fibrosis of the pancreas. *American Journal of Diseases of Childhood* 126, 22–26.

Allen, L.H., Lung'aho, M.S., Shaheen, M., Harrison, G. and Neuman, C. (1994) Maternal body mass index and pregnancy outcome in the Nutrition Collaborative Support Program. *European Journal of Clinical Nutrition* 48 (Suppl. 3), S68–S77.

Allison, M.C., Morris, A.J., Park, R.H.R. and Mills, P.R. (1992) Percutaneous endoscopic gastrostomy tube feeding may improve outcome of late rehabilitation following stroke. *Journal of the Royal Society of Medicine* 85, 147–149.

Allison, S.P. (1992) The uses and limitations of nutritional support. *Clinical Nutrition* 11, 319–330.

Allison, S.P. (1995) Cost-effectiveness of nutritional support in the elderly. *Proceedings of the Nutrition Society* 54, 693–699.

Allison, S.P. (1996) The management of malnutrition in hospital. *Proceedings of the Nutrition Society* 55, 855–862.

Allison, S.P. (1997) Impaired thermoregulation in malnutrition. In: Kinney, J.M. and Tucker, H.N. (eds) *Physiology, Stress and Malnutrition: Functional Correlates, Nutritional Intervention.* Lippincott-Raven, Philadelphia, pp. 571–593.

Allison, S.P. (1998) Outcomes from nutritional support in the elderly. *Nutrition* 14, 479–480.

Allison, S.P. (ed.) (1999) *Hospital Food as Treatment.* BAPEN, Maidenhead.

Allman, M.A., Stewart, P.M., Tiller, D.J., Horvath, J.S., Duggin, G.G. and Truswell, A.S. (1990) Energy supplementation and the nutritional status of hemodialysis patients. *American Journal of Clinical Nutrition* 51, 558–562.

Allman, R.M. (1989) Pressure ulcers among the elderly. *New England Journal of Medicine* 320, 850–854.

Allman, R.M. (1997) Pressure ulcer prevalence, incidence, risk factors, and impact. *Clinics in Geriatric Medicine* 13, 421–436.

Allman, R.M., Laprade, C.A., Noel, L.B., Walker, J.M., Moorer, C.A., Dear, M.R. and Smith, C.R. (1986) Pressure sores among hospitalised patients. *Annals of Internal Medicine* 105, 337–342.

Allman, R.M., Goode, P.S., Burst, N., Bartolucci, A.A. and Thomas, D.R. (1999) Pressure ulcers, hospital complications and disease severity: impact on hospital costs and length of stay. *Advances in Wound Care* 12, 22–30.

Almeida Santos, L., Ruza, F., Guerra, A.J.M., Alves, A., Dora, P., Garcia, S. and Santos, N.T. (1998) Evaluación nutricional de niños con insufiencia respiratoria (IR): antropometría al ingreso en cuidados intensivos pediátricos (Nutritional evaluation of children with respiratory failure (RF): anthropometric evaluation upon admission to the pediatric intensive care unit). *Anales Españoles de Pediatria* 49, 11–16.

Altman, D.G. (1995) *Practical Statistics for Medical Research.* Chapman & Hall, London.

Altman, D.G. and Schulz, K.F. (2001) Concealing treatment allocation in randomised trials. *British Medical Journal* 323, 446–447.

Alverdy, J.C. and Burke, D. (1992) Total parenteral nutrition: iatrogenic immunosuppression. *Nutrition* 8, 359–365.

Amadi, B., Kelly, P., Mwiya, M., Mulwazi, E., Sianongo, S., Changwe, F., Thomson, M., Hachungula, J., Watuka, A., Walker-Smith, J. and Chintu, C. (2001) Intestinal and systemic infection, HIV and mortality in Zambian children with persistent diarrhoea and malnutrition. *Journal of Pediatric Gastroenterology and Nutrition* 32, 550–554.

American Society for Parenteral and Enteral Nutrition (1989) Standards for nutrition support for residents of long-term care facilities. *Nutrition in Clinical Practice* 4, 148–153.

Anderson, C.F., Moxness, K., Meister, J. and Burritt, M.F. (1984) The sensitivity and specificity of nutrition related variables in relationship to the duration of hospital stay and the rate of complications. *Mayo Clinic Proceedings* 59, 477–483.

Anderson, M.D., Collins, G., Davis, G. and Bivins, B.A. (1985) Malnutrition and length of stay – a relationship? *Henry Ford Hospital Medical Journal* 33, 190–193.

Anderson, P. (2000) Tickling patients' taste buds. *Nursing Times* 96, 24–26.

Andersson, P., Persson, M., Vedin, I., Ljungqvist, I., Wretlind, B. and Cederholm, T. (2001) Inflammation, −308 TNF α promoter gene polymorphism and nutritional status in geriatric patients. *Clinical Nutrition* 20 (Suppl. 3), 48.

Andreyev, H.J.N., Norman, A.R., Oates, J. and Cunningham, D. (1998) Why do patients with weight loss have a worse outcome when undergoing chemotherapy for gastrointestinal malignancies? *European Journal of Cancer* 34, 503–509.

Anker, S.D., Ponikowski, P., Varney, S., Chua, T.P., Clark, A.L., Webb-Peploe, K.M., Harrington, D., Kox, W.J., Poole-Wilson, P.A. and Coats, A.J.S. (1997) Wasting as independent risk factor for mortality in chronic heart failure. *Lancet* 349, 1050–1053.

Anon. (1994) Position of the American Dietetic Association and the Canadian Dietetic Association: nutrition intervention in the care of persons with human immunodeficiency virus infection. *Journal of the American Dietetic Association* 94, 1042–1045.

Anon. (1998) XII. International comparisons of ESRD therapy. *American Journal of Kidney Diseases* 32, S136–S141.

Anon. (2001a) Consensus recommendations from the US summit on immune-enhancing enteral therapy. *Journal of Parenteral and Enteral Nutrition* 25, S61–S62.

Anon. (2001b) To feed or not to feed: tube feeding in patients with advanced dementia. *Nutrition Reviews* 59, 86–88.

Anthony, H., Bines, J., Phelan, P. and Paxton, S. (1998) Relation between dietary intake and nutritional status in cystic fibrosis. *Archives of Disease in Childhood* 78, 443–447.

Anthony, H., Paxton, S., Catto-Smith, A. and Phelan, P. (1999) Physiological and psychological contributors to malnutrition in children with cystic fibrosis: review. *Clinical Nutrition* 18, 327–335.

Antila, H., Salo, M., Nanto, V., Forssell, K., Salonen, M. and Kirvela, O. (1993) The effect of intermaxillary fixation on leukocyte zinc, serum trace elements and nutritional status of patients undergoing maxillofacial surgery. *Clinical Nutrition* 12, 223–229.

Aoun, J.P., Abousalby, M. and Geahchan, N. (1992) Prevalence of malnutrition in general medical patients. *Revue Médicale Libanaise* 4, 148–151.

Aoun, J.P., Baroudi, J. and Geahchan, N. (1993) Prevalence of malnutrition in general surgical patients. *Journal Médical Libanais* 4, 57–61.

Aparicio, M., Cano, N., Chauveau, P., Azar, R., Canaud, B., Flory, A., Laville, M., Leverve, X. and the French Study Group for Nutrition in Dialysis (FSG–ND). (1999) Nutritional status of haemodialysis patients: a French national cooperative study. *Nephrology, Dialysis and Transplantation* 14, 1679–1686.

Aparicio, M., Chauveau, P. and Combe, C. (2001) Low protein diets and outcome of renal patients. *Journal of Nephrology* 14, 433–439.

Aquino, V.M., Smyrl, C.B., Hagg, R., McHard, K.M., Prestridge, L. and Sandler, E.S. (1995) Enteral nutritional support by gastrostomy tube in children with cancer. *Journal of Pediatrics* 127, 58–62.

Aref, G., Badr El Din, M., Hassan, A. and Araby, I. (1970) Immunoglobulins in kwashiorkor. *Journal of Tropical Medicine and Hygiene* 73, 186–190.

Arnold, C. and Richter, M. (1989) The effect of oral nutritional supplements on head and neck cancer. *International Journal of Radiation Oncology, Biology and Physics* 16, 1595–1599.

Arnold, J., Wybrew, L., Rollins, H., Smith, A. and Simmonds, N. (2001) Audit of nutritional screening and weight change in patients in an acute hospital trust. *Proceedings of the Nutrition Society* 60, 110A.

Arnott, I.D.R., Kingstone, K. and Ghosh, S. (2000) Abnormal intestinal permeability predicts relapse in inactive Crohn's disease. *Scandinavian Journal of Gastroenterology* 35, 1163–1169.

Arora, N.S. and Rochester, D.F. (1982a) Effect of body weight and muscularity on human diaphragm muscle mass, thickness, and area. *Journal of Applied Physiology: Respiratory and Environmental Exercise Physiology* 52, 64–70.

Arora, N.S. and Rochester, D.F. (1982b) Respiratory muscle strength and maximal voluntary ventilation in undernourished patients. *American Review of Respiratory Disease* 126, 5–8.

Arpadi, S.M., Horlick, M.N.B., Wang, J., Cuff, P., Bamji, M. and Kotler, D.P. (1998) Body composition in prepubertal children with human immunodeficiency virus type 1 infection. *Archives of Pediatric and Adolescent Medicine* 152, 688–693.

Ashley, C. and Howard, L. (2000) Evidence base for specialized nutrition support. *Nutrition Reviews* 58, 282–289.

Ashton, W., Nanchahal, K. and Wood, D. (2001) Body mass index and metabolic risk factors for coronary heart disease in women. *European Heart Journal* 22, 46–55.

Ashworth, F., McAlweenie, A., Williams, S., Hodson, M., Poole, S. and Westaby, D. (1996) Overnight percutaneous endoscopic gastrostomy (PEG) feeding using an elemental formula in adolescents and adults with cystic fibrosis. *Proceedings of the Nutrition Society* 56, 200A.

ASPEN (1988) Standards for home nutrition support. *Nutrition in Clinical Practice* 3, 202–205.

ASPEN (1995) Standards for nutrition support: hospitalised patients. *Nutrition in Clinical Practice* 10, 208–219.

ASPEN (1993a) Guidelines for the use of parenteral and enteral nutrition in adult and pediatric patients. *Journal of Parenteral and Enteral Nutrition* 17, 1SA–52SA.

ASPEN (1993b) Section II: Rationale for adult nutrition support guidelines. *Journal of Parenteral and Enteral Nutrition* 17, 5SA–6SA.

ASPEN (2002) Guidelines for the use of parenteral and enteral nutrition in adult and pediatric patients. *Journal of Parenteral and Enteral Nutrition* 26, 1SA–138SA.

Association of Community Health Councils for England and Wales (1997) *Hungry in Hospital?* Community Health Councils for England and Wales, London.

Athlin, E., Norberg, A., Axelsson, K., Moller, A. and Nordstrom, G. (1989) Aberrant eating behavior in elderly Parkinsonian patients with and without dementia: analysis of video-recorded meals. *Research in Nursing and Health* 12, 41–51.

Atkinson, S., Sieffert, E. and Bihari, D. (1998) A prospective, randomized, double-blind, controlled clinical trial of enteral immunonutrition in the critically ill. Guy's Hospital Intensive Care Group. *Critical Care Medicine* 26, 1164–1172.

Audivert, S., Jimenez, G., Conde, M., Luque, S., Echenique, M., Castella, M., Portabella, C.P. and Planas, M. (2000) Nutritional status in hospitalized patients. *Clinical Nutrition* 19 (Suppl.), 3.

Ausobosky, J.R., Bean, P., Proctor, J. and Pollock, A.V. (1982) Delayed hypersensitivity testing for the prediction of postoperative complications. *British Journal of Surgery* 69, 346–348.

Avenell, A. (1994) Starvation in hospital: ethically indefensible and expensive (letter). *British Medical Journal* 308, 1369.

Avenell, A. and Handoll, H.H.G. (2001) Nutritional supplementation for hip fracture aftercare in the elderly. In: *The Cochrane Library*, Issue 1. Update Software, Oxford.

Avenell, A., Handoll, H.H. and Grant, A.M. (2001) Lessons for search strategies from systematic reviews, in the Cochrane Library, of nutritional supplementation in patients after hip fracture. *American Journal of Clinical Nutrition* 73, 505–510.

Axelsson, K., Norberg, A. and Asplund, K. (1984) Eating after a stroke – towards an integrated view. *International Journal of Nursing Studies* 21, 93–99.

Axelsson, K., Asplund, K., Norberg, A. and Alafuzoff, I. (1988) Nutritional status in patients with acute stroke. *Acta Medica Scandinavica* 224, 217–224.

Axelsson, K., Asplund, K., Norberg, A. and Eriksson, S. (1989) Eating problems and nutritional status during hospital stay of patients with severe stroke. *Journal of the American Dietetic Association* 89, 1092–1096.

Azad, N., Murphy, J., Amos, S.S. and Toppan, J. (1999) Nutrition survey in an elderly population following admission to a tertiary care hospital. *Canadian Medical Association Journal* 161, 511–515.

Baarends, E.M., Schols, A.M.W.J., Pannemans, D.L.E., Westerterp, K.R. and Wouters, E.F.M. (1997) Total free living energy expenditure in patients with severe chronic obstructive pulmonary disease. *American Journal of Respiratory and Critical Care Medicine* 155, 549–554.

Babineau, T.J. and Blackburn, G.L. (1994) Time to consider early gut feeding. *Critical Care Medicine* 22, 191–193.

Bachrach-Lindström, M., Unosson, M., Ek, A.C. and Jarnqvist, H. (2001) Assessment of nutritional status using biochemical and anthropometric variables in a nutritional intervention study of women with hip fracture. *Clinical Nutrition* 20, 217–223.

Baigire, R.J., Devitt, P.G. and Watkin, D.S. (1996) Enteral versus parenteral nutrition after oesophagogastric surgery: a prospective randomized comparison. *Australia and New Zealand Journal of Surgery* 66, 668–670.

Baines, M.J. (1997) Nausea, vomiting and intestinal obstruction: ABC of palliative care. *British Medical Journal* 315, 1148–1150.

Baker, F., Vitale, J., Elkort, R., Vavrousek-Jakuba, E. and Cordano, A. (1977) Nutritional enteral support of breast cancer patients. *Journal of Parenteral and Enteral Nutrition* 1, 18A.

Bakke, J., Lawrence, N., Bennett, J. and Robinson, S. (1975) Endocrine syndromes produced by neonatal hyperthyroidism, hypothyroidism, or altered nutrition and effects seen in untreated progeny. In: Fisher, D. and Burrow, G. (eds) *Perinatal Thyroid Physiology and Disease*. Raven Press, New York, pp. 79–116.

Baldwin, C., Parsons, T. and Logan, S. (2002) Dietary advice for illness-related malnutrition in adults (Cochrane Review). In: *The Cochrane Library*, Issue 2. Update Software, Oxford.

Balfe, J.W., Secker, D.J., Coulter, P.E., Balfe, J.A. and Geary, D.F. (1990) Tube feeding in children on chronic peritoneal dialysis. *Advances in Peritoneal Dialysis* 6, 257–261.

Ballinger, A. and Clark, M. (2001) Nutrition, appetite control and disease. In: Payne-James, J., Grimble, G. and Silk, D. (eds) *Artificial Nutrition Support in Clinical Practice*. Greenwich Medical Media, London, pp. 225–239.

Ballmer, P.E. (2001) Causes and mechanisms of hypoalbuminaemia. *Clinical Nutrition* 20, 271–273.

Banerjee, A.K., Brocklehurst, J.C., Wainwright, H. and Swindell, R. (1978) Nutritional status of long-stay geriatric in-patients: effects of a food supplement (Complan). *Age and Ageing* 7, 237–243.

Banerjee, A.K., Brocklehurst, J.C. and Swindell, R. (1981) Protein status in long-stay geriatric in-patients. *Gerontology* 27, 161–166.

Bannerman, E., Pendlebury, J., Phillips, F. and Ghosh, S. (1999) Health related quality of life and nutritional outcomes after percutaneous endoscopic gastrostomy: a prospective study. *Proceedings of the Nutrition Society* 58, 127A.

Bannerman, E., Davidson, I., Conway, C., Culley, D., Aldhous, M.C. and Ghosh, S. (2001) Altered subjective appetite parameters in Crohn's disease patients. *Clinical Nutrition* 20, 399–405.

Bansal, V.K., Popli, S., Pickering, J., Ing, T.S., Vertuno, L.L. and Hano, J.E. (1980) Protein–calorie malnutrition and cutaneous anergy in hemodialysis maintained patients. *American Journal of Clinical Nutrition* 33, 1608–1611.

Barber, M.D., McMillan, D.C., Donnelly, J., Slater, C., Ross, J.A., Fearon, K.C.H. and Preston, T. (1998) Liver export protein synthetic rates are increased by oral meal feeding in weight-losing cancer patients. *Clinical Nutrition* 17 (Suppl.), 15.

Barber, M.D., Ross, J.A., Preston, T., Shenkin, A. and Fearon, K.C.H. (1999a) Fish oil-enriched nutritional supplement attenuates progression of the acute-phase response in weight-losing patients with advanced pancreatic cancer. *Journal of Nutrition* 129, 1120–1125.

Barber, M.D., Ross, J.A., Voss, A.C., Tisdale, M.J. and Fearon, K.C.H. (1999b) The effect of an oral nutritional supplement enriched with fish oil on weight-loss in patients with pancreatic cancer. *British Journal of Cancer* 81, 80–86.

Barber, M.D., McMillan, D.C., Preston, T., Ross, J.A. and Fearon, K.C.H. (2000) Metabolic response to feeding in weight-losing pancreatic cancer patients and its modulation by a fish-oil-enriched nutritional supplement. *Clinical Science* 98, 389–399.

Barclay, R.P.C. and Shannon, R.S. (1975) Trial of artificial diet in treatment of cystic fibrosis of pancreas. *Archives of Diseases of Childhood* 50, 490–493.

Barer, D.H. (1989) The natural history and functional consequences of dysphagia after hemispheric stroke. *Journal of Neurology, Neurosurgery and Psychiatry* 52, 236–241.

Barkeling, B., Rossner, S. and Bjorvell, H. (1990) Effects of a high-protein meal (meat) and a high-carbohydrate meal (vegetarian) on satiety measured by automated computerized monitoring of subsequent food intake, motivation to eat and food preferences. *International Journal of Obesity* 14, 743–751.

Barker, D.J. and Fall, C.H. (1993) Fetal and infant origins of cardiovascular disease. *Archives of Diseases in Childhood* 68, 797–799.

Barle, H., Nyberg, B., Ramel, S., Essen, P., McNurlan, M., Wernerman, J. and Garlick, P. (1998) The synthesis rate of total liver protein, but not of albumin, decreases during a surgical trauma. *Clinical Nutrition* 17 (Suppl. 1), 15.

Barratt, J. (2000) A patient with Alzheimer's disease, fed via percutaneous endoscopic gastrostomy, with personal reflections on some of the ethical issues arising from this case [case study]. *Journal of Human Nutrition and Dietetics* 13, 51–54.

Barrett-Connor, E. (1995) The economic and human costs of osteoporotic fracture. *American Journal of Medicine* 98, 3S–8S.

Barrett-Connor, E., Edelstein, S., Corey-Bloom, J. and Wiederholt, W. (1998) Weight loss precedes dementia in community-dwelling older adults. *Journal of Nutrition, Health and Aging* 2, 113–114.

Bartlett, R.H., Allyn, P.A., Medley, T. and Wetmore, N. (1977) Nutritional therapy based on positive caloric balance in burn patients. *Archives of Surgery* 112, 974–980.

Barton, A.D., Beigg, C.L., Macdonald, I.A. and Allison, S.P. (2000a) High food wastage and low nutritional intakes in hospital patients. *Clinical Nutrition* 19, 445–449.

Barton, A.D., Beigg, C.L., Macdonald, I.A. and Allison, S.P. (2000b) A recipe for improving food intakes in elderly hospitalized patients. *Clinical Nutrition* 19, 451–454.

Bashir, Y., Graham, T.R., Torrance, A., Gibson, G.J. and Corris, P.A. (1990) Nutritional state of patients with lung cancer undergoing thoracotomy. *Thorax* 45, 183–186.

Bastow, M.D., Rawlings, J. and Allison, S.P. (1985) Overnight nasogastric tube feeding. *Clinical Nutrition* 4, 7–11.

Bastow, M.D., Rawlings, J. and Allison, S.P. (1983) Benefits of supplementary tube feeding after fractured neck of femur: a randomised controlled trial. *British Medical Journal* 287, 1589–1592.

Batchelor, J.A. (1999) Causal factors in FTT. In: *Failure to Thrive in Young Children*. The Children's Society, pp.34–55.

Baumgartner, D.T.G. (ed.) (1991) *Clinical Guide to Parenteral Micronutrition*. Lyphomed, Division of Fujisawa USA Inc.

Beach, R., Gershwin, M. and Hurley, L. (1982) Gestational zinc deprivation in mice: persistence of immunodeficiency for three generations. *Science* 218, 469–470.

Beale, R.J., Bryg, D.J. and Bihari, D.J. (1999) Immunonutrition in the critically ill: a systematic review of clinical outcome. *Critical Care Medicine* 27, 2799–2805.

Beattie, A.H., Prach, A.T., Baxter, J.P. and Pennington, C.R. (2000) A randomised controlled trial evaluating the use of enteral nutritional supplements postoperatively in malnourished surgical patients. *Gut* 46, 813–818.

Beaugerie, L., Carbonnel, F., Carrat, F., Rached, A.A., Maslo, C., Gendre, J.P., Rozenbaum, W. and Cosnes, J. (1998) Factors of weight loss in patients with HIV and chronic diarrhoea. *Journal of Acquired Immune Syndromes and Human Retrovirology* 19, 34–39.

Beaver, M.E., Matheney, K.E., Roberts, D.B. and Myers, J.N. (2001) Predictors of weight loss during radiation therapy. *Otolaryngology and Head and Neck Surgery* 125, 645–648.

Beck, M.A. (2001) Antioxidants and viral infections: host immune response and viral pathogenicity. *Journal of the American College of Nutrition* 20, 384S–388S.

Beck, A.M. and Ovesen, L. (1998) At which body mass index and degree of weight loss should hospitalised elderly patients be considered at nutritional risk? *Clinical Nutrition* 17, 195–198.

Beck, A.M., Ovesen, L. and Schroll, M. (2001a) A six months' prospective follow-up of 65+y-old patients from general practice classified according to nutritional risk by the Mini Nutritional Assessment. *European Journal of Clinical Nutrition* 55, 1028–1033.

Beck, A.M., Balknäs, U.N., Fürst, P., Hasunen, K., Jones, L., Keller, U., Melchior, J.C., Mikkelsen, B.E., Schauder, P., Sivonen, L., Zinck, O., Øien, H. and Ovesen, L. (2001b) Food and nutritional care in hospitals: how to prevent undernutrition – report and guidelines from the Council of Europe. *Clinical Nutrition* 20, 455–460.

Behnke, A.R., Feen, B.G. and Welham, W.C. (1942) The specific gravity of healthy men. *Journal of the American Medical Association* 118, 495–501.

Behrman, R.E. and Kliegman, R.M. (1998) *Nelson Essentials of Pediatrics*. W.B. Saunders, Philadelphia.

Beier-Holgersen, R. and Boesby, S. (1996) Influence of postoperative enteral nutrition on postsurgical infections. *Gut* 39, 833–835.

Bell, E.A. and Rolls, B.J. (2001) Energy density of foods affects energy intake across multiple levels of fat content in lean and obese women. *American Journal of Clinical Nutrition* 73, 1010–1018.

Bell, S.C., Bowerman, A.R., Davies, C.A., Campbell, I.A., Shale, D.J. and Elborn, J.S. (1998) Nutrition in adults with cystic fibrosis. *Clinical Nutrition* 17, 211–215.

Belli, D.C., Seidman, E., Bouthiliier, L., Weber, A.M., Roy, C.C., Pletincx, M., Beaulieu, M. and Morin, C.L. (1988) Chronic intermittent elemental diet improves growth failure in children with Crohn's disease. *Gastroenterology* 94, 603–610.

Bengmark, S. (1998) Progress in perioperative enteral tube feeding. *Clinical Nutrition* 17, 145–152.

Bengmark, S., Andersson, R. and Mangiante, G. (2001) Uninterrupted perioperative enteral nutrition. *Clinical Nutrition* 20, 11–19.

Bennegard, K., Eden, E., Ekman, L., Schersten, T. and Lundholm, K. (1983) Metabolic response of whole body and peripheral tissues to enteral nutrition in weight-losing cancer and noncancer patients. *Gastroenterology* 85, 92–99.

Benton, D. and Parker, P.Y. (1998) Breakfast, blood glucose and cognition. *American Journal of Clinical Nutrition* 67, 772S–778S.

Berg, R.D. (1983) Translocation of indigenous bacteria from the intestinal tract. In: Hentges, D.J. (ed.) *Human Intestinal Microflora in Health and Disease*. Academic Press, New York, pp. 333–352.

Berger, M.M., Chiolero, R.L., Pannatier, A., Cayeux, M.C. and Tappy, L. (1997) A 10-year survey of nutritional support in a surgical ICU: 1986–1995. *Nutrition* 13, 870–877.

Bergstrom, J. (1995) Why are dialysis patients malnourished? *American Journal of Kidney Diseases* 26, 229–241.

Bergstrom, J. (1999) Regulation of appetite in chronic renal failure. *Mineral and Electrolyte Metabolism* 25, 291–297.

Bergstrom, J. and Lindholm, B. (1993) Nutrition and adequacy of dialysis: how do hemodialysis and CAPD compare? *Kidney International* 43, S39–S50.

Bergstrom, J. and Lindholm, B. (1998) Malnutrition, cardiac disease, and mortality: an integrated point of view. *American Journal of Kidney Diseases* 32, 834–841.

Bergstrom, N. and Braden, B. (1992) A prospective study of pressure sore risk among institutionalized elderly. *Journal of the American Geriatric Society* 40, 747–758.

Berhane, R., Bagenda, D., Marum, L., Aceng, E., Ndugwa, C., Bosch, R.J. and Olness, K. (1997) Growth failure as a prognostic indicator of mortality in pediatric HIV infection. *Pediatrics* 100, E7.

Berkman, D.S., Lescano, A.G., Gilman, R.H., Lopez, S.L. and Black, M.M. (2002) Effects of stunting, diarrhoeal disease and parasitic infection during infancy on cognition in late childhood: a follow up study. *The Lancet* 359, 564–571.

Berlowitz, D.R. and Wilking, S.V. (1989) Risk factors for pressure sores: a comparison of cross-sectional and cohort-derived data. *Journal of the American Geriatric Society* 37, 1043–1050.

Bermudez, O.L., Becker, E.K. and Tucker, K.L. (1999) Development of sex-specific equations for estimating stature of frail elderly Hispanics living in the northeastern United States. *American Journal of Clinical Nutrition* 69, 992–998.

Bernard, S., LeBlanc, P., Whittom, F., Carrier, G., Jobin, J., Belleau, R. and Maltais, F. (1998) Peripheral muscle weakness in patients with chronic obstructive pulmonary disease. *American Journal of Respiratory and Critical Care Medicine* 158, 629–634.

Berneis, K., Battegay, M., Bassetti, S., Nuesch, R., Leisibach, A., Bilz, S. and Keller, U. (2000) Nutritional supplements combined with dietary counselling diminish whole body protein catabolism in HIV-infected patients. *European Journal of Clinical Investigation* 30, 87–94.

Bernstein, L., Bachman, T.E., Meguid, M., Ament, M., Baumgartner, T., Kinosian, B., Martindale, R. and Spilekerman, M. (1995) Prealbumin in Nutritional Care Consensus Group: measurement of visceral protein status in assessing protein and energy malnutrition: standard of care. *Nutrition* 11, 169–171.

Berry, H.K., Kellogg, F.W., Hunt, M.M., Ingberg, R.L., Richter, L. and Gutjahr, C. (1975) Dietary supplement and nutrition in children with cystic fibrosis. *American Journal of Diseases of Childhood* 129, 165–171.

Bertrand, J.M., Morin, C.L., Lasalle, R., Patrick, J. and Coates, A.L. (1984) Short-term clinical, nutritional, and functional effects of continuous elemental enteral alimentation in children with cystic fibrosis. *Journal of Pediatrics* 104, 41–46.

Bingham, S. (1987) The dietary assessment of individuals; methods, accuracy, new techniques and recommendations. *Nutrition Abstracts and Reviews* 57, 705–742.

Binkin, N.J., Yip, R., Fleshood, L. and Trowbridge, F.L. (1988) Birth weight and childhood growth. *Pediatrics* 82, 828–834.

Bishop, C.W., Bowen, P.E. and Ritchey, S.J. (1981) Norms for nutritional assessment of American adults by upper arm anthropometry. *American Journal of Clinical Nutrition* 34, 2530–2539.

Bistrian, B.R., Blackburn, G.L., Vitale, J., Cochran, D. and Naylor, J. (1976) Prevalence of malnutrition in general medical patients. *Journal of the American Medical Association* 235, 1567–1570.

Bistrian, B.R. and Khaodhiar, L. (1999) The systemic inflammatory response and its impact on iron nutriture in end-stage renal disease. *American Jounal of Kidney Diseases* 34, S35–S39.

Blackburn, G.L. and Harvey, K.B. (1982) Nutritional assessment as a routine in clinical medicine. *Postgraduate Medicine* 71, 46–63.

Blackburn, G., Bistrian, G.L., Maini, B.S., Schlamm, H.T. and Smith, M.F. (1977) Nutritional and metabolic assessment of the hospitalized patient. *Journal of Parenteral and Enteral Nutrition* 1, 11–22.

Blanshard, C., Francis, N. and Gazzard, B.G. (1996) Investigation of chronic diarrhoea in acquired immunodeficiency syndrome. A prospective study of 155 patients. *Gut* 39, 824–832.

Blundell, J.E. and Stubbs, R.J. (1999) High and low carbohydrate and fat intakes: limits imposed by appetite and palatability and their implications for energy balance. *European Journal of Clinical Nutrition* 53, S148–S165.

Blundell, J.E., Burley, V.J., Cotton, J.R. and Lawton, C.L. (1993) Dietary fat and the control of energy intake: evaluating the effects of fat on meal size and postmeal satiety. *American Journal of Clinical Nutrition* 57, 772S–778S.

Bobel, L.M. (1987) Nutritional implications in the patient with pressure sores. *Nursing Clinics of North America* 22, 379–390.

Bodger, K. and Heatley, R.V. (2001) The immune system and nutrition support. In: Payne-James, J., Grimble, G. and Silk, D. (eds) *Artificial Nutrition Support in Clinical Practice*. Greenwich Medical Media, London, pp. 137–148.

Boelens, P.G., van Hoorn, D.E., van Norren, K., Nijveldt, R.J., Prins, H.A., M'Rabet, L., Hofman, Z. and van Leeuwen, P.A.M. (2001) Feeding before ischemia reperfusion of the intestine reduces oxidative stress in both kidney and lung and preserves vitality of kidney, heart and liver. *Clinical Nutrition* 20 (Suppl. 3), 2–3.

Bøhmer, T. and Mowé, M. (2000) The association between atrophic glossitis and protein–calorie malnutrition in old age. *Age and Ageing* 29, 47–50.

Boland, M.P., Stoski, D.S., MacDonald, N.E., Soucy, P. and Patrick, J. (1986) Chronic jejunostomy feeding with a non-elemental formula in undernourished patients with cystic fibrosis. *Lancet* i, 232–234.

Bolton, J., Shannon, L., Smith, V., Abbott, R., Bell, S.J., Stubbs, L. and Slevin, M.L. (1990) Comparison of short-term and long-term palatability of six commercially available oral supplements. *Journal of Human Nutrition and Dietetics* 3, 317–321.

Bolton, J., Abbott, R., Kiely, M., Alleyne, M., Bell, S., Stubbs, L. and Slevin, M. (1992) Comparison of three oral sip-feed supplements in patients with cancer. *Journal of Human Nutrition and Dietetics* 5, 79–84.

Bonjour, J.-P., Schurch, M.-A. and Rizzoli, R. (1996) Nutritional aspects of hip fractures. *Bone* 18, 139S–144S.

Bonnefont-Rousselot, D., Jaudon, M.C., Issad, B., Cacoub, P., Congy, F., Jardel, C., Delattre, J. and Jacobs, C. (1997) Antioxidant status of elderly chronic renal patients treated by continuous ambulatory peritoneal dialysis. *Nephrology, Dialysis and Transplantation* 12, 1399–1405.

Booth, D.A., Chase, A. and Campbell, A.T. (1970) Relative effectiveness of protein in the late stages of appetite suppression in man. *Physiology and Behavior* 5, 1299–1302.

Booth, K., Morgan, S. and Hindle, T. (1995) *Financial Issues for Clinical Nutrition in NHS Hospitals*. Nutricia Clinical Care, Trowbridge.

Bories, P.N. and Campillo, B. (1994) One-month regular oral nutrition in alcoholic cirrhotic patients: changes of nutritional status, hepatic function and serum lipid pattern. *British Journal of Nutrition* 72, 937–946.

Borlase, B.C., Bell, S.J., Lewis, E.J., Swails, W., Bistrian, B.R., Forse, R.A. and Blackburn, G.L. (1992) Tolerance of enteral tube feeding diets in hypoalbuminemic critically ill geriatric patients. *Surgery, Gynecology and Obstetrics* 174, 181–188.

Bos, C., Benamouzig, R., Bruhat, A., Roux, C., Mahe, S., Valensi, P., Gaudichon, C., Ferriere, F.,

Rautureau, J. and Tome, D. (2000) Short-term protein and energy supplementation activates nitrogen kinetics and accretion in poorly nourished elderly subjects. *American Journal of Clinical Nutrition* 71, 1129–1137.

Bosaeus, I., Daneryd, P., Svanberg, E. and Lundholm, K. (2001) Dietary intake and resting energy expenditure in relation to weight loss in unselected cancer patients. *International Journal of Cancer* 93, 380–383.

Bosch, X. (2002) Two billion people older than 60 years by 2050, warns UN Secretary General. *Lancet* 359, 1321.

Bounous, G. (1989) Elemental diets in the prophylaxis and therapy for intestinal lesions: an update. *Surgery* 105, 571–575.

Bounous, G., Gentile, J.M. and Hugon, J. (1971) Elemental diet in the management of the intestinal lesion produced by 5-fluorouracil in man. *Canadian Journal of Surgery* 14, 312–324.

Bounous, G., Tahan, W., Shuster, J., Gold, P., Cousineau, L., Rochon, M. and Lebel, E. (1973) The use of an elemental diet during abdominal radiation. *Clinical Research* 21, 1066.

Bounous, G., Le Bel, E., Shuster, J., Gold, P., Tahan, W.T. and Bastin, E. (1975) Dietary protection during radiation therapy. *Strahlentherapie* 149, 476–483.

Bourdel-Marchasson, I., Barateau, M., Rondeau, V., Dequae-Merchadou, L., Salles-Montaudon, N., Emeriau, J.-P., Manciet, G., Dartigues, J.-F. and for the GAGE Group (2000) A multi-center trial of the effects of oral nutritional supplementation in critically ill older inpatients. *Nutrition* 16, 1–5.

Bourdel-Marchasson, I., Joseph, P.A., Dehail, P., Biram, M., Faux, P., Rainfray, M., Emerian, J.-P., Canioni, P. and Thiaudière, E. (2001) Functional and metabolic early changes in calf muscle occurring during nutritional repletion in malnourished elderly patients. *American Journal of Clinical Nutrition* 73, 832–838.

Bouritius, H., Middelaar, M.C., Boelens, P.G., van Hoorn, D.E., Nijveldt, R.J., M'Rabet, L., Hofman, Z., van Leeuwen, P.A. and Van Norren, K. (2001) Fasting dramatically increases susceptibility of the intestine to ischemia reperfusion injury. *Clinical Nutrition* 20 (Suppl. 3), 55–56.

Bours, G.J.J.W., Halfens, R.J.G., Lubbers, M. and Haalboom, J.R.E. (1999) The development of a national registration form to measure the prevalence of pressure ulcers in the Netherlands. *Ostomy/Wound Management* 45, 28–40.

Bower, R.H., Talamini, M.A., Sax, H.C., Hamilton, F. and Fischer, J.E. (1986) Postoperative enteral versus parenteral nutrition: a randomised controlled trial. *Archives of Surgery* 121, 1040–1045.

Bower, R.H., Cerra, F.B., Bershadsky, B., Licari, J.J., Hoyt, D.B., Jensen, G.L., Van Buren, C.T., Rothkopf, M.M., Daly, J.M. and Adelsberg, B.R. (1995) Early enteral administration of a formula (IMPACT) supplemented with arginine, nucleotides, and fish oil in intensive care unit patients: results of a multicenter, prospective, randomized, clinical trial. *Critical Care Medicine* 23, 436–449.

Bowling, T.E. (1995) The Sir David Cuthbertson Medal Lecture. Enteral-feeding-related diarrhoea: proposed causes and possible solutions. *Proceedings of the Nutrition Society* 54, 579–590.

Boyce, W.J. and Vessey, M.P. (1985) Rising incidence of fracture of the proximal femur. *Lancet* i, 150–151.

Boyle, P. (1997) Global burden of cancer. *Lancet* 349, sii23–sii26.

Bozzetti, F. (1992) Nutritional support in the adult cancer patient. *Clinical Nutrition* 11, 167–179.

Bozzetti, F. and The Committee of the European Association for Palliative Care (1996) Guidelines on artificial nutrition versus hydration in terminal cancer patients. *Nutrition* 12, 163–167.

Bozzetti, F., Terno, G. and Longoni, C. (1975) Parenteral hyperalimentation and wound healing. *Surgery, Gynecology and Obstetrics* 141, 712–714.

Bozzetti, F., Braga, M., Gianotti, L., Gavazzi, C. and Mariani, L. (2001) Postoperative enteral versus parenteral nutrition in malnourished patients with gastrointestinal cancer: a randomised multi-centre trial. *Lancet* 358, 1487–1492.

Braga, M., Gianotti, L., Vignali, A., Cestari, A., Bisagni, P. and Di Carlo, V. (1998) Artificial nutrition after major abdominal surgery: impact of route of administration and composition of the diet. *Critical Care Medicine* 26, 24–30.

Braga, M., Gianotti, L., Radaelli, G., Vignali, A., Mari, G., Gentilini, O. and Di Carlo, V. (1999) Perioperative immunonutrition in patients undergoing cancer surgery: results of a randomized double-blind phase 3 trial. *Archives of Surgery* 134, 428–433.

Braga, M., Gianotti, L., Cestari, A., Vignali, A., Pellegatta, F., Dolci, A. and Di Carlo, V. (1996) Gut function and immune and inflammatory responses in patients perioperatively fed with supplemented enteral formulas. *Archives of Surgery* 131, 1257–1265.

Braga, M., Gianotti, L., Gentilini, O., Parisi, V., Salis, C. and Di Carlo, V. (2001) Early postoperative enteral nutrition improves gut oxygenation and reduces costs compared with total parenteral nutrition. *Critical Care Medicine* 29, 242–248.

Brantsma, A., Kelson, K. and Malcom, J. (1991) Percutaneous endoscopic gastrostomy feeding in HIV disease. *Australian Journal of Advanced Nursing* 8, 36–41.

Braulio, V.B., Castro, C.L., Vaisman, F., Cavalcanti, A.C., Conti, L.A., Emigdio, R.F. and Marschhausen, N. (2001) Nutritional status in patients with COPD candidates to pulmonary rehabilitation. *Clinical Nutrition* 20 (Suppl.), 3.

Braun, S.R., Dixon, R.M., Keim, N.L., Luby, M., Anderegg, A. and Shrago, E.S. (1984a) Predictive clinical value of nutritional assessment factors in COPD. *Chest* 85, 353–357.

Braun, S.R., Keim, N.L., Dixon, R.M., Clagnaz, P., Anderegg, A. and Shrago, E.S. (1984b) The prevalence and determinants of nutritional changes in chronic obstructive pulmonary disease. *Chest* 86, 558–563.

Braunschweig, C., Gomez, S. and Sheean, P.M. (2000) Impact of declines in nutritional status on outcomes in adult patients hospitalized for more than 7 days. *Journal of the American Dietetic Association* 100, 1316–1322.

Braunschweig, C.L., Levy, P., Sheean, P.M. and Wang, X. (2001) Enteral compared with parenteral nutrition: a meta-analysis. *American Journal of Clinical Nutrition* 74, 534–542.

Breslow, R. (1991) Nutritional status and dietary intake of patients with pressure ulcers: review of research literature 1943 to 1989. *Decubitus* 4, 16–21.

Breslow, R.A. and Bergstrom, N. (1994) Nutritional prediction of pressure ulcers. *Journal of the American Dietetic Association* 94, 1301–1304.

Breslow, R.A., Hallfrisch, J. and Goldberg, A.P. (1991) Malnutrition in tubefed nursing home patients with pressure sores. *Journal of Parenteral and Enteral Nutrition* 15, 663–668.

Breslow, R.A., Hallfrisch, J., Guy, D.G., Crawley, B. and Goldberg, A.P. (1993) The importance of dietary protein in healing pressure ulcers. *Journal of the American Geriatric Society* 41, 357–362.

Briassoulis, G.Z., Zavras, N. and Hatzis, T. (2001) Malnutrition, nutritional indices, and early enteral feeding in critically ill children. *Nutrition* 17, 548–557.

Briet, F., Twomey, C. and Jeejeebhoy, K.N. (1999) Refeeding malnourished patients increases mitochondrial complex I activity: evidence for a sensitive nutritional marker. *Clinical Nutrition* 18 (Suppl.), 2–3.

Briet, F., Twomey, C. and Jeejeebhoy, K.N. (2000) Inflammatory bowel disease (IBD) does not alter reduction in lymphocyte mitochondrial complex I activity (CI) associated with malnutrition. *Clinical Nutrition* 19, 4.

British Dietetic Association (1994) The assessment of nutritional status in clinical situations. In: Thomas, B. (ed.) *Manual of Dietetic Practice*. Blackwell Scientific Publications, for the British Dietetic Association, Oxford, pp. 52–57.

Broadhead, E.E., Hughes, P.M., Kelly, C.G. and Seal, C.J. (2001a) Effects of radiotherapy treatment on dietary intake, appetite and quality of life in patients with cancer of the head and neck. *Proceedings of the Nutrition Society* 60, 55A.

Broadhead, E.E., Hughes, P.M., Kelly, C.G. and Seal, C.J. (2001b) Changes in taste, appetite and quality of life in patients with cancer of the head and neck during radiotherapy treatment. *Proceedings of the Nutrition Society* 60, 55A.

Brookes, G.B. (1982) Nutritional status in head and neck cancer: observation and implication. *Clinical Otolaryngology and Allied Sciences* 8, 211–220.

Brookes, G.B. and Clifford, P. (1981) Nutritional status and general immune competence in patients with head and neck cancer. *Journal of the Royal Society of Medicine* 74, 132–139.

Brooks, A.D., Hochwaald, S.N., Heslin, M.J., Harrison, L.E., Burt, M. and Brennan, M.F. (1999) Intestinal permeability after early postoperative enteral nutrition in patients with upper gastrointestinal malignancy. *Journal of Parenteral and Enteral Nutrition* 23, 75–79.

Broqvist, M., Arnqvist, H., Dahlstrom, U., Larsson, J., Nylander, E. and Permert, J. (1994) Nutritional assessment and muscle energy metabolism in severe chronic congestive heart failure – effects of long-term dietary supplementation. *European Heart Journal* 15, 1641–1650.

Brough, W., Horne, G., Blount, A., Irving, M.J. and Jeejeebhoy, K.N. (1986) Effects of nutrient intake, surgery, sepsis and long term administration of steroids on muscle function. *British Medical Journal* 293, 983–988.

Brown, K.H., Sanchez-Grinan, M., Perez, F., Peerson, J.M., Ganoza, L. and Stern, J.S. (1995) Effects of dietary energy density and feeding frequency on total daily energy intakes of recovering malnourished children. *American Journal of Clinical Nutrition* 62, 13–18.

Brown, K.M. and Seabrook, N.A. (1992) Nutritional influences on recovery and length of hospital stay in elderly women following femoral fracture. *Proceedings of the Nutrition Society* 51, 132A.

Brown, M.S., Buchanan, R.B. and Karran, S.J. (1980) Clinical observations on the effects of elemental diet supplementation during irradiation. *Clinical Radiology* 31, 19–20.

Brown, R., Bancewicz, J., Hamid, J., Patel, N.J., Ward, C.A., Farrand, R.J., Pumphrey, R.S.H. and Irving, M. (1982) Failure of delayed hypersensitivity skin testing to predict postoperative sepsis and mortality. *British Medical Journal* 284, 851–853.

Brown, R.O., Schlegel, K., Hall, N.H., Bernard, S. and Heizer, W.D. (1986) Taste preferences for nutritional supplements: comparison of cancer patients and healthy controls using a wine-tasting scale. *Journal of Parenteral and Enteral Nutrition* 10, 490–493.

Brown, R.O., Hunt, H., Mowatt-Larssen, C.A., Wojtysiak, S.L., Henningfield, M.F. and Kudsk, K.A. (1994) Comparison of specialized and standard enteral formulas in trauma patients. *Pharmacotherapy* 14, 314–320.

Browne, K. and Moloney, M. (1998) Assessment of energy content of menus, energy intakes and wastage of food in two Irish teaching hospitals. *Proceedings of the Nutrition Society* 57, 144A.

Brozek, J. (1990) Effects of generalized malnutrition on personality. *Nutrition* 6, 389–396.

Bruce, S.A., Newton, D. and Woledge, R.C. (1989) Effect of subnutrition on normalized muscle force and relaxation rate in human subjects using voluntary contractions. *Clinical Science* 76, 637–641.

Bruins, M.J., Hallemeesch, M.M., Deutz, N.E.P. and Soeters, P.B. (1998) Increase in intestinal permeability after endotoxin challenge is due to fluid load. *Clinical Nutrition* 17, 66.

Bruning, P.F., Halling, A., Hilgers, F.J.M., Kappner, G., Poelhus, E.K., Kobashi-Schoot, A.M. and Schouwenburg, P.F. (1988) Postoperative nasogastric tube feeding in patients with head and neck cancer: a prospective assessment of nutritional status and well-being. *European Journal of Cancer and Clinical Oncology* 24, 181–188.

Bruun, L.I., Bosaeus, I., Bergstad, I. and Nygaard, K. (1999) Prevalence of malnutrition in surgical patients: evaluation of nutritional support and documentation. *Clinical Nutrition* 18, 141–147.

Brynes, A.E., Stratton, R.J., Wright, L. and Frost, G.S. (1998) Energy intakes fail to meet requirements on texture modified diets. *Proceedings of the Nutrition Society* 57, 117A.

Buchman, A.L. (1998) Comment: alterations in intestinal barrier function do not predispose to translocation of enteric bacteria in gastroenterologic patients. *Journal of Parenteral and Enteral Nutrition* 22, 399–400.

Buchman, A.L., Moukarzel, A.A., Bjuta, S., Belle, M., Ament, M.E., Eckhert, C.D., Hollander, D., Gornbein, J., Kopple, J.D. and Vijayaroghavan, S.R. (1995a) Parenteral nutrition is assocated with intestinal morphologic and functional changes in humans. *Journal of Parenteral and Enteral Nutrition* 19, 453–460.

Buchman, A.L., Mestecky, J., Moukarzel, A. and Ament, M.E. (1995b) Intestinal immune function is unaffected by parenteral nutrition in man. *Journal of the American College of Nutrition* 14, 656–661.

Buckler, D.A., Kelber, S.T. and Goodwin, J.S. (1994) The use of dietary restrictions in malnourished nursing home patients. *Journal of the Amerian Geriatric Society* 42, 1100–1102.

Buggy, D. (2000) Can anaesthetic management influence surgical wound-healing? *Lancet* 356, 399–400.

Bunker, V.W., Stansfield, M.F., Deacon-Smith, R., Marzil, R.A., Hounslow, A. and Clayton, B.E. (1994) Dietary supplementation and immunocompetence in housebound elderly subjects. *British Journal of Biomedical Science* 51, 128–135.

Bunout, D., Aicardi, V., Hirsch, S., Petermann, M., Kelly, M., Silva, G., Garay, P., Ugarte, G. and Iturriaga, H. (1989) Nutritional support in hospitalized patients with alcoholic liver disease. *European Journal of Clinical Nutrition* 43, 615–621.

Bunting, J. and Weaver, L.T. (1997) Staff use and quality of anthropometric measures in a children's hospital. *Proceedings of the Nutrition Society* 55, 254A.

Burger, B., Wessel, D., Junger, H., Ollenschlager, G., Schwenk, A. and Schrappe, M. (1992) Prospective study on the outcome of nutritional therapy including formula diets in malnourished HIV-infected. *Clinical Nutrition* 11, S15.

Burger, B., Ollenschlager, G., Schrappe, M., Stute, A., Fischer, M., Wessel, D., Schwenk, A. and Diehl, V. (1993) Nutrition behavior of malnourished HIV-infected patients and intensified oral nutritional intervention. *Nutrition* 9, 43–44.

Burger, B., Schwenk, A., Junger, H., Ollenschlager, G., Wessl, D., Diehl, V. and Schrappe, M. (1994) Oral supplements in HIV-infected patients with chronic wasting: a prospective trial. *Medizinische Klinik* 89, 579–581.

Burness, R., Horne, G. and Purdie, G. (1996) Albumin levels and mortality in patients with hip fractures. *New Zealand Medical Journal* 109, 56–57.

Burns, A., Marsh, A. and Bender, D.A. (1989) Dietary intake and clinical, anthropometric and biochemical indices of malnutrition in elderly demented patients and non-demented subjects. *Psychological Medicine* 19, 383–391.

Burrin, D.G., Stoll, B., Jiang, R., Chang, X., Hartmann, B., Holst, J.J., Greeley, G.H. and Reeds, P.J. (2000) Minimal enteral nutrient requirements for intestinal growth in neonatal piglets: how much is enough? *American Journal of Clinical Nutrition* 71, 1603–1610.

Buzby, G.P., Mullen, J.L., Matthews, D.C., Hobbs, C.L. and Rosato, E.F. (1980) Prognostic nutritional index in gastrointestinal surgery. *American Journal of Surgery* 139, 160–167.

Cabre, E. and Gassull, M.A. (1993) Nutritional aspects of chronic liver disease. *Clinical Nutrition* 12, S52–S63.

Cabre, E., Gonzalez-Huix, F., Abad-Lacruz, A., Esteve, M., Acero, D., Fernandez-Banares, F., Xiol, X. and Gassull, M.A. (1990) Effect of total enteral nutrition on the short-term outcome of severely malnourished cirrhotics: a randomized controlled trial. *Gastroenterology* 98, 715–720.

Cainzos, M., Potel, J. and Puente, J.L. (1989) Anergy in patients with biliary lithiasis. *British Journal of Surgery* 76, 169–172.

Calder, P.C. and Yaqoob, M.A. (2000) The level of protein and type of fat in the diet of pregnant rats both affect lymphocyte function in the offspring. *Nutrition Research* 20, 995–1005.

Calvaresi, E. and Bryan, J. (2001) B vitamins, cognition and aging: a review. *Journal of Gerontology Series B, Psychological Sciences and Social Sciences* 56, 327–339.

Calvey, H., Davis, M. and Williams, R. (1984) Prospective study of nasogastric feeding via East Grinstead or Viomedex tubes compared with oral dietary supplementation in patients with cirrhosis. *Clinical Nutrition* 3, 63–66.

Cameron, J.W., Rosenthal, A. and Olson, A.D. (1995) Malnutrition in hospitalized children with congenital heart disease. *Archives of Pediatric and Adolescent Medicine* 149, 1098–1102.

Campbell, I.T., Morton, R.P., Cole, J.A., Raine, C.H., Shapiro, L.M. and Stell, P.M. (1983) A comparison of the effects of intermittent and continuous nasogastric feeding on the oxygen consumption and nitrogen balance of patients after major head and neck surgery. *American Journal of Clinical Nutrition* 38, 870–878.

Campos, A.C.L. and Meguid, M.M. (1992) A critical appraisal of the usefulness of perioperative nutritional support. *American Journal of Clinical Nutrition* 55, 117–130.

Cappell, M.S. and Godil, A. (1993) A multicenter case-controlled study of percutaneous endoscopic gastrostomy in HIV-seropositive patients. *American Journal of Gastroenterology* 88, 2059–2066.

Carbonnel, F., Maslo, C., Beaugerie, L., Carrat, F., Wirbel, E., Aussel, C., Gobert, J.G., Girard, P.M., Gendre, J.P., Cosnes, J. and Rozenbaum, W. (1998) Effect of Indinavir on HIV-related wasting. *AIDS* 12, 1777–1784.

Caroline Walker Trust (1995) *Eating Well for Older People. Practical and Nutritional Guidelines for Food in Residential and Nursing Homes and for Community Meals. A Report of an Expert Working Group.* Wordworks, London.

Carr, A. and Cooper, D.A. (2000) Adverse effects of antiretroviral therapy. *Lancet* 356, 1423–1430.

Carr, A., Miller, J., Eisman, J.A. and Cooper, D.A. (2001) Osteopenia in HIV-infected men: association with asymptomatic lactic acidemia and lower weight pre-antiretroviral therapy. *AIDS* 15, 703–709.

Carr, C.S., Ling, K.D.E., Boulos, P. and Singer, M. (1996) Randomised trial of safety and efficacy of immediate postoperative enteral feeding in patients undergoing gastrointestinal resection. *British Medical Journal* 312, 869–871.

Carver, A.D. and Dobson, A.M. (1995) Effects of dietary supplementation of elderly demented hospital residents. *Journal of Human Nutrition and Dietetics* 8, 389–394.

Case, T. and Gilbert, L. (1997) Dietary and dining expectations of residents of long term care facilities. *Nutrition* 13, 703–704.

Castaldo, A., Tarallo, L., Palomba, E., Albano, F., Russo, S., Zuin, G., Buffardi, F. and Guarino, A. (1996) Iron deficiency and intestinal malabsorption in HIV disease. *Journal of Pediatric Gastroenterology and Nutrition* 22, 359–363.

Castetbon, K., Kadio, A., Bondurand, A., Boka Yao, A., Barouan, C., Coulibaly, Y., Anglaret, X., Msellati, P., Malvy, D. and Dabis, F. (1997) Nutritional status and dietary intakes in human immunodeficiency virus (HIV) infected outpatients in Abidjan, Côte D'Ivoire 1995. *European Journal of Clinical Nutrition* 51, 81–86.

Caughey, P., Seaman, C., Parry, D., Farquhar, D. and Maclennan, W.J. (1994a) Nutrition of old people in sheltered housing. *Journal of Human Nutrition and Dietetics* 7, 263–268.

Caughey, P., Seaman, C., Parry, D., Farquhar, D. and Maclennan, W.J. (1994b) Factors affecting dietary intake and nutritional status of tenants in sheltered housing. *Journal of Human Nutrition and Dietetics* 7, 269–273.

Cederholm, T. and Gyllenhammar, H. (1999) Impaired granulocyte formylpeptide-induced superoxide generation in chronically ill, malnourished, elderly patients. *Journal of Internal Medicine* 245, 475–482.

Cederholm, T. and Hellström, K. (1992) Nutritional status in recently hospitalised and free-living elderly subjects. *Gerontology* 38, 105–110.

Cederholm, T., Jägrén, C. and Hellström, K. (1993) Nutritional status and performance capacity in internal medical patients. *Clinical Nutrition* 12, 8–14.

Cederholm, T., Jägrén, C. and Hellström, K (1995) Outcome of protein–energy malnutrition in elderly medical patients. *American Journal of Medicine* 98, 67–74.

Cederholm, T.E. and Hellström, K.H. (1995) Reversibility of protein–energy malnutrition in a group of chronically-ill elderly outpatients. *Clinical Nutrition* 14, 81–87.

Ceesay, S.M., Prentice, A.M., Cole, T.M., Ford, F., Weaver, C.T., Poskitt, E.M. and Whitehead, R.G. (1997) Effects on birthweight and perinatal mortality of maternal dietary supplements in rural Gambia: 5 year randomised controlled trial. *British Medical Journal* 315, 786–790.

Cerra, F.B., McPherson, J.P., Konstantinides, F.N., Konstantinides, N.N. and Teasley, K.M. (1988) Enteral nutrition does not prevent multiple organ failure syndrome (MOFS) after sepsis. *Surgery* 104, 727–733.

Chadwick, S.J.D., Sim, A.J.W. and Dudley, H.A.F. (1986) Changes in plasma fibronectin during acute nutritional deprivation in healthy human subjects. *British Journal of Nutrition* 55, 7–12.

Chan, M.F., Weaver, K.E., Cello, J.P., Merkel, K.L. and Akrabawi, S.S. (1994) Benefits of outpatient nutritional supplementation in patients with AIDS (PWA) and fat malabsorption. *Gastroenterology* 106, A600.

Chandra, R.K. (1975) Antibody formation in first and second generation offspring of nutritionally deprived rats. *Science* 190, 289–290.

Chandra, R.K. (1986) Serum levels and synthesis of IgG subclasses in small for gestation low birth weight infants and in patients with selective IgA deficiency. In: Hanson, L.A., Soderstrom, T. and Oxelius, V.A. (eds) *Immunoglobulins Subclass Deficiencies*. Kruger, Basel, pp. 90–99.

Chandra, R.K. (1988) Immunity and infection. In: Kinney, J.M., Jeejeebhoy, K.N., Hill, G. and Owen, O.E. (eds) *Nutrition and Metabolism in Patient Care*. pp.598–604.

Chandra, R.K. (1999) Nutrition and immunology: from the clinic to cellular biology and back again. *Proceedings of the Nutrition Society* 58, 681–683.

Chandra, R.K. (2000) Food allergy and nutrition in early life: implications for later health. *Proceedings of the Nutrition Society* 59, 273–277.

Chandra, R.K. and Puri, S. (1985) Nutritional support improves antibody response to influenza virus vaccine in the elderly. *British Medical Journal* 291, 705–706.

Chandra, R.K., Ali, K.M., Kutty, K.M. and Chandra, S. (1977) Thymus-dependent lymphocytes and delayed hypersensitivity in low birth weight infants. *Biology of the Neonate* 31, 15–18.

Chandra, R.K., Joshi, P., Au, B., Woodford, G. and Chandra, S. (1982) Nutrition and immunocompetence of the elderly: effect of short-term nutritional supplementation on cell-mediated immunity and lymphocyte subsets. *Nutrition Research* 2, 223–232.

Chang, H.R., Dulloo, A.G. and Bistrian, B.R. (1998) Role of cytokines in AIDS wasting. *Nutrition* 14, 853–863.

Chapman-Novakofski, K., Brewer, S., Riskowski, J., Burkowski, C. and Winter, L. (1999) Alterations in taste thresholds in men with chronic obstructive pulmonary disease. *Journal of the American Dietetic Association* 99, 1536–1541.

Charles, R., Mulligan, S. and O'Neill, D. (1999) The identification and assessment of undernutrition in patients admitted to the age related health care unit of an acute Dublin General Hospital. *Irish Journal of Medical Science* 168, 180–185.

Charlton, K.E. (1997) The nutrient intake of elderly men living alone and their attitudes towards nutrition education. *Journal of Human Nutrition and Dietetics* 10, 343–352.

Chazot, C., Laurent, G., Charra, B., Blanc, C., Vo Van, C., Jean, G., Vanel, T., Terrat, J.C. and Ruffet, M. (2001) Malnutrition in long-term haemodialysis survivors. *Nephrology, Dialysis and Transplantation* 16, 61–69.

Chellis, M.J., Sanders, S.V., Webster, H., Dean, M. and Jackson, D. (1996) Early enteral feeding in the pediatric intensive care unit. *Journal of Parenteral and Enteral Nutrition* 20, 71–73.

Chernoff, R.S., Milton, K.Y. and Lipschitz, D.A. (1990) The effect of a high protein formula (Replete) on decubitus ulcer healing in long term tube fed institutionalized patients. *Journal of the American Dietetic Association* 90, A130.

Cherubini, S., Russo, M., Fanfarillo, F., Faviano, A., Muscaritoli, M., Cascino, A., Pandolfi, C. and Rossi Fanelli, F. (2000) Plasma tryptophan levels and the anorexia of sepsis. *Clinical Nutrition* 19 (suppl.), 44.

Chiarelli, A., Enzi, G., Casadei, A., Baggio, B., Valerio, A. and Mazzoleni, F. (1990) Very early nutrition supplementation in burned patients. *American Journal of Clinical Nutrition* 51, 1035–1039.

Chima, C.S., Barco, K., Dewitt, M.L.A., Maeda, M., Teran, J.C. and Mullen, K.D. (1997) Relationship of nutritional status to length of stay, hospital costs, and discharge status of patients hospitalized in the medicine service. *Journal of the American Dietetic Association* 97, 975–978.

Chima, C.S., Barco, K. and Smith, R. (1998) Use of practice guidelines by clinical dietitians impacts the route of nutrition support resulting in cost savings. *Journal of the American Dietetic Association* 98, A89.

Chin, S.E., Shepherd, R.W., Cleghorn, G.J., Patrick, M., Ong, T.H., Wilcox, J., Lynch, S. and Strong, R. (1990) Pre-operative nutritional support in children with end-stage liver disease accepted for liver transplantation: an approach to management. *Journal of Gastroenterology and Hepatology* 5, 566–572.

Chin, S.E., Shepherd, R.W., Thomas, B.J., Cleghorn, G.J., Patrick, M.K., Wilcox, J.A., Ong, T.H., Lynch, S.V. and Strong, R. (1992) The nature of malnutrition in children with end-stage liver disease awaiting orthotopic liver transplantation. *American Journal of Clinical Nutrition* 56, 164–168.

Chiolero, R. and Kinney, J.M. (2001) Metabolic and nutritional support in critically ill patients: feeding the whole body or individual organs? *Current Opinion in Clinical Nutrition and Metabolic Care* 4, 127–130.

Chlebowski, R.T., Grosvenor, M.B., Bernhard, N.J., Morales, L.S. and Bulcavage, L.M. (1989) Nutritional status, gastrointestinal dysfunction and survival in patients with AIDS. *American Journal of Gastroenterology* 84, 1288–1293.

Chlebowski, R.T., Tai, V., Novak, D., Cope, F., Minor, C., Kruger, S. and Beall, G. (1992) Adherence to an enteral supplement program in patients with HIV infection. *Clinical Nutrition* 11, S14.

Chlebowski, R.T., Beall, G., Grosvenor, M., Lillington, L., Weintraub, N., Ambler, C., Richards, E.W., Abbruzzese, B.C., McCamish, M.A. and Cope, F.O. (1993) Long-term effects of early nutritional support with new enterotropic peptide-based formula vs. standard enteral formula in HIV-infected patients: randomised, prospective trial. *Nutrition* 9, 507–512.

Chlebowski, R.T., Grosvenor, M., Lillington, L., Sayre, J. and Beall, G. (1995) Dietary intake and counseling, weight maintenance, and the course of HIV infection. *Journal of the American Dietetic Association* 95, 428–432, 435.

Choileáin, F.N., Moriarty, M., Gibney, M.J. and Moloney, M. (1995) The effect of intensive dietary counselling on the nutritional status of patients with head and neck cancer undergoing radiotherapy. *Proceedings of the Nutrition Society* 54, 163A.

Christensen, T. and Kehlet, H. (1984) Postoperative fatigue and changes in nutritional status. *British Journal of Surgery* 71, 473–476.

Christensson, L., Unosson, M. and Ek, A.C. (1999) Malnutrition in elderly people newly admitted to community resident home. *Journal of Nutrition, Health and Aging* 3, 133–139.

Christie, M.L., Sack, D.M., Pomposelli, J. and Horst, D. (1985) Enriched branched-chain amino acid formula versus a casein-based supplement in the treatment of cirrhosis. *Journal of Parenteral and Enteral Nutrition* 9, 671–678.

Christou, N. (1990) Perioperative nutritional support: immunologic defects. *Journal of Parenteral and Enteral Nutrition* 14, 186S–191S.

Chumlea, W.C., Roche, A.F. and Steinbaugh, M.L. (1985) Estimating stature from knee height for persons 60 to 90 years of age. *Journal of the American Geriatric Society* 33, 116–120.

Chumlea, W.M.C., Guo, S.S. and Steinbaugh, M.L. (1994) Prediction of stature from knee height for black and white adults and children with application to mobility-impaired or handicapped persons. *Journal of the American Dietetic Association* 94, 1385–1388.

Chuntrasakul, C., Sithamr, S., Chinswangwatankul, V., Pongprasobchai, T., Chockvivatanavanit, S. and Bunnak, A. (1996) Early nutritional support in severe traumatic patients. *Journal of the Medical Association of Thailand* 79, 21–26.

Church, J.M., Choong, S.Y. and Hill, G.L. (1984) Abnormalities in muscle metabolism and histology in malnourished patients awaiting surgery: effects of a course of intravenous nutrition. *British Journal of Surgery* 71, 563–569.

Cianciaruso, B., Brunori, G., Traverso, G., Panarello, G., Enia, G., Strippoli, P., De Vecchi, A., Querques, M., Vigilino, E., Vonesh, E. and Maiorca, R. (1995) Nutritional status in the elderly patient with uraemia. *Nephrology, Dialysis and Transplantation* 10, 65–68.

Ciocon, J.O., Galindo-Ciocon, D.J., Tiessen, C. and Galindo, D. (1992) Continuous compared with intermittent tube feeding in the elderly. *Journal of Parenteral and Enteral Nutrition* 16, 525–528.

Clark, M.A., Hentzen, B.T.H., Plank, L.D. and Hill, G.L. (1996) Sequential changes in insulin-like growth factor 1, plasma proteins and total body protein in severe sepsis and multiple injury. *Journal of Parenteral and Enteral Nutrition* 20, 363–370.

Clark, M.A., Plank, L.D. and Hill, G.L. (2000) Wound healing associated with severe surgical illness. *World Journal of Surgery* 24, 648–654.

Clarke, D.M., Wahlqvist, M.L. and Strauss, B.J.G. (1998) Undereating and undernutrition in old age: integrating bio-psychosocial aspects. *Age and Ageing* 27, S27–S34.

Clifton, G.L., Robertson, C.S. and Contant, C.F. (1985) Enteral hyperalimentation in head injury. *Journal of Neurosurgery* 62, 186–193.

Cluskey, M. and Dunton, N. (1999) Serving meals of reduced portion size did not improve appetite among elderly in a personal-care section of a long-term-care community. *Journal of the American Dietetic Association* 99, 733–735.

Cluskey, M. and Kim, Y.-K. (2001) Use and perceived effectiveness of strategies for enhancing food and nutrient intakes among elderly persons in long term care. *Journal of the American Dietetic Association* 101, 111–114.

Coats, K.G., Morgan, S.L., Bartolucci, A.A. and Weinsier, R.L. (1993) Hospital-associated malnutrition: a re-evaluation 12 years later. *Journal of the American Dietetic Association* 93, 27–33.

Cockram, D.B., Hensley, M.K., Rodriguez, M., Agarwal, G., Wennberg, A., Ruey, P., Ashbach, D., Hebert, L. and Kunau, R. (1998) Safety and tolerance of medical nutritional products as sole sources of nutrition in people on hemodialysis. *Journal of Renal Nutrition* 8, 25–33.

Cohen, J. (1988) *Statistical Power Analysis for the Behavioral Sciences*, 2nd edn. Laurence Erlbaum Associates, New Jersey.

Cohendy, R., Gros, T., Arnaud-Battandier, F., Tran, G., Plaze, J.M. and Eledjam, J.-J. (1999) Preoperative nutritional evaluation of elderly patients: the Mini Nutritional Assessment as a practical tool. *Clinical Nutrition* 18, 345–348.

Cohn, S.H., Vartsky, D., Vaswani, A.N., Sawitsky, A., Rai, K., Gartenhaus, W., Yasumura, S. and Ellis, K.J. (1982) Changes in body composition of cancer patients following combined nutritional support. *Nutrition and Cancer* 4, 107–119.

Cole, J.J. (1994) Do growth charts need a new face lift? *British Medical Journal* 308, 641–642.

Cole, T.J. and Stanfield, J.P. (1981) Weight-for-height indices to assess nutritional status – a new index on a slide rule. *American Journal of Clinical Nutrition* 34, 1934–1943.

Cole, T.J., Freeman, J.V. and Preece, M.A. (1995) Body mass index reference curves for the UK, 1990. *Archives of Diseases in Childhood* 73, 25–29.

Cole, T.J., Freeman, J.V. and Preece, M.A. (1998) British 1990 growth reference centiles for weight, height, body mass index and head circumference fitted by maximum penalized likelihood. *Statistics in Medicine* 17, 407–429.

Collins, M.M., Wight, R.G. and Partridge, G. (1999) Nutritional consequences of radiotherapy in early laryngeal carcinoma. *Annals of the Royal College of Surgeons of England* 81, 376–381.

Collins, S. (1995) The limit of human adaptation to starvation. *Nature Medicine* 1, 810–814.

Comi, M.M., Palmo, A., Brugnani, M., D'Amicis, A., Costa, A., D'Andrea, F., Del Toma, E., Domeniconi, D., Fusco, M.S., Gatti, E., Lesi, C. and Lucchin, L. (1998) The hospital malnutrition Italian study. *Clinical Nutrition* 17 (Suppl.), 2.

Commission on the Nutrition Challenges of the 21st Century (2000) Ending malnutrition by 2020: an agenda for change in the millennium. *Food and Nutrition Bulletin* 21 (suppl.), 1–88.

Compan, B., Di Castri, A., Plaze, J.M. and Arnaud-Battandier, F. (1999) Epidemiological study of malnutrition in elderly patents in acute, sub-acute and long-term care using the MNA. *Journal of Nutrition, Health and Ageing* 3, 146–151.

Congleton, J. (1999) The pulmonary cachexia syndrome: aspects of energy balance. *Proceedings of the Nutrition Society* 58, 321–328.

Connors, A.F., Dawson, N.V., Thomas, C., Harrell, F.E., Desbiens, N., Fulkerson, W.J., Kussin, P., Bellamy, P., Goldman, L. and Knaus, W.A. (1996) Outcomes following acute exacerbation of severe chronic obstructive lung disease. *American Journal of Respiratory and Critical Care Medicine* 154, 959–967.

Constans, T., Bacq, Y., Bréchot, J.F., Guilmot, J.L., Choutet, P. and Lamisse, F. (1992) Protein–energy malnutrition in elderly medical patients. *Journal of the American Geriatric Society* 40, 263–268.

Consumers' Association (1996) Malnourished inpatients: overlooked and undertreated. *Drugs and Therapeutics Bulletin* 8, 57–60.

Consumers' Association (1999) Helping undernourished adults in the community. *Drugs and Therapeutics Bulletin* 37, 93–95.

Conway, S.P., Morton, A. and Wolfe, S. (2002) Enteral tube feeding for cystic fibrosis (Cochrane Review). In: *The Cochrane Library*, Issue 2. Update Software, Oxford.

Cooper, C. and Beaven, S. (1993) Protein and energy content of diets of patients undergoing haemodialysis for treatment of chronic renal failure – a short report. *Journal of Human Nutrition and Dietetics* 6, 521–523.

Corey, M., McLaughlin, F.J., Williams, M. and Levison, H. (1988) A comparison of survival, growth and pulmonary function in patients with cystic fibrosis in Boston and Toronto. *Journal of Clinical Epidemiology* 41, 583–591.

Corish, C., Flood, P., Reynolds, J.V. and Kennedy, N.P. (1998) Nutritional characteristics of Irish patients undergoing resection of major carcinoma. *Proceedings of the Nutrition Society* 57, 145A.

Corish, C.A., Flood, P., Mulligan, S. and Kennedy, N.P. (2000a) Apparent low frequency of undernutrition in Dublin hospital inpatients: should we review the anthropometric thresholds for clinical practice? *British Journal of Nutrition* 84, 325–335.

Corish, C., Flood, P. and Kennedy, N.P. (2000b) Prevalence of undernutrition and obesity among elderly inpatients using old and new reference data. *Proceedings of the Nutrition Society* 59, 174A.

Corrêa Leite, M.L., Nicolosi, A., Cristina, S., Hauser, W.A. and Nappi, G. (2001) Nutrition and cognitive deficit in the elderly: a population study. *European Journal of Clinical Nutrition* 55, 1053–1058.

Correia, I.D. and Waitzberg, D.L. (1999) Malnutrition increases morbidity, mortality and hospital costs in 25 public hospitals. *Clinical Nutrition* 18 (Suppl.), 13.

Cosgrove, M. and Jenkins, H.R. (1997) Experience of percutaneous endoscopic gastrostomy in children with Crohn's disease. *Archives of Diseases in Childhood* 76, 141–143.

Cotterill, A.M., Majrowski, W.H., Hearn, S., Jenkins, S., Preece, M.A. and Savage, M.O. (1996) The potential effect of the UK 1990 height centile charts on community growth surveillance. *Archives of Diseases in Childhood* 74, 452–454.

Cotton, E., Zinober, B. and Jessop, J. (1996) A nutritional assessment tool for older patients. *Professional Nurse* 11, 609–612.

Coulston, A.M., Craig, L. and Voss, A.C. (1996) Meals-on-wheels applicants are a population at risk for poor nutritional status. *Journal of the American Dietetic Association* 96, 570–573.

Council of Europe (2001) *Food and Nutrition Care in Hospitals: How to Prevent Undernutrition.* Council of Europe, April.

Covinsky, K.E., Martin, G.E., Beyth, R.J., Justice, A.C., Sehgal, A.R. and Landefeld, C.S. (1999) The relationship between clinical assessments of nutritional status and adverse outcomes in older hospitalised medical patients. *Journal of the American Geriatric Society* 47, S32–S38.

Cox, B.D., Huppert, F.A. and Whickelow, M.J. (1993) *The Health and Lifestyle Survey. Seven Years On.* Dartmouth Publishing, Aldershot.

Craig, C.B., Weinsier, R.L., Saag, M.S., Darnell, B., Epps, L., Mullins, L. and Akrabawi, S.S. (1994) Specialized enteral nutrition with medium chain triglycerides (MCT) in people with AIDS (PWA) and fat malabsorption. *Journal of Parenteral and Enteral Nutrition* 18, 26S.

Craig, L.D., Nicholson, S., Silverstone, F.A. and Kennedy, R.D. (1998) Use of a reduced-carbohydrate, modified-fat enteral formula for improving metabolic control and clinical outcomes in long-term care residents with type 2 diabetes: results of a pilot trial. *Nutrition* 14, 529–534.

Creutzberg, E.C., Schols, A.M.W.J., Weling-Scheepers, C.A.P.M., Buurman, W.A. and Wouters, E.F.M. (2000) Characterization of nonresponse to high caloric oral nutritional therapy in depleted patients with chronic obstructive pulmonary disease. *American Journal of Respiratory and Critical Care Medicine* 161, 745–752.

Crossland, S.G. and Higgins, G.C. (1977) Nutritional supplement in head and neck radiation therapy. *Journal of Parenteral and Enteral Nutrition* 1, 27A.

Cruickshank, A.M. (1989) Effect of nutritional status on acute phase protein response to elective surgery. *British Journal of Surgery* 76, 165–168.

Cruickshank, A.M., Jennings, G., Fearon, K.H., Elia, M. and Shenkin, A. (1991) Serum interleukin 6 (IL-6)-effect of surgery and undernutrition. *Clinical Nutrition* 10 (suppl.), 65–69.

Cummings, S.R., Kelsey, J.L., Nevitt, M.C. and O'Dowd, O.J. (1985) Epidemiology of osteoporosis and osteoporotic fractures. *Epidemiological Reviews* 7, 178–208.

Cummins, A., Chu, G., Faust, L., Chandy, G., Argyrides, J., Robb, T. and Wilson, P. (1995) Malabsorption and villous atrophy in patients receiving enteral feeding. *Journal of Parenteral and Enteral Nutrition* 19, 193–198.

Cunha, D.F., Cunha, S.F.C., Ferreira, T.P.S., Sawan, Z.T.E., Rodrigues, L.S., Prata, S.P. and Silva-Vergara, M.L. (2001) Prolonged QTc intervals on the electrocardiograms of hospitalized malnourished adults. *Nutrition* 17, 370–372.

Cunningham-Rundles, S. (1998) Analytical methods for evaluation of immune response in nutrient intervention. *Nutrition Reviews* 56, S27–S37.

Cuppari, L., Medeiros, F.A.M., Papini, H.F., Neto, M.C., Canziani, M.E.F., Martini, L., Ajzen, H. and Draibe, S.A. (1994) Effectiveness of oral energy–protein supplementation in severely malnourished hemodialysis patients. *Journal of Renal Nutrition* 4, 127–135.

Dahl, M. and Gebre-Medhin, M. (1993) Feeding and nutritional problems in children with cerebral palsy and myelomeningocoele. *Acta Paediatrica* 82, 816–820.

Dahl, M., Thommessen, M., Rasmussen, M. and Selberg, T. (1997) Feeding and nutritional characteristics in children with moderate or severe cerebral palsy. *Acta Paediatrica* 85, 697–701.

Daly, J.M., Hearne, B., Dunaj, J., LePorte, B., Vikram, B., Strong, E., Green, M., Muggio, F., Goshen, S. and DeCosse, J.J. (1984) Nutritional rehabilitation in patients with advanced head and neck cancer receiving radiation therapy. *American Journal of Surgery* 148, 514–520.

Daly, J.M., Reynolds, J., Thom, A., Kinsley, L., Dietrick-Gallagher, M., Shou, J. and Ruggieri, B. (1988) Immune and metabolic effects of arginine in the surgical patient. *Annals of Surgery* 208, 512–523.

Daly, J.M., Weintraub, F.N., Shou, J., Rosato, E.F. and Lucia, M. (1995) Enteral nutrition during multimodality therapy in upper gastrointestinal cancer patients. *Annals of Surgery* 221, 327–338.

Daly, J.M., Fry, W.A., Little, A.G., Winchester, D.P., McKee, R.F., Stewart, A.K. and Fremgen, A.M. (2000) Esophageal cancer: results of an American College of Surgeons' Patient Care Evaluation Study. *Journal of the American College of Surgeons* 190, 562–573.

Dalzell, A.M., Shepherd, R.W., Dean, B., Cleghorn, G.J., Holt, T.L. and Francis, P.J. (1992) Nutritional rehabilitation in cystic fibrosis: a 5 year follow-up study. *Journal of Pediatric Gastroenterology and Nutrition* 15, 141–145.

Daniels, A. and Wright, J. (1997) Hospitals with nutrition support teams are more likely to have a nutritional assessement policy and ward nurses who identify 'at risk' patients than those that do not. *Proceedings of the Nutrition Society* 56, 254A.

Daniels, L., Davidson, G.P., Martin, A.J. and Pouras, T. (1989) Supplemental nasogastric feeding in cystic fibrosis patients during treatment for acute exacerbation of chest disease. *Australian Paediatric Journal* 25, 164–167.

Dannhauser, A., Van Zuyl, J.M. and Nel, C.J.C. (1995a) Preoperative nutritional status and prognostic nutritional index in patients with benign disease undergoing abdominal operations – Part I. *Journal of the American College of Nutrition* 14, 80–90.

Dannhauser, A., VanZuyl, J.M. and Nel, C.J.C. (1995b) Preoperative nutritional status and prognostic nutritional index in patients with benign disease undergoing abdominal operations – Part II. *Journal of the American College of Nutrition* 14, 91–98.

Dardaine, V., Dequin, P.F., Ripault, H., Constans, T. and Giniès, G. (2001) Outcome of older patients requiring ventilatory support in intensive care: impact of nutritional status. *Journal of the American Geriatric Society* 49, 564–570.

Davalos, A., Ricart, W., Gonzalez-Huix, F., Soler, S., Marrugat, J., Molins, A., Suner, R. and Genis, D. (1996) Effect of malnutrition after acute stroke on clinical outcome. *Stroke* 27, 1028–1032.

Dave, K., O'Boyle, C.J., Nargis, B., Buckley, P., Mitchell, C.J. and Macfie, J. (1996) Changes in mucosal morphology do not affect intestinal permeability (IP) and do not predispose to bacterial translocation. *Clinical Nutrition* 15 (Suppl.), 38.

Davidson, H.I.M., Pattison, R.M. and Richardson, R.A. (1998) Clinical undernutrition states and their influence on taste. *Proceedings of the Nutrition Society* 57, 633–638.

Davidson, H.I.M., Richardson, R.A., Sutherland, D. and Garden, O.J. (1999) Macronutrient preference, dietary intake, and substrate oxidation among stable cirrhotic patients. *Hepatology* 29, 1380–1386.

Davies, H.A., Didcock, E., Didi, M., Oglivy-Stuart, A., Wales, J.K.H. and Shalet, S.M. (1995) Growth, puberty and obesity after treatment for leukaemia. *Acta Paediatrica* 411, 45–50.

Davies, J., Leeder, P., Dobbins, B., Miller, G.V., Sue-Ling, H.M., Martin, I.G. and Johnston, D. (1997) Early enteral feeding preserves intestinal permeability following gastro-oesophageal resection: use of a novel differential polyethylene gylcol absorption technique. *Clinical Nutrition* 16 (Suppl.), 40.

Davis, A.M. and Bristow, A. (1999) Managing nutrition in hospital. *British Medical Journal* 318, 1098.

Davison, C. and Stables, I. (1996) Nutrition screening of acute in-patients. *Proceedings of the Nutrition Society* 55, 144A.

Debnam, E.S. and Grimble, G.K. (2001) Methods for assessing intestinal absorptive function in relation to enteral nutrition. *Current Opinion in Clinical Nutrition and Metabolic Care* 4, 355–367.

Dechelotte, P., Jusserand, D., Merle, V., Carpentier, M.C., Petit, J., Hellot, M.F., Czernichow, P. and Lerebours, E. (2001) Prevalence of malnutrition and nosocomial infections in 881 hospitalized patients. *Clinical Nutrition* 20 (Suppl.), 72.

De Deuxchaisnes, C.N. and Devogelaer, J.-P. (1988) Increase in the incidence of hip fractures and of the ration of trochanteric to cervical hip fractures in Belgium. *Calcified Tissue International* 42, 201–203.

Deeg, H.J., Seidel, K., Bruemmer, B., Peope, M.S. and Appelbaum, F.R. (1995) Impact of patient weight on non-relapse mortality after marrow transplantation. *Bone Marrow Transplantation* 15, 461–468.

Deems, R.O., Friedman, M.I., Friedman, L.S., Munoz, S.J. and Maddrey, W.C. (1993) Chemosensory function, food preferences and appetite in human liver disease. *Appetite* 20, 209–216.

de Graaf, C., Hulshof, T., Weststrate, J.A. and Jas, P. (1992) Short-term effects of different amounts of protein, fats and carbohydrates on satiety. *American Journal of Clinical Nutrition* 55, 33–38.

de Groot, L.C.P.G.M., Sette, S., Zajkas, G., Carbajal, A., Amorin Cruz, J.A. and Euronut SENECA Investigators (1991) Nutritional status: anthropometry. *European Journal of Clinical Nutrition* 45, 31–42.

de Jong, N., de Groot, C.P.G.M., de Graaf, C., Chin, A., Paw, J.M.M. and van Staveren, W.A. (1998) Assessment of dietary intake and appetite in frail elderly. *European Journal of Clinical Nutrition* 53 (suppl., 2), S37.

de Jong, N., Chin, A., Paw, M.J.M., de Groot, L.C.P.G.M., de Graaf, C., Kok, F.J. and van Staveren, W.A. (1999) Functional biochemical and nutrient indices in frail elderly people are partly affected by dietary supplements but not by exercise. *Journal of Nutrition* 129, 2028–2036.

de Jong, P.C.M., Wesdorp, R.I.C., Volovics, A., Roufflart, M., Greep, J.M. and Soeters, P.B. (1985) The value of objective measurements to select patients who are malnourished. *Clinical Nutrition* 4, 61–66.

de Ledinghen, V., Beau, P., Labat, J. and Ingrand, P. (1995) Compared effects of enteral nutrition by percutaneous endoscopic gastrostomy in cancer and in non-cancer patients: a long-term study. *Clinical Nutrition* 14, 17–22.

de Ledinghen, V., Beau, P., Mannant, P.-R., Borderie, C., Ripault, M.-P., Silvain, C. and Beauchant, M. (1997) Early feeding or enteral nutrition in patients with cirrhosis after bleeding from esophageal varices? *Digestive Diseases and Sciences* 42, 536–541.

Delmi, M., Rapin, C.H., Bengoa, J.M., Delmas, P.D., Vasey, H. and Bonjour, J.P. (1990) Dietary supplementation in elderly patients with fractured neck of femur. *Lancet* 335, 1013–1016.

Demling, R.H. and DeSanti, L. (1998) Increased protein intake during the recovery phase after severe burns increases body weight gain and muscle function. *Journal of Burn Care and Rehabilitation* 19, 161–168.

Dempsey, D.T., Mullen, J.L. and Buzby, G.P. (1988) The link between nutritional status and clinical outcome: can nutritional intervention modify it? *American Journal of Clinical Nutrition* 47, 352–356.

den Broeder, E., Lippens, R.J.J., van 't Hof, M.A., Tolboom, J.J.M., van Staveren, W.A., Hofman, Z. and Sengers, R.C.A. (1998) Effects of naso-gastric tube feeding on the nutritional status of children with cancer. *European Journal of Clinical Nutrition* 52, 494–500.

den Broeder, E., Lippens, R.J.J., van't Hof, M.A., Tolboom, J.J.M., Sengers, R.C.A., van den Berg, A.M.J., van Houdt, N.B.M., Hofman, Z. and van Staveren, V.A. (2000) Nasogastric tube feeding in children with cancer: the effect of two different formulas on weight, body composition, and serum protein concentration. *Journal of Parenteral and Enteral Nutrition* 24, 351–360.

de Onis, M., Villar, J. and Gulmezoglu, M. (1998) Nutritional interventions to prevent intrauterine growth retardation. *European Journal of Clinical Nutrition* 52, S83–S93.

Department of Health (1991) *Report on Health and Social Subjects 41. Dietary Reference Values for Food Energy and Nutrients for the United Kingdom.* HMSO, London.

Department of Health (1991–1998) *Prescription Cost Analysis.* Government Statistical Service, Department of Health, London.

Department of Health (1992) *Report on Health and Social Subjects: 43. The Nutrition of Elderly People.* HMSO, London.

Department of Health (1998) *NHS Hospital Statistics: England 1987–88 to 1997–98. Statistical Bulletin 1998/31 30th September 1998.* Government Statistical Service.

Department of Health (1999) *Saving Lives. Our Healthier Nation.* Government White Paper, Stationery Office, London.

Department of Health (2001) *National Service Framework for Older People.* Department of Health, London.

Desport, J.C., Preux, P.M., Tuong, T.C., Vallat, J.M., Sautereau, D. and Couratier, P. (1999) Nutritional status is a prognostic factor for survival in ALS patients. *Neurology* 53, 1059–1063.

Desseigne, P., Bizouarn, P. and Le Teurnier, Y. (2001) Morbidity after cardiac surgery: impact of body-mass index and albumin. *Clinical Nutrition* 20, 15–16.

Detsky, A.S., McLaughlin, J.R., Baker, J.P., Johnston, N., Whittaker, S., Mendelson, R.A. and Jeejeebhoy, K.N. (1987) What is Subjective Global Assessment of nutritional status? *Journal of Parenteral and Enteral Nutrition* 11, 8–13.

de Vree, J.M.L., Romijn, J.A., Mok, K.S., Mathus-Vliegen, L.M.H., Stoutenbeek, C.P., Ostrow, J.D., Tytgat, G.N.J., Sauerwein, H.P., Elferink, R.P.J.O. and Groen, A.K. (1999) Lack of enteral nutrition during critical illness is associated with profound decrements in biliary lipid concentrations. *American Journal of Clinical Nutrition* 70, 70–77.

de Vries, E.G.E., Mulder, N.H., Houwen, B. and de Vries-Hospers, H.G. (1982) Enteral nutrition by nasogastric tube in adult patients treated with intensive chemotherapy for acute leukemia. *American Journal of Clinical Nutrition* 35, 1490–1496.

DeWys, W.D. (1986) Weight loss and nutritional abnormalities in cancer patients: incidence, severity and significance. *Clinics in Oncology* 5, 251–257.

DeWys, W.D., Begg, C., Lavin, P.T., Band, P.R., Bennett, J.M., Bertino, J.R., Cohen, M.H., Douglass, H.O., Engstrom, P.F., Ezdinli, E.Z., Horton, J., Johnson, G.J., Moertel, C.G., Oken, M.M., Perlia, C., Rosenbaum, C., Silverstein, M.N., Skeel, R.T., Sponzo, R.W. and Tormey, D.C. (1980) Prognostic effect of weight loss prior to chemotherapy in cancer patients. *American Journal of Medicine* 69, 491–497.

Dhanraj, P., Chacko, A., Mammen, M. and Bharathi, R. (1997) Hospital-made diet versus commercial supplement in postburn nutritional support. *Burns* 23, 512–514.

Dhoot, M.K., Gerogieva, C., Grottrup, T., Mahdavian, R. and Hindle, T. (1996) The management of clinical nutrition in NHS hospitals [MBA project]. *Journal of Clinical Nursing* 5, 399–400.

Dibley, M.J., Goldsby, J.B., Staehling, N.W. and Trowbridge, F.L. (1987) Development of normalised curves for the international growth reference: historical and technical considerations. *American Journal of Clinical Nutrition* 46, 736–748.

Dickersin, K., Scherer, R. and Lefebvre, C. (1994) Identifying relevant studies for systematic reviews. *British Medical Journal* 309, 1286–1291.

Dickson, T.M.C., Kusnierz-Glaz, C.R., Blume, K.G., Negrin, R.S., Hu, W.W., Shizuru, J.A., Johnston, L.L., Wong, R.M. and Stockerl-Goldstein, K.E. (1999) Impact of admission body weight and chemotherapy dose adjustment on the outcome of autologous bone marrow transplantation. *Biology of Blood and Marrow Transplantation* 5, 299–305.

Dietary Guidelines for Americans (1990) Government Printing Office (Publication no. 1990.261-463/2044), Washington, DC.

Dietary Guidelines for Americans (1995) Government Printing Office (Publication no. 1995.402.519). Washington, DC.

Doekel, R.C., Zwillich, C.W., Scoggin, C.H., Kryger, M. and Weil, J.V. (1976) Clinical semi-starvation: depression of hypoxic ventilatory response. *New England Journal of Medicine* 295, 358–361.

Dominioni, L. and Dionigi, R. (1987) Immunological function and nutritional assessment. *Journal of Parenteral and Enteral Nutrition* 11, 70S–72S.

Donahoe, M. and Rogers, R.M. (1990) Nutritional assessment and support in chronic obstructive pulmonary disease. *Clinics in Chest Medicine* 11, 487–504.

Donahoe, M., Rogers, R.M., Openbrier, D.R. and Wilson, D.O. (1989) Effect of calorie intake on muscle strength and walking distance in malnourished COPD. *American Reviews of Respiratory Disease* 139, A334.

Donahoe, M., Mancino, J., Costantino, J., Lebow, H. and Rogers, R.M. (1994) The effect of an aggressive nutritional support regimen on body composition in patients with severe COPD and weight loss. *American Journal of Respiratory and Critical Care Medicine* 149, A313.

Donaldson, S.S. (1984) Nutritional support as an adjunct to radiation therapy. *Journal of Parenteral and Enteral Nutrition* 8, 302–310.

Doshi, M.K., Lawson, R., Ingoe, L.E., Colligan, J.M., Barton, J.R. and Cobden, I. (1998) Effect of nutritional supplementation on clinical outcome in post-operative orthopaedic patients. *Clinical Nutrition* 17 (Suppl.), P05.

Douglass, H.O., Milliron, S., Nava, H., Eriksson, B., Thomas, P., Novick, A. and Holyoke, E.D. (1978) Elemental diet as an adjuvant for patients with locally advanced gastrointestinal cancer receiving radiation therapy: a prospectively randomized study. *Journal of Parenteral and Enteral Nutrition* 2, 682–686.

Dowd, P.S., Kelleher, J., Walker, B.E. and Guillou, P.J. (1986) Nutrition and cellular immunity in hospital patients. *British Journal of Nutrition* 55, 515–527.

Dowling, S., Mulcahy, F. and Gibney, M.J. (1990) Nutrition in the management of HIV antibody positive patients: a longitudinal study of dietetic out-patient advice. *European Journal of Clinical Nutrition* 44, 823–829.

Dreblow, D.M., Anderson, C.F. and Moxness, K. (1981) Nutritional assessment of orthopedic patients. *Mayo Clinical Proceedings* 56, 51–54.

Dresler, C.M., Jeevanandam, M. and Brennan, M.F. (1987) Metabolic efficacy of enteral feeding in malnourished cancer and noncancer patients. *Metabolism* 36, 82–88.

Dreyfuss, M.L., Msamanga, G.I., Spiegelman, D., Hunter, D.J., Urassam, E.J.N., Hertzmark, E. and Fawzi, W.W. (2001) Determinants of low birth weight among HIV-infected pregnant women in Tanzania. *American Journal of Clinical Nutrition* 74, 814–826.

Druml, W. (1993) Nutritional support in acute renal failure. *Clinical Nutrition* 12, 196–207.

Duche, M., Habes, D., Lababidi, A., Chardot, C., Wenz, J. and Bernard, O. (1999) Percutaneous endoscopic gastrostomy for continuous feeding in children with chronic cholestasis. *Journal of Pediatric Gastroenterology and Nutrition* 29, 42–45.

Duff, E.N. and Livingstone, M.B.E. (1997) A survey of nutrition knowledge, practice, attitudes and behaviour of general practitioner trainees in Ireland. *Journal of Human Nutrition and Dietetics* 10, 219–228.

Dulloo, A.G. (1997a) Human pattern of food intake and fuel-partitioning during weight recovery after starvation: a theory of autoregulation of body composition. *Proceedings of the Nutrition Society* 56, 25–40.

Dulloo, A.G. (1997b) Regulation of body composition during weight recovery: integrating the control of energy partitioning and thermogenesis. *Clinical Nutrition* 16, 25–35.

Dulloo, A.G., Jacquet, J. and Girardier, L. (1996) Autoregulation of body composition during weight recovery in humans: the Minnesota Experiment revisited. *International Journal of Obesity* 20, 393–405.

Dumler, F., Falla, P., Butler, R., Wagner, C. and Fancisco, K. (1999) Impact of dialysis modality and acidosis on nutritional status. *ASAIO Journal* 45, 413–417.

Dworkin, B.M., Wormser, G.P., Axelrod, F., Pierre, N., Schwarz, E. and Seaton, T. (1990) Dietary intake in patients with acquired immunodeficiency syndrome (AIDS), patients with AIDS-related complex and serologically positive human immunodeficiency virus patients: correlations with nutritional status. *Journal of Parenteral and Enteral Nutrition* 14, 605–609.

Eastwood, C., Davies, G.J. and Dettmar, P.W. (2001) The dietary intake of free-living and institutionalized elderly people. *Proceedings of the Nutrition Society* 60, 184A.

Eastwood, M. (1997) Hospital food [letter]. *New England Journal of Medicine* 336, 1261.

Edington, J., McMaster, C. and Macklin, J. (1994) Evaluation of a semi-elemental enteral feed in patients with malabsorption and/or disease-related malnutrition. *Journal of Human Nutrition and Dietetics* 7, 417–424.

Edington, J., Kon, P. and Martyn, C.N. (1996) Prevalence of malnutrition in patients in general practice. *Clinical Nutrition* 15, 60–63.

Edington, J., Kon, P. and Martyn, C.N. (1997) Prevalence of malnutrition after major surgery. *Journal of Human Nutrition and Dietetics* 10, 111–116.

Edington, J., Winter, P.D., Coles, S.J., Gale, C.R. and Martyn, C.N. (1999) Outcomes of undernutrition in patients in the community with cancer or cardiovascular disease. *Proceedings of the Nutrition Society* 58, 655–661.

Edington, J., Boorman, J., Durrant, E.R., Perkins, A., Giffin, C.V., James, R., Thomson, J.M., Oldroyd, J.C., Smith, J.C., Torrance, A.D., Blackshaw, V., Green, S., Hill, C.J., Berry, C., McKensie, C., Vicca, N., Ward, J.E. and Coles, S.J. (2000) Prevalence of malnutrition on admission to four hospitals in England. *Clinical Nutrition* 19, 191–195.

Efthimiou, J., Fleming, J., Gomes, C. and Spiro, S.G. (1988) The effect of supplementary oral nutrition in poorly nourished patients with chronic obstructive pulmonary disease. *American Review of Respiratory Disease* 137, 1075–1082.

Egger, M., Smith, G.D. and Altman, D.G. (2001) *Systematic Reviews in Health Care. Meta-analysis in Context*. British Medical Journal Books, London.

Ek, A.-C., Larsson, J., von Schenck, H., Thorslund, S., Unosson, M. and Bjurulf, P. (1990) The correlation between anergy, malnutrition and clinical outcome in an elderly hospital population. *Clinical Nutrition* 9, 185–189.

Ek, A.-C., Unosson, M., Larsson, J., Von Schenck, H. and Bjurulf, P. (1991) The development and healing of pressure sores related to the nutritional state. *Clinical Nutrition* 10, 245–250.

Elbers, M., Awwad, E., Scharfstadt, A., Drucke, D. and Lohlein, D. (1997) Effekte einer postoperativen, oralen, supplementaren, proteinreichen Substratzufuhr auf Korperzusammensetzung, Proteinstatus und Lebensqualitat bei Magenkarzinom-Patienten. *Aktuelle Ernaehrungsmedizin* 22, 69–75.

Elia, M. (1992a) Effect of starvation and very low calorie diets on protein–energy interrelationships in lean and obese subjects. In: Scrimshaw, N.S. and Schurch, B. (eds) *Protein–energy Interactions*. IDECG, Lausanne, pp. 249–284.

Elia, M. (1992b) An evaluation of two and more than two component models of body composition. *Clinical Nutrition* 11, 114–127.

Elia, M. (1993) Artificial nutritional support in clinical practice in Britain. *Journal of the Royal College of Physicians, London* 27, 8–15.

Elia, M. (1995) Changing concepts of nutrient requirements in disease: implications for artificial nutritional support. *Lancet* 345, 1279–1284.

Elia, M. (1996a) Special nutritional problems and the use of enteral and parenteral nutrition. In: Weatherall, D.J., Ledingham, J.G.G. and Warrell, D.A. (eds) *Oxford Textbook of Medicine*. Oxford Medical Publications, Oxford, pp. 1314–1326.

Elia, M. (Chairman and Editor) (1996b) *Report of the British Artificial Nutritional Survey (BANS)*. BAPEN, Maidenhead, Berkshire.

Elia, M. (1997a) Tissue distribution and energetics in weight loss and undernutrition. In: Kinney, J.M. and Tucker, H.N. (eds) *Physiology, Stress and Malnutrition: Functional Correlates and Nutritional Intervention*. Lippincott–Raven, Philadelphia, pp. 383–412.

Elia, M. (Chairman and Editor) (1997b) *Report of the British Artificial Nutritional Survey (BANS)*. BAPEN, Maidenhead.

Elia, M. (1999) *Malnutrition in the Community*. Malnutrition Advisory Group (an associate group of BAPEN), London.

Elia, M. (2000a) Hunger disease. *Clinical Nutrition* 19, 379–386.

Elia, M. (Chairman and Editor) (2000b) *Guidelines for Detection and Management of Malnutrition*. Malnutrition Advisory Group (MAG), Standing Committee of BAPEN, Maidenhead.

Elia, M. (2001a) Metabolic response to starvation, injury and sepsis. In: Payne-James, J., Grimble, G. and Silk, D. (eds) *Artificial Nutrition Support in Clinical Practice*. Greenwich Medical Media, London, pp. 1–24.

Elia, M. (2001b) Obesity in the elderly. *Obesity Research* 9 (Suppl. 4), 244S–248S.

Elia, M. and Jebb, S.A. (1992) Changing concepts of energy requirements in critically ill patients. *Current Medical Literature – Clinical Nutrition* 1, 35–38.

Elia, M. and Lunn, P.G. (1996) Biological markers of protein–energy malnutrition. *Clinical Nutrition* 16, 1–46.

Elia, M., Goren, A., Behrens, R., Barber, R.W. and Neale, G. (1987) Effect of total starvation and very low calorie diets on intestinal permeability in man. *Clinical Science* 73, 205–210.

Elia, M., Cottee, S., Holden, C., Micklewright, A., Pennington, C., Plant, J., Shaffer, J., Wheatley, C. and Wood, S. (1994) *Enteral and Parenteral Nutrition in the Community*. A report by a working party of the British Association for Parenteral and Enteral Nutrition, Maidenhead.

Elia, M. (Chairman and Editor), Micklewright, A., Russell, C.A., Stratton, R.J., Holden, C., Thomas, A., Wood, S., Shaffer, J., Meadows, N., Wheatley, C. and Scott, D. (1998) *Annual Report of the British Artificial Nutrition Survey*. BAPEN, Maidenhead.

Elia, M., Stubbs, R.J. and Henry, C.J.K. (1999) Differences in fat, carbohydrate, and protein metabolism between lean and obese subjects undergoing total starvation. *Obesity Research* 7, 597–604.

Elia, M. (Chairman), Russell, C.A., Stratton, R.J., Scott, D.W., Shaffer, J.L., Micklewright, A., Wood, S.R., Wheatley, C., Holden, C.E., Meadows, N.J., Thomas, A.G. and Jones, B.J.M. (2000a) *Trends in Home Artificial Nutrition Support in the UK during 1996–1999*. BAPEN, Maidenhead.

Elia, M., Ritz, P. and Stubbs, R.J. (2000b) Total energy expenditure in the elderly. *European Journal of Clinical Nutrition* 54, S92–S103.

Elia, M., Stratton, R.J., Holden, C., Meadows, N., Micklewright, A., Russell, C., Scott, D., Thomas, A., Shaffer, J., Wheatley, C. and Woods, S. Committee of the British Artifical Nutrition Survey (2001a) Home enteral tube feeding following cerebrovascular accident. *Clinical Nutrition* 20, 27–30.

Elia, M. (Chairman and Editor), Russell, C.A. (Editor) and Stratton, R.J. (Editor) (2001b) *Trends in Artificial Nutrition Support in the UK during 1996–2000*. Committee of the British Artificial Nutrition Survey, BAPEN, Maidenhead.

Elkort, R.J., Baker, F.L., Vitale, J.J. and Cordano, A. (1981) Long-term nutritional support as an adjunct to chemotherapy for breast cancer. *Journal of Parenteral and Enteral Nutrition* 5, 385–390.

Elmore, M.F., Gallagher, S.C., Jones, J.G., Koons, K.K., Schmalhausen, A.W. and Strange, P.S. (1989) Esophagogastric decompression and enteral feeding following cholecystectomy: a controlled, randomized prospective trial. *Journal of Parenteral and Enteral Nutrition* 13, 377–381.

Elmstahl, S. (1987) Energy expenditure, energy intake and body composition in geriatric long-stay patients. *Comprehensive Gerontology* 1, 118–125.

Elmstahl, S. and Steen, B. (1987) Hospital nutrition in geriatric long-term care medicine: II. Effects of dietary supplements. *Age and Ageing* 16, 73–80.

Elmstahl, S., Blabolil, V., Fex, G., Kuller, R. and Steen, B. (1987) Hospital nutrition in geriatric long-term care medicine I. Effects of a changed meal environment. *Comprehensive Gerontology* 1, 29–33.

Elmstahl, S., Persson, M., Andren, M. and Blabolil, V. (1997) Malnutrition in geriatric patients: a neglected problem? *Journal of Advanced Nursing* 26, 851–855.

Elwood, P.C. (1982) Randomised controlled trials: sampling. *British Journal of Clinical Pharmacology* 13, 631–636.

Eneroth, M., Apelqvist, J., Larsson, J. and Persson, B.M. (1997) Improved wound healing in trans-tibial amputees receiving supplementary nutrition. *International Orthopaedics* 21, 104–108.

Engel, B., Kon, P. and Raftery, M.J. (1995) Strategies to identify and correct malnutrition in hemodialysis patients. *Journal of Renal Nutrition* 5, 62–66.

Engelen, M.P.K.J., Schols, A.M.W.J., Baken, W.C., Wesseling, G.J. and Wouters, E.F.M. (1994) Nutritional depletion in relation to respiratory and peripheral skeletal muscle function in out-patients with COPD. *European Respiratory Journal* 7, 1793–1797.

Engelen, M.P.K.J., Schols, A.M.W.J., Lamers, R.J.S. and Wouters, E.F.M. (1999) Different patterns of chronic tissue wasting among patients with chronic obstructive pulmonary disease. *Clinical Nutrition* 18, 275–280.

Erens, B. and Primatesta, P. (1999) *Health Survey for England. Cardiovascular Disease '98*. Stationery Office, London.

Eriksson, J.G., Forsen, T., Tuomilehto, J., Winter, P.D., Osmond, C. and Barker, D.J.P. (1999) Catch-up growth in childhood and death from coronary heart disease: longitudinal study. *British Medical Journal* 318, 426–431.

Eriksson, L.I. and Sandin, R. (1996) Fasting guidelines in different countries. *Acta Anaesthesiologica Scandinavica* 40, 971–974.

European Commission (2001) *Key Data on Health 2000*. European Commission, Luxembourg.

Evans, W.K., Nixon, D.W., Daly, J.M., Ellenberg, S.S., Gardner, L., Wolfe, E., Shepherd, F.A., Feld, R., Gralla, R., Fine, S., Kemeny, N., Jeejeebhoy, K.N., Heymsfield, S. and Hoffman, F.A. (1987) A randomized study of oral nutritional support versus ad lib nutritional intake during chemotherapy for advanced colorectal and non-small cell lung cancer. *Journal of Clinical Oncology* 5, 113–124.

Everitt, B.S. and Pickles, A. (1999) *Statistical Aspects of the Design and Analysis of Clinical Trials*. Imperial College Press, London.

Fahal, I.H., Amad, R. and Edwards, R.H.T. (1995) Muscle weakness in continuous ambulatory peritoneal dialysis patients. *Peritoneal Dialysis International* 16, S419–S423.

Faintuch, J., Soriano, F.G., Ladeira, J.P., Janiszewski, M., Velasco, I.T. and Gama-Rodrigues, J.J. (2001) Refeeding procedures after 43 days of total fasting. *Nutrition* 17, 100–104.

Falch, J.A., Ilebekk, A. and Slungaard, U. (1985) Epidemiology of hip fractures in Norway. *Acta Orthopaedica Scandinavica* 56, 12–16.

Falconer, J.S., Fearon, K.C., Plester, C.E., Ross, J.A. and Carter, D.C. (1994) Cytokines, the acute-phase response, and resting energy expenditure in cachectic patients with pancreatic cancer. *Annals of Surgery* 219, 325–331.

Falconer, J.S., Fearon, K.C., Ross, J.A., Elton, R., Wigmore, S.J., Garden, O.J. and Carter, D.C. (1995) Acute-phase protein response and survival duration of patients with pancreatic cancer. *Cancer* 75, 2077–2082.

Fallowfield, L. (1996) Quality of quality-of-life data. *Lancet* 348, 421–422.

Fan, S.-T., Lo, C.-M., Lai, E.C.S., Chu, K.-M., Liu, C.-L. and Wong, J. (1994) Perioperative nutritional support in patients undergoing hepatectomy for hepatocellular carcinoma. *New England Journal of Medicine* 331, 1547–1552.

FAO/WHO/UNU (1985) *Energy and Protein Requirements*. Technical Report Series 724, WHO, Geneva.

Farthing, M. (1994) Malnutrition in the wards of the world. *Nutrition* 10, 424–425.

Faxén Irving, G.E., Olsson, B.A. and Cederholm, T. (1999) Nutritional and cognitive status in elderly subjects living in service flats and the effect of nutrition education on personnel. *Gerontology* 45, 187–194.

Faxén Irving, G.E., Basun, H., Wahlund, L.O. and Cederholm, T. (2000) Associations between changes in weight and in mini mental state examination in patients undergoing examination of the cognitive function. *Clinical Nutrition* 19 (Suppl.), 7.

Faxén Irving, G., Andrén-Olsson, B., af Geijerstam, A., Basun, H. and Cederholm, T. (2002) The effect of nutritional intervention in elderly subjects residing in group-living for the demented. *European Journal of Clinical Nutrition* 56, 221–227.

Fearon, K.C., Falconer, J.S., Slater, C., McMillan, D.C., Ross, J.A. and Preston, T. (1998) Albumin synthesis rates are not decreased in hypoalbuminemic cachectic cancer patients with an ongoing acute-phase protein response. *Annals of Surgery* 227, 249–254.

Fedje, L., Moore, L. and McNeely, M. (1996) A role for oral nutrition supplements in the malnutrition of renal disease. *Journal of Renal Nutrition* 6, 198–202.

Feilhauer, K., Schall, H. and Butters, M. (2000) Early postoperative nutrition in colorectal surgery: jejunal vs. parenteral feeding – a prospective randomised trial. *Clinical Nutrition* 19 (Suppl.), 57.

Feitelson Winkler, M., Gerrior, S.A., Pomp, A. and Albina, J.E. (1989) Use of retinol-binding protein and prealbumin as indicators of the response to nutrition therapy. *Journal of the American Dietetic Association* 89, 684–687.

Fell, J.M.E., Paintin, M., Arnaud-Battandier, F., Beattie, R.M., Hollis, A., Kitching, P., Donnet-Hughes, A., MacDonald, T.T. and Walker-Smith, J.A. (2000) Mucosal healing and a fall in mucosal pro-inflammatory cytokine mRNA induced by a specific oral polymeric diet in paediatric Crohn's disease. *Alimentary Pharmacology and Therapy* 14, 281–289.

Fellows, I.W., Macdonald, I.A., Bennett, T. and Allison, S.P. (1985) The effect of undernutrition on thermoregulation in the elderly. *Clinical Science* 69, 525–532.

Felson, D.T., Anderson, J.J. and Meenan, R.F. (1990) The comparative efficacy and toxicity of second-line drugs in rheumatoid arthritis. *Arthritis Rheumatism* 33, 1449–1461.

Fenton, J., Eves, A., Kipps, M. and O'Donnell, C. (1995) Menu changes and their effects on the nutritional content of menus and nutritional status of elderly, hospitalised, mental health patients. *Journal of Human Nutrition and Dietetics* 8, 395–409.

Ferguson, A. (1994) Immunological functions of the gut in relation to nutritional state and mode of delivery of nutrients. *Gut* (Suppl.1), S10–S12.

Ferguson, M. and Capra, S. (1998) Quality of life in patients with malnutrition. *Journal of the American Dietetic Association* 98, A-22.

Ferraris, R.P. and Carey, H.V. (2000) Intestinal transport during fasting and malnutrition. *Annual Review of Nutrition* 20, 195–219.

Ferreira, I.M., Brooks, D., Lacasse, Y. and Goldstein, R.S. (2000) Nutritional support for individuals with COPD: a meta-analysis. *Chest* 117, 672–678.

Ferro-Luzzi, A., Branca, F. and Pastore, G. (1994) Body mass index defines the risk of seasonal energy stress in the Third World. *European Journal of Clinical Nutrition* 48, S165–S178.

Fettes, S. (2000) An audit of the provision of parenteral nutrition in two acute hospitals: team v. non-team. *Proceedings of the Nutrition Society* 59, 155A.

Fettes, S.B., Richardson, R.A., Chen, R. and Pennington, C.R. (2001a) Nutritional status of elective gastrointestinal surgical patients pre- and post-operatively. *Proceedings of the Nutrition Society* 60, 118a.

Fettes, S.B., Richardson, R.A., Davidson, H.I. and Pennington, C.R. (2001b) Influence of gender on changes in nutritional status following major electrive gastrointestinal surgery. *Clinical Nutrition* 20 (Suppl.), 71.

Fiatarone, M.A., O'Neill, E.F., Doyle, N., Clements, K.M., Roberts, S.B., Kehayias, J.J., Lipsitz, L.A. and Evans, W.J. (1993) The Boston FICSIT study: the effects of resistance training and nutritional supplementation on physical frailty in the oldest old. *Journal of the American Geriatric Society* 41, 333–337.

Fiatarone, M.A., O'Neill, E.F., Ryan, N.D., Clements, K.M., Solares, G.R., Nelson, M.E., Roberts, S.B., Kehayias, J.J., Lipsitz, L.A. and Evans, W.J. (1994) Exercise training and nutritional supplementation for physical frailty in very elderly people. *New England Journal of Medicine* 330, 1769–1775.

Fiatarone Singh, M.A., Bernstein, M.A., Ryan, N.D., O'Neill, E.F., Clements, K.M. and Evans, W.J. (2000) The effect of oral nutritional supplements on habitual dietary quality and quantity in frail elders. *Journal of Nutrition, Health and Ageing* 4, 5–12.

Field, J., Stanga, Z., Lobo, D.N. and Allison, S.P. (2001) The effect of nutritional management on the mood of undernourished patients. *Proceedings of the Nutrition Society* 60, 82A.

Fietkau, R., Thiel, H.J., Iro, H., Ritcher, B., Senft, M., Robler, C., Kolb, S. and Sauer, R. (1989) Comparison between oral nutrition and enteral nutrition by percutaneous endoscopically guided gastrostomy (PEG) in patients with head and neck tumors treated by radiotherapy. *Strhlentherapie Onkologie* 165, 844–851.

Fietkau, R., Iro, H., Sailer, D. and Sauer, R. (1991) Percutaneous endoscopically guided gastrostomy in patients with head and neck cancer. *Recent Results Cancer Research* 121, 269–282.

Finch, H.E. and Lawson, M.S. (1993) Clinical trial of a paediatric enteral feed. *Journal of Human Nutrition and Dietetics* 6, 399–409.

Finch, S., Doyle, W., Lowe, C., Bates, C.J., Prentice, A., Smithers, G. and Clarke, P.C. (1998) *National Diet and Nutrition Survey*. Stationery Office, London.

Finestone, H.M., Greene-Finestone, L.S., Wilson, E.S. and Teasell, R.W. (1995) Malnutrition in stroke patients on the rehabilitation service and at follow-up: prevalence and predictors. *Archives of Physical Medicine and Rehabilitation* 76, 310–316.

Finocchiaro, C., Galletti, R., Rovera, G., Ferrari, A., Todros, L., Vuolo, A. and Balzola, F. (1997) Percutaneous endoscopic gastrostomy: a long term follow-up. *Nutrition* 13, 520–523.

Finucane, T.E., Christmas, C. and Travis, K. (1999) Tube feeding in patients with advanced dementia: a review of the evidence. *Journal of the American Medical Association* 282, 1365–1370.

Fischer, J. and Johnson, M.A. (1990) Low body weight and weight loss in the aged. *Journal of the American Dietetic Association* 90, 1697–1706.

Fiske, J. (1999) The National Diet and Nutrition Survey: people aged 65 years and over. Volume 2: Report of the Oral Health Survey. *Journal of Human Nutrition and Dietetics* 12, 467–468.

Flanagan, M. (2000) The physiology of wound healing. *Journal of Wound Care* 9, 299–300.

Fleck, A., Hawker, F., Wallace, P.I., Raines, G., Trotter, J., Ledingham, I.M. and Calman, K.C. (1985) Increased vascular permeability: a major cause of hypoalbuminaemia in disease and injury. *Lancet* i, 781–783.

Fletcher, J.P. and Little, J.M. (1986) A comparison of parenteral nutrition and early postoperative enteral feeding on the nitrogen balance after major surgery. *Surgery* 100, 21–24.

Flodin, L., Svensson, S. and Cederholm, T. (2000) Body mass index as a predictor of 1 year mortality in geriatric patients. *Clinical Nutrition* 19, 121–125.

Flynn, M.B. and Leightty, F.F. (1987) Preoperative outpatient nutritional support of patients with squamous cancer of the upper aerodigestive tract. *American Journal of Surgery* 154, 359–362.

Fogaca, H., Souza, H., Carneiro, A.J., Carvalho, A.T., Pimentel, M.L., Papelbaum, M., Elia, P. and Elia, C. (2000) Effects of oral nutritional supplementation on the intestinal mucosa of patients with AIDS. *Journal of Clinical Gastroenterology* 30, 77–80.

Fontana, M., Zuin, G., Plebani, A., Bastoni, K., Visconti, G. and Principi, N. (1999) Body composition in HIV-infected children: relations with disease progression and survival. *American Journal of Clinical Nutrition* 69, 1282–1286.

Ford, E., Williamson, D. and Liu, S. (1997) Weight change and diabetes incidence: findings from a national cohort of US adults. *American Journal of Epidemiology* 146, 214–222.

Foschi, D., Cavagna, G., Callioni, F., Morandi, E. and Rovati, V. (1986) Hyperalimentation of jaundiced patients on percutaneous transhepatic biliary drainage. *British Journal of Surgery* 73, 716–719.

Foskett, M., Kapembwa, M., Sedgwick, P. and Griffin, G.E. (1991) Prospective study of food intake and nutritional status in HIV infection. *Journal of Human Nutrition and Dietetics* 4, 149–154.

Foster, K.J., Brown, M.S., Alberti, K.G.M.M., Buchanan, R.B., Dewar, P., Karran, S.J., Price, C.P. and Wood, P.J. (1980) The metabolic effects of abdominal irradiation in man with and without dietary therapy with an elemental diet. *Clinical Radiology* 31, 13–17.

Foudraine, N.A., Weverling, G.J., van Gool, T., Roos, M.T.L., de Wolf, F., Koopmans, P.P., van den Broek, P.J., Meenhorst, P.L., van Leeuwen, R., Lange, J.M.A. and Reiss, P. (1998) Improvement of chronic diarrhoea in patients with advanced HIV-1 infection during potent antiretroviral therapy. *AIDS* 12, 35–41.

Franch-Arcas, G. (2001) The meaning of hypoalbuminaemia in clinical practice. *Clinical Nutrition* 20, 265–269.

Frankel, A.M. and Horowitz, G.D. (1989) Nasoduodenal tubes in short-stay cholecystectomy. *Surgery, Gynecology and Obstetrics* 168, 433–436.

Fraser, D., Keegan, M., Harvic, M., Venning, M.C. and Campbell, I.T. (1999) Energy balance in chronic haemodialysis. *Proceedings of the Nutrition Society* 58, 514–521.

French, A.M. and Merriman, S.H. (1999) Nutritional status of a brain-injured population in a long-stay rehabilitation unit: a pilot study. *Journal of Human Nutrition and Dietetics* 12, 35–42.

Friedenberg, F., Jensen, G., Gujral, N., Braitman, L.E. and Levine, G.M. (1997) Serum albumin is predictive of 30-day survival after percutaneous endoscopic gastrostomy. *Journal of Parenteral and Enteral Nutrition* 21, 72–74.

Friedmann, J.M., Jensen, G.L., Smiciklas-Wright, H. and McCamish, M.A. (1997) Predicting early nonelective hospital readmission in nutritionally compromised older adults. *American Journal of Clinical Nutrition* 65, 1714–1720.

Frost, P. and Bihari, D. (1997) The route of nutritional support in the critically ill: physiological and economical considerations. *Nutrition* 13, 58S–63S.

FSPEN (1996) Consensus statement and comments: perioperative artificial nutrition in elective adult surgery. *Clinical Nutrition* 15, 223–258.

Fuenzalida, C.E., Petty, T.L., Jones, M.L., Jarrett, S., Harbeck, R.J., Terry, R.W. and Hambidge, K.M. (1990) The immune response to short-term nutritional intervention in advanced chronic obstructive pulmonary disease. *American Review of Respiratory Disease* 142, 49–56.

Fuller, N.J., Jebb, S.A., Goldberg, G.R., Pullicino, E., Adams, C., Cole, T.J. and Elia, M. (1991) Inter-observer variability in the measurement of body composition. *European Journal of Clinical Nutrition* 45, 43–49.

Fung, E.B., Samson-Fang, L., Stallings, V.A., Conaway, M., Liptak, G., Henderson, R.C., Worley, G., O'Donnell, M., Calvert, R., Rosenbaum, P., Chumlea, W. and Stevenson, R.D. (2002) Feeding dysfunction is associated with poor growth and health status in children with cerebral palsy. *Journal of the American Dietetic Association* 102, 361–368, 373.

Gaare, J., Singer, P., Katz, D., Kirvela, O., Martinez, K. and Askanazi, J. (1991) Enteral supplementation in AIDS: an open trial. *FASEB Journal* 5, A1668.

Gabe, S.M. (2001) Gut barrier function and bacterial translocation in humans. *Clinical Nutrition* 20, 107–112.

Gabe, S.M., Patel, M., Grimble, G.K., Barclay, G.R., Williams, R., Bjarnason, I. and Silk, D.B.A. (1998a) Intestinal permeability in critical illness: relationship with severity of illness, splanchnic ischaemia and endotoxaemia. *Clinical Nutrition* 17 (Suppl.), 6.

Gabe, S.M., Patel, M., Grimble, G.K., Barclay, G.R., Williams, R., Bjarnason, I. and Silk, D.B.A. (1998b) Intestinal permeability in acute liver failure: relationship with severity of illness, splanchnic ischaemia and endotoxaemia. *Clinical Nutrition* 17 (Suppl.), 18–19.

Gabe, S.M., Patel, M., Grimble, G.K., Barclay, G.R., Williams, R., Bjarnason, I. and Silk, D.B.A. (1998c) Small bowel and colonic permeability in general ICU and acute liver failure patients: association with endotoxaemia. *Clinical Nutrition* 17 (Suppl.), 67.

Gadek, J.E., DeMichele, S.J., Karlstad, M.D., Pacht, E.R., Donahoe, M., Albertson, T.E., Hoozen, C.V., Wennberg, A.K., Nelson, J.L., Noursalehi, M. and Enteral Nutrition in ARDS Study Group (1999) Effect of enteral feeding with eicosapentaenoic acid, gamma-linolenic acid, and antioxidants in patients with acute respiratory distress syndrome. *Critical Care Medicine* 27, 1409–1420.

Galanos, A.N., Pieper, C.F., Cornoni-Huntley, J.C., Bales, C.W. and Fillenbaum, G.G. (1994) Nutrition and function: is there a relationship between body mass index and functional capabilities of community-dwelling elderly? *Journal of the American Geriatric Society* 42, 368–373.

Galanos, A.N., Pieper, C.F., Kussin, P.S., Winchell, M.T., Fulkerson, W.J., Harrell, F.E., Teno, J.M., Layde, P., Connors, A.F., Phillips, R.S. and Wenger, N.S. (1997) Relationship of body mass index to subsequent mortality among seriously ill hospitalized patients. *Critical Care Medicine* 25, 1962–1968.

Gales, B. and Gales, M. (1994) Nutritional support teams: a review of comparative trials. *Annals of Pharmacotherapy* 28, 227–235.

Galkowski, J., Silverstone, F.A., Brod, M. and Isaac, R.M. (1989) Use of a low carbohydrate with fiber enteral formula as a snack for elderly patients with type 2 diabetes. *Clinical Research* 37, Abstract.

Gall, M., Grimble, G., Reeve, N. and Thomas, S. (1998) Effect of providing fortified meals and between-meal snacks on energy and protein intake of hospital patients. *Clinical Nutrition* 17, 259–264.

Gallagher-Allred, C.R., Voss, A.C., Finn, S.C. and McCamish, M.A. (1996) Malnutrition and clinical outcomes: the case for medical nutrition therapy. *Journal of the American Dietetic Association* 96, 361–366, 369.

Galloway, P., McMillan, D.C. and Sattar, N. (2000) Effect of the inflammatory response on trace element and vitamin status. *Annals of Clinical Biochemistry* 37, 289–297.

Ganzoni, A., Heilig, P., Schonenberger, K., Hugli, O., Fitting, J.W. and Brandli, O. (1994) Hochkalorische Ernahrung bei chronischer obstruktiver Lungenkrankheit. *Schweizerische. Rundschau Medizin.* 83, 13–16.

Gariballa, S.E. (2000) Nutritional factors in stroke. *British Journal of Nutrition* 84, 5–17.

Gariballa, S.E. (2001) Malnutrition in hospitalized elderly patients: when does it matter? *Clinical Nutrition* 20, 487–491.

Gariballa, S.E., Parker, S.G., Taub, N. and Castleden, C.M. (1998a) A randomized, controlled, single-blind trial of nutritional supplementation after acute stroke. *Journal of Parenteral and Enteral Nutrition* 22, 315–319.

Gariballa, S.E., Parker, S.G., Taub, N. and Castleden, M. (1998b) Nutritional status of hospitalized acute stroke patients. *British Journal of Nutrition* 79, 481–487.

Garrel, D.R., Davignon, I. and Lopez, D. (1991) Length of care in patients with severe burns with or without early enteral nutritional support. *Journal of Burn Care and Rehabilitation* 12, 85–90.

Garrow, J.S. (1988) *Obesity and Related Diseases.* Churchill Livingstone, Edinburgh.

Garrow, J. (1994) Starvation in hospital. *British Medical Journal* 308, 934.

Gassull, M.A. (2001) New insights in nutritional therapy in inflammatory bowel disease. *Clinical Nutrition* 20 (Suppl.), 113–121.

Gebhardt, B.M. and Newberne, P.M. (1974) Nutrition and immunologic responsiveness: T-cell function in the offspring of lipotrope and protein-deficient rats. *Immunology* 26, 489–495.

Geerling, B., Badart-Smook, A., Stockbrugger, R. and Brummer, R. (1998a) Comprehensive nutritional status in patients with long-standing Crohn's disease currently in remission. *American Journal of Clinical Nutrition* 67, 919–926.

Geerling, B.J., Russel, M.G.V.M., Stockbrugger, R.W. and Brummer, R.-J.M. (1998b) Quality of life in patients with Crohn's disease in a double blind placebo controlled nutritional intervention study. *Gastroenterology* 114, G4031.

Geerling, B.J., van Deursen, C., Stockbrugger, R.W. and Brummer, R.-J.M. (1998c) Restoration of muscle strength after nutritional supplementation in patients with Crohn's disease in a double blind placebo controlled study. *Gastroenterology* 114, G4032.

Geerling, B., Badart-Smook, A., Stockbrugger, R. and Brummer, R. (2000a) Comprehensive nutritional status in recently diagnosed patients with inflammatory bowel disease compared with population controls. *European Journal of Clinical Nutrition* 54, 514–521.

Geerling, B.J., Badart-Smook, A., van Deursen, C., van Houwelingen, A.C., Russel, M.G.V.M., Stockbrugger, R.W. and Brummer, R.-J.M. (2000b) Nutritional supplementation with N-3 fatty acids and antioxidants in patients with Crohn's disease in remission: effects on antioxidant status and fatty acid profile. *Inflammatory Bowel Disease* 6, 77–84.

Geerlings, S. and Hoepelman, A. (1999) Immune dysfunction in patients with diabetes mellitus. *FEMS Immunology and Medical Microbiology.* 26, 259–265.

Gegerie, P., Bengoa, J.-M., Delmi, M., Rapin, C.-H., Loizeau, E. and Vasey, H. (1986) Enquête alimentaire après fracture du col du fémur: effet d'un supplement diététique sur les apports nutritionnels. *Schweizerische Rundschau Medizin (PRAXIS)* 75 (Suppl.), 933–935.

Geliebter, A.A. (1979) Effects of equicaloric loads of protein, fat, and carbohydrate on food intake in the rat and man. *Physiology and Behavior* 22, 267–273.

Gentile, M.G., Corradi, E., Manna, G.M. and Ciceri, R. (2000) Enteral nutrition in severely ill patients with anorexia nervosa. *Clinical Nutrition* 19, 44.

George, L. (1994) Starvation in hospital: screen patients on admission [letter]. *British Medical Journal* 308, 1369.

Gertner, J.M., Kaufman, F.R., Donfield, S.M., Sleeper, L.A., Shapiro, A.D., Howard, C., Gomperts, E.D. and Hilgartner, M.W. (1994) Delayed somatic growth and pubertal development in human immunodeficiency virus-infected hemophiliac boys: hemophilia growth and development study. *Journal of Pediatrics* 124, 896–902.

Ghignone, M. and Quintin, L. (1986) Malnutrition and respiratory function. *International Anesthesiology Clinics* 24, 65–74.

Gianotti, L., Braga, M., Radaelli, G., Mariani, L., Vignali, A. and Di Carlo, V. (1995) Lack of improvement of prognostic weight loss when combined with other parameters. *Nutrition* 11, 12–16.

Gianotti, L., Braga, M., Fortis, C., Soldini, L., Vignali, A., Colombo, S., Radaelli, G. and Di Carlo, V. (1999) A prospective, randomized clinical trial on perioperative feeding with arginine-, omega-3 fatty acid-, and RNA-enriched enteral diet: effect on host response and nutritional status. *Journal of Parenteral and Enteral Nutrition* 23, 314–320.

Gibert, C.L., Wheeler, D.A., Collins, G., Madans, M., Muurahainen, N., Raghavan, S.S. and Bartsch, G. (1999) Randomized, controlled trial of caloric supplements in HIV infection. *Journal of Acquired Immune Deficiency Syndromes* 22, 253–259.

Gibney, E.R. (2002) The physical, psychological and metabolic effects of nutritional depletion and subsequent repletion. PhD thesis, University of Cambridge, Cambridge.

Gibney, E., Elia, M., Jebb, S.A., Murgatroyd, P.R. and Jennings, G. (1997) Total energy expenditure in patients with small-cell lung cancer: results of a validated study using the bicarbonate-urea method. *Metabolism* 46, 1412–1417.

Gibney, E.R., Johnstone, A.M., Faber, P., Stubbs, R.J. and Elia, M. (2002a) Effect of different rates of weight loss in healthy lean men on total energy expenditure and physical activity. *Proceedings of the Nutrition Society* 61, 3A.

Gibney, E.R., Johnstone, A.M., Faber, P., Stubbs, R.J. and Elia, M. (2002b) Effect of different degrees of energy restriction on subjective and objective measurements of fatigue in healthy lean males. *Proceedings of the Nutrition Society* 61, 6A.

Gibney, E.R., Stratton, R.J., Johnstone, A.M., Faber, P., Stubbs, R.J. and Elia, M. (2002c) Effect of starvation and a very low energy diet (VLED) on subjective feelings of hunger in healthy lean males. *Proceedings of the Nutrition Society* 61, 27A.

Gillick, M.R. (2000) Rethinking the role of tube feeding in patients with advanced dementia. *New England Journal of Medicine* 342, 206–210.

Gillin, J.S., Shike, M., Alcock, N., Urmacher, C., Krown, S., Kurtz, R.C., Lightdale, C.J. and Winawer, S.J. (1985) Malabsorption and mucosal abnormalities of the small intestine in the acquired immunodeficiency syndrome. *Annals of Internal Medicine* 102, 619–622.

Giner, M., Laviano, A., Meguid, M.M. and Gleason, J.R. (1996) In 1995 a correlation between malnutrition and poor outcome in critically ill patients still exists. *Nutrition* 12, 23–29.

Godfrey, K.M., Barker, D.J.P. and Osmond, C. (1994) Disproportionate fetal growth and raised IgE concentration in adult life. *Clinical and Experimental Allergy* 24, 641–648.

Godoy, I., Castro E Silva, M.H., Togashi, R.H., Geraldo, R.R.C. and Campana, A.O. (2000) Is chronic hypoxemia in patients with chronic obstructive pulmonary disease associated with more marked nutritional deficiency? *Journal of Nutrition, Health and Aging* 4, 102–108.

Gogos, C.A., Ginopoulos, P., Salsa, B., Apostolidou, E., Zoumbos, N.C. and Kalfarentzos, F. (1998) Dietary omega-3 polyunsaturated fatty acids plus vitamin E restore immunodeficiency and prolong survival for severely ill patients with generalized malignancy. *Cancer* 82, 395–402.

Goldner, M.G. and Spergel, G. (1972) On the transmission of alloxan diabetes and other influences. *Advances in Metabolic Disorders* 6, 57–72.

Goldstein, S.A., Thomashow, B.M., Kvetan, V., Askanazi, J., Kinney, J.M. and Elwyn, D.H. (1988) Nitrogen and energy relationships in malnourished patients with emphysema. *American Review of Respiratory Disease* 138, 636–644.

Gomez, F., Ramos-Galvan, R., Frenk, S., Munoz, J.C., Chavez, R. and Vasquez, J. (1956) Mortality in second and third degree malnutrition. *Journal of Tropical Paediatrics* 8, 1–5.

González-Gross, M., Marcos, A. and Pietrzik, K. (2001) Nutrition and cognitive impairment in the elderly. *British Journal of Nutrition* 86, 313–321.

Gonzalez-Huix, F., de Leon, R., Fernandez-Banares, F., Esteve, M., Cabre, E., Acero, D., Abad-Lacruz, A., Figa, M., Guilera, M., Planas, R. and Gassull, M.A. (1993) Polymeric enteral diets as primary treatment of active Crohn's disease: a prospective steroid controlled trial. *Gut* 34, 778–782.

Goode, H.F., Burns, E. and Walker, B.E. (1992) Vitamin C depletion and pressure sores in elderly patients with femoral neck fracture. *British Medical Journal* 305, 925–926.

Goodson, W.H., Jensen, J.A., Granja-Mena, L., Lopez-Sarmiento, A., West, J. and Chavez-Estrella, J. (1987) The influence of a brief pre-operative illness on post-operative healing. *Annals of Surgery* 205, 250–255.

Goodwin, J.S. (1989) Social, psychological and physical factors affecting the nutritional status of elderly subjects: separating cause and effect. *American Journal of Clinical Nutrition* 50, 1201–1209.

Gopalan, S., Saran, S. and Sengupta, R. (2000) Practicalities of nutrition support in chronic liver disease. *Current Opinion in Clinical Nutrition and Metabolic Care* 3, 227–229.

Gorsky, R.D. and Calloway, D.H. (1983) Activity pattern changes with decrease in food energy intake. *Human Biology* 55, 577–586.

Gosker, H.R., Wouters, E.F.M., van der Vusse, G.J. and Schols, A.M.W.J. (2000) Skeletal muscle dysfunction in chronic obstructive pulmonary disease and chronic heart failure: underlying mechanisms and therapy perspectives. *American Journal of Clinical Nutrition* 71, 1033–1047.

Gosling, P., Shearman, C.P., Gwynn, B.R., Simms, M.H. and Bainbridge, E.T. (1988) Microproteinuria: response to operation. *British Medical Journal* 296, 338–339.

Gottschlich, M.M., Jenkins, M., Warden, G.D., Baumer, T., Havens, P., Snook, J.T. and Alexander, J.W. (1990) Differential effects of three enteral dietary regimens on selected outcome variables in burn patients. *Journal of Parenteral and Enteral Nutrition* 14, 225–236.

Götzsche, P.C., Podenphant, J., Olesen, M. and Halberg, P. (1992) Meta-analysis of second-line antirheumatic drugs: sample size bias and uncertain benefit. *Journal of Clinical Epidemiology* 45, 587–594.

Gower-Rousseau, C., Salomez, J.L., Dupas, J.L., Marti, R., Nuttens, M.C., Votte, A., Lemahieu, M., Lemaire, B., Colombel, J.F. and Cortot, A. (1994) Incidence of inflammatory bowel disease in northern France (1988–1990). *Gut* 35, 1433–1438.

Grahm, T.W., Zadrozny, D.B. and Harrington, T. (1989) The benefits of early jejunal hyperalimentation in the head-injured patient. *Neurosurgery* 25, 729–735.

Grant, A.D. and De Cock, K.M. (2001) HIV infection and AIDS in the developing world: ABC of AIDS. *British Medical Journal* 322, 1475–1478.

Grantham-McGregor, S. (2002) Linear growth retardation and cognition. *Lancet* 359, 542.

Grantham-McGregor, S.M., Waker, S.P. and Chang, S. (2000) Nutritional deficiencies and later behavioural development. *Proceedings of the Nutrition Society* 59, 47–54.

Grau Carmona, T., Calvo Herranz, E., Zubillaga Munoz, S., Casado Hoces, S., Blas Obispo, B. and Ayuso Murillo, D. (1996) Influence of gastrointestinal complications of enteral nutrition on caloric intake in critically ill patients. *Clinical Nutrition* 15, 47.

Gray-Donald, K. (1995) The frail elderly: meeting the nutritional challenges. *Journal of the American Dietetic Association* 95, 538–540.

Gray-Donald, K., Gibbons, L., Shapiro, S.H. and Martin, J.G. (1989) Effect of nutritional status on exercise performance in patients with chronic obstructive pulmonary disease. *American Review of Respiratory Disease* 140.

Gray-Donald, K., Payette, H., Boutier, V. and Page, S. (1994) Evaluation of the dietary intake of home-bound elderly and the feasibility of dietary supplementation. *Journal of the American College of Nutrition* 13, 277–284.

Gray-Donald, K., Payette, H. and Boutier, V. (1995) Randomized clinical trial of nutritional supplementation shows little effect on functional status among free-living elderly. *Journal of Nutrition* 125, 2965–2971.

Gray-Donald, K., Gibbons, L., Shapiro, S.H., Macklem, P.T. and Martin, J.G. (1996) Nutritional status and mortality in chronic obstructive pulmonary disease. *American Journal of Respiratory and Critical Care Medicine* 153.

Gray-Donald, L. K., Carrey, Z. and Martin, J.G. (1998) Postprandial dyspnea and malnutrition in patients with chronic obstructive pulmonary disease. *Clinical and Investigative Medicine* 21, 135–141.

Green, C.J. (1995) Nutritional support in HIV infection and AIDS. *Clinical Nutrition* 14, 197–212.

Green, C.J. (1999) Existence, causes and consequences of disease-related malnutrition in the hospital and the community, and clinical and financial benefits of nutritional intervention. *Clinical Nutrition* 18 (Suppl. 2), 3–28.

Green, C.J. (2001a) The cost effectiveness of nutritional support. In: Payne-James, J., Grimble, G.K. and Silk, D.B.A. (eds) *Artificial Nutrition Support in Clinical Practice*, 2nd edn. Greenwich Medical Media, London, pp.733–757.

Green, C.J. (2001b) Fibre in enteral nutrition. *Clinical Nutrition* 20 (Suppl.), 23–39.

Green, C.J., Campbell, I., McClelland, P., Hutton, J., Ahmed, M., Helliwell, T., Wilkes, R., Gilbertson, A. and Bone, J. (1995) Energy and nitrogen balance and changes in mid upper-arm circumference with multiple organ failure. *Nutrition* 11, 739–746.

Green, J.H. and Muers, M.F. (1991) The thermic effect of food in underweight patients with emphysematous chronic obstructive pulmonary disease. *European Respiratory Journal* 4, 813–819.

Green, S.M., Winterberg, H., Franks, P.J., Moffatt, C.J., Eberhardie, C. and McLaren, S. (1999) Dietary intake of adults, with and without pressure sores, treated by community nursing staff. *Proceedings of the Nutrition Society* 58, 140A.

Greene, H.L., Slonim, A.E. and Burr, I.M. (1980) Type I glycogen storage disease: five years of management with nocturnal intragastric feeding. *Journal of Pediatrics* 96, 590–595.

Greene, H.L., Helinek, G.L., Folk, C.C., Courtney, M., Thompson, S., MacDonell, R.C. and Lukens, J.N. (1981) Nasogastric tube feeding at home: a method for adjunctive nutritional support of malnourished patients. *American Journal of Clinical Nutrition* 34, 1131–1138.

Greer, A., McBride, D.H. and Shenkin, A. (1986) Comparison of the nutritional state of new and long-term patients in a psychogeriatric unit. *British Journal of Psychiatry* 149, 738–741.

Gregory, J., Foster, K., Tyler, H. and Wiseman, M. (1990) *The Dietary and Nutritional Survey of British Adults*. Office of Population Censuses and Surveys, Her Majesty's Stationery Office, London.

Gregory, J., Lowe, S., Bates, C.J., Prentice, A., Jackson, L.V., Smithers, G., Wenlock, R. and Farron, M. (1994) *National Diet and Nutrition Survey: People Aged 4 to 18 Years.* Stationery Office, London.

Gretebeck, R.J. and Boileau, R.A. (1998) Self-reported energy intake and energy expenditure in elderly women. *Journal of the American Dietetic Association* 98, 574–576.

Griep, M., van der Niepen, P., Sennesael, J., Mets, T., Massart, D. and Verbeelen, D. (1997) Odour perception in chronic renal disease. *Nephrology, Dialysis and Transplantation* 12, 2093–2098.

Griep, M.I., Mets, T.F., Collys, K., Ponjaert-Kristoffersen, I. and Massart, D.L. (2000) Risk of malnutrition in retirement homes elderly persons measured by the 'Mini-Nutritional Assessment'. *Journal of Gerontology* 55A, M57–M63.

Griffiths, A.M., Ohlsson, A., Sherman, P.M. and Sutherland, L.R. (1995) Meta-analysis of enteral nutrition as a primary treatment of active Crohn's disease. *Gastroenterology* 108, 1056–1067.

Griffiths, R.D., Jones, C. and Palmer, T.E.A. (1997) Six-month outcome of critically ill patients given glutamine-supplemented parenteral nutrition. *Nutrition* 13, 295–302.

Groos, S., Hünefeld, G. and Luciano, L. (1996) Parenteral versus enteral nutrition: morphological changes in human adult intestinal mucosa. *Journal of Submicroscopic Cytology and Pathology* 28, 62–74.

Groot-Loonen, J.J., Otten, B.J., van't Hof, M.A., Lippens, R.J.J. and Stoelinga, G.B.A. (1995) Chemotherapy plays a major role in the inhibition of catch-up growth during maintenance therapy for childhood acute lymphoblastic leukaemia. *Pediatrics* 96, 693–695.

Grunfeld, C. (1995) What causes wasting in AIDS? *New England Journal of Medicine* 333, 123–124.

Grunfeld, C., Pang, M., Shimizu, L. and Shigenaga, J.K. (1992) Resting energy expenditure, caloric intake and short-term weight change in human immunodeficiency virus infection and the acquired immunodeficiency syndrome. *American Journal of Clinical Nutrition* 55, 455–460.

Guedon, C., Schmitz, J., Lerebours, E., Metayer, J., Audran, E., Hemet, J. and Colin, R. (1986) Decreased brush border hydrolase activities without gross morphologic changes in human intestinal mucosa after prolonged total parenteral nutrition of adults. *Gastroenterology* 90, 373–378.

Guedon, C., Ducrotte, P., Hochain, P., Zalar, A., Dechelotte, P., Denis, P. and Colin, R. (1996) Does percutaneous endoscopic gastrostomy prevent gastro-oesophageal reflux during the enteral feeding of elderly patients? *Clinical Nutrition* 15, 179–183.

Guenter, P., Muurahainen, N., Simons, G., Kosok, A., Cohan, G.R., Rudenstein, R. and Turner, J.L. (1993) Relationships among nutritional status, disease progression and survival in HIV infection. *Journal of Acquired Immune Deficiency Syndromes* 6, 1130–1138.

Guigoz, Y. and Vellas & Garry, P. (1994) Mini Nutritional Assessment (MNA): a practical tool for grading the nutritional state of elderly patients. *Facts and Research in Gerontology* (Suppl 2.), 15–59.

Guinard, J.-X. and Brun, P. (1998) Sensory-specific satiety: comparison of taste and texture effects. *Appetite* 31, 141–157.

Gungor, E.T., Aydintug, S., Arat, M., Demirer, S., Balci, D. and Akan, H. (2001) Identifying malnutrition and its effects in patients who are to receive hematopoietic stem cell transplantation. *Clinical Nutrition* 20 (Suppl.), 61.

Guo, C.-B. (1994) Applicability of the general nutritional status score to patients with oral and maxillofacial malignancies. *International Journal of Oral and Maxillofacial Surgery* 23, 167–169.

Gupta, A. (1999) The treatment of pressure ulcers. *Geriatric Medicine* 12, 35–37.

Ha, T.K.K., Sattar, N., Talwar, D., Cooney, J., Simpson, K., O'Reilly, D.S.T. and Lean, M.E.J. (1996) Abnormal antioxidant vitamin and carotenoid status in chronic renal failure. *Quarterly Journal of Medicine* 89, 765–769.

Haalboom, J.R.E. (2000a) A new century without pressure ulcers? *British Journal of Nursing* 9, S4, S6.

Haalboom, J.R.E. (2000b) The Dutch experience of pressure ulcers – a personal view. *Journal of Wound Care* 9, 121–122.

Hackett, A.F., Yeung, C.K. and Hill, G.L. (1979) Eating patterns in patients recovering from major surgery – a study of voluntary food intake and energy balance. *British Journal of Surgery* 66, 415–418.

Hadfield, R.J., Sinclair, D.G., Houldsworth, P.E. and Evans, T.W. (1995) Effects of enteral and parenteral nutrition on gut mucosal permeability in the critically ill. *American Journal of Respiratory and Critical Care Medicine* 152, 1545–1548.

Hadley, M.N., Grahm, T.W., Harrington, T., Schiller, W.R., McDermott, M.K. and Ponillico, D.B. (1986) Nutritional support and neurotrauma: a critical review of early nutrition in forty-five acute head injury patients. *Neurosurgery* 19, 367–373.

Haffejee, A.A. and Angorn, I.B. (1977) Oral alimentation following intubation for esophageal carcinoma. *Annals of Surgery* 186, 759–761.

Haffejee, A.A. and Angorn, I.B. (1979) Nutritional status and the nonspecific cellular and humoral immune response in esophageal carcinoma. *Annals of Surgery* 189, 475–479.

Hak, L.J., Leffell, M.S., Lamanna, R.W., Teasley, K.M., Bazzarre, C.H. and Mattern, W.D. (1982) Reversal of skin test anergy during maintenance hemodialysis by protein and calorie supplementation. *Americal Journal of Clinical Nutrition* 36, 1089–1092.

Hall, C. and Myers, A. (2000) Does the input of a hospital/community liaison nurse improve the quality of care for home parenteral nutrition patients? *Proceedings of the Nutrition Society* 59, 170A.

Hall, D.B.M. (1996) *Health for All Children*, 3rd edn. Oxford University Press, Oxford.

Hall, K., Whiting, S.J. and Comfort, B. (2000) Low nutrient intake contributes to adverse clinical outcomes in hospitalized elderly patients. *Nutrition Reviews* 58, 214–217.

Hallameesch, M.M., Deutz, N.E.P. and Soeters, P.B. (1998) Increased lactulose/rhamnose ratio during fluid administration is caused by increased renal lactulose excretion. *Clinical Nutrition* 17 (Suppl.), 1.

Haller, J. (1999) The vitamin status and its adequacy in the elderly: an international overview. *International Journal for Vitamin and Nutrition Research* 69, 160–168.

Hamaoui, E., Lefkowitz, R., Olender, L., Krasnopolsky-Levine, E., Favale, M., Webb, H. and Hoover, E.L. (1990) Enteral nutrition in the early postoperative period: a new semi-elemental formula versus total parenteral nutrition. *Journal of Parenteral and Enteral Nutrition* 14, 501–507.

Hammerlid, E., Wirblad, B., Sandin, C., Mercke, C., Eström, S., Kaasa, S., Sullivan, M. and Westin, T. (1998) Malnutrition and food intake in relation to quality of life in head and neck cancer patients. *Head and Neck* 20, 540–548.

Hanger, H.C., Smart, E.J., Merrilees, M.J. and Frampton, C.M. (1999) The prevalence of malnutrition in elderly hip fracture patients. *New Zealand Medical Journal* 112, 88–90.

Hankard, R., Bloch, J., Martin, P., Randrianasolo, H., Bannier, M.F., Machinot, S. and Cézard, J.P. (2001) État et risque nutritionnel de l'enfant hospitalisé. *Archives de Pédiatrie* 8, 1203–1208.

Hankey, C. and Wynne, H. (1996) An audit of meal provision in an elderly care hospital. *International Journal of Quality of Health Care* 8, 375–382.

Hankey, C.R., Summerbell, J. and Wynne, H.A. (1993) The effect of dietary supplementation in continuing-care elderly people: nutritional, anthropometric and biochemical parameters. *Journal of Human Nutrition and Dietetics* 6, 317–322.

Hanning, R.M., Blinkie, C.J.R., Bar-Or, O., Lands, L.C., Moss, L.A. and Wilson, W.M. (1993) Relationships among nutritional status and skeletal and respiratory muscle function in cystic fibrosis: does early dietary supplementation make a difference? *American Journal of Clinical Nutrition* 57, 580–587.

Hansbrough, W.B. and Hansbrough, J.F. (1993) Success of immediate intragastric feeding of patients with burns. *Journal of Burn Care and Rehabilitation* 14, 512–516.

Harley, J.R., Pohl, S.L. and Isaac, R.M. (1989) Low carbohydrate with fiber versus high carbohydrate without fiber enteral formulas: effect on blood glucose excursion in patients with type II diabetes. *Clinical Research* 37, 141A.

Harries, A.D., Jones, L.A., Danis, V., Fifield, R., Heatley, R.V., Newcombe, R.G. and Rhodes, J. (1983) Controlled trial of supplemented oral nutrition in Crohn's disease. *Lancet* i, 887–890.

Harries, A.D., Danis, V.A. and Heatley, R.V. (1984) Influence of nutritional status on immune functions in patients with Crohn's disease. *Gut* 25, 465–472.

Harris, C.E., Griffiths, R.D., Freestone, N., Billington, D., Atherton, S.T. and Macmillan, R.R. (1992) Intestinal permeability in the critically ill. *Intensive Care Medicine* 18, 38–41.

Harrison, J., McKiernan, J. and Neuberger, J.M. (1997) A prospective study on the effect of recipient nutritional status on outcome in liver transplantation. *Transplantation International* 10, 369–374.

Harrison, L. (1997) Nutritional status of patients admitted for elective surgery. *Proceedings of the Nutrition Society* 56, 265A.

Hart, J. and Reeves, J. (1996) *Adult Enteral and Parenteral Nutrition Guidelines for Dietitians in Training*. British Dietetic Association, Birmingham.

Hartley, G.H. (2001) Nutritional status, delaying progression and risks associated with protein restriction. *EDTNA ERCA Journal* 27, 101–104.

Hartley, G.H., Lawrence, I.R., Brown, A.L., Tapson, J.S. and Wilkinson, R. (1997) The nutritional assessment of renal patients. *Proceedings of the Nutrition Society* 56, 272A.

Hartwell, H. and Edwards, J. (2002) Comparison of mean energy intake between eating situations in a NHS hospital – a pilot study. *Proceedings of the Nutrition Society* (in press).

Harty, J., Boulton, H., Heelis, N., Uttley, L., Venning, M. and Gokal, R. (1993) Limitations of kinetic models as predictors of nutritional and dialysis adequacy in continuous ambulatory peritoneal dialysis patients. *American Journal of Nephrology* 13, 454–463.

Harvard School of Public Health, on behalf of the WHO and the World Bank (1996) *Global Health Statistics: a Compendium of Incidence, Prevalence and Mortality Estimates for over 200 Conditions.* Harvard University Press, Boston.

Hasse, J., Strong, S., Gorman, M.A. and Liepa, G. (1993) Subjective global assessment: alternative nutrition-assessment technique for liver-transplant candidates. *Nutrition* 9, 339–343.

Hasse, J.M., Blue, L.S., Liepa, G.U., Goldstein, R.M., Jennings, L.W., Mor, E., Husberg, B.S., Levy, M.F., Gonwa, T.A. and Klintmalm, G.B. (1995) Early enteral nutrition support in patients undergoing liver transplantation. *Journal of Parenteral and Enteral Nutrition* 19, 437–443.

Hattevig, G., Kjellman, B., Sigurs, N. and Kjellman, N.-I. (1989) The effect of maternal avoidance of eggs, cow's milk and fish during lactation upon allergic manifestations in infants. *Clinical Allergy* 19, 27–32.

Hausel, J., Nygren, J., Lagerkranser, M., Hellström, P.M., Hammarqvist, F., Almström, C., Lindh, A., Thorell, A. and Ljungqvist, O. (2001) A carbohydrate-rich drink reduces preoperative discomfort in elective surgery patients. *Anesthesia Analgesia* 93, 1344–1350.

Hawkins, C. (2000) Anorexia and anxiety in advanced malignancy: the relative problem. *Journal of Human Nutrition and Dietetics* 13, 113–117.

Haydock, D.A. and Hill, G.L. (1986) Impaired wound healing in surgical patients with varying degrees of malnutrition. *Journal of Parenteral and Enteral Nutrition* 10, 550–554.

Haydock, D.A. and Hill, G.L. (1987) Improved wound healing response in surgical patients receiving intravenous nutrition. *British Journal of Surgery* 74, 320–323.

Hayes, R., Kanga, J.F., Craigmyle, L. and D'Angelo, S. (1995) Nocturnal oral supplementation (NOS) in patients with cystic fibrosis (CF). *Pediatric Pulmonology 20* (Suppl). 12, 266.

Heald, A.E. and Schiffman, S.S. (1997) Taste and smell: neglected senses that contribute to the malnutrition of AIDS. *North Carolina Medical Journal* 58, 100–104.

Health Advisory Service 2000 (1998) *Not Because They Are Old – An Independent Inquiry into the Care of Older People on Acute Wards in General Hospitals.* Health Advisory Service, London.

Hearne, B.E., Dunaj, J.M., Daly, J.M., Strong, E.W., Vikram, B., LePorte, B.J. and DeCosse, J.J. (1985) Enteral nutrition support in head and neck cancer: tube vs. oral feeding during radiation therapy. *Continuing Education* 85, 669–675.

Hebuterne, X., Broussard, J.-F. and Rampal, P. (1995) Acute renutrition by cyclic enteral nutrition in elderly and younger patients. *Journal of American Medical Association* 273, 638–643.

Hebuterne, X., Schneider, S., Peroux, J.L. and Rampal, P. (1997) Effects of refeeding by cyclic enteral nutrition on body composition: comparative study of elderly and younger patients. *Clinical Nutrition* 16, 283–289.

Heel, K.A., Kong, S.E., Maccauley, R.D., Erber, W.N. and Hall, J.C. (1998) The effect of minimum luminal nutrition on mucosal cellularity and immunity of the gut. *Journal of Gastroenterology and Hepatology* 13, 1015–1019.

Heffernan, A. and Moloney, M. (2000) Patient satisfaction and food wastage in private hospital: a comparison with two public hospitals. *Proceedings of the Nutrition Society* 59, 74A.

Heibert, J.M., Brown, A., Anderson, R.G., Halfacre, S., Rodeheaver, G.T. and Edlich, R.F. (1981) Comparison of continuous vs. intermittent tube feedings in adult burn patients. *Journal of Parenteral and Enteral Nutrition* 5, 73–76.

Heilbronn, L.K., Noakes, M. and Clifton, P.M. (2001) Energy restriction and weight loss on very-low-fat diets reduce C-reactive protein concentrations in obese, healthy women. *Arteriosclerosis, Thrombosis and Vascular Biology* 21, 968–970.

Heimburger, O., Qureshi, A.R., Blaner, W.S., Berglund, L. and Stenvinkel, P. (2000) Hand-grip muscle strength, lean body mass, and plasma proteins as markers of nutritional status in patients with chronic renal failure close to start of dialysis therapy. *American Journal of Kidney Diseases* 36, 1213–1225.

Heithoff, K.A., Cuffel, B.J., Kennedy, S. and Peters, J. (1997) The association between body mass and health care expenditure. *Clinical Therapeutics* 19, 811–820.

Hellerstein, M.K., Pelfini, A., Hoa, R., Clinton, R., Faix, R., Richards, E.W., Abbruzzese, B.C., McCamish, M.A. and Cope, F.O. (1994) A fully randomised, prospective, double-blind short-term trial contrasting the use of a novel enterotropic peptide-based formula and the current standard of practice enteral formula in HIV and AIDS patients: evaluation of multiple clinical parameters. *Journal of Parenteral and Enteral Nutrition* 18, 25S.

Henderson, R.A. and Saavedra, J.M. (1995) Nutritional considerations and management of the child with human immunodeficiency virus infection. *Nutrition* 11, 121–128.

Henderson, R.A., Saavedra, J.M., Perman, J.A., Hutton, N., Livingston, R.A. and Yolken, R.H. (1994) Effect of enteral tube feeding on growth of children with symptomatic human immunodeficiency virus infection. *Journal of Pediatric Gastroenterology and Nutrition* 18, 429–434.

Hendricks, K.M., Duggan, C., Gallagher, L., Carlin, A.C., Richardson, D.S., Collier, S.B., Simpson, W. and Lo, C. (1995) Malnutrition in hospitalised pediatric patients. *Archives of Pediatric and Adolescent Medicine* 149, 1118–1122.

Hendrikse, W.H., Reilly, J.J. and Weaver, L.T. (1997) Malnutrition in a children's hospital. *Clinical Nutrition* 16, 13–18.

Henry, C., Sayoum, T., Lightowler, H. and Woo, J. (2001) Effect of flavour enhancers on food intake in hospitalized elderly patents in Hong Kong. *Proceedings of the Nutrition Society* 60, 237A.

Henry, C.J.K. (2001) The biology of human starvation: some new insights. *British Nutrition Foundation Nutrition Bulletin* 26, 205–211.

Henry, C.J.K. and Ulijaszek, S.J. (1996) *Long-term Consequences of Early Environment: Growth, Development and the Lifespan Developmental Perspective.* Press Syndicate of the University of Cambridge, Cambridge.

Herselman, M., Moosa, M.R., Kotze, T.J., Kritzinger, M., Wuister, S. and Mostert, D. (2000) Protein–energy malnutrition as a risk factor for increased morbidity in long-term hemodialysis patients. *Journal of Renal Nutrition* 10, 7–15.

Heslin, M.J. and Brennan, M.F. (2000) Advances in perioperative nutrition: cancer. *World Journal of Surgery* 24, 1477–1485.

Heslin, M.J., Latkany, L., Leung, D., Brooks, A.D., Hochwald, S.N., Pisters, P.W.T., Shike, M. and Brennan, M.F. (1997) A prospective, randomized trial of early enteral feeding after resection of upper gastrointestinal malignancy. *Annals of Surgery* 226, 567–580.

Hess, M. (1997) Taste: the neglected nutritional factor. *Journal of the American Dietetic Association* 97, S205–S207.

Hessov, I. (1977) Energy and protein intake in elderly patients in an orthopedic surgical ward. *Acta Chirurgica Scandinavica* 43, 145–149.

Hessov, I. (2000) Oral dietary supplements before and after surgery [letter]. *Nutrition* 16, 776.

Hetherington, M.M. (1998) Taste and appetite regulation in the elderly. *Proceedings of the Nutrition Society* 57, 625–631.

Heuschkel, R.B., Menache, C.C., Megerian, J.T. and Baird, A.E. (2000) Enteral nutrition and corticosteroids in the treatment of acute Crohn's disease in children. *Journal of Pediatric Gastroenterology and Nutrition* 31, 8–15.

Hey, S. (1996) Pressure sore care and cure [letter]. *Lancet* 348, 1511.

Heyland, D.K., MacDonald, S., Keefe, L. and Drover, J.W. (1998) Total parenteral nutrition in the critically ill patient: a meta-analysis. *Journal of the American Medical Association* 280, 2013–2019.

Heyland, D.K., Montalvo, M., MacDonald, S., Keefe, L., Yao Su, X. and Drover, J.W. (2001a) Total parenteral nutrition in the surgical patient: a meta-analysis. *Canadian Journal of Surgery* 44, 102–111.

Heyland, D.K., Novak, F., Drover, J.W., Jain, M., Su, X. and Suchner, U. (2001b) Should immunonutrition become routine in critically ill patients? A systematic review of the evidence. *Journal of the American Medical Association* 286, 944–953.

Heylen, A.M., Lybeer, M.B., Penninckx, F.M., Kerremans, R.P. and Frost, P.G. (1987) Parenteral versus needle jejunostomy nutrition after total gastrectomy. *Clinical Nutrition* 6, 131–136.

Heyligenberg, R., Romijn, J.A., Hommes, M.J.T., Endert, E., Eeftinck Schattenkerk, J.K.M. and Sauerwein, H.P. (1993) Insulin mediated and non-insulin mediated glucose uptake in HIV-infected men. *Clinical Science* 84, 209–216.

Heymsfield, S.B., Bethel, R.A., Ansley, J.D., Gibbs, D.M., Felner, J.M. and Nutter, D.O. (1978) Cardiac abnormalities in cachectic patients before and during nutritional repletion. *American Heart Journal* 95, 584–593.

Heymsfield, S.B., Hoff, R.D., Gray, T.F., Galloway, J. and Casper, K. (1988) Heart disease. In: Kinney, J., Jeejeebhoy, K., Hill, G. and Owen, O. (eds) *Nutrition and Metabolism in Patient Care*. W.B. Saunders, Philadelphia, pp. 477–509.

Heys, S.D. and Wahle, K.W.J. (2001) Targeted nutrition in the critically ill: a therapeutic modality for the new millenium. *Nutrition* 17, 57–58.

Heys, S.D., Walker, L.G., Smith, I. and Eremin, O. (1999) Enteral nutritional supplementation with key nutrients in patients with critical illness and cancer: a meta-analysis of randomised, controlled clinical trials. *Annals of Surgery* 229, 467–477.

Hill, G.L., Blackett, R.L., Pickford, I., Burkinshaw, L., Young, G.A., Warren, J.V., Schorah, C.J. and Morgan, D.B. (1977) Malnutrition in surgical patients: an unrecognised problem. *Lancet* i, 689–692.

Hill, S.A., Nielsen, M.S. and Lennard-Jones, J.E. (1995) Nutritional support in intensive care units in England and Wales: a survey. *European Journal of Clinical Nutrition* 49, 371–378.

Hirsch, S., de Obaldia, N., Petermann, M., Rojo, P., Barrientos, C., Iturriaga, H. and Bunout, D. (1991) Subjective global assessment of nutritional status: further validation. *Nutrition* 7, 35–38.

Hirsch, S., Bunout, D., De La Maza, P., Iturriaga, H., Petermann, M., Icazar, G., Gattas, V. and Ugarte, G. (1993) Controlled trial on nutrition supplementation in outpatients with symptomatic alcoholic cirrhosis. *Journal of Parenteral and Enteral Nutrition* 17, 119–124.

Hodgson, L., Ghattas, H., Pritchitt, H., Schwenk, A. and Macallan, D. (2001) Nutritional demographics in an HIV outpatients clinic. *Clinical Nutrition* 20 (Suppl.), 72.

Hoensch, H.P., Steinhardt, H.J., Weiss, G., Haug, D., Maier, A. and Malchow, H. (1984) Effects of semisynthetic diets on xenobiotic metabolizing enzyme activity and morphology of small intestinal mucosa in humans. *Gastroenterology* 86, 1519–1530.

Hogarth, M.B., Marshall, P., Lovat, L.B., Palmer, A.J., Frost, C.G., Fletcher, A.E., Nicholl, C.G. and Bulpitt, C.J. (1996) Nutritional supplementation in elderly medical in-patients: a double-blind placebo-controlled trial. *Age and Ageing* 25, 453–457.

Hogg, R.S., Zadra, J.N., Chan-Yan, C., Voigt, R., Craib, K.J.P., Korosi-Ronco, J., Montaner, J.S.G. and Schechter, M.T. (1995) Analysis of nutritional intake in a cohort of homosexual men. *Journal of Acquired Immune Syndromes and Human Retrovirology* 9, 162–167.

Hoh, R., Pelfini, A., Neese, R.A., Chan, M., Cello, J.P., Cope, F.O., Abbruzese, B.C., Richards, E.W., Courtney, K. and Hellerstein, M.K. (1998) De novo lipogenesis predicts short-term body composition response by bioelectrical impedance analysis to oral nutritional supplements in HIV-associated wasting. *American Journal of Clinical Nutrition* 68, 154–163.

Holden, C.E., Puntis, J.W.L., Charlton, C.P.L. and Booth, I.W. (1991) Nasogastric feeding at home: acceptability and safety. *Archives of Diseases in Childhood* 66, 148–151.

Hollander, D., Vadheim, C.M., Brettholz, E., Petersen, G.M., Delahunty, T. and Rotter, J.I. (1986) Increased intestinal permeability in patients with Crohn's disease and their relatives: a possible etiologic factor. *Annals of Internal Medicine* 105, 883–885.

Hollis, J. and Henry, C. (2001) 7-day food intake in an Oxfordshire residential home for the elderly. *Proceedings of the Nutrition Society* 60, 226A.

Holmes, S. (1993) Food avoidance in patients undergoing cancer chemotherapy. *Support Care Cancer* 1, 326–330.

Holmes, S. and Dickerson, J. (1991) Food intake and quality of life in cancer patients. *Journal of Nutritional Medicine* 2, 359–368.

Hommes, M.J.T., Romijn, J.A., Godfried, M.H., Eeftinck Schattenkerk, J.K.M., Buurman, W.A., Endert, E. and Sauerwein, H.P. (1990) Increased resting energy expenditure in HIV-infected men. *Metabolism* 39, 1186–1190.

Hommes, M.J.T., Romijn, J.A., Endert, E. and Sauerwein, H.P. (1991a) Resting energy expenditure and substrate oxidation in human immunodeficiency virus (HIV)-infected asymptomatic men: HIV affects host metabolism in the early asymptomatic stage. *American Journal of Clinical Nutrition* 54, 311–315.

Hommes, M.J.T., Romijn, J.A., Endert, E., Eeftinck Schattenkerk, J.K.M. and Sauerwein, H.P. (1991b) Basal fuel homeostasis in symptomatic immunodeficiency virus (HIV) infection. *Clinical Science* 80, 359–365.

Hommes, M.J.T., Romijn, J.A., Endert, E., Eeftinck Schattenkerk, J.K.M. and Sauerwein, H.P. (1991c) Insulin sensitivity and insulin clearance in HIV infected men. *Metabolism* 40, 651–656.

Hoover, H.C., Ryan, J.A., Anderson, E.J. and Fischer, J.E. (1980) Nutritional benefits of immediate postoperative jejunal feeding of an elemental diet. *American Journal of Surgery* 139, 153–159.

Howard, J., Jonkers, C., Lochs, H., Lerebours, W., Meier, R., Messing, B. and Soeters, P. (1999) Survey to establish the current status of artificial nutritional support in Europe. *Clinical Nutrition* 18, 179–188.

Howard, L., Ament, M., Fleming, C.R., Shike, M. and Steiger, E. (1995) Current use and clinical outcome of home parenteral and enteral nutrition therapies in the United States. *Gastroenterology* 109, 355–365.

Howard, P. and Bowen, N. (2001) The challenges of innovation in the organization of home enteral tube feeding. *Journal of Human Nutrition and Dietetics* 14, 3–11.

Howell, D.C. (1997) *Statistical Methods for Psychology*, 4th edn, pp. 490–493.

Howell, W.H. (1998) Anthropometry and body composition analysis. In: Matarese, L.E. and Gottschlich, M.M. (eds) *Contemporary Nutrition Support Practice. A Clinical Guide.* W.B. Saunders, Philadelphia, pp. 33–46.

Huang, Y.C. (2001) Malnutrition in the critically ill. *Nutrition* 17, 263–264.

Huang, Y.C., Yen, C.E., Cheng, C.H., Jih, K.S. and Kan, M.N. (2000) Nutritional status of mechanically ventilated critically ill patients: comparison of different types of nutritional support. *Clinical Nutrition* 19, 101–107.

Hubsch, S., Volkert, D., Oster, P. and Schlief, G. (1994) [Benefits and limits of liquid nutritional supplements in the treatment of malnutrition in geriatric patients]. *Aktuelle Ernaehrungsmedizin* 19, 109–114.

Hugli, O., Schutz, Y. and Fitting, J.W. (1996) The daily energy expenditure in stable chronic obstructive pulmonary disease. *American Journal of Respiratory and Critical Care Medicine* 153, 294–300.

Huitema, B.A. (1980) *The Analysis of Covariance and Alternatives.* John Wiley & Sons, New York.

Hull, M.A., Rawlings, J., Murray, F.E., Field, J., McIntyre, A.S., Mahida, Y.R., Hawkey, C.J. and Allison, S.P. (1993) Audit of outcome of long-term enteral nutrition by percutaneous endoscopic gastrostomy. *Lancet* 341, 869–872.

Hulshof, T., de Graaf, C. and Westrate, J.A. (1993) The effects of preloads varying in physical state and fat content on satiety and energy intake. *Appetite* 21, 273–286.

Hulst, J.M., Albers, M.J., Meinardi, M., Tibboel, D. and Joosten, K.F. (2001) Assessment of nutritional status of pediatric intensive care patients: a national cross-sectional study. *Clinical Nutrition* 20 (Suppl.), 22.

Hunt, D.R., Rowlands, B.J. and Johnston, D. (1985) Hand grip strength – a simple prognostic indicator in surgical patients. *Journal of Parenteral and Enteral Nutrition* 9, 701–704.

Huxley, R.R., Shiell, A.W. and Law, C.M. (2000) The role of size at birth and postnatal catch-up growth in determining systolic blood pressure: a systematic review of the literature. *Journal of Hypertension* 18, 815–831.

Iida, K., Kadota, J., Kawakami, K., Shirai, R., Abe, K., Yoshinaga, M., Iwashita, T., Matsubara, Y., Ishimatsu, Y., Ohmagari, K. and Ohno, S. (1999) Immunological function and nutritional status in patients with hepatocellular carcinoma. *Hepato-Gastroenterology* 46, 2476–2482.

Ikizler, T.A., Wingard, R.L., Harvell, J., Shyr, Y. and Hakim, R.M. (1999) Association of morbidity with markers of nutrition and inflammation in chronic hemodialysis patients: a prospective study. *Kidney International* 55, 1945–1951.

Incalzi, R.A., Gemma, A., Capparella, O., Cipriani, L., Landi, R. and Carbonin, P. (1996) Energy intake and in-hospital starvation: a clinically relevant relationship. *Archives of Internal Medicine* 156, 425–429.

Incalzi, R.A., Pedone, C., Onder, G., Pahor, M. and Carbonin, P.U., for the GIFA. (2001) Predicting length of stay of older patients with exacerbated chronic obstructive pulmonary disease. *Aging Clinical Experimental Research* 13, 49–57.

Inelmen, E.M., Jiminez, G.F., Gatto, M.R.A., Miotto, F., Sergi, G., Maccari, T., Gonzalez, A.M., Maggi, S., Peruzza, S., Pisent, C. and Enzi, G. (2000) Dietary intake and nutritional status in Italian elderly subjects. *Journal of Nutrition, Health and Aging* 4, 91–101.

Institute of Medicine (1990) *Nutrition During Pregnancy.* National Academy of Sciences Press, Washington, DC.

Iovinelli, G., Marsili, I. and Varrassi, G. (1993) Nutrition support after total laryngectomy. *Journal of Parenteral and Enteral Nutrition* 17, 445–448.

Iqbal, T.H., Lewis, K.O., Gearty, J.C. and Cooper, B.T. (1996) Small intestinal permeability to mannitol and lactulose in the three ethnic groups resident in West Birmingham. *Gut* 39, 199–203.

Irwin, M.M. and Openbrier, D.R. (1985) Effects of supplemental nasoenteric tube feeding in patients with COPD: a pilot study. *American Review of Respiratory Disease* 131, 165A.

Ivanovic, D.M., Leiva, B.P., Perez, H.T., Inzunza, N.B., Almagia, A.F., Toro, T.D., Urrutia, M.S.C., Cervilla, J.O. and Bosch, E.O. (2000) Long-term effects of severe undernutrition during the first year of life on brain development and learning in Chilean high-school graduates. *Nutrition* 16, 1056–1063.

Jackson, A. (2001) Human nutrition in medical practice: the training of doctors. *Proceedings of the Nutrition Society* 60, 257–263.

Jackson, H.S., Wicks, V.C., Forbes, G. and Williams, R. (1996) Nutritional assessment and status of liver transplant candidates. *Proceedings of the Nutrition Society* 56, 187A.

Jackson, W.D. and Grand, R.J. (1991) The human intestinal response to enteral nutrients: a review. *Journal of the American College of Nutrition* 10, 500–509.

Jadad, A.R., Moore, A., Carroll, D., Jenkinson, C., Reynolds, D.J.M., Gavaghan, D.J. and McQuay, H.J. (1996) Assessing the quality of reports of randomized clinical trials: is blinding necessary? *Controlled Clinical Trials* 17, 1–12.

Jager, K.J., Merkus, M.P., Huisman, R.M., Boeschoten, E.W., Dekker, F.W., Korevaar, J.C., Tijssen, J.G.P. and Kredict, R.T. (2001) Nutritional status over time in hemodialysis and peritoneal dialysis. *Journal of the American Society of Nephrology* 12, 1272–1279.

Jager-Wittenaar, H., Vork, F.C., Van Loon, A.J. and Klingenberg, J. (2000) Protocol for home treatment of hyperemesis gravidarum with nasogastric tube feeding. *Clinical Nutrition* 19 (Suppl.), 59.

Jagoe, R.T., Goodship, T.H.J. and Gibson, G.J. (2001a) Nutritional status of patients undergoing lung cancer operations. *Annals of Thoracic Surgery* 71, 929–935.

Jagoe, R.T., Goodship, T.H.J. and Gibson, G.J. (2001b) The influence of nutritional status on complications after operations for lung cancer. *Annals of Thoracic Surgery* 71, 936–943.

Jallut, D., Tappy, L., Kohut, M., Bloesch, D., Munger, R., Schutz, Y., Chiolero, R., Felber, J.-P., Livio, J.-J. and Jequier, E. (1990) Energy balance in elderly patients after surgery for a femoral neck fracture. *Journal of Parenteral and Enteral Nutrition* 14, 563–568.

James, W.P.T. and Ralph, A. (eds) (1992) *The Functional Significance of Low Body Mass Index.* Nestlé Foundation, Rome, Italy.

James, W.P.T., Ferro-Luzzi, A. and Waterlow, J.C. (1988) Definition of chronic energy deficiency in adults. *European Journal of Clinical Nutrition* 42, 969–981.

James, W.P.T., Leach, R., Kalamara, E. and Shayeghi, M. (2001) The worldwide obesity epidemic. *Obesity Research* 9 (Suppl. 4), 228S–233S.

Jamieson, C.P., Norton, B., Day, T., Lakeman, M. and Powell-Tuck, J. (1997) The quantitative effect of nutrition support on quality of life in outpatients. *Clinical Nutrition* 16, 25–28.

Jamieson, C.P., Obeid, O.A. and Powell-Tuck, J. (1999) The thiamin, riboflavin and pyridoxine status of patients on emergency admission to hospital. *Clinical Nutrition* 18, 87–91.

Januszkiewicz, A., Essen, P., McNurlan, M.A., Garlick, P.J., Ringden, O. and Wernerman, J. (1998) Stress hormone infusion decreases protein synthesis of circulating human T lymphocytes. *Clinical Nutrition* 17 (Suppl.), 2.

Jawaheer, G., Shaw, N.J., Lloyd, D.A. and Pierro, A. (1996) Minimal enteral feeding promotes gallbladder contractility in neonates. *Proceedings of the Nutrition Society* 56, 148A.

Jawaheer, G., Shaw, N.J. and Pierro, A. (2001) Continuous enteral feeding impairs gallbladder emptying in infants. *Journal of Pediatrics* 138, 822–825.

Jebb, S. (1997) Energy metabolism in cancer and human immunodeficiency virus infection. *Proceedings of the Nutrition Society* 56, 763–775.

Jeejeebhoy, K.N. (1984) Nutrition and serum albumin levels. *Nutrition* 10, 353.

Jeejeebhoy, K.N. (1988a) Bulk or bounce – the object of nutritional support. *Journal of Parenteral and Enteral Nutrition* 12, 539–549.

Jeejeebhoy, K.N. (1988b) The functional basis of assessment. In: Kinney, J.M., Jeejeebhoy, K.N., Hill, G.L. and Owen, O.E. (eds) *Nutrition and Metabolism in Patient Care.* W.B. Saunders, Philadelphia, pp. 739–751.

Jeejeebhoy, K.N. and Sole, M. (2001) Nutrition and the heart. *Clinical Nutrition* 20 (Suppl. 1), 181–186.

Jelalian, E., Stark, L.J., Reynolds, L. and Seifer, R. (1998) Nutrition intervention for weight gain in cystic fibrosis: a meta analysis. *Journal of Pediatrics* 132, 486–492.

Jenkins, M.E., Gottschlich, M.M. and Warden, G.D. (1994) Enteral feeding during operative procedures in thermal injuries. *Journal of Burn Care and Rehabilitation* 15, 199–205.

Jennings, G. and Elia, M. (1991) Independent effects of protein and energy deficiency on acute-phase protein response in rats. *Nutrition* 7, 430–434.

Jennings, G. and Elia, M. (1994) Effect of dietary restriction on the response of α_2-macroglobulin during an acute phase response. *Journal of Parenteral and Enteral Nutrition* 18, 510–515.

Jennings, G., Bourgeouis, C. and Elia, M. (1992a) The magnitude of the acute phase protein response, and its relationship to the degree of protein deficiency in the rat. *Journal of Nutrition* 22, 1325–1331.

Jennings, G., Cruickshank, A.M., Shenkin, A., Wight, D.G. and Elia, M. (1992b) Effect of aseptic abscesses in protein deficient rats on the relationship between interleukin-6 and the acute phase protein α_2-macroglobulin. *Clinical Science* 83, 731–735.

Jensen, J.E., Jensen, T.G., Smith, T.K., Johnston, S.A. and Dudrick, S.J. (1982) Nutrition in orthopaedic surgery. *Journal of Bone and Joint Surgery* 64A, 1263–1272.

Jensen, M.B. and Hessov, I.B. (1997) Dietary supplementation at home improves the regain of lean body mass after surgery. *Nutrition* 13, 422–430.

Jensen, S. (1985) Clinical effects of enteral and parenteral nutrition preceding cancer surgery. *Medical Oncology and Tumor Pharmacotherapy* 2, 225–229.

Jensen, T.T. and Juncker, Y. (1987) Pressure sores common after hip operations. *Acta Orthopaedica Scandinavica* 58, 209–211.

Jiminez-Exposito, M.J., Garcia-Lorda, P., Alonso-Villaverde, C., De Virgala, C.M., Sola, R., Masana, L., Arija, V., Iacquierdo, V. and Salas-Salvado, J. (1998) Effect of malabsorption on nutritional status and resting energy expenditure in HIV-infected patients. *AIDS* 12, 1965–1972.

Johansen, K.L., Chertow, G.M., Ng, A.V., Mulligan, K., Carchy, S., Schoenfeld, P.Y. and Kent-Braun, J.A. (2000) Physical activity levels in patients on hemodialysis and healthy sedentary controls. *Kidney International* 57, 2564–2570.

Johnson, R., Smiciklas-Wright, H., Soucy, I. and Rizzo, J. (1995) Nutrient intake of nursing-home residents receiving puréed foods of a regular diet. *Journal of American Geriatric Society* 43, 344–348.

Johnston, J.D., Harvey, C.J., Menzies, I.S. and Treacher, D.F. (1996) Gastrointestinal permeability and absorptive capacity in sepsis. *Critical Care Medicine* 24, 1144–1149.

Jones, A. (2001) Causes and effects of chronic obstructive pulmonary disease. *British Journal of Nursing* 10, 845–850.

Jones, E., Hughes, R.E. and Davies, H.E.F. (1988) Intake of vitamin C and other nutrients by elderly patients receiving a hospital diet. *Journal of Human Nutrition and Dietetics* 1, 347–353.

Joosten, E., Vanderelst, B. and Pelemans, W. (1999) The effect of different diagnostic criteria on the prevalence of malnutrition in a hospitalized geriatric population. *Aging Clinical and Experimental Research* 11, 390–394.

Jose, D.G., Stutman, O. and Good, R.A. (1973) Long term effects on immune function of early nutritional deprivation. *Nature* 241, 57–58.

Joy, M.B. and Halling, J.F. (1998) Factors related to the absence or presence of pressure ulcers and the degree of pressure ulcer involvement in long term care. *Journal of the American Dietetic Association* 98, A93.

Juni, P., Witschi, A., Bloch, R. and Egger, M. (1999) The hazards of scoring the quality of clinical trials for meta analysis. *Journal of the American Medical Association* 282, 1064–1060.

Kalfarentzos, F., Kehagias, J., Mead, N., Kokkinis, K. and Gogos, C.A. (1997) Enteral nutrition is superior to parenteral nutrition in severe acute pancreatitis: results of a randomized prospective trial. *British Journal of Surgery* 84, 1665–1669.

Kalfarentzos, F., Tsamandas, A. and Lymperopoulou, D. (1999) Apoptosis in cases of malnutrition: the beneficial effect of artificial nutrition. *Clinical Nutrition* 18 (Suppl. 1), 4.

Kalnins, D., Durie, P.R., Corey, M., Ellis, L., Pencharz, P. and Tullis, E. (1996) Are oral dietary supplements effective in the nutritional management of adolescents and adults with CF? *Pediatric Pulmonology* 22 (Suppl. 11), 314–315.

Kamath, S.K., Lawler, M., Smith, A.E., Kalat, T. and Olson, R. (1986) Hospital malnutrition: a 33-hospital screening study. *Journal of the American Dietetic Association* 86, 203–206.

Kaminski, M.V.J., Haase, T.J., Rosas, M. and Butler, G. (1990) [Letter – response to McGeer, Detsky and O'Rourke (1990)] Parenteral nutrition in cancer patients undergoing chemotherapy – a meta-analysis. *Nutrition* 6, 336–337.

Kaminsky, V.M. and Deitel, M. (1975) Nutritional support in the management of external fistulas of the alimentary tract. *British Journal of Surgery* 62, 100–103.

Kang, A., Zamora, S.A., Scott, R.B. and Parsons, H.G. (1998) Catch-up growth in children treated with home enteral nutrition. *Pediatrics* 102, 951–955.

Kanwar, S., Elhasani, S., Murchan, P.M., Perry, S., Windsor, A.C.J., Somers, S.S., Guillou, P.J. and Reynolds, J.V. (1998a) Effect of malnutrition on gut permeability and septic outcome following major surgery. *Journal of Parenteral and Enteral Nutrition* 22 (Suppl.), S3.

Kanwar, S., Elhasani, S., Murchan, P.M., Perry, S., Windsor, A.C.J., Somers, S.S., Guillou, P.J. and Reynolds, J.V. (1998b) Lack of correlation between failure of gut barrier function and septic complications following major upper gastro-intestinal surgery. *Journal of Parenteral and Enteral Nutrition* 22 (Suppl.), S3.

Kapembwa, M.S., Bridges, C., Joseph, A.E.A., Fleming, S.C., Batman, P. and Griffin, G.E. (1990) Ileal and jejunal absorptive function in patients with AIDS and enterococcidial infection. *Journal of Infection* 21, 43–53.

Karlsson, A. and Nordstrom, G. (2001) Nutritional status, symptoms experienced and general state of health in HIV-infected patients. *Journal of Clinical Nursing* 10, 609–617.

Kashirskaja, N., Hill, C.M., Ilangovan, P., Kapranov, N., Simonova, O., Shabalova, L. and Rolles, C.J. (1996) The relative contribution of optimal nutritional support in cystic fibrosis. *Journal of the Royal Society of Medicine* 89, 48–50.

Katakity, M., Webb, J.F. and Dickerson, J.W.T. (1983) Some effects of a food supplement in elderly hospital patients: a longitudinal study. *Human Nutrition: Applied Nutrition* 37A, 85–93.

Kauffman, C.A., Jones, P.G. and Kluger, M.J. (1986) Fever and malnutrition: endogenous pyrogen/interleukin-1 in malnourished patients. *American Journal of Clinical Nutrition* 44, 449–452.

Kaysen, G.A. (1999) Inflammation nutritional state and outcome in end stage renal disease. *Mineral and Electrolyte Metabolism* 25, 242–250.

Keane, E.M., Healy, M., O'Moore, R., Coakley, D. and Walsh, J.B. (1995) Hypovitaminosis D in the healthy elderly. *British Journal of Clinical Practice* 49, 301–303.

Kearns, P.J., Young, H., Garcia, G., Blaschke, T., O'Hanlon, G., Rinki, M., Sucher, K. and Gregory, P. (1992) Accelerated improvement of alcoholic liver disease with enteral nutrition. *Gastroenterology* 102, 200–205.

Keating, J., Bjarnason, I., Somasundaram, S., Macpherson, A., Francis, N., Price, A.B., Sharpstone, D., Smithson, J., Menzies, I.S. and Gazzard, B.G. (1995) Intestinal absorptive capacity, intestinal permeability and jejunal histology in HIV and their relation to diarrhoea. *Gut* 37, 623–629.

Keele, A.M., Bray, M.J., Emery, P.W., Duncan, H.D. and Silk, D.B.A. (1997) Two phase randomised controlled clinical trial of postoperative oral dietary supplements in surgical patients. *Gut* 40, 393–399.

Keim, N.L., Luby, M.H., Braun, S.R., Martin, A.M. and Dixon, R.M. (1986) Dietary evaluation of outpatients with chronic obstructive pulmonary disease. *Journal of the American Dietetic Association* 86, 902–906.

Keith, M.E. and Jeejeebhoy, K.N. (1997) Immunonutrition. *Baillière's Clinical Endocrinology and Metabolism* 11, 709–738.

Keithley, J.K. and Swanson, B. (2001) Oral nutritional supplements in human immunodeficiency virus disease: a review of the evidence. *Nutrition in Clinical Practice* 16, 98–104.

Keithley, J.K., Zeller, J.M., Szeluga, D.J. and Urbanski, P.A. (1992) Nutritional alterations in persons with HIV infection. *Image: Journal of Nursing Scholarship* 24, 183–189.

Kelleher, J., Mascie-Taylor, B.J., Davison, A.M., Bruce, G. and Losowsky, M.S. (1983) Vitamin status in patients on maintenance haemodialysis. *International Journal of Vitamin and Nutrition Research* 53, 330–337.

Keller, H.H. (1993) Malnutrition in institutionalized elderly: how and why? *Journal of American Geriatric Society* 41, 1212–1218.

Kelly, I.E., Tessier, S., Cahill, A., Morris, S.E., Crumley, A., McLaughlin, D., McKee, R.F. and Lean, M.E.J. (2000) Still hungry in hospital: identifying malnutrition in acute hospital admissions. *Quarterly Journal of Medicine* 93, 93–98.

Kelly, L. (1999) Audit of food wastage: differences between a plated and bulk system of meal provision. *Journal of Human Nutrition and Dietetics* 12, 415–424.

Kelly, S.M., Rosa, A., Field, S., Coughlin, M., Shizgal, H.M. and Macklem, P.T. (1984) Inspiratory muscle strength and body composition in patients receiving total parenteral nutrition therapy. *American Review of Respiratory Diseases* 130, 33–37.

Kemen, M., Senkal, M., Homann, H.-H., Mumme, A., Dauphin, A.-K., Baier, J., Windeler, J., Neumann, H. and Zumtobel, V. (1995) Early postoperative enteral nutrition with arginine, omega-3 fatty acids and ribonucleic acid-supplemented diet versus placebo in cancer patients: an immunologic evaluation of Impact. *Critical Care Medicine* 23, 652–659.

Kendell, B.D., Fonseca, R.J. and Lee, M. (1982) Postoperative nutritional supplementation for the orthognathic surgery patient. *Journal of Oral and Maxillofacial Surgery* 40, 205–213.

Kennedy, M., McCombie, L., Dawes, P., McConnell, K.N. and Dunnigan, M.G. (1997) Nutritional support for patients with intellectual disability and nutrition/dysphagia disorders in community care. *Journal of Intellectual Disability Research* 41, 430–436.

Keohane, P.P., Attrill, H., Grimble, G., Spiller, R., Frost, P., Path, M.R.C. and Silk, D.B.A. (1983) Enteral nutrition in malnourished patients with hepatic cirrhosis and acute encephalopathy. *Journal of Enteral and Parenteral Nutrition* 7, 346–350.

Kerr, J., Butterworth, R. and Bath, P. (1996) Speech and language therapists should have participated in study [letter]. *British Medical Journal* 312, 972.

Keys, A., Henschel, A. and Taylor, H.L. (1947) The size and function of the human heart at rest in semi-starvation and in subsequent rehabilitation. *American Journal of Physiology* 50, 153–169.

Keys, A., Brozek, J., Henschel, A., Michelsen, O. and Taylor, H.L. (1950) *The Biology of Human Starvation*. University of Minnesota Press, Minneapolis.

Kiecolt-Glaser, J.K., Marucha, P.T., Malarkey, W.B., Mercado, A.M. and Glaser, R. (1995) Slowing of wound healing by psychological stress. *Lancet* 346, 1194–1196.

Kim, J.H., Spiegelman, D., Rimm, E. and Gorbach, S.L. (2001) The correlates of dietary intake among HIV-positive adults. *American Journal of Clinical Nutrition* 74, 852–861.

King, T.S., Woolner, J.T. and Hunter, J.O. (1997) The dietary management of Crohn's disease. *Alimentary Pharmacology and Therapy* 11, 17–31.

Kinsella, T.J., Malcolm, A.W., Bothe, A.J., Valerio, D. and Blackburn, G.L. (1981) Prospective study of nutritional support during pelvic irradiation. *International Journal of Radiation, Oncology, Biology and Physics* 7, 543–548.

Kirby, D.F., Marder, R.J., Craig, R.M., Eskildsen, R. and Middaugh, P. (1985) The clinical evaluation of plasma fibronectin as a marker for nutritional depletion and repletion and as a measure of nitrogen balance. *Journal of Parenteral and Enteral Nutrition* 9, 705–708.

Kirby, D.F., Clifton, G.L., Turner, H., Marion, D.W., Barrett, J. and Gruemer, H.-D.F. (1991) Early enteral nutrition after brain injury by percutaneous endoscopic gastrojejunostomy. *Journal of Parenteral and Enteral Nutrition* 15, 298–302.

Kirschner, B.S., Klich, J.R., Kalman, S.S., DeFavaro, M.V. and Rosenberg, I.H. (1981) Reversal of growth retardation in Crohn's disease with therapy emphasizing oral nutritional restitution. *Gastroenterology* 80, 10–15.

Kissileff, H.R. (1985) Effects of physical state (liquid–solid) of foods on food intake: procedural and substantive contributions. *American Journal of Clinical Nutrition* 42, 956–965.

Klebanoff, M.A. and Yip, R. (1987) Influence of maternal birth weight on rate of fetal growth and duration of gestation. *Journal of Paediatrics* 111, 287–292.

Klein, S., Simes, J. and Blackburn, G. (1986) Total parenteral nutrition and cancer clinical trials. *Cancer* 58, 1378–1386.

Klein, S., Kinney, J., Jeejeebhoy, K., Alpers, D., Hellerstein, M., Murray, M. and Twomey, P. (1997) Nutrition support in clinical practice: review of published data and recommendations for future research directions. *American Journal of Clinical Nutrition* 66, 683–706.

Klidjian, A.M., Foster, K.J., Kammerling, R.M., Cooper, A. and Karran, S.J. (1980) Relation of anthropometric and dynamometric variables to serious postoperative complications. *British Medical Journal* 281, 899–901.

Klipstein-Grobusch, K., Reilly, J.J., Potter, J., Edwards, C.A. and Roberts, M.A. (1995) Energy intake and expenditure in elderly patients admitted to hospital with acute illness. *British Journal of Nutrition* 73, 323–334.

Klipstein-Grobusch, K., Witteman, J.C.M., den Breeijen, J.H., Goldbohm, R.A., Hofman, A., de John, P.T.V.M., Pols, H.A. and Grobbee, D.E. (1999) Dietary assessment in the elderly: application of a two-step semi-quantitative food frequency questionnaire for epidemiological studies. *Journal of Human Nutrition and Dietetics* 12, 361–373.

Knowles, J.B., Fairbarn, M.S., Wiggs, B.J., Chan-Yan, C. and Pardy, R.L. (1988) Dietary supplementation and respiratory muscle performance in patients with COPD. *Chest* 93, 977–983.

Ko, G.T.C., Chan, J.C.N., Cockram, C.S. and Woo, J. (1999) Prediction of hypertension, diabetes, dyslipidaemia or albuminuria using simple anthropometric indexes in Hong Kong Chinese. *International Journal of Obesity* 23, 1136–1142.

Kobayashi, A., Yoneda, T., Yoshikawa, M., Ikuno, M., Fukuoka, A., Narita, N. and Nezu, K. (2000) The relation of fat-free mass to maximum exercise performance in patients with chronic obstructive pulmonary disease. *Lung* 178, 119–127.

Koch, J., Garcia-Shelton, Y.L., Neal, E.A., Chan, M.F., Wever, K.E. and Cello, J.P. (1996) Steatorrhea: a common manifestation in patients with HIV/AIDS. *Nutrition* 121, 507–510.

Koch, J.D., Schauder, P., Koch, S. and Ochler, G. (2001) Prevalence of malnutrition in child liver cirrhosis: a controlled study. *Clinical Nutrition* 20 (Suppl.), 18.

Koehler, J. and Buhl, K. (1991) Percutaneous endoscopic gastrostomy for postoperative rehabilitation after maxillofacial tumor surgery. *International Journal of Oral and Maxillofacial Surgery* 20, 38–39.

Kohout, P. (2001) Small-bowel permeability after ingestion of test solution per os and through nasojejunal tube. *Clinical Nutrition* 20, 94–96.

Kompan, L., Kremzar, B., Gadzijev, E. and Prosek, M. (1999) Effects of early enteral nutrition on intestinal permeability and the development of multiple organ failure after multiple injury. *Intensive Care Medicine* 25, 157–161.

Kondrup, J. (2001) Can food intake in hospitals be improved? *Clinical Nutrition* 20 (Suppl. 1), 153–160.

Kong, C.K., Tse, P.W.T. and Lee, W.Y. (1999) Bone age and linear skeletal growth of children with cerebral palsy. *Developmental Medicine and Child Neurology* 41, 758–765.

Kopple, J.D., Lew, N.L. and Lowrie, E.G. (1999) Body weight-for-height relationships predict mortality in maintenance hemodialysis patients. *Kidney International* 56, 1136–1148.

Koretz, R.L. (1994) Is nutritional support worthwhile? In: Heatley, R.V., Green, J.H. and Lasowsky, M.S. (eds) *Consensus in Clinical Nutrition*. Cambridge University Press, Cambridge.

Koretz, R.L., Lipman, T.O. and Klein, S. (2001) AGA technical review on parenteral nutrition. *Gastroenterology* 121, 970–1001.

Kotler, D.P., Wang, J. and Pierson, R.N. (1985) Body composition studies in patients with the acquired immunodeficiency syndrome. *American Journal of Clinical Nutrition* 42, 1255–1265.

Kotler, D.P., Tierney, A.R., Wang, J. and Pierson, R.N. (1989) Magnitude of body cell mass depletion and timing of death from wasting in AIDS. *American Journal of Clinical Nutrition* 50, 444–447.

Kotler, D.P., Tierney, A.R., Brenner, S.K., Couture, S., Wang, J. and Pierson, R.N. (1990) Preservation of short-term energy balance in clinically stable patients with AIDS. *American Journal of Clinical Nutrition* 51, 7–13.

Kotler, D.P., Tierney, A.R., Ferraro, R., Cuff, P., Wang, J., Pierson, R.N. and Heymsfield, S.B. (1991) Enteral alimentation and repletion of body cell mass in malnourished patients with acquired immunodeficiency syndrome. *American Journal of Clinical Nutrition* 53, 149–154.

Koval, K.J., Maurer, S.G., Su, E.T., Aharonoff, G.B. and Zuckerman, J.D. (1999) The effects of nutritional status on outcome after hip fracture. *Journal of Orthopaedic Trauma* 13, 164–169.

Kramer, J.A. (1999) A longitudinal study of nutritional status, body function and quality of life in inoperable lung cancer. PhD thesis, University of Cambridge, Cambridge.

Kramer, J., Crowe, E., Dewit, O. and Elia, M. (1998) Relationships between physical activity, disease activity and quality of life in inoperable lung cancer. *Proceedings of the Nutrition Society* 57, 106A.

Kramer, M.S. (1987) Detriments of low birth weight: methodological assessment and meta-analysis. *Bulletin of the World Health Organization* 65, 633–637.

Krassie, J., Smart, C. and Roberts, D.C.K. (2000) A review of the nutritional needs of meals on wheels consumers and factors associated with the provision of an effective meals on wheels service – an Australian perspective. *European Journal of Clinical Nutrition* 54, 275–280.

Krick, J. and Van Duyn, M.A. (1984) The relationship between oral–motor involvement and growth: a pilot study in a pediatric population with cerebral palsy. *Journal of the American Dietetic Association* 84, 555–559.

Krondl, M., Coleman, P.H., Bradley, C.L., Lau, D. and Ryan, N. (1999) Subjectively healthy elderly consuming a liquid nutrition supplement maintained body mass index and improved some nutritional parameters and perceived well being. *Journal of the American Dietetic Association* 99, 1542–1548.

Kruizenga, H., Van Bokhorst-de van der Schueren, M. and de Jonge, P. (2001) Prevalence and treatment of malnutrition in medical inpatients of 17 European counties. *Clinical Nutrition* 20 (Suppl. 3), 71.

Krynski, M.D., Tymchuk, A.J. and Ouslander, J.G. (1994) How informed can consent be? New light on comprehension among elderly people making decisions about enteral tube feeding. *Gerontologist* 34, 36–43.

Kubena, K.S. and McMurray, D.N. (1996) Nutrition and the immune system: a review of nutrient-nutrient interactions. *Journal of the American Dietetic Association* 96, 1156–1164.

Kuby, J. (1992) *Immunology*. W.H. Freeman, New York.

Kudsk, K.A., Campbell, S.M., O'Brien, T. and Fuller, R. (1990) Postoperative jejunal feedings following complicated pancreatitis. *Nutrition in Clinical Practice* 5, 14–17.

Kudsk, K.A., Croce, M.A., Fabian, T.C., Minard, G., Tolley, E.A., Poret, A., Kuhl, M.R. and Brown, R.O. (1992) Enteral versus parenteral feeding: effects on septic morbidity after blunt and penetrating abdominal trauma. *Annals of Surgery* 215, 503–511.

Kudsk, K.A., Minard, G., Croce, M.A., Brown, R.O., Lowrey, T.S., Pritchard, F.E., Dickerson, R.N. and Fabian, T.C. (1996) A randomized trial of isonitrogenous enteral diets after severe trauma: an immune enhancing diet reduces septic complications. *Annals of Surgery* 224, 531–543.

Kuhlmann, M.K., Schmidt, F. and Kohler, H. (1997) Oral nutritional support in malnourished HD-patients: preliminary results of a randomised controlled study. *Journal of the American Society of Nephrology* 8, SS A0924.

Kulkarni, J. (1994) Pressure sores: not considered a priority by medical staff [letter]. *British Medical Journal* 309, 1436.

Kurugöl, Z., Egemen, A., Çetingül, N., Kavakli, K., Nisli, G. and Öztop, S. (1997) Early determination of nutritional problems in pediatric cancer patients. *Turkish Journal of Pediatrics* 39, 325–334.

Kurz. A., Sessler, D.I. and Lenhardt, R. (1996) Perioperative normothermia to reduce the incidence of surgical-wound infection and shorten hospitalization: study of the wound infection and temperature group. *New England Journal of Medicine* 334, 1209–1215.

Kusin, J.A., Kardjati, S. and Renqvist, U.H. (1994) Maternal body mass index: the functional significance during reproduction. *European Journal of Clinical Nutrition* 48 (Suppl. 3), S56–S67.

Kwoun, M.O., Ling, P.R., Lydon, E., Imrich, A., Qu, Z., Palombo, J. and Bistrian, B.R. (1997) Immunologic effects of acute hyperglycemia in nondiabetic rats. *Journal of Parenteral and Enteral Nutrition* 21, 91–95.

Kyle, U.G., Morabia, A., Slosman, D.O., Nensi, N., Unger, P. and Pichard, C. (2001) Contribution of body composition to nutritional assessment at hospital admission in 995 patients: a controlled population study. *British Journal of Nutrition* 86, 725–731.

Laaban, J.P., Kouchakji, B., Dore, M.F., Orvoen-Frijia, E., David, P. and Rochemaure, J. (1993) Nutritional status of patients with chronic obstructive pulmonary disease and acute respiratory failure. *Chest* 103, 1362–1368.

Ladeira, J.P., Janiszewski, M., Soriano, F.G., Faintuch, J. and Velasco, I.T. (1999) Clinical and haematological abnormalities during prolonged fasting. *Clinical Nutrition* 18 (Suppl.), 33.

Lai, H.C., Corey, M., FitzSimmins, S., Kosorok, M.R. and Farrell, P.M. (1999) Comparison of growth status of patients with cystic fibrosis between the United States and Canada. *American Journal of Clinical Nutrition* 69, 531–538.

Lai, H.C., Kosorok, M.R., Sondel, S.A., Chen, S.T., Fitzsimmons, S.C., Green, C.G., Shen, G., Walker, S. and Farrell, P.M. (1998) Growth status in children with cystic fibrosis based on the National Cystic Fibrosis Patients' Registry data: evaluation of various criteria used to identify malnutrition. *Journal of Pediatrics* 132, 478–485.

Lamy, M., Mojon, P., Kalykakis, G., Legrand, R. and Butz-Jorgensen, A. (1999) Oral status and nutrition in the institutionalized elderly. *Journal of Dentistry* 27, 443–448.

Landbo, C., Prescott, E., Lange, P., Vestbo, J. and Almdal, T.P. (1999) Prognostic value of nutritional status in chronic obstructive pulmonary disease. *American Journal of Respiratory and Critical Care Medicine* 160, 1856–1861.

Landi, F., Onder, G., Gambassi, G., Pedone, C., Cabonin, P. and Bernabei, R. (2000) Body mass index and mortality among hospitalized patients. *Archives of Internal Medicine* 160, 2641–2644.

Langhans, W. (2000) Anorexia of infection: current prospects. *Nutrition* 16, 996–1005.

Langkamp-Henken, B., Kudsk, K.A. and Proctor, K.G. (1995a) Fasting-induced reduction of intestinal reperfusion injury. *Journal of Parenteral and Enteral Nutrition* 19, 127–132.

Langkamp-Henken, B., Donovan, T.B., Pate, L.M., Maull, C.D. and Kudsk, K.A. (1995b) Increased intestinal permeability following blunt and penetrating trauma. *Critical Care Medicine* 23, 660–664.

Langley, S.C., Seakins, M., Grimble, R.F. and Jackson, A.A. (1994) The acute phase response of adult rats is altered by *in utero* exposure to maternal low-protein diets. *Journal of Nutrition* 124, 1588–1596.

Lara, T.M. and Jacobs, D.O. (1998) Effect of critical illness and nutritional support on mucosal mass and function. *Clinical Nutrition* 17, 99–105.

Larsson, J., Unosson, M., Ek, A., Nilsson, L., Thorslund, S. and Bjurulf, P. (1990) Effect of dietary supplement on nutritional status and clinical outcome in 501 geriatric patients – a randomised study. *Clinical Nutrition* 9, 179–184.

Larsson, J., Akerlind, I., Permerth, J. and Hornqvist, J.-O. (1994a) The relation between nutritional state and quality of life in surgical patients. *European Journal of Surgery* 160, 329–334.

Larsson, J., Andersson, M., Askelöf, N. and Bark, T. (1994b) Undernäring valigt vid svenska sjukhus: risken för komplitationer och förlängd vårdtid ökar. *Nordisk Medicin* 109, 292–295.

Lasheras, C., Ganzalez, C., Garcia, A., Patterson, A. and Fernandez, S. (1999) Dietary intake and biochemical indicators of nutritional status in an elderly institutionalized and non-institutionalized population. *Nutrition Research* 19, 1299–1312.

Lauque, S., Arnaud-Battandier, F., Mansourian, R., Guigoz, Y., Paintin, M., Nourhashemi, F. and Vellas, B. (2000) Protein–energy oral supplementation in malnourished nursing-home residents: a controlled trial. *Age and Ageing* 29, 51–56.

Lavernia, C.J., Sierra, R.J. and Baerga, L. (1999) Nutritional parameters and short term outcome in arthroplasty. *Journal of the American College of Nutrition* 18, 274–278.

Laviano, A. and Meguid, M.M. (1996) Nutritional issues in cancer management. *Nutrition* 12, 358–371.

Laws, R.A., Tapsell, L.C. and Kelly, J. (2000) Nutritional status and its relationship to quality of life in a sample of chronic hemodialysis patients. *Journal of Renal Nutrition* 10, 139–147.

Lawson, J.A., Lazarus, R. and Kelly, J.J. (2001) Prevalence and prognostic significance of malnutrition in chronic renal insufficiency. *Journal of Renal Nutrition* 11, 16–22.

Lawson, R.M., Doshi, M.K., Ingoe, L.E., Colligan, J.M., Barton, J.R. and Cobden, I. (2000) Compliance of orthopaedic patients with postoperative oral nutritional supplementation. *Clinical Nutrition* 19, 171–175.

Lean, M. (1996) Nutrition in the medical undergraduate curriculum. *Proceedings of the Nutrition Society* 55, 139A.

Le Cornu, K.A., McKiernan, F.J., Kapadia, S.A. and Neuberger, J.M. (2000) A prospective randomized study of preoperative nutritional supplementation in patients awaiting elective orthotopic liver transplantation. *Transplantation* 69, 1364–1369.

Lee, L., Kang, S.A., Lee, H.O., Lee, B.H., Park, J.S., Kim, J.H., Jung, I.K., Park, Y.J. and Lee, J.E. (2001) Relationship between dietary intake and cognitive function level in Korean elderly people. *Public Health* 115, 133–138.

Lee, P. and Cunningham, K. (1990) *Irish National Nutrition Survey*. Irish Nutrition and Dietetic Institute, Dublin.

Lees, J. (1999) Incidence of weight loss in head and neck cancer patients on commencing radiotherapy treatment at a regional oncology centre. *European Journal of Cancer Care* 8, 133–136.

Lefevre, C. and Clarke, M.J. (2001) *Identifying Randomised Trials*, 2nd edn. BMJ Publishing Group, London.

Legaspi, A., Roberts, J.P., Albert, J.D., Tracey, K.J., Shires, T. and Lowry, S.F. (1988) The effect of starvation and total parenteral nutrition on skeletal muscle amino acid content and membrane potential difference in normal man. *Surgery, Gynecology and Obstetrics* 166, 233–240.

Leite, H.P. and Fantozzi, G. (1998) Metabolic assessment and enteral tube feeding usage in children with acute neurological diseases. *Revista Paulista de Medicina* 116, 1858–1865.

Leizorovicz, A., Haugh, M.C., Chapuis, F.-R., Samama, M.M. and Boissel, J.-P. (1992) Low molecular weight heparin in prevent of perioperative thrombosis. *British Medical Journal* 1992, 913–920.

Lengyel, C., Whiting, S. and Zello, G. (2001) Nutrition adequacy of food consumed by elderly residents in long term care facilities. *Journal of the American Dietetic Association* 101, A49.

Lennard-Jones, J.E. (1992) *A Positive Approach to Nutrition as Treatment*. King's Fund Centre, London.

Lennard-Jones, J.E. (1998) *Ethical and Legal Aspects of Clinical Hydration and Nutritional Support*. BAPEN, Maidenhead.

Lennard-Jones, J.E., Arrowsmith, H., Davison, C., Denham, A.F. and Micklewright, A. (1995) Screening by nurses and junior doctors to detect malnutrition when patients are first assessed in hospital. *Clinical Nutrition* 14, 336–340.

Lennmarken, C., Sandstedt, S., Schenck, H.V. and Larsson, J. (1986) The effect of starvation on skeletal muscle function in man. *Clinical Nutrition* 5, 99–103.

Leroy, V., Newell, M.L., Dabis, F., Peckham, C., Van de Perre, P., Bulterys, M., Kind, C., Simmonds, R.J., Wiktor, S. and Msellati, P. (1998) International multicentre pooled analysis of late postnatal mother-to-child transmission of HIV-1 infection. *Lancet* 352, 597–600.

Lesourd, B. (1999) Immune response during disease and recovery in the elderly. *Proceedings of the Nutrition Society* 58, 85–98.

Lesourd, B.M. and Mazari, L. (1997) Immune responses during recovery from protein–energy malnutrition. *Clinical Nutrition* 16, 37–46.

Lesourd, B. and Mazari, L. (1999) Nutrition and immunity in the elderly. *Proceedings of the Nutrition Society* 58, 685–695.

Levine, J. and Morgan, M. (1994) Self-selected dietary composition in ten hospitalized patients with cancer cachexia and in ten control patients. *Nutrition* 10, 495.

Levine, J.A. and Morgan, M.Y. (1996) Weighed dietary intakes in patients with chronic liver disease. *Nutrition* 12, 430–435.

Levine, J.M. and Totolos, E. (1995) Pressure ulcers: a strategic plan to prevent and heal them. *Geriatrics* 50, 32–37.

Levy, L.D., Durie, P.R., Pencharz, P.B. and Corey, M.L. (1985) Effects of long-term nutritional rehabilitation on body composition and clinical status in malnourished children and adolescents with cystic fibrosis. *Journal of Pediatrics* 107, 225–230.

Lew, E.A. and Garfinkel, L. (1979) Variation in mortality by weight among 750,000 men and women. *Journal of Chronic Diseases* 12, 563–576.

Lewis, A.F. (1981) Fracture of the neck of femur: changing incidence. *British Medical Journal* 283, 1217–1219.

Lewis, B., Hitchings, H. and Harding, K. (1993) Nutritional status of elderly patients with venous ulceration of the leg – report of a pilot study. *Journal of Human Nutrition and Dietetics* 6, 509–515.

Lewis, M.I., Belman, M.J. and Dorr-Uyemura, L. (1987) Nutritional supplementation in ambulatory patients with chronic obstructive pulmonary disease. *American Review of Respiratory Disease* 135, 1062–1068.

Lewis, S.J., Egger, M., Sylvester, P.A. and Thomas, S. (2001) Early enteral feeding versus 'nil by mouth' after gastrointestinal surgery: systematic review and meta-analysis of controlled trials. *British Medical Journal* 323, 773–776.

Leyton, G.B. (1946) The effects of slow starvation. *Lancet* ii, 73–79.

Lin, E., Kotani, J.G. and Lowry, S.F. (1998) Nutritional modulation of immunity and the inflammatory response. *Nutrition* 14, 545–550.

Lindahl, S.G.E. (2001) Not only towards enhanced preoperative comfort. *Anesthesia Analgesia* 93, 1091–1092.

Lindor, K.D., Fleming, C.R., Burnes, J.U., Nelson, J.K. and Ilstrup, D.M. (1992) A randomized prospective trial comparing a defined formula diet, corticosteroids, and a defined formula diet plus corticosteroids in active Crohn's disease. *Mayo Clinic Proceedings* 67, 328–333.

Linn, B.S. (1984) Outcomes of older and younger malnourished and well-nourished patients one year after hospitalization. *American Journal of Clinical Nutrition* 39, 66–73.

Lipman, T.O. (1991) Clinical trials of nutritional support in cancer: parenteral and enteral therapy. *Hematology/Oncology Clinics of North America* 5, 91–102.

Lipman, T.O. (1995) Bacterial translocation and enteral nutrition in humans: an outsider looks in. *Journal of Parenteral and Enteral Nutrition* 19, 156–165.

Lipman, T.O. (1998) Grains or veins: is enteral nutrition really better than parenteral nutrition? A look at the evidence. *Journal of Parenteral and Enteral Nutrition* 22, 167–182.

Lipschitz, D.A. (1991) Malnutrition in the elderly. *Seminars in Dermatology* 10, 273–281.

Lipschitz, D.A. and Mitchell, C.O. (1980) Enteral hyperalimentation and hematopoietic toxicity caused by chemotherapy of small cell lung cancer. *Journal of Parenteral and Enteral Nutrition* 4, 593.

Lipschitz, D.A. and Mitchell, C.O. (1982) The correctability of the nutritional, immune, and hematopoietic manifestations of protein calorie malnutrition in the elderly. *Journal of the American College of Nutrition* 1, 17–25.

Lipschitz, D.A., Mitchell, C.O., Steele, R.W. and Milton, K.Y. (1985) Nutritional evaluation and supplementation of elderly subjects participating in a 'Meals on Wheels' program. *Journal of Parenteral and Enteral Nutrition* 9, 343–347.

Lissauer, T. and Clayden, G. (1997) Pediatric emergencies. In: *Illustrated Textbook of Paediatrics.* Harcourt Publishers, London, pp. 29–40.

Livingston, D.H. and Deitch, E.A. (1995) Multiple organ failure: a common problem in surgical intensive care unit patients. *Annals of Medicine* 27, 13–20.

Ljungqvist, O., Nygren, J., Thorell, A., Brodin, U. and Efendic, S. (2001) Pre-operative nutrition – elective surgery in the fed or overnight fasted state. *Clinical Nutrition* 20, 167–171.

Llop, J.M., Muñoz, C., Badia, M.B., Virgili, N., Tubau, M., Ramón, J.M., Pita, A. and Jódar, J.R. (2001) Serum albumin as indicator of clinical evolution in patients on parenteral nutrition: multivariable study. *Clinical Nutrition* 20, 77–81.

Lobo, D.N., Bostock, K.A., Neal, K.R., Perkins, A.C., Rowlands, B.J. and Allison, S.P. (2001) Effect of salt and water balance on gastrointestinal function and outcome after abdominal surgery: a prospective randomised controlled study. *Clinical Nutrition* 20, 35–36.

Lochs, H., Steinhardt, H.J., Klaus-Wentz, B., Zeitz, M., Vogelsang, H., Sommer, H., Fleig, W.E., Bauer, P., Schirrmeister, J. and Malchow, H. (1991) Comparison of enteral nutrition and drug treatment in active Crohn's disease: results of the European cooperative Crohn's disease study IV. *Gastroenterology* 101, 881–888.

Lock, M. and Vald, V. (1994) Starvation in hospital: refer early to a dietitian [letter]. *British Medical Journal* 308, 1369–1370.

Logan, R.F.A., Gillon, J., Ferrington, C. and Ferguson, A. (1981) Reduction of gastrointestinal protein loss by elemental diet in Crohn's disease of the small bowel. *Gut* 22, 383–387.

Lolley, D.M., Myers, W.O., Ray, J.F.D., Sautter, R.D. and Tewksbury, D.A. (1985) Clinical experience with preoperative myocardial nutrition management. *Journal of Cardiovascular Surgery* 26, 236–243.

Longe, R.L. (1986) Current concepts in clinical therapeutics: pressure sores. *Clinical Pharmacology* 5, 669–681.

Lopes, J., Russell, D., Whitwell, J. and Jeejeebhoy, K.N. (1992) Skeletal muscle function in malnutrition. *American Journal of Clinical Nutrition* 36, 602–610.

Lord, K. (2002) Effect on patient energy intakes of adding snacks to the patient menu at a district general hospital. *Proceedings of the Nutrition Society* 61, 23A.

Lorefalt, B., Unosson, M. and Ek, A.-C. (1998) Protein–energy-rich diet increases energy intake in elderly patients. *European Journal of Clinical Nutrition* 52, S31.

Lorenzo, V., de Bonis, E., Ruffino, M., Hernandez, D., Rebollo, S.G., Rodriguez, A.P. and Torres, A. (1995) Caloric rather than protein deficiency predominates in stable chronic haemodialysis patients. *Nephrology, Dialysis and Transplantation* 10, 1885–1889.

Losser, M.R., Bernard, C., Beaudeux, J.L., Pison, C. and Payen, D. (1997) Glucose modulates hemodynamic, metabolic, and inflammatory responses to lipopolysaccharide in rabbits. *Journal of Applied Physiology* 83, 1566–1574.

Louw, J.A., Werbeck, A., Louw, M.E., Kotze, T.J., Cooper, R. and Labadarios, D. (1992) Blood vitamin concentrations during the acute-phase response. *Critical Care Medicine* 20, 934–941.

Lowik, M.R., van den Berg, H., Schrijver, J., Odink, J., Wedel, M. and van Houten, P. (1992) Marginal nutritional status among institutionalized elderly women as compared to those living more independently (Dutch Nutrition Surveillance System). *Journal of the American College of Nutrition* 11 (6), 673–681.

Lucas, A., Bloom, S.R. and Aynsley-Green, A. (1986) Gut hormones and 'minimal enteral feeding'. *Acta Paediatrica Scandinavica* 75, 719–723.

Luder, E., Godfrey, E., Godbold, J. and Simpson, D.M. (1995) Assessment of nutritional, clinical and immunologic status of HIV-infected, inner-city patients with multiple risk factors. *Journal of the American Dietetic Association* 95, 655–660.

Lumbers, M., Driver, L.T., Howland, R.J., Older, M.W.J. and Williams, C.M. (1996) Nutritional status and clinical outcome in elderly female surgical orthopaedic patients. *Clinical Nutrition* 15, 101–107.

Lumbers, M., Murphy, M., Pither, C., Creedon, M., Older, M. and New, S. (1998) Differences in dietary intake and food selection between hospital patients and day-centre visitors: implications for supplementation. *Proceedings of the Nutrition Society* 57, 56A.

Lumbers, M., New, S.A., Gibson, S. and Murphy, M.C. (2001) Nutritional status in elderly female hip fracture patients: comparison with an age-matched home living group attending day centres. *British Journal of Nutrition* 85, 733–740.

Lunn, P.G. (2000) The impact of infection and nutrition on gut function and growth in childhood. *Proceedings of Nutrition Society* 59, 147–154.

Lynch, K., Henry, D.A., Roberts, C. and Coburn, J.W. (1983) Clinical trial with oral carbohydrate supplement in hemodialysis patients: a nutritional evaluation. *Dialysis and Transplantation* 12, 566–568.

Maaravi, Y., Berry, E.M., Ginsberg, G., Cohen, A. and Stessman, J. (2000) Nutrition and quality of life in the aged: the Jerusalem 70-year-olds longitudinal study. *Ageing: Clinical and Experimental Research* 12, 173–179.

Macallan, D.C. (1996) Metabolic abnormalities and the 'Wasting Syndrome' in HIV infection. *Nutrition* 2, 641–642.

Macallan, D.C. (1998) Sir David Cuthbertson Prize Medal Lecture: Metabolic abnormalities and wasting in human immunodeficiency virus infection. *Proceedings of the Nutrition Society* 57, 323–330.

Macallan, D.C., Noble, C., Baldwin, C., Foskett, M., McManus, T. and Griffin, G.E. (1993) Prospective analysis of patterns of weight change in stage IV human immunodeficiency virus infection. *American Journal of Clinical Nutrition* 58, 417–424.

Macallan, D., Noble, C., Baldwin, C., Jebb, S., Prentice, A., Coward, W., Sawyer, M., McManus, T. and Griffin, G. (1995) Energy expenditure and wasting in human immunodeficiency virus infection. *New England Journal of Medicine* 333, 83–88.

McArdle, A.H., Wittnich, C., Freeman, C.R. and Duguid, W.P. (1985) Elemental diet as prophylaxis against radiation injury. *Archives of Surgery* 120, 1026–1032.

McAtear, C.A. (1999) *Current Perspectives on Enteral Nutrition in Adults*. BAPEN, Maidenhead.

McAtear, C.A. and Wright, C. (1996) *Dietetic Standards for Nutritional Support*. British Dietetic Association, Birmingham.

McBean, L.D., Smith, J.C., Berne, B.H. and Halsted, J.A. (1974) Serum zinc and alpha2-macroglobulin concentration in myocardial infarction, decubitus ulcer, multiple myeloma, prostatic carcinoma, Down's syndrome and nephrotic syndrome. *Clinica Chimica Acta* 50, 43–51.

McCafferty, P. (1994) *A Study of the Home Needs of Elderly and Disabled People*. Department of the Environment, London.

McCarey, D.W., Buchanan, E., Gregory, M., Clark, B.J. and Weaver, L.T. (1996) Home enteral feeding of children in the west of Scotland. *Scottish Medical Journal* 41, 147–149.

McCargar, L.J., Hotson, B.L. and Nozza, A. (1995) Fibre and nutrient intakes of chronic care elderly patients. *Journal of Nutrition for the Elderly* 15, 13–30.

McCarter, M.D., Gentilini, O.D., Gomez, M.E. and Daly, J.M. (1998) Preoperative oral supplement with immunonutrients in cancer patients. *Journal of Parenteral and Enteral Nutrition* 22, 206–211.

McCarthy, H. and McIvor, H.R.M. (2001) Nutritional status of children on admission to a children's hospital. *Proceedings of the Nutrition Society* 60, 82A.

McClave, S.A., Lowen, C.C. and Snider, H.L. (1992) Immunonutrition and enteral hyperalimentation of critically ill patients. *Digestive Diseases and Sciences* 37, 1153–1161.

McClave, S.A., Greene, L.M., Snider, H.L., Makk, L.J.K., Cheadle, W.G., Owens, N.A., Dukes, L.G. and Goldsmith, L.J. (1997) Comparison of the safety of early enteral vs. parenteral nutrition in mild acute pancreatitis. *Journal of Parenteral and Enteral Nutrition* 21, 14–20.

McClure, R.J. and Newell, S.J. (2000) Randomised controlled study of clinical outcome following trophic feeding. *Archives of Diseases in Childhood* 82, F29–F33.

McCollum, K. (2000) Appetite and nutritional intake in patients with chronic liver disease. *Journal of Human Nutrition* 13, 363–371.

McDowell, K. (1997) Knowledge of nutrition and its application within a children's hospital. *Proceedings of the Nutrition Society* 56, 263A.

McEvoy, A.W. and James, O.F. (1982) The effect of a dietary supplement (Build-Up) on nutritional status in hospitalized elderly patients. *Human Nutrition: Applied Nutrition* 36A, 374–376.

MacFie, J. (2000a) Enteral versus parenteral nutrition. *British Journal of Surgery* 97, 1121–1122.

MacFie, J. (2000b) Enteral versus parenteral nutrition: the significance of bacterial translocation and gut-barrier function. *Nutrition* 16, 606–611.

MacFie, J., Woodcock, N.P., Palmer, M.D., Walker, A., Townsend, S. and Mitchell, C.J. (2000) Oral dietary supplements in pre- and post operative surgical patients: a prospective and randomized clinical trial. *Nutrition* 16, 723–728.

MacLennan, W.J., Martin, P. and Mason, B.J. (1975) Causes for reduced dietary intake in a long-stay hospital. *Age and Ageing* 4, 175–180.

McGeer, A.J., Detsky, A.S. and O'Rourke, K. (1990) Parenteral nutrition in cancer patients undergoing chemotherapy: a meta-analysis. *Nutrition* 6, 233–240.

McGlone, P.C., Dickerson, J.W.T. and Davies, G.J. (1996) Provision of Asian foods in hospital. *Proceedings of the Nutrition Society* 55, 74A.

McGlone, P.C., Davies, G.J., Murcott, A., Powell-Tuck, J. and Dickerson, J.W.T. (1997) Foods consumed by a Bengali population in a British hospital. *Proceedings of the Nutrition Society* 56, 28A.

McGrath, S.J., Splaingard, M.I., Alba, H.M., Kaufman, B.H. and Glicklick, M. (1992) Survival and functional outcome of children with severe cerebral palsy following gastrostomy. *Archives of Physical Medicine and Rehabilitation* 73, 133–137.

McGuire, J.S. and Austin, J.E. (1987) Beyond survival: children's growth for national development. *Assignment Children* 2, 3–52.

Machin, D. and Campbell, M.J. (1987) *Statistical Tables for the Design of Clinical Trials.* Blackwell, Oxford.

Macia, E., Moran, J., Santos, J., Blanco, M., Mahedero, G. and Salas, J. (1991) Nutritional evaluation and dietetic care in cancer patients treated with radiotherapy: prospective study. *Nutrition* 7, 205–209.

MacIntosh, C., Morley, J.E. and Chapman, I.M. (2000) The anorexia of aging. *Nutrition* 16, 983–995.

McIntyre, P.B., Wood, S.R., Powell-Tuck, J. and Lennard-Jones, J.E. (1983) Nocturnal nasogastric tube feeding at home. *Postgraduate Medical Journal* 59, 767–769.

McIntyre, P.B., Powell-Tuck, J., Wood, S.R., Lennard-Jones, J.E., Lerebours, E., Hecketsweiler, P., Galmiche, J.-P. and Colin, R. (1986) Controlled trial of bowel rest in the treatment of severe acute colitis. *Gut* 27, 481–485.

McKenna, S.P. and Thörig, L. (1995) Nutrition and quality of life. *Nutrition* 11, 308–309.

McKinney, R.E., Wilfert, C. and the Aids Clinical Trials Group, Protocol 043 Study Group (1994) Growth as a prognostic indicator in children with human immunodeficiency virus infection treated with zidovudine. *Journal of Pediatrics* 125, 728–733.

McLaren, D.S. and Read, W.W.C. (1972) Classification of nutritional status in early childhood. *Lancet* ii, 146–148.

McLaren, D.S. and Read, W.W.C. (1975) Weight/length classification of nutritional status. *Lancet* ii, 219–220.

McLeod, R.S., Taylor, B.R., O'Connor, B.I., Greenberg, G.R., Jeejeebhoy, K.N., Royall, D. and Langer, B. (1995) Quality of life, nutritional status and gastrointestinal hormone profile following the Whipple Procedure. *American Journal of Surgery* 169, 179–185.

McMillan, D.C., Sattar, N., Talwar, D., O'Reilly, D.S.J. and McArdle, C.S. (2000) Changes in micronutrient concentrations following anti-inflammatory treatment in patients with gastrointestinal cancer. *Nutrition* 16, 425–428.

McNamara, E.P. and Kennedy, N.P. (2001) Tube feeding patients with advanced dementia: an ethical dilemma. *Proceedings of the Nutrition Society* 60, 179–185.

McNamara, E.P., Flood, P. and Kennedy, N.P. (2000) Enteral tube feeding in the community: survey of adult patients discharged from a Dublin hospital. *Clinical Nutrition* 19, 15–22.

McNaughton, S.A., Shepherd, R.W., Greer, R.G., Cleghorn, G.J. and Thomas, B.J. (2000) Nutritional status of children with cystic fibrosis measured by total body potassium as a marker of body cell mass: lack of sensitivity of anthropometric measures. *Journal of Pediatrics* 136, 188–194.

Macqueen, C.E. and Frost, G. (1998) Visual analogue scales: a screening tool for assessing nutritional need in head and neck radiotherapy patients. *Journal of Human Nutrition and Dietetics* 11, 115–124.

McWhirter, J.P. and Pennington, C.R. (1994) Incidence and recognition of malnutrition in hospital. *British Medical Journal* 308, 945–948.

McWhirter, J.P. and Pennington, C.R. (1996) A comparison between oral and nasogastric nutritional supplements in malnourished patients. *Nutrition* 12, 502–506.

McWhirter, J.P., Hambling, C.E. and Pennington, C.R. (1994a) The nutritional status of patients receiving home enteral feeding. *Clinical Nutrition* 13, 207–211.

McWhirter, J.P., Hill, K. and Pennington, C.R. (1994b) The nutritional status of patients with gastrointestinal disease. *Nutrition* 10, 495.

McWhirter, J.P., Hill, K., Richards, J. and Pennington, C.R. (1995) The use, efficacy and monitoring of artificial nutritional support in a teaching hospital. *Scottish Medical Journal* 40, 179–183.

Madapallimkattam, A., Law, L. and Jeejeebjoy, K. (2000) Effect of hypocaloric feeding on mitochondrial respiratory chain activity. *Clinical Nutrition* 19 (Suppl.), 23.

Madden, A.M., McCormick, P.A., Davidson, B., Rolles, K., Burroughs, A.K. and Morgan, M.Y. (1994) Nutritional status and survival of patients after liver transplant. *Nutrition* 10, 504.

Madden, A., Bradvury, W. and Morgan, M. (1997) Taste perception in cirrhosis: its relationship to circulating micronutrients and food preferences. *Hepatology* 26, 40–48.

Madill, J., Guttierrez, C., Grossman, J., Allard, J., Chan, C., Hutcheon, M., Keshavee, S.H. and the Toronto Lung Transplant Program. (2001) Nutritional assessment of the lung transplantation patient: body mass index as a predictor of 90-day mortality following transplantation. *Journal of Heart and Lung Transplantation* 20, 288–296.

Maffulli, N., Dougall, T.W., Brown, M.T.F. and Golden, M.H.N. (1999) Nutritional differences in patients with proximal femoral fractures. *Age and Ageing* 28, 458–462.

Maggi, P., Larocca, A.M., Quarto, M., Serio, G., Brandonisio, O., Angarano, G. and Pastore, G. (2000) Effect of antiretroviral therapy on cryptosporidiosis and microsporidiosis in patients infected with human immunodeficiency virus type 1. *European Journal of Clinical Microbiology and Infectious Diseases* 19, 213–217.

Main, A.N.H., Morgan, R.J., Hall, M.J., Russell, R.I., Shenkin, A. and Fell, G.S. (1980) Home enteral tube feeding with a liquid diet in the long term management of inflammatory bowel disease and intestinal failure. *Scottish Medical Journal* 25, 312–314.

Malavé, I., Vethencourt, M.A., Pirela, M. and Cordero, R. (1998) Serum levels of thyroxine-binding prealbumin, C-reactive protein and interleukin-6 in protein-energy undernourished children and normal controls without or with associated clinical infections. *Journal of Tropical Pediatrics* 44, 256–262.

Malvy, D., Thiébaut, R., Marimoutou, C., Dabis, F. and Groupe d'Epidémiologie Clinique du Sida en Aquitaine (2001) Weight loss and body mass index as predictors of HIV disease progression to AIDS in adults. Aquitaine Cohort, France, 1985–1997. *Journal of the American College of Nutrition* 20, 609–615.

Mancey-Jones, B., Palmer, D., Townsend, S., Mitchell, C.J. and MacFie, J. (1994) Inadequate oral intake in surgical patients. *Nutrition* 10, 494.

Mansell, P.I., Fellows, I.W., MacDonald, I.A. and Allison, S.P. (1990a) Defect in thermoregulation in malnutrition reversed by weight gain: physiological mechanisms and clinical importance. *Quarterly Journal of Medicine New Series* 76, 817–829.

Mansell, P.I., Rawlings, J., Allison, S.P., Bendall, M.J., Pearson, M., Bassey, E.J. and Bastow, M. (1990b) Low anthropometric indices in elderly females with fractured neck of femur. *Clinical Nutrition* 9, 190–194.

Mansfield, J.C., Giaffer, M.H. and Holdsworth, C.D. (1995) Controlled trial of oligopeptide versus amino acid diet in treatment of active Crohn's disease. *Gut* 36, 60–66.

Marckmann, P. (1988) Nutritional status of patients on hemodialysis and peritoneal dialysis. *Clinical Nephrology* 29, 75–78.

Marckmann, P. (1989) Nutritional status and mortality of patients in regular dialysis therapy. *Journal of Internal Medicine* 226, 429–432.

Marcos, A. (1997) The immune system in eating disorders: an overview. *Nutrition* 13, 853–862.

Marcus, E.-L. and Berry, E.M. (1998) Refusal to eat in the elderly. *Nutrition Reviews* 56, 163–171.

Marechova, O., Schuck, O., Teplan, V., Dedicova, L., Kaslikova, J., Ruzickova, J. and Matl, I. (1995) [A nutritionally defined liquid diet for hemodialyzed patients]. *Casopis Lekaru Ceskych* 134, 77–79.

Margetts, B.M., Thompson, R.L., Elia, M. and Jackson, A.A. (2002) Prevalence of risk of undernutrition is associated with poor health status in older people in the UK. *European Journal of Clinical Nutrition* 56, 1–6.

Marik, P.E. and Zaloga, G.P. (2001) Early enteral nutrition in acutely ill patients: a systematic review. *Critical Care Medicine* 29, 2264–2270.

Marin, O.E., Glassman, M.S., Schoen, B.T. and Caplan, D.B. (1994) Safety and efficacy of percutaneous endoscopic gastrostomy in children. *American Journal of Gastroenterology* 89, 357–361.

Maroni, B.J. (1998) Protein restriction in the pre-end-stage renal disease (ESRD) patient: who, when, how, and the effect on subsequent ESRD outcome. *Journal of the American Society of Nephrology* 9, S100–S106.

Martin, C.A., Walsh, G.L. and Moreland, K. (1999) Relationship of weight loss and postoperative nutritional complications in esophagogastrectomy patients. *Journal of Parenteral and Enteral Nutrition* 23, S20.

Martin, S., Neale, G. and Elia, M. (1985) Factors affecting maximal momentary grip strength. *Human Nutrition. Clinical Nutrition* 39C, 137–147.

Martindale, R.G. and Cresci, G.A. (2001) Use of immune-enhancing diets in burns. *Journal of Parenteral and Enteral Nutrition* 25, S24–S26.

Marton, K.I., Sox, H.C. and Krupp, J.R. (1981) Involuntary weight loss: diagnostic and prognostic significance. *Annals of Internal Medicine* 95, 568–574.

Martyn, C.N., Winter, P.D., Coles, S.J. and Edington, J. (1998) Effect of nutritional status on use of health care resources by patients with chronic disease living in the community. *Clinical Nutrition* 17, 119–123.

Maskell, C., Daniels, P. and Johnson, C. (1999) Dietary intake after pancreatectomy. *British Journal of Surgery* 86, 323–326.

Matarese, L.E. and Gottschlich, M.M. (1998) *Contemporary Nutrition Support Practice. A Clinical Guide*. W.B. Saunders, Philadelphia.

Mathey, M., Vanneste, V., de Graaf, C., de Groot, L. and van Staveren, W. (2001a) Health effect of improved meal ambiance in a Dutch nursing home: a 1-year intervention study. *Preventative Medicine* 32, 416–423.

Mathey, M., Siebeling, E., de Graaf, C. and van Staveren, W. (2001b) Flavour enhancement of food improves dietary intake and nutritional status of elderly nursing home residents. *Journal of Gerontology A Biological Science and Medical Science* 56, M200–M205.

Mathus-Vliegen, E.M.H. (2001) Nutritional status, nutrition and pressure ulcers. *Nutrition in Clinical Practice* 16, 286–291.

Mattern, W.D., Hak, L.J., Lamanna, R.W., Teasley, K.M. and Laffell, M.S. (1982) Malnutrition, altered immune function and the risk of infection in maintenance hemodialysis patients. *American Journal of Kidney Diseases* 1, 206–218.

Mattila, K., Haavisto, M. and Rajala, S. (1986) Body mass index and mortality in the elderly. *British Medical Journal* 292, 867–868.

Maurer, J., Weinbaum, F., Turner, J., Brady, T., Pistone, B. and D'Addario, V., Lun, W. and Ghazali, B. (1996) Reducing the inappropriate use of parenteral nutrition in an acute care teaching hospital. *Journal of Parenteral and Enteral Nutrition* 20, 272–274.

Maxfield, D., Geehan, D. and Van Way, C.W. (2001) Perioperative nutritional support. *Nutrition in Clinical Practice* 16, 69–73.

Maxton, D.G., Menzies, I.S., Slavin, B. and Thompson, R.P.H. (1989) Small-intestinal function during enteral feeding and starvation in man. *Clinical Science* 77, 401–406.

Mazolewski, P., Turner, J.F., Baker, M., Kurtz, T. and Little, A.G. (1999) The impact of nutritional status on the outcome of lung volume reduction surgery: a prospective study. *Chest* 116, 693–696.

Mears, E. (1996) Outcomes of continuous process improvement of a nutritional care program incorporate serum prealbumin measurements. *Nutrition* 12, 479–484.

Meaume, S. and Senet, P. (1999) Prevention of pressure sores in the elderly. *Press-Médicale* 28, 1846–1853.

Meguid, M.M. (1993) An open letter to Hillary Rodham Clinton. *Nutrition* 9, ix–xi.

Meguid, M.M., Mughal, M.M., Debonis, D., Meguid, V. and Terz, J.J. (1986) Influence of nutritional status on the resumption of adequate food intake in patients recovering from colorectal cancer operations. *Surgical Clinics of North America* 66, 1167–1176.

Meguid, M.M., Campos, A.C.L., Meguid, V., Debonis, D. and Terz, J.J. (1988) IONIP, a criterion of surgical outcome and patient selection for perioperative nutritional support. *British Journal of Clinical Practice* 42, 8–14.

Mehta, P.L., Alaka, K.J., Filo, R.S., Leapman, S.B., Milgrom, M.L. and Pescovitz, M.D. (1994) Comparison of enteral vs. parenteral nutritional support in postoperative liver transplant recipients. *Journal of Parenteral and Enteral Nutrition* 18, 26S.

Meier, P. (1981) Stratification in the design of clinical trials. *Controlled Clinical Trials* 1, 355–361.

Meier, A. (1988) Nutrient metabolism. In: Jeejeebhoy, M.B., Kinney, J.M., Hill, G.L. and Owen, O.E. (eds) *Nutrition and Metabolism in Patient Care*. W.B. Saunders, Philadelphia, pp. 60–88.

Mejía-Aranguré, J.M., Fajardo-Gutiérrez, A., Reyes-Ruíz, N.I., Bernáldez-Ríos, R., Mejía-Domínguez, A.M., Navarrete-Navarro, S. and Martínez-García, M.D. (1999) Malnutrition in childhood lymphoblastic leukaemia: a predictor of early mortality during the induction-to-remission phase of the treatment. *Archives of Medical Research* 30, 150–153.

Melchior, J.C., Raguin, G., Boulier, A., Bouvet, E., Rigaud, D., Matheron, S., Casalino, E., Vilde, J.L., Vachon, F., Coulaud, J.P. and Apfelbaum, M. (1993) Resting energy expenditure in human immunodeficiency virus-infected patients: comparison between patients with and without secondary infections. *American Journal of Clinical Nutrition* 57, 614–619.

Melchior, J.C., Niyongabo, T., Henzel, D., Durack-Bown, I., Henri, S.C. and Boulier, A. (1999) Malnutrition and wasting, immunodepression and chronic inflammation as independent predictors of survival in HIV-infected patients. *Nutrition* 15, 865–869.

Melling, A.C., Ali, B., Scott, E.M. and Leaper, D.J. (2001) Effects of pre-operative warming on the incidence of wound infection after clean surgery: a randomised controlled trial. *Lancet* 358, 876–880.

Mendenhall, C.L., Anderson, S., Garcia-Pont, P., Goldberg, S., Kiernan, T., Seeff, L.B., Sorrell, M., Tamburro, C., Weesner, R., Zetterman, R., Chedid, A., Chen, T. and Rabin, L. (1984a) Short-term and long-term survival in patients with alcoholic hepatitis treated with oxandrolone and prednisolone. *New England Journal of Medicine* 311, 1464–1470.

Mendenhall, C.L., Anderson, S., Weesner, R.E., Goldberg, S.J. and Crolic, K.A. (1984b) Protein–calorie malnutrition associated with alcoholic hepatitis. *American Journal of Medicine* 76, 211–222.

Mendenhall, C., Bongiovanni, G., Goldberg, S., Miller, B., Moore, J., Rouster, S., Schneider, D., Tamburro, C., Tosch, T., Weesner, R. and Veterans Affairs Cooperative Study Group on Alcoholic Hepatitis (1985) VA Cooperative Study on alcoholic hepatitis III: Changes in protein–calorie malnutrition associated with 30 days of hospitalization with and without enteral nutritional therapy. *Journal of Parenteral and Enteral Nutrition* 9, 590–596.

Mendenhall, C.L., Moritz, T.E., Roselle, G.A., Morgan, T.R., Nemchausky, B.A., Tamburro, C.H., Schiff, E.R., McClain, C.J., Marsano, L.S., Allen, J.I., Samanta, A., Weesner, R.E., Henderson, W., Gartside, P., Chen, T.S., French, S.W., Chedid, A. and Veterans Affairs Cooperative Study Group (1993) A study of oral nutritional support with oxandrolone in malnourished patients with alcoholic hepatitis: results of a Department of Veterans Affairs Cooperative Study. *Hepatology* 17, 564–576.

Mendez, M.A. and Adair, L.S. (1999) Severity and timing of stunting in the first two years of life affect performance on cognitive tests in late childhood. *Journal of Nutrition* 129, 1555–1562.

Menzies, I.S., Zuckerman, M.J., Nukaham, W.S., Somasundaram, S.G., Murphy, B., Jenkins, A.P., Crane, R.S. and Gregory, G.G. (1999) Geography of intestinal permeability and absorption. *Gut* 44, 483–489.

Meredith, C.N., Frontera, W.R., O'Reilly, K.P. and Evans, W.J. (1992) Body composition in elderly men: effect of dietary modification during strength training. *Journal of the American Geriatric Society* 40, 155–162.

Merli, M., Riggio, O., Dally, L. and Policentrica Italiana Nutrizione Cirrosi (1996) Does malnutrition affect survival in cirrhosis? *Hepatology* 23, 1041–1046.

Messori, A., Trallori, G., D'Albasio, G., Milla, M., Vannozzi, G. and Pacini, F. (1996) Defined-formula diets versus steroids in the treatment of active Crohn's disease: a meta-analysis. *Scandinavian Journal of Gastroenterology* 31, 267–272.

Metropolitan Life Insurance Company (1959) *Statistical Bulletin.* Metropolitan Life Insurance Company.

Meydani, M. (2001) Antioxidants and cognitive function. *Nutrition Reviews* 59, S75–S82.

Meyer, N.A., Muller, M.J. and Herndon, D.N. (1994) Nutrient support of the healing wound. *New Horizons* 2, 202–214.

Middleton, M.H., Nazarenko, G., Nivison-Smith, I. and Smederly, P. (2001) Prevalence of malnutrition and 12-month incidence of mortality in two Sydney teaching hospitals. *Internal Medicine Journal* 31, 455–461.

Middleton, R.A. and Allman-Farinelli, M.A. (1999) Taste sensitivity is altered in patients with chronic renal failure receiving continuous ambulatory peritoneal dialysis. *Journal of Nutrition* 129, 122–125.

Migliorati, C.A. and Migliorati, E.K. (1997) Oral lesions and HIV. An approach to the diagnosis of oral mucosal lesions for the dentist in private practice. *Schweizer Monatsschrift fur Zahnmedizin* 107, 860–871.

Miján, A., Pérez-Garcia, A., Lorenzo, J.F. and Locutura, J. (1997) Malnutrition (PEM): an independent factor in predicting mortality length among advanced HIV+ in-patients. *Clinical Nutrition* 16 (Suppl.), 18.

Miján, A., Pérez-Garcia, A., Lorenzo, J.F. and Locutura, J. (1998) Malnutrition (PEM): an independent factor to predict length of stay (LoS) among HIV+ in-patients. *Clinical Nutrition* 17 (Suppl.), 7.

Miján, A., Ruiz, P., Juarros, C., Velasco, J.L. and de Mateo, B. (2000) The effects of undernutrition and age on cardiac muscle structure in eating disorders (ED) in patients. *Clinical Nutrition* 19 (Suppl.), 5.

Milano, M.C., Cusumano, A.M., Navarro, E.T. and Turin, M. (1998) Energy supplementation in chronic hemodialysis patients with moderate and severe malnutrition. *Journal of Renal Nutrition* 8, 212–217.

Miller, A.R.O., Griffin, G.E., Batman, P., Farquar, C., Forster, S.M., Pinching, A.J. and Harris, J.R.W. (1988) Jejunal mucosal architecture and fat absorption in male homosexuals infected with human immunodeficiency virus. *Quarterly Journal of Medicine* 69, 1009–1119.

Miller, J. and O'Hara, C. (2000) Observational audit of mealtime care. *Proceedings of the Nutrition Society* 59, 169A.

Miller, P. and Schencker, S. (2000) Does the NHS need celebrity chefs to spice up hospital food? *Nursing Times* 96, 18.

Miller, S. and Miller, J.M. (1994) Starvation in hospital: malnutrition goes unnoticed before surgery [letter]. *British Medical Journal* 308, 1369.

Miller, T.L. (2000) Nutrition in paediatric human immunodeficiency virus infection. *Proceedings of the Nutrition Society* 59, 155–162.

Miller, T.L. (2002) Nutritional interventions in pediatric HIV: it's hard to hit a moving target. *Journal of Pediatric Gastroenterology and Nutrition* 34, 353–356.

Miller, T.L., Awnetwant, E.L., Evans, S., Morris, V.M., Vazquez, I.M. and McIntosh, K. (1995) Gastrostomy tube supplementation for HIV-infected children. *Pediatrics* 96, 696–702.

Miller, T.L., Orav, E.J., Colan, S.D. and Lipshultz, S.E. (1997) Nutritional status and cardiac mass and function in children infected with the human immunodeficiency virus. *American Journal of Clinical Nutrition* 66, 660–664.

Miller, T.L., Mawn, B.E., Orav, E.J., Wilk, D., Weinberg, G.A., Nicchitta, J., Furuta, L., Cutroni, R., McIntosh, K., Burchett, S.K. and Gorbach, S.L. (2001a) The effect of protease inhibitor therapy on growth and body composition in human immunodeficiency virus type 1-infected children. *Pediatrics* 107, E77.

Miller, T.L., Easley, K.A., Zhang, W., Orav, E.J., Bier, D.M., Luder, E., Ting, A., Shearer, W.T., Vargas, J.H. and Lipshultz, S.E. (2001b) Maternal and infant factors associated with failure to thrive in children with vertically transmitted human immunodeficiency virus-1 infection: the Prospective, P2C2 Human Immunodeficiency Virus Multicenter Study. *Pediatrics* 108, 1287–1296.

Milne, A.C., Potter, J.M. and Avenell, A. (2001) Do routine oral protein and energy supplements improve survival in elderly people: a systematic review for the Cochrane Collaboration. *Proceedings of the Nutrition Society* 61, 18A.

Minard, G., Kudsk, K.A., Melton, S., Patton, J.H. and Tolley, E.A. (2000) Early versus delayed feeding with an immune-enhancing diet in patients with severe head injuries. *Journal of Parenteral and Enteral Nutrition* 24, 145–149.

Mindel, A. and Tenant-Flowers, M. (2001) Natural history and management of early HIV infection: ABC of AIDS. *British Medical Journal* 322, 1290–1293.

Mizock, B.A. (1999) Nutritional support in hepatic encephalopathy. *Nutrition* 15, 220–228.

Moher, D., Jahad, A.R., Nichol, G., Penman, M., Tugwell, P. and Walsh, S. (1995) Assessing the quality of randomized controlled trials: an annotated bibliography of scales and checklists. *Clinical Trials* 16, 62–73.

Moher, D., Jahad, A.R. and Tugwell, P. (1996) Assessing the quality of randomised clinical trials. *Journal of Technology Assessment in Health Care* 12, 195–208.

Moiniche, S., Bulow, S., Hesselfeldt, P., Hestbaek, A. and Kehlet, H. (1995) Convalescence and hospital stay after colonic surgery with balanced analgesia, early oral feeding, and enforced mobilisation. *European Journal of Surgery* 161, 283–288.

Mojon, P., Budtz-Jorgensen, E. and Rapin, C.H. (1999) Relationship between oral health and nutrition in very old people. *Age and Ageing* 28, 463–468.

Moller-Madsen, B., Tottrup, A., Hessov, I. and Jensen, J. (1988) Nutritional intake and nutritional status of patients with a fracture of the femoral neck: value of oral supplements. *Acta Orthopaedica Scandinavica* 59, 48.

Moncure, M., Samaha, E., Moncure, K., Mitchell, J., Rehm, C., Cypel, D., Eydelman, J. and Ross, S.E. (1999) Jejunostomy tube feedings should not be stopped in the perioperative patient. *Journal of Parenteral and Enteral Nutrition* 23, 356–359.

Monso, E., Fiz, J.M., Izquierdo, J., Alonso, J., Coll, R., Rosell, A. and Morera, J. (1998) Quality of life in severe chronic obstructive pulmonary disease: correlation with lung and muscle function. *Respiratory Medicine* 92, 221–227.

Montecalvo, M.A., Steger, K.A., Farber, H.W., Smith, B.F., Dennis, R.C., Fitzpatrick, G.F., Pollack, S.D., Korsberg, T.Z., Birkett, D.H., Hirsch, E.F., Craven, D.E. and The Critical Care Research Team (1992) Nutritional outcome and pneumonia in critical care patients randomised to gastric versus jejunal tube feedings. *Critical Care Medicine* 20, 1377–1387.

Montejo, J.C. for the National and Metabolic Working Group of the Spanish Society of Intensive Care Medicine and Coronary Units (1999) Enteral nutrition-related gastrointestinal complications in critically ill patients: a multicenter study. *Critical Care Medicine* 27, 1447–1453.

Moody, C., Seal, C.J. and Regnard, C.F.B. (1998) Taste and appetite in patients with advanced cancer. *Proceedings of the Nutrition Society* 57, 85A.

Moore, A.A., Siu, A.L., Partridge, J.M., Hays, R.D. and Adams, J. (1997) A randomised trial of office-based screening for common problems in older persons. *American Journal of Medicine* 102, 371–378.

Moore, E.E. and Jones, T.N. (1986) Benefits of immediate jejunostomy feeding after major abdominal trauma – a prospective randomised study. *Journal of Trauma* 26, 874–881.

Moore, E.E. and Moore, F.A. (1991) Immediate enteral nutrition following multisystem trauma: a decade perspective. *Journal of the American College of Nutrition* 10, 633–648.

Moore, F.A., Feliciano, D.V., Andrassy, R.J., McArdle, A.H., Booth, F.V.M., Morgenstein-Wagner, T.B., Kellum, J.M., Welling, R.E. and Moore, E.E. (1992) Early enteral feeding, compared with parenteral, reduces postoperative septic complications: the results of a meta-analysis. *Annals of Surgery* 216, 172–183.

Moore, F.A., Moore, E.E., Kudsk, K.A., Brown, R.O., Bower, R.M., Koruda, M.J., Baker, C.C. and Barbul, A. (1994) Clinical benefits of an immune-enhancing diet for early postinjury enteral feeding. *Journal of Trauma* 37, 607–615.

Moore, M.C., Greene, H.L., Donald, W.D. and Dunn, G.D. (1986) Enteral-tube feeding as adjunct therapy in malnourished patients with cystic fibrosis: a clinical study and literature review. *American Journal of Clinical Nutrition* 44, 33–41.

Moore, S.E., Cole, T.J., Poskitt, E.M.E., Sonko, B.J., Whitehead, R.G., McGregor, I.A. and Prentice, A.M. (1997) Season of birth predicts mortality in rural Gambia. *Nature* 388, 434.

Moore, S.E., Collinson, A.C. and Prentice, A.M. (2001) Moderate levels of undernutrition have little impact on immune function in rural Gambian children. *Proceedings of the Nutrition Society* 60, 20A.

Mooser, V. and Carr, A. (2001) Antiretroviral therapy-associated hyperlipidaemia in HIV disease. *Current Opinion in Lipidology* 12, 313–319.

Morais, J., Horsman, R., Richardson, A. and Middleton, C. (2000) The impact of a formal enteral feeding policy when introduced in the intensive care unit. *Proceedings of the Nutrition Society* 59, 168A.

Moran, B.J. and Jackson, A.A. (1995) Nutrition education: the attitude and involvement of clinicians in nutritional support. *Clinical Nutrition* 14, 191–192.

Morgan, D.B., Newton, H.M.V., Schorah, C.J., Jewitt, M.A., Hancock, M.R. and Hullin, R.P. (1986) Abnormal indices of nutrition in the elderly: a study of different clinical groups. *Age and Ageing* 15, 65–76.

Morgan, G. (1997) What, if any, is the effect of malnutrition on immunological competence? *Lancet* 349, 1693–1695.

Morin, C.L., Roulet, M., Roy, C.C. and Weber, A. (1980) Continuous elemental enteral alimentation in children with Crohn's disease and growth failure. *Gastroenterology* 79, 1205–1210.

Morison, S., Dodge, J.A., Cole, T.J., Lewis, P.A., Coles, E.C., Geddes, D., Russell, G., Littlewood, J.M., Scott, M.T. and the UK Cystic Fibrosis Survey Management Committee (1997) Height and weight in cystic fibrosis: a cross sectional study. *Archives of Diseases in Childhood* 77, 497–500.

Morley, J.E. (1991) Why do physicians fail to recognize and treat malnutrition in older persons? *Journal of the American Geriatric Society* 39, 1139–1140.

Morley, J.E. (1996) Anorexia in older persons: epidemiology and optimal treatment. *Drugs and Ageing* 8, 134–155.

Morley, J.E. (1998) Protein-energy malnutrition in older subjects. *Proceedings of the Nutrition Society* 57, 587–592.

Morley, J.E. and Kraenzle, D. (1994) Causes of weight loss in a community nursing home. *Journal of American Geriatric Society* 42, 583–585.

Morley, J.E., Mooradian, A.D., Silver, A.J., Heber, D. and Alfin-Slater, R.B. (1988) Nutrition in the elderly (UCLA conference). *Annals of Internal Medicine* 109, 890–904.

Morris, R., Hart, K., Smith, V., Shannon, L., Bolton, J., Abbott, R., Alleyne, M., Plant, H. and Slevin, M.L. (1990) A comparison of the energy supplements Polycal and Duocal in cancer patients. *Journal of Human Nutrition and Dietetics* 3, 171–176.

Moses, A.G., Slater, C., Barber, M.D., Preston, T. and Fearon, K.C. (2000) The energy expenditure of activity, physical activity level, and Karnofsky performance score in patients with pancreatic cancer cachexia. *Clinical Nutrition* 19 (Suppl.), 29.

Mostert, R., Goris, A., Weling-Scheepers, C., Wouters, E.F. and Schols, A.M. (2000) Tissue depletion and health related quality of life in patients with chronic obstructive pulmonary disease. *Respiratory Medicine* 94, 859–867.

Mowatt-Larssen, C.A., Brown, R.O., Wojtysiak, S.L. and Kudsk, K.A. (1992) Comparison of tolerance and nutritional outcome between a peptide and a standard enteral formula in critically ill, hypoalbuminemic patients. *Journal of Parenteral and Enteral Nutrition* 16, 20–24.

Mowé, M. and Bøhmer, T. (1991) The prevalence of undiagnosed protein-calorie undernutrition in a population of hospitalised elderly patients. *Journal of the American Geriatric Society* 39, 1089–1092.

Mowé, M. and Bøhmer, T. (2000) Increased 5-year mortality in aged undernourished patients. *Clinical Nutrition* 19 (Suppl.), 8.

Mowé, M., Bøhmer, T. and Kindt, E. (1994) Reduced nutritional status in an elderly population (> 70 y) is probable before disease and possibly contributes to the development of disease. *American Journal of Clinical Nutrition* 59, 317–324.

Moy, R.J.D., Smallman, S. and Booth, I.W. (1990) Malnutrition in a UK children's hospital. *Journal of Human Nutrition and Dietetics* 3, 93–100.

Moye, J., Rich, K.C., Kalish, L.A., Sheon, A.R., Diaz, C., Cooper, E.R., Pitt, J. and Handelsman, E. (1998) Natural history of somatic growth in infants born to women infected by human immunodeficiency virus. *Journal of Pediatrics* 128, 58–69.

MCR Vitamin Study Research Group (1991) Prevention of neural tube defects: results of the Medical Research Council vitamin study. *The Lancet* 338, 131–137.

Mughal, M.M. and Meguid, M.M. (1987) The effect of nutritional status on morbidity after elective surgery for benign gastrointestinal disease. *Journal of Parenteral and Enteral Nutrition* 11, 140–143.

Muhlethaler, R., Stuck, A.E., Minder, C.E. and Frey, B.M. (1995) The prognostic significance of protein–energy malnutrition in geriatric patients. *Age and Ageing* 24, 193–197.

Muldoon, M.F., Barger, S.D., Flory, J.D. and Manuck, S.B. (1998) What are quality of life measurements measuring? *British Medical Journal* 316, 542–545.

Mulholland, J.H., Tui, C., Wright, A.M. and Vinci, V.J. (1943) Nitrogen metabolism, caloric intake and weight loss in postoperative convalescence. *Annals of Surgery* 117, 512–534.

Müller, M.J. (1998) Hepatic energy and substrate metabolism: a possible metabolic basis for early nutritional support in cirrhotic patients. *Nutrition* 14, 30–38.

Müller, M.J., Loyal, S., Schwarze, M., Lobers, J., Selberg, O., Ringe, B. and Pichlmayr, R. (1994) Resting energy expenditure and nutritional state in patients with liver cirrhosis before and after liver transplantation. *Clinical Nutrition* 13, 145–152.

Mulligan, J., Voss, L.D., McCaughey, E.S., Bailey, B.J.R. and Betts, P.R. (1998) Growth monitoring: testing the new guidelines. *Archives of Diseases in Childhood* 79, 318–322.

Mulligan, K., Tai, V.W. and Schambelan, M. (1997) Cross-sectional and longitudinal evaluation of body composition in men with HIV infection. *Journal of Acquired Immune Deficiency Syndromes and Human Retrovirology* 15, 43–48.

Murchan, P.M., Bradford, I., Palmer, P., Townsend, S., Harrison, J.D., Mitchell, C.J. and Macfie, J. (1995) Value of preoperative and postoperative supplemental enteral nutrition in patients undergoing major gastrointestinal surgery. *Clinical Nutrition* 14 (Suppl.), O22.

Murciano, D., Rigaud, D., Pingleton, S., Armengaud, M.H., Melchior, J.C. and Aubier, M. (1994) Diaphragmatic function in severely malnourished patients with anorexia nervosa: effects of renutrition. *American Journal of Respiratory and Critical Care Medicine* 150, 1569–1574.

Murphy, J., Cameron, D.W., Garber, G., Conway, B. and Denomme, N. (1992) Dietary counselling and nutritional supplementation in HIV infection. *Journal of the Canadian Dietetic Association* 53, 205–208.

Murphy, J., Badaloo, V.A., Cawood, A., Chambers, B., Forrester, T.E., Wootton, S.A. and Jackson, A.A. (2001a) Gastrointestinal handling of vitamin A in severely malnourished children at admission and following treatment. *Proceedings of the Nutrition Society* 60, 173A.

Murphy, J.L., Badaloo, V.A., Chambers, B., Hounslow, A., Forrester, T.E., Wootton, S.A. and Jackson, A.A. (2001b) Lipid digestion and absorption during rehabilitation from severe childhood malnutrition. *Proceedings of the Nutrition Society* 60, 235A.

Murphy, M.C., Brooks, C.N., New, S.A. and Lumbers, M.L. (2000) The use of the Mini-Nutritional Assessment (MNA) tool in elderly orthopaedic patients. *European Journal of Clinical Nutrition* 54, 555–562.

Murphy, P.M., Cawdery, E.C. and Lewis, W.G. (2001) Energy and protein in hospital patients after oesophagogastrectomy for oesophageal cancer. *Proceedings of the Nutrition Society* 60, 118A.

Murray, C.P., Sitzia, J., Smits, M. and McLaren, S.M. (2000) Nutritional risk and its association with stroke variables. *Proceedings of the Nutrition Society* 59, 173A.

Murray, M.J. and Murray, A.B. (1977) Starvation suppression and refeeding activation of infection. *Lancet* i, 123–125.

Murray, M.J. and Murray, A.B. (1979) Anorexia of infection as a mechanism of host defense. *American Journal of Clinical Nutrition* 32, 593–596.

Murray, M., Murray, A., Murray, M. and Murray, C. (1978) The adverse effect of iron repletion on the course of certain infections. *British Medical Journal* 2, 1113–1115.

Murray, M., Murray, A., Murray, N. and Murray, M. (1995) Infections during severe primary undernutrition and subsequent refeeding: paradoxical findings. *Australia and New Zealand Journal of Medicine* 25 (5), 507–511.

Mussolino, M.E., Looker, A.C., Madans, J.H., Langlois, J.A. and Orwell, E.S. (1998) Risk factors for hip fracture in white men: the NHANES 1 epidemiologic follow-up study. *Journal of Bone and Mineral Research* 13, 918–924.

Mutlu, E.A. and Mobarhan, S. (2000) Nutrition in the care of the cancer patient. *Nutrition in Clinical Care* 3, 3–23.

Myers, S.A., Takiguchi, S. and Yu, M. (1994) Stature estimated from knee height in elderly Japanese Americans. *Journal of American Geriatric Society* 42, 157–160.

Naber, T.H.J., Schermer, T., de Bree, A., Nusteling, K., Eggink, L., Kruimel, J.W., Bakkeren, J., van Heereveld, H. and Katan, M.B. (1997) Prevalence of malnutrition in nonsurgical hospitalized patients and its association with disease complications. *American Journal of Clinical Nutrition* 66, 1232–1239.

Nagata, T., Tobitani, W., Kiriike, N., Iketani, T. and Yamagami, S. (1999) Capacity to produce cytokines during weight restoration in patients with anorexia nervosa. *Psychosomatic Medicine* 61, 371–377.

Nagel, M.R. (1993) Nutrition screening: identifying patients at risk for malnutrition. *Nutrition in Clinical Practice* 8, 171–175.

Naidu, A.N. and Rao, N.P. (1994) Body mass index: a measure of the nutritional situation in Indian populations. *European Journal of Clinical Nutrition* 48, S131–S140.

Nataloni, S., Gentili, P., Marini, B., Guidi, A., Marconi, P., Busco, F. and Pelaia, P. (1999) Nutritional assessment in head injured patients through the study of rapid turnover visceral proteins. *Clinical Nutrition* 18.

National Audit Office, N.E.N. (2000) *Inpatient Admissions and Bed Management in NHS Acute Hospitals*. Stationery Office, London.

National Institutes of Health (1998) Clinical guidelines on the identification, evaluation, and treatment of overweight and obesity in adults – the evidence report (published correction appears in *Obesity Research* (1998) 6, 464). *Obesity Research* 6 (Suppl. 2), 51S–209S.

National Prescribing Centre (1998) Oral nutritional support (part 1). *MeReC Bulletin* 9, 25–30.

National Pressure Ulcer Advisory Panel (NPUAP) (1989) Pressure ulcers prevalence, costs and risk assessment: consensus development conference statement. *Decubitus* 2, 24.

National Research Council (1989) *Diet and Health*. Academy Press, Washington, DC.

Navarro, J., Cezard, J.P. and Vargas, J. (1981) Nasogastric tube feeding at home in gastroenterological pediatric practice [letter]. *American Journal of Clinical Nutrition* 35, 408–409.

Nayel, H., El-Ghoneimy, E. and El-Haddad, S. (1992) Impact of nutritional supplementation on treatment delay and morbidity in patients with head and neck tumours treated with irradiation. *Nutrition* 8, 13–18.

Newell, M.L. and Peckham, C. (1994) Vertical transmission of HIV infection. *Acta Paediatrica* 400, 43–45.

Newton, R. (2001) Changes in parenteral nutrition supply when the nutrition support team control prescribing. *Nutrition* 17, 347–350.

Nezu, K., Yoshikawa, M., Yoneda, T., Kushibe, T., Kawaguchi, T., Kimura, M., Kobayashi, A., Takenaka, H., Fukuoka, A., Narita, N. and Taniguchi, S. (2001) The effect of nutritional status on morbidity in COPD patients undergoing bilateral lung reduction surgery. *Thoracic and Cardiovascular Surgery* 49, 216–220.

Ng, D.H., Timmis, L. and Bowling, T.E. (2001) A two year audit on percutaneous endoscopic gastrostomy: is the nutrition support team generating more work? *Proceedings of the Nutrition Society* 60, 123A.

Nguyen, L.T., Bedu, M., Caillaud, D., Beaufrere, B., Beaujon, G. and Vasson, M.P. (1999) Increased resting energy expenditure is related to plasma TNF-α concentration in stable COPD patients. *Clinical Nutrition* 18, 269–274.

Nicolas, A.S., Faisant, C., Lanzmann-Petithory, D., Tome, D. and Vellas, B. (2000) The nutritional intake of a free-living healthy French population: a four-year follow-up. *Journal of Nutrition, Health and Ageing* 4, 77–80.

Nielsen, F. (1998) Ultratrace elements – physiology. In: *Encyclopaedia of Human Nutrition*. Harcourt Brace, pp. 1884–1897.

Nielsen, K., Kondrup, J., Martinsen, L., Stilling, B. and Wikman, B. (1993) Nutritional assessment and adequacy of dietary intake in hospitalized patients with alcoholic liver cirrhosis. *British Journal of Nutrition* 69, 665–679.

Nielsen, K., Kondrup, J., Martinsen, L., Dossing, H., Larsson, B., Stilling, B. and Jensen, M.G. (1995) Long-term oral refeeding of patients with cirrhosis of the liver. *British Journal of Nutrition* 74, 557–567.

Nightingale, J.M.D. and Reeves, J. (1999) Knowledge about the assessment and management of undernutrition: a pilot questionnaire in a UK teaching hospital. *Clinical Nutrition* 18, 23–27.

Nightingale, J.M.D., Walsh, N., Bullock, M.E. and Wicks, A.C. (1996) Three simple methods of detecting malnutrition on medical wards. *Journal of the Royal Society of Medicine* 89, 144–148.

Nikolaus, T., Bach, M., Siezen, S., Volkert, D., Oster, P. and Schlierf, G. (1995) Assessment of nutritional risk in the elderly. *Annals of Nutrition and Metabolism* 39, 340–345.

Nitenberg, G. and Raynard, B. (2000) Nutritional support of the cancer patient: issues and dilemmas. *Critical Reviews in Oncology/Hematology* 34, 137–168.

Niyongabo, T., Bouchaud, O., Henzel, D., Melchior, J.C., Samb, B., Dazza, M.C., Ruggeri, C., Begue, J.C., Coulaud, J.P. and Larouzé, B. (1997) Nutritional status of HIV-seropositive subjects in an AIDS clinic in Paris. *European Journal of Clinical Nutrition* 51, 637–640.

Niyongabo, T., Henzel, D., Idi, M., Mnimubona, S., Gikora, E., Melchior, J.C., Matheron, S., Kamafu, G., Samb, B., Messing, B., Begue, J., Aubry, P. and Larouze, B. (1999) Tuberculosis, human immunodeficiency virus infection and malnutrition in Burundi. *Nutrition* 15, 289–293.

Nordenram, G., Ljunggren, G. and Cederholm, T. (2001) Nutritional status and chewing capacity in nursing home residents. *Aging Clinical and Experimental Research* 13, 370–377.

Norman, L.J., Coleman, J.E., Macdonald, I.A., Tomsett, A.M. and Watson, A.R. (2000) Nutrition and growth in relation to severity of renal disease in children. *Pediatric Nephrology* 15, 259–265.

Norregaard, O., Tottrup, A., Saaek, A. and Hessov, I. (1987) Effects of oral nutritional supplements to adults with chronic obstructive pulmonary disease. *Clinical and Research Physiology* 23, 388s.

Norton, B., Homer-Ward, M., Donnelly, M.T., Long, R.G. and Holmes, G.K.T. (1996) A randomised prospective comparison of percutaneous endoscopic gastrostomy and nasogastric tube feeding after acute dysphagic stroke. *British Medical Journal* 312, 13–16.

Nurmohamed, M.T., Rosendaal, F.R., Bueller, H.R., Dekker, E., Hommes, D.W., Vandenbrouche, J.P. and Briet, E. (1992) Low-molecular-weight heparin versus standard heparin in general and orthopaedic surgery: a meta-analysis. *Lancet* 340, 152–156.

Nutrition Screening Initiative (1996) *The Clinical and Cost Effectiveness of Medical Nutritional Therapy: Evidence and Estimates of Potential Medicare Savings from the Use of Selected Nutritional Interventions.* Nutrition Screening Initiative, Washington, DC.

Nygren, J., Thorell, A. and Ljungqvist, O. (2001) Preoperative oral carbohydrate nutrition: an update. *Current Opinion in Clinical Nutrition and Metabolic Care* 4, 255–259.

Nyswonger, G.D. and Helmchen, R.H. (1992) Early enteral nutrition and length of stay in stroke patients. *Journal of Neuroscience Nursing* 24, 220–223.

O'Boyle, C.J., Ziegler, D., Wadsworth, C., Mitchell, C.J. and Macfie, J. (1997) Clinical associations with bacterial translocation. *Clinical Nutrition* 16 (Suppl.), 48.

O'Boyle, C.J., Macfie, J., Dave, K., Sagar, P.S., Poon, P. and Mitchell, C.J. (1998) Alterations in intestinal barrier function do not predispose to translocation of enteric bacteria in gastroenterologic patients. *Nutrition* 14, 358–362.

O'Brien, P.M.S., Wheeler, T. and Barker, D.P.J. (1999) *Fetal Programming: Influences on Development and Disease in Later Life.* Royal College of Obstetrics and Gynaecology Press, London.

Ochoa, J.B., Magnuson, B., Swintowsky, M., Loan, T., Boulanger, B., McClain, C. and Kearney, P. (2000) Long-term reduction in the cost of nutritional intervention achieved by a nutrition support service. *Nutrition in Clinical Practice* 15, 174–180.

Ockenga, J., Suettmann, U., Bischoff, S.C., Wagner, S., Schlesinger, A., Muller, M.J., Deicher, H. and Manns, M. (1994) Outcome of long-term enteral nutrition by percutaneous endoscopic gastrostomy in HIV-infected patients. *Clinical Nutrition* 13 (Suppl.), 11.

Ockenga, J., Schlesinger, A., Süttmann, U., Seibt, C. and Manns, M.P. (1997) Dietary intake in asymptomatic HIV-infected outpatients: association to stage of disease and present of malnutrition. *Clinical Nutrition* 16 (Suppl.), 37.

O'Dea, K. (1995) The prevalence of pressure sores in four European countries. *Journal of Wound Care* 4, 192–195.

Odlund-Olin, A., Osterberg, P., Hadell, K., Armyr, I., Jerstrom, S. and Ljungqvist, O. (1996) Energy-enriched hospital food to improve energy intake in elderly patients. *Journal of Parenteral and Enteral Nutrition* 20, 93–97.

Odlund-Olin, A., Armyr, I., Soop, M., Ljungqvist, E., Jerstrom, S., Classon, I., Ljunggren, G. and Ljungqvist, O. (1998) Energy enriched meals improve energy intake in elderly residents in a nursing home. *Clinical Nutrition* 17 (Suppl.), P09

Office of Population Censuses and Surveys (1993) *Health Survey for England 1991.* Her Majesty's Stationery Office, London.

Office of Population Censuses and Surveys (1994) *Health Survey for England, 1992.* HMSO, London.

Ofman, J. and Koretz, R.L. (1997) Clinical economics review: nutritional support. *Alimentary Pharmacology and Therapy* 11, 453–471.

Ogilvy-Stuart, A.L. and Shalet, S.M. (1995) Effect of chemotherapy on growth. *Acta Paediatrica* 411, 52–56.

Ohri, S.K., Bjarnason, I., Pathi, V., Somasundaram, S., Bowles, C.T., Keogh, B.E., Khaghani, A., Menzies, I., Yacoub, M.H. and Taylor, K.M. (1993) Cardiopulmonary bypass impairs small intestinal transport and increases gut permeability. *Annals of Thoracic Surgery* 55, 1080–1086.

Okada, Y., Klein, N., van Saene, K.H.F., Reynolds, A. and Pierro, A. (1997) The immune response to invading bacteria is impaired in neonates receiving parenteral nutrition. *Proceedings of the Nutrition Society* 56, 218A.

Okada, Y., Klein, N., van Saene, H.K.F. and Pierro, A. (1998) Small volumes of enteral feedings normalise immune function in infants receiving parenteral nutrition. *Journal of Pediatric Surgery* 33, 16–19.

O'Keefe, S.J.D., Lemmer, E.R., Ogden, J.M. and Winter, T. (1998) The influence of intravenous infusions of glucose and amino acids on pancreatic enzyme and mucosal protein synthesis in human subjects. *Journal of Parenteral and Enteral Nutrition* 22, 253–258.

Okita, M., Watanabe, A. and Nagashima, H. (1985) Nutritional treatment of liver cirrhosis by branched-chain amino acid-enriched nutrient mixture. *Journal of Nutritional Science and Vitaminology* 31, 291–303.

Older, M.W.J., Edwards, D. and Dickerson, J.W.T. (1980) A nutrient survey in elderly women with femoral neck fractures. *British Journal of Surgery* 67, 884–886.

Oldfield, G.S., Commerford, P.J. and Opie, L.H. (1986) Effects of preoperative glucose–insulin–potassium on myocardial glycogen levels and on complications of mitral valve replacement. *Journal of Thoracic and Cardiovascular Surgery* 91, 874–878.

Olejko, T.D. and Fonseca, R.J. (1984) Preoperative nutritional supplementation for the orthognathic surgery patient. *Journal of Oral and Maxillofacial Surgery* 42, 573–577.

O'Loughlin, E., Forbes, D., Parsons, H., Scott, B., Cooper, D. and Gall, G. (1986) Nutritional rehabilitation of malnourished patients with cystic fibrosis. *American Journal of Clinical Nutrition* 43, 732–737.

O'Morain, C., Segal, A.W. and Levi, A.J. (1984) Elemental diet as primary treatment of acute Crohn's disease: a controlled trial. *British Medical Journal* 288, 1859–1862.

Onizuka, Y., Mizuta, Y., Isomoto, H., Takeshima, F., Murase, K. and Miyazaki, M. (2001) Sludge and stone formation in the gallbladder in bedridden elderly patients with cerebrovascular disease: influence of feeding method. *Journal of Gastroenterology* 36, 330–337.

Openbrier, D.R., Irwin, M.M., Rogers, R.M., Gottlieb, G.P., Dauber, J.H., Van Thiel, D.H. and Pennock, B.E. (1983) Nutritional status and lung function in patients with emphysema and chronic bronchitis. *Chest* 83, 17–22.

Openbrier, D.R., Irwin, M.M., Dauber, J.H., Owens, G. and Rogers, R.M. (1984) Factors affecting nutritional status and the impact of nutritional support in patients with emphysema. *Chest* 85, 67S–69S.

O'Regan, S. and Garel, L. (1990) Percutaneous gastrojejunostomy for caloric supplementation in children on peritoneal dialysis. *Advances in Peritoneal Dialysis* 6, 273–275.

Orenstein, S.R. (1986) Enteral versus parenteral therapy for intractable diarrhea of infancy: a prospective, randomized trial. *Journal of Pediatrics* 109, 277–286.

Oriishi, T., Sata, M., Toyonaga, A., Sasaki, E. and Tanikawa, K. (1995) Evaluation of intestinal permeability in patients with inflammatory bowel disease using lactulose and measuring antibodies to lipid A. *Gut* 36, 891–896.

Ortiz, A., Parra, E.G., Rodeles, M. and Mendez, A. (1992) [Complementary artificial nutrition in kidney failure]. *Nutricion Hospitalaria* 7, 393–399.

Ott, M., Lembcke, B., Fischer, H., Jäger, R., Polat, H., Geier, H., Rech, M., Staszeswki, S., Helm, E.B. and Caspary, W.F. (1993) Early changes of body composition in human immunodeficiency virus infected patients: tetrapolar body impedance analysis indicates significant malnutrition. *American Journal of Clinical Nutrition* 57, 15–19.

Ott, M., Fischer, H., Polat, H., Helm, E.B., Frenz, M., Caspary, W.F. and Lembcke, B. (1995) Bioelectrical impedance analysis as a predictor of survival in patients with human immunodeficiency virus infection. *Journal of Acquired Immune Deficiency Syndromes and Human Retrovirology* 9, 20–25.

Otte, K.E., Ahlburg, P., D'Amore, F. and Stellfeld, M. (1989) Nutritional repletion in malnourished patients with emphysema. *Journal of Parenteral and Enteral Nutrition* 13, 152–156.

Ouslander, J.G., Tymchuk, A.J. and Krynski, M.D. (1993) Decisions about enteral tube feeding among the elderly. *Journal of the American Geriatric Society* 41, 70–77.

Ovesen, L. (1992) The effect of a supplement which is nutrient dense compared to standard concentration on the total nutritional intake of anorectic patients. *Clinical Nutrition* 11, 154–157.

Ovesen, L. and Allingstrup, L. (1992) Different quantities of two commercial liquid diets consumed by weight-losing cancer patients. *Journal of Parenteral and Enteral Nutrition* 16, 275–278.

Ovesen, L., Hannibal, J., Sorensen, M. and Allingstrup, L. (1991) Food intake, eating-related complaints and smell and taste sensations in patients with cancer of the lung, ovary and breast undergoing chemotherapy. *Clinical Nutrition* 10, 336–341.

Ovesen, L., Hannibal, J. and Mortensen, E.L. (1993) The interrelationship of weight loss, dietary intake and quality of life in ambulatory patients with cancer of the lung, breast and ovary. *Nutrition and Cancer* 19, 159–167.

Pacelli, F., Bossola, M., Papa, V., Malerba, M., Modesti, C., Sgadari, A., Bellantone, R. and Doglietto, G.B. (2001) Enteral vs. parenteral nutrition after major abdominal surgery. *Archives of Surgery* 136, 933–936.

Paillaud, E., Bories, P.-N., Le Parco, J.-C. and Campilo, B. (2000) Nutritional status and energy expenditure in elderly patients with recent hip fracture during a 2-month follow up. *British Journal of Nutrition* 83, 97–103.

Palella, F.J., Delaye, K.M., Moorman, A.C., Loveless, M.O., Fuhrer, J., Satten, G.A., Aschman, D.J., Holmberg, S.D. and HIV Outpatient Study Investigators (1998) Declining morbidity and mortality among patients with advanced human immunodeficiency virus infection. *New England Journal of Medicine* 338, 853–860.

Palenicek, J.P., Graham, N.M., He, Y.D., Hoover, D.A., Oishi, J.S., Kingsley, L. and Saah, A.J. (1995) Weight loss prior to clinical AIDS as a predictor of survival. Multicenter AIDS Cohort Study Investigators. *Journal of Acquired Immune Deficiency Syndromes and Human Retrovirology* 10, 366–373.

Palomares, M.R., Sayre, J.W., Shekar, K.C., Lillington, L.M. and Chlebowski, R.T. (1996) Gender influence on weight-loss pattern and survival of nonsmall cell lung carcinoma patients. *Cancer* 78, 2119–2126.

Papadopoulou, A., Holden, C.E., Paul, L., Sexton, E. and Booth, I.W. (1995) The nutritional response to home enteral nutrition in childhood. *Acta Paediatrica* 84, 528–531.

Pape, H.C., Dwenger, A., Regel, G., Auf'm'Kolch, M., Gollub, F., Wisner, D., Sturm, J.A. and Tsherne, H. (1994) Increased gut permeability after multiple trauma. *British Journal of Surgery* 81, 850–852.

Pardy, R.L., Knowles, J.L., Fairbarn, M.S. and Chan-Yan, C. (1986) Supplemental nutrition does not alter respiratory muscle strength (RMS) or endurance (RME) in ambulatory COPD patients. *American Review of Respiratory Disease* 133, A204.

Pareira, M.D., Conrad, E.J., Hicks, W. and Elman, R. (1954) Therapeutic nutrition with tube feeding. *Journal of the American Medical Association* 156, 810–816.

Parisien, C., Gélinas, M.D. and Cossette, M. (1993) Comparison of anthropometric measures of men with HIV: asymptomatic, symptomatic and AIDS. *Journal of the American Dietetic Association* 93, 1404–1408.

Park, R.H.R., Allison, M.C., Lang, J., Spence, E., Morris, A.J., Danesh, B.J.Z., Russell, R.I. and Mills, P.R. (1992) Randomised comparison of percutaneous endoscopic gastrostomy and nasogastric tube feeding in patients with persisting neurological dysphagia. *British Medical Journal* 304, 1406–1409.

Parker, T., Neale, G., Cottee, S. and Elia, M. (1996a) Management of artificial nutrition in East Anglia: a community study. *Journal of the Royal College of Physicians of London* 30, 27–32.

Parker, T., Neale, G. and Elia, M. (1996b) Home enteral tube feeding in East Anglia. *European Journal of Clinical Nutrition* 50, 47–53.

Parkin, J. and Cohen, B. (2001) An overview of the immune system. *Lancet* 357, 1777–1789.

Parkinson, S.A., Lewis, J., Morris, R., Allbright, A., Plant, H. and Slevin, M.L. (1987) Oral protein and energy supplementation in cancer patients. *Human Nutrition: Applied Nutrition* 41A, 233–243.

Parsons, H.G., Beaudry, P., Dumas, A. and Pencharz, P.B. (1983) Energy needs and growth in children with cystic fibrosis. *Journal of Pediatric Gastroenterology and Nutrition* 2, 44–49.

Patek, A.J. and Post, J. (1941) Treatment of cirrhosis of the liver by a nutritious diet and supplements rich in vitamin B complex. *Journal of Clinical Investigation* 20, 481–505.

Patel, M.G. and Raftery, M.J. (1997) The use of dietary supplements in continuous ambulatory peritoneal dialysis patients. *Journal of Renal Nutrition* 7, 129–133.

Patel, M.G., Kitchen, S. and Miligan, P.J. (2000) The effect of dietary supplements on the nPCR in stable hemodialysis patients. *Journal of Renal Nutrition* 10, 69–75.

Patrick, J., Boland, M., Stoski, D. and Murray, G.E. (1986) Rapid correction of wasting in children with cerebral palsy. *Developmental Medicine and Child Neurology* 29, 734–739.

Patterson, B.M., Cornell, C.N., Carbone, B., Levine, B. and Chapman, D. (1992) Protein depletion and metabolic stress in elderly patients who have a fracture of the hip. *Journal of Bone and Joint Surgery* 74A, 251–260.

Pattison, D. and Young, A. (1997) Effect of a multi-disciplinary care team on the management of gastrostomy feeding. *Journal of Human Nutrition and Dietetics* 10, 103–109.

Pattison, R.M., Richardson, R.A., Dougan, H. and Davidson, H.I.M. (1997a) Impact of altered taste sensitivity on dietary intake of patients with advanced cancer. *Proceedings of the Nutrition Society* 56, 314A.

Pattison, R.M., Richardson, R.A., Dougan, H. and Davidson, H.I.M. (1997b) Biochemical correlates of altered taste perception in patients with advanced cancer. *Clinical Nutrition* 16 (Suppl.), 29.

Payette, H., Coulombe, C., Boutier, V. and Gray, D.K. (2000) Nutrition risk factors for institutionalization in a free-living functionally dependent elderly population. *Journal of Clinical Epidemiology* 53, 579–587.

Payne-James, J. and Silk, D. (1990) Clinical nutrition support: better control and assessment are needed. *British Medical Journal* 301, 1–2.

Payne-James, J., de Gara, C., Grimble, G., Rees, R., Bray, J., Rana, S., Cribb, R., Frost, P. and Silk, D. (1990) Nutritional support in hospitals in the United Kingdom: national survey 1988. *Health Trends* 221, 9–13.

Payne-James, J., de Gara, C., Grimble, G., Bray, J., Rana, S., Kapadia, S. and Silk, D. (1992) Artificial nutrition support in hospitals in the United Kingdom – 1991: second national survey. *Clinical Nutrition* 11, 187–192.

Peake, H.J., Evans, S.C., Malby, A.A., Bartram, J. and Frost, G.S. (2000) Determining the incidence of hospital trust malnutrition to plan and target nutritional support strategies. *Proceedings of the Nutrition Society* 59, 139A.

Peck, K. and Johnson, S. (1990) The role of nutrition in HIV infection: a report of the working party of the AIDS interest group of the BDA. *Journal of Human Nutrition and Dietetics* 3, 147–157.

Pedersen, N.W. and Pedersen, D. (1992) Nutrition as a prognostic indicator in amputations: a prospective study of 47 cases. *Acta Orthopaedica Scandinavica* 63, 675–678.

Peel, M. (1997) Hunger strikes: understanding the underlying physiology will help doctors provide proper advice. *British Medical Journal* 315, 829–830.

Peerless, J.R., Davies, A., Klein, D. and Yu, D. (1999) Skin complications in the intensive care unit. *Clinics in Chest Medicine* 20, 453–467.

Pelletier, D., Frongillo, E.A. and Habicht, J.-P. (1993) Epidemiologic evidence for a potentiating effect of malnutrition on child mortality. *American Journal of Public Health* 83, 1130–1133.

Pencharz, P.B. and Durie, P.R. (2000) Pathogenesis of malnutrition in cystic fibrosis, and its treatment. *Clinical Nutrition* 19, 387–394.

Pennington, C.R. (1996) Malnutrition in hospital practice. *Nutrition* 12, 56–57.

Pepys, M.B. and Baltz, M.L. (1983) Acute phase proteins with special reference to C-reactive protein and related proteins (pentaxins) and serum amyloid A protein. *Advances in Immunology* 34, 141–212.

Pereira, A.M., Hamani, N., Nogueira, P.C.K. and Carvalhaes, T.A.C. (2000) Oral vitamin intake in children receiving long-term dialysis. *Journal of Renal Nutrition* 10, 24–29.

Perissinotto, E., Pisent, C., Sergi, G., Grigoletto, F. and Enzi, G. (2002) Anthropometric measurements in the elderly: age and gender differences. *British Journal of Nutrition* 87, 177–186.

Perman, M., Crivelli, A. and Wyszynski, D.F. (2001) Prevalence of hospital malnutrition in Argentina: preliminary results of a population-based survey. *Journal of Parenteral and Enteral Nutrition* 25, S12.

Pernerstorfer-Schoen, H., Schindler, K., Parschalk, B., Schindl, A., Thoeny-Lampert, S., Wunderer, K., Emladfa, I., Tschachler, E. and Jilma, B. (1999) Beneficial effects of protease inhibitors on body composition and energy expenditure: a comparison between HIV-infected and AIDS patients. *AIDS* 13, 2389–2396.

Persson, C., Sjoden, P.-O. and Glimelius, B. (1999) The Swedish version of the patient-generated subjective global assessment of nutritional status: gastrointestinal vs. urological cancers. *Clinical Nutrition* 18, 71–77.

Persson, M., Elmstahl, S. and Westerterp, K.R. (2000a) Validation of a dietary record routine in geriatric patients using doubly labelled water. *European Journal of Clinical Nutrition* 54, 789–796.

Persson, M.D., Hytter, A. and Cederholm, T. (2000b) Effects of dietary counselling and liquid supplementation on weight, ADL function and serum lipids in malnourished geriatric out-patients. *Clinical Nutrition* 19 (Suppl.), 9.

Pescovitz, M.D., Mehta, P.L., Leapman, S.B., Milgrom, M.L., Jindal, R.M. and Filo, R.S. (1995) Tube jejunostomy in liver transplant recipients. *Surgery* 117, 642–647.

Peters, A.L., Davidson, M.B. and Isaac, R.M. (1989) Lack of glucose elevation after simulated tube feeding with a low-carbohydrate, high fat enteral formula in patients with type I diabetes. *American Journal of Medicine* 87, 178–182.

Pezner, R.D., Archambeau, J.O., Lipsett, J.A., Kokal, W.A., Thayer, W. and Hill, L.R. (1987) Tube feeding enteral nutritional support in patients receiving radiation therapy for advanced head and neck cancer. *International Journal of Radiation Oncology, Biology and Physiology* 13, 935–939.

Phillips, P. (1986) Grip strength, mental performance and nutritional status as indicators of mortality risk among female geriatric patients. *Age and Ageing* 15, 53–56.

Pichard, C. and Jeejeebhoy, K.N. (1988) Muscle dysfunction in malnourished patients. *Quarterly Journal of Medicine New Series* 69, 1021–1045.

Pichard, C., Sudre, P., Karsegard, V., Yerly, S., Slosman, D.O., Delley, V., Perrin, L., Hirschel, B. and Study, S.H.C. (1998) A randomized double-blind controlled study of 6 months of oral nutritional supplementation with arginine and omega-3 fatty acids in HIV-infected patients. *AIDS* 12, 53–63.

Piena, M., Albers, M.J.I.J., van Haard, P.M.M., Gischler, S. and Tibboel, D. (1998) Introduction of enteral feeding in neonates on extracorporeal membrane oxygenation after evaluation of intestinal permeability changes. *Journal of Pediatric Surgery* 33, 30–34.

Pietsch, J.B. and Ford, C. (2000) Children with cancer: measurements of nutritional status at diagnosis. *Nutrition in Clinical Practice* 15, 185–188.

Pinchcofsky-Devin, G.D. and Kaminski, M.V. (1985a) Increasing malnutrition during hospitalization: documentation by a nutritional screening program. *Journal of the American College of Nutrition* 4, 471–479.

Pinchcofsky-Devin, G.D. and Kaminski, M.V. (1985b) Visceral protein increase associated with interrupt versus continuous enteral hyperalimentation. *Journal of Parenteral and Enteral Nutrition* 9, 474–476.

Pinchcofsky-Devin, G.D. and Kaminski, M.V. (1986) Correlation of pressure sores and nutritional status. *Journal of the American Geriatric Society* 34, 435–440.

Pinilla, J.C., Samphire, J., Arnold, C., Liu, L. and Thiessen, B. (2001) Comparison of gastrointestinal tolerance to two enteral feeding protocols in critically ill patients: a prospective, randomised, controlled trial. *Journal of Parenteral and Enteral Nutrition* 25, 81–86.

Pires, A.L.G., da Silveira, T.R. and Scholl, J.G. (1999) Relationship between nutritional status and histologic findings in small bowel mucosa of children presenting with diarrhoea of more than 14 days duration. *Journal of Tropical Pediatrics* 45, 302–304.

Pirlich, M., Schuetz, T., Luhmann, N., Burmester, G., Lochs, H. and Plauth, M. (2000) Malnutrition in hospitalized GI patients: prevalence and severity. *Clinical Nutrition* 19 (Suppl.), 8.

Pironi, L. and Tognoni, G. (1995) Cost–benefit and cost-effectiveness analysis of home artificial nutrition: reappraisal of available data. *Clinical Nutrition* 14, 87–91.

Pironi, L., Paganelli, G.M., Miglioli, M., Biasco, G., Santucci, R., Ruggeri, E., Di Febo, G. and Barbara, L. (1994) Morphologic and cytoproliferative patterns of duodenal mucosa in two patients after long-term total parenteral nutrition: changes with oral refeeding and relation to intestinal resection. *Journal of Parenteral and Enteral Nutrition* 18, 351–354.

Planas, M., Audivert, S., Burgos, R., Puiggros, C., Perez-Portabella, C. and Casanellas, J.M. (2001) Nutritional status, length of stay and readmission rates in patients admitted to a university hospital. *Journal of Parenteral and Enteral Nutrition* 25, S9–S10.

Plata-Salaman, C. (1996) Anorexia during acute and chronic disease. *Nutrition* 12, 69–78.

Plauth, M., Gerstner, C., Schutz, T., Roske, A.E., Baehr, V., Volk, H.D. and Lochs, H. (1998) Pathogenesis of protein–energy-malnutrition in liver cirrhosis (LC): role of pro- and antiinflammatory cytokines. *Clinical Nutrition* 17 (Suppl.), 65.

Pliner, P.L. (1973) Effect of liquid and solid preloads on eating behavior of obese and normal persons. *Physiology and Behavior* 11, 285–290.

Pocock, S.J. (1983) *Clinical Trials: a Practical Approach*. John Wiley & Sons, Chichester.

Pocock, S.J. (1985) Current issues in the design and interpretation of clinical trials. *British Medical Journal* 290, 39–42.

Poehlman, E.T. and Dvorak, R.V. (2000) Energy expenditure, energy intake and weight loss in Alzheimer disease. *American Journal of Clinical Nutrition* 71, 650S–655S.

Pollack, H., Glasberg, H., Lee, E., Nirenberg, A., David, R., Krasinski, K., Borkowsky, W. and Oberfeld, S. (1997) Impaired early growth of infants perinatally infected with human immunodeficiency virus: correlation with viral load. *Journal of Pediatrics* 130, 915–922.

Pollack, M.M., Wiley, J.S. and Holbrook, P.R. (1981) Early nutritional depletion in critically ill children. *Critical Care Medicine* 9, 580–583.

Pollitt, E. (1995) The relationship between undernutrition and behavioural development in children (a report of the International Dietary Energy Consultative Group (IDECG) workshop on malnutrition and behavior). *Journal of Nutrition* 125 (Suppl.), 2211S–2284S.

Pollitt, E. and Mathews, R. (1998) Breakfast and cognition: an integrative summary. *American Journal of Clinical Nutrition* 67, 804S–813S.

Pollitt, E., Leibel, R.L. and Greenfield, D. (1981) Brief fasting, stress and cognition in children. *American Journal of Clinical Nutrition* 34, 1526–1533.

Pollitt, E., Gorman, K.S., Engle, P., Martorell, R. and Rivera, J. (1993) Early supplementary feeding and cognition: effect over two decades. *Monographs of the Society for Research in Child Development* 58, 1–116.

Pons Leite, H., Isatugo, M.K.I., Sawaki, L. and Fisberg, M. (1993) Anthropometric nutritional assessment of critically ill hospitalized children. *Revista Paulista de Medicina* 111, 309–313.

Ponzer, S., Tidermark, J., Brismar, K., Soderqvist, A. and Cederholm, T. (1999) Nutritional status, insulin-like growth factor-1 and quality of life in elderly women with hip fractures. *Clinical Nutrition* 18, 241–246.

Poppit, S.D. and Prentice, A.M. (1996) Energy density and its role in the control of food intake: evidence from metabolic and community studies. *Appetite* 26, 153–174.

Posner, B., Jette, A., Smigelski, C., Miller, D. and Mitchell, P. (1994) Nutritional risk in New England elders. *Journal of Gerontology* 49, M123–M132.

Posner, B.M., Jette, A.M., Smith, K.W. and Miller, D.R. (1993) Nutrition and health risks in the elderly: the nutrition screening initiative. *American Journal of Public Health* 83, 972–978.

Potter, J.F., Schafer, D.F. and Bohi, R.L. (1988) In-hospital mortality as a function of body mass index: an age-dependent variable. *Journal of Gerontology: Medical Sciences* 43, M59–M63.

Potter, J.M. (2001) Oral supplements in the elderly. *Current Opinion in Clinical Nutrition and Metabolic Care* 4, 21–28.

Potter, J.M., Klipstein, K., Reilly, J.J. and Roberts, M. (1995) The nutritional status and clinical course of acute admissions to a geriatric unit. *Age and Ageing* 24, 131–136.

Potter, J.M., Langhorne, P. and Roberts, M. (1998) Routine protein energy supplementation in adults: systematic review. *British Medical Journal* 317, 495–501.

Potter, J.M., Roberts, M.A., McColl, J.H. and Reilly, J.J. (2001) Protein energy supplements in unwell elderly patients – a randomized controlled trial. *Journal of Parenteral and Enteral Nutrition* 25, 323–329.

Potter, M.A. and Luxton, G. (1999) Prealbumin measurement as a screening tool for protein calorie malnutrition in emergency hospital admissions: a pilot study. *Clinical and Investigative Medicine* 22, 44–52.

Poustie, V.J., Smyth, R.L. and Watling, R.M. (2002) Oral protein calorie supplementation for children with chronic diesease. In: *The Cochrane Library*, Issue 2. Update Software, Oxford.

Pouw, E.M., ten Velde, G.P.M., Croonen, B.H.P.M., Kester, A.D.M., Schols, A.M.W.J. and Wouters, E.F.M. (2000) Early non-elective readmission for chronic obstructive pulmonary disease is associated with weight loss. *Clinical Nutrition* 19, 95–99.

Prentice, A.M. (1999) The thymus: a barometer of malnutrition. *British Journal of Nutrition* 81, 345–347.

Prentice, A.M., Black, A.E., Murgatroyd, P.R., Goldberg, G.R. and Coward, W.A. (1989) Metabolism or appetite: questions of energy balance with particular reference to obesity. *Journal of Human Nutrition and Dietetics* 2, 95–104.

Prentice, A.M., Goldberg, G. and Prentice, A. (1994) Body mass index and lactational performance. *European Journal of Clinical Nutrition* 48 (Suppl.), S78–S89.

Prentice, A.M., Cole, T.J., Moore, S.E. and Collinson, A. (1999) Programming the adult immune system. In: O'Brien, P., Wheeler, T. and Barker, D. (eds) *Fetal Programming: Influences on Development and Disease in Later Life*. Royal College of Obstetrics and Gynaecology Press, London.

Preston, K. (1991) Counting the cost of pressure sores. *Community Outlook* 9, 19–24.

Puntis, J.W.L. (2001) Nutritional support at home and in the community. *Archives of Diseases in Childhood* 84, 295–298.

Pupelis, G., Selga, G., Austrums, E. and Kaminski, A. (2001) Jejunal feeding, even when instituted late, improves outcomes in patients with severe pancreatitis and peritonitis. *Nutrition* 17, 91–94.

Quasim, T., McMillan, D.C., Kinsella, J. and Booth, M.G. (2000) Hypoalbuminaemia, the inflammatory response and survival in the critically ill surgical patient. *Proceedings of the Nutrition Society* 59, 167A.

Rabeneck, L., Palmer, A., Knowles, J.B., Seidehamel, R.J., Harris, C.L., Merkel, K.L., Risser, J.M.H. and Akrabawi, S.S. (1998) A randomized controlled trial evaluating nutrition counseling with or without oral supplementation in malnourished HIV-infected patients. *Journal of the American Dietetic Association* 98, 434–438.

Raber-Durlacher, J.E. (1999) Current practices for management of oral mucositis in cancer patients. *Support Care Cancer* 7, 71–74.

Rabinovitz, M., Pitlik, S.D., Leifer, M., Garty, M. and Rosenfeld, J.B. (1986) Unintentional weight loss: a retrospective analysis of 154 cases. *Archives of Internal Medicine* 146, 186–187.

Rademaker, J.W., Richards, C., Marsham, J., Wheeler, J., Batty, P., Summerell, J. and Williams, H. (1996) Management of malnutrition in the elderly: a clinical audit. *Proceedings of the Nutrition Society* 56, 175A.

Ragneskog, H., Brane, G., Karlsson, I. and Kihlgren, M. (1996) Influence of dinner music on food intake and symptoms common in dementia. *Scandinavian Journal of Caring Sciences* 10, 11–17.

Ramage, I.J., Simposon, R.M., Thomson, R.B. and Patersen, J.R. (1997) Letter: feeding difficulties in children with cerebral palsy [Letter]. *Acta Paediatrica* 86, 336.

Ramsey, B.W., Farrell, P.M., Pencharz, P. and Consensus Committee (1992) Nutritional assessment and management in cystic fibrosis: a consensus report. *American Journal of Clinical Nutrition* 55, 108–116.

Rana, S.K., Bray, J., Menzies-Gow, N., Jameson, J., Payne James, J., Frost, P. and Silk, D.B.A. (1992) Short term benefits of post-operative oral dietary supplements in surgical patients. *Clinical Nutrition* 11, 337–344.

Raouf, A.H., Hildrey, V., Daniel, J., Walker, R.J., Krasner, N., Elias, E. and Rhodes, J.M. (1991) Enteral feeding as sole treatment for Crohn's disease: controlled trial of whole protein vs. amino acid based feed and a case study of dietary challenge. *Gut* 32, 702–707.

Rasmussen, H.H., Kondrup, J., Ladefoged, K. and Staun, M. (1999) Clinical nutrition in Danish hospitals: a questionnaire-based intervention among doctors and nurses. *Clinical Nutrition* 18, 153–158.

Rassias, A., Marrin, C., Arruda, J., Whalen, P., Beach, M. and Yeager, M. (1999) Insulin infusion improves neutrophil function in diabetic cardiac surgery patients. *Anesthesia Analgesia* 88, 1011–1016.

Raul, F. and Schleiffer, R. (1996) Intestinal adaptation to nutritional stress. *Proceedings of the Nutrition Society* 55, 279–289.

Ravaglia, G., Forti, P., Maioli, F., Bastagli, L., Facchini, A., Mariani, E., Savarino, L., Sassi, S., Cucinotta, D. and Lenaz, G. (2000) Effect of micronutrient status on natural killer cell immune function in healthy free-living subjects aged $\geqslant$ 90 y. *American Journal of Clinical Nutrition* 71, 590–598.

Ravasco, P., Camilo, M.E., Gouveia-Oliveirea, A., Adam, S. and Brum, G. (2002) A critical approach to nutritional assessment in critically ill patients. *Clinical Nutrition* 21, 73–77.

Rayfield, E., Ault, M., Keusch, G., Brothers, M., Nechemias, C. and Smith, H. (1982) Infection and diabetes: the case for glucose control. *American Journal of Medicine* 72, 439–450.

Rea, I.M., Nelson, S.J., Murphy, A., Ward, M. and McNulty, H. (1998) The use of 24 hour dietary assessment in 70–96 year old subjects living in the community of Belfast urban area. *European Journal of Clinical Nutrition* 53 (Suppl. 2), S41.

Rees, R.G.P., Hare, W.R., Grimble, G.K., Frost, P.G. and Silk, D.B.A. (1992) Do patients with moderately impaired gastrointestinal function requiring enteral nutrition need a predigested nitrogen source? A prospective crossover controlled clinical trial. *Gut* 33, 877–881.

Reid, C. (2000) Immunological and metabolic features of multiple organ dysfunction syndrome: a study of their association and potential modification by 'immunonutrition'. PhD thesis, University of Manchester, Manchester.

Reid, C.L. and Campbell, I.T. (2001) High energy deficits in MODs patients are associated with prolonged ICU length of stay (LOS) but not mortality. *Clinical Nutrition* 20 (Suppl.), 52.

Reilly, H.M., Martineau, J.K., Moran, A. and Kennedy, H. (1995) Nutritional screening – evaluation and implementation of a simple nutrition risk score. *Clinical Nutrition* 14, 269–273.

Reilly, J.J., Hull, S.F., Albert, N., Waller, A. and Bringardener, S. (1988) Economic impact of malnutrition: a model system for hospitalized patients. *Journal of Parenteral and Enteral Nutrition* 12, 371–376.

Reilly, J.J., Mackintosh, M., Potter, J. and Roberts, M.A. (1995) An evaluation of the feasibility of sip-feed supplementation in undernourished, acutely sick, elderly patients. *Proceedings of the Nutrition Society* 54, 135A.

Reilly, J.J., Weir, J., McColl, J.H. and Gibson, B.E.S. (1999) Prevalence of protein-energy malnutrition at diagnosis in children with acute lymphoblastic leukaemia. *Journal of Pediatric Gastroenterology and Nutrition* 29, 194–197.

Reilly, S., Skuse, D. and Poblete, X. (1996) Prevalence of feeding problems and oral motor dysfunction in children with cerebral palsy: a community survey. *Journal of Pediatrics* 129, 877–882.

Rettamel, A.L., Marcus, M.S., Farrell, P.M., Sondel, S.A., Koscik, R.E. and Mischler, E.H. (1995) Oral supplementation with a high-fat, high-energy product improves nutritional status and alters serum lipids in patients with cystic fibrosis. *Journal of the American Dietetic Association* 95, 454–459.

Rey-Ferro, M., Castano, R., Orozco, O., Serna, A. and Moreno, A. (1997) Nutritional and immunologic evaluation of patients with gastric cancer before and after surgery. *Nutrition* 13, 878–881.

Reynolds, J.V., Kanwar, S., Welsh, F.K.S., Windsor, A.C.J., Murchan, P., Barclay, G.R. and Guillou, P.J. (1997) Does the route of feeding modify gut barrier function and clinical outcome in patients after major upper gastrointestinal surgery? *Journal of Parenteral and Enteral Nutrition* 21, 196–201.

Richards, A.M., Mitsou, J., Floyd, D.C., Terenghi, G. and McGrouther, D.A. (1997) Neural innervation and healing. *Lancet* 350, 339–340.

Richards, E.W., Hob, R., Pelfini, A., Reese, R., Clinton, R. and Hellerstein, M. (1996) Effects of enteral nutrition supplements on HIV disease. *FASEB Journal* 10, P4555.

Richardson, I., Nyulasi, I., Cameron, K., Ball, M. and Wilson, J. (2000) Nutritional status of an adult cystic fibrosis population. *Nutrition* 16, 255–259.

Richardson, R.A., Farden, O.J. and Davidson, H.I. (2001) Reduction in energy expenditure after liver transplantation. *Nutrition* 17, 585–589.

Rickard, K.A., Grosfeld, J.L., Kirksey, A., Ballantine, T.V.N. and Baehner, R.L. (1979) Reversal of protein-energy malnutrition in children during treatment of advanced neoplastic disease. *Annals of Surgery* 190, 771–781.

Rickard, K.A., Detamore, C.M., Coates, T.D., Grosfeld, J.L., Weetman, R.M., White, N.M., Provisor, A.J., Boxer, L.A., Loghmani, E.S., Oei, T.O., Yu, P.-L. and Baehner, R.L. (1983) Effect of nutrition staging on treatment delays and outcome in stage IV neuroblastoma. *Cancer* 52, 587–598.

Rigaud, D., Cosnes, J., LeQuintrec, Y., Rene, E., Gendre, J.P. and Mignon, M. (1991) Controlled trial comparing two types of enteral nutrition in treatment of active Crohn's disease: elemental vs. polymeric diet. *Gut* 32, 1492–1497.

Rigaud, D., Angel, L.A., Ceref, M., Carduner, M.J., Melchior, J.C., Sautier, C., Rene, E., Apfelbaum, M. and Mignon, M. (1994) Mechanisms of decreased food intake during weight loss in adult Crohn's disease patients without obvious malabsorption. *American Journal of Clinical Nutrition* 60, 775–781.

Rigaud, D., Moukaddem, M., Cohen, B., Malon, D., Reveillard, V. and Mignon, M. (1997) Refeeding improves muscle performance without normalization of muscle mass and oxygen consumption in anorexia nervosa patients. *American Journal of Clinical Nutrition* 65, 1845–1851.

Rikimaru, T., Taniguchi, K., Yartey, J.E., Kennedy, D.O. and Nkrumah, F.K. (1998) Humoral and cell-mediated immunity in malnourished children in Ghana. *European Journal of Clinical Nutrition* 52, 344–350.

Ritchie, C.S., Burgio, K.L., Locker, J.L., Cornwell, A., Thomas, D., Hardin, M. and Redden, D. (1997) Nutritional status of urban homebound older adults. *American Journal of Clinical Nutrition* 66, 815–818.

Ritz, P., Maillet, A., Blanc, S. and Stubbs, R.J. (1999) Observations in energy and macronutrient intake during prolonged bed-rest in a head-down tilt position. *Clinical Nutrition* 18, 203–207.

Robbins, L.J. (1989) Evaluation of weight loss in the elderly. *Geriatrics* 44, 31–37.

Roberge, C., Tran, M., Massoud, C., Poiree, B., Duval, N., Damecour, E., Frout, D., Malvy, D., Joly, F., Lebailly, P. and Henry-Amar, M. (2000) Quality of life and home enteral tube feeding: a French prospective study in patients with head and neck or oesophageal cancer. *British Journal of Cancer* 82, 263–269.

Roberts, M.F. and Levine, G.M. (1992) Nutrition support team recommendations can reduce hospital costs. *Nutrition in Clinical Practice* 7, 227–230.

Robinson, G., Goldstein, M. and Levine, G.M. (1987) Impact of nutritional status on DRG length of stay. *Journal of Parenteral and Enteral Nutrition* 11, 49–51.

Roediger, W.E.W. (1994) Famine, fiber, fatty acids and failed colonic absorption: does fiber fermentation ameliorate diarrhoea? *Journal of Parenteral and Enteral Nutrition* 18, 4–8.

Rogers, P.J. (2001) A healthy body, a healthy mind: long-term impact of diet on mood and cognitive function. *Proceedings of the Nutrition Society* 60, 135–143.

Rogers, R.M., Donahoe, M. and Costantino, J. (1992) Physiologic effects of oral supplemental feeding in malnourished patients with chronic obstructive pulmonary disease. *American Review of Respiratory Disease* 146, 1511–1517.

Rojas, A.I. and Phillips, T.J. (1999) Patients with chronic leg ulcers show diminished levels of vitamins A and E, carotenes and zinc. *Dermatologic Surgery* 25, 601–604.

Roland, M. and Torgerson, D. (1988) Understanding clinical trials: what outcomes should be measured. *British Medical Journal* 319, 279–283.

Rolandelli, R.H., DePaula, J.A., Guenter, P. and Rombeau, J.L. (1990) Critical illness and sepsis – enteral and tube feeding. In: Rombeau, J.L. and Caldwell, M.D. (eds) *Clinical Nutrition*. W.B. Saunders, Philadelphia, pp. 288–305.

Rollins, H., Arnold, J., Buckner, K. and Richardson, R.A. (2001) Benchmarking knowledge and understanding of clinical nutrition in an NHS trust. *Proceedings of the Nutrition Society* 60, 107A.

Rolls, B.J., Rolls, E.T., Rowe, E.A. and Sweeney, K. (1981) Sensory specific satiety. *Physiology and Behavior* 27, 137–142.

Rolls, B.J., Hetherington, M. and Burley, V.J. (1988) The specificity of satiety: the influence of foods of different macronutrient content on the development of satiety. *Physiology and Behavior* 43, 145–153.

Roob, J.M., Konrad, M., Sprinz, M., Holzer, H. and Winkelhofer-Roob, B.M. (1998) Dietary intake and plasma concentrations of beta-carotene in chronic hemodialysis (HD) patients. *Clinical Nutrition* 17 (Suppl.), 24.

Roongpisuthipong, C., Sobhonslidsuk, A., Nantiruj, K. and Songchitsomboon, S. (2001) Nutritional assessment in various stages of liver cirrhosis. *Nutrition* 17, 761–765.

Rooyackers, O., Myrenfors, P., Thorell, A., Nygren, J. and Ljungqvist, O. (2001) Effect of starvation on insulin stimulated glucose uptake by skeletal muscle assessed by combined microdialysis and tracer methodology. *Clinical Nutrition* 20 (Suppl.), 5.

Roselle, G.A., Mendenhall, C.L., Grossman, C.J. and Weesner, R.E. (1988) Lymphocyte subset alterations in patients with alcoholic hepatitis. *Journal of Clinical and Laboratory Immunology* 26, 169–173.

Rosenberg, I.H. (2001) B vitamins, homocysteine and neurocognitive function. *Nutrition Reviews* 59, S69–S74.

Rosenthal, R. (1979) The 'file drawer problem' and tolerance for null results. *Psychological Bulletin* 86, 638–641.

Rossi, A. and Confalonieri, M. (2000) Burden of chronic obstructive pulmonary disease. *Lancet* 356, s56.

Roubenoff, R., Roubenoff, R.A., Preto, J. and Balke, C.W. (1987) Malnutrition among hospitalized patients: a problem of physician awareness. *Archives of Internal Medicine* 147, 1462–1465.

Roumen, R.M.H., van der Viet, J.A., Wevers, R.A. and Goris, R.J.A. (1993) Intestinal permeability is increased after major vascular surgery. *Journal of Vascular Surgery* 17, 734–737.

Rous, P. (1914) The influence of diet on transplanted and spontaneous mouse tumors. *Journal of Experimental Medicine* 20, 433–451.

Royal College of Physicians (2002) *Nutrition and Medicine: a Doctor's Responsibility.* Royal College of Physicians, London.

Royall, D., Kahan, I., Baker, J.P., Allard, J.P., Habal, F.M., Jeejeebhoy, K.N. and Greenberg, G.R. (1994) Clinical and nutritional outcome of an elemental versus semi-elemental diet in active Crohn's disease. *Gastroenterology* 102, A576.

Royce, C. and Taylor, M. (1994) Starvation in hospital: identifying malnutrition benefits everybody [letter]. *British Medical Journal* 308, 1370.

Ruddock, N.R. (2000) Gastrostomy feeding in adults receiving peritoneal dialysis. *Proceedings of the Nutrition Society* 59, 185A.

Rudman, D. and Feller, A.G. (1989) Protein-calorie undernutrition in the nursing home. *Journal of the American Geriatric Society* 37, 173–183.

Rudman, D., William, J.M., Richardson, T.J., Bixler, T.J., Stackhouse, W.J. and McGarrity, W.C. (1975) Elemental balanced during intravenous hyperalimentation of underweight adult subjects. *Journal of Clinical Investigation* 55, 94–104.

Rudman, D., Feller, A.G., Nagraj, H.S., Jackson, D.L., Rudman, I.W. and Mattson, D.E. (1987) Relation of serum albumin concentrations to death rate in nursing home men. *Journal of Parenteral and Enteral Nutrition* 11, 360–363.

Ruggenenti, P., Schieppati, A. and Remuzzi, G. (2001) Progression, remission, regression of chronic renal diseases. *Lancet* 357, 1601–1608.

Rush, D. (1989) Effects of changes in protein and calorie intake during pregnancy on the growth of the human fetus. In: Chalmers, I. and Enkin, M. (eds) *Effective Care in Pregnancy and Childbirth.* Oxford University Press, Oxford.

Russell, D.M., Prendergast, P.J., Darby, P.L., Garfinkel, P.E., Whitwell, J. and Jeejeebhoy, K.N. (1983) A comparison between muscle function and body composition in anorexia nervosa: the effect of refeeding. *American Journal of Clinical Nutrition* 38, 229–237.

Ryan, C.M., Atkins, M.B., Mier, J.W., Gelfand, J.A. and Tompkins, R.G. (1995) Effects of malignancy and interleukin-2 infusion on gut macromolecular permeability. *Critical Care Medicine* 23, 1801–1806.

Ryan, J.A., Page, C.P. and Babcock, L. (1981) Early postoperative jejunal feeding of elemental diet in gastrointestinal surgery. *American Surgeon* 47, 393–403.

Saadia, R. (1995) Trauma and bacterial translocation. *British Journal of Surgery* 82, 1243–1244.

Saavedra, J.M., Henderson, R.A., Perman, J.A., Hutton, N., Livingston, R.A. and Yolken, R.H. (1995) Longitudinal assessment of growth in children born to mothers with human immunodeficiency virus infection. *Archives of Pediatric and Adolescent Medicine* 149, 497–502.

Sacks, G.S., Dearman, K., Replogle, W.H., Cora, V.L., Meeks, M. and Canada, T. (2000) Use of subjective global assessment to identify nutrition-associated complications and death in geriatric long-term care facility residents. *Journal of the American College of Nutrition* 19, 570–577.

Saffle, J.R., Wiebke, G., Jennings, K., Morris, S.E. and Barton, R.G. (1997) Randomized trial of immune-enhancing enteral nutrition in burn patients. *Journal of Trauma* 42, 793–800.

Sagar, P.M. and Macfie, J. (1994) Effect of preoperative nutritional status on the outcome of cardiac valve replacement. *Nutrition* 10, 490.

Sagar, P., Wai, D., Poon, P., Macfie, J. and Mitchell, C. (1994) The effects of major abdominal surgery, enteral and parenteral nutrition on pancreatic function and morphology. *Clinical Nutrition* 13, 314–318.

Sagar, S., Harland, P. and Shields, R. (1979) Early postoperative feeding with elemental diet. *British Medical Journal* 1, 293–295.

Sahebjami, H. and Sathianpitayakul, E. (2000) Influence of body weight on the severity of dyspnea in chronic obstructive pulmonary disease. *American Journal of Respiratory and Critical Care Medicine* 161, 469–474.

Sahebjami, H., Doers, J.T., Render, M.L. and Bond, T.L. (1993) Anthropometric and pulmonary function test profiles of outpatients with stable chronic obstructive pulmonary disease. *American Journal of Medicine* 94, 469–474.

Saini, N., Miller, A.M., Maxwell, S.M., Dugdill, L. and Hackett, A.F. (1998) Measurement of nutritional intake and nutritional status of free living elderly: a pilot study. *Proceedings of the Nutrition Society* 57, 56A.

Salas-Salvadó, J. and Garcia-Lorda, P. (2001) The metabolic puzzle during the evolution of HIV infection. *Clinical Nutrition* 20, 379–391.

Saletti, A., Johansson, L. and Cederholm, T. (1999) Mini nutritional assessment in elderly subjects receiving home nursing care. *Journal of Human Nutrition and Dietetics* 12, 381–387.

Saletti, A., Lindgren, E.Y., Johansson, L. and Cederholm, T. (2000) Nutritional status according to mini nutritional assessment in an institutionalized elderly population in Sweden. *Gerontology* 46, 139–145.

Salgueiro, M.J. and Boccio, J.R. (2001) Nutritional care in renal disease patients [letter]. *Nutrition* 17, 157–158.

Salmon, P. (1994) Nutrition, cognitive performance and mental fatigue. *Nutrition* 10, 427–428.

Saloojee, H. and Violari, A. (2001) HIV infection in children. *British Medical Journal* 323, 670–674.

Salusky, I.B., Fine, R.N., Nelson, P., Blumenkrantz, M.J. and Kopple, J.D. (1983) Nutritional status of children undergoing continuous ambulatory peritoneal dialysis. *American Journal of Clinical Nutrition* 38, 599–611.

Sanchez-Grinan, M.I., Peerson, J.M. and Brown, K.H. (1992) Effect of dietary energy density on total ad-libitum energy consumption by recovering malnourished children. *European Journal of Clinical Nutrition* 46, 197–204.

Sanders, H.N., Narvarte, J., Bittle, P.A. and Ramirez, G. (1991) Hospitalized dialysis patients have lower nutrient intakes on renal diet than on regular diet. *Journal of the American Dietetic Association* 91, 1278–1280.

Sandström, B., Alhaug, J., Einarsdottir, K., Simpura, E.-M. and Isaksson, B. (1985) Nutritional status, energy and protein intake in general medical patients in three Nordic hospitals. *Human Nutrition: Applied Nutrition* 39A, 87–94.

Sanz, A., Albero, R., Playan, J., Acha, F.J., Casamayor, L., Celaya, S. and Servet, M. (1994) Comparison of a high-complex carbohydrate enteral formula with a high-monounsaturated fat formula in patients with type II diabetes mellitus treated with insulin or sulphonylurea. *Journal of Parenteral and Enteral Nutrition* 18, 31S.

Saudny-Unterberger, H., Martin, J.G. and Gray-Donald, K. (1997) Impact of nutritional support on functional status during an acute exacerbation of chronic obstructive pulmonary disease. *American Journal of Respiratory Care Medicine* 156, 794–799.

Sax, H.C., Illig, K.A., Ryan, C.K. and Hardy, D.J. (1996) Low-dose enteral feeding is beneficial during total parenteral nutrition. *American Journal of Surgery* 171, 587–590.

Sayce, H.A., Rowe, P.A. and McGonigle, R.J.S. (2000) Percutaneous endoscopic gastrostomy feeding in haemodialysis out-patients. *Journal of Human Nutrition and Dietetics* 13, 333–341.

Scalfi, L., Laviano, A., Reed, L.A., Borrelli, R. and Contaldo, F. (1990) Albumin and labile-protein serum concentrations during very-low-calorie diets with different compositions. *American Journal of Clinical Nutrition* 51, 338–342.

Scalfi, L., Polito, A., Bianchi, L., Marra, M., Caldara, A., Nicolai and Contaldo, F. (2002) Body composition changes in patients with anorexia nervosa after complete weight recovery. *European Journal of Clinical Nutrition* 56, 15–20.

Scarlatti, G. (1996) Paediatric HIV infection. *Lancet* 348, 863–868.

Schena, F.P. (2000) Epidemiology of end-stage renal disease: international comparisons of renal replacement therapy. *Kidney International* 57, S39–S45.

Schenker, S. (2001) Better hospital food. *British Nutrition Foundation Nutrition Bulletin* 26, 195–196.

Schiffman, S.S. (1983) Taste and smell in disease. *New England Journal of Medicine* 308, 1275–1279.

Schiffman, S.S. and Graham, B.G. (2000) Taste and smell perception affect appetite and immunity in the elderly. *European Journal of Clinical Nutrition* 26, 195–196.

Schiffman, S.S. and Warwick, Z.S. (1993) Effect of flavor enhancement of foods for the elderly on nutritional status: food intake, biochemical indices, and anthropometric measures. *Physiology and Behavior* 53, 395–402.

Schlettwein-Gsell, D. (1992) Nutrition and the qualify of life: a measure for the outcome of nutritional intervention. *American Journal of Clinical Nutrition* 55, 1263S–1266S.

Schneider, S., Hebuterne, X., Benzaken, S., Hastier, P., Tran, A. and Rampal, P. (1996) Effects of cyclic enteral nutrition on the immunological status of malnourished patients. *Clinical Nutrition* 15, 189–195.

Schneider, S.M., Pouget, I., Staccini, P., Rampal, P. and Hebuterne, X. (2000a) Quality of life in long-term home enteral nutrition patients. *Clinical Nutrition* 19, 23–28.

Schneider, S.M., Raina, C., Pugliese, P., Pouget, I., Rampal, P. and Hebuterne, X. (2000b) Long-term outcome of patients treated with home enteral nutrition. *Clinical Nutrition* 19 (Suppl.), 52.

Schneider, S.M., Pouget, I., Pivot, X., Hardion, M., Rampal, P. and Hebuterne, X. (2000c) Improvement in quality of life in home enteral nutrition patients: a prospective study. *Clinical Nutrition* 19 (Suppl.), 56.

Schofield, W.N., Schofield, C. and James, W.P.T. (1985) Basal metabolic rate – review and prediction, together with annotated bibliography of source material. *Human Nutrition: Applied Nutrition* 39C, 5–41

Schols, A.M.W.J. (1999) TNF-α and hypermetabolism in chronic obstructive pulmonary disease. *Clinical Nutrition* 18, 255–257.

Schols, A.M.W.J. and Wouters, E.F.M. (1995) Nutritional considerations in the treatment of chronic obstructive pulmonary disease. *Clinical Nutrition* 14, 64–73.

Schols, A.M.W.J., Mostert, R., Soeters, P.B., Greve, L.H. and Wouters, E.F.M. (1989) Nutritional state and exercise performance in patients with chronic obstructive lung disease. *Thorax* 44, 937–941.

Schols, A.M., Soeters, P.B., Mostert, R., Saris, W.H. and Wouters, E.F. (1991) Energy balance in chronic obstructive pulmonary disease. *American Review of Respiratory Disease* 143, 1248–1252.

Schols, A.M.W.J., Soeters, P.B., Dingemans, A.M.C., Mostert, R., Frantzen, P.J. and Wouters, E.F.M. (1993) Prevalence and characteristics of nutritional depletion in patients with stable COPD eligible for pulmonary rehabilitation. *American Review of Respiratory Diseases* 147, 1151–1156.

Schols, A.M.W.J., Soeters, P.B., Mostert, R., Pluymers, R.J. and Wouters, E.F.M. (1995) Physiologic effects of nutritional support and anabolic steroids in patients with chronic obstructive pulmonary disease. *American Journal of Respiratory and Critical Care Medicine* 152, 1268–1274.

Schols, A.M.W.J., Volovics, L. and Wouters, E.F.M. (1998) Weight loss is a reversible factor in the prognosis of chronic obstructive pulmonary disease. *American Journal of Respiratory and Critical Care Medicine* 157, 1791–1797.

Schols, A.M.W.J., Creutzberg, E.C., Buurman, W.A., Campfield, L.A., Saris, W.H.M. and Wouters, E.F.M. (1999) Plasma leptin is related to proinflammatory status and dietary intake in patients with chronic obstructive pulmonary disease. *American Journal of Respiratory and Critical Care Medicine* 160, 1220–1226.

Schroeder, D., Gillanders, L., Mahr, K. and Hill, G.L. (1991) Effects of immediate postoperative enteral nutrition on body composition, muscle function, and wound healing. *Journal of Parenteral and Enteral Nutrition* 15, 376–383.

Schuetz, T., Priepke, S., Nitschkoff-Breitmann, M., Lochs, H. and Plauth, M. (2000) Food preferences in oncology patients: different patterns in patients with hepatocellular, cholangiocellular or colorectal carcinoma. *Clinical Nutrition* 19 (Suppl.), 25.

Schultz, K.F. and Grimes, D.A. (2002a) Generation of allocation sequences in randomised trials: chance, not choice. *Lancet* 359, 515–519.

Schultz, K.F. and Grimes, D.A. (2002b) Allocation concealment in randomised trials: defending against deciphering. *Lancet* 359, 614–618.

Schurch, B. and Scrimshaw, N.S. (eds) (1987) *Chronic Energy Deficiency: Consequences and Related Issues.* Nestlé Foundation, Lausanne, Switzerland.

Schürch, M.-A., Rizzoli, R., Slosman, D., Vadas, L., Vergaud, P. and Bonjour, J.-P. (1998) Protein supplements increase serum insulin-like growth factor-1 levels and attenuate proximal femur bone loss in patients with recent hip fracture. *Annals of Internal Medicine* 128, 801–809.

Schwartz, D.B. (1996) Enhanced enteral and parenteral nutrition practice and outcomes in an intersive care unit with a hospital-wide performance improvement process. *Journal of the American Dietetic Association* 96, 484–489.

Schwebel, C., Pin, I., Barnoud, D., Devouassoux, G., Brichon, P.Y., Chaffanjon, P., Chavanon, O., Sessa, C., Blin, D., Guignier, M., Leverne, X. and Pison, C. (2000) Prevalence and consequences of nutritional depletion in lung transplant candidates. *European Respiratory Journal* 16, 1050–1055.

Schwenk, A., Burger, B., Ollenschlager, G., Stutzer, H., Wessel, D., Diehl, V. and Schrappe, M. (1994) Evaluation of nutritional counselling in HIV-associated malnutrition. *Clinical Nutrition* 13, 212–220.

Schwenk, A., Höffer-Belitz, E., Hung, B., Kremer, G., Bürger, B., Salzberger, B., Diehl, V. and Schrappe, M. (1996) Resting energy expenditure, weight loss and altered body composition in HIV infection. *Nutrition* 12, 595–601.

Schwenk, A., Kremer, G., Cornely, O., Diehl, V., Fatkenheuer, G. and Salzberger, B. (1999a) Body weight changes with protease inhibitor treatment in undernourished HIV-infected patients. *Nutrition* 15, 453–457.

Schwenk, A., Steuck, H. and Kremer, G. (1999b) Oral supplements as adjunctive treatment to nutritional counselling in malnourished HIV-infected patients: randomized controlled trial. *Clinical Nutrition* 18, 371–374.

Scobie, I.N. (1987) *A Study of the Inter-relationships Between Ketosis and Leucine, Alanine and Glucose Metabolism in Normal and Obese Fasted Human Subjects Using Tracer Methodology.* University of Glasgow, Glasgow.

Scott, H.F., Smedley, F.J., Timmis, L., Beeck, R., Roffe, C. and Bowling, T.E. (2001) Does multidisciplinary nutrition team care in the first 6 months post-PEG have an impact on clinical course? An interim analysis. *Proceedings of the Nutrition Society* 60, 111A.

Scott, K.J., Thurnham, D.I., Hart, D.J., Bingham, S.A. and Day, K. (1996) The correlation between the intake of lutein, lycopene and beta-carotene from vegetables and fruits, and blood plasma concentrations in a group of women aged 50–65 years in the UK. *British Journal of Nutrition* 75, 409–418.

Scottish Office (1995) *Scottish Health Survey, 1995*, Vol. 2. HMSO, Edinburgh.

Scrimshaw, N.S. (1998) Malnutrition, brain development, learning and behaviour. *Nutrition Research* 18, 351–379.

Sedman, P.C., Macfie, J., Palmer, M.D., Mitchell, C.J. and Sagar, P.M. (1995) Preoperative total parenteral nutrition is not associated with mucosal atrophy or bacterial translocation in humans. *British Journal of Surgery* 82, 1663–1667.

Seligman, P.A., Fink, R. and Massy-Seligman, E.J. (1998) Approach to the seriously ill or terminal cancer patient who has a poor appetite. *Seminars in Oncology* 25, 33–34.

Sekhon, S. (2000) Chronic radiation enteritis: women's food tolerances after radiation treatment for gynecologic cancer. *Journal of the American Dietetic Association* 100, 941–943.

Sellden, E., Brundin, T. and Wahren, J. (1994) Augmented thermic effect of amino acids under general anaesthesia: a mechanism useful for prevention of anaesthesia. *Clinical Science* 86, 611–618.

Sellden, E., Branstrom, R. and Brundin, T. (1996) Pre-operative infusion of amino acids prevents post-operative hypothermia. *British Journal of Anaesthesia* 76, 227–234.

Seltzer, M.F., Slocum, B.A., Cetaldi-Belcher, M.L., Fileti, C. and Gerson, N. (1982) Absolute weight loss and surgical mortality. *Journal of Parenteral and Enteral Nutrition* 6, 218–221.

Semba, R.D., Shah, N. and Vlahov, D. (2001) Improvement of anemia among HIV-infected injection drug users receiving highly active antiretroviral therapy. *Journal of Acquired Immune Deficiency Syndromes* 26, 315–319.

Senapati, A., Slavin, B.M. and Thompson, R.P.H. (1990) Zinc depletion and complications of surgery. *Clinical Nutrition* 9, 341–346.

Senkal, M., Zumtobel, V., Bauer, K.H., Marpe, B., Wolfram, G., Frei, A., Eickhoff, U. and Kemen, M. (1999) Outcome and cost-effectiveness of perioperative enteral immunonutrition in patients undergoing elective upper gastrointestinal tract surgery: a prospective randomized study. *Archives of Surgery* 134, 1309–1316.

Sentongo, T.A., Semeao, E.J., Piccoli, D.A., Stallings, V.A. and Zemel, B.S. (2000) Growth, body composition, and nutritional status in children and adolescents with Crohn's disease. *Journal of Pediatric Gastroenterology and Nutrition* 31, 33–40.

Seri, S. and Aquilio, E. (1984) Effects of early nutritional support in patients with abdominal trauma. *Italian Journal of Surgical Sciences* 14, 223–227.

Sermet-Gaudelus, I., Poisson-Salomon, A.-S., Colomb, V., Brusset, M.-C., Mosser, F., Berrier, F. and Ricour, C. (2000) Simple pediatric nutritional risk score to identify children at risk of malnutrition. *American Journal of Clinical Nutrition* 72, 64–70.

Sessler, D.I. (1997) Mild perioperative hypothermia. *New England Journal of Medicine* 336, 1730–1737.

Sessler, D.I. and Kurz, A. (1996) Perioperative normothermia and surgical-wound infection. *New England Journal of Medicine* 335, 747–750.

Severinsen, T. and Munch, I.C. (1999) Body core temperature during food restriction in rats. *Acta Physiologica Scandinavica* 165, 299–305.

Shah, S., Whalen, C., Kotler, D.P., Mayanja, H., Namale, A., Melikian, G., Mugerwa, R. and Semba, R.D. (2001) Severity of human immunodeficiency virus infection is associated with decreased phase angle, fat mass and body cell mass in adults with pulmonary tuberculosis infection in Uganda. *Journal of Nutrition* 131, 2843–2847.

Shannon, M.L. and Skorga, P. (1989) Pressure ulcer prevalence in two general hospitals. *Decubitus* 2, 38–43.

Sharkey, S.J., Sharkey, K.A., Sutherland, L.R., Church, D.L. and Group, G.H.S. (1992) Nutritional status and food intake in human immunodeficiency virus infection. *Journal of Acquired Immune Deficiency Syndromes* 5, 1091–1098.

Shatenstein, B. and Ferland, G. (2000) Absence of nutritional or clinical consequences of decentralized bulk food portioning in elderly nursing home residents with dementia in Montreal. *Journal of the American Dietetic Association* 100, 1354–1360.

Shaver, H.J., Loper, J.A. and Lutes, R.A. (1980) Nutritional status of nursing home patients. *Journal of Parenteral and Enteral Nutrition* 4, 367–370.

Shaw, N.J., White, C.P., Fraser, W.D. and Rosenboom, L. (1994) Osteopenia in cerebral palsy. *Archives of Diseases in Childhood* 71, 235–238.

Shaw, V. and Lawson, M. (2001) *Clinical Paediatric Dietetics.* Blackwell Science, Oxford.

Shaw-Stiffel, T.A., Zarny, L.A., Pleban, W.E., Rosman, D.D., Rudolph, R.A. and Bernstein, L.H. (1993) Effect of nutrition status and other factors on length of hospital stay after major gastrointestinal surgery. *Nutrition* 9, 140–145.

Sheehan, L.A. and Macallan, D.C. (2000) Determinants of energy intake and energy expenditure in HIV and AIDS. *Nutrition* 16, 101–106.

Sheiham, A., Steele, J.G., Carcenes, W., Lowe, C., Finch, S., Bates, C.J., Prentice, A. and Walls, A.W.G. (2001) The relationship among dental status, nutrient intake, and nutritional status in older people. *Journal of Dental Research* 80, 408–413.

Shenkin, A. (2000) . . . and can now get training in it [Letter]. *British Medical Journal* 320, 1538.

Shenkin, A., Cederblad, G., Elia, M. and Isaksson, B. (1996) Laboratory assessment of protein–energy status. *Clinica Chimica Acta* 252, 1–56.

Shepherd, R.W., Thomas, B.J., Bennett, D., Cooksley, W.G.E. and Ward, L.C. (1983) Changes in body composition and muscle protein degradation during nutritional supplementation in nutritionally growth-retarded children with cystic fibrosis. *Journal of Pediatric Gastroenterology and Nutrition* 2, 439–446.

Shepherd, R.W., Holt, T.L., Thomas, B.J., Kay, L., Isles, A., Francis, P.J. and Ward, L.C. (1986) Nutritional rehabilitation in cystic fibrosis: controlled studies of effects on nutritional growth retardation, body protein turnover, and course of pulmonary disease. *Journal of Pediatrics* 109, 788–794.

Shepherd, R.W., Holt, T.L., Cleghorn, G., Ward, L.C., Isles, A. and Francis, P. (1988) Short-term nutritional supplementation during management of pulmonary exacerbations in cystic fibrosis: a controlled study, including effects of protein turnover. *American Journal of Clinical Nutrition* 48, 235–239.

Shetty, P.S. and James, W.P.T. (1994) Body mass index: a measure of chronic energy deficiency in adults. *FAO Food and Nutrition Paper* 56, 1–57.

Shike, M., Berner, Y.N., Gerdes, H., Gerold, F.P., Bloch, A., Sessions, R. and Strong, E. (1989) Percutaneous endoscopic gastrostomy and jejunostomy for long-term feeding in patients with cancer of the head and neck. *Otolaryngology and Head and Neck Surgery* 101, 549–554.

Shils, M.E. (1979) Principles of nutritional therapy. *Cancer* 43, 2093–2101.

Shirabe, K., Matsumata, T., Shimada, M., Takenaka, K., Kawahara, N., Yamamoto, K., Nishizaki, T. and Sugimachi, K. (1997) A comparison of parenteral hyperalimentation and early enteral feeding regarding systemic immunity after major hepatic resection – the results of a randomized prospective study. *Hepato-Gastroenterology* 44, 205–209.

Shirley, R. and Moloney, M. (2000) A comparison of energy, food and nutrient intakes between a private hospital and two public hospitals. *Proceedings of the Nutrition Society* 59, 74A.

Shopbell, J.M., Hopkins, B. and Shronts, E.P. (2001) Nutrition screening and assessment. In: Gottschlich, M.M. (ed.) *The Science and Practice of Nutrition Support. A Case-based Core Curriculum.* Kendall/Hunt, Dubuque, Iowa, pp. 107–140.

Shronts, E.P. (1993) Basic concepts of immunology and its application to clinical nutrition. *Nutrition in Clinical Practice* 8, 177–183.

Shukla, H.S., Raja Rao, R., Banu, N., Gupta, R.M. and Yadav, R.C. (1984) Enteral hyperalimentation in malnourished surgical patients. *Indian Journal of Medical Research* 80, 339–346.

Shulkin, D.J., Kinosian, B., Glick, H., Glen-Puschett, C., Daly, J. and Eisenberg, J.M. (1993) The economic impact of infections: an analysis of hospital costs and charges in surgical patients with cancer. *Archives of Surgery* 128, 449–452.

Sidenvall, B. and Ek, A.-C. (1993) Long-term care patients and their dietary intake related to eating ability and nutritional needs: nursing staff interventions. *Journal of Advanced Nursing* 18, 565–573.

Siebens, H., Trupe, E., Siebens, A., Cook, F., Anshen, S., Hanauer, R. and Oster, G. (1986) Correlates and consequences of eating dependency in institutionalised elderly. *Journal of the American Geriatric Society* 34, 192–198.

Silk, D. (2001) Enteral diets: clinical uses and formulation. In: Payne-James, J., Grimble, G. and Silk, D. (eds) *Artificial Nutrition Support in Clinical Practice*. Greenwich Medical Media, London, pp. 303–331.

Silk, D.B.A. (1994) *Organisation of Nutritional Support in Hospitals*. BAPEN, Maidenhead.

Silver, A.J., Morley, J.E., Strome, L.S., Jones, D. and Vickers, L. (1988) Nutritional status in an academic nursing home. *Journal of the American Geriatric Society* 36, 487–491.

Simeon, D.T. and Grantham-McGregor, S. (1989) Effects of missing breakfast on the cognitive functions of school children of differing nutritional status. *American Journal of Clinical Nutrition* 49, 646–653.

Simko, V. (1983) Long-term tolerance of a special amino acid oral formula in patients with advanced liver disease. *Nutrition Reports International* 27, 765–773.

Simon, S. (1991) A survey of the nutritional adequacy of meals served and eaten by patients. *Nursing Practice* 4, 7–11.

Singer, P., Katz, D.P., Askanazi, J., Lazarus, T., Berkowitz, L. and LiCari, J. (1992) Enteral nutritional support in patients with acquired immune deficiency syndrome (AIDS): effect of Impact versus Replete. *Clinical Nutrition* 11 (Suppl.), 88.

Singh, G., Ram, R.P. and Khanna, S.K. (1998) Early postoperative enteral feeding in patients with nontraumatic intestinal perforation and peritonitis. *Journal of the American College of Surgeons* 187, 142–146.

Sizer, T. (Chairman and Editor) (1996) *Standards and Guidelines for Nutritional Support of Patients in Hospitals: a Report by the Working Party of the British Association for Parenteral and Enteral Nutrition*. BAPEN, Maidenhead.

Skypala, I.J., Ashworth, F.A., Hodson, M.E., Leonard, C.H., Knox, A., Hiller, E.J., Wolfe, S.P., Littlewood, J.M., Morton, A., Conway, S., Patchell, C., Weller, P., McCarthy, H., Redmond, A. and Dodge, J. (1998) Oral nutritional supplements produce significant weight gain in cystic fibrosis patients. *Journal of Human Nutrition and Dietetics* 11, 95–104.

Slusarczyk, R. (1994) The influence of the human immunodeficiency virus on resting energy expenditure. *Journal of Acquired Immune Deficiency Syndromes* 7, 1025–1027.

Smathers, J.S., Moles, K. and Sandroni, S. (1992) Strategies to improve protein intake in peritoneal dialysis patients. *Journal of Renal Nutrition* 2, 33–36.

Smit, E., Graham, N.M.H., Tang, A., Flynn, C., Solomon, L. and Vlahov, D. (1996) Dietary intake of community-based HIV-1 seropositive and seronegative injecting drug users. *Nutrition* 12, 496–502.

Smith, A.E., Powers, C.A., Cooper-Meyer, R.A. and Lloyd-Still, J.D. (1986) Improved nutritional management reduces length of hospitalization in intractable diarrhea. *Journal of Parenteral and Enteral Nutrition* 10, 479–481.

Smith, D.E., Stevens, M.C.G. and Booth, I.W. (1990) Malnutrition in children with malignant solid tumours. *Journal of Human Nutrition and Dietetics* 3, 303–309.

Smith, D.E., Stevens, M.C.G. and Booth, I.W. (1991) Malnutrition at diagnosis of malignancy in childhood: common but mostly missed. *European Journal of Paediatrics* 150, 318–322.

Smith, D.E., Handy, D.J., Holden, C.E., Stevens, M.C.G. and Booth, I.W. (1992) An investigation of supplementary naso-gastric feeding in malnourished children undergoing treatment for malignancy: results of a pilot study. *Journal of Human Nutrition and Dietetics* 5, 85–91.

Smith, D.L., Clarke, J.M. and Stableforth, D.E. (1994) A nocturnal nasogastric feeding programme in cystic fibrosis adults. *Journal of Human Nutrition and Dietetics* 7, 257–262.

Smith, D.M. (1995) Pressure ulcers in the nursing home. *Annals of Internal Medicine* 123, 433–442.

Smith, G., Weidel, S.E. and Fleck, A. (1994) Albumin catabolic rate and protein-energy depletion. *Nutrition* 10, 335–341.

Smith, J., Horowitz, J., Henderson, J.M. and Heymsfield, S. (1982) Enteral hyperalimentation in under-nourished patients with cirrhosis and ascites. *American Journal of Clinical Nutrition* 35, 56–72.

Smith, R.C., Hartemink, R.J., Hollinshead, J.W. and Gillett, D.J. (1985) Fine bore jejunostomy feeding following major abdominal surgery: a controlled randomized clinical trial. *British Journal of Surgery* 72, 458–461.

Smithard, D.G. (1996) Gag reflex has no role in ability to swallow [letter]. *British Medical Journal* 312, 972.

Smyth, R. and Walters, S. (2002) *Oral Calorie Supplements for Cystic Fibrosis (Cochrane Review).* Cochrane Library, Oxford.

Snyderman, C.H., Kachman, K., Molseed, L., Wagner, R., D'Amico, F., Bumpous, J. and Rueger, R. (1999) Reduced postoperative infections with an immune-enhancing nutritional supplement. *Laryngoscope* 109, 915–921.

Soberon, S., Pauley, M.P., Duplantier, R., Fan, A. and Halsted, C.H. (1987) Metabolic effects of enteral formula feeding in alcoholic hepatitis. *Hepatology* 7, 1204–1209.

Sobotka, L., Westerterp, K., Chaloupka, J., Malá, H., Slemrová, M., Coufalová, V., Havel, E., Maňák, J. and Zadák, Z. (1999) The effect of starvation on body composition in obese patients. *Clinical Nutrition* 18 (Suppl.), 34.

Society of Actuaries and Association of Life Insurance Medical Doctors of America (1980) *Build Study 1979.* SA and ALIMD, Chicago.

Soeters, P.B., von Meyenfeldt, M.F., Meijerink, W.J.H., Fredrix, E.W.H.M., Wouters, E.F.M. and Schols, A.M.W.J. *et al.* (1990) Serum albumin and mortality [letters]. *Lancet* 335, 348–351.

Soeters, P.B., Dejong, C.H.C. and Deutz, N.E.P. (2001) Clinical nutrition: the future. *Clinical Nutrition* 20, 191–197.

Sokol, R.J. and Stall, C. (1990) Anthropometric evaluation of children with chronic liver disease. *American Journal of Clinical Nutrition* 52, 203–208.

Solem, L.D., Strate, R.G. and Fischer, R.P. (1979) Antacid therapy and nutritional supplementation in the prevention of Curling's ulcer. *Surgery, Gynecology and Obstetrics* 148, 367–370.

Solomons, N.W. (1998) Secondary malnutrition. In: Sadler, M.J., Strain, J.J. and Caballero, B. (eds) *Encyclopedia of Human Nutrition*, Vol. 2. Academic Press, San Diego, pp. 1254–1259.

Sondel, S.A., Parrell, S.W., Becker, D. and Mischler, E.H. (1987) Oral nutritional supplementation in cystic fibrosis. *Nutritional Support Services* 7, 20–22.

Soriano, F.G., Ladeira, J.P., Janiszewski, M., Faintuch, J. and Velasco, I.T. (1999) Body composition changes during fasting. *Clinical Nutrition* 18 (Suppl.), 35.

Spitz, J., Gandhi, S., Hecht, G. and Alverdy, J. (1993) The effects of total parenteral nutrition on gastrointestinal function. *Clinical Nutrition* 12, S33–S37.

Spurr, G.B. (1987) The effects of chronic energy deficiency on stature, work capacity and productivity. In: Schurch, B.S. and Scrimshaw, N.S. (eds) *Effects of Chronic Energy Deficiency on Stature, Work Capacity and Productivity.* International Dietary Consultancy Group, Lausanne.

Spurr, G.B., Barac-Nieto, M. and Maksud, M.G. (1977) Productivity and maximal oxygen consumption in sugar cane cutters. *American Journal of Clinical Nutrition* 30, 316–321.

Sridhar, M.K., Galloway, A., Lean, M.E.J. and Banham, S.W. (1994) An out-patient nutritional supplementation programme in COPD patients. *European Respiratory Journal* 7, 720–724.

Staal-van den Brekel, A.J., Schols, A.M.W.J., ten Velde, G.P.M. and Buurman, W.A. (1994) Analysis of the energy balance in lung cancer patients. *Cancer Research* 54, 6430–6433.

Stableforth, P.G. (1986) Supplement feeds and nitrogen and calorie balance following femoral neck fracture. *British Journal of Surgery* 73, 651–655.

Stack, J.A., Bell, S.J., Burke, P.A. and Forse, R.A. (1996) High-energy, high-protein, oral, liquid, nutrition supplementation in patients with HIV infection: effect on weight status in relation to incidence of secondary infection. *Journal of the American Dietetic Association* 96, 337–341.

Stahl, W.M. (1987) Acute phase protein response to tissue injury. *Critical Care Medicine* 15, 545–550.

Stallings, V.A., Charney, E.B., Davies, J.C. and Cronk, C.E. (1993) Nutritional status and growth of children with diplegic or hemiplegic cerebral palsy. *Developmental Medicine and Child Neurology* 35, 997–1006.

Stallings, V.A., Cronk, C.E., Zemel, B.S. and Charney, E.B. (1995) Body composition in children with spastic quadriplegic cerebral palsy. *Journal of Pediatrics* 126, 833–839.

Standen, J. and Bihari, D. (2000) Immunonutrition: an update. *Current Opinion in Clinical Nutrition and Metabolic Care* 3, 149–157.

Stapleton, D., Kerrm, D., Gurrin, L., Sherriff, J. and Sly, P. (2001) Height and weight fail to detect early signs of malnutrition in children with cystic fibrosis. *Journal of Pediatric Gastroenterology and Nutrition* 33, 319–325.

Stark, L.J., Bowen, A.M., Tyc, V.L., Evans, S. and Passero, M.A. (1990) A behavioral approach to increasing calorie consumption in children with cystic fibrosis. *Journal of Pediatric Psychology* 15, 309–326.

Stark, L.J., Knapp, L., Bowen, A.M., Powers, S.W., Jelalian, E., Evans, S., Passero, M.A., Mulvihill, M.M. and Hovell, M. (1993) Increasing calorie consumption in children with cystic fibrosis: replication with two year follow-up. *Journal of Applied Behavior Analysis* 26, 435–450.

Stark, L.J., Mulvihill, M.M., Powers, S.W., Jelalian, E., Keating, K., Creveling, S., Brynes-Collins, B., Harwood, I., Passero, M.A., Light, M., Miller, D.L. and Hovell, M.F. (1996) Behavioral intervention to improve calorie intake of children with cystic fibrosis: Treatment versus wait list control. *Journal of Pediatric Gastroenterology and Nutrition* 22, 240–253.

Statistics Netherlands (1995) *Vademecum of Health Statistics of the Netherlands*. Ministry of Health, Welfare and Sports, SDU-uitgeverij, 's-Gravenhage, 192pp.

Stauffer, J.L., Carbone, J.E. and Bendoski, M.T. (1986) Effects of diet supplementation on anthropometric and laboratory nutritional parameters in malnourished ambulatory patients with severe chronic obstructive pulmonary disease (COPD). *American Review of Respiratory Disease* 133, A204.

Steele, E.J., Lindley, R.A. and Blanden, R.V. (1998) *Lamarck's Signature. How Retogenes are Changing Darwin's Natural Selection Paradigm*. Allen & Unwin, St Leonards.

Steiger, U., Lippuner, K., Jensen, E.X., Montandon, A., Jacger, P. and Horber, F.F. (1995) Body composition and fuel metabolism after kidney grafting. *European Journal of Clinical Investigation* 25, 809–816.

Steinkamp, G. and von der Hardt, H. (1994) Improvement of nutritional status and lung function after long-term nocturnal gastrostomy feedings in cystic fibrosis. *Journal of Pediatrics* 124, 244–249.

Steinkamp, G., Rodeck, B., Seidenberg, J., Ruhl, I. and von der Hardt, H. (1990) Stabilisierung der Lungenfunktion bei zystischer Fibrose durch langzeitsondenernahrung uber eine perkutane endoskopische Gastrostomie. *Pneumologie* 44, 1151–1153.

Steinkamp, G., Demmelmair, H., Ruhl-Bagheri, I., von der Hardt, H. and Koletzko, B. (2000) Energy supplements rich in linoleic acid improve body weight and essential fatty acid status of cystic fibrosis patients. *Journal of Pediatric Gastroenterology and Nutrition* 31, 418–423.

Stenvinkel, P., Lindholm, B. and Heimburger, O. (2000) New strategies for management of malnutrition in peritoneal dialysis patients. *Peritoneal Dialysis International* 20, 271–275.

Stephenson, G.R., Moretti, E.W., El-Moalem, H., Clavien, P.A. and Tuttle-Newhall, J.E. (2001) Malnutrition in liver transplant patients. *Transplantation* 72, 666–670.

Sterne, J.A.C., Egger, M. and Smith, G.D. (2001) Investigating and dealing with publication and other biases in meta-analysis. *British Medical Journal* 323, 101–105.

Stettler, N., Kawchak, D.A., Boyle, L.L., Propert, K.J., Scanlin, T.F., Stallings, V.A. and Zemel, B.S. (2000) Prospective evaluation of growth, nutritional status and body composition in children with cystic fibrosis. *American Journal of Clinical Nutrition* 72, 407–413.

Stevens, J., Cai, J., Pamuk, E.R., Williamson, D.F., Thun, M.J. and Wood, J.L. (1998) The effect of age on the association between body-mass index and mortality. *New England Journal of Medicine* 338, 1–7.

Stewart, R.J., Sheppart, H., Preece, R. and Waterlow, J.C. (1980) The effect of rehabilitation at different stages of development of rats marginally malnourished for ten to twelve generations. *British Journal of Nutrition* 43, 403–412.

Stokes, M.A. (1992) Crohn's disease and nutrition. *British Journal of Surgery* 79, 391–394.

Stokes, M.A. and Hill, G.L. (1993) Total energy expenditure in patients with Crohn's disease: measurement by the combined body scan technique. *Journal of Parenteral and Enteral Nutrition* 17, 3–7.

Stotts, N.A. and Wipke-Tevis, D. (1996) Nutrition, perfusion and wound healing: an inseparable triad. *Nutrition* 12, 733–734.

Stotts, N.A., Deosaransingh, K., Roll, R.J. and Newman, J. (1998) Underutilization of pressure ulcer risk assessment in hip fracture patients. *Advances in Wound Care* 11, 32–38.

Strain, A.J. (1979) Cancer cachexia in man: a review. *Investigative Cell Pathology* 2, 181–193.

Strain, N.C., Wright, C.E., Ward, K. and Shaffer, J.L. (1999) Can the true prevalence of malnutrition be assessed at admission to hospital? *Proceedings of the Nutrition Society* 58, 112A.

Stratton, R.J. (1994) *Nutritional Assessment of the Meals Served to and Consumed by Twelve Elderly Patients.* University of Surrey, Guildford.

Stratton, R.J. (1999) Artificial nutrition, appetite and food intake in health and disease. PhD thesis, University of Cambridge, Cambridge.

Stratton, R.J. and Elia, M. (1999a) A critical, systematic analysis of the use of oral nutritional supplements in the community. *Clinical Nutrition* 18 (Suppl. 2), 29–84.

Stratton, R.J. and Elia, M. (1999b) The effects of enteral tube feeding and parenteral nutrition on appetite sensations and food intake in health and disease. *Clinical Nutrition* 18, 63–70.

Stratton, R.J. and Elia, M. (2000) How much undernutrition is there in hospitals? *British Journal of Nutrition* 84, 257–259.

Stratton, R.J. and Elia, M. (2002) Concurrent validity of three nutrition screening tools for use in the community. *Proceedings of the Nutrition Society* 61, 19A.

Stratton, R.J., Dewit, O., Crowe, E., Jennings, G., Villar, R.N. and Elia, M. (1997) Plasma leptin, energy intake and hunger following total hip replacement surgery. *Clinical Science* 93, 113–117.

Stratton, R.J., Stubbs, R.J. and Elia, M. (1998) Appetite and food intake during artificial nutrition. *Proceedings of the Nutrition Society* 57, 96A.

Stratton, R.J., Thompson, R.L., Margetts, B.M., Stroud, M., Jackson, A.A. and Elia, M. (2002) Health care utilisation according to malnutrition risk in the elderly: an analysis of data from the National Diet and Nutrition Survey. *Proceedings of the Nutrition Society* 61, 20A.

Strauss, D., Kastner, T., Ashwal, S. and White, J. (1997) Tubefeeding and mortality in children with severe disabilities and mental retardation. *Pediatrics* 99, 358–362.

Strologo, L.D., Principato, F., Sinibaldi, D., Appiani, A.C., Terzi, F., Dartois, A.M. and Rizzoni, G. (1997) Feeding dysfunction in infants with severe chronic renal failure after long-term nasogastric tube feeding. *Pediatric Nephrology* 11, 84–86.

Stubbs, R.J. and Elia, M. (2001) Macronutrients and appetite control with implications for the nutritional management of the malnourished. *Clinical Nutrition* 20, 129–139.

Stubbs, R.J., Harbron, C.G., Murgatroyd, P.R. and Prentice, A.M. (1995) Covert manipulation of dietary fat and energy density: effect on substrate flux and food intake in men eating ad libitum. *American Journal of Clinical Nutrition* 62, 316–329.

Stubbs, R.J., Johnstone, A.M., O'Reilly, L.M., Barton, K. and Reid, C. (1998) The effect of covertly manipulating the energy density of mixed diets on ad libitum food intake in 'pseudo free-living' humans. *International Journal of Obesity* 22, 980–987.

Studley, H.O. (1936) Percentage of weight loss as a basic indicator of surgical risk in patients with chronic peptic ulcer disease. *Journal of the American Medical Association* 106, 458–460.

Suchner, U., Senftleben, U., Eckart, T., Scholz, M.R., Beck, K., Murr, R., Enzenbach, R. and Peter, K. (1996) Enteral versus parenteral nutrition: effects on gastrointestinal function and metabolism. *Nutrition* 12, 13–22.

Sullivan, D.H., Moriarty, M.S., Chernoff, R. and Lipschitz, D.A. (1989) Patterns of care: an analysis of the quality of nutritional care routinely provided to elderly hospitalized veterans. *Journal of Parenteral and Enteral Nutrition* 13, 249–254.

Sullivan, D.H., Patch, G.A., Walls, R.C. and Lipschitz, D.A. (1990) Impact of nutrition status on morbidity and mortality in a select population of geriatric rehabilitation patients. *American Journal of Clinical Nutrition* 51, 749–758.

Sullivan, D.H., Walls, R.C. and Lipschitz, D.A. (1991) Protein–energy undernutrition and the risk of mortality within 1 y of hospital discharge in a select population of geriatric rehabilitation patients. *American Journal of Clinical Nutrition* 53, 599–605.

Sullivan, D.H., Nelson, C.L., Bopp, M.M., Puskarich-May, C.L. and Walls, R.C. (1998) Nightly enteral nutrition support of elderly hip fracture patients: a phase I trial. *Journal of the American College of Nutrition* 17, 155–161.

Sullivan, D.H., Sun, S. and Walls, R.C. (1999) Protein-energy undernutrition among elderly hospitalized patients: a prospective study. *Journal of the American Medical Association* 281, 2013–2019.

Sullivan, P.B., Lambert, B., Rose, M., Ford-Adams, M., Johnson, A. and Griffiths, P. (2000) Prevalence and severity of feeding and nutritional problems in children with neurological impairment: Oxford Feeding Study. *Developmental Medicine and Child Neurology* 42, 674–680.

Summerbell, C.D., Perrett, J.P. and Gazzard, B.G. (1993) Causes of weight loss in human immunodeficiency virus infection. *International Journal of STD & AIDS* 4, 234–236.

Süttmann, U., Müller, M.J., Hoogestraat, L., Coldewey, R., Schedel, I. and Deicher, H. (1991) Malnutrition and immune dysfunction in patients infected with human immunodeficiency virus. *Klinische Wochenschrift* 69, 156–162.

Süttmann, U., Selberg, O., Muller, M.J., Schlesinger, A., Gebel, M., Manns, M.P. and Deicher, H. (1993) Home enteral nutrition in patients with acquired immunodeficiency syndrome. *Clinical Nutrition* 12, 287–292.

Süttmann, U., Ockenga, J., Schneider, H., Selberg, O., Schlesinger, A., Gallati, H., Wolfram, G., Deicher, H. and Muller, M.J. (1996) Weight gain and increased concentrations of receptor proteins for tumor necrosis factor after patients with symptomatic HIV infection received fortified nutrition support. *Journal of the American Dietetic Association* 96, 565–569.

Symreng, T., Anderberg, B., Kagedal, B., Norr, A., Schildt, B. and Sjodahl, R. (1983) Nutritional assessment and clinical course in 112 elective surgical patients. *Acta Chirurgica Scandinavica* 149, 657–662.

Szeluga, D.J., Stuart, R.K., Brookmeyer, R., Utermohlen, V. and Santos, G.W. (1987) Nutritional support of bone marrow transplant recipients: a prospective, randomised clinical trial comparing total parenteral nutrition to an enteral feeding program. *Cancer Research* 47, 3309–3316.

Tandon, S.P., Gupta, S.C., Sinha, S.N. and Naithani, Y.P. (1984) Nutritional support as an adjunct therapy of advanced cancer patients. *Indian Journal of Medical Research* 80, 180–188.

Tang, N.L.S., Chung, M.L., Elia, M., Hui, E., Lum, C.M., Luk, J.K.H., Jones, M.G. and Woo, J. (2002) Total daily energy expenditure in wasted chronic obstructive pulmonary disease patients. *European Journal of Clinical Nutrition* 56, 282–287.

Tanner, J.M., Whitehouse, R.H. and Takaishi, M. (1966) Standards from birth to maturity for height, weight, height velocity, and weight velocity: British children. *Archives of Diseases in Childhood* 1966, 613–645.

Task Force on Nutrition Support in AIDS (1989) Guidelines for nutrition support in AIDS. *Nutrition* 5, 39–46.

Taskinen, M. and Saarinen-Pihkala, U.M. (1998) Evaluation of muscle protein mass in children with solid tumors by muscle thickness measurement with ultrasonography, as compared with anthropometric methods and visceral protein concentrations. *European Journal of Clinical Nutrition* 52, 402–406.

Taylor, S.J. (1993) Audit of nasogastric feeding practice at two acute hospitals: is early enteral feeding associated with reduced mortality and hospital stay? *Journal of Human Nutrition and Dietetics* 6, 477–489.

Taylor, S.J., Fettes, S.B., Jewkes, C. and Nelson, R.J. (1999) Prospective, randomized controlled trial to determine the effect of early enhanced enteral nutrition on clinical outcome in mechanically ventilated patients suffering head injury. *Critical Care Medicine* 27, 2525–2531.

Tchekmedyian, N.S. (1995) Costs and benefits of nutrition support in cancer. *Oncology* 9, 79–84.

Teahon, K., Somasundaram, S., Smith, T., Menzies, I. and Bjarnason, I. (1996) Assessing the site of increased intestinal permeability in coeliac and inflammatory bowel disease. *Gut* 38, 864–869.

Tepaske, R., te Velthuis, H., Oudemans-van Straaten, H.M., Heisterkamp, S.H., van Deventer, S.J.H., Ince, C., Eysman, L. and Kesecioglu, J. (2001) Effect of preoperative oral immune-enhancing nutritional supplement on patients at high risk of infection after cardiac surgery: a randomised placebo-controlled trial. *Lancet* 358, 696–701.

Tessier, S., Kelly, I.E., Cahill, A., Morris, S.E., Crumley, A., McLaughlin, D., McKee, R.F. and Lean, M.E.J. (2000) Still hungry in hospital: identifying malnutrition in acute hospital admissions. *Proceedings of the Nutrition Society* 59, 94A.

Testa, M.A. and Simonson, D.C. (1996) Assessment of quality-of-life outcomes. *New England Journal of Medicine* 334, 835–840.

Thomas, A.J. and Gill, C.L. (1998) Malnutrition in the elderly. *Prescriber's Journal* 38, 249–254.

Thomas, A.J., Bunker, V.W., Brennan, E. and Clayton, B.E. (1986) The trace element content of hospital meals and potential low intake by elderly patients. *Human Nutrition: Applied Nutrition* 40A, 440–446.

Thomas, B. (1994) *Manual of Dietetic Practice*, 2nd edn. Blackwell Scientific Publications, Oxford.

Thomas, B.E. (2001) *Manual of Dietetic Practice*, 3rd edn. Blackwell Scientific Publications, Oxford.

Thomas, D.R. (1997) The role of nutrition in prevention and healing of pressure ulcers. *Clinics in Geriatric Medicine* 13, 497–511.

Thomas, D.R., Verdery, R.B., Fardner, L., Kant, A. and Lindsay, J.A. (1991) A prospective study of outcome from protein-energy malnutrition in nursing home residents. *Journal of Parenteral and Enteral Nutrition* 15, 400–404.

Thomas, M.K., Lloyd-Jones, D.M., Thadhani, R.I., Shaw, A.C., Deraska, D.J., Kitch, B.T., Vamvakas, E.C., Dick, I.M., Prince, R.L. and Finkelstein, J.S. (1998) Hypovitaminosis D in medical inpatients. *New England Journal of Medicine* 338, 777–783.

Thomas, S., Bender, S.A., Sharkey, S. and Horn, S. (1998) Preliminary nutrition findings from the long term care pressure ulcer study. *Journal of the American Dietetic Association* 98, A93.

Thommessen, M., Kase, B.F., Riis, G. and Heiberg, A. (1991) The impact of feeding problems on growth and energy intake in children with cerebral palsy. *European Journal of Clinical Nutrition* 45, 479–487.

Thompson, R.L., Margetts, B.M. and Jackson, A.A. (2001) Prevalence of malnutrition in people aged 65 years and over in Great Britain. *Proceedings of the Nutrition Society* 60, 223A.

Thomson, M.A., Carver, A.D. and Sloan, R.L. (2001) Nutritional status of traumatic and anoxic brain injured patients on admission to rehabilitation. *Proceedings of the Nutrition Society* 60, 83A.

Thorngren, K.G. and Werner, C.O. (1979) Normal grip strength. *Acta Orthopaedica Scandinavica* 50, 255–259.

Thorsdottir, I. and Gunnarsdottir, I. (2002) Energy intake must be increased among recently hospitalized patients with chronic obstructive pulmonary disease to improve nutritional status. *Journal of the American Dietetic Association* 102, 247–249.

Thorsdottir, I., Eriksen, B. and Eysteinsdottir, S. (1999) Nutritional status at submission for dietetic services and screening for malnutrition at admission to hospital. *Clinical Nutrition* 18, 15–21.

Thorsdottir, I., Gunnarsdottir, I. and Eriksen, B. (2001) Screening method evaluated by nutritional status measurements can be used to detect malnourishment in chronic obstructive pulmonary disease. *Journal of the American Dietetic Association* 101, 648–654.

Thorslund, S., Toss, G., Nilsson, I., Schenck, H., Symreng, T. and Zetterqvist, H. (1990) Prevalence of protein-energy malnutrition in a large population of elderly people at home. *Scandinavian Journal of Primary Health Care* 8, 243–248.

Thuluvath, P.J. and Triger, D.R. (1994) Evaluation of nutritional status by using anthropometry in adults with alcoholic and non-alcoholic liver disease. *American Journal of Clinical Nutrition* 60, 269–273.

Thunberg, B.J., Swamy A.P. and Cestero, R.V.M. (1981) Cross-sectional and longitudinal nutritional measurements in maintenance hemodialysis patients. *American Journal of Clinical Nutrition* 34, 2005–2012.

Tierney, A.J. (1996) Undernutrition and elderly hospital patients: a review. *Journal of Advanced Nursing* 23, 228–236.

Tkatch, L., Rapin, C.-H., Rizzoli, R., Slosman, D., Nydegger, V., Vasey, H. and Bonjour, J.-P. (1992) Benefits of oral protein supplementation in elderly patients with fracture of the proximal femur. *Journal of the American College of Nutrition* 11, 519–525.

Todd, A.J., Dickinson, P.J., Brynes, A.E. and Frost, G.S. (2000) The effect of enteral nutrition in allogeneic bone marrow transplant patients on length of hospital stay, pyrexia, diarrhoea, nausea and vomiting. *Proceedings of the Nutrition Society* 59, 157A.

Todd, J.A., Farquharson, C.A., Koulentaki, M., Fettes, S. and Pennington, C.R. (2000) Increased QT dispersion during refeeding. *Clinical Nutrition* 19, 43.

Toigo, G., Aparicio, M., Attman, P.-O., Cano, N., Cianciaruso, B., Engel, B., Fouque, D., Heidland, A., Teplan, V. and Wanner, C. (2000) Expert working group report on nutrition in adult patients with renal insufficiency (Part 2 of 2). *Clinical Nutrition* 19 (Suppl.), 281–291.

Tolia, V. (1995) Very early onset nonorganic failure to thrive in infants. *Journal of Pediatric Gastroenterology and Nutrition* 20, 73–80.

Tomorrow's Guides Limited (1997) *A–Z Care Homes Guide.* Tomorrow's Guides Ltd, London.

Torosian, M.H. (1999) Perioperative nutrition support for patients undergoing gastrointestinal surgery: critical analysis and recommendations. *World Journal of Surgery* 23, 565–569.

Torun, B., Flores, R., Viteri, F., Immink, M. and Diaz, E. (1989) Energy supplementation and work performance: summary of Incap studies. In: *Proceedings XIV International Congress of Nutrition*, pp. 306–309.

Treber, L.A. and Harris, M.A. (1996) Effect of early nutrition intervention on patient length of stay. *Journal of the American Dietetic Association* 96, A29.

Tretli, S. and Gaard, M. (1996) Lifestyle changes during adolescence and risk of breast cancer: an ecologic study of the effect of World War II in Norway. *Cancer Causes and Control* 7, 507–512.

Trick, L.M.J. (2000) A study of nutritional intake in surgical patients, pre- and post-operatively. *Journal of Human Nutrition and Dietetics* 13, 366–367.

Tripp, F. (1997) The use of dietary supplements in the elderly: current issues and recommendations. *Journal of the American Dietetic Association* 97, S181–S183.

Trousseau, A. (1872) True and false chlorosis. In: *Lectures on Clinical Medicine.* Philadelphia, pp. 95–117.

Trujillo, E.B. (1993) Effects of nutritional status on wound healing. *Journal of Vascular Nursing* 11, 12–18.

Trujillo, E.B., Borlase, B.C., Bell, S.J., Guenther, K.J., Swails, W., Queen, P.M. and Trujillo, J.R. (1992) Assessment of nutritional status, nutrient intake and nutrition support in AIDS patients. *Journal of the American Dietetic Association* 92, 477–478.

Tucker, H.N. (1996) Cost containment through nutrition intervention. *Nutrition Reviews* 54, 111–121.

Turic, A., Gordon, K.L., Craig, L.D., Ataya, D.G. and Voss, A.C. (1998) Nutrition supplementation enables elderly residents of long-term-care facilities to meet or exceed RDAs without displacing energy or nutrient intakes from meals. *Journal of the American Dietetic Association* 98, 1457–1459.

Tuten, M.B., Wogt, S., Dasse, F. and Leider, Z. (1985) Utilization of prealbumin as a nutritional parameter. *Journal of Parenteral and Enteral Nutrition* 9, 709–711.

Twiston Davies, C.W., Moody Jones, D. and Shearer, J.R. (1984) Hand grip – a simple test for morbidity after fracture of the neck of femur. *Journal of the Royal Society of Medicine* 77, 833–836.

Twomey, C., Briet, F. and Jeejeebhoy, K.N. (1999) Adverse effect of malnutrition on lymphocyte mitochondrial complex I activity in humans. *Clinical Nutrition* 18 (Suppl.), 5.

Twomey, C., Briet, F. and Jeejeebhoy, K.N. (2000) One month of refeeding normalized mitochondrial complex I activity (CI) in malnourished patients while other nutritional assessment parameters remained abnormal. *Clinical Nutrition* 19 (Suppl.), 3–4.

Twomey, P.L. and Patching, S.C. (1985) Cost-effectiveness of nutritional support. *Journal of Parenteral and Enteral Nutrition* 9, 3–10.

Ulander, K., Jeppsson, B. and Grahn, G. (1998) Postoperative energy intake in patients after colorectal cancer surgery. *Scandinavian Journal of Caring Sciences* 12, 131–138.

Ulivieri, F.M., Piodi, L.P., Aroldi, A. and Cesana, B.M. (2002) Effect of kidney transplantation on bone mass and body composition in males. *Transplantation* 73, 612–615.

Ullrich, R., Zeitz, M., Heise, W., L'age, M., Höffken, G. and Riecken, E.O. (1989) Small intestinal structure and function in patients with human immunodeficiency virus (HIV): evidence for HIV-induced enteropathy. *Annals of Internal Medicine* 111, 15–21.

Umpleby, A.M., Scobie, I.N., Boroujerdi, M.A. and Sonksen, P.H. (1995) The effect of starvation on leucine, alanine and glucose metabolism in obese subjects. *European Journal of Clinical Investigation* 25, 619–626.

United States Department of Agriculture, The Human Development Network of the World Bank, UNICEF and United Nations Children's Fund (2002) *Technical Consultation on Low Birthweight.* New York.

Unosson, M., Larsson, J., Ek, A.-C. and Bjurulf, P. (1992) Effects of dietary supplement on functional condition and clinical outcome measured with a modified Norton scale. *Clinical Nutrition* 11, 134–139.

Unosson, M., Ek, A.-C., Bjurulf, P., von Schenck, H. and Larsson, J. (1994) Feeding dependence and nutritional status after acute stroke. *Stroke* 25, 366–371.

Unosson, M., Ek, A.-C., Bjurulf, P., Von Schenck, H. and Larsson, J. (1995) Influence of macronutrient status on recovery after hip fracture. *Journal of Nutritional and Environmental Medicine* 5, 23–34.

Utley, R. (1992) Nutritional factors associated with wound healing in the elderly. *Ostomy/Wound Management* 38, 22, 24, 26–27.

Vailas, L.I., Nitzke, S.A., Becker, M. and Gast, J. (1998) Risk indicators for malnutrition are associated inversely with quality of life for participants in meal programs for older adults. *Journal of the American Dietetic Association* 98, 548–553.

Valla, C., Schneider, S.M., Stalins, S. and Hebuterne, X. (2000) Food intake in medical and surgical hospitalized patients. *Clinical Nutrition* 19 (Suppl. 1), 1.

Van Acker, B.A.C., Hulsewé, K.W.E., Wagenmakers, A.J.M., Deutz, N.E.P., von Meyenfeldt, M.F. and Soeters, P.B. (1998) Effect of surgery on albumin synthesis rate in humans. *Clinical Nutrition* 17 (Suppl.), 14–15.

Van Acker, B.A.C., Hulsewé, K.W.E., Wagenmakers, A.J.M., von Meyenfeldt, M.F. and Soeters, P.B. (2000) Response of glutamine-supplemented parenteral nutrition. *American Journal of Clinical Nutrition* 72, 790–795.

Van Asselt, D.Z., Pasman, J.W., van Lier, H.J., Vingerhoets, D.M., Poels, P.J., Kuin, Y., Blom, H.J. and Hoefnagels, W.H. (2001) Cobalamin supplementation improves cognitive and cerebral function in older cobalamin-deficient persons. *Journal of Gerontology Series A Biological Science and Medical Science* 56, M775–M779.

Van Bokhorst-de van der Schueren, M.A.E., van Leeuwen, P.A.M., Sauerwein, H.P., Kuik, D.J., Snow, G.B. and Quak, J.J. (1997) Assessment of malnutrition parameters in head and neck cancer and their relation to postoperative complications. *Head and Neck* 19, 419–425.

Van Bokhorst-de van der Schueren, M.A.E., von Blomberg-van der Flier, B.M.E., Riezebos, R.K., Scholten, P.E.T., Quak, J.J., Snow, G.B. and van Leeuwen, P.A.M. (1998) Differences in immune status between well-nourished and malnourished head and neck cancer patients. *Clinical Nutrition* 17, 107–111.

Van Bokhorst-de van der Schueren, M.A.E., van Leeuwen, P.A.M., Kuik, D.J., Klop, W.M.C., Sauerwein, H.P., Snow, G.B. and Quak, J.J. (1999) The impact of nutritional status on the prognoses of patients with advanced head and neck cancer. *Cancer* 86, 519–527.

Van Bokhorst-de van der Schueren, M.A.E., von Blomberg-van der Flier, B.M.E., Kuik, D.J., Scholten, P.E.T., Siroen, M.P.C., Snow, G.B., Quak, J.J. and van Leeuwen, P.A.M. (2000a) Survival of malnourished head and neck cancer patients can be predicted by human leukocyte antigen-DR expression and interleukin-6/tumor necrosis factor – a response of the monocyte. *Journal of Parenteral and Enteral Nutrition* 24, 329–336.

Van Bokhorst-de van Der Schueren, M.A.E., Langendoen, S.I., Vondeling, H., Kuik, D.J., Quak, J.J. and van Leeuwen, P.A.M. (2000b) Perioperative enteral nutrition and quality of life of severely malnourished head and neck cancer patients: a randomized clinical trial. *Clinical Nutrition* 19, 437–444.

Van Bokhorst-de van der Schueren, M.A.E., Quak, J.J., von Blomberg-van der Flier, B.M.E., Kuik, D.J., Langendoen, S.I., Snow, G.B., Green, C.J. and van Leeuwen, P.A.M. (2001) Effect of perioperative nutrition, with and without arginine supplementation, on nutritional status, immune function, postoperative morbidity and survival in severely malnourished head and neck cancer patients. *American Journal of Clinical Nutrition* 73, 323–332.

Van den Berghe, G., Wouters, P., Weekers, F., Verwaest, C., Bruyninckx, F., Schetz, M., Vlasserlaers, D., Ferdinande, P., Lauwers, P. and Bouillon, R. (2001) Intensive insulin therapy in critically ill patients. *New England Journal of Medicine* 345, 1359–1367.

Van der Hulst, R.R.W.J., van Kreel, B.K., von Meyenfeldt, M.F., Brummer, R.-J.M., Arends, J.-W., Deutz, N.E.P. and Soeters, P.B. (1993) Glutamine and the preservation of gut integrity. *Lancet* 341, 1363–1365.

Van der Hulst, R.R.W.J., von Meyenfeldt, M.F., van Kreel, B.K., Thunnissen, B.J.M., Brummers, R.J.M., Arends, J.W. and Soeters, P.B. (1998) Gut permeability, intestinal morphology and nutritional depletion. *Nutrition* 14, 1–6.

Van der Linden, C.J., Buurman, W.A., Spronken, E.E.M. and Soeters, P.B. (1986) Fibronectin levels in stressed and septic patients fed with total parenteral nutrition. *Journal of Parenteral and Enteral Nutrition* 10, 360–363.

Van der Wielen, R.P.J., de Wold, G.M., de Groot, L.C.P.G.M., Hoefnagels, W.H.L. and van Staveren, W.A. (1996) Dietary intakes of energy and water-soluble vitamins in different categories of aging. *Journal of Gerontology: Biological Science* 51A, B100–B107.

Vanek, V.W. (1998) The use of serum albumin as a prognostic or nutritional marker and the pros and cons of IV albumin therapy. *Nutrition in Clinical Practice* 13, 110–122.

Van Nes, M.-C., Herrmann, F.R., Gold, G., Michel, J.-P. and Rizzoli, R. (2001) Does the Mini Nutritional Assessment predict hospitalization outcomes in older people? *Age and Ageing* 30, 221–226.

Van Rijswijk, L. and Polansky, M. (1994) Predictors of time to healing deep pressure ulcers. *Ostomy/Wound Management* 40, 40–42, 44, 46–48.

Vellas, B., Baumgartner, R.N., Wayne, S.J., Conceicao, J., Lafont, C., Albarede, J.-L. and Garry, P.J. (1992) Relationship between malnutrition and falls in the elderly. *Nutrition* 8, 105–108.

Ventham, J., Reilly, J.J., Donaldson, M. and Gibson, B.E.S. (1998) Pattern and timing of excess weight gain in Scottish children treated for acute lymphoblastic leukaemia. *Proceedings of the Nutrition Society* 57, 133A.

Venugopalan, P., Akinbami, F.O., Al-Hinai, K.M. and Agarwal, A.K. (2001) Malnutrition in children with congenital heart defects. *Saudi Medical Journal* 22, 964–967.

Verboeket-van de Venne, W.P.H.G., Westerterp, K.R., Van Hoek, B. and Swart, G.R. (1993) Habitual pattern of food intake in patients with liver disease. *Clinical Nutrition* 12, 293–297.

Vermeeren, M.A., Schols, A.M. and Wouters, E.F. (1997) Effects of an acute exacerbation on nutritional and metabolic profile of patients with COPD. *European Respiratory Journal* 10, 2264–2269.

Vermeeren, M.A.P., Wouters, E.F., Nelissen, L.H., van Lier, A., Hofman, Z. and Schols, A.M. (2001) Acute effects of different nutritional supplements on symptoms and functional capacity in patients with chronic obstructive pulmonary disease. *American Journal of Clinical Nutrition* 73, 295–301.

Versluyen, M. (1985) Pressure sores in elderly patients: the epidemiology related to hip operations. *Journal of Bone and Joint Surgery* 67, 10–13.

Verweel, G., van Rossum, A.M.C., Hartwig, N.G., Wolfs, T.F.W., Scherpbier, H.J. and de Groot, R. (2002) Treatment with highly active antiretroviral therapy in human immunodeficiency virus type-1 infected children is associated with a sustained effect on growth. *Pediatrics* 109, E25.

Veterans Affairs TPN Cooperative Study Group (1991) Perioperative total parenteral nutrition in surgical patients. *New England Journal of Medicine* 325, 525–532.

Vetta, F., Ronzoni, S., Taglieri, G. and Bollea, M.R. (1999) The impact of malnutrition on the quality of life in the elderly. *Clinical Nutrition* 18, 259–267.

Vickers, A.J. and Altman, D.G. (2001) Analysing controlled trials with baseline and follow up measurements. *British Medical Journal* 323, 1123–1124.

Viola, S., Boule, M., Hyun Thi Hong, L., Medjadhi, Tounian, P. and Girardet, J.P. (2000) Interrelationship of nutrition and pulmonary function in children with chronic obstructive pulmonary disease. *Clinical Nutrition* 19 (Suppl.), 48.

Vir, S.C. and Love, A.H.G. (1979) Nutritional status of institutionalized and noninstitutionalized aged in Belfast Northern Ireland. *American Journal of Clinical Nutrition* 32, 1934–1947.

Vlaming, S., Biehler, A., Chattopadhyay, S., Jamieson, C., Cunliffe, A. and Powell-Tuck, J. (1999) Nutritional status of patients on admission to acute services of a London teaching hospital. *Proceedings of the Nutrition Society* 58, 119A.

Vlaming, S., Biehler, A., Hennessey, E.M., Jamieson, C.P., Chattophadhyay, S., Obeid, O.A., Archer, C., Farrell, A., Durman, K., Warrington, S. and Powell-Tuck, J. (2001) Should the food intake of patients admitted to acute hospital services be routinely supplemented? A randomized placebo controlled trial. *Clinical Nutrition* 20, 517–526.

Vohra, R.K. and McCollum, C.N. (1994) Pressure sores. *British Medical Journal* 309, 853–857.

Volkert, D. and Stehle, P. (1999) Vitamin status of elderly people in Germany. *International Journal for Vitamin and Nutrition Research* 69, 154–159.

Volkert, D., Kruse, W., Oster, P. and Schlierf, G. (1992) Malnutrition in geriatric patients: diagnostic and prognostic significance of nutritional parameters. *Annals of Nutrition and Metabolism* 36, 97–112.

Volkert, D., Hubsch, S., Oster, P. and Schlierf, G. (1996) Nutritional support and functional status in undernourished geriatric patients during hospitalization and 6-month follow-up. *Aging: Clinical and Experimental Research* 8, 386–395.

Von Herz, U., Rzehak, P., Kuechler, T., Mueller, M.J. and Loeser, C. (2000) Prospective evaluation of nutritional status and quality of life during long-term enteral feeding via percutaneous endoscopic gastrostomy (PEG). *Clinical Nutrition* 19 (Suppl.), 58.

Von Meyenfeldt, M.F., Fredrix, E.W.H.M., Haagh, W.A.J.J.M., Van Der Aalst, A.C.M.J. and Soeters, P.B. (1988) The aetiology and management of weight loss and malnutrition in cancer patients. *Baillière's Clinical Gastroenterology* 2, 869–885.

Von Meyenfeldt, M.F., Meijerink, W.J.H., Rouflart, M.M., Builmaassen, M.T. and Soeters, P.B. (1992) Perioperative nutritional support: a randomised clinical trial. *Clinical Nutrition* 11, 180–186.

Wagenmakers, A.J.M. (2001) Muscle function in critically ill patients. *Clinical Nutrition* 20, 451–454.

Waite, M.L., Aneiros, S., Hudson, D.I. and Cartwright, A.F. (2000) Ward hostess study at Basildon and Thurrock General Hospitals NHS Trust. *Proceedings of the Nutrition Society* 59, 183A.

Waitzberg, D.L., Caiaffa, W.T. and Correia, I.T.D. (2001) Hospital malnutrition: the Brazilian national survey (IBRANUTRI): a study of 4000 patients. *Nutrition* 17, 573–580.

Wallace, J.I., Schwartz, R.S., LaCroix, A.Z., Uhlmann, R.F. and Pearlman, R.A. (1995) Involuntary weight loss in older outpatients: incidence and clinical significance. *Journal of the American Geriatric Society* 43, 329–337.

Wallner, P.E., Endersbe, L.A. and Marlin, R.L. (1990) Nutritional supplementation in two high-risk cancer populations. *Current Therapeutic Research* 47, 924–932.

Waltman, N.L., Bergstrom, N., Armstrong, N., Norvell, K. and Braden, B. (1991) Nutritional status, pressure sores and mortality in elderly patients with cancer. *Oncology Nursing Forum* 18, 867–873.

Wandall, J.H., Hylander, E., Kappel, M. and Hage, E. (1992) Malabsorption and effect of enteral nutrition in HIV/AIDS patients without gastrointestinal infections. *Clinical Nutrition* 11 (Suppl.), 14.

Wang, H.X., Wahlin, Å., Basun, H., Fastbom, J., Winblad, B. and Fratiglioni, L. (2001) Vitamin B_{12} and folate in relation to the development of Alzheimer's disease. *Neurology* 56, 1188–1194.

Wanke, C.A., Pleskow, D., Degirolami, P.C., Lambl, B.B., Merkel, K. and Akrabawi, S. (1996) A medium chain triglyceride-based diet in patients with HIV and chronic diarrhea reduces diarrhea and malabsorption: a prospective, controlled trial. *Nutrition* 12, 766–771.

Wanke, C.A., Silva, M., Knox, T.A., Forrester, J., Speigelman, D. and Gorbach, S.L. (2000) Weight loss and wasting remain common complications in individuals infected with human immunodeficiency virus in the era of highly active antiretroviral therapy. *Clinical Infectious Diseases* 31, 803–805.

Wanklyn, P., Cox, N. and Belfield, P. (1995) Outcome in patients who require a gastrostomy after stroke. *Age and Ageing* 24, 510–514.

Wara, P. and Hessov, I. (1985) Nutritional intake after colorectal surgery: a comparison of a traditional and a new post-operative regimen. *Clinical Nutrition* 4, 225–228.

Warady, B.A., Kriley, M., Belden, B. and Hellerstein, S. (1990) Nutritional and behavioural aspects of nasogastric tube feeding in infants receiving chronic peritoneal dialysis. *Advances in Peritoneal Dialysis* 6, 265–268.

Warady, B.A., Weis, L. and Johnson, L. (1996) Nasogastric tube feeding in infants on peritoneal dialysis. *Peritoneal Dialysis International* 16, S521–S525.

Ward, E. (2001) Nutritional support: leukaemias, lymphomas and solid tumours. In: Shaw, V. and Lawson, M. (eds) *Clinical Paediatric Dietetics*. Blackwell Science, Oxford, pp. 351–360.

Ward, K., Strain, N.C., Wright, C., James, M. and Makin, A.J. (2000) A prospective economic evaluation of the cost of a catheter related sepsis: best case scenario vs. worst case scenario and the impact of a nutrition support team on cost savings. *Proceedings of the Nutrition Society* 59, 170A.

Ward, K., Burden, S.T., Wright, C.E., Moran, N.C., Brierley, E.R., Leslie, F. *et al.* (2001a) Prospective cost effectiveness analysis of a nutritional support team. *Proceedings of the Nutrition Society* 60, 84A.

Ward, K., Burden, S.T., Wright, C.E., Moran, N.C., Brierley, E.R., Leslie, F., Waters, K. and Makin, A.J. (2001b) A study to evaluate the effectiveness of a nutrition support team within a university teaching hospital. *Proceedings of the Nutrition Society* 60, 111A.

Ware, L.J., Wootton, S.A., Morlese, J.M., Gazzard, B.G. and Jackson, A.A. (2002) The paradox of improved antiretroviral therapy in HIV: potential for nutritional modulation? *Proceedings of the Nutrition Society* 61, 131–136.

Warnold, I. and Lundholm, K. (1984) Clinical significance of preoperative nutritional status in 215 noncancer patients. *Annals of Surgery* 199, 299–305.

Waterlow, J.C. (1972) The classification and definition of protein-calorie malnutrition. *British Medical Journal* 3, 566–569.

Waterlow, J.C. (1992) Effects of PEM on structure and functions of organs. In: Waterlow, J.C., Tomkins, A.M. and Grantham-McGregor (eds) *Protein Energy Malnutrition.* Edward Arnold, London

Watson, J.L. (1999) The prevalence of malnutrition in patients admitted to Care of the Elderly wards. *Proceedings of the Nutrition Society* 58, 139A.

Watters, J.M., Kirkpatrick, S.M., Norris, S.B., Shamji, F.M. and Wells, G.A. (1997) Immediate postoperative enteral feeding results in impaired respiratory mechanics and decreased mobility. *Annals of Surgery* 226, 369–380.

Weekes, E. and Elia, M. (2002) Identifying patients with nutritional problems: a comparison of two nutrition screening tools. *Proceedings of the Nutrition Society* 61, 4A.

Weekes, E. (1999) The incidence of malnutrition in medical patients admitted to a hospital in south London. *Proceedings of the Nutrition Society* 58, 126A.

Weekes, E. and Elia, M. (1996) Observations on the patterns of 24-hour energy expenditure changes in body composition and gastric emptying in head-injured patients receiving nasogastric tube feeding. *Journal of Parenteral and Enteral Nutrition* 20, 31–37.

Weekes, E., Cottee, S.M. and Elia, M. (1992) Home artificial nutritional support in Cambridge Health District – 1988–1990. *Journal of Human Nutrition and Dietetics* 5, 139–146.

Weigley, E.S. (1984) Average? Ideal? Desirable? A brief review of height-weight tables in the United States. *Journal of the American Dietetic Association* 84, 417–423.

Weiler, P.G., Franzi, C. and Kecskes, D. (1990) Pressure sores in nursing home patients. *Aging (Milano)* 2, 267–275.

Weindruch, R. and Walford, R.L. (1988) *The Retardation of Aging and Disease by Dietary Restriction.,* Charles C. Thomas, Springfield.

Weinsier, R.L., Hunker, E.M., Krumdieck, C.L. and Butterworth, C.E. (1979) Hospital malnutrition: a prospective evaluation of general medical patients during the course of hospitalization. *American Journal of Clinical Nutrition* 32, 418–426.

Weisdorf, S., Lysne, J., Wind, D., Haake, R.J., Sharp, H.L., Goldman, A., Schissel, K., McGlave, P.B., Ramsay, N.K. and Kersey, J.H. (1987) Influence of prophylactic total parenteral nutrition on long-term outcome of bone marrow transplantation. *Transplantation* 43, 833–838.

Weiss, R. (2001) AIDS: unbeatable 20 years on. *Lancet* 357, 2073–2074.

Welch, P.K., Dowson, M. and Endres, J.M. (1991) The effect of nutrient supplements on high risk long term care residents receiving puréed diets. *Journal of Nutrition for the Elderly* 10, 49–62.

Welsh, F.K.S., Farmery, S.M., Ramsden, C., Guillou, P.J. and Reynolds, J.V. (1996) Reversible impairment in monocyte major histocompatability complex class II expression in malnourished surgical patients. *Journal of Parenteral and Enteral Nutrition* 20, 344–348.

Welsh, F.K.S., Farmery, S.M., Maclennan, K., Sheridan, P.M., Barclay, G.R., Guillou, P.J. and Reynolds, J.V. (1997) Impaired gut barrier function in clinical protein-calorie malnutrition. *Journal of Parenteral and Enteral Nutrition* 21, S4.

Westwood, A.T. and Saitowitz, R. (1999) Growth and nutrition in South African children with cystic fibrosis. *South African Medical Journal* 89, 1276–1278.

Whicher, J. and Spence, C. (1987) When is serum albumin worth measuring? *Annals of Clinical Biochemistry* 24, 572–580.

White, J.V. (1997) *The role of Nutrition in Chronic Disease Care. Nutrition Screening Initiative: a Project of the American Academy of Family Physicians, the American Dietetic Association, and the National Council on Aging.* Nutrition Screening Initiative, Washington, DC.

White, R. and Ashworth, A. (2000) How drug therapy can affect, threaten and compromise nutritional status. *Journal of Human Nutrition and Dietetics* 13, 119–129.

Whitfield, M.D., Kaltenthaler, E.C., Akehurst, R.L., Walters, S.J. and Paisley, S. (2000) How effective are prevention strategies in reducing the prevalence of pressure ulcers? *Journal of Wound Care* 9, 261–266.

Whittaker, J.S., Ryan, C.F., Buckley, P.A. and Road, J.D. (1990) The effects of refeeding on peripheral and respiratory muscle function in malnourished chronic obstructive pulmonary disease patients. *American Review of Respiratory Disease* 142, 283–288.

Wicks, C., Gimson, A., Vlavianos, P., Lombard, M., Panos, M., Macmathuna, P., Tudor, M., Andrews, K. and Westaby, D. (1992) Assessment of the percutaneous endoscopic gastrostomy feeding tube as part of an integrated approach to enteral feeding. *Gut* 33, 613–616.

Wicks, C., Somasundaram, S., Bjarnason, I., Menzies, I.S., Routley, D., Potter, D., Tan, K.C. and Williams, R. (1994) Comparison of enteral feeding and total parenteral nutrition after liver transplantation. *Lancet* 344, 837–840.

Wicks, C., Bray, G.P. and Williams, R. (1995) Nutritional assessment in primary biliary cirrhosis: the effect of disease severity. *Clinical Nutrition* 14, 29–34.

Widhalm, K., Lackner, B. and Bauernfried, M. (1997) Medical education in nutrition in Europe. *Annals of Nutrition and Metabolism* 41, 66–68.

Widhalm, K., Pokorny, J., Virtanen, S.M., Oberritter, H., McKenna, B., Gronowska-Senger, A., Correa, F., Ellegard, L.H. and Vries, P.J.F. (1999) FENS program for nutrition education in medical schools. *Annals of Nutrition and Metabolism* 43, 66–68.

Wiedemann, B., Steinkamp, G., Sens, B. and Stern, M. (2001) The German cystic fibrosis quality assurance project: clinical features in children and adults. *European Respiratory Journal* 17, 1187–1194.

Wigmore, S.J., Plester, C.E., Richardson, R.A. and Fearon, K.C.H. (1997) Changes in nutritional status associated with unresectable pancreatic cancer. *British Journal of Cancer* 75, 106–109.

Willett, W.C., Dietz, W.H. and Colditz, G.A. (1999) Guidelines for healthy weight. *New England Journal of Medicine* 341, 427–434.

Williams, C.M., Lines, C.M. and McKay, E.C. (1988) Iron and zinc status in multiple sclerosis patients with pressure sores. *European Journal of Clinical Nutrition* 42, 321–328.

Williams, C.M., Driver, L.T., Older, J. and Dickerson, J.W.T. (1989) A controlled trial of sip-feed supplements in elderly orthopaedic patients. *European Journal of Clinical Nutrition* 43, 267–274.

Williams, E.A., Powers, H.J. and Rumsey, R.D.E. (1995) Morphological changes in the rat small intestive in response to riboflavin deprivation. *British Journal of Nutrition* 73, 141–146.

Williams, E.A., Rumsey, R.D.E. and Powers, H.J. (1996) An investigation into the reversibility of the morphological and cytokinetic changes seen in the small intestine of riboflavin deficient rats. *Gut* 39, 220–225.

Wilschanski, M., Sherman, P., Pencharz, P., Davis, L., Corey, M. and Griffiths, A. (1996) Supplementary enteral nutrition maintains remission in paediatric Crohn's disease. *Gut* 38, 543–548.

Wilson, A., Evans, S. and Frost, G. (2000) A comparison of the amount of food served and consumed according to meal service system. *Journal of Human Nutrition and Dietetics* 13, 271–275.

Wilson, B., Fernandez-Madrid, A., Hayes, A., Hermann, K., Smith, J. and Wassell, A. (2001) Comparison of the effects of two early intervention strategies on the health outcomes of malnourished hemodialysis patients. *Journal of Renal Nutrition* 11, 166–171.

Wilson, D.O., Rogers, R.M., Sanders, M.H., Pennock, B.E. and Reilly, J.J. (1986) Nutritional intervention in malnourished patients with emphysema. *American Review of Respiratory Disease* 134, 672–677.

Wilson, D.O., Rogers, R.M., Wright, E.C. and Anthonisen, N.R. (1989) Body weight in chronic obstructive pulmonary disease: the National Institutes of Health Intermittent Positive-Pressure Breathing Trial. *American Review of Respiratory Disease* 139, 1435–1438.

Wilson, D.O., Donahoe, M., Rogers, R.M. and Pennock, B.E. (1990) Metabolic rate and weight loss in chronic obstructive lung disease. *Journal of Parenteral and Enteral Nutrition* 14, 7–11.

Wilson, L., Devine, E.B. and So, K. (2000) Direct medical costs of chronic obstructive pulmonary disease: chronic bronchitis and emphysema. *Respiratory Medicine* 94, 204–213.

Wilson, M.G., Purushothaman, R. and Morley, J.E. (2002) Effect of liquid dietary supplements on energy intake in the elderly. *American Journal of Clinical Nutrition* 75, 944–947.

Wilson, M.M.G. and Morley, J.E. (1988) Undernutrition. In: Sadler, M.J., Strain, J.J. and Caballero, B. (eds) *Encyclopedia of Human Nutrition*. Academic Press, San Diego, pp. 1485–1495.

Wilson, N.L., Wilson, R.H.L. and Farber, S.M. (1964) Nutrition in pulmonary emphysema. *Journal of the American Dietetic Association* 45, 530–536.

Windsor, A.C.J., Kanwar, S., Li, A.G.K., Barnes, E., Guthrie, J.A., Spark, J.I., Welsh, F., Guillou, P.J. and Reynolds, J.V. (1998) Compared with parenteral nutrition, enteral feeding attenuates the acute phase response and improves disease severity in acute pancreatitis. *Gut* 42, 431–435.

Windsor, J.A. and Hill, G. (1988) Weight loss with physiologic impairment: a basic indicator of surgical risk. *Annals of Surgery* 207, 290–296.

Windsor, J.A., Knight, G.S. and Hill, G.L. (1988) Wound healing response in surgical patients: recent food intake is more important than nutritional status. *British Journal of Surgery* 75, 135–137.

Winer, B.J., Brown, D.R. and Michels, K.M. (1991) *Statistical Principles in Experimental Design,* 3rd edn. McGraw-Hill, New York.

Wing, E.J. and Young, J.B. (1980) Acute starvation protects mice against *Listeria monocytogenes. Infection and Immunity* 28, 771–776.

Winick, M. (1994) Hunger disease. *Nutrition* 10, 365–380.

Winograd, C.H. and Brown, E.M. (1990) Aggressive oral refeeding in hospitalized patients. *American Journal of Clinical Nutrition* 52, 967–968.

Winter, T.A. (2001) Cardiac consequences of malnutrition – Ancel Keys revisited! *Nutrition* 17, 422–423.

Winter, T.A., Lemmer, E.R., O'Keefe, S.J.D. and Ogden, J.M. (2000) The effect of severe undernutrition and subsequent refeeding on digestive function in human patients. *European Journal of Gastroenterology and Hepatology* 12, 191–196.

Wissing, U. and Unosson, M. (1999) The relationship between nutritional status and physical activity, ulcer history and ulcer-related problems in patients with leg and food ulcers. *Scandinavian Journal of Caring Sciences* 13, 123–128.

Wolf, C., Spaniol, U., Korber, J. and Lichtenegger, W. (2001) Body mass index (BMI), bioelectrical impedance analysis (BIA) and adverse events under chemotherapy. *Clinical Nutrition* 20 (Suppl.), 60.

Wolfe, B.M. and Mathiesen, K.A. (1997) Clinical practice guidelines: can they be based on randomized clinical trials? *Journal of Parenteral and Enteral Nutrition* 21, 1–6.

Woo, J., Ho, S.C., Mak, Y.T., Law, L.K. and Cheung, A. (1994) Nutritional status of elderly patients during recovery from chest infection and the role of nutritional supplementation assessed by a prospective randomized single-blind trial. *Age and Ageing* 23, 40–48.

Wood, S. (1995) *Home Parenteral Nutrition.* BAPEN, Maidenhead.

Woodcock, N.P., Zeigler, D., Palmer, D., Buckley, P., Mitchell, C.J. and MacFie, J. (2001) Enteral versus parenteral nutrition: a pragmatic study. *Nutrition* 17, 1–12.

Woods, M.N., Spiegelman, D., Knox, T.A., Forrester, J.E., Connors, J.L., Skinner, S.C., Silva, M., Kim, J.H. and Gorbach, S.L. (2002) Nutrient intake and body weight in a large HIV cohort that includes women and minorities. *Journal of the American Dietetic Association* 102, 203–211.

World Health Organization (1992) *International Statistical Classification of Diseases and Health Related Problems*, Vol. 1, 10th revision. WHO, Geneva.

World Health Organization (1995) *Physical Status: the Use and Interpretation of Anthropometry.* WHO Technical Report Series 854, WHO, Geneva.

Wouters-Wesseling, W., Wouters, A.E.J., Kleijer, C.N., Bindels, J.G., de Groot, C.P.G.M. and van Staveren, W.A. (2002) Study of the effect of a liquid nutrition supplement on the nutritional status of psycho-geriatric nursing home patients. *European Journal of Clinical Nutrition* 56, 245–251.

Wu, D., Hockenbery, D.M., Brentnall, T.A., Baehr, P.H., Ponec, R.J., Kuver, R., Tzung, S.P., Todaro, J.L. and McDonald, G.B. (1998) Persistent nausea and anorexia after marrow transplantation: a prospective study of 78 patients. *Transplantation* 66, 1319–1324.

Wylie, C., Copeman, J. and Kirk, S.F.L. (1999) Health and social factors affecting the food choice and nutritional intake of elderly people with restricted mobility. *Journal of Human Nutrition and Dietetics* 12, 375–380.

Wynn, M. and Wynn, A. (2001) Reducing waiting lists for hospital admission: community nutrition services reduce the need for hospital beds. *Nutrition and Health* 15, 3–16.

Yahav, J., Avigad, S., Frand, M., Shem-Tov, A., Barzilay, Z., Linn, S. and Jonas, A. (1985) Assessment of intestinal and cardiorespiratory function in children with congenital heart disease on high-caloric formulas. *Journal of Pediatric Gastroenterology and Nutrition* 4, 778–785.

Yamaguchi, L.Y., Coulston, A.M., Lu, N.C., Dixon, L.B. and Craig, L.D. (1998) Improvement in nutrient intake by elderly meals-on-wheels participants receiving a liquid nutrition supplement. *Nutrition Today* 33, 37–44.

Yamazaki, K., Maiz, A., Moldawer, L.L., Bistrian, B.R. and Blackburn, G.L. (1986) Complications associated with overfeeding of infected animals. *Journal of Surgical Research* 40, 152–158.

Yariş, N., Akyüz, C., Coskunm, T., Kutluk, T. and Büyükpamukçu, M. (2002) Nutritional status of children with cancer and its effect on survival. *Turkish Journal of Pediatrics* 44, 35–39.

Yassa, J.G., Prosser, R. and Dodge, J.A. (1978) Effects of an artificial diet on growth of patients with cystic fibrosis. *Archives of Diseases in Childhood* 53, 777–783.

Yates, C.A., Evans, G.S. and Powers, H.J. (1997) Very early changes in gastrointestinal morphology in response to riboflavin depletion. *Proceedings of the Nutrition Society* 56, 96A.

Yeoh, E., Horowitz, M., Russo, A., Muecke, T., Robb, T., Waddox, A. and Chatterton, B. (1993) Effect of pelvic irradiation on gastrointestinal function: a prospective longitudinal study. *American Journal of Medicine* 95, 397–406

Yeung, C.K., Smith, R.C. and Hill, G.L. (1979a) Effect of an elemental diet on body composition. *Gastroenterology* 77, 652–657.

Yeung, C.K., Young, G.A., Hackett, A.F. and Hill, G.L. (1979b) Fine needle jejunostomy – an assessment of a new method of nutritional support after major gastrointestinal surgery. *British Journal of Surgery* 66, 727–732.

Yoshikawa, M., Yoneda, T., Kobayashi, A., Fu, A., Takenaka, H., Narita, N. and Nezo, K. (1999) Body composition analysis by dual energy X-ray absorptiometry and exercise performance in underweight patients with COPD. *Chest* 115, 371–375.

Young, B., Ott, L., Twyman, D., Norton, J., Rapp, R., Tibbs, P., Haack, D., Brivins, B. and Dempsey, R. (1987) The effect of nutritional support on outcome from severe head injury. *Journal of Neurosurgery* 67, 668–676.

Young, G.A., Oli, H.I., Davidson, A.M., and Parsons, F.M. (1978) The effects of calorie and essential amino acid supplementation on plasma proteins in patients with chronic renal failure. *American Journal of Clinical Nutrition* 31, 1802–1807.

Young, G.A., Kopple, J.D., Lindholm, B., Vonesh, E.F., De Vecchi, A., Scalamogna, A., Castelnova, C., Oreopoulos, D.G., Anderson, G.H., Bergstrom, J., DiChiro, J., Gentile, D., Nissenson, A., Sakhrani, L., Brownjohn, A.M., Nolph, K.D., Prowant, B.F., Algrim, C.E., Martis, L. and Serkes, K.D. (1991) Nutritional assessment of continuous ambulatory peritoneal dialysis patients: an international study. *American Journal of Kidney Diseases* 17, 462–471.

Young, J.B. and Dobrzanski, S. (1992) Pressure sores: epidemiology and current management concepts. *Drugs and Aging* 2, 42–57.

Young, L., Scheltinga, M., Bye, R. and Wilmore, D. (1992) Can tests of patients' well-being be used to evaluate nutritional efficacy? An affirmative answer. *Journal of Parenteral and Enteral Nutrition* 16, 20S.

Yulo, N., Fishbane, S., Scalza, H., DiGiacomo, A., Lostrappo, D. and Kowalski, E.A. (1997) Nutritional supplementation during the hemodialysis treatment in malnourished hemodialysis patients. *Journal of the American Society of Nephrology* 8, SS A1193.

Zachos, M., Tondeur, M. and Griffiths, A.M., (2001) Enteral nutritional therapy for inducing remission of Crohn's disease (Cochrane Review). *Cochrane Database System Review* 3, CD000542.

Zaloga, G.P. (1998) Immune-enhancing enteral diets: where's the beef? *Critical Care Medicine* 26, 1143–1146.

Zeiderman, M.R. and McMahon, M.J. (1989) The role of objective measurement of skeletal muscle function in the pre-operative patient. *Clinical Nutrition* 8, 161–166.

Zemel, B.S., Jawad, A.F., FitzSimmons, S. and Stallings, V.A. (2000) Longitudinal relationship among growth, nutritional status and pulmonary function in children with cystic fibrosis: analysis of the Cystic Fibrosis Foundation National CF Patient Registry. *Journal of Pediatrics* 137, 374–380.

Ziegler, T.R., Smith, R.J., O'Dwyer, S.T., Demling, R.H. and Wilmore, D.W. (1988) Increased intestinal permeability associated with infection in burn patients. *Archives of Surgery* 123, 1313–1319.

Zimmerman, J.E., Knaus, W.A., Wagner, D.P., Sun, X., Hakim, R.B. and Nystrom, P.O. (1996) A comparison of risks and outcomes for patients with organ system failure: 1982–1990. *Critical Care Medicine* 24, 1633–1641.

Glossary*

Bias: Systematic distortion of the estimated intervention effect away from the 'truth', caused by inadequacies in the design, conduct or analysis of a trial. An example is *ascertainment bias*, which is the systematic distortion of results of a randomized trial that occur from knowledge of the group assignment by the person assessing outcome, whether an investigator or the participant. Another example is *selection bias*, which is the systematic error in creating intervention groups, such that they differ with respect to prognosis. That is, the groups differ in the way participants were selected or assigned. Selection bias is also used to mean that the participants are not representative of the population of all possible participants. *Performance bias* refers to systematic differences in the care provided to the participants in the comparison groups other than the intervention under investigation. *Attrition bias* arises from protocol deviations and loss of patients to follow up.

Blinding (masking): The practice of keeping the trial participants, care providers, those collecting data, and even those analysing the data, unaware of which intervention is being administered to the participants. Blinding is intended to prevent bias arising from study personnel. A common form of blinding is '*double blinding*', in which participants, caregivers and those assessing outcome are blinded to the intervention assignment. If only one of the parties involved is aware of which subjects are receiving the treatment, the study is '*single blind*'.

Concealment (allocation concealment): A technique used to prevent selection bias by concealing the allocation sequences from those assigning participants to intervention groups, until the moment of assignment. Allocation concealment prevents researchers from consciously or unconsciously influencing the assignment of participants to particular groups.

Cross-sectional study: A study in which data are collected from subjects at one point in time, e.g. assessment of nutritional status on admission to hospital.

Effect size (treatment effect): A measure of the difference in outcome between intervention groups. It may be expressed in different ways, such as a difference between means, proportions or ratios of risks (e.g. odds ratio or relative risk).

Endpoint: A clearly defined outcome in a trial, such as mortality or complication rates.

Incidence: The number of new diseases (conditions or characteristics) that develop during a specified time period (often 1 year).

*Partly based on Consort.

Intention-to-treat analysis: A strategy of analysing data in which all participants are included in the group to which they were assigned, whether or not they completed the intervention.   Intention-to-treat analysis prevents bias caused by the loss of participants, which may disrupt the baseline equivalence established by random assignment and which may reflect violation of the protocol.

Interim analysis: Analysis comparing intervention groups at any time before the formal completion of the trial, usually before recruitment is complete. Information from the interim analysis can be used to enforce the *'stopping rule'*, to avoid putting patients at risk unnecessarily or because the intervention effect is so strong that further data collection is unnecessary. The timing and frequency of the interim analyses should be specified in the protocol (planned interim analyses). The criteria for enforcing the stopping rule are based on planned statistical measures. Data from an interim analysis may also be used to (re)calculate the sample size of study, which may be of particular value if no prior experience exists.

Longitudinal study: A study in which subjects are measured or assessed repeatedly through time, e.g. assessment of nutritional status during hospital stay.

Meta-analysis: A statistical procedure that integrates the results of two or more independent studies to provide a single quantitative estimate of a treatment effect. The rationale for this analysis is to provide more power than is provided by the studies individually. Essential requirements for meta-analyses are that inclusion criteria for studies are defined in advance, and wherever possible, attempts are made to ensure that all eligible studies are identified.

Minimization: An assigned strategy, similar in intention to stratification (see randomization, stratified), that ensures a very good balance between intervention groups for specified prognostic factors. The next participant is assigned to whichever group would minimize the imbalance between groups on specified prognostic factors. Minimization is an acceptable alternative to random assignment.

Odds ratio: Odds is defined as the number of patients who fulfil the criteria for a given endpoint divided by the number of patients who do not.   The odds of dying during a treatment in a group of 10 patients may be 2 to 8 (2 dying divided by 8 not dying, 0.25) compared with 4 to 8 (0.5) in a control group.   The odds ratio of the treatment to control group would be $0.25/0.5 = 0.5$.

Open trial: A randomized trial in which both participants and investigators are aware of the treatments assigned.

Planned analyses (a priori analyses): Statistical analyses specified in the trial protocol (that is planned in advance of data collection).   These analyses contrast with unplanned analyses (also called *exploratory, data-derived, or post hoc analyses*), which are analyses suggested by the data.

Power: The probability that a trial will detect, as statistically significant, an intervention effect of a specified size. The pre-specified trial size is often chosen to give the trial the desired power.

Precision: A quantification of the certainty in an estimate, such as an effect size, usually expressed as the 95% confidence interval around the estimate. Imprecision, which is the opposite of precision, also refers more generally to other sources of uncertainty, such as measurement error.

Prevalence: The number of persons with a particular condition present within a population either at a point in time (point prevalence) or a period of time (period prevalence). It may be expressed as a percentage (division by the total population) or per 1000 or multiple of 1000 of the population.

Prognostic variable: A baseline variable that predicts outcome.

Prospective study: Investigation and categorization of a sample of individuals who are then followed over a period of time to determine specified outcomes.

Randomization (random allocation; random assignment): In a randomized trial, the process of assigning participants to groups such that each participant has a known and usually equal chance of being assigned to a given group. Randomization aims to ensure that the group assignment cannot be predicted. *Simple randomization* (*non-restricted randomization*) is randomization without restriction. In a trial with two groups, it is equivalent to tossing a coin. *Block randomization* (*block design; blocking; permutated block design*) is a method for generating an allocation sequence in which the number of assignments to intervention groups satisfies a specified allocation ratio (e.g. 1:1 or 2:1) after every 'block' (see text for example). *Stratified randomization* is carried out separately within each of two or more subsets of participants (e.g. according to study centre or disease activity) to ensure that the patient characteristics are closely balanced within each intervention group. Stratified and block randomization are restricted forms of randomization (*restricted randomization*).

Reliability: The extent to which the same measurement can be reproduced e.g. inter-observer agreement about severity of malnutrition.

Retrospective study: A study that collects information about past events with a view to testing a hypothesis or establishing incidence/prevalence or other relevant characteristic.

Rosenthals' fail safe score: A measure of the robustness of data in a meta-analysis. The fail-safe score is the number of non-significant, missing or unpublished studies that would need to be added to a meta-analysis in order to change a significant result to a non-significant result. If the number is large ($5n+10$ or more (n number of trials in meta-analysis)), there is greater confidence that the observed result, even with some publication bias, is likely to be a reliable estimate of the true effect.

Sample size (intended and achieved): The number of participants in a trial. The intended sample size is the number of participants planned to be included in the trial, usually determined using a statistical power calculation. The sample size should be adequate to provide a high probability of detecting a significant effect size of a given magnitude if such an effect actually exists. The achieved sample size is the number of participants enrolled, treated and analysed.

Sensitivity: The proportion of patients with a disease (condition or characteristic) who are correctly classified as having the disease.

Specificity: The proportion of patients without a disease (condition or characteristic) who are correctly classified as not having the disease.

Systematic review: A critical objective appraisal of evidence, conducted according to explicit and reproducible methodology in order to minimize biases and random errors.

Type 1 (alpha) error: Rejection of the null hypothesis when it is true (i.e. a conclusion that there is an effect, when in reality there is no effect). More stringent criteria for rejecting the null hypothesis (e.g. $P < 0.001$) will reduce the likelihood of a type 1 error, but increase the likelihood of a type 2 error.

Type 2 (beta) error: Acceptance of the null hypothesis when it is incorrect (i.e. a conclusion that there is no effect, when in reality there is). As sample size increases, the probability of a type 2 error decreases.

Validity: The extent to which a method provides a true assessment of that which it purports to measure. *Internal validity* is the extent to which the design and conduct of the trial minimizes bias. *External validity* (*generalizability; applicability*) is the extent to which the results of a trial can be extrapolated more widely or more generally to other circumstances.

z score: The number of standard deviations. In a normal distribution, 1 SD below and above the mean (z score of ±1) accounts for 68% of the observations. A z score of ±2 accounts for 95% of the observations (see Fig. 1.4, Chapter 1). Z scores can be used instead of centiles to assess growth (e.g. in weight-for-age, weight-for-height and height-for-age).

Index

Entries in *italic* refer to information that is presented in tabular form or otherwise outside of the main text.

The following abbreviations are used throughout the index: ETF = enteral tube feeding, ONS = oral nutritional supplements, PN = parenteral nutrition.